Clinical
Laboratory
Management

Clinical Laboratory Management

LYNNE S. GARCIA, EDITOR IN CHIEF
LSG & Associates, Santa Monica, California

EDITORS

VICKIE S. BASELSKI
Department of Pathology
University of Tennessee Health Science Center
at Memphis
Memphis, Tennessee

M. DESMOND BURKE
Department of Pathology and Laboratory Medicine
Cornell University Medical College
New York Presbyterian Hospital
New York, New York

DALE A. SCHWAB
Microbiology
Nichols Institute, Quest Diagnostics, Inc.
San Juan Capistrano, California

DAVID L. SEWELL
Pathology and Laboratory Medicine Service
Veterans Affairs Medical Center and
Oregon Health and Science University
Portland, Oregon

JOHN C. H. STEELE, JR.
Department of Pathology
Medical College of Georgia
Augusta, Georgia

ALICE S. WEISSFELD
Microbiology Specialists Incorporated
Houston, Texas

DAVID S. WILKINSON
Department of Pathology
Virginia Commonwealth University
Richmond, Virginia

WASHINGTON C. WINN, JR.
Department of Pathology
University of Vermont College of Medicine
Burlington, Vermont

ASM PRESS

WASHINGTON, D.C.

Library of Congress Cataloging-in-Publication Data

Clinical laboratory management / Lynne S. Garcia, editor in chief ; [edited by] Vickie
S. Baselski ... [et al.].
    p. ; cm.
  Includes index.
  ISBN 1-55581-279-1
    1. Medical laboratories—Administration. 2.   Pathological laboratories—
Administration.
    [DNLM: 1.   Laboratories—organization & administration. 2.   Clinical Laboratory
Techniques. QY 23
C6405 2004] I. Garcia, Lynne Shore.

  R860.C56 2004
  610′.28′4—dc22

                              2003028290

Address editorial correspondence to: ASM Press, 1752 N St., N.W., Washington, DC
20036-2904, U.S.A.

Send orders to: ASM Press, P.O. Box 605, Herndon, VA 20172, U.S.A.
Phone: 800-546-2416; 703-661-1593
Fax: 703-661-1501
Email: books@asmusa.org
Online: www.asmpress.org

Contents

I OVERVIEW OF LABORATORY MANAGEMENT AND CURRENT HEALTHCARE ENVIRONMENT 1

4   Current Challenges to Financial Stability within the Diagnostic Laboratory 67

Thomas J. Dilts and David S. Wilkinson

5   The Impact of Regulatory Requirements 79

Susan D. Roseff, Ann L. Harris, and Carol H. Rodgers

6   The Changing Practice of Medicine 135

Susan D. Roseff, Brenda G. Nichols, and Margaret M. Grimes

II   MANAGERIAL LEADERSHIP   193

14   Managing Change 267

Christopher S. Frings

III   PERSONNEL MANAGEMENT 275

15   Employee Selection 277

Anthony S. Kurec

16   Performance Appraisals and Competency Assessment 291

Diane C. Halstead and Donna L. Oblack

17   Staffing and Scheduling 326

Patti Medvescek

IV   REQUIREMENTS FOR EFFECTIVE LABORATORY MANAGEMENT   367

V FINANCIAL MANAGEMENT 491

32 Financial Decision Making: the Endgame of the Planning and Analytical Process 551

Washington C. Winn, Jr.

VI GENERATION OF REVENUE 555

33 Correct Coding of Billable Services in the Clinical Laboratory 557

Vickie S. Baselski, Alice S. Weissfeld, and Fran Sorrell

34 Approaches to Billing Laboratory Services 567

Vickie S. Baselski, Alice S. Weissfeld, and Fran Sorrell

35 Charges and Fees for Laboratory Services 574

Vickie S. Baselski, Alice S. Weissfeld, and Fran Sorrell

IX DEFINING AND MEASURING STANDARDS FOR SUCCESS 721

X THE FUTURE OF CLINICAL LABORATORIES 761

Contributors

Paul Bachner
Department of Pathology and Laboratory Medicine, University of Kentucky Chandler Medical Center, 800 Rose St., Room MS 119, Lexington, KY 40536-0298

Daniel D. Bankson
Clinical Chemistry and STAT Laboratories, Veterans Affairs Puget Sound Health Care System, and Department of Laboratory Medicine, University of Washington, 1660 S. Columbia Way (S-113), Seattle, WA 98108

Vickie S. Baselski
University of Tennessee Health Science Center at Memphis, Clinical Microbiology, 349 Riverbluff Place, Memphis, TN 38103-4132

James W. Bishop
New Mexico State University, 5165 Hunters Chase Rd., Las Cruces, NM 88011

Michael G. Bissell
Ohio State University College of Medicine and Public Health, Room N337 Doan Hall, 410 W. 10th Ave., Columbus, OH 43210

M. Desmond Burke
Department of Laboratory Medicine and Pathology, Weill Medical College of Cornell University, F-715 Weill Cornell Center, New York Presbyterian Hospital, 525 East 68th St., New York, NY 10021

Joseph M. Campos
Microbiology Laboratory and Laboratory Informatics, Department of Laboratory Medicine, Children's National Medical Center, Washington, DC 20010, and Departments of Pediatrics, Pathology, and Microbiology/Tropical Medicine, George Washington University Medical Center, Washington, DC 20037

Jeffrey Casterline
Department of Pathology, Virginia Commonwealth University, P.O. Box 980662, Richmond, VA 23298-0662

George Cembrowski
Division of Medical Biochemistry, 4B1.24 Mackenzie Health Sciences Centre, Edmonton, Alberta, Canada T6G 2R7

Beth H. Deaton
Sentara Lab Services, 600 Gresham Dr., Norfolk, VA 23507

Thomas J. Dilts
Department of Pathology, Virginia Commonwealth University Health System, P.O. Box 980258, Richmond, VA 23298-0258

Jean Egan
Jean Egan Associates, 64 Wren Dr., Suffield, CT 06078; Asnuntuck Community College, Enfield, CT 06082

Christopher S. Frings
Chris Frings & Associates, 633 Winwood Dr., Birmingham, AL 35226; University of Alabama at Birmingham

Lynne S. Garcia
LSG & Associates, 512 12th St., Santa Monica, CA 90402

Margaret M. Grimes
Virginia Commonwealth University Health System and School of Medicine, Richmond, VA 23298

Diane C. Halstead
North Florida Pathology, P.A., and Clinical Laboratory Services, Baptist Medical Center, Jacksonville, FL 32207

Ann L. Harris
Department of Pathology, Virginia Commonwealth University Health System, P.O. Box 980258, Richmond, VA 23298-0258

Charlene H. Harris
Regional Lab Outreach, 413 Jasmine Trail, Athens, GA 30606; Corpus-Sanchez International, Toronto, Ontario, Canada

Glen L. Hortin
Department of Laboratory Medicine, National Institutes of Health, Bldg. 10, Room 2C-407, Bethesda, MD 20892

Rebecca Katsaras
Sonora Quest Laboratories, Tempe, AZ 85281

Adarsh K. Khalsa
Laboratory Sciences of Arizona, Banner Samaritan Medical Center, Phoenix, AZ 85006

Frederick L. Kiechle
Department of Clinical Pathology and Beaumont Reference Laboratory, William Beaumont Hospital, 3601 West 13 Mile Rd., Royal Oak, MI 48073-6769

Anthony S. Kurec
University Pathologists Laboratories, LLP, State University of New York-Upstate Medical University, 250 Harrison St., Suite 502, Syracuse, NY 13202

Ronald B. Lepoff
Pathology, University of Colorado Health Sciences Center, Denver, CO 80262

Carmen Mariano
Quincy Public Schools, 70 Coddington St., Quincy, MA 02169

Diana Mass
Clinical Laboratory Sciences Program, School of Life Sciences, Arizona State University, P.O. Box 874501, Tempe, AZ 85287-4501

Michael D. D. McNeely
MDS Metro Laboratory Services, 4489 Viewmont Ave., Victoria, British Columbia, Canada V8Z 5K8

Patti Medvescek
3007 Earl Dr., Indianapolis, IN 46227

Sheshadri Narayanan
Department of Pathology and Laboratory Medicine, Weill Medical College of Cornell University, New York Presbyterian Hospital, Clinical Laboratory Administration, 525 East 68th St., New York, NY 10021

Brenda G. Nichols
Virginia Commonwealth University Health System, Richmond, VA 23298

Donna L. Oblack
Pathology and Laboratory Medicine Service, Veterans Affairs Medical Center, and Department of Pathology and Laboratory Medicine, University of Cincinnati, Cincinnati, OH 45220

Elissa Passiment
American Society for Clinical Laboratory Science, 6701 Democracy Blvd., Suite 300, Bethesda, MD 20817

Gary W. Procop
Clinical Microbiology Laboratory and Department of Pathology, Cleveland Clinic, Cleveland, Ohio

L. Barth Reller
Clinical Microbiology Laboratory and Departments of Medicine and Pathology, Duke University Medical Center, Durham, North Carolina

Carol H. Rodgers
Department of Pathology, VCU Health System, 403 N. 13th St., CSC-611, Box 980258, Richmond, VA 23298-0258

Susan D. Roseff
Department of Pathology, Virginia Commonwealth University School of Medicine, VCU Health System, 403 N. 13th St., CSC-611, P.O. Box 980258, Richmond, VA 23298-0258

Michael A. Saubolle
Department of Clinical Pathology, Banner Good Samaritan Medical Center, 1111 E. McDowell Rd., Phoenix, AZ 85006

Ron B. Schifman
Diagnostics Service Line, Southern Arizona Veterans Affairs Healthcare System, 3601 South 6th Ave. (6-113), Tucson, AZ 85723; Department of Pathology, University of Arizona College of Medicine

David L. Sewell
Pathology and Laboratory Medicine Service, Veterans Affairs Medical Center, and Department of Pathology, Oregon Health and Sciences University, Portland, OR 97239

Riley M. Sinder
John F. Kennedy School of Government, Harvard University, 79 JFK St., Cambridge, MA 02138

Joseph E. Skrisson
Department of Clinical Pathology and Beaumont Reference Laboratory, William Beaumont Hospital, 3601 West 13 Mile Rd., Royal Oak, MI 48073-6769

Rebecca A. Smith
Sonora Quest Laboratories, Tempe, AZ 85281

John R. Snyder
The Ohio State University at Lima, 4240 Campus Dr., Lima, OH 45804

Fran Sorrell
Memphis Pathology Laboratory, Memphis, Tennessee

Geoffrey C. Tolzmann
Department of Network Development and Department of Pathology and Laboratory Medicine, Fletcher Allen Health Care, 111 Colchester Ave., Burlington, VT 05041

Diane C. Turnbull
Medical College of Georgia, 407 Wade Plantation Dr., Martinez, GA 30907

Paul Valenstein
Pathology and Laboratory Management Associates, P.C., 5301 East Huron River Dr., Ann Arbor, MI 48106-3058

Laurence P. Vetter
Department of Pathology, Virginia Commonwealth University, P.O. Box 980662, Richmond, VA 23298-0662

Richard J. Vincent
Department of Network Development and Department of Pathology and Laboratory Medicine, Fletcher Allen Health Care, 111 Colchester Ave., Burlington, VT 05041

Lei Wang
New Mexico State University, 5165 Hunters Chase Rd., Las Cruces, NM 88011

Alice S. Weissfeld
Microbiology Specialists Incorporated, 8911 Interchange Dr., Houston, TX 77054

Lionelle D. Wells
VA New England Healthcare, Director, Network Consolidated Laboratory, VA Brockton Medical Center, Brockton, MA 02301-5596

Fred Westenfeld
Department of Pathology and Laboratory Medicine, University of Vermont College of Medicine, and Microbiology Laboratory, Fletcher Allen Health Care, Burlington, VT 05401

David S. Wilkinson
Department of Pathology, Virginia Commonwealth University, P.O. Box 980662, Richmond, VA 23298-0662

Dean Williams
John F. Kennedy School of Government, Harvard University, 79 JFK St., Cambridge, MA 02138

Michael L. Wilson
Department of Pathology and Laboratory Medicine, Denver Health Medical Center, and Department of Pathology, University of Colorado School of Medicine, Denver, Colorado

Washington C. Winn, Jr.
Microbiology Laboratory, Fletcher Allen Health Care, 1 South Prospect St., Burlington, VT 05401; Department of Pathology and Laboratory Medicine, University of Vermont College of Medicine, Burlington

Donna Wolk
Clinical Pathology, University of Arizona; Director, Molecular Diagnostics & Research Laboratories, Southern Arizona Veterans Affairs Healthcare System, Tucson, AZ 85723

Preface

The current environment for laboratory medicine and pathology continues to undergo dramatic transformation, influenced by significant changes in the legislative, regulatory, reimbursement, technological, sociological, economic, communication, and business sectors. The practice of all aspects of medicine and allied healthcare requires new approaches and a much broader range of managerial expertise. Areas which a laboratory director, manager, or supervisor is expected to understand, and to perform well in, include fiscal and human resources, patient care testing and quality performance issues, and overall accountability to the facility's administration.

It is very important that individuals working within the healthcare environment learn to hear, speak, and thoroughly understand the operational language of healthcare administration. During the past few years, the fields of laboratory medicine and pathology management have seen many dramatic changes, including those related to quality assurance, communication, data storage and retrieval, point-of-care testing, test management, automation, safety and emergency preparedness, regulatory requirements, information confidentiality, billing and coding requirements, physical space changes, laboratory consolidation, shortage of training programs and trained personnel, competency testing, specimen handling and shipping requirements, decrease in reimbursement, demand for increased productivity, and increased need for consultation and educational initiatives for clients.

The purpose of this text is to provide comprehensive, practical information and guidelines for healthcare management in the 21st century to laboratory directors; managers; chief technologists; supervisors; trainees in schools of healthcare administration, medical laboratory technology, and other allied health disciplines; those training for leadership positions; and those studying for board or registry certification in management. This book is designed both for those who are training to enter these fields and for those who are already actively working in clinical pathology and clinical laboratory management. It contains a comprehensive overview of management principles and how they apply to the clinical laboratory. In-depth analysis of the financial challenges facing clinical laboratories is included, as are discussions on good business practices. There is extensive information on the impact of the regulatory environment on every aspect of clinical laboratory practice, as well as specific personnel issues related to all relevant job classifications.

The authors are all practicing laboratorians, many of whom have had extensive "hands-on" experience in all facets of clinical laboratory practice, including both technical and managerial responsibilities. Each section is edited by experienced professionals and includes comprehensive coverage, both didactic and practical, of all issues related to clinical laboratory operations.

This book is a single resource for extensive laboratory management information, including practical examples and numerous summary tables to serve as guidelines for relevant documentation. Various management tools are provided, particularly related to personnel, technical, regulatory, and financial responsibilities. The information is relevant for all job levels within the laboratory, as well as for all healthcare management and technical training courses. Each chapter follows a consistent format that is designed to flow easily from one section to another. When appropriate, chapters contain checklists, work sheets, forms, abbreviations/acronyms, diagrams, figures, photographs, and specific practical examples of relevant material. A compilation of the terminology glossaries from every chapter is presented at the back of the book.

It is important for readers to understand that there are many different laboratory settings; not every laboratory will handle managerial responsibilities the same way, nor will every option be applicable to every situation. The key to quality and clinically relevant laboratory management approaches requires a thorough understanding of the pros and cons of each approach and how various options may or may not be relevant for one's particular laboratory size and range of expertise, client base, number and type of patients seen, personnel expertise and availability, equipment availability, educational initiatives, and communication requirements.

The use of product or program names is not intended to endorse specific products or programs or to exclude substitute products or programs. Every effort has been made to ensure accuracy; however, ASM Press and the Editors encourage you to submit to us any suggestions, comments, and information on errors found.

Acknowledgments

As editors, we would like to express our thanks to the many teachers, colleagues, and students who have helped shape our perspectives regarding the field of clinical laboratory and pathology management. If the information contained in this book provides help to those in these or related healthcare fields, we will have succeeded in passing on this composite knowledge to the next generation of students and teachers.

Our special thanks go to the authors, all of whom were juggling many other responsibilities during the preparation of this book, for their outstanding contributions. We appreciate their efforts and know the readers will also appreciate the time and energy it took to produce such a comprehensive volume.

We thank the staff of ASM Press, including Ellie Tupper, Susan Birch, Jeff Holtmeier (Director), and our copyeditors; they are outstanding professionals and made our job not only challenging but also enjoyable. Their encouragement led to the completion of this project, one that had been "perking" for several years.

Above all, our special thanks go to our families and colleagues for their support during this extensive project. We could never have undertaken this challenge without their help and understanding.

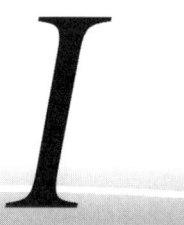

I

Overview of Laboratory Management and Current Healthcare Environment

(Section Editor, *David S. Wilkinson*)

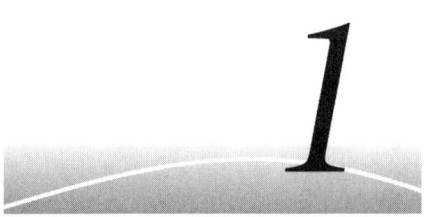

1

Principles of Management

Jeffrey Casterline and John R. Snyder

OBJECTIVES

To familiarize the reader with the concepts of leadership, management, and administration

To place modern management ideas in their historical context

To review in general terms the variety of management concepts and philosophy in such a way that the reader will feel familiar enough to apply the concepts or know where to turn for more information

To discuss in general terms the process of decision making and how a decision-making style is a reflection of one's leadership style

To consider the issue of management ethics and their positive impact on the workplace

"The new technology will not render managers superfluous or replace them by more technicians. On the contrary, it will demand many more managers. It will greatly extend the management area; many people now considered rank-and-file will have to become capable of doing management work."

PETER DRUCKER (14)

THE HISTORY OF HUMANS COULD BE CHARACTERIZED as the story of our attempts and methods to organize ourselves. Our ability to create often exceeds our ability to manage the fruits of our collective and individual genius. It is unclear in the historical record just who was the first person to think through the questions of how to get a job done through other people and how to convey that message. Intuitively we can think of cave dwellers in prehistoric times, working together to hunt for food or to protect themselves from other marauding bands of primitive people. Villages became towns, which grew into large cities. Amalgamations of people and buildings provide one of the basic challenges of management, and urban management is one of those areas where the problems humankind can create often exceed the abilities of those charged with keeping the order.

Modern times require modern solutions. As society has become more complex, the solutions have become equally complex and sophisticated. The beginning of this chapter is devoted to the consideration of leadership versus management. What do these terms mean? Are they truly different or is it just semantics? Once these points are made clear, the chapter briefly covers the history of management thought, to illustrate that as society and organizations have become more complex, the theories to explain group behaviors have become similarly complex.

One of the main tasks of management is to decide what to do and then provide the roadmap on how to get it done. The chapter devotes several pages to the issues surrounding decision making and decision theory.

Finally, the chapter devotes itself to ethics and questions managers now face on deciding what is appropriate behavior, not just on the shop floor but also in the boardroom.

Peter Drucker's quote raises several interesting questions and provides a basic theme for the chapter. Is our progressively more technological society eliminating the need for managers? Is the mechanization of the workplace and our society rendering management unnecessary? On the contrary, many more people will absorb basic management function into their work lives. Perhaps this can be looked upon as a form of self-empowerment. Individuals will have some measure of control over their own work life and what they will do on a day-to-day basis. We are the managers of the machines we operate, and we decide what role they will play. This is not to say that higher authority will lose its prominence. Rather, strategic direction will become the primary focus of upper management, as opposed to hands-on direction of precisely what we are doing and how we do it. Maybe another way to say this is as follows: upper management must exercise leadership in the modern enterprise if it is to meet its goals and objectives.

Leadership, Management, and Administration

Leadership

As kids we used to play the game "follow the leader." Politicians often talk about the need for leadership or the lack thereof. On the job we hear of individuals who take a leadership position on an issue or in that organization. We always talk about what is important to us, and considering the amount of print space we devote to this concept, clearly it is a key concern to many people. Leadership is at once something that people do and a key driving force for humankind.

A leader is also a piece of fishing line. This may seem a silly analogy, but the role of the leader with bait and tackle is very similar to the role of the leader in an organization. What does a fishing leader do? In some instances, it is designed to be a near-invisible connection between the heavier fishing line and the lure. Its lack of weight and heft makes it easier to cast out to where the fish are, and near invisibility makes it less likely that the fish will see the lure as anything other than a tasty morsel. In other cases the leader is designed to be an indestructible connection between the hook and the fishing line. Its toughness means that the catch will not be able to bite through it and coral and rocks will not destroy it. Some "human" leaders maintain near invisibility, letting those tasked with getting the job done go forward without any distraction. Some leaders present themselves as an unbreakable connection between those doing the work and the ultimate goal.

Starting at the beginning, what precisely is leadership? Or perhaps the question to ask is, what is a leader? More often than not, the definition of leadership is phrased in comparative terms, comparable to what is leadership versus what is management? For example, managers are persons appointed to positions of authority who enable others to do their work effectively. Leadership is one of the roles that a manager needs to exercise. By executing the leadership role, managers get things done through people. Leadership is modeling the behavior, attitudes, and values that inspire others to work together enthusiastically (31). Managers do things right. Leaders do the right things. Managers direct, where leaders model and coach. The list goes on.

We live in a rapidly changing business world which probably requires more leadership, and less managing, than in past decades. But organizations must still strike a balance between change and stability, which means that anyone in a position to influence or direct others must exhibit a balance between leading and managing. If you want to manage, you've got to lead. And if you want to lead, you've got to manage. It is important to make the distinction between leadership and management and for the reader to understand that at any given point he or she may be involved in tasks associated with either or both simultaneously.

A "leader" can be defined as someone who occupies a position in a group, influences others in accordance with the role expectation of the position, and coordinates and directs the group in maintaining itself and reaching its goal (60). Leadership, when viewed this way, is a function of the use of power. The leader has power over his group. Followers follow because of the perceived power of the leader.

Power, as exercised in a leadership model, comes in a variety of types. One's leadership style in part is a function of the type of power one chooses to use. Expert and informational power relate to those skills and knowledge the leader may have and can use to gain influence over others. Reward and coercive power relate to the ability to reward or punish as a means to gain compliance. Legitimate power is that which is confirmed by the group or the organization itself, such as the elected leadership. And finally, referent power is influence by and identification with the leader. An example here might be the power of a rock star or other notable personality (46).

Most leaders use a combination of the various types of power, depending upon their leadership style or what is needed at that moment. For example, an authoritarian leader would use more reward and coercive power than the participative leader, who would use more legitimate or referent power (47). But no one leader has or uses the same style at all times. Leadership is responsive to the needs of the moment. One's leadership style will match what is needed for the group to succeed (48).

It is said that great leaders are made, not born (6). There is considerable evidence and commentary in the literature to support this notion and the opposite. If you believe that leaders are born, you accept more or less that there are certain inborn qualities, such as initiative, courage, and intelligence, which might predestine someone to leadership. Alternatively, one could accept the idea that a leader is a person who was in the right place at the right time.

Leadership theory can support either concept. The great man/great woman theory suggests that major events in the world both draw out and mold the leader or that major events are influenced by persons of power (73). The trait theory expands on the personal characteristics of the leader. However, knowing that leaders come in all varieties and often are as dissimilar as they are similar, one can only think that some traits merely increase the probability that an individual will rise to a position of leadership and power (7). Thus, a situational view is now accepted as a predominate theory, that historical forces drive great events and leaders either rise or do not rise to that occasion. The characteristic of the individual and the situation that presents itself determine who will be the leader (2).

Management

What of the leader as a manager? Is management truly a different task or merely something a leader must attend to in order to be successful? Is management a separate and distinct behavior? Managers in general provide four separate but equally important functions: planning, organizing, controlling, and leading (20). Each of these concepts is covered in depth in subsequent chapters. It should be noted that the manager is not necessarily the group's leader. One can influence a group toward reaching its goals and not be the manager, and the manager can succeed by letting the informal leader of any group carry on with the task of motivating the group (70). Managers can be very task specific. For example, financial managers focus on generating and reinvesting financial capital. Human resource managers help recruit staff and oversee labor law vis-à-vis the organization where they work.

One of the basic definitions of management is getting things done through other people. Managers prefer to work with others. Managers provide the resources and the direction to accomplish the task. Managers decide upon goals based on necessity and are therefore strongly tied to the organization as it currently exists (56). Management has no meaning apart from its goals. Managers therefore keep organizational goals in mind at all times. Management produces predictability and order. Managers emphasize rationality and control. Managers solve problems. In short, management is an activity that provides structure. Management in some ways provides the "what" that needs to be done. In the Financial Management Network website article by Lorin Woolfe, he explains how often the words "managers" and "management" have been used interchangeably (http://www.fmnonline.com/publishing/article.cfm?article_id=545 [last accessed 28 April 2003]). This was purposeful, to emphasize the meaning behind the basic management definition. What managers do and what management is are often one in the same.

Is there such a thing as a management style? Referring back to the discussion on leadership, largely this is a function of the situation at hand. One of the more prevalent perspectives on management style comes from Blake and Mouton, who as a result of their studies were able to create what is known as the Managerial Grid (11). This grid places "concern for people" on the vertical axis and "concern for task" on the horizontal one. Most people fall somewhere in the middle. But Blake and Mouton derived four types of leaders who fall near the extremes of the grid, as shown in Fig. 1.1.

The Authoritarian Manager is highly task oriented, with low concern for people. There is little allowance for cooperation or collaboration. Heavily task-oriented people are strong on scheduling and expect people to do what they are told with little discussion or debate. When something goes wrong, they tend to focus on blame rather than on the problem.

Conversely, the Country Club Manager has a low level of task orientation, with a high concern for people. This manager uses reward power to maintain discipline and to encourage his or her team to achieve its goals. This manager is incapable of using coercive powers, because doing so would jeopardize that manager's relationship with the group.

The Impoverished Manager, with a low level of task orientation and a low concern for people, uses delegation as the primary management tool and for the most part is not committed to the accomplishment of the task or maintenance of the group. The team does what it wishes.

Finally, the Team Manager is highly task oriented and maintains a high concern for people. This manager leads by example and works at creating an environment where

Figure 1.1 The Managerial Grid. Adapted from R. R. Blake and J. S. Mouton, *The Managerial Grid* (Gulf Publishing Company, Houston, Tex., 1974), and J. R. Snyder and D. S. Wilkinson, *Management in Laboratory Medicine*, 3rd ed. (Lippincott-Raven Publishers, Philadelphia, Pa., 1998).

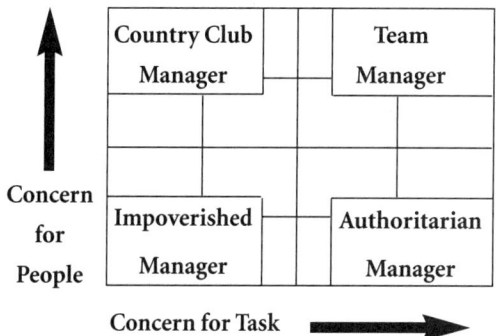

all team members may prosper. The manager works with the team to reach its goals as effectively as possible, while also working to strengthen the bonds among the team members. By grid design this is the most effective manager and leads to the most effective teams.

But as has been discussed before, management, like leadership, is situational (55). The lieutenant tasked with taking a hill may not have the luxury of acting like a Team Manager. There is a time where discussion and debate have no place. Alternatively, while we might look down at the Impoverished Manager as singularly ineffective, using this model may lead to more self-reliance on the part of the team.

Administration

We have talked about leadership and management. What of administration? Is it something different from the above or merely a different word for what managers and leaders do? A *Webster's* definition of "administer" lists first "to act as manager. . ." and second "to furnish help or be of service" (65). Based on the second definition, it is possible to think of administration as an action apart from leadership and management, in that it focuses one's effort on assistance and service as opposed to the specific acts that a manager or leader might undertake. A manager and/or leader may have as his charge the requirement to serve others. But that becomes a task specific to that individual, rather than a general charge to managers at large.

One of the primary definitions of administrator refers to government and public sector jobs (65). Administration by that definition becomes a public service job, much like one would see in academia or healthcare. Thus, administrators might in fact do different things than a manager. This is to say, administration is a subset of management. Administrators do all those things that make one a manager. Administrators have a public service requirement and commitment that would not necessarily be found in the portfolio of all working managers.

We have covered quickly some of the basics of leadership and management and touched briefly on administration. The above topics have been the focus of many books and academic treatises. It is left to the reader to explore these topics further, either elsewhere in this text or in the multitude of available reference materials.

Management Concepts

Above was the sentence, "Modern times require modern solutions." While this is often heard, the reality is that for the most part we are using old solutions and methods to deal with current problems. Generals are said always to be fighting the last war. The technology we buy today is already outdated. The feedback loop we work in is retrospective. We cannot fully plan for or project what the future will be or what it will bring. The concept of cultural lag is derived from these notions.

Cultural Lag

What is cultural lag? Here is a basic definition: "the failure of one element of a culture to keep pace with changes in other aspects of the culture; e.g. a situation in which rapid technological change is not accompanied by change in the non-material culture" (1). Clearly, technological advance moves at a pace much faster than the majority of humankind can absorb it. The scale is global. Sometimes it is referred to as a computerized giant leap forward; those who have a technological edge will move forward, whereas those who do not will be left behind. By inference one can see this applying with individual urban centers, with national economies, or within global regions. The definition of haves and have-nots will be focused not so exclusively on material goods so much as access to knowledge and the power that goes with it.

This is not a new issue, however. Such has been the case in one form or another since medieval times and more pointedly with the beginning of the current industrial era. Much of the basis of management thought has been how to organize ourselves to match the advances in technology and how best to exploit those advances to the betterment of all.

Review of Management Thought

Classical theory. The earliest perspectives on management and management theory were described by a group loosely called classical theorists. Most notably this group includes Frederick Taylor and his work on scientific management theory. Additionally, this group includes Henri Fayol and his work on what he referred to as administrative management and Max Weber and his research into the nature of bureaucracy. This group and others laid the foundation for management theory, in part by identifying the key managerial processes and skills a manager needs to succeed. Perhaps most importantly, their work made management a valid subject for academic inquiry.

Taylor was one of the first to create a science of management (69). He is best known for his attempts to systematically analyze human behavior at work. His model was a machine made of cheap interchangeable parts. Taylor attempted to do to complex organizations what engineers had done to machines. This involved breaking down each task into the smallest identifiable unit and then figuring out the best way to do that part of the job. He felt that productivity would improve if each aspect of work was carefully studied and the alternatives facing each worker were restricted. He was correct, but he has been criticized for dehumanizing the workplace and reducing human beings to little more than machine cogs in the production process. But the principles of scientific management had been well defined. Describe and break down each task into its smallest component and study that task until the best way to do that task is fully defined. Remove uncertainty and alternatives facing each employee and reward productivity with incentives. Use experts, for example, industrial engineers, to define optimal work outputs and plan for optimal results.

Fayol identified the four basic management functions: planning, organizing, leading, and controlling. His work focused on management more than task and production. He identified 14 principles of management, universal truths that he thought could be taught (21):

- Division of work
- Authority
- Discipline
- Unity of command
- Unity of direction
- Subordination of individual interest
- Remuneration
- Centralization
- Chain of command
- Order
- Equity
- Stability
- Initiative
- Esprit de corps

We do not discuss each principle individually, leaving that for the reader to explore. These are still taught as the basics of management, and Fayol's work remains as pertinent today as it did early in the 20th century.

Max Weber embellished the scientific management theories with his views on bureaucracy and organizational theory (72). He focused on dividing organizations into hierarchies and on the establishment of lines of authority and control. He suggested that organizations develop comprehensive and detailed standard operating procedures for all routine tasks. Where Fayol before him had laid out his principles of management, Weber identified the core elements of the new organization, the bureaucracy:

- Formal rules and behavior defined by those rules
- Uniformity of operations despite changes in personnel
- Division of labor based on functional specialization
- Rational allocation of tasks
- Impersonal orientation
- Membership constitutes a career
- Promotion based on technical competence
- Employment based on merit
- Qualifications are tested
- Legally defined, proscribed lines of authority
- Limited discretion of senior management and officers
- Specific spheres of competence
- Legally based organizational tenure (72)

Emphasizing order, rationality, and uniformity, he believed, would lead to more equitable treatment of the workers. He is faulted in some circles for his authoritarian views and the concept that authority is position based and not focused on the individual. Clearly, however, his work moved beyond that of Taylor and Fayol and laid the groundwork for the next generation of management thought.

Behavioral theory. Despite the economic progress brought about by the implementation of scientific management, and as noted above, many critics were pointing to the dehumanization of the workplace. Labor and management conflict ensued, and worker apathy and boredom were believed to be widespread. These concerns, along with developments in the field of psychology and economics, brought to the forefront challenges to the assumptions of the scientific management school.

The Hawthorne studies at a Western Electric plant were a straightforward attempt to determine if there was a relationship between the work environment and productivity (43). In one famous experiment, the illumination in one work area was adjusted and another area acted as a control. The productivity levels of the two groups were compared. Curiously, the productivity of each group increased, challenging the assumption that mere physical environmental changes were the key. Elton Mayo and his associates, those who performed the experiments, felt that the increase in productivity was a result of increased attention paid to both sets of workers. Other studies performed by Mayo illustrated that workers will perform at a level informally set by the work group and that external management often will have little impact on those decisions. Thus, Mayo concluded that social processes played a major role in determining worker attitudes and behavior, far from the previously accepted notions that workers and tasks could be parsed out like parts of a machine (43). This led to the development of the human relations movement, which is based on the idea that a manager's concern for his workers will lead to increased worker satisfaction and improved performance.

Shifting the focus from strictly organizational needs, the human relations movement sought to bring the wants and needs of the individual worker into the discussion. American psychologist Abraham Maslow devised his six-level hierarchy of needs that, according to his theory, determines human behavior (42). He ranked them as follows:

- Physiological
- Security and safety
- Love and feelings of belonging
- Prestige and esteem
- Self-fulfillment
- Curiosity and the need to understand

As one level of needs is met, we are able to work towards meeting the next level. If management wants solid, productive employees, motivated to work at their best, then every individual must be compensated and supported to the point where the basic needs are fulfilled and no longer seem to be a concern. Crucial, of course, is the understanding that what would fulfill one person may not address another's perceived needs. Hence, individual attention to each worker is a requirement for management to succeed.

Douglas McGregor developed his own theory of motivation and management, which is referred to as theory X and theory Y (45). In short, behind every management decision and action are assumptions about human nature and human behavior. Theory X ascribes to the more negative and perhaps Taylorism concept, that people need direction and control and are incapable of taking responsibility. Every individual needs financial inducements and threats to make them work. Theory Y, on the other hand, presumes that people want their work to be fulfilling, that they seek self-respect and self-development. Theory Y suggests that work is a natural human enterprise and that the average person does not dislike work. Effort on the job need not come as a result of threats, but rather comes if the individual is committed to the organization and its objectives. Satisfaction on the job and self-actualization can be directed toward the objectives of the organization. Additionally, theory Y proponents accept that imagination, ingenuity, and creativity are not restricted to a narrow group within the organization, but are widespread and only need to be tapped.

Both behavioralist models emerged because previous management theory was far too simplistic and did not address the needs of the individual. Maslow and McGregor tried to address individual needs and their relation to the needs of the organization (42, 45). From these theories we were able to gain some insights into group process and interpersonal relationships among the workers, and the theories focused management on the needs of employees as people, not just as part of the production process. But therein lies some of the limitations of this view. People are complex beings and it is never easy to predict what anyone will want at any given moment. Managers themselves often find it easier to focus on process than people. Organizational goals and objectives are frequently stated in other than human relations terms. Nonetheless, these theories remain at the core of modern human resource management and are robust still in their insights and perspectives.

Quantitative theory. As the world moved out of World War II and industrial production shifted its focus from military hardware and support of national causes to consumer-desired goods and services, so did the corporation move from a cost-is-no-object to a cost containment, profit-driven mind-set. The legions of industrial engineers, previously focused on industrial efficiency to support the war effort, were now charged with improving corporate efficiency. Who said it first is lost in history, but the adage "if it can be measured, it can be managed" took hold and strong quantitative approaches were adopted.

Management science focused very specifically on the development of mathematic models (49). Early computer applications in this direction centered on helping managers find the best way to do things and how to save money. Linear programming models and inventory management and control, which are difficult mathematical concepts and often beyond the ability of a person to compute within rational time limits, become trivial questions when the power of even the simplest of computers is employed. But this also looked very much like the pendulum was swinging back into Taylorism and the dehumanization of the organization. Much of senior management in the post-World War II period was made of former officers and military, who placed their focus on accomplishment of the task at hand, often at the expense of the welfare of their employees. Employee work groups could not readily convert to a mathematic problem; hence, a new concept of management needed to be developed to bring together the needs of the corporation and the needs of the individual.

Operations management was that attempt to develop a set of tools, applied mathematics and human resource management, to develop techniques to produce products and services more efficiently (49). Operations management often includes substantial measurement and analysis of internal processes. Ultimately, the nature of how operations management is carried out in an organization depends very much on the nature of products or services in the organization, for example, retail, manufacturing, or wholesale. As with management science, though, the focus was away from the individual and related more toward the organization at large and how it interacted within the larger business environment (24).

Management by objectives tried to integrate the concept of managing what can be measured and bringing the individual into focus (15, 59). At its simplest, every employee will have a set of objectives to achieve, which together with all other employees in the organization will pull the enterprise toward its overall objectives. All targets will be quantifiable and easily recognizable for their value to the company. But the reality is that most performance cannot be measured and is evaluated based on the supervisor's own biases and personal agenda. Key points here are that objectives must be clearly defined, plans for achieving the objective must be detailed and clear, and there must be ongoing monitoring to see if the plans are moving forward (15).

Thus, the quantitative perspective did push the development of mathematic techniques for decision making and the setting of objectives. This modeling methodology dramatically increased the awareness of organizational processes and assisted greatly in organizational planning. Much like with the previous theories, however, human behavior is unpredictable, and following the dictate "garbage in, garbage out," mathematic models based on faulty information or assumptions will not lead to better management.

Integrated theory. With the failure of mathematic modeling to fully address management problems, a new, more holistic view of the organization developed (50). Speaking generally, the integrated systems approach to management tried to incorporate the best of all that came before it while trying to maintain a human focus (30). Systems theory represents the merger of many ideas from scientific management and the human relations movement. It is project based and strives toward organizational synergy. There are those who would nest systems theory under the heading of quantitative management. Such an approach misses the point that systems theory is all encompassing, whereas the basics of quantitative management are pure mathematics.

A system here is defined as an organized unit composed of two or more interdependent parts, subsystems perhaps, where the whole can be identified as something separate and apart from its surrounding environment (51). Consider an organization to be a system. It will experience problems, and issues will need to be addressed. The systems-oriented manager, rather than merely trying to manage the problem away, will look at the opportunities a problem might bring and will try to bring all available resources from his organization to bear on the situation.

Much of systems theory resembles the scientific method. You see a problem to be examined. You hypothesize a solution. You design a controlled experiment to test that hypothesis. You collect and analyze the data. The key here is to maintain your focus and attention on the organization as a whole (30). You cannot change one part of the system without affecting all the others. Systems theory might seem quite basic. Yet it is extremely difficult to examine the whole of an entity. We are used to breaking down problems into identifiable and workable parts. It should be noted that the information system tools to allow a real-time focus on an entire organization have only recently become available.

Into this mix, and possibly in part as a result of the difficulty in trying to manage the whole, a contingency theory of management emerged. At its most basic, contingency theory asserts that when managers make decisions, they must take into account all aspects of the current situation and then act only on those aspects that are most crucial (39). You keep the entire entity in mind but focus only on that which seems most important. You acknowledge that you will be impacting the entire system, but you keep your attention directed at that which seems most pressing at that moment. Thus, there is no one "best way" to manage an organization. The contingency perspective would say that universal theories do not apply to every organization, because every organization is unique. This falls under the subheading of an integrated theory, because it presupposes that the decision maker involved will keep in mind that even though his concern might be on a subsystem of the larger organization it is still nested in that larger system.

As powerful as the above integrated approaches might be, they soon were dwarfed by the emergence of the various total quality management (TQM) and continuous quality improvement (CQI) models.

W. Edwards Deming is often referred to as the founder of the modern quality movement (52). While an American whose ideas were developed based on western management theory, he gained wide prominence through the acceptance of his theories by the Japanese. The Japanese themselves will say that the application of his ideas led in great measure to their postwar economic success. His theories by themselves are very basic and deceptively simple to implement. To start, Deming believed that TQM begins at the corporate level (63). The entire enterprise must have a deep and wide-ranging commitment to the continuing improvement of products and services (27). You can never stand still and say, figuratively, that what you have is good enough. Don't bother with postproduction inspection as the place to identify errors. Inspection and review must be ongoing. Build quality into the production process and the product. Do not rely on low-cost bidding by suppliers. Instead, require true quality, measure quality, and be willing to pay the price for that result. And finally, initiate training programs and leadership models to help people do a better job and to empower them to speak out and respond when problems are detected (61). Deming says do this and you'll produce a better product.

More than 40 years after their adoption, these concepts seem obvious and basic to modern industrial management. At the time, however, they were very revolutionary, and their very adoption by the Japanese changed the meaning of the phrase "made in Japan" from cheap and poorly made to solid and reliably built (62).

TQM, one of the first so-named theories of the quality movement, is a structured system for satisfying internal and external customers by integrating the business environment, continuous improvement, and technological and production breakthroughs (9). "Structured" means that it is a strategy driven by identification of customer wants and needs that have been determined through ongoing interaction with those clients. TQM is a description of the culture, attitudes, and organization of a company that aims to provide, and continue to provide, its customers with products and services that satisfy their identified needs. It is a corporate culture that requires quality in all aspects of the company's operation, with things done right the first time and defects and waste removed from operations. The products are designed to be quality output, and the manufacturing and product systems follow through to meet that goal.

Consider the differences. Ford Motor Company strove to become the number one producer of automobiles by determining first what price the consumer would accept and then working toward making a car that could be produced for that price. The challenge was not quality. The challenge was production efficiency and unit cost (53). More or less you could look at the production of Ford cars as a "Taylorism" experiment. Divide the work into its smallest parts, make each part as efficiently as possible, and ramp up production to get quantity pricing. On the other hand, consider the production of a Toyota in 1975. Via marketing research, the focus was on what level of quality the customer expected for every unit of cost (63). Design the product to meet those quality demands. Focus not on throughput but on quality production at each step. Acknowledge that the customer does not want the cheapest car, but rather the best value for the selling price. The attitude shift is from car production at whatever the market will bear to getting the best-quality product onto the market as the best value to be found.

Many organizations have trouble integrating a TQM model into their operations. Less than half of those who have tried a TQM approach report any improvement in quality, productivity, competitiveness, or financial return (10). But that percentage may be deceiving. The focus should be on successful operations, where much more than 50% rely upon TQM to maintain their success.

A subset of the TQM movement is often referred to as CQI. What separates CQI from TQM is the focus on the employee (29). A CQI approach forces the organization to look at its employees and their work as part of a continuous process. CQI is thought to have a more human face than TQM. We find it hard to see the distinction.

Whatever acronym you choose to use, the quality management approach to production changed forever the way manufacturers looked at their world. The focus on cost reduction and profit improvement has been replaced forever by a focus on the customer and the production of a quality product at a reasonable price that meets the customer's needs.

New concepts. Management theory and thought continue to move forward, with ongoing work in the behavioral and individual employee world, as well as a focus on the organization and production processes.

Above it was noted that management by objectives was one of the most widespread approaches to dealing with individual employees. Taking that notion a step farther is the current interest in lifelong learning, also known as continuous lifelong learning (32). The continuous lifelong learning process starts by identifying where a person is at that moment and where a person needs or wants to be. Assessment of the individual is an essential part of this self-identification, so that person can move to the next phase of the process. Phase two has individuals taking over and leading themselves to their desired performance level and to the amount of change they wish to achieve. There are several key factors. First, the employer recognizes that crucial to lifelong learning is the concept that no one individual will necessarily stay in their job or with that employer forever. As people learn and grow they move on to new jobs and experiences. Second, individuals can take charge of their life to reach their full potential. Self-empowerment is both a result and an employee need. Third, individuals are accountable for and responsible for their individual progress. One might have a mentor. But that mentor is not responsible for the individual's growth.

The connection to the employer and management is that learning-inspired and driven employees do better work and absorb the TQM message much more effectively (32). TQM and CQI require the employee to think and to consider the options available, to work better and more efficiently. Dialogue between management and worker is enhanced when the employee thinks in terms of the job as part of a lifelong journey and is learning and working toward a better life. This is almost a utopian vision but nonetheless the direction in which much of the industrial world is heading.

Similarly, while on an individual basis the organization actively develops their employees so that they evolve and grow, on a product and process basis modern corporations are starting to work towards a total product life cycle management concept. This theory suggests that more than merely focusing on a product as a unit at a point in time, that the organization needs to consider whether that product is in the ascendancy or is fading and adjust the product to the customer needs accordingly (8, 26). The marketplace is always moving forward, and the organization must move forward with it. Product design and production must think through the issues of product introduction and placement in the marketplace, ultimately the disposal and replacement of that product, and planning for the next generation of product to meet the customer's demands and needs. Similar in many ways to TQM, in which a product design defines its quality and use, the life cycle management theory goes a step farther to plan for product demise and redefinition as the customers change their focus to something new. At some point the organization will decide to stop making or doing one thing and to move on to another. Life cycle management forces an enterprise early in a product life to plan for its replacement (8). Thus, engineering is always thinking ahead and employee education always works toward preparing the workforce for the future.

Also similarly, process reengineering forces the organization to rethink how it does its work and how it can be done better (66). Again, this is an extrapolation on TQM and CQI. The difference is that with TQM and CQI you are always trying to improve what you already do. Process reengineering suggests that you entirely abandon what you are doing now in favor of something entirely new and different (67). In the extreme, process reengineering assumes the current process to be irrelevant. Thus, you should start over with a clean slate and see what you can do. Those subscribing to this theory think in terms of vision and the future (12). What must we look like at some future point to meet the needs of our customers? What technological changes have taken place that we should incorporate to make us better and more responsive? What will our customers expect of us in the future that we must plan and build toward now?

A reengineering given is that technological change has negated all that we do now. Thus, it is not merely a desire on our part to change what we do to improve ourselves. Changes in technology by themselves have invalidated all that we do. Hence, we must rebuild from the beginning to utilize all that is new. Competition in the marketplace says that new organizations, those which have never used outdated methods, are there to surpass you. Thus, finding new ways to do things, redesigning processes around new technology, is central to organizational survival.

Finally, it is believed by many that the customer base we work with now is much more quality sensitive and driven. Only the best will survive. Defining what is the best is a current challenge. Six Sigma is one of those approaches. What is Six Sigma? A very thorough coverage of Six Sigma may be found at the Six Sigma website, which covers in depth all aspects of Six Sigma. That site defines Six Sigma as a highly disciplined process to focus on developing and delivering near-perfect products and services (http://www.isixsigma.com/library/content/six-sigma-newbie.asp [last accessed 28 April 2003]). The word "sigma" is a statistical term that measures how far a given process deviates from perfection. Knowing that deviation, you can predict how many errors and defects you will have in a process; thus, you can systematically try to find and remove them.

The Six Sigma website states the following: "Six-Sigma by definition is not more than 3.4 defects per million events" (http://www.isixsigma.com/library/content/six-sigma-newbie.asp [last accessed 28 April 2003]). A Six Sigma defect is further defined as anything outside of customer specifications (3). Thus, it is not merely an operational or production defect. A process can function perfectly. But if the end result is outside of what the customer wants, it is a product defect.

Six Sigma talks of product and process improvement. It incorporates many of the features of TQM and CQI and also of process reengineering. Loosely the theory proponents refer to two different acronyms: DMAIC (define, measure, analyze, improve, control) and DMADV (define, measure, analyze, design, verify) (4). Six Sigma process implementation staff are often referred to as Green Belts and

Black Belts, suggesting a special, trained status and the aggressive nature by which the measurement and improvement processes are implemented (5).

What is Six Sigma? It is another in the many process and product review methodologies, all with the aim of giving the customers what they want. Six Sigma has raised the bar on the definition of product and process quality. Like all management techniques, commitment at all levels of the organization is required and if nothing else this is the primary message carried in all of the above-listed modern and new theories.

Decision Making

Most everyone makes many decisions every day. Granted, many decisions are small and made almost unconsciously. Other decisions are more significant and require more conscious effort, time to study, and consideration of the potential consequences. Regardless of the nature of the decision, every decision encompasses elements of a basic decision-making process.

Decision making by laboratory managers is an everyday activity. Decision making is a core administrative action (68). It is a common process that pervades all healthcare organizations and is essential to the managerial functions of planning, organizing, directing, and controlling as shown in Fig. 1.2. Sometimes referred to as the "brain work" of organizations, decision making affects both efficiency and effectiveness in delivering laboratory products and services. The best decisions are made based on "cost-effectiveness (tests we perform or outsource), productivity (employees we hire), service quality (how we organize services), technology (equipment and methods we purchase), and outcomes (what we accomplish for patients)" (28).

Decisions are made by all levels of management with resource responsibility. In addition, decisions are made by staff. The latter can also affect efficiency and effectiveness in an organization. In fact, sometimes decisions should involve staff in either data gathering or actually making the decision instead of the manager. A common rule of thumb is that decisions should be made at the lowest possible level in an

Figure 1.2 Decision making: integral to management functions.

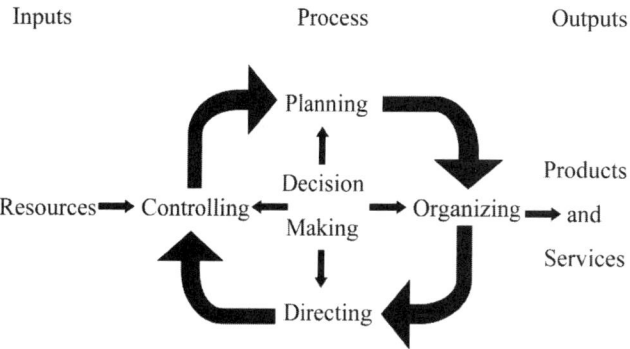

organization. The closer one is to the information and effects of a decision, the higher the quality of that decision.

This section on decision making begins with a definition and review of the leadership role in decision making. Different types of decisions are described and contrasted, followed by a discussion of group involvement in decision making. Steps in the decision-making/problem-solving process are dissected to avoid pitfalls and improve skills. Finally, the element of risk in decision making is explored.

What Is It?

Concisely, decision making is the act of choosing one alternative from among a set of alternatives. This act is complex, however. Inherent in this definition is an awareness that a decision needs to be made, that alternatives need to be developed and considered, and that one "best" alternative is chosen and implemented. Consequently, the "act" of decision making is more appropriately termed a "process," as is described later.

The science of decision making, as described in the literature, applies models based on deductive, inductive, analytical, and simulation approaches. These note that decision making is a deliberate process, differentiating managerial decisions from habit and reflex. Decision making also has an artistic side, drawing on the decision maker's creativity and judgment. In addition, managers often base their decisions on personal or organizational value systems and philosophies.

Recent reports have looked at decision making as a window into leadership style and leadership effectiveness. Indeed, the distinctions between managers' and leaders' decision making as shown in Table 1.1 point to important philosophical and practical differences (57). Embodied in these differences is an understanding of the five crucial elements of leadership:

1. Leadership, like decision making, is a process.
2. The locus of leadership is a person, the "leader."
3. The focus of leadership is other individuals or groups (followers).
4. Leadership entails influencing.
5. The objective of leadership is good accomplishment (64).

Pickett's differences between leaders and managers in Table 1.1 point to an empowerment of individuals in an organization so that they are better able to participate in decision making. He notes that empowerment requires "stretching, coaching, training giving authority, and implying permission to make mistakes (obviously, this must be judiciously applied)" (57). When people in an organization are empowered decision makers, they think differently, act differently, and are more energetic.

During an interview, a reporter once asked a successful executive what the secret to his success was. "Two words," the executive replied, "Right decisions." The reporter probed for more information, asking, "How are right decisions made?" The executive replied, "One word—experience." "But how did you get this experience?" asked the reporter. "Two words," replied the executive, "Wrong decisions." Experience is a powerful teacher.

Types of Decisions

Decisions can be studied and classified from a number of perspectives (13). Some decisions are strategic or tactical, the former focusing on the means to reach a goal, the latter focusing on steps or objectives to be accomplished. Some decisions are administrative, requiring substantial resource commitment; other decisions are operational, dealing with the day-to-day activities. Some decisions are termed programmed because they are more routine and repetitive in nature. Other decisions are termed nonprogrammed because they are novel and unstructured. Still other decisions are individual or group, differentiated by who makes the decision.

Strategic decisions are concerned with an organization's relationships with the external environment, the choice of a competitive posture, and the formulation of major policies (41). The goal is to arrive at the best plan for the organization given operational, economic, logistical, and political constraints. Examples include mergers, expansions into new markets, or off-site testing facilities.

Tactical decisions are, as the name implies, tactics or steps for implementing the organizational strategy. These can be categorized further as administrative decisions or

Table 1.1 Decision-making differences between leaders and managers[a]

Characteristic	Leader	Manager
Vision	Search for long-term opportunities	Maximize current opportunities
Communication	Tell people why we are doing something	Tell people what to do; listen to have an effect; listen for understanding
Question(s) asked	Why?	How? What?
Planning	An opportunity to excite, educate, prepare for future	A path to follow
Power	Something to share and use for the goal of the group	Something to have and use
Problem-solving style	Something to learn from, opportunity for growth	Something to solve, to fix
Perceived role	Integrator; maker of decision makers	Controller or decision maker

[a]Adapted from Pickett (57)

operational decisions. Administrative decisions deal with authority, responsibility, and accountability relationships. Operational decisions handle the routine, day-to-day problems in accomplishing work.

Decisions may also be classified as programmed or nonprogrammed. Programmed decisions are fairly structured and recur with some frequency (13). For example, the decision to reorder supplies and reagents for the laboratory is a programmed decision. Structure exists in terms of quantity to order, purchase requisition process, etc. This decision is made on a recurring basis. Programmed decisions are guided by rules, policies, and procedures.

By contrast, nonprogrammed decisions are relatively unstructured, in part because these occur infrequently (13). Situations which have never arisen exactly like the present or are very complex usually do not have procedures to guide the decision-making process. Some years ago when the concept of core laboratories was introduced, the decisions necessary to plan these high-volume, cross-specialty facilities were unstructured, hence nonprogrammed. A decision today to purchase experimental equipment is a nonprogrammed decision. Nonprogrammed decisions require intuition, creativity, and a tolerance for ambiguity.

A manager's natural tendency toward decision making prompts two more decision types: intuitive decisions and judgmental decisions. Intuitive decisions are made using hunches, subjective values, and personal or emotional factors. A manager who becomes impatient with the time it takes to gather information and sort through details may make an intuitive decision. The manager's decision cannot be readily explained by looking for details but is more likely rationalized by a perception of the "big picture," a holistic view of the situation. Individuals who tend to make intuitive decisions believe that creativity comes from inspiration rather than perspiration.

Most laboratory managers with education and experience in clinical laboratory science tend to make judgmental decisions. These decisions are reached after data are gathered, facts are analyzed, and concrete examples are explored. Judgmental decisions rely on objective analysis and rational procedures. For those decision makers who tend to make judgmental decisions predominate, creativity is really perspiration. The potential danger of "analysis paralysis" is a real threat.

Individual versus Group Decision Making

Individual versus group decision making has received much attention in the management literature. By appointment to a position, the manager has the authority and power to make certain decisions. If managers were all-knowing and highly creative, and if the workplace were not a complex environment, perhaps the involvement of subordinates in decision making would be less important. But all managers have limitations, the work environment

is complex, and some of the necessary information and creativity to reach a high-quality decision reside with the subordinates.

The involvement of groups in decision making adds both benefits and liabilities. Groups tend to make decisions that are more accurate than individual decisions, although reaching a group decision is slower. Social interaction in group decision making tends to foster competition for respect among members, provide social support, and self-correct errors that might occur when an individual is making the decision alone. Group decision-making dynamics sometimes are counterproductive, however. When not constrained by a mandate to reach a group decision, individuals tend to produce more ideas, more unique ideas, and better ideas. Generally, people accept better decisions reached by a group versus an individual if they feel that their participation in the decision was considered and valued. Obviously, acceptance of a decision is key to commitment and implementation.

Insight into the question of whether a decision should be made by the individual manager or with involvement of the affected group of employees has been shared by Vroom and Jago (71). Originally researched by Vroom and Yetton, these insights take into account three criteria: (i) quality or rationality of the decision, (ii) acceptance or commitment of subordinates to implement the decision, and (iii) time required to make a decision.

Vroom and Yetton's decision-making model identified seven rules to protect the quality and acceptance of a decision as shown in Table 1.2. Adherence to these rules and guidance about when to involve groups in decision making are aided by the corresponding questions shown in this table. Before considering each rule, it is important to answer the first question, "Does the problem possess a quality requirement?" Management decisions are rarely right or wrong in a "black or white" sense. Many decisions are simply better than others; hence, they are higher-quality decisions. For example, a manager can make the fairly simple decision of who will staff which holidays simply on the basis of who is available and the number of staff needed. But is this the best decision, the highest-quality decision? Likely not, since certain holidays are more important to some employees than to others. Decisions affecting employees directly often have a quality element, which carries over to affect both acceptance and commitment.

Each of Vroom and Yetton's seven rules to protect quality and acceptance identify specific concerns in decision making (71):

1. The leader information rule raises the question of whether the manager has sufficient information or expertise to solve the problem himself. Some level of group involvement, even if the group is only seeking information, may be necessary to protect the quality of the decision.

Table 1.2 Concerns in decision making (71)

Parameter	Rule	Question(s)
Quality	1. Leader information rule	Does the problem possess a quality requirement? Do I have sufficient information to make a high-quality decision?
	2. Unstructured problem rule	Is the problem structured?
Acceptance	3. Acceptance rule	Is acceptance of the decision by subordinates important for effective implementation?
	4. Acceptance priority rule	If I were to make the decision by myself, am I reasonably certain that it would be accepted by my subordinates?
Quality and acceptance	5. Goal congruence rule	Do subordinates share the organizational goals to be attained in solving the problem?
	6. Conflict rule	Is conflict among subordinates likely in a preferred solution?
	7. Fairness rule	

2. The unstructured-problem rule asks whether this is a programmed or nonprogrammed decision: i.e., has it been solved before and are there already rules, policies, and procedures to guide decision making?
3. The acceptance rule asks whether subordinates' commitment to the decision is key to implementation.
4. The acceptance priority rule asks whether subordinates will be committed to the decision if the manager makes it autocratically.
5. The goal congruence rule queries whether subordinates share (agree with and hence will be committed to) organizational goals to be reached by solving the problem.
6. The conflict rule poses the question of whether there will be disagreement among subordinates about which is the best solution.
7. The fairness rule considers how subordinates will perceive their involvement and opportunity to air and resolve differences in reaching a decision.

Decision styles illustrated in Fig. 1.3 show Vroom and Yetton's continuum from total management prerogative when an autocratic decision is made, through group involvement in a consultative process, to more employee prerogative in the group having responsibility for a decision. A review of the code descriptions, AI and AII for autocratic, CI and CII for consultative, and GI and GII for group, reveals the subtle differences in approaches. For example, the consultative approach may be done by the manager sharing the problem with employees one at a time to seek their input or all employees at the same time. The latter approach will experience both the benefits and limitations of group social interaction.

Figure 1.3 also attempts to capture the essence of acceptance or commitment and time criteria. When a decision is made predominately through management prerogative, resistance to acceptance and commitment is highest, but the decision is made in the least amount of time. By contrast, the greater the employee prerogative in making a group decision, the more time is needed to reach the decision but the less resistance is met.

In healthcare, group involvement in decision making has become popular as a form of participative management, or shared governance. Shared-governance models, ranging from interdisciplinary committees to self-directed work teams, attempt to develop group structures where members have "power, authority, accountability and final decision-making capacity" (58). Often these groups are created around functions, such as patient care or practice opera-

Figure 1.3 Continuum of decision styles. AI, you solve the problem or make the decision yourself, using information available to you. AII, you solve the problem or make the decision yourself, using information from subordinates. They may or may not be aware of the decision-making process and their role in it. CI, you share the problem with relevant subordinates individually, getting their ideas. Then you make the decision yourself, accepting or rejecting advice from subordinates. CII, you share the problem with relevant subordinates at a group meeting, getting their ideas. Then you make the decision yourself, accepting or rejecting advice from subordinates. GI, you share the problem with subordinates individually, and together you analyze the problem and arrive at a mutual solution. You both contribute. GII, you share the problem with relevant subordinates at a group meeting, and together you analyze the problem and arrive at a group decision. You do not try to influence the group, and you are willing to accept and implement what the group recommends. DI (not shown), you delegate the problem to a subordinate, providing him relevant information and giving him responsibility for the problem alone.

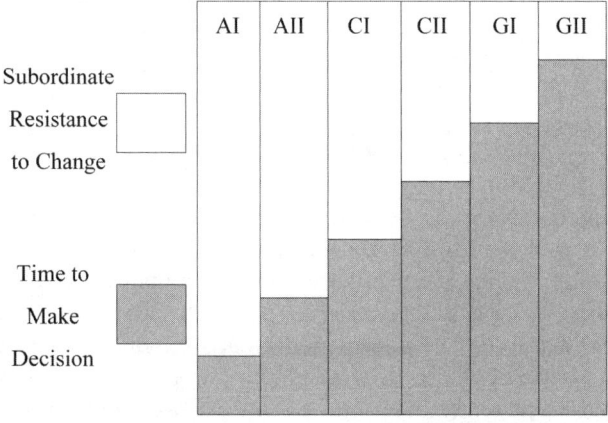

tions, or education. Gill points out that it is important for the manager to understand how different groups interact, communicate, and influence individuals within the group, to effectively facilitate group decision making (22). Moreover, it is important for the manager to have a level of understanding about individual preferences and strengths as a contributor to group decision making. Drucker points out that "a great many people perform best as advisors, but cannot take the burden and pressure of the decision. A good many people, by contrast, need an advisor to force themselves to think, but then they can take the decision and act on it with speed, self-confidence, and courage" (19).

The Problem-Solving/Decision-Making Process

While it is true that decisions are choices, decision making and problem solving are indeed a process of steps as shown in Fig. 1.4. Definition of these steps, a dissection of the anatomy of a decision if you will, points to the value and potential pitfalls in reaching a high-quality decision whether made by an individual or a group (44). True, many decisions can be made quickly with little attention to the steps along the process. The more complex the problem, the more mission critical the objectives are and the more important each step is to reaching a successful, high-quality decision. McConnell notes that "one of the greatest trouble spots in decision-making exists because of the human tendency to move from observation to conclusion on limited information" (44).

- *Step 1: Identify the problem or determine the objectives.* Identifying the problem requires a manager to first diagnose the situation. Too often a symptom of the problem is misidentified as the root cause. For example, a manager who identifies poor morale in the laboratory has misdiagnosed the situation. Poor morale is a symptom of an underlying problem. The range of root causes could include low pay, unappreciative supervi-

sors, and lack of respect by coworkers, among other causes. Failure to define the problem in step 1 will negate all subsequent steps to solve the problem. Similarly, clear definition of objectives for a decision provides a constant point of reference when subsequently gathering information and developing alternatives.

- *Step 2: Gather facts and evaluate information.* At this step, the manager will learn whether he is dealing with a programmed or nonprogrammed decision. Are there rules, policies, and procedures which need to be followed? Has someone already solved this problem, and if so, how similar are the characteristics to this situation? Is there a need to get group input, and if so, individually or collectively, and from whom? Figure 1.4 shows the influence of the manager's perceptions of information gathered as data are evaluated. The natural tendencies to either rely on the five senses to identify factual detail (sensing) or to use hunches and a more holistic view (intuition) will be part of this step.

- *Step 3: Develop and evaluate alternative solutions and options.* Some possible solutions will be obvious; other solutions will be more creative. The tendency to quickly adopt the first viable solution may be time efficient but lead to a lesser-quality decision or solution. In general, the more important the decision, the more alternatives should be developed. At this step, as shown in Fig. 1.4, evaluation of options will be influenced by judgments of the decision maker. The use of both subjective values and objective analysis will lead to a better sort among potential options.

- *Step 4: Select the best alternative.* After considering each option in light of the situation or objectives to be achieved, the manager chooses the one most likely to be the highest quality with the greatest acceptance within the time available for decision making.

Figure 1.4 Problem-solving/decision-making process.

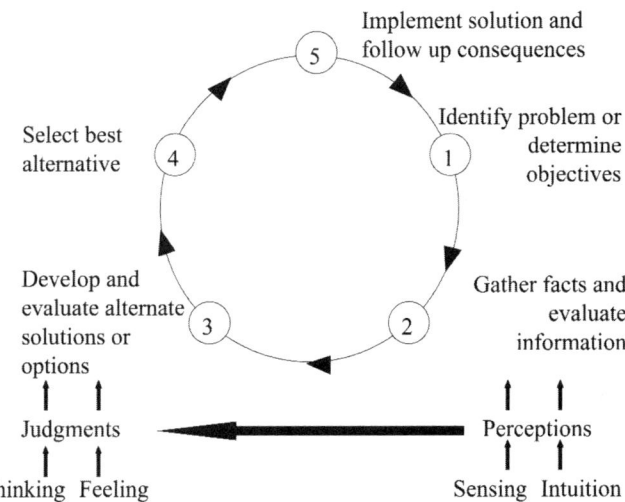

- *Step 5: Implement solution and follow up on consequences.* The chosen alternative is implemented, and over time the manager determines if the problem has been solved or the objectives met. It is imperative for the manager to ensure that once the chosen alternative is implemented, the process is complete. Two key questions need to be answered: (i) did the chosen alternative work? and (ii) are there unintended consequences to the decision which now must be addressed?

The problem-solving/decision-making process described is illustrated as a continuous circle of events (68). First, because the steps often overlap in practice, a manager may be simultaneously gathering information while still identifying the problem, or evaluating information while developing alternatives, for example. Second, the connection of all steps leading back to solving the identified problem or meeting the intended objectives is important to "closing the loop."

Risk

All decisions have some element of risk involved. Risk is based on uncertainty. The greater the uncertainty of outcome from the alternative chosen, the greater the risk. Managers must carefully weigh both the tangible and intangible elements of risk to arrive at a comfortable level of certainty. Often there are competing elements, which contribute to risk. A manager who recognizes a staff salary inequity chooses between the risk of alienating upper administration by pressing for equity or incurring cost from employee turnover.

A manager's decisions can be influenced significantly by both his own and his organization's propensity for risk. A manager with a high propensity for taking risks with decisions in an organizational culture with a low propensity for risk will likely experience problems. Both a personal and organizational comfort level must be achieved. Clearly, the manager must be aware of his own personal attribute regarding risk level: one's propensity for risk may lead to an underestimate of the actual risk or overconfidence to overcome the risk.

Time available or consumed in decision making can be viewed as a risk. For some, there is never enough information to reach a comfortable level of risk, leading to what some call "analysis paralysis." For others, making a quick decision "because they are in charge" increases the risk of a less-than-high-quality decision.

Some elements of risk lie in the behavioral factors of risk makers. Hammond et al. identify these as psychological traps (25):

- *Anchoring trap.* Placing disproportionate weight on the first or more superficial information found during information gathering.

- *Status quo trap.* Bias toward doing what we've always done despite better alternatives.
- *Sunk-cost trap.* Tendency to perpetuate mistakes of the past.
- *Confirming-evidence trap.* Bias toward information and judgment that support existing predilection.
- *Framing trap.* Misstating the problem, focusing on a symptom.
- *Overconfidence trap.* Overestimation of accuracy of information.
- *Prudence trap.* Being overcautious of degree of risk.
- *Recallability trap.* Placing undue weight on recent, dramatic experiences.

Good decision making relies on knowledge of both the importance and components of the process. It requires an awareness of personal skills to determine the best way to reach the highest-quality decision with the greatest acceptance in the amount of time available. Good decision making requires experience and learning from one's mistakes (33). Good decision making requires the ability to reflect on information and then decide (23, 40).

Management Ethics

It is far too easy in these complex times to presume that you or your employees will always know how to do the right thing. Dictates that we have often heard, e.g., follow the Golden Rule, or that Druckerism, "do the right things," are hard to follow when the issues we face are not that easy to understand or do not readily gel with our value systems. Most discussions of ethics and morals are couched in philosophical or sociological terms. Indeed, the study of ethics remains for the most part an academic discipline, and thus the management literature on the subject is sparse. That literature that can be found is often simplistic, since many business leaders until recently thought the topic irrelevant.

It is very relevant, nonetheless, that we think through many issues and concerns surrounding business and management ethics, in that the moral conduct a modern organization must espouse must be clear, set a high standard, and echo the best in everyone. *The Complete Guide to Ethics,* an Internet-based guide, provides an excellent resource for all matters relating to business and managerial ethics (http://www.managementhelp.org/ethics/ethxgde. htm [last accessed 28 April 2003]).

Definitions

Ethics, speaking simply, involves learning what is right and wrong. At an early age each of us learned these lessons from parents and other caregivers (54). Much of the argument one would hear about ethics revolves around absolutism versus relativism. Is there always the right thing to do based on moral principle, or does the situation drive the ethics question? Above, part of the discussion on management theory referred to the contingency theory in management, that there is no one right way to approach a problem (39). One must focus on the situation at hand, and that will lead to a resolution of that particular problem. A relativistic approach to ethics would say the same thing. There are no moral absolutes, only the most ethical approach to a situation at that moment.

Is the definition of "business ethics" any different? Perhaps not. Business ethics would refer to doing what is right or wrong in the workplace, and doing what is right in relation to products, services, and the various stakeholders (16). Business ethics most directly connects to one's customers, rather than abstractions such as the community, an open question, or a political issue. It is this direct connection to the practical aspects of running an enterprise that makes business ethics different and worthy of separate consideration.

Speaking generally, business ethics problems center around two main themes, managerial mischief and "moral mazes" (34). Managerial mischief would refer to illegal or questionable practices of individual managers or organizations, as well as the causes of those behaviors. Note that it is individuals, and not organizations, that are the issue. An individual cannot hide behind the cloak of an organizational policy. Organizations are groups of people, and people decide what is to be done or not done (34). Most of the focus on ethics has centered on this issue and how to approach these problems. Whistleblower policies and laws most likely spring from this area of concern. Perhaps it is comparatively easy to legislate and regulate business behavior to meet ethical standards. Indeed, the law and the generation of regulation are in some ways a societal method of imposing standards of action and behavior on the organization and its individuals.

Moral mazes, on the other hand, are not so clear and not so easily handled. A moral maze refers to the numerous and unclear ethical issues a manager would face in everyday work life (17). Examples here might be perceived as real conflicts of interest, wrongful use of resources, or mismanagement of contracts. What is right and what is wrong are not always clear in a competitive work environment. Seeking competitive advantage might mean bending the rules in accounting for expenses or in researching a competitor's products and services. Are accounting standards flexible or inflexible? Is it unethical to stretch the boundaries of accounting principles if it fits your economic model? Is industrial espionage unethical? As you can see, moral absolutes in these situations are not easy to find. A random group of managers, employees, or other stakeholders might read these questions from very different perspectives and hence derive very different answers (18).

None of the answers would be wrong, necessarily, but the differences of opinion, like political questions, would raise many issues beyond the questions at hand.

Conflict of interest can be seen as a version of moral maze. Most everyone would want to help those close to him or her. When does a form of aid prove to be a bad choice? Generically, conflict of interest is a situation in which a person, such as a public official, an employee, or a professional, has a private or personal interest sufficient to appear to influence the objective exercise of his or her duties. Conflict of interest can involve anyone and is not limited to officials or politicians. Obligation to your organization and its stakeholders must be viewed as superceding any personal gain you might derive from your work or gain you might pass on to another connected and interested party. For example, everyone would want a family member to succeed in business. As a manager, however, it would be unethical to show favoritism to that family member by passing business in their direction in a noncompetitive manner. Similarly, accepting personal gain for your decisions, like sending business to a company you own or accepting bribes to do the same, is a form of conflict of interest.

Characteristics of High-Ethics Organizations

In the same manner that a successful organization would lay out its mission, goals, and objectives, its ethical guidelines would be laid out and understood (34). First and foremost, an ethical organization would have a clear vision of right and wrong. Above, the question of relativism versus absolutism was raised. By design, an ethical organization would clarify to the greatest extent possible what is acceptable behavior versus what is not. Obviously, not every question can be addressed. But the organization can state clearly that ethical behavior in all areas and in all activities is what is expected and that failure to meet this standard will have its consequences.

Organizational vision most often comes from the top (34). The organization's chief executive must support and underwrite an ethics program. Failure on the part of top management to actively and enthusiastically support an ethics program will be noted by the rank and file. The executive officer should champion its development and foster a climate that encourages ethical behavior. From the start, the senior officers must espouse honesty and integrity as primary operational traits.

Everyone in an ethical organization will understand its ethical stance. Training in organizational ethics will be a part of new employee orientation and part of an organizational ongoing training program. All employees will receive this training, and all will understand the need to stay vigilant and sensitive to ethics issues. Ethical behavior in this context is good behavior, and the ethical organization will design its reward system around good behaviors. For example, employees can be measured on adherence to policy and their participation in ethics committees and management groups.

Benefits of Strong Workplace Ethics

Aside from the desire to do what is right, and perhaps that is a good enough reason in itself, why should an organization devote so much time and energy to an ethics program? To start, business ethics has improved society for all of us (35). Thinking back to the period of the business robber barons, where anything and everything were and could be done to promote one's competitive edge, worker safety was often compromised, sweatshops were everywhere, price fixing among the major corporate powers was rampant, and workers had no rights. Think now of the situation as it exists today. Perhaps the work environment can be better, but child labor has largely vanished, and there are laws to protect the consumer and the worker. All of this comes at a cost, however, but as a society we have determined that the cost of good and ethical business is one we should bear (36).

Mission and vision statements tell the employee and those outside of an organization who you are and what you are trying to do. For the employee, it helps foster teamwork and a sense of place in that organization (37). Teamwork leads to productivity and organizational success. Maintaining a strong ethical stance helps one's employees work through questions of what is right and wrong and what they are to do in difficult situations. For the employer, a strong ethics program can reduce some of the problems associated with risk management and conflict of interest. And of course, a strong ethics program can mesh with the entire strategic planning and quality management process, where trust among individuals and strong communication skills are needed to promote organization success and attention to what should be done and how the organization is to accomplish its goals.

Additionally, the ethical organization displays a positive public image (38). Positive images often translate into marketability and improvement in the bottom line for the enterprise. This cannot be one of the primary reasons for adopting strong and open ethical practices. But there is nothing wrong in strongly stating one's ethical position in a public forum, so that all will know where you stand and what you value. It may set you apart from the mainstream, and that is not a bad thing.

Within the healthcare environment, compliance is an often-heard word. Compliance refers to a variety of operational issues: billing, the Health Insurance Portability and Accountability Act, the Occupational Safety and Health Agency, the Joint Commission for Accreditation of Hospitals and Health Care Organizations, and the Clinical Laboratory Improvement Amendment regulations, to name a few. Compliance programs should be viewed as a regulatory enforced form of ethical behavior. The rules and regulations around all of these issues are complex, are at times difficult to implement and enforce, and many times add layers of complication to already tough working situations. The positive attribute of all, however, is the clarity they provide to the employee and the organization on what is acceptable behavior and what is not. Shades of gray are disappearing, and everyone is learning what is perceived as right and wrong.

Management Roles and Responsibilities

Restating what was said above, the most important step management must take with regard to an ethics program is to fully promote it and never waiver from the tenets that are accepted as organizational guidelines (34). Beyond that, however, management must recognize that ethics and the maintenance of an ethical organization require an ongoing and ever-renewed commitment to its success. Much like strategic or financial planning, an ethics program must be an ongoing process. It will be difficult to measure program success. But nonetheless it must be a continuous evaluation of where the organization stands and where its values have moved.

Management can take a strong lead in the development of ethical policies and codes of conduct. A staff fully educated on organizational ethics is less likely to stray into illegal and unethical behavior. The best way to avoid managerial mischief and the moral maze is to state at the outset what is expected in moral and ethical behavior and what activities to avoid that might lead to difficult working situations.

While the initiation and promotion of an ethics program must come from the top of the organization, there must be support from and ongoing interaction with all levels of that enterprise (34). It is the role of management to make sure that everyone is involved and that all understand the reasons for and the need for prescribed ethical behavior. Employee teams can be put into place for the purposes of policy development and review, and as forums for employee guidance when ethics issues arise. Ethics issues and decisions should be public and known, and it remains a responsibility of management to make sure that happens.

Finally, and perhaps a characteristic of the ethical organization, it is better to try and fail, often openly and publicly, than to not try at all. As ethics programs are fully integrated into an organizational culture, the increased communication that results among employees, and between management and staff, can lead to embarrassing disclosures and discussions of inappropriate behavior. The intent of an ethics program is not to develop an organization of finger-pointers. Rather, knowing that bad behavior will be found and exposed, the entire organization will move in a more ethical direction and repeat episodes hopefully will be less frequent.

Summary

When it comes to the management of an organization, there is no right or wrong way to get the job done. So long as they stay within the boundaries of ethics, legalities, and moral behavior, managers can and must choose their own path to success. Many studies have been completed and articles written describing what managerial behavior works best and what does not. For the most part the question is situational and focuses on the manager and what he must do at that moment to help his organization achieve positive results and move forward. We study the past to learn from notable successes and failures. We live in the present, moving forward ever faster it seems, where the decisions we make must come quickly and the issues we face are more complex and pressing. The best managers remain thoughtful about their avocation, always seeking new answers to the questions they face.

KEY POINTS

- Leadership, management, and administration are not one and the same. At any given moment, any one person may fill any of those roles, however. Learning what style fits you is a process of self-discovery and is shaped by the needs of the moment.

- The body of research and literature on management theory is large, both from a historical context and from the number of those interested in the topic. There is no consensus on what theories present the best and most accurate picture of how to manage groups of people. As humankind moves forward and our technology advances, management theory likewise expands and adapts to the new workplace.

- The ability to make good decisions often separates the best leaders and managers from the rest. Knowing how to work through to a good decision, bearing in mind the elements of time and risk, will provide one of the solid bases for managerial success.

- A strong ethical framework must be one of the guiding tenets for the modern organization. The benefits of building one are many, whereas the downside can be severe. From the top to the bottom, every employee must accept and live the positive values their organization espouses, thus removing any uncertainty of where they stand with any moral dilemma.

GLOSSARY

Administration Managerial work with a service orientation.

Bureaucracy Organizational hierarchies and defined lines of control.

Business ethics Learning and doing the right thing in the workplace, directly relating to products, services, and stakeholders.

Conflict of interest A situation in which a person has a private or personal interest sufficient to appear to influence the objective exercise of his duties.

Continuous/lifelong learning A self-empowering theory that the employee will throughout his or her life learn and strive to improve and move on to new things.

Continuous quality improvement A more human-focused quality management theory, relying heavily on worker involvement in the product improvement process.

Cultural lag The gap between technologic advances and the ability of society to control and work with them.

Decision theory The study of how decisions are made and what guides a manager to a good decision.

Hierarchy of needs Defined by Maslow, from the most basic to the highest level, these are needs that must be addressed to motivate the employee.

Human relations movement An approach to management focusing on the worker and his individual needs.

Intuitive decisions Utilization of hunches, subjective values, and personal or emotional factors in deciding what actions to take.

Judgmental decisions Conclusions reached after data are gathered, facts are analyzed, and concrete examples are explored.

Leadership Influencing others to attain group, organizational, and societal goals.

Management Getting things done through other people.

Management by objectives Setting goals for the individual to achieve, dovetailing with larger organizational objectives.

Management science Management techniques based on mathematic models.

Nonprogrammed decisions Unusual or atypical situational solutions.

Operations management Applied management technique utilizing mathematic modeling and industrial engineering to promote efficiency and effectiveness.

Situational management Acting only on what needs to be addressed at that moment and recognizing that there is no best way to get a job done.

Six Sigma A highly disciplined process focusing on developing and delivering near-perfect products and services.

Strategic decision Focus on an organization's relationship with the external environment, competitive posture, and major policies.

Tactical decision Steps toward the implementation of organizational strategy.

Taylorism and scientific management An approach to work and the workplace where every job is divided into the smallest possible segments and each segment is examined and improved.

Theory X and theory Y Defined by McGregor, a theory highlighting the difference between those who believe that people need to be forced to work and those who believe that people want to work.

Total quality management Designed-in product quality, with the focus on customer wants and needs as the key drivers in product and process improvement.

REFERENCES

1. Academic Press. 2002. *Academic Press Dictionary of Science and Technology.* Harcourt Press, Orlando, Fla.

2. Adair, J. 1984. *The Skills of Leadership*, p. 8. Gower Press, London, England.

3. Adams, C., P. Gupta, and C. Wilson. 2002. *Six Sigma Deployment*, p. 184–202. Butterworth Heinemann, New York, N.Y.

4. Adams, C., P. Gupta, and C. Wilson. 2002. *Six Sigma Deployment*, p. 329. Butterworth Heinemann, New York, N.Y.

5. Adams, C., P. Gupta, and C. Wilson. 2002. *Six Sigma Deployment*, p. 125–145. Butterworth Heinemann, New York, N.Y.

6. Adler, R. B., and G. Rodman. 1991. *Understanding Human Communication*, p. 4. Holt, Rinehart and Winston, Fort Worth, Tex.

7. Adler, R. B., and G. Rodman. 1991. *Understanding Human Communication*, p. 267. Holt, Rinehart and Winston, Fort Worth, Tex.

8. Berkowitz, E. N., R. A. Kerin, S. W. Hartley, and W. Rudelius. 2000. *Marketing*, 6th ed., p. 315–402. McGraw-Hill, New York, N.Y.

9. Berry, T. 1991. *Managing the Total Quality Transformation*, p. 15–37. McGraw Hill, New York, N.Y.

10. Berry, T. 1991. *Managing the Total Quality Transformation*, p. 6. McGraw Hill, New York, N.Y.

11. Blake, R. R., and J. S. Mouton. 1964. *The Managerial Grid*, p. 7–148. Gulf Publishing Company, Houston, Tex.

12. Burlton, R. T. 2001. *Business Process Management*, p. 81–97. Sams Publishing, Indianapolis, Ind.

13. Charns, M. P., and M. J. Shaefer. 1983. *Health Care Organizations: a Model for Management*, p. 223–249. Prentice-Hall, Inc., Englewood Cliffs, N.J.

14. Drucker, P. F. 1954. *The Practice of Management*, p. 22. Harper and Row, New York, N.Y.

15. Drucker, P. F. 1954. *The Practice of Management*, p. 126–127. Harper and Row, New York, N.Y.

16. Drucker, P. F. 1973. *Management: Tasks, Responsibilities, Practices*, p. 366. Harper and Row, New York, N.Y.

17. Drucker, P. F. 1973. *Management: Tasks, Responsibilities, Practices*, p. 347–348. Harper and Row, New York, N.Y.

18. Drucker, P. F. 1973. *Management: Tasks, Responsibilities, Practices*, p. 348. Harper and Row, New York, N.Y.

19. Drucker, P. F. 1999. *Management Challenges for the 21st Century*, p. 174–175. Harper Collins Publishers, Inc., New York, N.Y.

20. Fayol, H. 1949. *General and Industrial Management*, p. 5–6. Pitman Publishing, New York, N.Y.

21. Fayol, H. 1949. *General and Industrial Management*, p. 20–41. Pitman Publishing, New York, N.Y.

22. Gill, S. L. 1995. Groups and decision-making. *Clin. Lab. Manag. Rev.* **9:**464–476.

23. Giuliani, R. W. 2002. *Leadership*, p. 123–154. Miramax Books, New York, N.Y.

24. Gulick, L. 1965. Management is a science. *Acad. Manag. J.* **18**(1):7–13.

25. Hammond, J. S., R. L. Keeney, and H. Raiffa. 1999. The hidden traps in decision-making. *Clin. Lab. Manag. Rev.* **13:**39–47.

26. Harvard Business Review. 1991. *Managing Product Life Cycles: from Start to Finish*, p. 8–91. Harvard Business Review paperback series. McGraw Hill, New York, N.Y.

27. Hatvany, N., and V. Tucik. 1981. Japanese management practices and productivity. *Organ. Dyn.* **4**(2): 10–23.

28. Jones, H. 1999. Bayesian analysis: an objective, scientific approach to better decisions. *Clin. Lab. Manag. Rev.* **13:**148–153.

29. Juran, J. M. 1995. *Managerial Breakthrough*, p. 402–403. McGraw-Hill, New York, N.Y.

30. Kast, F. E., and J. E. Rosenzweig. 1972. General systems theory. *Acad. Manag. J.* **15**(4): 447–465.

31. Kouzes, J. M., and B. Z. Posner. 1995. *The Leadership Challenge*, p. 30–31. Jossey-Bass, Inc., San Francisco, Calif.

32. Kouzes, J. M., and B. Z. Posner. 1995. *The Leadership Challenge*, p. 332–336. Jossey-Bass, Inc., San Francisco, Calif.

33. Kouzes, J. M., and B. Z. Posner. 1995. *The Leadership Challenge*, p. 66–68. Jossey-Bass, Inc., San Francisco, Calif.

34. Kouzes, J. M., and B. Z. Posner. 1995. *The Leadership Challenge*, p. 255. Jossey-Bass, Inc., San Francisco, Calif.

35. Kouzes, J. M., and B. Z. Posner. 1995. *The Leadership Challenge*, p. 339. Jossey-Bass, Inc., San Francisco, Calif.

36. Kouzes, J. M., and B. Z. Posner. 1995. *The Leadership Challenge*, p. 212. Jossey-Bass, Inc., San Francisco, Calif.

37. Kouzes, J. M., and B. Z. Posner. 1995. *The Leadership Challenge*, p. 213. Jossey-Bass, Inc., San Francisco, Calif.

38. Kouzes, J. M., and B. Z. Posner. 1995. *The Leadership Challenge*, p. 20–23. Jossey-Bass, Inc., San Francisco, Calif.

39. Luthans, F. 1973. The contingency theory of management: a path out of the jungle. *Bus. Horiz.* **6:**62–72.

40. Mackoff, B., and G. Wenet. 2001. *The Inner Work of Leaders*, p. 81–103. AMACOM, New York, N.Y.

41. Martin, A. L. 1988. Information systems for human resources management, p. 151–152. *In* M. D. Fottler, S. A. Hernandez, and C. L. Joiner (ed.), *Strategic Management of Human Resources in Health Services Organizations.* John Wiley and Sons, Inc., New York, N.Y.

42. Maslow, A. 1943. A theory of human motivation. *Psychol. Rev.* **50:**376–396.

43. Mayo, E. 1933. *The Human Problems of an Industrial Civilization*, p. 48–97. McMillan Publishing, New York, N.Y.

44. McConnell, C. R. 2000. The anatomy of a decision. *Health Care Manag.* **18**(4):63–74.

45. McGregor, D. 1960. *The Human Side of Enterprise*, p. 33–48. McGraw Hill, New York, N.Y.

46. Mescon, M. H., M. Albert, and F. Khedouri. 1985. *Management: Individual and Organizational Effectiveness*, 2nd ed., p. 465–466. Harper and Row Publishers, Inc., New York, N.Y.

47. Mescon, M. H., M. Albert, and F. Khedouri. 1985. *Management: Individual and Organizational Effectiveness*, 2nd ed., p. 490–492. Harper and Row Publishers, Inc., New York, N.Y.

48. Mescon, M. H., M. Albert, and F. Khedouri. 1985. *Management: Individual and Organizational Effectiveness,* 2nd ed., p. 489. Harper and Row Publishers, Inc., New York, N.Y.

49. Mescon, M. H., M. Albert, and F. Khedouri. 1985. *Management: Individual and Organizational Effectiveness,* 2nd ed., p. 49–52. Harper and Row Publishers, Inc., New York, N.Y.

50. Mescon, M. H., M. Albert, and F. Khedouri. 1985. *Management: Individual and Organizational Effectiveness,* 2nd ed., p. 56–57. Harper and Row Publishers, Inc., New York, N.Y.

51. Mescon, M. H., M. Albert, and F. Khedouri. 1985. *Management: Individual and Organizational Effectiveness,* 2nd ed., p. 58. Harper and Row Publishers, Inc., New York, N.Y.

52. Mescon, M. H., M. Albert, and F. Khedouri. 1985. *Management: Individual and Organizational Effectiveness,* 2nd ed., p. 622. Harper and Row Publishers, Inc., New York, N.Y.

53. Mescon, M. H., M. Albert, and F. Khedouri. 1985. *Management: Individual and Organizational Effectiveness,* 2nd ed., p. 130–131. Harper and Row Publishers, Inc., New York, N.Y.

54. Mescon, M. H., M. Albert, and F. Khedouri. 1985. *Management: Individual and Organizational Effectiveness,* 2nd ed., p. 86. Harper and Row Publishers, Inc., New York, N.Y.

55. Metcalf, H. C., and L. Urwick. 1941. *Dynamic Administration,* p. 277. Harper and Row, New York, N.Y.

56. Mintzberg, H. 1973. *The Nature of Managerial Work,* p. 31. Harper and Row, New York, N.Y.

57. Pickett, R. B. 2001. What does all this leadership stuff mean to me? *Clin. Leadersh. Manag. Rev.* **15:**395–400.

58. Porter-O'Grady, T., and R. Hess. 1996. Perspectives on shared governance. *J. Shar. Gov.* **2**(4):11–15.

59. Raia, A. 1974. *Management by Objectives,* p. 11. Scott, Foresman, Glenview, Ill.

60. Raven, B. H., and J. E. Rubin. 1976. *Social Psychology: People in Groups,* p. 37. John Wiley and Sons, New York, N.Y.

61. Riggs, J. L., and G. H. Felix. 1983. *Productivity by Objectives,* p. 129. Prentice-Hall, Englewood Cliffs, N.J.

62. Riggs, J. L., and G. H. Felix. 1983. *Productivity by Objectives,* p. 98–99. Prentice-Hall, Englewood Cliffs, N.J.

63. Ringle, W. M. 1981. The American who remade "Made in Japan." *Nat. Bus.* **69:**67–70.

64. Shortell, S. M., and A. D. Kaluzny. 2000. *Health Care Management: Organization, Design and Behavior,* 4th ed., p. 109. Delmar Thomson Learning, Albany, N.Y.

65. Simon and Schuster. 1982. *Webster's New World Dictionary.* Simon and Schuster, New York, N.Y.

66. Smith, H., and P. Fingar. 2002. *Business Process Management: the Third Wave,* p. 103–129. Meghan-Kiffer Press, Tampa, Fla.

67. Smith, H., and P. Fingar. 2002. *Business Process Management: the Third Wave,* p. 174–192. Meghan-Kiffer Press, Tampa, Fla.

68. Snyder, J. R., and B. R. Hendrix. 1998. *Problem-Solving—the Decision-Making Process,* p. 61–78. *In* J. R. Snyder and D. S. Wilkinson (ed.), *Management in Laboratory Medicine,* 3rd ed., Lippincott-Raven Publishers, Philadelphia, Pa.

69. Taylor, F. W. 1912. *Principles of Scientific Management,* p. 23–75. D. Van Nostrand, New York, N.Y.

70. Vecchio, R. P., G. Hearn, and G. Southey. 1988. *Organisational Behavior: Life at Work in Australia,* p. 334. Harcourt Brace Jovanovich, Sydney, Australia.

71. Vroom, V. H., and A. G. Jago. 1978. On the validity of the Vroom-Yetton model. *J. Appl. Psychol.* **69:**151–162.

72. Weber, M. 1921. *Theory of Social and Economic Organization* (translated by A. M. Henderson and T. Parsons), p. 328–333. The Free Press, Simon and Schuster, New York, N.Y.

73. Wrightsman, L. S. 1977. *Social Psychology,* 2nd ed., p. 638. Brooks and Cole, Monterey, Calif.

APPENDIX 1.1 Websites

Complete Guide to Ethics Management: an Ethics Toolkit for Managers
(http://www.managementhelp.org/ethics/ethxgde.htm)

The Financial Management Network
(http://www.fmnonline.com/publishing/article.cfm?article_id=545)
"Management versus Leadership," by Lorin Woolfe.

Six Sigma
(http://www.isixsigma.com/library/content/six-sigma-newbie.asp)
"New to Six Sigma," an introduction to Six Sigma and discussion of product and process improvement.

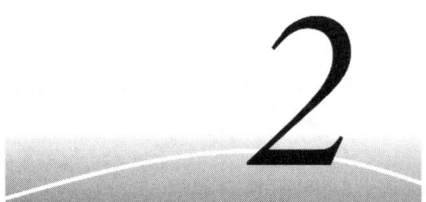

2

Management Functions

Laurence P. Vetter

OBJECTIVES

To provide an overview of basic management functions in simple, straightforward language, for use as a primer for laboratory managers and supervisors

To provide specific examples that demonstrate the application of management functions to a laboratory or clinical setting

To give the reader insight into the strategic planning process

To point the reader toward significant writings on the functions of management through citations and a bibliography

---

If we do not succeed, then we run the risk of failure.

DAN QUAYLE

ON THE SURFACE, DAN QUAYLE'S STATEMENT, "If we do not succeed, then we run the risk of failure," may seem somewhat obvious. In clinical laboratory science, however, many operations languish in the gray area of mediocrity that exists between true success and glaring failure. Specimens move, cash flows, staffing is adequate, payroll is met, and supplies get ordered, so the laboratory is by no means a failure. Still, there are unused capacity, untapped potential for enhanced revenue, unexplored opportunities for employee growth, and an overriding lack of enthusiasm among the staff, so the laboratory cannot be called a true success either. An engaged and thoughtful laboratory manager can be an agent of change, the key catalyst in moving a laboratory from mediocrity to excellence.

Laboratory managers are highly specialized employees, often performing numerous important but quite distinct roles within the healthcare system. A laboratory manager's primary role is chief laboratorian, providing specialized technical expertise within the medical laboratory. They are "extenders" of the physician directors in providing patient care through laboratory service. As such, they must remain abreast of wide-ranging federal regulations, credentialing and compliance issues, new technologies, and advancements in testing.

In addition to those very important technical responsibilities, however, laboratory managers must also oversee the business, personnel supervision, and human resources aspects of the laboratory. This multifaceted role—as healthcare provider, laboratory expert, accountant, business manager, and personnel supervisor—places a laboratory manager in a unique situation. Still, basic management functions in the clinical laboratory setting are very similar to management functions in any other complex organization. There are some fundamental practices and principles that must be applied to the oversight of the laboratory to ensure that the laboratory's operations are carried out with maximum efficiency. A manager will be more effective, and ultimately more successful, when he or she takes a systematic approach. Without taking action to ensure success, the laboratory manager, true to Mr. Quayle's observation, runs the risk of failure.

A manager's primary responsibility is directing the day-to-day (and often minute-to-minute) affairs of the laboratory. It will serve a manager well to be aware of the environment in which the laboratory functions. Anticipation of potential problems allows a manager to avoid costly mistakes in staffing, scheduling, purchasing, and budgeting.

The best managers know how to balance their many responsibilities, functioning in a well-organized manner. They are always looking to the future and thinking about how major trends affect the operation of the laboratory. They see changes in the operational environment as opportunities to make needed improvements in staffing, technology, and processes. This progressive approach requires insight, commitment, and the ability to teach the staff how to identify and solve problems.

> A good manager is a "high-performance" manager. The high-performance manager is:
> **A strategist**—One who looks to the future, makes educated guesses about the major forces and trends he or she can see, and interprets them in terms of opportunities for growth and progress.
> **A problem solver**—One who clearly perceives the differences between the anticipated future and the unfolding present and who decides what must be done with those factors under his or her control to influence the environment or to adapt to it most effectively.
> **A teacher**—One who guides others and helps them to identify and solve problems, so that they can perform their tasks effectively and can develop themselves as individuals as well as workers. (15)

In this chapter, management is broken into four primary areas: planning, organizing, directing, and controlling. This section provides an overview of those management functions, presented in basic, practical language.

Planning

Strategic Planning

The surest path to success in any enterprise is careful and committed strategic planning.

> Planning is the process of formulating objectives and determining the steps, which will be employed in obtaining them. No modern healthcare organization can be effective without an overall plan of action. (5)

Strategic planning is a methodical and structured process whereby an organization defines its mission, identifies directions, develops a unified approach, prioritizes long- and short-term goals, assigns accountabilities, and allocates financial resources. Therefore, a manager must plan to plan. A strategic plan helps the organization develop an action-oriented approach and identify the pieces needed to build a successful laboratory operation.

Good strategic planning is a structured process. It is "structured" because the plans of individual laboratory sections must fit into an overall plan that covers the entire laboratory operation. It is a "process" because good plans are not produced in isolation according to some predefined formula.

There are many books offering expert advice on how to develop a strategic plan. These can be useful tools. However, managers should not get caught up in a by-the-book approach. Managers should be flexible enough to use a process that fits their particular organization. Several points should be considered when planning:

- Involve staff at every level in developing a strategic plan. Solicit feedback from individuals who really know what's going on and who will be responsible for executing the plan. You will get great ideas and critical buy-in by getting staff at the bench level to offer input.

- Be flexible in developing a plan by circulating drafts and allowing people to provide feedback.

- Ensure that everyone knows their responsibility for deployment of the plan and that feedback mechanisms are implemented. The most carefully written plan will fail if those responsible for its execution do not know their roles, deadlines, and resource allocations. A defined feedback mechanism will ensure that the plan does not get lost in the daily crises.

Strategic planning always presents a challenge, regardless of the size and scope of an organization. The more far-reaching the laboratory's mission is defined, the greater the challenge. One constant, whenever the paramount resource of an organization is the experience of its people, is the absolute necessity to include the input of the staff (22).

The objective of planning is to set an achievable course of action by establishing long- and short-term goals, monitoring progress, and establishing an environment where day-to-day activities are well controlled, measurable, and thoroughly understood.

Selecting a Planning Group

A small, knowledgeable, and motivated group from within the laboratory should be assembled by the senior leader in order to participate in strategic planning. The group must contain key people from all areas of the laboratory. In a large and comprehensive pathology laboratory, there should be executive-level representatives from all functional areas (for example, hematology, microbiology, chemistry, and immunology), as well as key administrative and support leaders (for example, from sales, marketing, accounting, and billing). Since physician directors, laboratory managers, and supervisors are ultimately accountable for meeting the goals and objectives of the plan, they should make up the core of the planning group. Other key people in the laboratory who possess a strong working knowledge of policies, procedures, technology, and processes should also be included. As planning progresses, there will be occasions where facilitation must be utilized to tactfully assist the participants through the material in a logical and structured way. The role of the designated facilitator is to encourage constructive dialogue while remaining unbiased as to the outcome.

Environmental Analysis

It is critical for managers to be aware of the changes that routinely occur in the operational environment. Awareness of these changes is necessary during the planning process because it keeps decisions realistic and expectations achievable. This awareness stems from active involvement and participation.

Management cannot be accomplished in a vacuum. The manager must have professional affiliations to gain the insight and perspective of peers in other organizations. Some examples include the Clinical Laboratory Management Association, American Society for Microbiology, American Association of Blood Banks, American Association for Clinical Chemistry, American College of Physician Executives, American Society of Hematology, American Society of Clinical Pathology, and the NCCLS. There are unique professional organizations for almost every subspecialty of clinical laboratory science.

Laboratory managers must also regularly read laboratory-specific literature and trade journals. While most professional organizations have some type of regular publication, some examples with an emphasis on management topics include *Clinical Leadership and Management Review, Advance,* and *The Dark Report.* Professional involvement allows the manager to remain abreast of trends, knowing which questions to ask and where to find pertinent information in order to answer those questions.

This investigative process at the beginning of the strategic planning activity is often called an environmental analysis— a systematic review of the internal and external factors that influence the operation of the laboratory. A thorough, honest environmental analysis forces an organization to face reality, setting a tone for the planning process.

> In this analysis, the administrative staff seeks to answer questions such as: what kinds of services should we be offering the community five years from now? How will these services be different from those offered currently? What kinds of resources (machinery, equipment, buildings,

patient rooms, employee personnel) will we have to acquire in order to provide these future services? How will we finance the purchase of these resources? (6)

A thorough environmental analysis should be performed at the very beginning of the planning process. Accurate data should be gathered from every possible source. These data should include financial information (trends, current fiscal situation, and projections), capital equipment inventories, quantifiable personnel data, and laboratory-specific performance data. In some cases, a simple survey can be developed to gauge satisfaction and expectations of clients and employees. The most important consideration in performing an environmental analysis is to be completely realistic. The planning process must begin from a point firmly grounded in reality. If assumptions are not accurate, the resulting strategic plan will be fatally flawed.

SWOT Analysis

A necessary component of an environmental analysis is the careful consideration of the laboratory's strengths, weaknesses, opportunities, and threats, often called a SWOT analysis.

> The modern healthcare organization must appraise its strengths and weaknesses so that it can determine its future opportunities and environmental threats. (7)

By comparing the laboratory's existing strengths to known opportunities, concrete strategies can be put in place to capitalize on those opportunities. Using the same approach, matching the laboratory's known weaknesses to actual environmental threats will be useful in avoiding costly mistakes and bad decisions.

Vision and Mission Statements

At some point during the planning process, a vision statement should be written to articulate what the organization seeks to become. An example of a vision statement is from the Virginia Commonwealth University (VCU) Department of Pathology, which states, "Our vision is to become a preeminent Department of Pathology in the United States, which is recognized for excellence in biomedical research, the education of healthcare professionals, and the innovative application of science and technology to the diagnosis and management of human disease."

A statement of mission for the laboratory should also be developed. A mission statement answers certain fundamental questions about the organization, such as, What is our purpose? In what activities will we be engaged in order to accomplish that purpose?, and What are our basic values and shared beliefs? An example of a mission statement, also from the VCU Department of Pathology, states: "The mission of the Department of Pathology is to provide high-quality, cost-effective pathology services in a manner that supports the patient care, education, and research missions of the VCU Health System Academic Medical

Center and the Virginia Commonwealth University School of Medicine." Note that this statement clearly defines what the organization is and the clientele which it serves. As planning progresses, people should look to the mission statement for guiding principles in the decision-making process.

Goals, Objectives, and Strategies

> If you do not know where you are going, any road will get you there. Hence, goals for direction and objectives for steps are crucial to an organization. (3)

Planning seeks to produce a list of goals, objectives, and strategies that will guide laboratory management decisions for a predetermined period of time. For practical purposes, a planning horizon that is too distant will result in dramatic changes in technology and the economy before the planning period is complete. For the medical laboratory, a planning horizon of 18 months to 2 years is practical.

A goal is an end or an outcome that one hopes to attain. Through discussion and negotiation, the planning group should develop a list of goals for the laboratory. An example of a goal is to "enhance revenue by increasing referral testing from external sources." This is a clear statement of something that the laboratory will try to achieve.

An objective is a specific aim taken toward achieving a goal. An example of an objective related to the above goal would be to "build an outreach program."

A strategy is an artful means to a defined end. For this example, a strategy relevant to the above goal and objective might be to "hire a marketing director to develop business and increase referrals from community hospitals."

Prioritization

In planning, as in all other aspects of effective management, it is necessary to assign priority by weighing the importance of the tasks at hand to determine which have the highest level of immediate precedence. Therefore, planning is often a struggle between "must-do" and "want-to-do" decisions. Certain clinical activities are at the center of the laboratory's existence. Planning for these situations will always revolve around how to perform those activities better. A hematology laboratory should not plan to stop handling bone marrow specimens, as that decision would put the laboratory out of business. Handling bone marrow specimens is the laboratory's reason for existence. Instead, the laboratory should consider how to handle bone marrow specimens more effectively.

Accountability

A plan must have built-in accountability for all objectives and strategies. This amounts to assigning a specific individual to be responsible for each action. If "supervisors" is listed on the accountability line, no one is specifically responsible. Accountability, by definition, is the obligation of a person to be responsible for his own actions. Therefore, individuals must be assigned to implement specific actions in order to ensure follow-through.

Measuring Success (Metrics)

Progress on planning objectives must be monitored by making specific, quantifiable measurements, called metrics. A regular reporting mechanism must be established to review progress, impediments, and changes in environment. This is where persons accountable for specific action items are asked to report upon the progress made on their assignments. A regular reporting forum helps to maintain momentum by removing the human inclination to procrastinate. Monthly, or perhaps even weekly, meetings should be scheduled to discuss progress toward stated goals and objectives (Appendix 2.1).

Organizing

> Organizing is the process of structuring activities, materials, and personnel for accomplishing predetermined objectives. (8)

A key management task is to organize the activities of the laboratory in such a way that effort and expenditures are minimized and output is maximized. Organization consists of knowing the tasks that must be performed, understanding what knowledge and expertise the employees must possess in order to perform the tasks, and understanding the physical and capital requirements that must be assembled to accomplish the desired results. This is an ongoing process, since tests, equipment, and personnel are in a constant state of flux.

Knowledge and technologies are constantly evolving. The educational base of the employees is also dynamic, changing with personnel turnover. Improvements in technology further impact staffing needs. Therefore, a manager must be prepared to lead in a constantly changing environment where different pieces of the equation are forever being transformed by external factors.

Time Management

Every hour of a manager's day is occupied with urgent concerns and pressing issues. Without a structured and disciplined time management system, a manager might easily be overwhelmed. There are many different time management approaches and tools. Some are formal, store-bought day-planning systems. Some are as informal as "sticky notes" affixed to the computer screen. There is no universally prescribed time management system. An experienced manager must find a system that works best for his or her own unique needs and then use it all of the time. If a manager is using a time management system but still feels pressured by time constraints, he should experiment with different approaches until he gains control of time issues.

It is conceivable in a modern laboratory for a manager to be fully engaged 12 to 16 h a day. This is not desirable, even for the most dedicated executive, and more time spent on the job should only be considered in times of crisis. In all other circumstances, a manager should set and adhere to a reasonable schedule, building enough time into the day for essential meetings, interaction, and completion of necessary paperwork.

A time management system allows a manager to do the following:

- Minimize time wasted on nonproductive issues
- Be prepared for meetings
- Be aware of existing commitments
- Understand his or her capacity to take on new assignments and when to say no
- Plan each day's work efficiently and effectively
- Make certain that no project (large or small) is neglected

Conscious use of a time management system will help a manager to be well organized and well prepared.

Organizational Chart

An important management tool is the organizational chart. An organizational chart shows hierarchical relationships between functional areas in an organization. An organizational chart helps to clarify work flow, reporting lines, and areas of responsibility by explicitly listing delineated work areas, be it by division, laboratory, or medical specialty (Appendix 2.2).

The chart specifically indicates positional authority. Authority implicitly accompanies a position on the organizational chart, and its location on the chart implies a degree of consent by those who directly report to the person(s) in authority. The organizational chart is a contract of sorts, as it unambiguously illustrates the structure of the organization and the relationships among the people within it.

> A laboratory manager possesses authority within the organization if he has the right to issue instructions that others are expected to follow. The organizational chart serves as a visual aid for evaluating each of these basics. The organizational chart also attempts to show relationships between line and staff. In this organizational concept, a line position is one in which a superior exercises direct supervision over a subordinate. (19)

Policies

Policies are the "laws" of the laboratory. Little different from laws in a society, policies must be fair and equally applied to everyone in the organization. Every laboratory should have an open, accessible, and easy-to-understand set of policies. These policies must be made known to each employee. The manager and employees should review

policies regularly as part of an annual review process, and policies should be communicated to all employees at the time of hire. Policies should be reviewed regularly to ensure that they are current and realistic within the environment. Outdated policies should be rescinded or replaced. In large laboratories, a committee may manage policy writing and review. The committee should be populated by supervisors and key employees who are knowledgeable about how the laboratory functions. Policies are a contract between the employees and the managers.

> All policies have seven basic characteristics: they must be well thought out; flexible enough to be applied to both normal and unusual situations; acceptable to those who apply them; consistent; objective; clear and communicated to those individuals to whom they apply; and continuously reevaluated and changed when necessary. (16)

A representative example of a table of contents for an administrative policy manual is provided as Appendix 2.3.

Procedures

Where policies are rules to codify employee conduct, procedures are formal steps to guide an employee through a specific task. A procedure is a written, sequential course of action. A laboratory manager must maintain current, concise procedure manuals for all processes that are performed in the laboratory. As with policies, the book of laboratory procedures should be continuously updated by a team of experts.

The standard operating procedures (SOP) manual is a very important tool in the laboratory. An up-to-date SOP ensures that procedures performed by the technical staff are consistent and of the highest quality. Managers use the procedure manuals to train the laboratory technologists, and technologists use the procedure manuals as a reference source when performing laboratory tasks. Laboratory methods and technologies constantly change, and the SOP manuals must be updated to reflect the technical activities in the laboratory.

Work Flow

A laboratory manager must be aware of all of the interconnected processes within the laboratory. This is known as work flow, or tasks organized in a particular way to accomplish a specified result. Analysis of work flow within a laboratory will quite often identify inefficiencies that can be corrected, resulting in a more productive process. This analysis should include evaluating equipment, technology, information services, computer systems, physical layout, and location of resources.

An important tool for analyzing work flow is the flowchart. Process design flowcharting is a fact-gathering technique used to make the effort of a task visible by writing down what is done. A flowchart graphically illustrates the relationships among necessary tasks. By writing down the steps in a task, you can often identify areas of overlap, redundant effort, and opportunities for improvement (Fig. 2.1).

Once the elements of work are identified, it is necessary to determine how they fit together to form a coherent whole: to determine for each element of work the other elements essential to its effective performance. At one extreme are elements that can be performed independently of each other. In contrast, successful performance of other types of work requires that different work elements occur in sequence or that one element affects a second element, which, in turn, acts upon the first element. At the most complex level, elements of work affect each other simultaneously. The concept of interconnectedness of work is critical to effective work design. When different people perform interconnected elements of work, components must be coordinated to ensure effective performance. (18)

Staffing and Scheduling

Each laboratory has an ideal number of employees based upon the number of specimens that it handles and the level of automation in the laboratory. A manager must ensure that efficient staffing is maintained. The best-equipped laboratory will not function at top efficiency if it is improperly staffed. Too many full-time employees can result in excess capacity and unduly high overhead expenses. Too few full-time employees can result in excessive need for overtime. Overworked employees, regardless of how well they are paid, will eventually burn out.

Accurate staffing must be directly linked to the organizational chart, taking into consideration how each laboratory component serves the ultimate mission of the laboratory as a whole. A well-thought-out strategic plan will enable a manager to make long-term predictions about future staffing needs. When making staffing decisions, the laboratory manager should always refer to the strategic plan. Plan-based staffing decisions remove much of the guesswork. This allows a manager to stay ahead of staffing issues, providing lead time to hire and train efficiently.

Only with efficient staffing and scheduling can management make the best use of personnel, supplies, instrumentation, and facilities in a prompt and cost-effective manner.

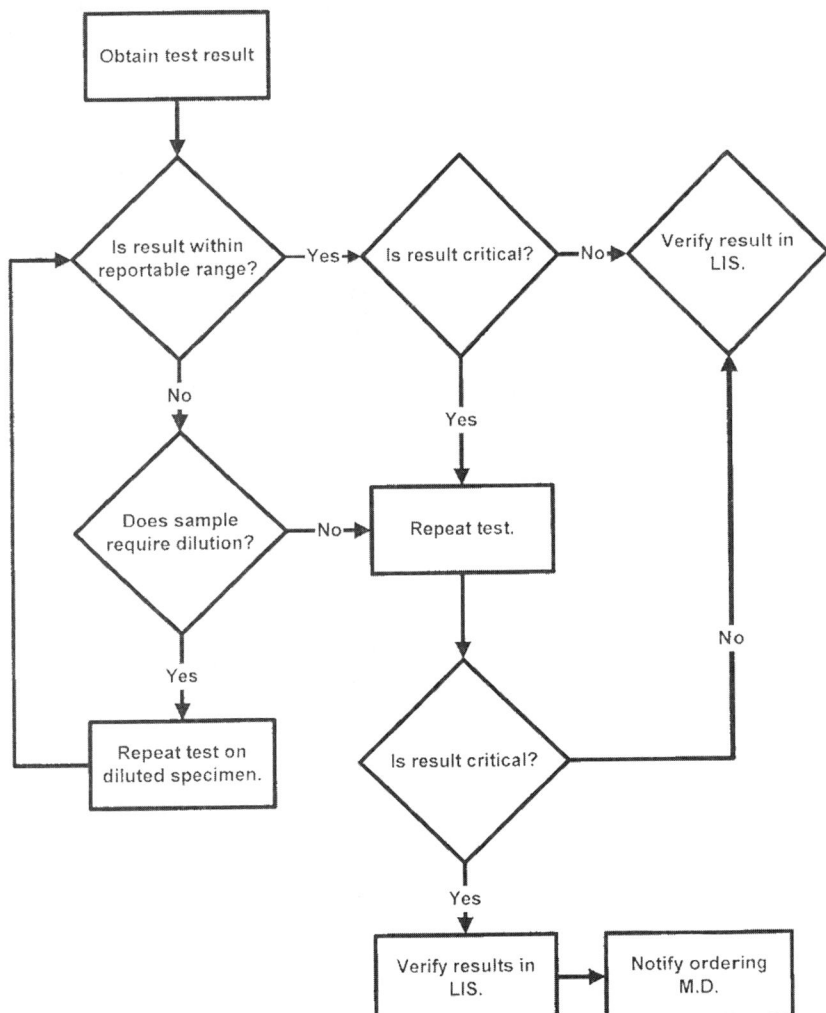

Figure 2.1 Flowchart showing steps involved in handling the reporting of critical values. LIS, laboratory information system.

By definition, "to staff" is to provide a group of workers for the purpose of securing united and cohesive performance. Specifically, staffing of a clinical laboratory is a two-step process. The initial step is to set up a table of organization denoting laboratory structure and chain of command. It is important to clearly define what the function of the laboratory is and how it fits into the overall organization. Once the mission and purpose of the laboratory have been determined, decisions in efficient utilization of personnel and equipment can be made with accuracy. After thought is given to the need for present and future numbers of positions, a comparison can be made between predicted demand and supply. Differences can then be assessed and finally a plan formulated to recruit, train, and meet suitable staffing needs. (13)

Directing

Directing is the process of influencing people to attain predetermined objectives. (5)

There are several key elements in this process. Communicating, delegating, motivating, and coaching are discussed here.

Communicating

Communication is among the most important components of management. Without clear written and oral communication from manager to employee, and among peers, there is no effective way of articulating expectations, expressing concerns, providing feedback, and ensuring that policies are implemented. Communication must flow in all directions. It must be concise, clear, and continuous. Employees rely upon regular feedback, training, and mentoring from their supervisors. Supervisors rely upon their employees to inform them of their needs. People at all levels of authority within the laboratory rely upon communication with their peers to remain aware of changes in policy.

> In every healthcare organization, there are four basic communication flows through which messages can be passed: downward, upward, lateral, and diagonal. Downward communications travel from the superior to the immediate subordinate. Downward communications are used to transmit information and instruct employees in the performance of their jobs. Upward communication travels from the subordinate to the immediate supervisor, and it is used to provide feedback on how things are going. Lateral communication takes place between people on the same level of authority within an organization, and it is used for promoting coordination and teamwork. Diagonal communication occurs between people who are neither in the same department nor on the same level of authority within the organization. Diagonal communication is used for cutting across organizational boundaries in an effort to save time. (9)

Without structured communication, a manager cannot expect employees to act as a coordinated unit. Employees require direction, and they need to know what is expected of them. An organization cannot allow important decisions and information to be disseminated in a haphazard or informal way. It is the manager's responsibility to develop and adhere to a regular, formal communication system.

> Individuals cannot act in a coordinated, organized fashion in the absence of a communications network that both stimulates and controls the flow of information needed to make and disseminate decisions. (17)

Communication is a job skill that can be developed and improved. A manager can ask certain fundamental questions to make communication within the organization more focused and productive.

- What information do you receive on a regular basis?
- What does your team need to know?
- What are the ideal methods of communication (formal meetings, e-mail, memos, conference calls, video conferencing)?
- How often should meetings be held, what subject matter will be discussed, and who should attend?
- With regard to communication, what do your employees want you to start doing?
- What do your employees want you to stop doing?
- What do they want you to continue doing?

Some basic attributes of quality communication include attention, acceptance, and empathy. Attention is the thoughtful consideration of others. When speaking to someone, be considerate of his or her concerns, needs, and experiences. Actively listen to what the person is saying. Ask questions to clarify his or her concerns. Affirm your understanding by paraphrasing and restating the concerns until there is no room for misunderstandings.

There are some aspects of active listening that should always be incorporated when communicating with staff members. Acceptance means simply to receive someone's thoughts and opinions favorably. This does not imply tacit agreement but instead that you understand the concerns and will keep an open mind.

> Successful listening is an active, dynamic process. Alertness at every point of the communication encounter is a prerequisite for the supervisor, as well as for the subordinate. (10)

Empathy is the ability to share another's feelings. It is the projection of your own personality onto the personality of another in order to understand him or her better.

> A clinical supervisor can show concern for a subordinate by standing in the subordinate's position, identifying with the subordinate's frame of reference, and helping to meet the subordinate's objectives. From this standpoint, empathy is an exceptionally strong component of effective communication. (11)

Delegating

Another critical aspect of management is the delegation of responsibilities to others. Delegation is the process of selecting qualified people to perform various tasks. A manager must understand the desired results and then make informed decisions about who is best qualified to meet these performance expectations. When a manager delegates, he or she is making a prediction that the person selected will follow through to the desired conclusion. The manager must be well informed about what needs to be done before a wise decision can be made about how responsibilities are best delegated.

> Delegation is the process of selecting people from a very limited pool (current job incumbents) to perform a task. When a manager delegates work to someone, that manager is predicting that the employee will meet performance expectations. The more clearly we know what we are looking for someone to do and how we want it done, the easier it will be to choose the right person for the right tasks. (1)

Motivating

Employees require motivation in order to consistently give their best effort. Motivation is both internally and externally derived. The best employees are the ones who come equipped with a good deal of enthusiasm and self-direction. They are self-motivated. They want to do a good job. They take pride in their work. They ask questions when they are in doubt. If they see an opportunity for improvement, there is no hesitation to "take the ball and run with it." Motivated employees have very few problems with absenteeism, tardiness, and poor work habits.

Even the most self-motivated employees, however, must be given positive feedback and encouragement on a regular basis. Positive reinforcement is always a motivating factor. Many organizations offer financial incentives of one kind or another to serve as a motivator and a reward system for excellent performance. These financial rewards are a powerful stimulator, giving people a clear incentive to do their best work. Even in difficult financial times, when there is no extra money in the budget for these types of incentives, there are other programs that can be established to build enthusiasm and reward excellence. A certificate or letter of appreciation in the personnel file is an easy and inexpensive motivator. Recognition in the form of a public "pat on the back" has incalculable benefits in motivating employees.

A successful manager understands the art of motivation. Every individual has professional strengths and limitations, activities that they find exciting and tasks that are drudgery. A. H. Maslow, who developed a theory about what motivates people, performed a classic psychological study of motivation. This "hierarchy of needs" provides some insight into the complexity of human motivation and the importance of providing an environment where the most complex of these needs are met (14).

We may expect that discontent and restlessness will soon develop unless the individual is doing that for which he is most fit. A musician must make music, an artist must paint, a poet must write, if a person is to be truly at peace. This need is called self-actualization (14). A manager must therefore understand the individual strengths and interests of the staff and find ways to tap into those strengths, where possible, in the performance of daily activities.

> Because the art of management is getting things done through others, it is important, not only to know the fine points of delegation, but also to be able to *motivate* people to want to achieve. A basic understanding of the psychological needs of the individual is a helpful way to match organizational expectations with the individual's capabilities. A. H. Maslow's work *Motivation and Personality* (1954) is a prime study for understanding motivation. His hierarchy of basic needs is well known.
> Physiological Needs—The essentials, such as food, sleep, and air.
> Safety Needs—Based on human preference for a safe, orderly, predictable, organized world that can be relied upon to be free of danger or unexpected happenings.
> Belongingness and Love Needs—If both physiological and safety needs are fairly well gratified, the love and affection and belongingness needs will emerge. A person will hunger for affectionate relations and will look for a secure place in his or her group.
> Esteem Needs—The desire or need for a stable, firmly based evaluation of himself or herself for self-respect or self-esteem.
> Need for Self-Actualization—If all of the above needs are satisfied, a new discontent may develop unless the individual is doing what he or she is fitted to do. In other words, what a person can be, he or she must be—coming from a desire for self-fulfillment. (2)

Coaching

Many employees require active, hands-on development to realize the best of their abilities. The best managers are teachers and coaches, always engaging their employees in a productive and ongoing process of continuing education. This is accomplished through traditional teaching, such as standing at the bench and actually showing an employee how a process is run. It also involves encouraging an employee to try new things and to strive for a higher level of accomplishment. This is done in a supportive way meant to develop self-confidence. Of course, each employee has his or her own temperament and sensitivities, and everyone should be handled as an individual. Everyone has unique talents and limitations. As a coach, the manager should always be mindful of each person's needs and desires.

> **Coaching** is providing a person or group with the **guidance, support,** and **confidence** to enable them to enhance their performance **continuously.**
> • **Guidance** enables someone to develop his or her skills and knowledge appropriately. Through skillful

guidance a coach can also help another person develop useful insights into their work and character.

- **Support** means being there only when you're needed.
- **Confidence** means believing in someone so that they can believe in themselves and perform effectively.
- **Continuously** means all the time! Coaching is not something which is turned on and off like a tap. Successful coaching depends on planning coaching assignments and developing supportive relationships over time. (4)

Controlling

Controlling is the process of determining that everything is going according to plan. (5)

A manager must constantly and consistently review the current situation in the laboratory to ensure that there are no unattended details. Being mindful of the daily activities of the laboratory is one of a manager's most important responsibilities. There is no substitute for engaged leadership.

Evaluating Employee Performance and Setting Performance Standards

A basic obligation of a manager is to make each employee aware of his or her performance at regular, scheduled intervals. When a new employee is brought into the laboratory, there should be a written and signed agreement concerning the responsibilities of the position. This formal job description is a contract that lets the employee know in specific terms what he or she should be doing. It should also be directly linked to the organizational chart, giving the employee a clear understanding of the lines of authority. The job description should include a job title, a compensation classification if appropriate, the name of the supervisor who will review performance, a specific and detailed listing of responsibilities, and a schedule for performance evaluation.

This is a contract, of sorts, and it is good for the employee, for the manager, and for the organization. It spells out where the employee fits in the larger picture, and it forces the manager to look critically at what role the employee will play in the laboratory operation. It also articulates the expectation for performance by providing a baseline standard of performance. During the appraisal period, it helps the manager make decisions about pay raises, promotion, and areas where the employee should concentrate on improvement, and it helps identify training needs.

Regardless of the purpose or format of an appraisal, there are a few critical elements without which an appraisal system will not function. These include:

- Standards and criteria of performance—Performance standards must be specified for performance to be evaluated meaningfully. One possible source of standards is the job description. When job descriptions are short and not very specific, a more exacting set of standards may be derived from a job analysis. In this process, someone who is currently fulfilling the responsibilities of a job writes down or reports all the different tasks the job includes. Another possible source of standards is mutual consent to specified goals where the subordinate and manager agree upon certain tasks that the subordinate is to perform during the evaluation period.
- Communication of these standards and criteria to the subordinate—Once performance standards and criteria have been specified, the subordinate to be evaluated must be aware of them. The manager or personnel department may communicate standards and criteria during the initial job orientation session, during the subordinate's first meeting with the manager, or by means of a written document, such as a detailed job description along with the performance appraisal form.
- Sufficient frequency of appraisal—The most common interval for appraisal is every 12 months; this is usually adequate for salary and promotion decisions. However, formal review of progress toward goals might be required at more frequent intervals, depending on the nature of the job.
- Clear communication of appraisal results—A final vital element in effective performance appraisals is communication of the results to the subordinate. These results must be clear and indicate that the purpose of the performance appraisal was fulfilled. (20)

Performance evaluations must be fairly administered and consistent among all employees. In other words, the same set of criteria must be applied to all employees performing similar responsibilities throughout the laboratory. All phlebotomists working in a laboratory section must be held to consistent standards of performance and behavior; otherwise, the appraisal system is implicitly unfair and flawed.

Performance appraisals are formalized manager-employee encounters. They should be conducted at scheduled, preordained intervals. A new hire is usually given a probationary evaluation at a preordained point (for example, 90 days after the initial hiring date). This probationary review provides the manager with an opportunity to decide if the employee has made satisfactory progress to warrant continued, permanent employment. A probationary period, usually 6 months or 1 year in duration from the time of hire, is the time when the manager should be critically observant of performance. This should be treated as an orientation process when a great deal of teaching, coaching, and mentoring must take place to ensure that the new employee is given every opportunity to succeed. During a probationary period, an employee can usually be dismissed without cause if he or she has not performed to expectation and there is reason to believe that performance deficiencies cannot be rectified. Once the organization makes a commitment to keep a new employee beyond the probationary period, it becomes much more difficult to dismiss an employee because of performance problems, poor attendance record, and work behavior issues.

The purpose of a performance appraisal is to provide the employee with written feedback about how he or she is progressing toward specific employment objectives. This is a manager's opportunity to put into writing an employee's level of competence measured against the stated requirements of the position. An appraisal also provides a forum for discussion about the employee's training needs, salary expectations, professional deportment, and career progress. A properly conducted performance appraisal is a two-way conversation, with the manager actively listening to the employee's feedback.

While some companies conduct formal reviews at least once a year, there should really be an informal and continuous process. A sound review system, fairly administered, can be beneficial to a company and its employees. On the other hand, one that is not properly administered can result in lower performance, greater mistrust, and legal problems. Some of the benefits of regular reviews are:
- Keeping good people from getting buried in the system and exposing nonproductive people who disrupt the system.
- Corrections of deficiencies and improved performance.
- Providing helpful data for promotion decisions, as well as being a basis for salary and wage adjustments, bonuses, and other financial rewards.
- Establishing a baseline against which people can measure their own progress and encouraging them to take affirmative action to work toward more challenging goals.
- Forcing communication between manager and staff.
- Giving managers a sense of how people are coming along.
- Letting people sort out their problems.
- Providing an opportunity for managers to ask themselves what they have done to improve employees' performance. (12)

Performance criteria require clear definitions of what constitutes poor, fair, and excellent performance. If the definition is left to the individual, performance appraisals will be inconsistent from rater to rater and from the same rater at different times. Providing criteria that are based on observable behaviors may increase the validity of a rating system. If a criterion gives the rater a clear choice among alternatives A, B, and C, with minimal judgment involved, that criterion is more likely to contribute to a successful performance appraisal (23).

Problem Solving

A laboratory manager is a problem solver. Every day, there will be situations that require executive-level decisions. Some will involve employees, some will involve interpretation of procedures, and some will involve application of technical expertise. A manager must approach problem solving in a structured way. Problem solving is a skill that improves with practice.

The manager should approach problem resolution through creative thinking, much the same way a scientist applies novel techniques to get past existing problems. Problem solving is a process that contains several key elements. The manager must be able to ascertain the exact source and nature of the problem, which is often difficult in complex situations where many people or processes are involved. In the laboratory setting, root problems in technique or procedure often compound at each ensuing step, causing amplified impact further downstream. In these situations, the true cause of the problem is not obvious, since it becomes visible at a point that is far removed from the source. Therefore, the manager must be a dedicated detective, gathering evidence and pulling together as much information as possible in order to identify the root cause of the flawed process.

Once the cause of a problem is known, a manager has to come up with a solution. If a machine is not functioning because it is unplugged, there is only one solution: plug it back in. Problems in the laboratory are rarely so simple, however, that there is only one obvious solution. More often than not, there will be a range of alternatives that should be carefully considered. Through consultation with bench level experts, the manager should create a list of possible actions directed toward a problem. This step often requires the human touch, bringing people together in an unbiased way to discuss the range of options that are available. Implementing the best solution will often involve some level of compromise, usually requiring the cooperation of many affected individuals. A skillful manager will make his or her employees feel that they are part of the solution instead of making them feel that they are responsible for the problem.

The final phase of problem solving is follow-up. Once the solution is implemented, it is absolutely necessary to measure outcomes. The manager must gauge the effectiveness of the solution in a structured way at prescribed intervals to make sure that the problem was truly corrected. The fix might create a new set of unanticipated problems. Monitoring the situation to ensure that the desired results have been achieved is an essential final step. Monitors are as unique as the problems, but they should be consciously considered and applied.

An example of a scientific approach to problem solving is provided here. The following seven-step checklist offers a systematic approach to identifying a problem and making a clear and rational decision in order to solve it:

The simple, seven-step approach described here allows the manager the flexibility to modify when necessary but still have some basic guidelines to follow.

Step One: Definition of the Problem—One pitfall many managers encounter as they begin a problem-solving process is the temptation to hypothesize about what should have been done earlier so the problem would not have developed. Some problems will be inherited, some resulting from decisions made elsewhere in the organizational hierarchy, and still others from one's own doing. Regardless of the origin of the problem, the solution must still be made within the framework of the situation.

Step Two: Fact Gathering—Once the problem has been identified, the manager can begin to gather information needed for developing alternative solutions.

Step Three: Development of Alternative Solutions—The generation of possible solutions calls for creative thinking. Often when faced with this step, a manager will draw on his past experience; in most cases this will be adequate. Today's manager must supplement his creativity by seeking information from others who have solved a similar problem or from individuals directly involved in the situation. It is wise to keep an open mind and not prejudge ideas as they are generated.

Step Four: Weighing of Alternative Solutions—This step requires the analysis of alternative solutions by stating the advantages and disadvantages of each possible course of action. The manager must consider the ramifications of each potential solution. Consideration should be given to the question of whether a chosen alternative will eliminate recurrence of the problem or generate another in its place.

Step Five: Selection of Solutions—Choosing the best possible course of action is an integrated process. Considerable fact gathering and planning have already occurred. Even though alternatives have been scrutinized, any single approach is not always the "best." There is generally more than one way to solve a problem.

Step Six: Implementation of the Solution—Of all the steps in the problem-solving process, the implementation step is usually the most time-consuming. At the same time, even the best decision, if not properly implemented, is useless. As in the decision-making process, implementation must involve those who are directly affected by the solution.

Step Seven: Measurement of the Consequences—Not all decisions rendered will have the effect that was planned. An analysis of what occurred, whether predicted or not, provides an ever-increasing basis of experience from which future problems can be solved. (21)

Decision Making

Managers are frequently required to make decisions. It is in many ways an extension of the problem-solving process. A manager's effectiveness often hinges upon the consistency and quality of the decisions that are made. As in problem solving, there is a scientific approach that enables a manager to make the best possible decisions. Certain factors affect the decision-making process, and they should be carefully considered:

Before attempting to make any management decisions, there are several general areas of concern to which a laboratory manager must be sensitive:

- Quality of the Decision—In order to make a quality decision, a manager must determine if he has all of the appropriate information available. The manager may need to seek out information regarding specific skills necessary to complement a given alternative.
- Acceptance of Commitment to the Decision—It is important to consider not only the degree of acceptance by the subordinates affected directly by the decision but also the degree of acceptance at other levels of management within the organization.
- Speed of the Decision—The time element must be considered. Even if it is not essential that the decision be a quick one, the laboratory manager must consider the length of time it will take to involve appropriate parties.
- The Nature of the Value Judgments of the Decision—All decisions involve a value judgment in terms of what is beneficial or nonbeneficial and important or not important in projecting the probable outcomes of the decision. (20)

The decisions that a manager makes will have a profound impact on how the laboratory functions. Decision making is a conscious process that requires rational consideration of cause and effect. The quality of decisions will ultimately be the mark of a manager's success or failure. In most cases, decisions are made in order to create improvement in a given situation. If the manager has a lucid understanding of what needs to be accomplished through the decision-making process, and furthermore takes into consideration a wide range of possible actions, the resulting decisions will be quality ones.

When presented with a big decision-making opportunity, it is often helpful to write down the problem and make a list of possible solutions, intended outcomes, and potential problems. Most importantly, never panic. A rushed decision is rarely the optimal decision. Step away from the situation long enough to perform a factual analysis before making any decision.

Sometimes factual analysis leads to a single obvious decision. More often than not, however, there are numerous possible decisions whose outcomes must be weighed. A manager must rely on input from others in the laboratory who are positioned to offer sound advice, not only on the factors that are causing the problem but also on the possible far-ranging effects of the decision. Still, seasoned managers learn to trust their gut instincts and listen to the wisdom of their own experience.

Many internal factors have an adverse impact on the decision-making process, including stress, self-doubt, lack of self-awareness, pressure to act too quickly, and procrastination to avoid difficult decisions. As a manager gains experience and confidence, many of these internal barriers will fall away.

Summary

A laboratory manager is a uniquely skilled employee with a very high level of daily responsibility that spans all areas of the organization. The technical aspects of running a laboratory are codified and tightly regulated. When technical problems arise, there is very often a manual to help guide the solution. When it comes to managing the human side of the laboratory, there are daily challenges for which there are no obvious solutions. There does exist, however, a set of time-tested management tools for use by laboratory managers in addressing these daily challenges. A laboratory manager must become familiar with these tools and use them on a daily basis to gain confidence and experience in managing the human side of the laboratory. Some consequences of neglecting basic management functions are listed in Appendix 2.4.

A program of regular, committed strategic planning helps an organization to predict and avoid problems while maximizing opportunities.

KEY POINTS

- The manager must develop and utilize a system to organize the work flow, policies, and staffing of the laboratory.

- The manager must provide direction to the laboratory by communicating, delegating, motivating, and coaching.

- A manager must control the activities of the laboratory, constantly reviewing the current situation to ensure that there are no unattended details. There is no substitute for engaged leadership.

GLOSSARY

Accountability The obligation of a person to be responsible for his or her own actions.

Coaching Providing an employee with the direction, support, and self-assurance to improve performance on the job.

Communication The exchange of information, flowing in all directions within the organization. It can be written or spoken, verbal or nonverbal, formal or informal.

Delegation Assigning a specific task to an accountable subordinate.

Directing Planning specific action and actively overseeing the execution of a plan.

Environmental analysis A thorough and systematic review of the external and internal factors that affect the functioning and performance of the laboratory.

Facilitation The process of assisting participants to move through material in a logical and structured way.

Goal An outcome that the organization hopes to attain.

Metrics Specific, quantifiable measurements used as an indicator of progress.

Mission statement A written statement that clearly defines what the organization does and why it is important.

Motivation Inspiration or stimulation to perform in a desired way or to achieve a desired result.

Objective A specific aim directed toward achieving a goal.

Organizational chart A diagram that shows hierarchical and authority relationships among functional areas in an organization.

Organizing The process of structuring resources and activities in a way that promotes the accomplishment of specific activities.

Performance evaluation Feedback regarding current performance on job tasks and responsibilities that is used as a guide for future performance.

Policies Internally generated rules that set expectations for behaviors within the laboratory.

Priority Weighing the importance of the tasks at hand to determine which have the highest level of immediate precedence.

Standard operating procedures (SOP) A written set of instructions that codify technical and administrative activity in the laboratory.

Strategic planning A methodical and structured process whereby an organization defines its mission, identifies directions, develops a unified approach, prioritizes long- and short-term goals, assigns accountabilities, and allocates financial resources.

Strategy An artful means to a defined objective or goal.

SWOT analysis A careful consideration of the laboratory's strengths, weaknesses, opportunities, and threats (SWOT). In most analyses, strengths and weaknesses are internal to the organization, while opportunities and threats derive externally.

Vision statement A written statement that defines not what an organization is but what the organization expects to become. A vision statement should inspire the organization to achieve its mission.

Workflow Tasks organized in a particular way to accomplish a specified result.

REFERENCES

1. Camp, R., M. E. Vielhaber, and J. L. Simonetti. 2001. *Strategic Interviewing: How To Hire Good People,* p. 65. Jossey-Bass, San Francisco, Calif.

2. Hardwick, D. F., and J. I. Morrison. 1990. *Directing the Clinical Laboratory,* p. 133–134. Field and Wood Medical Publishers, New York, N.Y.

3. Henry, J. B. (ed.). 2001. *Clinical Diagnosis and Management by Clinical Methods,* 20th ed., p. 5. W. B. Saunders Co., Philadelphia, Pa.

4. Hill, J. 1997. *Managing Performance,* p. 87. Gower Publishing, Aldershot, United Kingdom.

5. Hodgettes, R. M., and D. M. Cascio. 1983. *Modern Health Care Administration,* p. 30. Academic Press, New York, N.Y.

6. Hodgettes, R. M., and D. M. Cascio. 1983. *Modern Health Care Administration,* p. 54. Academic Press, New York, N.Y.

7. Hodgettes, R. M., and D. M. Cascio. 1983. *Modern Health Care Administration,* p. 84. Academic Press, New York, N.Y.

8. Hodgettes, R. M., and D. M. Cascio. 1983. *Modern Health Care Administration,* p. 136. Academic Press, New York, N.Y.

9. **Hodgettes, R. M., and D. M. Cascio.** 1983. *Modern Health Care Administration,* p. 211–214. Academic Press, New York, N.Y.

10. **Johnson, E. A.** 1989. Managerial-organizational communications, p. 86. *In* J. R. Snyder and D. A. Senhauser (ed.), *Administration and Supervision in Laboratory Medicine,* 2nd ed. J. B. Lippincott Company, Philadelphia, Pa.

11. **Johnson, E. A.** 1989. Managerial-organizational communications. p. 87. *In* J. R. Snyder and D. A. Senhauser (ed.), *Administration and Supervision in Laboratory Medicine,* 2nd ed. J. B. Lippincott Company, Philadelphia, Pa.

12. **Krieff, A.** 1996. *Manager's Survival Guide: How To Avoid the 750 Most Common Mistakes When Dealing with People,* p. 110. Prentice Hall, Englewood Cliffs, N.J.

13. **Martin, B. G., and A. S. Kurec.** 1989. Staffing and scheduling of laboratory personnel, p. 199. *In* J. R. Snyder and D. A. Senhauser (ed.), *Administration and Supervision in Laboratory Medicine,* 2nd ed. J. B. Lippincott Company, Philadelphia, Pa.

14. **Maslow, A. H.** 1954. *Motivation and Personality.* Harper Collins, New York, N.Y.

15. **McClatchey, K. D.** 1994. *Clinical Laboratory Medicine,* p. 5. Williams and Wilkins, Baltimore, Md.

16. **Rakich, J. S., B. B. Longest, and T. R. O'Donovan.** 1977. *Managing Health Care Organizations,* p. 127–129. W. B. Saunders, Philadelphia, Pa.

17. **Reinke, W.** 1988. *Health Planning for Effective Management,* p. 187. Oxford University Press, New York, N.Y.

18. **Shortell, S. M., and A. D. Kaluzny.** 1994. *Health Care Management—Organization, Design and Behavior,* 3rd ed., p. 172. Delmar Publishers, Albany, N.Y.

19. **Snyder, J. R., and D. A. Senhauser (ed.).** 1989. *Administration and Supervision in Laboratory Medicine,* 2nd ed., p. 34. J. B. Lippincott Company, Philadelphia, Pa.

20. **Snyder, J. R.** 1989. Problem solving—the decision-making process, p. 45–46. *In* J. R. Snyder and D. A. Senhauser (ed.), *Administration and Supervision in Laboratory Medicine,* 2nd ed. J. B. Lippincott Company, Philadelphia, Pa.

21. **Snyder, J. R., and D. S. Wilkinson.** 1998. *Management in Laboratory Medicine,* 3rd ed., p. 66–68. Lippincott-Raven, Philadelphia, Pa.

22. **Vetter, L. P., R. Carden, and D. S. Wilkinson.** 2001. Strategic planning in a clinical environment. *Clin. Leadersh. Manag. Rev.* **15:**34–38.

23. **Wolfgang, J. W., and L. M. Brigando.** 1989. Standards and appraisal of laboratory performance, p. 217–219. *In* J. R. Snyder and D. A. Senhauser (ed.), *Administration and Supervision in Laboratory Medicine,* 2nd ed. J. B. Lippincott Company, Philadelphia, Pa.

APPENDIX 2.1 Laboratory Strategic Plan

Goal/objective/strategy	Comments/metrics	Target date	Accountability	Cost
1. Improve cost control				
a. Consolidate vendor relationships				
Increase use of capital equipment leases and reagent rental agreements	Track incremental dollar savings	Jul 03	Jones	
Develop RFP[a] for automation of front-end specimen management		Jan 04	James	
b. Acquisition of satellite labs when cost-effective for health system				
Develop feasibility study for cytogenetics lab (human genetics)	Working group formed	Apr 03	Shaw	
c. Improve test utilization control				
Develop a better understanding of physician ordering patterns	Track tests per discharge, tests per patient day	Ongoing	White	
	Form a task force	Mar 03	James	
Decrease volume of intensive care unit testing, esoteric testing, and send-outs	Track test volume	Ongoing	James	
d. Use information services to improve operational efficiency				
Create management databases as needed, centralized through laboratory information system (LIS)	Hire database programmer	Jul 03	White	50,000
Increase informatics skill level of existing personnel	Provide informatics training opportunities		Jones	
2. Increase revenue				
a. Improve billing effectiveness				
Increase physician understanding and awareness of billing (Part A and Part B)	Develop an educational program	Feb 03	Brown	
Widen compliance training	Schedule teleconference	Apr 03	Williams	200
Appoint a billing "expert" for each lab or section	List of billing experts for each lab section	Mar 03	Brown	
Improve physician access to reimbursement information	Obtain fee schedules for major payors	Feb 03	Mays	
Improve front-end registration training	Focus on outreach accounts	Dec 02	Mays	
b. Consultations				
Improve reimbursement mechanism for consultative services	Form a working group	May 03	Gray	
c. Increase outreach volume				
Increase marketing of "niche" specialties	Hire additional sales personnel	Mar 03	Mays	50,000
Automate Service Master maintenance		June 03	White	

(continued)

APPENDIX 2.1   Laboratory Strategic Plan *(continued)*

Goal/objective/strategy	Comments/metrics	Target date	Accountability	Cost
3. Improve work environment				
a. Physical environment				
Encourage employees to take personal responsibility for cleanliness of environment	Add routine maintenance and cleanliness to safety checklist	Jan 03	Williams	
b. Improve recruitment and retention				
Deploy existing retention/recruitment plan within 12 months		Jan 04	Jones	200,000
Develop a career ladder for all employees (communication, compensation, development, professional growth opportunity)	Assemble a working group	Jul 03	Jones	
Create opportunities for internal staff presentations	Track number of presentations	Ongoing	Jones	
More one-on-one interaction between managers and staff outside of annual review	Develop a 360° feedback	Ongoing	Jones	
4. Improve customer service				
a. Acknowledge receipt of specimens, possibly in LIS	Message back to customers for consultative cases	Apr 03	White	
b. Develop a dial-in process for outreach customers	LIS vendor or third party	Sep 03	White	50,000
Cross train surgical pathology laboratory/client services personnel		Jul 03	Mays	

*ª*RFP, requested for proposal.

APPENDIX 2.2   Laboratory Organizational Chart

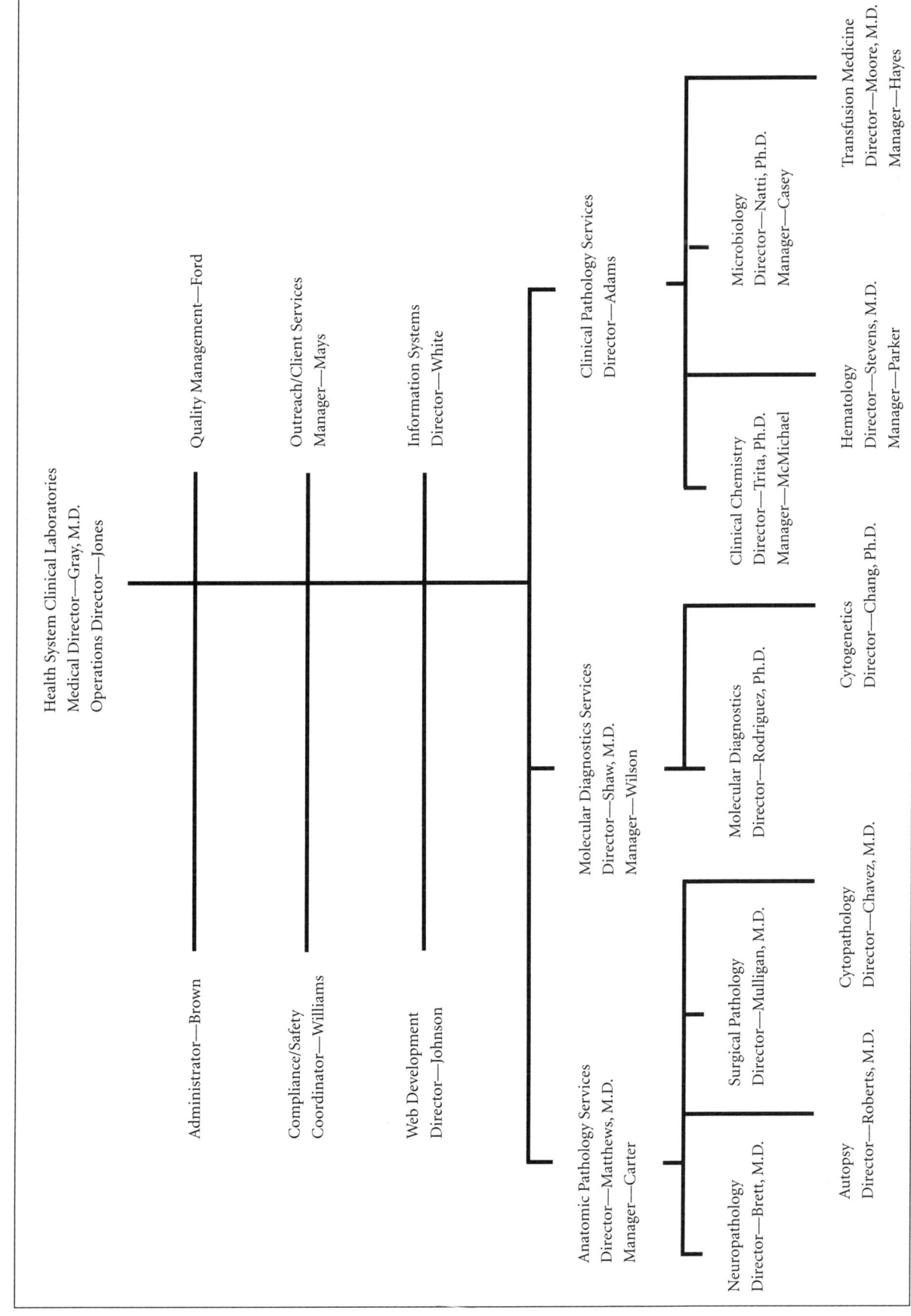

APPENDIX 2.3   Administrative Policy and Procedure Manual table of contents

Policy no.ᵃ	Title	Initial effective date	Release/revised date
Administrative—001 to 199 Series			
100.002	Formulation and Distribution Policies and Procedures	12/07/98	04/01/00
107.001	Inclement Weather Policy	12/05/96	01/09/01
Laboratory—200 to 299 Series			
209.001	Unacceptable Laboratory Specimens (see compliance policies also)	06/19/97	10/01/98
210.001	Request for Release of Pathology Records, Slides, and/or Blocks	01/09/97	03/13/01
213.002	Waste Disposal	12/01/96	08/04/98
214.000	Guidelines for the Retention, Storage and Disposal of Laboratory Records and Materials	04/03/96	01/25/97
215.000	Handling of External Quality Control Materials	01/25/97	01/25/97
216.000	External Survey Reports	01/25/97	01/25/97
217.000	Procedures for Review of Policies and Procedures (for compliance with regulatory guidelines)	01/27/97	01/27/97
218.000	Specimen Collection Boxes	03/12/97	03/12/97
219.000	Faxing of Confidential Patient Information	02/27/97	03/10/97
220.000	Reagent Labeling Policy	12/08/99	05/15/00
233.001	Reagent Grade Water	10/02/98	06/01/01
234.000	Client Access to Current Test Methods	11/18/97	11/18/97
235.000	Notification of Delay in Testing	10/19/98	10/09/98
236.000	Guidelines For Assuring Proper Authorization Prior To Performing Autopsies	03/01/00	03/01/00
237.000	Guidelines For Accepting Autopsies From Outside Institutions	03/01/00	03/01/00
238.000	Release of Biological Specimens to the Medical Examiner's Office	07/11/00	06/01/01
239.000	Anatomic Pathology Support of Research Projects	12/18/00	01/09/00
241.000	Latex Allergy Abatement	07/15/02	07/15/02
242.000	Reference Laboratory Validation and Monitoring	11/22/00	11/22/00
Information systems—400 to 499 Series			
401.005	Computer Downtime Procedure	12/06/88	01/22/02
405.001	Verification of Test Results Transmittal Accuracy Between Test Performance and Computer Output	10/07/98	06/06/02
406.000	Electronic Mail (E-Mail) and Internet Access/Usage	09/12/00	01/09/01
Personnel—600 to 699 Series			
602.001	Standards of Personnel Attire (While on Duty)	11/22/93	03/23/00
611.003	Approval Process for Overtime to Ensure Proper Staffing	07/28/98	05/10/99
614.002	Leave Policies and Procedures	01/31/97	07/22/98
615.000	Leave Request Procedure	09/20/00	01/09/01
617.000	Compliance as an Element of Performance Plans (see compliance policies)	01/01/99	01/01/99

(continued)

APPENDIX 2.3　Administrative Policy and Procedure Manual table of contents *(continued)*

Policy no.[a]	Title	Initial effective date	Release/revised
Safety and security—700 to 799 Series			
701.000	Shipping of Hazardous Materials	07/15/02	07/15/02
Physician re-credentialing—1000 to 1199 Series			
1000.002	Criteria for Physician Appointment and Reappointment to Medical Staff	06/01/93	07/01/02
Compliance			
Hospital Policy	Advance Beneficiary Notice	01/01/99	01/01/99
Hospital Policy	Laboratory Compliance in the Outpatient Ambulatory Setting	01/01/99	01/01/99
Hospital Policy	Laboratory Services Non-Compliance	01/01/99	01/01/99
	Department of Pathology Compliance Plan	01/01/99	01/01/02
209.001	Unacceptable Laboratory Specimens	06/19/97	10/01/98
617.000	Compliance as an Element of Performance Plans	01/01/99	01/01/99
1200.000	Laboratory Billing	10/01/98	10/01/98
1201.000	Technical Update Notifications	10/01/98	10/01/98
1202.000	Health Fairs	10/01/98	10/01/98
1203.000	Compliance in Sales and Marketing	10/01/98	10/01/98
1204.000	Order Entry for Laboratory Tests	10/01/98	10/01/98
Hospital Policy	Accounts Missing Diagnosis at Time of Billing	01/01/99	01/01/99
Hospital Policy	Preprocessor Maintenance	01/01/99	01/01/99

[a]Revision number (e.g., 209.001 is first revision).

APPENDIX 2.4   Consequences of Neglecting Basic Management Functions

Management function	Type of neglect	Consequences of neglect
Planning		
Strategic planning	Planning for the future is considered casually or not at all.	Laboratory will be ill-prepared to handle crises and changes in the environment, resulting in economic and staffing problems.
Selecting a planning group	Failure to include a representative planning group	Needs of some laboratory sections will not be addressed.
Environmental analysis	Current issues in healthcare are not fully considered when planning.	Strategic plan will not deliver realistically achievable recommendations.
SWOT analysis	Inadequate thought is given to internal and external strengths, weaknesses, opportunities, and threats.	Missed chances for enhanced revenue, cost savings, and staff development
Vision and mission statements	The organization's employees are not presented with a clearly articulated statement of purpose.	Plans made in the absence of a compelling vision are likely to be vague, misdirected, and poorly implemented.
Goals, objectives, and strategies	Planning is completed without creating an itemized list of clearly stated strategic objectives.	Resulting plan will not be truly strategic, but will instead resemble a "to-do" list of operational details.
Prioritization	A plan is made without consideration to which objectives have the highest impact.	Resources will be misdirected toward objectives that are not of paramount importance.
Accountability	The strategic plan fails to make individuals specifically accountable for action items.	If everybody is responsible, then nobody is responsible, and the details of the plan will not be carried forth.
Measuring success	The plan does not contain a mechanism to monitor progress made toward objectives.	Failure to measure will result in wasted time and lost resources as effort is expended upon flawed objectives.
Organizing		
Time management	No systematic time management system is used by the manager in the course of daily business.	Lack of structure will result in increasing amounts of time spent at work and decreasing productivity during that time.
Organizational chart	The structure of the laboratory is not formally mapped out.	Employees will be vague about reporting lines and work flow will be adversely affected due to lack of clarity.
Policies	Policies are not written out and catalogued in an orderly way.	Manager will not have the benefit of written rules to maintain desired and orderly behavior in the workplace, resulting in loss of control.
Procedures	Procedures are not written out and catalogued in an orderly way.	Very serious consequences related to patient care, regulatory compliance, safety, and employee health
Work flow	Consideration is not given to the management of work flow within the laboratory.	Lost efficiency, wasted time, duplicated processes, and redundancy in effort
Staffing and scheduling	The schedule does not give proper consideration to staffing needs at critical times.	Understaffing during busy periods and overstaffing during slack periods affect throughput and productivity.
Directing		
Communicating	The manager does not hold regularly scheduled staff meetings.	Staff are uninformed about important matters, often leading to low morale, disengagement, and high turnover.
Delegating	The manager does not make subordinates responsible for executing assignments.	Manager becomes stressed/burned out and staff feel undervalued.
Motivating	The manager does not put energy into motivation of the staff.	Many on the staff will stagnate as professional growth is halted.
Coaching	Employees are not provided with regular coaching.	Employees require the benefit of managerial experience. Without it, there will be morale problems and turnover.
Controlling		
Evaluating performance	Individual employee performance is not regularly reviewed.	Employees not aware of deficiencies cannot improve.
Decision making	Manager fails to employ a systematic decision making process.	Quality of decisions will lack consistency, and underlying problems will be ignored.

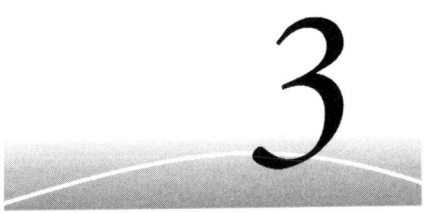

3

Relevant Economic and Business Concepts

Ann L. Harris

OBJECTIVES

To define relevant economic issues that influence the delivery of healthcare services and their relevance to the practice of laboratory medicine

To outline the key concepts and principles (for example, supply, demand, and competition) that drive the business decisions faced by laboratory directors, managers, pathologists, and hospital administrators

To relate relevant global economy concerns to changes in healthcare policies

To identify marketing, sales, and customer service tools used to formulate a business plan to respond to the service requirements and economic needs of the healthcare delivery system

---

In our free enterprise system, business traditionally has been held responsible for quantities—for the supply of goods and jobs, for costs, prices, wages, hours of work, and for standards of living. Today, however, business is being asked to take on responsibility for the quality of life in our society. The expectation is that business, in addition to its traditional accountability for economic performance and results—will concern itself with the health of society, that it will come up with the cures for the ills that currently beset us and, indeed, will find ways of anticipating and preventing future problems in these areas.

R. F. BARKER (2)

Introduction

Overview of Laboratory Industry Trends during the Past Decade

Following several decades of profitability created by low direct costs, favorable inpatient reimbursement, hospital-based outpatient reimbursement, and physician utilization, the clinical laboratory industry suffered a severe setback in the 1990s. Increased regulatory requirements and the expansion of managed care were the change drivers for many trends in the healthcare and clinical laboratory industries, as listed in Table 3.1 (23). The industry as a whole suffered a loss of several billion dollars in reimbursements from the impact on test utilization patterns. Faced with possible loss of market share during the mid-1990s, commercial laboratories engaged in fierce competitive bidding for managed-care contracts, further decreasing laboratory reimbursement. Reimbursements began to improve by the end of the decade as commercial laboratories sought more profitable contracts. At the same time, hospital laboratories faced excess testing capacity created by shifting STAT testing to near-patient testing and shortened inpatient lengths of stay. Laboratory managers changed their focus

Table 3.1 Change drivers during the 1990s[a]

Driver	Change
Tighter quality and documentation requirements (CLIA '88[b])	Reduced test volume
	Increased cost of production
Increased coding and claim requirements	Reduced collections
	Increased denials
Reduced Medicare fee schedule	Reduced reimbursements
Managed-care enrollments more than doubled	Shift from fee-for-service to capitated-reimbursement model
Fierce competitive bidding among commercial laboratories	Prices and reimbursements reached plateau and then decreased in the 1990s.

[a]See reference 24.

[b]CLIA '88, Clinical Laboratory Improvement Amendments of 1988.

from evaluating technical proficiency to analyzing and controlling costs. Successful managers strengthened their skills in human resource management, money management, and process management. Operations managers used their business savvy and experience to create business plans. The industry observed record numbers of laboratory consolidations, mergers, acquisitions, and joint ventures during the decade. Laboratory restructuring often followed hospital or healthcare system reorganization. The concept of laboratory regionalization, first developed in the 1980s, focused on standardizing policies and procedures and providing improved continuity of care across multiple facilities and sites of care. Enhancing income by expanding the geographic market and lowering costs through economy of scale became the primary goals.

Managed care, pricing pressure, and advances in medicine and technology have created a constant state of change. Table 3.2 contains the typical paradigm shifts encountered by the laboratory industry over the past decade. Adding to a growing population of uninsured patients, employees in their fifties are taking early retirement as employers balk at continuing to pay escalating premiums for healthcare coverage. The baby boomer generation retirement will peak in the year 2010. Neither the government nor the private sector yet seems willing to meet these demands. A growing number of patients will not be able to pay their medical bills, and bad-debt write-offs will continue to rise. The downward trends in reimbursement will continue with even greater controls and limitations on utilization, forcing further reductions in the unit cost of medical services (34).

Forecast for the New Millennium

To compensate for the changes of the past decade, hospital laboratories have become competitive players in the local market by developing their outreach business to capture new revenue from market segments like physician offices and long-term-care facilities. Hospital laboratories have formed networks to enable them to compete for managed-care contracts. With the trend to consolidate hospitals and

Table 3.2 Industry trends during the past decade

Old paradigm	New paradigm
Centralized laboratory testing	POCT (point-of-care testing)
	Near-patient and bedside testing
Physician office testing	Home testing kits
	Direct-access testing
Lab-supervised phlebotomy	Patient care technician at nursing stations
Inpatient procedures	Outpatient invasive procedures
Fee-for-service reimbursement	Global payment systems
	Diagnosis-related groups
	Ambulatory payment classification
Skilled hospital beds	SNF (skilled-nursing facility) beds
Prospective payment system for SNFs	Consolidated billing: services reimbursed under resource utilization groups
Standing orders	Patient care plans
Preventative healthcare screening and diagnosis V codes	Medically necessary testing
	Local medical review policies
	Advanced beneficiary notices
Routine testing	Specialized esoteric testing
Top-down hierarchy	Bottom-up customer focus

develop core laboratories to keep more tests in-house, there is now competition to perform esoteric testing among hospital-based laboratories. National commercial laboratories also compete for referral testing in the esoteric market, where the profit margin is more attractive. New advances in point-of-care testing (POCT) instruments are stimulating an increase in the number of physician office laboratories. Both academic medical centers and independent commercial laboratories are focusing on research and development of specialized testing to augment the routine testing performed in hospital core laboratories. Successful centralization may involve robotics and increased automation. Standardization and centralization of data management, methods, facilities, equipment, quality assurance, education, and information systems are fundamental to the implementation of responsive business strategies (48). Healthcare administrators and laboratory managers must develop the skills needed to deal with the logistical and cultural changes required to develop strategic business plans. They must realize that customers are every organization's most valuable resource. Ultimately, customer satisfaction will be the critical strategic weapon for any enterprise (26).

Strategic Business Planning Overview

Market Assessment

The development of a strategic business plan begins with a market assessment of consumer needs. The primary purpose is to perform market research (market assessment) and a feasibility study to determine the impact of a project on laboratory production, estimate the potential new revenue in the market, evaluate sales and service requirements, perform a competitive analysis, and then develop strategies and goals that will enable the company to implement the plan (33, 37).

The Four Environmental Variables

Before a product or service reaches the consumer, the development strategies should be evaluated against four environmental variables: legal (regulatory), competitive, economic, and societal environments (5). These four variables influence both the business development strategies and the consumer's perceptions about product value. The legal climate attempts to maintain a competitive environment while at the same time regulating specific marketing practices. The economic environment influences consumer behavior. As society has become more educated and interdependent, more emphasis has been placed on the marketing strategies for the societal environment, both domestically and globally.

Key Strategies

Strategy can be defined as the approach or techniques developed by the management team to facilitate the organization's ability to perform successfully. The strategic planning process functions best when formulated in an open and inclusive atmosphere. The goals established for product and service delivery should be innovative and visionary (4). A business plan has four key strategies that must be carefully weighed against each of the four environmental variables cited above along with customer perceptions (6).

- *Production (product planning) strategies.* Production strategies include decisions about research and development, production times for new products, and branding.
- *Service (distribution) strategies.* Service strategies define how the products and services will be delivered.
- *Marketing and sales (promotional) strategies.* Promotional strategies include market research, sales management, customer service, communication, marketing, sales support, and the approach to advertising (publications and promotions).
- *Pricing strategies.* Pricing strategies are typically the most difficult and are often dependent on the complexity of regulatory oversight and public scrutiny. Prices must always be profitable and defendable.

The key to success is being able to align and blend these four strategies into a dynamic business plan as depicted in Fig. 3.1 (5). In most cases, one or more of the environmental variables are beyond management's control, ultimately putting pressure on every organization to continuously reevaluate the basic business strategies being used. Society (or the consumer) generally supports businesses as long as the business is perceived to be a contributing partner. Economists refer to the satisfying of this need as utility (7). In medicine it is more commonly referred to as clinical utility.

Perform a Competitive Analysis

Another vital step in the development of the business planning process is to define each of the organization's strengths and weaknesses to measure how the operation stacks up against the competition. This process, known as a SWOT analysis (strengths, weaknesses, opportunities, and threats), is covered in chapter 2. After performing a competitive analysis, hospital laboratories are equipped to identify the opportunities for new business and the threats to the operation while formulating the marketing and sales strategies to be implemented as a part of the strategic business plan.

Competitive Environment

Clinical Laboratory Competitive Market

The competitive environment is created by interaction among businesses that offer similar products and services. In the clinical laboratory industry, the competition changes in response to other environmental influences, such as the regulatory environment. Over the past three

Figure 3.1 Strategic business planning. The four key strategies (pricing, production, marketing, and service) serve as the cornerstones in the framework for the development of a successful business plan. The strategies must be carefully weighed against the influences of the four variable environmental factors and the market research information on consumer needs for the products and services.

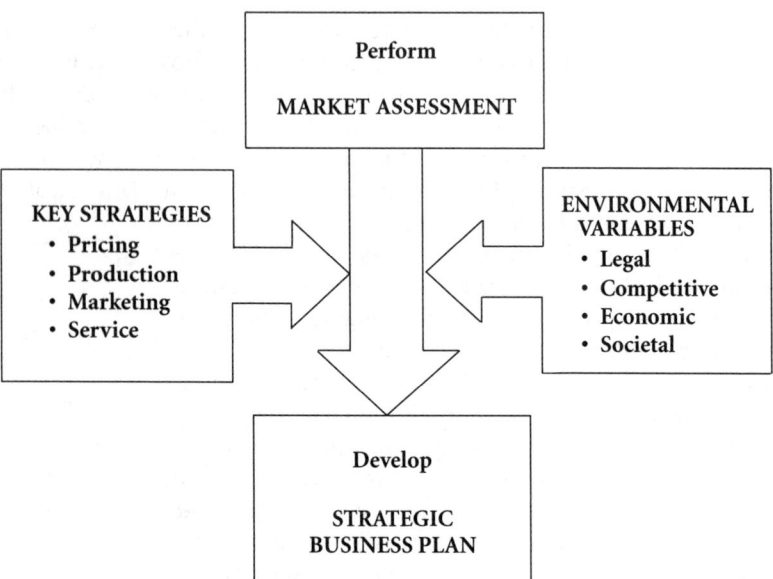

decades, competition among commercial laboratories resulted in many mergers and acquisitions. Regional laboratories and local independent laboratories consolidated in an effort to increase market share and offset the declining revenue base. However, new technology is now driving the growth of smaller, independent specialty laboratories focusing on specific niche markets like clinical trials, genetic testing, molecular diagnostics, flow cytometry, coagulation and hemostasis, substance abuse testing, and pathology support services. The smaller specialty companies have formed strategic alliances among themselves in order to compete with the two major players and offer a wider scope of services to their customers. Regulations for patients with end-stage renal disease created the need for dialysis centers to own and manage central laboratories for testing covered under the Medicare composite rate for the care of chronic renal failure patients. Physician office laboratories are now expanding the test offerings as new POCT integrates the tests onto robust, near-patient testing platforms. As POCT technology improves, we are likely to witness home healthcare agencies and patients opting for home testing.

Business Entities, Strategic Alliances, Joint Ventures, Mergers and Acquisitions, and Integrated Networks

Healthcare facilities typically respond to the pressures created by the financial constraints of healthcare reform by solidifying their current market share, expanding their geographic service area, and implementing better cost controls. Industry restructuring is unpredictable and often includes relationships between unlikely business partners. The arrangements include physician practice organizations, physician management groups, physician hospital

business organizations (health systems), integrated delivery systems, independent provider associations, and provider networks. The type of business entity that institutions typically form is based on tax status. Tax-exempt status is sometimes difficult to obtain when more than 20% of the healthcare organization's board members are physicians. Individuals, sole proprietors, corporations, and trusts are all taxpayers.

Types of business entities. The following types of business entities are presented below:

- *Corporations* are required by state laws to file articles of incorporation as a for-profit or a not-for-profit organization. A corporation's owners have limited liabilities based on their individual investments in the company.

- *Partnerships* are not considered taxable entities and do not pay taxes. The general partners are personally liable for financial obligations and are taxed on their earnings. Partners in a limited partnership are only liable for the amount equal to their investment.

- A *limited liability company (LLC)* is a legal entity treated like a corporation, but the owner's liability is limited to its investment and the company is treated like a partnership for federal income tax purposes. An LLC may or may not have centralized management. To gain classification as a partnership, the LLC must have at least two members (43).

Strategic alliances. Faced with increasingly complex technologies and more intense global competition, strategic alliances enable companies to combine their resources to share risk, reduce costs, and solidify customer and supplier relationships. When properly planned and managed, an alliance can significantly strengthen competitive advantage through technology exchange, reduction in time to market, opening new markets, securing investment capital, and sharing costs of research and development. Equity investments, cooperative ventures, research and development contracts, licensing agreements, and sales and marketing agreements fall under the umbrella term of strategic partnering. Whenever the income from the venture can be referred to as unrelated business income, the entities should consider restructuring the affiliation agreement. The parties should execute due diligence or confidentiality agreements at the onset of the negotiation process (15).

Strategic partnerships are typically formed by corporations with strategic objectives that complement one another for a variety of reasons. The partners agree to mutual and open communication that supports long-term, multiyear preferential relationships that share risk and reduce cost. These partnerships allow laboratories to deal with fewer suppliers, streamline, standardize, automate purchasing practices, reduce inventories, and measure both quality and financial outcome (4).

Less formal alliances allow for the creation of cooperative databases that support information sharing so that the partners can make business decisions with current, detailed information about the healthcare environment. There is a growing need for healthcare providers and insurers to share information across databases. The resulting network server is generally referred to as a community health information network. Roundtable discussions provide another mechanism to discuss mutual problems and share case studies.

More formal equity partnerships create a business arrangement with shared ownership and interlocking boards. Franchise alliances link the partners through exclusive license agreements that provide training, products, systems, and marketing in exchange for the financial investment. A shared clinical service alliance allocates the costs for specialized clinical services, such as magnetic resonance imaging, among multiple sponsors. A joint venture brings two or more entities together to share an investment (13).

Joint venture. A joint venture is formed for economic purposes to achieve mutual or common financial goals. The arrangement may include partnerships, corporations, trusts, LLCs, leases, and contracts. Joint venture is the terminology used to describe management agreements, partnerships, strategic laboratory arrangements, or outsourcing. Such ventures are not legal entities with legal protection. Facilities entering into a joint venture arrangement should first seek the advice of counsel to ensure that the partnership does not violate Internal Revenue Service guidelines, antikickback statutes, fraud and abuse, Stark, or safe harbor regulations (43). These regulations are discussed in more detail in chapter 5.

Mergers and acquisitions. Performing due diligence in the merger process includes an examination of the financial and legal records of the parties involved. The process identifies the scope of liabilities that will be assumed and the legal impediments and provides a comprehensive understanding of the merging parties' business operations (1). Typical structures used in mergers are as follows:

- *Statutory merger.* The stock in the merging company is combined with the stock in the surviving company.
- *Stock acquisition.* The stock in the merging company is acquired by the surviving entity, and the merging company continues to operate as a subsidiary corporation of the surviving company.
- *Asset acquisition.* The surviving company acquires some or all of the assets of the merging entity in return for stock in the surviving company. The merging company continues to exist as a legally distinct corporation.

Integrated delivery systems. An integrated delivery system is formed when payors and healthcare providers (including acute-care providers, physicians, home healthcare agencies, nursing homes, primary care offices, and others) combine forces to extend their service lines to improve the coordination and quality of care while controlling costs. Financing an integrated delivery system requires a basic understanding of capital markets and the ability to adapt to the changing market demands.

The business structures and associated risks for each of the partners in an integrated delivery system vary widely. Hospitals are managed on fixed assets with cost centers and are considered to be high risk for capital investment. Physician group administrators, who manage the services provided by individual physicians, are generally perceived to have the lowest risk. Managed-care organizations deal with healthcare insurance and are moderate risks for capital investment (30).

Integrated delivery systems measure their success using outcome data like patient satisfaction surveys, readmission rates, costs for emergency care, and patient compliance to prescription refills. The creation of integrated delivery systems is a business strategy used to facilitate the change from treating chronic disease and acute episodes to the practice of preventative and predictive medicine.

Emerging network models. There are at least seven loosely connected organizational models emerging with changing partners linked by contracts, not ownership. Each one takes a slightly different approach to organizing governance and directorship (32). Table 3.3 discusses various emerging network models (13).

Regional network outreach programs. Healthcare facilities developing regional laboratory networks have encountered a number of difficulties along the way. It is

Table 3.3 Emerging network models[a]

Description of network	Network organization and governance
Medical clinics	Physician-governed and medically dominated clinics form their own managed-care organizations or start joint ventures with managed-care plans.
Hub and spoke	Academic medical center forms networks with large regional hospitals. The academic medical center serves as the network hub, and most decisions favor it.
Multicenter network	A network that is composed of strong regional hospitals and tertiary-care centers without the expense of the academic medical center
Public system	Urban hospitals form networks to capture Medicaid contract work to compete with managed-care and medical center networks.
Enterprise corporation	Corporations offer stock to physician and hospital partners, but the parent maintains control.
Provider-insurer partnerships	Networks formed by physicians and insurers are difficult to operate due to differences in culture and leadership styles.
Community partnerships	Community-based healthcare systems or community care networks differ according to the locality and its needs. These networks are focused on financial risk, continuum of care, integration, outcome data, and clinical protocols.

[a]See reference 13.

never easy to overcome long-standing rivalry and antagonism among local competitors. Obtaining capital funding for outreach often takes a backseat to capital funding for information systems, acquisitions, and replacing aging facilities. Managers face difficult inequities in salary and benefit structures among the systems. Start-up costs, inaccurate estimates of specimen volume, and inferior information and billing systems often leave managers unable to demonstrate increased revenue, income, or profit in the outreach market (24).

Managed competition. As hospital outreach programs develop relationships with community healthcare providers, commercial laboratories argue that hospital-based laboratories have an unfair advantage in the physician market segment, where physicians may feel obligated to patronize the hospital. Hospitals have also become aggressive in buying physician office practices in an effort to capture more referrals. In many areas, hospitals are developing their own managed-care programs in conjunction with the physicians. This approach is known as managed competition. The physician hospital organization negotiates contracts with third-party payors in order to provide full scope of services under a managed-care arrangement.

The Economic Environment

Four Stages of the Business Cycle

There are two main categories of economics. Microeconomics focuses on individual behavior and the interaction of companies. Macroeconomics examines the interaction of income, employment, and inflation on the economy as a whole. More information is available from Wikipedia,

the free encyclopedia. Wikipedia is an international, open-content, collaboratively developed encyclopedia found at http://www.wikipedia.org/ (last accessed April 2003).

Businesses operate in a complex environment. The business cycle fluctuates through four dynamic stages that follow a cyclic pattern, as demonstrated in Fig. 3.2. Many economists argue that society can avoid future depression by intelligent utilization of economic and fiscal policies. In this model, the business cycle would move directly from recession to recovery (8).

The National Economy: Fiscal and Monetary Policies

A variable economic factor that influences marketing strategies is inflation. The federal government uses two basic approaches to counter the effects of inflation on the economy. Fiscal policies target the government's receipts and expenditures, while monetary policies refer to the management of

Figure 3.2 The four stages of the economy. The economy is cyclic and progresses through four stages. There are cycles when the economic environment supports the move from recession directly to recovery, bypassing an economic depression.

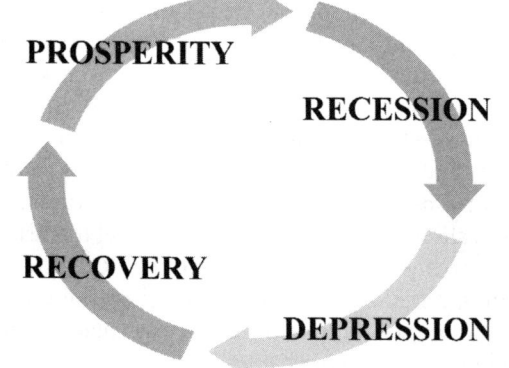

the money supply and the market interest rates. During periods of inflation, the government's fiscal policy changes could include reduced spending, increased taxes, or a price freeze. A monetary action plan might be to decrease the money supply or to raise the prime interest rate to curtail spending. Consumers generally do not take notice of modest price increases over time. This pricing phenomenon is known as creeping inflation. As customers perceive erosion of their buying power, they will modify their behavior for major purchases to either buy now, believing that the price will be higher later, or reallocate their funds, postponing their purchase until later. Each of these results in a decline in demand for goods and services and creates a supply surplus and an excess capacity on the production line (8).

Most laboratory expenses, including fixed and variable costs, are impacted by inflation. Inflation factors are not typically applied to expenses associated with depreciation, interest, rent or leases (except by contract), or bad debt. Inflation factors should be applied to an annual budget on a month-to-month accrual basis, rather than at the first of the year, so as not to overstate the cost (21).

Global economy. In the global economy, businesses are forced to shift from being multinational (a national company with foreign subsidiaries) to being transnational (where the world is one economic unit). Sales, service, public relations, and legal affairs are local. Parts, machines, planning, research, finance, marketing, pricing, and management are obtained from a world market perspective (17). (Additional information can be found at http://www.mtholyoke.edu/acad/intrel/drucker.html [last accessed January 2003].) The neoclassical concept of the global economy implies that the free mobility of products and factors of production across national boundaries will maximize efficiency through forced competition. Since the wider the market, the greater the possibilities for specialization, it follows that the most efficient market is the global market. Additional information on global economy can be found at Howard Richard's website (http://www.Howardri.org/Trade.html [last accessed January 2003]). Richards is a professor of global economy at Earlham College.

Principles of Supply and Demand

The laws of supply and demand are the foundation of a market system. There are certain characteristic behaviors that form the market norms. Companies that sell products and deliver services are in business to yield a profit. Customers typically purchase products and services with the expectation of getting the best value and service for their money. When the price of an item purchased on a regular basis increases, the buyer may order a smaller quantity, based on its relationship to the budget or the relationship of the purchased product to other products. When the

price of a regularly purchased item decreases, the buyer may buy more of the items with the same investment. Change in consumer tastes also affects demand, but trying to measure the effect is difficult. This behavior is known as the law of demand. Changes in price not only affect consumer behavior but also influence supplier behavior. Price has a powerful, predictable, and measurable effect on the quantity purchased.

Supply is also affected by price, but in the opposite way. There is a tendency for the production of a good or service to increase when the price goes up and to decrease when the price goes down. In order to demonstrate a profit when production increases, the other variables that affect the cost of production like labor, consumables, and the availability of and access to competitive products and services must remain unchanged. Market price is the actual price at which a commodity (product or service) is commonly purchased. In a market economy, price is determined by the interaction of supply and demand. A free-market economy is usually driven by the consumer, not the manufacturer. The market value for products and services is ultimately determined by their perceived value to the consumer. At the individual level, companies generally continue to manufacture a product or service as long as the market price is equal to or greater than the cost to deliver it. When the buyer and the seller agree, a quantity is purchased for a price, and the supply and demand at that point are in equilibrium (Fig. 3.3). Additional information is available from the website of Keystone Marketing Services, a leader in commodity market training (http://tfc-charts.w2d.com/learning/supply_and_demand.html [last accessed April 2003]).

When either the supply or the demand changes the equilibrium, market price also changes. Technology is another key factor that drives price. In the long run, as costs

Figure 3.3 Product price is a result of the interaction of supply and demand. Products and services are not sold until the buyer and seller agree on a price. Equilibrium price is the price at which buyers are willing to buy the same quantity as suppliers are willing to supply. Adapted from http://tfc-charts.w2d.com/learning/supply_and_demand.html from material provided by Keystone Marketing Services (site last accessed April 2003).

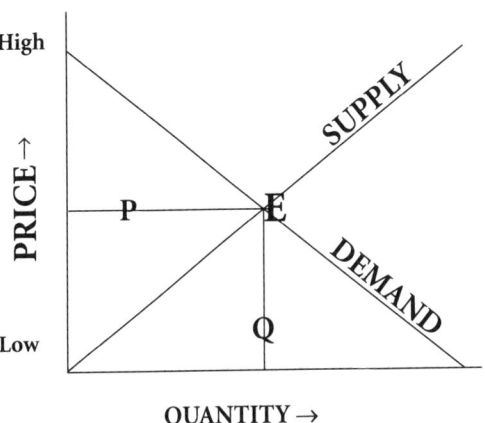

of production are reduced, the market price for the goods also goes down.

Assess Infrastructure and Develop Production Strategies

Developing a business plan to pursue new business opportunities always includes an assessment of the existing infrastructure, facilities, equipment, and human resources and a realistic assessment of the laboratory's excess capacity, using robust benchmarking tools.

- *Physical location.* Determine whether the present location of the laboratory is adequate for convenient access for patients and couriers. Evaluate the space requirements for the anticipated increase in test volumes.
- *Testing personnel.* Analyze the personnel required to support accessioning, testing, reporting, courier, and billing functions for the anticipated test volumes by shift.
- *Instrumentation/equipment.* Work with laboratory managers to assess the existing equipment's age, reliability, throughput, and cost per test. If new instrumentation is indicated, consider both capital funding and reagent rental. Does the proposed volume justify front-end automation or robotics?
- *Production strategies.* Develop a detailed test schedule. Evaluate setup times and turnaround time (TAT) needs for the customers. Move batched testing to the most efficient shift for optimal TAT.

Cost Accounting Principles

Laboratory costs. Traditional cost accounting methods focus on unit cost per test. Today, laboratory managers must also take into consideration other environmental factors, such as test performance site, for example, near-patient testing versus STAT laboratory to shorten TAT or length of stay for inpatients. Developing financial management skills is requisite to a manager's ability to make sound business decisions. In order to establish the price for a laboratory procedure, managers must first understand the factors affecting the cost to perform the test. Laboratory costs are typically divided into four groups (22).

- *Preanalytical.* The cost of obtaining the specimen, transporting it to the laboratory, and accessioning and processing the sample for testing.
- *Analytical.* The costs of reagents, labor, equipment purchase, depreciation, or lease.
- *Postanalytical.* The costs associated with reporting results and billing for the services.
- *Quality assurance/quality control.* The associated costs for monitoring and maintaining test quality.

Table 3.4 lists terms frequently used in cost and price analysis.

Activity-based costing is a method being used by some laboratories that assigns a cost to every activity throughout the organization. It captures associated costs for specimen collection, transportation, handling, usage, and disposal and assigns costs to bottlenecks, scheduling delays, and other process costs traditionally not captured in healthcare accounting systems.

By performing a larger volume of tests in one location, laboratories spread the fixed costs over a larger number of tests, reducing the average fixed cost per test. If the output is increased without increasing the cost on the same scale, the laboratory has achieved economy of scale. Laboratories generally experience a decrease in cost per reportable result created by increased purchasing power for reagents, consumables, and kits. Laboratory managers must recognize that there is a point of diminishing return. When additional volume reaches a point that instruments and people are performing at their maximum throughput, the operational efficiency achieved by economy of scale begins to decline. An infinite number of tests cannot be performed in a finite amount of time and space (47).

Return on investment. Capital budgeting is the process of planning for the expenditures expected to generate income to flow into the organization. The analysis for capital budgeting should include the following steps (12):

1. Identify the needed initial cash outflow using bids and proposals from vendors.
2. Forecast the anticipated net cash flows over the life of the project.
3. Evaluate the financial risks associated with the project.
4. Measure the required rate of return for projects of similar risk levels.
5. Compute the net present value (NPV) and/or the internal rate of return (IRR) and assess project feasibility.

First, determine the total gross revenue, or market potential, for the anticipated increase in volume of services over the life of the project. Then estimate the anticipated market share of the specific territory that is being targeted for growth. In order to estimate the cash flows of the new venture, laboratory managers must know their fixed costs and the changes in variable costs for the anticipated growth. The fifth step is a simple arithmetic operation, but steps 1 through 4 may become quite complex and require significant effort.

After determining the cash flows, the laboratory management team can determine whether the financial benefit of the capital investment exceeds the cost; for example, compute the NPV and IRR (18). The logic behind the NPV and IRR analysis is to determine if the annual after-tax cash flow generated over the life of the project will be enough to justify the initial cash outlay needed for the

Table 3.4 Commonly used terms in cost and price analysis[a]

Term	Definition
Direct costs	The costs incurred to perform analysis and produce test results for a specimen in the laboratory
	Technical labor
	Reagents
	Depreciation of equipment
Indirect costs	The costs to acquire specimens and bill for tests
	Billing
	Courier service
	Office supplies and administrative costs (telephone)
Fixed costs	Costs that do not fluctuate with volume changes. Fixed costs per test decrease as test volume increases.
	Lease/rent
	Administrative overhead (client service, sales, marketing)
	Depreciation on capital expenditures like cars, instrumentation, and LIS (laboratory information system)
Variable costs	Costs that fluctuate proportionately with volume changes
	Collection supplies
	Processing labor
	Vehicle maintenance and expenses
	Printer, fax, telephone lines for clients
Fully loaded costs	The total cost to perform a test. All elements of expense from front-end registration and specimen collection to back-end reporting, billing, and collection.
	Direct and indirect
	Fixed and variable
Allocation of indirect expenses	Distribution of indirect costs across the department as a percentage of testing volumes
Incremental cost	The cost to perform an additional test once the direct cost of the assay is derived; also referred to as marginal cost

[a]See reference 20.

project. An NPV formula used by David Upton, professor of finance at Virginia Commonwealth University, follows:

$$NPV = PV - \Sigma \frac{Y_n}{(1+r)^n} + \frac{FV}{(1+r)^N} + \frac{(FV - NBV_N)t}{(1+r)^N}$$

where PV is initial cash outlay, Y_n is net annual cash flow (discussed below), r is rate of return for investments of similar risk, t is tax rate, n is a subscript indicating year, N is final year of project, FV is future value of the assets of the project when sold (or salvage value), and NBV is net book value of the assets of the project after depreciation. NPV can be roughly interpreted as the difference between the cost of the project and the amount that, if invested at the discount rate (r), would provide the anticipated cash flows. When the NPV is positive, the project generates the cash flows more cheaply than alternatives of the same risk and should be accepted. When the NPV is negative, the cash flows can be generated more cheaply through investing elsewhere in projects of similar risk, and the project should not be accepted.

Care must be taken to include the effect of depreciation when computing Y_n, the net annual cash flow. Accounting income and cash flows may differ substantially. For instance, depreciation is deducted when calculating taxes and net income. Depreciation is, however, the result of allocating original expense over periods of use and does not constitute a direct cash flow. The only effect of depreciation on cash flows is indirect: it reduces the tax outlays. The depreciation tax shield (depreciation $\times t$) is sometimes added to net income to approximate cash flows, but this approach ignores other differences between accounting income and cash flows.

The formula can be broken into three parts:

- PV represents the initial cash outlay required to initiate the project. This would include not only the cost of physical assets but also any other costs required to initiate the project.

- $\Sigma \frac{Y_n}{(1+r)^n}$ is the sum of the present values of the future cash flows, for example, the amount that, if invested at the required rate of return, would generate the future cash flows.

- $\frac{FV}{(1+r)^N} + \frac{(FV - NBV_N)t}{(1+r)^N}$ is the present value of the cash flow which is recaptured when the project is ended. The first term is the salvage value of the assets, while the second term reflects the tax effects of differences between book value and sale price.

An alternative approach is to use the computed IRR as the discount rate that, when substituted for r in the formula, results in an NPV of 0. This is the rate of return on the investment and can be compared to the rate of return.

System-Wide Approach to Establishing a Fee Schedule

The development of a laboratory fee schedule is more successful when a system-wide focus on all of the factors related to laboratory economics is used. Communication must be open among accounting, patient reimbursements, finance, budgeting, production, and administration. The pricing formulas used and fees established must be able to accommodate discounting policies that are based on sound business rules but have the flexibility to remain competitive. The individual fees should be reviewed to ensure that maximum reimbursement across the spectrum of payors is achieved.

Pricing Strategies

Hospital laboratories typically have two fee schedules, one for inpatients and one for outpatients. Laboratories should have input in the development of the hospital's inpatient and outpatient fee schedules. Fees for outpatient testing should never be higher than the inpatient fees. Most hospitals use rate-modeling programs that compare their charges with those of other healthcare providers in the local market. Hospitals with community-based outreach programs must determine the pricing strategies necessary to be competitive with each laboratory providing services in the designated service area. Table 3.5 includes tools and techniques frequently used in developing pricing strategies. Pricing strategies must give careful consideration and weight to the im-

pact of competitive market forces and contract negotiations with customers, suppliers, and insurers (35).

Price is defined as the exchange value for a product or service, or the value of an item. Pricing objectives typically fall into one of three groups:

- *Profitability.* The goal is to maximize profits and target new income. Profits are a function of income and expense. Profit = income − expense.
- *Volume.* Volume strives to maximize sales or market share. Gross revenue is determined by the sales price and the volume of the items purchased. Gross revenue = (unit price) (volume).
- *Status quo versus prestige pricing.* Status quo minimizes competitive pricing wars and allows the company to focus its efforts on product improvement or product promotion. Prestige pricing goals set a relatively high price to create an image of quality or prestige in the mind of the buyer.

List price is the term used when the current rate is quoted to the potential buyer. List price is usually determined using a cost-plus formula. Market price is the actual amount the customer pays. Laboratory pricing strategies and policies depend on the types of customers served and their needs.

Account billing strategies. Strategies for billing accounts on an itemized invoice often include using a combination of across-the-board percentage discounts and special prices to meet the customer's needs. When designing pricing options to accommodate customer needs, carefully review the fees to ensure that they are never below incremental costs. When selling to a customer, the best practice is to sell value rather than price.

Table 3.5 Tools and techniques used in developing pricing strategies

Tool	Technique for use
Reimbursement data	Use patient demographic information gathered in the market assessment in conjunction with hospital statistics on patient mix.
	Work with the patient accounting or decision support to establish the average reimbursement per patient encounter.
Billing procedures	Establish pricing policies for accounts that are consistent and are based on anticipated monthly dollar volume.
	Maintain signed service agreements with customers that outline compliance issues.
Billing systems	Does the hospital patient accounting office or the LIS produce client invoices?
	For direct account billing, does the invoice format provide corporate accounting, line item discounting, special pricing, and monthly test utilization summaries?
	Can the billing system generate both a CMS (formerly HCFA) 1500 and UB-92 billing format? (See chapter 5.)
	How are accounts-receivable, aged trial balance reports, revenue reports for third-party payors, feedback on remittance advice and denials, past-due balances, and collections handled?
Revenue tracking	Work with decision support and financial systems to generate monthly net revenue statements.
	Prepare monthly revenue reports that show net revenue after expense.
Business planning	Monitor net revenue per test compared to sales projections.
	Track progress and revise financial projection-based data.
	Revise the financial pro forma for the 3-year business plan quarterly.
	Work with finance to prepare a return on investment that rolls the outreach program revenues up into the laboratory operational budget.

- *Discounting strategies*
  - *Cash discounts* are reductions in the list price that are given in return for prompt payment of a bill. Such discounts are legal provided they are offered to all customers on the same terms.
  - *Quantity (volume) discounts* are reductions in price based on volume purchases and may be a one-time transaction or a cumulative volume discount. Laboratories may give accounts higher discounts on certain high-volume tests and offer a standard percentage discount referred to as an across-the-board discount for all other test procedures ordered on a monthly basis.
  - *Nondiscountable prices* are usually established for tests that are not performed by the laboratory directly but are sent to a reference lab. Esoteric testing may also be nondiscountable, as start-up costs and initial production costs are higher and the profit margin is lower than for the typical high-volume, routine tests. This strategy, referred to as stratified pricing, targets certain procedures as carve outs or exclusions from the rate negotiations with insurers. Pricing is stratified according to the test description or service line (for example, surgical and cyto-pathology, molecular diagnostics and cytogenetic testing), based on cost and technical expertise.
- *Rate negotiation strategies for third-party insurers.* Rate negotiation with insurers in most hospitals for inpatient, outpatient, and managed-care patient reimbursements is generally conducted by the hospital administrative contract or managed-care department. The contract fees may be a combination of prospective payments (paid on a per-day or per-case basis), fee-for-service payments (billed after the service), or capitation (a fixed fee or rate per member per month). Test utilization information on the patient population is critical in negotiating an equitable agreement that includes a stop-loss threshold for overutilization.
- *Market positioning strategies.* Low option pricing maximizes the sales effort and is used when the goal is to gain market share from the competition or when trying to penetrate a new territory. It is sometimes referred to as marginal pricing.
- *Defensive pricing to maintain market share.* Defensive pricing is a low option pricing strategy used to maintain market share and defend against the competitors pricing strategy. It is not always necessary to match the competition's lowest price when the customer is loyal and agrees that using the hospital laboratory service has a value-added benefit.
- *Value-added pricing.* Value-added pricing is a high option pricing strategy used whenever value-added product or service differentiation from the competition is demonstrated (20).

Promotional (Marketing and Sales) Strategies

Market Research

Companies utilize market research to identify product or service needs in new and existing markets. The inside-out approach develops the product first and then identifies the market. The method employed most frequently is the outside-in (or market pull) approach, which identifies the needs in the marketplace first and then develops the product or service to meet the need. Primary sources for market research include customers, manufacturers, competitors, and consultants who are familiar with the market. Secondary sources are from a literature search. Three techniques typically used to obtain primary market information are mail surveys, telephone surveys (telemarketing), and personal interviews. Direct observation is the fastest and most reliable means of doing market research. Gathering accurate, up-to-date information on the competition is best accomplished on a daily basis while making sales calls. Effective sales representatives routinely take note of the office procedures, hours of operation, type of practice and medical school affiliations. They collect examples of competitors' literature and request slips. The sales team must always be aware of the competitive activities at the local, regional, and national levels. Customers and prospects will provide most of the market intelligence needed. Competitive information and literature should be reported and filed in a central repository in the laboratory's marketing office.

Before entering a new market, it should be standard practice to perform a market survey asking a few specific questions about the customer, the customer's laboratory needs, and the competition. Knowledge about a prospect or a market segment increases your success rate in developing interest in laboratory services. Market surveys can be performed using a written questionnaire that is mailed with return postage. The response rate for this approach generally is around 5%. It is best to have the sales representative make an appointment to survey the office on-site. Telemarketing can also be incorporated into the duties of the client service group. This response rate is improved to an estimated 20% if your team has the time to dedicate to this activity. The newly acquired market information is used in conjunction with knowledge about finance and the other environmental factors to develop sound marketing strategies (11).

Marketing Strategies

Performing a market assessment ensures that the revenue projections and sales forecasts are realistic. Each of the following factors should be considered:

- *Market demographics.* The statistics related to the size of the market within the geographic boundaries served are called demographics. Population statistics can be obtained by contacting the bureau of census in the state or county. Frequently, the healthcare facility's managed-care department has these population and geographic data readily available. The healthcare system utilizes data from the decision support systems to generate useful information related to patient and third-party payor mix and relevant reimbursement rates for both inpatient and outpatient procedures. Healthcare systems can extract the detailed laboratory revenue reports necessary to make sound business decisions.

- *Provider base.* The market assessment should also include a thorough knowledge of the total number and distribution of healthcare providers by specialty in the market. Traditionally, the physician has been the gatekeeper to most medical services, including laboratory testing. Even though the trend is toward sharing the responsibility with the payor, doctors will always play a significant role in the determination of preventative health appraisals and medically necessary testing.

- *Employer base.* The market assessment should research the major Fortune 500 companies in the defined service area. Fortune 500 companies are considered to be the largest, most profitable, and most powerful companies in America. Commonly referred to as the "blue chips," they represent vast holdings and revenues in the billions and include firms like Exxon, General Electric, and Philip Morris. Employers purchase healthcare for their employees as a form of compensation, to enhance wellness, and to increase productivity on the job. Surveying the employer's need for executive physicals, preemployment health assessments, drug screening, and insurance benefit packages for their employees is useful in developing strategies for the industrial market segment, as well as for understanding how many employees in the service area are tied to capitated managed-care contracts. With the escalating costs of healthcare, employers are searching for ways to reduce expenditures for healthcare. In late 1996, commercial laboratories introduced new programs that allowed employers to provide maximum benefit coverage for contracted outpatient and nonemergency laboratory services when the company's employees sought the laboratory testing at the contracted commercial laboratory directly. Direct contracting offers increased net revenue to the commercial laboratory, bypassing the major health plans that realize margins from squeezing down laboratory reimbursements.

- *Insurer base.* Traditional indemnity companies, third-party administrators, and managed-care organizations offer a variety of programs to employers and private individuals for healthcare coverage. Obtaining a working knowledge of the terms and conditions related to insurance coverage will aid the laboratory in surveying the needs of the insurer for contracting with a community-based provider. Increasingly third-party payors, including federally funded programs, continue to move toward global reimbursements, like diagnosis-related groups for hospital inpatients, consolidated billing for skilled-nursing facilities (SNFs), and composite rates for end-stage renal disease patients.

- *Access to laboratory services.* Develop a marketing strategy that includes convenient access to laboratory service through strategic placement of patient service centers in the service area.

- *Laboratory infrastructure.* Assess the production and service needs in terms of equipment and human resources.

Out-of-pocket expenses. As employers and insurers negotiate benefit packages, the beneficiary's copays, noncovered services, and utilization limitations are increasing. Medical-necessity guidelines shift the responsibility for payment of noncovered services to the beneficiary. The number of underinsured Americans continues to rise. Over time, more patients will not be able to pay their medical bills and write-offs will increase. The downward trends in insurance reimbursement will force reductions in the unit cost of laboratory services in order for the laboratory to remain profitable (34).

Decision makers and their buying preferences. Providers have multiple options for choosing a laboratory. Physicians are the constant targets of high-powered sales representatives from regional and national commercial laboratories offering features and benefits that enhance their basic laboratory services. Customers base the decision to use a particular laboratory on a combination of the following factors:

- Professional relationship with a local representative
- Scope of services offered
- Convenient and consistent level of service
- Reputation of the laboratory
- Personal or professional attachment to an academic institution laboratory
- Price

Customers are not motivated to switch laboratories because they desire the product or service. The decision to change either eliminates a problem or is perceived to have a value-added benefit compared to the competitor. Identifying the prospect's "hot-button" or buying motivators is a necessary step for closing the sale. Table 3.6 includes the more typical motivators encountered.

Differentiated marketing strategies. Companies that produce numerous separate and distinct products and services directed at different market segments develop differentiated marketing strategies. The objective is to match a specific product or service to the customer's needs. Costs to serve multiple market segments are typically greater than those for serving a single market segment due to

Table 3.6 Buying motivators (hot buttons)

TAT (turnaround time)

Courier service (7 days per week)

Convenient access to technical support (client services, pathology consultation)

Educational support

Quality assurance support

Computer and telecommunication support

Full scope of services (patient service centers, clinical and anatomic pathology)

Price

---

higher production costs, increased space needs, expanded record keeping, and promotion. Product or service acceptance occurs in a series of steps.

1. The consumer is aware of the product but has little information about its utility.
2. When his or her interest is piqued, the consumer seeks more information.
3. The consumer evaluates the product.
4. The consumer makes a trial purchase or agrees to use of the product.
5. If the trial proves satisfactory, then the consumer decides to continue to purchase the product.

Concentrated marketing strategies. Concentrated marketing strategies are used when companies focus their efforts on servicing a single niche market segment. This strategy is self-limiting, and companies may end up in financial difficulty when buying preferences change to a competitive product (9).

Assess laboratory market potential and estimate market revenue. The best market estimates are based on historical and competitive price data. If the customer will share the information, then you can accurately assess the potential profitability of the new business opportunity. If this information is not available, there are several established models for estimating the market:

- *Population model.* The population model will provide an estimate of the gross revenue potential in a geographic area. Calculate the anticipated outpatient gross revenue for a new geographic service area by multiplying the current gross revenue per capita by the population of the prospective market.

  Calculated gross revenue = (current gross revenue per capita) (population in proposed new service area)

  The flaw in this formula is the assumption that the economic, political, reimbursement, and competitive conditions are similar in both markets.

- *Test mix model.* Most clients order a standard battery of tests on their patients. Laboratories that monitor the average number of tests ordered per requisition report an average of 2.5 to 3.0 tests per requisition. To calculate the average reimbursement per test, laboratories should divide the total reimbursement for the outpatient book of business by the total number of outpatient billed tests. The outpatient market typically operates 5 days per week, which averages 22 business days per month.

  Calculated reimbursement per month = (average number of requisitions per day) (average number of tests per requisition) (average reimbursement per test) (22)

- *Practice type model.* The practice type model requires estimates of revenue from similar practices (both by specialty and by number of physicians). For example,

  Calculated reimbursement per month) = (average reimbursement per physician) (number of physicians)

  This formula can be used to build estimated-revenue models for each physician specialty based on actual reimbursement experiences.

- *Hospital model.* Hospital revenue models can be formulated using existing hospital clients with similar characteristics, like number of beds, urban or rural setting, and general, specialty, or tertiary services. Other factors that have an impact on the accuracy of these models are the inpatient-outpatient mix and the actual referral test menu. The focus for hospital prospects must be on those clients whose test mix meets the laboratory's targeted tests where excess capacity exists.

  Calculated reimbursement per month = (average daily census of prospective hospital) (average laboratory reimbursement per patient day) (30)

Targeted market segments and prospecting. Resources that are useful in preparing prospect lists are local telephone directories and the yellow pages, state and local medical society directories, the American Hospital Association listing by state, nursing home directories by state, managed-care provider lists, the Clinical Laboratory Management Association directory, and classified and other advertisements for new office locations or physicians joining practices in local newspapers as shown in Table 3.7.

Recruiting the laboratory sales team. One of the keys to a successful hospital outreach program is selecting the best candidates for your marketing and sales representatives. Successful salespeople are self-motivated, self-confident individuals who always seem to maintain a positive attitude. Their enthusiasm is contagious. Customers can sense when a salesperson is sincere and genuinely believes in their services. Salespeople must be thick-skinned and very persistent. The customer's first encounter with a sales representative is crucial. The first impression must be a good one. Sales rep-

Table 3.7 Target market segments for clinical laboratories

Market segment	Specific type
Hospitals	Academic
	Affiliated
	Community
	Rural
Independent laboratories and physician office labs	Niche business specialty laboratories (drug testing and pharmaceutical)
	Group practices (family practice and internal medicine)
Physician offices	Family physicians
	Internal medicine specialties
	Obstetrics and gynecology
	Pediatrics
	Surgical specialties
	Dermatologists
Nursing homes	SNFs (skilled-nursing facilities)
	Intermediate-care facilities
	Assisted-living facilities
	Home health agencies
Public sector (federal, state, and local governments)	Veterans Administration Medical Centers
	State and local mental health facilities
	Prisons
	Health departments
Clinical trials	Phase I–IV trials, pharmaceutical companies, investigator, independent research
Industrial	Preemployment, employee health services, health fairs
Other	Veterinarians, chiropractors, podiatrists, dentists

resentatives must look and act like professionals whenever in the presence of current and prospective customers. Product knowledge is essential when trying to close a sale. Sales representatives must know the features and benefits of each of the services being offered by the laboratory in order to handle indifference or objections from the customer.

Sales forecasting. The process of measuring sales success actually begins with the department's administrative strategic planning goals and objectives. Combined with the marketing team's strategies, revenue projections, target markets, and prospect lists are the metrics used to measure the laboratory's success.

The Rule of 78 is a formula used in forecasting revenue based on the premise that a new account sold in the first month of the fiscal year will add revenue for 12 months, while an account sold in the second month will only add revenue for 11 months, and so on.

The sum of $12 + 11 + 10 + 9 + 8 + 7 + 6 + 5 + 4 + 3 + 2 + 1$ is 78.

The Rule of 78 assigns weighted values to each month during the fiscal year (Table 3.8).

Sales incentives. Many studies have shown that outreach programs operating from regional or hospital-based facilities select seasoned sales representatives who have exceptional skills in developing rapport with customers and for

forming a stable long-term relationship while acting as a laboratory consultant. Most often these sales representatives are offered a base salary in line with other laboratory management staff with little in terms of incentives or commissions. Incentives, commissions, and bonuses reward people for productivity. The decision to offer bonuses and incentives must be weighed carefully. If everyone on staff who is asked to improve productivity is not included in the incentive process, it can be detrimental to employee morale throughout the entire laboratory operation.

Territory management. Sales representatives are extremely competitive. Establishing territory boundaries allows the laboratory to manage the sales effort from a team approach. Sales territory assignments can be defined using several techniques:

- *Geography.* A sales territory can be defined by using geographic boundaries specific to county or city lines or by using the postal service zip code boundaries.

- *Account type.* Another method of defining territories is by account type. For example, individual representatives can focus on specific strategies to bring on family practices or internal medicine or obstetric practices.

- *Market segment.* Focusing on the special needs for each market segment offers another option for sales representatives to become experts in areas of hospital reference testing, physician office testing, clinical trials, in-

Table 3.8 Rule of 78[a]

Experience level of sales representative	Revenue/month												
	Jan.	Feb.	Mar.	Apr.	May	Jun.	Jul.	Aug.	Sept.	Oct.	Nov.	Dec.	Total
New, with sales quota (net revenue) of $3,500/month	$3,500	$7,000	$10,500	$14,000	$17,500	$21,000	$24,500	$28,000	$31,500	$35,000	$38,500	$42,000	$273,000
Experienced with sales quota (net revenue) of $5,000/month	$5,000	$10,000	$15,000	$20,000	$25,000	$30,000	$35,000	$40,000	$45,000	$50,000	$55,000	$60,000	$390,000
Total sales revenue	$8,500	$17,000	$25,500	$34,000	$42,500	$51,000	$59,500	$68,000	$76,500	$85,000	$93,500	$102,000	$663,000

[a]This formula is based on the premise that when a new account is sold in the first month of the fiscal year, it will add revenue for 12 months. An account that is brought on board in the second month will only add revenue for 11 months and so on. 12 + 11 + 10 + 9 + 8 + 7 + 6 + 5 + 4 + 3 + 2 + 1 = 78.

fectious diseases, long-term care facilities, substance abuse testing, and public-sector contracting.

- *Combination.* Some laboratories ask the representative to create a detailed prospect list from the laboratory's service area each quarter. The representatives use the prospect list to make their daily call plan. If a prospect is not closed within 90 days, another representative can then add the targeted account to his or her prospect list for the next quarter.

Sales Strategies

Sales strategies are used to position the company and product before the sale begins. The key to a successful sales strategy is to identify prospective customers who are not satisfied with their present product or service. Long-term sales goals are focused on account cultivation and retention by developing a "customer for life" relationship with the accounts. Short-term sales goals include identifying and closing as many deals as possible.

Sales planning. Successful salespersons use a combination of preparation, planning, and just plain luck to place themselves in the right place at the right time. The sales plan should include some flexibility in order to take advantage of unanticipated opportunities as they present themselves. Sales objectives can be adjusted for a sudden change in competitive activity. Identifying changes in the environment and ranking their relevance assist sales representatives in defining the sales objective for the call. Effective representatives constantly evaluate the laboratory's position in order to reposition the product or service based on need and perception. Thorough planning enables sales representatives to concentrate the call activity within a small geographic area, avoiding excess travel time. Making appointments is the most efficient way to plan a day working in the field. Good time and territory management is vital for the success of the salesperson. As the adage goes, plan your work, and work your plan. Daily activities should be prioritized, making it possible for the salesperson to always act with a sense of urgency. Maintaining a daily call itinerary that lists each prospective call to be made, including updates and reminders from a tickler file, allows the representative to function more effectively and provide timely follow-up with prospective customers. Hugh Gouldthorpe, Jr., vice president of Owens and Minor, a Fortune 500 medical supply company, and a master of customer service strategies, reminds his world-class organization to "DWYPYWD," which simply translates to "Do what you promised you would do."

Sales techniques and strategies. A number of different sales techniques and strategies are seen below:

1. *Precall strategy.* Sales representatives, much like a teacher preparing a lesson plan, should prepare for their calls in advance (Table 3.9). The customer's first encounter

Table 3.9 Steps of call preparation and rehearsal

1. Identify the needs of the prospect, short term and long term.
2. How do the customer's needs relate to the perceived needs?
3. List the distinctive features of the laboratory services that meet these needs.
4. How are these needs currently being met?
5. Identify the testing area with the greatest opportunity for new or increased business.
6. Is the prospective customer knowledgeable about the hospital laboratory service?
7. Evaluate ahead of time the degree of indifference the customer may have to the laboratory services.
8. List the specific benefits that the prospect may be skeptical about.
9. Gather appropriate proof sources to handle the anticipated indifferences and skepticism.
10. Think through the process to handle objections due to misunderstandings or perceived drawbacks to the services.
11. Plan your tactics to identify the decision maker.
12. List the objectives for each call before you begin.

with a sales representative is crucial. First impressions are lasting and must be good. Sales representatives must look and act like professionals whenever in the presence of current and prospective customers.

2. *Cold calling.* Even after an exhausting planning process, most prospecting takes place by knocking on doors, making the often dreaded and first-time, face-to-face, cold call (see Table 3.10).

3. *Making the sales call.* Sales representatives should always present a positive impression. They build rapport by showing interest and enthusiasm in the client. As salespersons gain experience, they learn to pace the rhythm of the call.

4. *Sales techniques* are the tactics or actions used during the sales call to deal with customer attitudes of

Table 3.10 The cold call: information gathering

Customer type (hospital, physician, nursing home)
Customer demographic information (number of beds, number of physicians, number of patients)
Gather office staff member business cards.
Develop key contacts.
Identify office billing system and procedures.
Third-party payor mix
Commercial laboratory pricing arrangements
Number of patients per day with laboratory orders
Most frequently ordered test menu
Identify the decision maker.
Gather information about the competition.
Understand office logistics and service needs.
Reporting and telecommunication system
Ask what else they need, or what they would change.
Take notes.
Schedule a follow-up appointment to present a proposal.

indifference and skepticism and to handle objections. **Features** are characteristics of your product or service. **Benefits** are the value the features bring to the customer. One must listen actively and courteously to identify key points and perceived drawbacks. Use simple **probing** with prospective customers to clarify their objections. Always restate the features and benefits of the product or service being promoted that support the customer need or that counter a misunderstanding and ultimately resolve the concerns identified. Since most customers generally think they are satisfied, they aren't aware of a better product or service. Creativity is usually necessary. Good salespeople identify a need or dissatisfaction. Then, they convert the need into a potential problem in the customer's mind. Next, they create a desire to have the problem solved, which leads to introducing a feature of the laboratory service that will satisfy the need and bring a benefit to the customer. Make sure the customer agrees that the stated benefit solves a need or problem, and then ask for the business. Over time the experienced sales representative is recognized as a laboratory consultant and a partner in providing quality healthcare and gains added respect from the client for his or her professional and capable contributions (25, 49).

5. *Opening.* After making the initial introduction, always thank the customer for the opportunity to meet with him or her. Asking about the customer's operation and needs for a reference laboratory helps break the ice. A sales call should begin by using an initial feature or benefit statement about the laboratory service that supports a specific customer need.

6. *Postcall evaluation.* The key to success is getting in to see the decision maker.

- Unless the representative is sitting face-to-face with a prospect, the representative's selling skills, product knowledge, and enthusiasm have very little relevance.
- Unless the sales call includes spending time with the decision maker or someone who can influence the decision, a sales representative is probably wasting valuable time.

7. *Close/trial close.* After the customer acknowledges product approval and is in agreement, ask for a commitment to use the product or service. To close a sale, the sales representative summarizes the benefits and outlines a plan to initiate using the product or service. The following actions by a prospective customer indicate a commitment:

- Agrees to have a presentation or in-service training program for the office,
- Accepts an invitation to take the staff on a facility tour, or

- Authorizes an appointment with the office manager to gather or discuss billing details.

8. *Call/close ratio.* Many companies with an aggressive sales operation expect sales representatives to make a minimum of eight calls per day, or an average of one productive call per hour. Making 35 to 40 sales calls a week, or at least 200 calls per month, provides adequate interaction to close three or four accounts by month's end, another three or four accounts within 2 months, and three or four accounts within 3 months. Maintaining the momentum of the selling cycle requires that the sales representative adhere to a regular sales schedule. One of the most important characteristics of a successful sales representative's style is persistence, as is demonstrated in the statistics that follow:

- Eighty percent of all closes are made during the fifth call on a prospect
- Fifty percent of sales representatives quit after one call
- Twenty-five percent more quit after two calls
- Ten percent more quit after three calls
- The 20% that keep selling close 80% of their prospects and bring in the most revenue.

Decision makers. A key element in the development of sales strategies is the ability to identify the relevant players. Strategic selling concentrates on the things that remain constant from one customer to another. A complex sale is one that requires more than one signature to authorize approval or involves more than one decision maker. In the corporate business world, each sale is complex and has four distinct buying influencers who must be identified early in the sales process. The "user" buying influencer is primarily concerned about the reliability of the product or service. The "technical" buying influencer acts as the gatekeeper and is responsible for measuring the value of the product or service. The "economic" buying influencer is the one person who gives the critical, final approval to the sale, is usually the most difficult to identify, and is typically very difficult to convince. The fourth buying influencer is a champion or "coach," an experienced, trustworthy person from either the purchaser or seller's organization who assists, guides, and directs the salesman through the difficult sale. Maintain written records of the decision makers and buying influencers for each customer, remembering that the names and faces change periodically along with the hats that they may wear (31).

Advertising Strategies

Products and services are identified through the use of brand names, symbols, logos, and distinctive packaging. A brand is a name, term, sign, symbol, design, or some combination thereof to differentiate a firm from the competition.

A trademark is a brand that has received legal protection for the exclusive use of the sole owner. Brands vary widely in consumer familiarity and acceptance. Brand acceptance goes through three stages of development: (i) recognition, (ii) preference, and (iii) insistence. Establishing a product or service that reaches brand insistence is the goal of every company . . . to be the healthcare provider of choice (10)

Building a reputation and image for the laboratory outreach program depends on the laboratory operation and the healthcare facility as an enterprise. Communicating with the marketing director or public relations coordinator in hospital administration is essential. There are usually policies related to the use of a hospital logo in conjunction with other printed materials. It is important to link the program to the organization from a branding perspective. Successful marketing and sales strategies depend on having printed publications that clearly identify the laboratory services. In developing a needs assessment for the marketing and sales program, laboratories must allocate sufficient funds for publications and advertising costs to ensure that the sales effort has the tools necessary to meet revenue projections (Table 3.11).

Customer-Focused Concepts and Service Strategies

Who is the Customer?

Customer satisfaction is the critical strategic weapon for every organization. The laboratory must treat each customer as a valuable and irreplaceable resource. World-class customer service organizations are successful because they are able to consistently exceed the customer's expectations. Their primary strategic and structural focus on the external customer includes rewards, recognition, and promotion and treats the customer like a king (27). Table 3.12 defines "who is the customer."

Understanding Customer Behavior

Customer behavior results from personal preferences and pressures exerted from forces in the outside environment. A customer is not motivated to act unless there is an unsatisfied need for a product or service. Selling is the process of uncovering and satisfying customer needs. Identifying an area of dissatisfaction with a competitive product or service becomes an opportunity. The manner in which products and services are presented influences customer perception.

Once customers form an opinion, they become indifferent or skeptical. If they have an objection or attitude about a product, effecting a change is difficult (Table 3.13). When this happens, the product and service strategies must be modified in one of two ways:

- Change the product or service to more closely match customer opinion or to overcome the basic objections.

Table 3.11 Marketing publication and advertising needs

Marketing tool	Needs associated with marketing tool
Publications	Directory of services—test procedure manuals
	Fee schedules
	Requisitions
	Supply order forms
	Procedure updates
	Telephone result pads
	Confidential-result envelopes
	Letterhead, envelopes, stamps
Advertising	Business cards
	Tabletop displays and exhibits
	Allocate costs to exhibit by number of conventions.
	Yellow pages
	Specimen lock boxes
	Promotional giveaway items
	Entertainment
	Holiday greetings, laboratory week recognition

Table 3.12 Who is the customer?[a]

A customer is the most important person in any business.

A customer is not dependent on us. We are dependent on them.

A customer is not an interruption of our work. They are the purpose of our work.

A customer does us a favor when they call. We are not doing them a favor by serving them.

A customer is not a cold statistic. They are human beings with feelings and emotions like our own.

A customer is not someone with whom to argue or match wits.

A customer is a person with needs. It is up to us to meet their needs.

A customer is deserving of the most courteous and attentive treatment we can give them.

A customer is the person that makes it possible to pay our salaries.

A customer is the life blood of this and every other business.

[a]See reference 26.

Table 3.13 Customer attitudes[a]

Customer acceptance occurs when a feature or benefit of the product or service is received with general approval or agreement.

Skeptical customers question or doubt that the product or service will satisfy their need. Providing a reference source or a demonstration offers proof of the benefits.

Indifferent customers display a lack of interest in the product when they do not perceive a need or when they are satisfied with a competitive product or an internal service. Seek first to understand the customer's attitude by using probing techniques.

Objectionable customers relay some degree of dissatisfaction, lack of trust, or dislike of the product or service based on perceptions. Misunderstandings occur when customers lack enough information about the product or service to make a decision. Whenever a misunderstanding cannot be clarified it becomes a drawback to the sale. It is critical that the drawback be reduced to the minimum by restating other features that offer benefits to the customer.

[a]See references 25 and 49.

- Attempt to change customer attitudes and opinions about the product or service.

Key Concepts and Recognized Customer Service Strategies

There is a quality revolution emerging in the service industry. Keeping customers satisfied takes a real commitment from management. During the 1980s companies learned that quality does not improve unless you can measure it. Quality became more than a slogan; it was recognized as the most profitable way to run a business. The following concepts and strategies represent various approaches to customer service used by many blue-chip market leaders.

Zero defections. Losing a customer over quality or service issues carries a high cost. Lost business impacts a company's profitability more than unit costs and market share. Performing defection analysis is the process of gathering feedback from defecting customers and acting on the information to reengineer the products and services. Typically companies lose 15 to 20% of their customer base annually. By striving for zero defections (keeping every customer the company can serve and empowering the organization to achieve it), companies can document double the average growth rate and increased profits from their loyal customers for each year that they stay. After all, loyal customers are the best form of advertisement and new customer referrals. However, the goal of achieving service quality does not mean retaining customers at all costs. Focus on retaining the most profitable customers; then, manage for zero defections. There are some customers you may not want to serve. The quality of the laboratory's customer is more important than the quantity of customers (40).

New customer development carries a price tag. Profitability is directly impacted by customer retention. Bringing on new business is more costly than maintaining a current customer. Customer loyalty is the main driver of revenue growth. Satisfied clients are easier to up-sell on new products and services and are more likely to generate referrals. Companies find that the Pareto Principle has application to customers and revenue. The top 20% of a company's customer base typically represents 80% of the revenue generated. Cultivating relationships with these customers, who are often referred to as "cash cows" in the marketplace, is invaluable. It is well recognized in the industry that the customers that generate the least revenue and are in the lowest tier of your customer base require the most resources to manage and service, ultimately representing a net loss to the bottom line (46). (Additional information can be found at http://www.quickbooks.com/ [last accessed November 2002].)

Consistently exceed the customer's expectations. Systematic approaches to providing service are 80% of customer service. The key is to create systems that allow the laboratory to do it right the first time every time. Success hinges on having a plan for when things fail. When it comes to service, it is always best to underpromise and then overdeliver. People inherently like doing business with people who keep their word. Customer satisfaction is about exceeding our customers' needs and expectations to the point of "delighting" them (28).

Create customers for life. According to C. Sewell and P. Brown in their book *Customers for Life,* there are 10 basic commandments for successful organizations to empower employees to create a company of service superstars who turn buyers into lifelong customers (41).

- Ask what customers want, and give it to them. If you don't keep your customers happy, someone else will.

- When the customer asks, the answer is always yes, up to a point. Quality customers are more valuable and profitable than business based on customer quantity.

- Do it right the first time every time. Employees are held accountable for their mistakes. Repeating tasks is costly and lowers productivity. Using a systematic approach is 80% of good customer service.

- Keep your promise for service. Simply DWYPYWD: *do what you promised you would do.* When you underpromise and then overdeliver, the customer is delighted.

- Train and empower every employee to be a customer service representative.

- No news is not good news. Encourage the customer to tell you when something is wrong. Be proactive and probe to uncover flaws in the systems.

- Measure everything that is relevant to performance. Set a target. Post the results. People are naturally competitive and will try to exceed whatever goals are set for them. Employees must be able to relate to the indicator being monitored. Typical indicators used are quantity, quality, cost, and timeliness. Just being good is not enough. The goals established must also be congruous with the best interests of the laboratory operation.

- Recognize employee performance. Pay employees like they are business partners.

- Lead by example, offering equal respect to both internal and external customers. If the organization expects employees to be polite to the customers, the employees must be treated courteously.

- Just like the Japanese, organizations should be students of the best customer service companies. Copy them, and then improve on their systems (42).

Creating value. Quality and value are generally measured by the end user of the product or service. Identifying how value is created in a business environment is critical to competitive success. Determining the cost associated with creating, delivering, and maintaining the customer's perceived value and quality becomes fundamental. The more complex processes require more activities and overhead expense for staffing, equipment, information, and communication systems and ultimately increase the possibility for error. Every process in a company eventually affects the external customer's perception about the product or service and determines whether they will make a buying decision. Creating an environment based on pay for performance has never been so important. The manner in which products and services are presented influences customer perception. Value is perceived to be quality divided by price.

There are two types of value:

- Customer-perceived value is the major driver of revenue. There are four drivers (function or utility, convenience, price, and exchange value of competitive products and services) that influence value perception.

- Process value is defined by the relative cost of value-added tasks and services and is influenced by accuracy, speed, consistency, conciseness, and relevance.

Cost/benefit analysis. Performing a cost/benefit analysis to identify the nonessential steps in the process, or process waste, enables companies to control the cost and price of a product or service. Managers must be cautious not to overinvest in technology. The focus should be on eliminating unnecessary work, not just speeding up the process (39). When an entire organization focuses on delivering what the customers really want, companies reduce costs by eliminating the processes that don't add any value to the product.

Relevant, meaningful, and quantifiable information. Customer service is more than a theory. In *Making Customer Service Happen,* Roderick McNealy writes, "By defining it, we can measure it. After measuring it, we can analyze it. If we analyze it, we can control it. If we can control it, we can improve it" (27). To ensure optimal proactive customer satisfaction, avoid taking the reactionary, quick-fix approach to customer complaints. Search out the root cause and eliminate it and the resulting downstream effects at the same time. Moments of truth occur when customers develop an impression or perception about products, services, and the organization through encounters that happen over time. Even though the impressions may have been incorrect, all that matters is the customer's perceptions. Perceptions are real (29). When organizations first uncover the customer's negative impression or perception about their product or service, it becomes a moment of truth.

Service Delivery Strategies

Service delivery strategies encompass the nontechnical operational support services necessary to deliver laboratory services to the customer (for example, courier services, supplies, information services and communications, customer service, specimen accessioning, and billing services).

Logistics and distribution service considerations. Developing a dependable courier network to support the customers' needs is fundamental to the laboratory's success. The service strategy must do or consider each of the following before developing the service:

- Decide whether to utilize in-house couriers or outsource to a contract courier.
- What type of vehicle will meet your needs?
- Evaluate options for capital purchase or lease agreements on vehicles.
- Identify daily and on-call stops based on customer needs, hours, and volume.
- Develop a logistical plan to meet the needs of each customer.
- Calculate the average cost per stop.
- Calculate the impact of adding new customers to a route.
- Review the number of stops, mileage, travel time, and specimen arrival to determine needs for additional vehicles and couriers.
- Include the associated costs of the impact from the recent International Air Transportation Associations regulatory changes for dangerous and infectious goods on specimen transportation decisions, costs of training, and handling. These regulations are discussed in more detail in chapter 5.

Customer supply policies. The support service strategies include the costs of setting up a new account with the supplies necessary for specimen collection, handling, and transportation to the laboratory.

- Establish a standard list of items supplied to customers.
- Develop policies and procedures for placing equipment like centrifuges, printers, and computer interfaces that meet compliance guidelines and are based on measurable parameters, like daily specimen volume.
- Develop a distribution system and supply audit process to monitor service and avoid possible charges of inducement.
- Use the anticipated test volume for clients to calculate the time needed to recoup the start-up expenses.
- Include the expense of providing and training for supplies compliant with the Occupational Safety and Health Administration's regulations for blood-borne pathogen and needle stick safety.

Customer service call center. Implementing a customer service communication center requires a detailed analysis of the phone calls related to service for the entire laboratory operation.

- Track the number and type of calls during each hour to determine the need for a dedicated group to free technical staff for testing.
- Investigate systems that automate data collection and measure call wait time and lost calls.
- Evaluate the skill sets and personnel level needed to handle the inquiries.
- Consider having the group support calls for nonscheduled pickups, quality assurance functions, and printing of custom requests.
- Establish quality assurance monitors, and develop a scorecard to report performance.

Outreach registration and specimen processing and accessioning. In order to sell the laboratory services, it is critical that a directory of laboratory services be available to customers. The directory should be a compendium of the test offerings listing specific information about specimen collection, storage, and transportation. The laboratory's test requisition forms should be easy to read and complete. The ability to customize the client's request forms to include the most frequently ordered tests is important. The request should have ample room and clear instructions for completion of billing information. Clients should be able to easily refer to a current medical-necessity guide and reference manual for tests ordered on patients covered by federally funded programs. The laboratory must also have a plan and process developed once the samples arrive.

- Develop a plan to handle the anticipated increase in specimen volume for each shift.

- Train the processing team annually regarding laboratory compliance and medical-necessity guidelines.
- Make sure that the registration, information, and billing systems can accommodate a short registration pathway for third-party billing to facilitate timely sample accessioning, testing, and reporting.
- Consider moving data entry for billing to the day shift to allow the staff to interact directly with the customer for any missing data elements required for clean claim submission.
- Have a procedure to track specimen handling errors and data entry errors by employee and shift as a quality monitor.

Billing systems and revenue tracking services. Most hospitals lack accounting systems to adequately measure and track cost or net revenue at a per-test level. Success depends on having a clear understanding of the hospital revenue systems and processes, including patient registration, coding requirements and regulations, reimbursement by test and payor, patient accounting system, preprocessor claim scrubbers for the electronic data interface with insurers, and decision support capabilities. Flowcharting the process often uncovers problematic areas that need attention in order to streamline the processes. The need to flowchart the billing process is dependent on the complexity and number of systems used for registration, billing, claim processing, accounts receivable, and decision support. The ability to generate accurate and timely monthly invoices, third-party insurance claim forms, and patient statements is a key component of the laboratory service and is essential to maintaining satisfied customers.

Laboratory information system (LIS) management. Laboratories have become information brokers that provide the majority of the clinical information used by healthcare providers in disease management. In order to create value, the results must be accurate and timely. During the past decade, proficiency testing, continuing-education programs, oversight by accrediting and regulatory agencies, and more sophisticated instrumentation were the change drivers that forced laboratories to exceed the standards for reproducibility and technical accuracy of the past (4).

Result reporting. External customers expect timely results reported to offices via remote printer or facsimile. Include these expenses when calculating new-account start-up costs. Evaluate equipment costs to support remote order entry and online test requests and inquiry. Calculate the impact that the Health Insurance Portability and Accountability Act (HIPAA) security regulations will have on the cost of reporting.

Knowledgeable consumers. According to Christine Diehl with MDS Laboratories, Inc., the world economy has transitioned from the Industrial Age into the Information Age during the recent technological revolution. Healthcare providers rely on laboratory testing to diagnose disease. Randall Spratt, Vice President of Product Planning and Development for Advanced Laboratory Group, a division of HBO & Co., has said that "laboratory data accounts for 60 to 70% of the data in the medical record and that physicians perceive that it accounts for as much as 80% of the diagnostic information they utilize." The laboratory has migrated from providing information about diagnostic detection and treatment to prognostic prediction and prevention (16). Personal computers and the Internet have provided a platform for computer-savvy healthcare providers and patients to communicate and seek information via access to the World Wide Web. E-mail and Internet server access provide means for on-line ordering and result reporting with appropriate security encryptions to ensure that HIPAA privacy regulations are maintained. Healthcare facilities and laboratories now have a mechanism to publish promotional materials and to advertise services by developing user-friendly websites (36).

Create a service delivery report card. Laboratory services are integral to the provision of healthcare. While laboratory test results influence nearly 80% of all treatment decisions, they represent only 3% of the total cost of healthcare. Many stakeholders make purchasing decisions primarily using four key service parameters in the order listed: quality, cost, access, and service. Organizations that align behaviors with goals and values achieve excellence in customer service through being accountable to the customer (19). Laboratories should develop a quality monitor and scoring system to measure and report the effectiveness and utility of these elements for each service line (patient service centers, customer service center, courier services, billing services, and information services). The highly competitive healthcare environment, historically focused on costs, is increasingly being driven by the need for meaningful information in order to make informed decisions. Service report cards have become a standard tool to assist in the negotiation of equitable contracts and demonstrate value to customers (38).

Summary
Survival of the Fittest

In the past the use of the term "healthcare system" to describe the delivery of services was somewhat of an oxymoron, since multiple organizations provided fragmented services while competing for the same customer. The laboratory manager's responsibilities include three categories of resources: physical infrastructure (space and equipment), financial (operating budget), and human resources (technical and support staff). Even though human resources constitute more than half of the operational expenses, focus on the physical and financial responsibilities now demands increasing attention. In the current market, consumers (linked by geography, employer group, or managed-care plan) have increased the demand for cooperation among the stakeholders, setting the stage for the unprecedented wave of consolidations, mergers, acquisitions, and partnerships witnessed in the past decade. Striving to coordinate a patient's episode of care, healthcare is vertically integrating across inpatient and outpatient service lines and from home testing to self-testing. Simultaneously, healthcare is integrating horizontally across communities and regions to achieve these goals (45).

After enjoying several decades of lucrative fee-for-service reimbursements and high-volume testing that supported duplication of services without collaboration among providers, the nation's healthcare system and the clinical laboratory industry were forced to reinvent the approach to providing healthcare. In 1984, government regulations aimed at cutting the escalating costs for federally funded programs paved the way for reimbursement to shift from traditional fee-for-service reimbursement to global reimbursements, like diagnosis-related groups and other prospective payment models. Hospital laboratories, formerly considered revenue centers, became cost centers. They responded to decreasing reimbursements and shifts in volume by using strategic techniques like reengineering, downsizing, rightsizing, consolidation, and regionalization. Following the emergence of managed care, the healthcare industry was forced to seek alternative treatment settings and to shift its focus to health promotion and prevention of disease. Manufacturers and suppliers responded to these environmental factors by introducing new technological advances in products and services to support genetic testing, near-patient testing, home testing, and promotion of direct access testing (14).

Both laboratories and manufacturers have developed new products and services to meet the changing market needs, targeting new markets and focusing on value-added customer service strategies to outperform the competition and to meet and exceed the customer's expectations. During the same period, the Internet developed and became the platform for knowledgeable consumers to access information and demand more value from the services related to their healthcare.

Today, healthcare providers realize that the patient is the client and consumer. They now recognize the importance of including the patient in the development of the care plan and the decision-making process. Ultimately, the greatest opportunity for creating added value in healthcare hinges on the interface between the patient and the caregiver. When technology contributes to the quality of that relationship, it becomes more valuable (3). The laboratory should expect even more significant changes in diagnostic testing in the future as the industry changes its focus to the following:

- Utilization management through elimination of unnecessary testing

- Implementation of practice guidelines and standards of practice
- Continued standardization of instrumentation and methodology
- Increased automation and robotics
- Increased testing in molecular diagnostics, genetics, and proteomics
- Using patient clinical outcome to measure laboratory quality (14)

The increasing importance of access to the most advanced technology must be tempered against the ethical and humane concerns for the use of laboratory information. The efficacy, safety, cost-effectiveness, and clinical outcomes of diagnostic and treatment strategies link utilization of resources and economics (45).

KEY POINTS

- Customers are every organization's most valuable resource.
- Customer satisfaction is the most critical strategic weapon for any organization.
- Customer service is more than a theory.
- Moments of truth occur when customers develop an impression or perception about products, services, and the organization through encounters that happen over time.
- The top 20% of the customers represent 80% of the revenues.
- Laboratory data account for 80% of the diagnostic information utilized by healthcare providers. The clinical utility of laboratory data is migrating from diagnostic detection and treatment to prognostic prediction and prevention.
- While laboratory test results influence nearly 80% of all treatment decisions, they represent only 3% of healthcare costs.

GLOSSARY

Activity-based costing A method being used by some laboratories that assigns a cost to every activity throughout the organization.

Benefit The value a feature of the product or service brings to the customer.

Brand A name, term, sign, symbol (logo), design, or combination used to identify and differentiate the products of one firm from the competition.

Capital budgeting The process of planning for the expenditures expected to generate income to flow into the organization.

Clinical utility Economists refer to the ability to satisfy needs as utility. In medicine, it is more commonly referred to as clinical utility.

Community health information network A network formed among community healthcare providers and insurers to maintain healthcare information for patient management purposes.

Competitive bidding The process used by buyers to request price quotations from suppliers to get the best product and service at the lowest price.

Complex sale A complex sale is one that requires more than one signature/authorization for approval or more than one decision maker.

Creeping inflation A pricing strategy that uses modest price increases over time that are typically not noticeable to the consumer.

Demand The relationship between the price and the quantity needed for a particular product or service. Demand is the quantity of goods that the customers are willing to buy at a given price.

Diminishing return When additional volume reaches a point that instruments and people are performing at their maximum throughput, the operational efficiency achieved by economy of scale begins to decline. An infinite number of tests cannot be performed in a finite amount of time and space without ultimately reaching the point of diminishing return.

Direct observation A marketing research technique that yields the fastest and most reliable information about the prospective market segments, customer base, and competition.

Due diligence A confidentiality agreement exercised between two competing businesses during discussions related to partnership and joint ventures.

DWYPYWD A customer service phrase: do what you promised you would do.

Economy of scale Whenever output is increased without increasing the cost of production, economy of scale is achieved.

Feature Characteristic of your product or service that adds value or benefit to the end user.

Fiscal polices Use of taxation and government spending as a means of controlling the economy.

General rule of supply The production of a good or service increases when the price goes up and decreases when the price goes down.

Global economy In a global economy, businesses are forced to shift from being multinational (a national company with foreign subsidiaries) to being transnational (where there is one economic unit, the world).

Gross revenue Gross revenue is derived by multiplying the volume or quantity of services used by the unit price for the service. Gross revenue is the actual billed charges or fees for products and services before applying any adjustment for contractual arrangements for volume discounts, third-party limits of allowance, or direct and indirect expenses.

Independent provider association An independent association of multiple healthcare providers organized to negotiate contracts with an insurer for the provision of healthcare services within a specified service area at a negotiated cap rate or fee schedule.

Inflation Inflation is the result of increases in the price of goods that reduce the consumer's purchasing power.

Inside-out approach A product development strategy in which the product is developed first and then the market is identified.

Integrated delivery system A system that is formed when payors and healthcare providers (including acute-care providers, physicians, home healthcare agencies, nursing homes, primary care offices, and others) combine forces to extend their service lines to improve the coordination and quality of care while controlling costs.

Joint venture Term used to describe management agreements, partnerships, strategic laboratory arrangements, or conglomerates formed to share risk or expertise.

Law of demand As the price for a product or service increases, the demand for the product decreases.

Length of stay Statistical measure of time used to describe the length of a hospital inpatient stay from admission to discharge.

Macroeconomics Macroeconomics examines the interaction of income, employment, and inflation on the economy as a whole.

Managed-care organization An organization formed by a third-party insurer as an alternative healthcare delivery system in an attempt to control the escalating costs of healthcare to large employer groups and the government.

Market potential The total anticipated revenue potential for volume of services during a defined period.

Market price The actual price at which a commodity is commonly purchased.

Market research A marketing strategy utilized by companies to identify the need for new products and services in new and existing markets.

Market share The estimate of the expected share of the specific market or territory that you expect to capture.

Market surveys Techniques typically used to obtain valuable market information, for example, direct-mail surveys, telephone surveys (telemarketing), and personal interviews.

Microeconomics Economic information that focuses on individual behavior and the interaction of companies.

Moment of truth The moment when a business recognizes that the customer has developed an impression or perception about their products and services and the organization through encounters that happen over time.

Monetary policies Policies related to the management of the money supply and the market rates of interest.

Net revenue Gross revenue minus contractual allowances and sales discounts is net revenue.

Outside-in approach A frequently utilized product development method that first identifies a need in the marketplace and then develops the product or service to meet the need.

Pareto Principle (Law) A total quality management principle used by W. Edwards Deming that demonstrates that cause and effect are not linearly related; for example, approximately 20% of the causes account for 80% of the effect (44).

Patient service centers Phlebotomy sites or draw stations located off-site in service areas convenient to medical office buildings are referred to as patient service centers. The employees are often cross trained to offer a variety of services, including electrocardiograms and chain-of-custody drug abuse screening collections for private industry.

Physician hospital organization An organization formed by hospitals and physicians to negotiate managed-care contracts with third-party payors.

Physician office laboratory A clinical laboratory operation located on-site in a healthcare provider's office. The testing performed by a physician office laboratory is regulated by the Clinical Laboratory Improvements Amendment and is limited to waived, moderate, or complex test services.

Point-of-care testing (POCT) An industry term used to describe user-friendly instrumentation developed for use in near-patient testing or bedside testing sites versus traditional laboratory sites.

Probing A sales technique used to gather information and uncover customer needs. An open probe asks a direct question, while a closed probe limits a customer's answers to yes or no and helps to confirm a need.

Profit Earnings above the expenditures for salaries, benefits, and direct and indirect costs.

Promotion The function of informing, persuading, or otherwise influencing the consumer's buying decision.

Return on investment The tangible and intangible returns received from an investment, minus the fixed, variable, and capital expenditures for the venture.

Rule of 78 A formula used in sales projections based on the premise that a new account sold in the first month of the fiscal year will add revenue for 12 months, while an account brought on board in the second month will only add revenue for 11 months, and so on. The sum of $12 + 11 + 10 + 9 + 8 + 7 + 6 + 5 + 4 + 3 + 2 + 1$ is 78.

Strategic alliance/partnership An arrangement that enables companies to combine their resources to share risks, reduce cost, and solidify customer and supplier relationships.

Strategy The technique, approach, or mechanics developed by the management team in order to facilitate the organization's ability to perform successfully.

Supply The quantity of goods and services that a company is willing to produce and sell at a specific price.

SWOT analysis An assessment of the strengths, weaknesses, opportunities, and threats for an organization, taking the market and the competition into account. See chapter 2 for a detailed description.

Telemarketing A market research technique employed by representatives using a predefined list of questions to gather vital information on the market potential. The survey, conducted by telephone, is directed to a specific staff member in a prospect's office.

Third-party administrator An unrelated third-party entity that administers and pays claims for multiple small insurers in a geographic region.

Trademark A brand that has received legal protection for the exclusive use of the sole owner.

Utility The satisfaction derived from using a product or service.

Zero defections A customer service strategy that strives for no lost customers, or zero defections. The goal is to keep every customer the company can serve, and this strategy empowers the organization to achieve the goal.

REFERENCES

1. Aaron, H. E. 1995. Physician practice mergers: part I. The merger process. *Va. Med. Q.* **122:**194–197.

2. Barker, R. F. 1971. Are profits and social concern incompatible? *Pittsburgh Bus. Rev.* **1971:**2.

3. Beckham, J. D. 2001. What to watch for in the next three years as Internet transforms the healthcare landscape. *Clin. Leadersh. Manag. Rev.* **15:**107–113.

4. Beckwith, D. G., and B. Rokus. 1997. Creating win-win partnerships. *Adv. Admin. Lab.* **6(8):** 64–71.

5. Boone, L., and D. Kurtz. 1977. The economic environment, p. 29. *In* P. Kotler and P. E. Green (ed.), *Contemporary Marketing,* 2nd ed. The Dryden Press, Hinsdale, Ill.

6. Boone, L., and D. Kurtz. 1977. The marketing process: an overview, p. 19. *In* P. Kotler and P. E. Green (ed.), *Contemporary Marketing,* 2nd ed. The Dryden Press, Hinsdale, Ill.

7. Boone, L., and D. Kurtz. 1977. The marketing process, p. 6. *In* P. Kotler and P. E. Green (ed.), *Contemporary Marketing,* 2nd ed. The Dryden Press, Hinsdale, Ill.

8. Boone, L., and D. Kurtz. 1977. The economic environment, p. 47–48. *In* P. Kotler and P. E. Green (ed.), *Contemporary Marketing,* 2nd ed. The Dryden Press, Hinsdale, Ill.

9. Boone, L., and D. Kurtz. 1977. The elements of product strategy, p. 202–205. *In* P. Kotler and P. E. Green (ed.), *Contemporary Marketing,* 2nd ed. The Dryden Press, Hinsdale, Ill.

10. Boone, L., and D. Kurtz. 1977. The elements of product strategy, p. 221–225. *In* P. Kotler and P. E. Green (ed.), *Contemporary Marketing,* 2nd ed. The Dryden Press, Hinsdale, Ill.

11. Bregman, M., and R. Greene. 1980. You and your job. Careers in industrial marketing research. *Chem. Eng.* **12:**61–63.

12. Butros, F. 1997. The manager's financial handbook, laboratory administration-capital budgeting. *Clin. Lab. Manag. Rev.* **11:**410–411.

13. Coile, R. 1997. *Probe,* Module 4: *Laboratory Networks and Alliances,* p. 7–8. CLMA, Wayne, Pa.

14. Counts, J. M. 2001. Washington Clinical Laboratory Initiative: a vision for collaboration and strategic planning for an integrated laboratory system. *Clin. Leadersh. Manag. Rev.* **15:**97–99.

15. DeBower, L. 1996. High technology industries: from courtship to union: making a strategic alliance work. *Knowledge Line. Solutions for Business.* Client newsletter, Coopers L.L.P. (now PricewaterhouseCoopers), New York, N.Y.

16. Diehl, C. 2001. The role of the laboratory in the integrated health-care system. Presented at the CLMA Leadership in Clinical Systems Management Annual Convention and Exhibition, St. Louis, Mo.

17. Drucker, P. F. 1997. The global economy and the nation-state. *Foreign Aff.* **76**(5):1–7.

18. Dye, J. 2002. Template topics. Business planning: a template for success. *Clin. Leadersh. Manag. Rev.* **16**:39–43.

19. Eckhart, J. 2002. Best practices in customer service report cards. *Clin. Leadersh. Manag. Rev.* **16**:98–100.

20. Fantus, J. E. 1996. *Cost-Based Pricing Strategies for Clinical Laboratories—An Interactive Financial Guide,* p. 103–107. Washington G-2 Reports, Washington, D.C.

21. Fantus, J. E. 1997. *Laboratory Industry Report,* p. 1–4. Washington G-2 Reports, Washington, D.C.

22. Hoerger, T. J., J. L. Eggleston, R. C. Lindroth, and E. Basker. 1997. *Background Report on the Clinical Laboratory Industry,* p. 1–105. Center for Economics Research, Research Triangle Park, N.C.

23. Klipp, J. 2000. Overview of clinical laboratory industry trends, p. 1–5. *In* D. J. Curren (ed.), *Laboratory Industry Strategic Outlook 2000 Market Trends & Analysis.* Washington G-2 Reports, Washington, D.C.

24. Klipp, J. 2000. Hospitals: laboratory outreach programs, networks and partnerships, p. 111–139. *In* D. J. Curren (ed.), *Laboratory Industry Strategic Outlook 2000 Market Trends & Analysis.* Washington G-2 Reports, Washington, D.C.

25. Learning International, Inc. 1983. *Xerox Professional Skills III.* Learning International, Inc., Stamford, Conn.

26. McNealy, R. M. 1996. *Making Customer Service Happen,* p. ix–xii, 23. Chapman and Hall, London, United Kingdom.

27. McNealy, R. M. 1996. *Making Customer Service Happen,* p. 26. Chapman and Hall, London, United Kingdom.

28. McNealy, R. M. 1996. *Making Customer Service Happen,* p. 45–47. Chapman and Hall, London, United Kingdom.

29. McNealy, R. M. 1996. *Making Customer Service Happen,* p. 61–75. Chapman and Hall, London, United Kingdom.

30. Mieling, T., and J. Keshner. 1996. Accessing capital for integrated delivery systems. *Health. Financ. Manag.* **1**:32–35.

31. Miller, R., S. Heiman, and T. Tuleja. 1985. *Strategic Selling,* p. 69–99. Warner Books, New York, N.Y.

32. Monahan, C. 1997. It's a done deal: the changing role of traditional medicine, what is a network. *Clin. Lab. Manag. Rev.* **11**:276–283.

33. Nigon, D. 1998. *Marketing in Your Laboratory,* 2nd ed., p. 25–43. Clinical Laboratory Management Association, Inc., Wayne, Pa.

34. Nigon, D. 1998. *Marketing in Your Laboratory,* 2nd ed., p. 170. Clinical Laboratory Management Association, Inc., Wayne, Pa.

35. Nigon, D. 1998. *Marketing in Your Laboratory,* 2nd ed., p. 133. Clinical Laboratory Management Association, Inc., Wayne, Pa.

36. Nigon, D. 1998. *Marketing in Your Laboratory,* 2nd ed., p. 130–131. Clinical Laboratory Management Association, Inc., Wayne, Pa.

37. Nigon, D., L. Shaw, and J. Barnes. 2000. A case study in laboratory outreach program development. *Clin. Leadersh. Manag. Rev.* **14**:97–108.

38. Otto, C. 2002. Utility scores for dimensions of clinical laboratory testing services from two purchaser perspectives. *Clin. Leadersh. Manag. Rev.* **16**:70–76.

39. Quevedo, R. 1991. Quality, waste, and value in white collar environments. *Qual. Prog.* **1991**(1):33–37.

40. Reichheld, F., and W. E. Sasser, Jr. 1990. Zero defections: quality comes to services. *Harv. Bus. Rev.* **1990**(9/10):105–111.

41. Sewell, C., and P. Brown. 1990. *Customers for Life,* p. xix–xx. Pocketbooks, a Division of Simon & Schuster, Inc., New York, N.Y.

42. Sewell, C., and P. Brown. 1990. *Customers for Life,* p. 6, 23, 17, 34, 11, 60, 32, 55, 118, 126, 147. Pocketbooks, a Division of Simon & Schuster, Inc., New York, N.Y.

43. Shepard, D. 1995. Strategic restructuring for healthcare organizations: choosing a business structure. *Prognosis* **1995**(11):1–11.

44. Smythe, M. H. 1997. Management in action. Low cost, high payoff solutions! *Clin. Lab. Manag. Rev.* **11**:236–242.

45. Snyder, J. R., and M. Best. 1997. Managing human resources in a changing healthcare environment. *Clin. Lab. Manag. Rev.* **11**:285–289.

46. Treacy, P. 2000. Ideas to help your business. *Effective Customer Relationship Management,* p. 1–5. *QuickBooks.com Newsletter,* November 2000.

47. Wilkinson, I. 1999. Dollar$ and ene: part II, the cost of adding value. *Clin. Lab. Manag. Rev.* **13**:219–222.

48. Wisler, P. W. 1997. Module 2: money and finance: strategic planning consideration in a dynamic marketplace by Coopers and Lybrand L.L.P. Presented at The Dark Report's Strategic Business Plans for Laboratory/Pathology Consolidation and Restructuring, New Orleans, La.

49. Xerox Learning Systems. 1976. Xerox Corporation, Stamford, Conn.

ADDITIONAL READING

Besley, S., and E. F. Brigham. 2003. *Principles of Finance,* 2nd ed. Southwestern Publishing/Thomson Learning, Mason, Ohio.

Block, S. B., and G. A. Hirt. 2002. *Foundations of Financial Management,* 10th ed. McGraw-Hill, New York, N.Y.

Clinical Leadership and Management Review. 2001. Template Topics. Calculating costs. *Clin. Leadersh. Manag. Rev.* **15**:124–127.

Degrote, L. 2002. Lowering bad debt in healthcare: the cure is easier than you think. *Clin. Leadersh. Manag. Rev.* **16**:59–62.

Emery, D. R., J. D. Finnerty, and J. D. Stowe. 2004. *Corporate Financial Management,* 2nd ed. Prentice-Hall, Englewood Cliffs, N.J.

Fantus, J. E. 1999. Business strategies for hospital outreach programs. *Clin. Lab. Manag. Rev.* **13**:188–196.

Hanford, W. C. 1997. Financial skills for the non-financial manager. Breakout session VI. Clinical Laboratory Management Association Annual Conference and Exhibit, Toronto, Ontario, Canada.

Nigon, D. 2000. Evaluating your laboratory outreach program. *Clin. Leadersh. Manag. Rev.* **14**:153–159.

Paxton, A. 2001. In the news—bean counting basics for laboratories, using ABC to show cost savings. *CAP Today* at http://www.cap.org/captoday/archive/2001 (last accessed August 2002).

Porter, M. 1996. What is strategy? *Harv. Bus. Rev.*

Seybold, P. B., R. T. Marshak, and J. M. Lewis. 2001. *The Customer Revolution: How To Thrive When Customers Are in Control.* Crown Business, New York, N.Y.

Seybold, P. B., and R. T. Marshak. 1998. *Consumers.com: How To Create a Profitable Business Strategy for the Internet and Beyond.* Crown Business, New York, N.Y.

Statland, B. 1995. The commercialization of lab services. . .or make no mistake about it, lab testing is big business. *MLO Med. Lab. Obs.* **27**(10):33–37.

Van Horne, J. 2002. *Financial Management and Policy,* 12th ed. Prentice-Hall, Englewood Cliffs, N.J.

Wilkinson, I. 1995. Economics 101: exploring the land of costs. *MLO Med. Lab. Obs.* **27**(12):39–43.

Ziegler, B. 1997. Will history repeat itself? *Vantage Point* **1**(20/21):1–5.

APPENDIX 3.1   Websites

http://www.Howardri.org/Trade.html: Howard Richards is a professor of global economy at Earlham College. Site last accessed 20 January 2003.

http://www.Labtestsonline.net: Lab tests on line is an American Association of Clinical Chemistry's vendor-sponsored website that provides test information written especially for use by the public. Site last accessed January 2003.

http://www.mtholyoke.edu/acad/intrel/drucker.html: Peter Drucker, faculty member at Mount Holyoke College. Site last accessed 20 January 2003.

http://www.quickbooks.com/newsletters/00: Paul Treacy at QuickBooks.com; newsletter, November 2000, p. 1–5. Site last accessed November 2002.

http://tfc-charts.w2d.com/learning/supply_and_demand.html: Keystone Marketing Services, a leader in commodity market training. Site last accessed April 2003.

http://www.wikipedia.org/: Wikipedia is an international, open-content, collaboratively developed encyclopedia. Site last accessed April 2003.

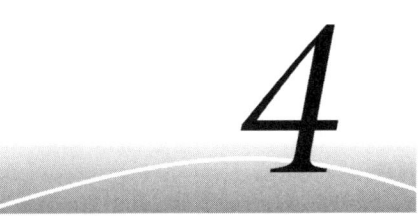

Current Challenges to Financial Stability within the Diagnostic Laboratory

Thomas J. Dilts and David S. Wilkinson

OBJECTIVES

To discuss the staffing shortage environment for laboratory medicine

To describe methods for recruiting and retaining laboratory staff

To describe advantages and disadvantages of different organizational structures for laboratory operations

To illustrate the effect of reimbursement on laboratory operations

To review the regulatory agencies that interact with different laboratory operations

Chance favors only the prepared mind.

L. PASTEUR

THE ECONOMICS OF HEALTHCARE TODAY challenge clinical laboratories nationwide to provide quality service and patient results in spite of decreasing resources. Decreasing reimbursement for patient testing and dwindling staff resources require the laboratorian to "do more with less." One must be aware of one's professional environment and be creative to utilize the existing resources effectively and efficiently. In many cases, this will require a laboratory environment of constant and major change. This chapter addresses some of these issues and their financial implications.

Workforce

Availability of Personnel

Medical laboratories across the nation are experiencing short staffing and significant problems with recruiting qualified personnel. One contributing cause is the closing of training programs for clinical laboratory scientists (CLS) and medical laboratory technicians (MLT). Since 1983 more than 57% of CLS programs have closed their doors (see Fig. 4.1). The production of certified laboratory professionals is decreasing and is not able to meet the demand (18). There also has been a concomitant decrease in the number of medical technologists (MT) certified by the American Society for Clinical Pathology (Table 4.1).

Professional groups and employers of laboratory professionals recognize this shortage (19). They have organized efforts to interest middle school, high

Figure 4.1 Number of National Accrediting Agency for Clinical Laboratory Sciences (NAACLS)-accredited CLS programs by year.

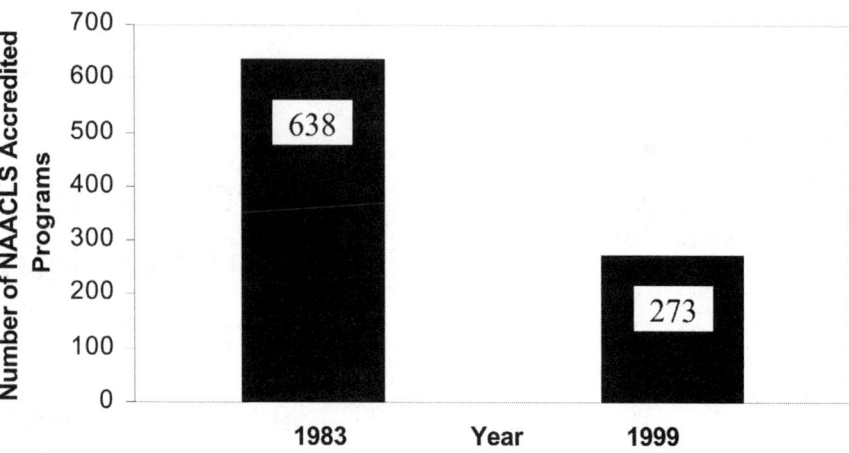

school, and college students in pursuing careers in clinical laboratory science. Some states are even planning to open new CLS and MLT programs.

Another significant reason for an inadequate supply of clinical laboratory staff is more job opportunities for people with the skills of a laboratorian. Computer technology firms, pharmaceutical companies, and laboratory instrument manufacturers and distributors all offer laboratory scientists challenging positions with good salaries and benefits. Entry-level positions in the clinical laboratory, such as specimen processing and phlebotomy, often pay less than entry-level positions in some large home appliance stores and fast-food outlets. Laboratory management must continually monitor how their staff salaries compare to surrounding competition.

Within the next 5 to 10 years we will see a shortage of CLS and MLT personnel on the order of 4,000 to 5,000 nationally due to schools closing and current staff retiring (18). Unless this trend can be reversed, the clinical laboratory industry is facing a critical shortage of personnel for the future.

Training Programs

There are several types of formal training programs for the clinical laboratory field.

- Phlebotomy at the high school degree level
- Histotechnician at the high school or associate degree level

Table 4.1 Annual certification of MTs by the American Society for Clinical Pathology[a]

Year	No.
1983	6,000
1989	3,000
1999	2,100

[a] See reference 18.

- MLT at the high school diploma or associate degree level
- Histotechnology at the bachelor of science degree level
- Cytotechnology at the bachelor of science degree level
- MT or CLS at the bachelor of science degree level
- Ph.D.-level training in the specialty areas such as clinical chemistry, microbiology, immunology, and toxicology
- Postdoctoral training programs in the specialty areas

There have been recent indications that the trend of closing programs may be reversing, and new or previously inactive programs have been returned to active status. If the number of laboratory trainees increases, there will be a need for more clinical training sites.

Most programs start with didactic courses in the first half and rotate students through the major areas of an operational clinical laboratory to give them clinical experience in the second half. Some CLS and MLT schools have difficulty arranging the clinical rotations because of the short staffing in the clinical laboratory. If the shortage of laboratory professionals is to be resolved, the profession as a whole must support the training programs.

On-the-Job Training

Some laboratories have developed training programs that allow individuals with a non-CLS degree to become qualified under the Clinical Laboratory Improvement Amendments of 1988 (CLIA '88) standards to perform laboratory procedures at the high complexity level. On-the-job laboratory training programs can also qualify individuals with high school diplomas to perform laboratory procedures at the CLIA '88 moderate complexity level. The on-the-job training programs must be approved by the director of the laboratory (CLIA '88 regulations).

Many laboratories have training programs that provide high school graduates an opportunity to become

Table 4.2 Comparison between accredited training programs and on-the-job training programs

Feature	Accredited training programs	On-the-job training programs
Breadth of training	Laboratory generalist	Usually limited to one laboratory specialty
Length of training	1- to 2-yr program	3–6 months of training
Salary potential	CLS-level salary	May be lower salary than certified CLS
Application pool	Pool of certified CLS applicants	Source of applicants to fill open positions decreasing
Didactic content	General didactic knowledge of laboratory	Limited didactic knowledge of laboratory
Flexibility	Can be cross trained easily, more flexible	Difficult to cross train, less flexible

phlebotomists (24). There are accreditation and certification programs for phlebotomy.

One advantage of an on-the-job training program is that it can provide applicants for vacant laboratory positions. However, some clinical laboratories will only hire CLS, MLT, and phlebotomists who have graduated from nationally accredited programs. Some states, such as California, Florida, and New York, require a state license for CLS and MLT positions, making on-the-job training more difficult. The salaries for on-the-job-trained positions may be lower in some laboratories than for certified MT and MLT positions.

There are two disadvantages of on-the-job training. First, it takes considerably longer to train a new employee who has not completed a formal CLS or MLT program. This can result in the removal of some staff from the laboratory bench area to do training, resulting in staffing shortages. Second, someone trained on the job is usually trained to function in only one section of the laboratory, such as chemistry. This limits the use of personnel resources to cross cover into other areas such as hematology or microbiology. The more on-the-job-trained technical staff you have, the less flexibility you will have. On-the-job training programs can also help a CLS or MLT who has not worked in a clinical laboratory for many years regain experience and confidence. Table 4.2 compares the features of accredited and on-the-job training programs.

Recruitment and Retention

As recruitment becomes more difficult, there are strategies to increase the number of applicants (Table 4.3).

Table 4.3 Recruitment benefits options

Sign-on bonus
Relocation expenses funded
Interview expenses funded
Referral bonus
Parking expenses funded
Flexible hours
Tuition benefits
Competitive salary

- *Sign-on bonus*—usually a lump sum (for example, $3,000) paid when someone accepts a specific position. The new employee must stay in the position for a specified period of time to retain the complete bonus.
- *Relocation expenses*—partial or full coverage by the employer for expenses related to relocation
- *Interview expenses*—partial or full coverage by the potential employer to an applicant for expenses incurred to travel for an interview
- *Referral bonus*—usually a lump sum (for example, $1,000) to any employee of an organization who refers a qualified applicant who accepts the position
- *National advertising*—using a medium such as professional publications or the Internet to advertise a position nationally

The cost of recruiting can be significant if you advertise nationally or in large urban newspapers, pay a sign-on bonus, and pay relocating expenses. It is not unusual to incur a cost of $10,000 or more to recruit and train a single new employee. The cost of filling a vacancy can be even greater. The additional overtime, agency staff, and burnout of existing staff to cover vacant positions may soar as high as $20,000.

Recruitment and retention issues and the resulting short staffing can lead to operational problems in a clinical laboratory. Turnaround times for patient test results may increase. Mistakes may increase due to overwork and stress. Outreach contracts may be at risk if the necessary quality of services cannot be provided. The morale and proficiency of staff may be negatively affected (see Table 4.4).

It is important that laboratory management monitor performance indicators to identify retention and recruitment problems. Table 4.5 lists a few common indicators for this purpose. Comparing the rise or fall of each indicator allows one to measure retention and recruitment activity. Each laboratory should have a recruitment and retention plan as part of their ongoing strategic plan. It is better to be proactive than to wait for a crisis. The development of any retention plan should include input from the laboratory staff to facilitate buy-in of the plan. The staff can give feedback on the root causes of retention problems and provide great ideas for improvement.

Table 4.4 Potential problems from staffing shortages

Increased turnaround time for test results
Increased errors
Decreased staff morale
Staff burnout
Increased staffing turnover
Increased overtime expenses
Increased expenses for agency staff
Decreased service, e.g., limited test menu, batching of tests
Decreased quality of laboratory operation
Increased stress to staff and management
Loss of outreach contracts

Table 4.5 Recruitment and retention indicators

Turnover rate (new hires/total FTE)
Vacancies (number)
Overtime (overtime hours/pay period)
Agency staff (hours/pay period)
Staff feedback (comments)

Generational Diversity

One of the challenges of laboratory medicine today is the mixture of age generations that make up the workforce. Each generation of people has different needs, wants, and interests. Management must be aware of this if a strong work team is to be developed and retained. Recruitment efforts must take this into consideration, since different recruiting tools will attract each generation. Younger generations may be interested in salary and perhaps tuition benefits for further educational opportunities. Older generations may be more interested in benefits such as healthcare and retirement plans. Competition for workforce resources requires laboratory facilities to provide benefit packages that meet the needs of available applicants.

Workplace

Centralized versus Decentralized Operations

The implementation of the diagnostic related group (DRG) payment methodology by the Medicare program, the massive growth of managed care, and the cut-back of Medicare fee schedules have resulted in a downward trend of reimbursements for healthcare facilities, including clinical laboratories (31). This has led to a constant pressure for laboratories to cut their operating budget and to adopt a "do-more-with-less" philosophy since the early 1980s.

Figure 4.2 shows a laboratory organizational structure that was very common in medium and large hospital laboratories until the 1980s. It was not uncommon to have a satellite laboratory in the emergency room, intensive care units, or large outpatient clinics throughout a medical center.

Many of these satellite laboratories functioned 24 h a day, 7 days a week. They usually performed stat hematology, chemistry, urinalysis, and even immunochemistry procedures. Procedures they did not perform were conducted in the main central laboratory of the facility. Even though test menus were limited in these satellite laboratories, there was a duplication of equipment and personnel since the main laboratory also performed the same procedures.

Convenience and fast turnaround times were the driving factors for the establishment of these satellite laboratories. The cost of one full-time equivalent (FTE) to staff satellite laboratories 7 days a week and 24 h a day could easily exceed $130,000 a year. If you add equipment, maintenance, reagents, and supplies, each satellite laboratory was very expensive.

The pressure to cut operating costs, use of automated transport systems such as pneumatic tube systems, and redesign of the main laboratory have resulted in a more centralized approach to laboratory testing in many institutions. This automated centralized approach has decreased costs (elimination of satellite laboratories) while still providing rapid turnaround times. A "stat" core laboratory within the main central laboratory of a medical facility can successfully and efficiently provide quality laboratory services. Many of these core laboratories have a combination of chemistry, hematology, and coagulation instrumentation in one area and trained staff capable of operating each instrument (6).

The development of point-of-care testing (POCT) instrumentation has led to another decentralized-laboratory approach (Fig. 4.3). Satellite laboratories in many cases

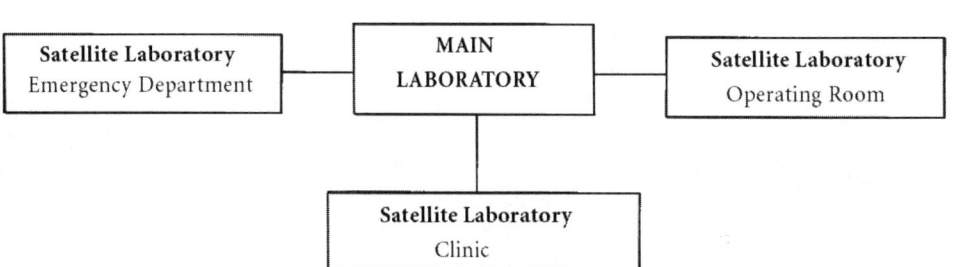

Figure 4.2 Relationship of satellite laboratories to the main laboratory. Turnaround time-sensitive tests are performed near the patient and providers. High-volume, more complex, and less time-sensitive tests are performed in the main (central) laboratory.

Figure 4.3 Deployment of POCT. It may be possible to achieve rapid turnaround of key laboratory test results by using POCT technology under the supervision of the main (or central) laboratory in lieu of satellite laboratories. Consolidation of key testing into a "core" laboratory may facilitate rapid turnaround time for most analytes, with only a few critical areas needing POCT capability.

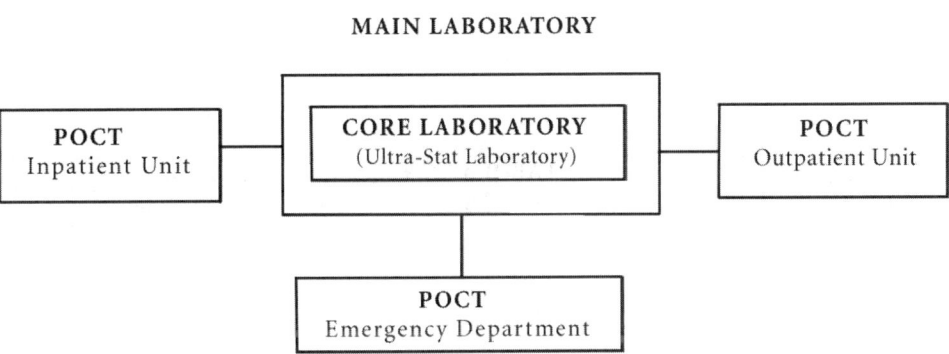

have been replaced with POCT instrumentation, especially for blood glucose testing.

POCT instrumentation has an increasing menu of available tests (Table 4.6). POCT may decrease the turnaround time for results, decrease the volume of blood collected from patients, and help improve medical management for the patient. However the cost to provide POCT may exceed the cost of central laboratory testing on a cost-per-test basis, and management of POCT can be a compliance challenge for the main laboratory (25). One must analyze the need for laboratory support for the particular patient population and each facility and then decide which approach is best for the quality, service, and cost of the operation.

Local and Regional Integration of Laboratory Services

The past two decades have seen the development of multiple hospital systems. Within a geographical area one hospital may purchase multiple hospitals, or several hospitals may merge into a single hospital system. One major driver of this is cost savings by eliminating duplication and consolidating services (15). Figure 4.4 shows a typical laboratory network that can result from the merger of multiple hospitals into a single healthcare delivery system. Usually the larger hospital laboratory serves as the core, or the main, laboratory performing the bulk of testing. The remaining smaller hospital laboratories become rapid-response laboratories performing procedures requiring a

fast turnaround time. These rapid-response laboratories send all other testing to the core laboratory (29).

A network structured as in Fig. 4.4 can result in significant operational cost savings in labor, reagents, supplies, and major equipment maintenance (probably 10 to 20% compared to the total cost of operating each laboratory independently). The development of rapid-response laboratories reduces duplication of equipment since the core laboratory will perform the majority of the high-volume routine testing (22).

Hospital laboratories may work together to form a network with larger geographical coverage. This network may allow a group of unrelated hospital laboratories to service statewide contracts for laboratory services. Commercial laboratories, also referred to as reference laboratories, all have wide geographic, often nationwide, networks to provide laboratory testing services (27).

A third network example is a joint venture with a commercial laboratory and a separate hospital or hospital system laboratory (11). The commercial laboratory can provide already existing state and nationwide courier services for specimen transport. Usually the hospital laboratory can provide local stat testing with fast turnaround times and some esoteric testing capabilities that the commercial laboratory cannot provide.

All networks are driven by an economic need to either lower operating costs or increase net revenue by increasing testing volume (11).

Work Flow

New Technology

Four critical tools that help the clinical laboratory industry meet the economic challenges of today are automation, computerization, POCT, and robotics. Technology in each of these areas continues to advance rapidly, allowing laboratories to do more with less.

Perhaps automation has had the greatest influence on laboratory productivity. Virtually every section of the laboratory benefits from automation, including molecular diagnostics, transfusion medicine, microbiology, and

Table 4.6 POCT procedures

Electrolytes	Pregnancy test
Blood urea nitrogen	Urinalysis dipsticks
Glucose	Strep screen
Blood gases	Occult blood
Hematocrit	Troponin
Hemoglobin	Activated clotting time
Creatinine	Prothrombin time
Calcium	Activated partial thrombin time
Lactate	Clotting time
Magnesium	Bleeding time

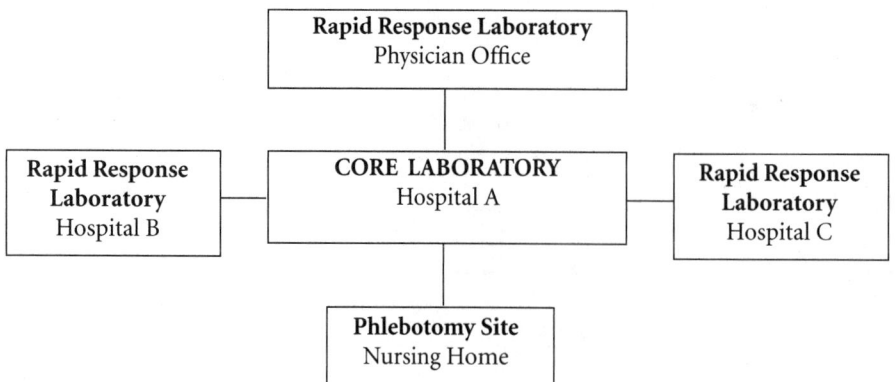

Figure 4.4 Organization of an integrated laboratory services delivery network. Several healthcare service delivery sites developed an integrated network to deliver laboratory services. The bulk of high-volume testing is consolidated at one site, the core laboratory. Other sites may offer rapid response testing or just phlebotomy services.

surgical pathology. Chemistry and hematology usually have the greatest level of automation. Automated instruments allow efficiencies in labor resources (10). One person may be sufficient to perform hundreds or even thousands of tests in 1 day. If the capacity of the automated system has not been reached, it may be easy to add new testing volume to the automated system without the need for additional personnel. The additional reagent and supply costs are usually minimal compared to adding labor costs (28).

Automation enables reengineering the laboratory. A core, automated laboratory where hematology, coagulation, chemistry, and immunochemistry instrumentation are grouped together with a staff cross trained on each instrument may be very cost-effective. Rapid turnaround times for results obtained on automated instruments allow laboratories to provide results quickly to clinicians. One may best appreciate the efficiency of higher automated instruments when they are not operational. The only reasonable backup system for automation is another automated system.

The large national laboratory conferences, such as Clinical Laboratory Management Association and the American Association of Clinical Chemists, exhibit the large number of automated instruments available. When choosing automation, laboratories need to understand the specific needs of their operation and do the necessary homework to determine which instrument is best for them. Three elements that should be considered are quality, service, and cost. If the first two are equivalent among the instruments being considered, then cost may be the deciding factor. Many times the right automation leads to major dollar savings in operational costs.

Computers have permeated all industries and even our personal lives. They play a major role in laboratory medicine today. The combination of a laboratory information system (LIS), hospital information system (HIS), and laboratory automation can facilitate a highly efficient and cost-effective laboratory operation (8). Automated instrumen-

tation interfaced to an LIS eliminates the labor of manual data entry. This allows immediate availability of results via the HIS to any location within the facility with access to HIS. It also eliminates the need for manual delivery of reports. Computer-generated work lists, pending test lists, and quality control data reduce laboratory personnel requirements.

Two additional capabilities of some computer systems are autoverification and rules (26). Autoverification allows the computer to automatically check certain parameters, such as reference values, delta checks, and quality control results. If everything is within a defined range, the computer will automatically release patient results. This eliminates the need for a technologist to review this information manually. This reduces turnaround time and reduces some labor requirements.

Rule-based systems are software programs allowing the computer to perform such functions as ordering a repeat test or ordering a confirmation test as a follow-up if certain circumstances (rules) prevail. Additionally, a prompt may come up on the computer screen when someone is ordering a laboratory test questioning the necessity of the test if certain circumstances (rules) prevail; for example, the same test was ordered 30 min ago. Rule-based systems can help the laboratory work with medical staff to improve the utilization of laboratory services. As with automation, one must understand one's needs before choosing one of the many computer systems available.

One of the most rapidly growing technologies is POCT. The standards of medical practice, especially in the emergency room and intensive care areas, require a rapid turnaround time. Even with automation, computerization, and pneumatic tubes, it is not always possible in some facilities to achieve an acceptable turnaround time in a central laboratory (7). Bringing the stat laboratory testing to the bedside of the patient through POCT instrumentation has become more and more popular as a means to achieve an acceptable goal. One must consider the cost/benefit analysis of POCT, as there are issues concerning operational costs, quality control, billing, accountability, and management of the system (4, 10, 12).

While robotics have been one of the core technologies in industrial automation for years, one of the more recent developments for the clinical laboratory is robotic automation of front-end, back-end, and workstation-linking processes. Total robotic systems exist that allow a barcoded specimen to be placed on a track system that does the following:

1. Logs specimen into LIS
2. Decaps, mixes, and centrifuges specimen (if necessary)
3. Aliquots specimen into daughter tubes if not using primary tube sampling
4. Loads specimen onto automated instruments (chemistry, hematology, and coagulation)
5. Stores specimen
6. Retrieves specimen for repeat or add-on tests

Front-end or linking robotic systems are usually installed in larger laboratory operations and are very expensive (23). Robotics can be approached in a modular fashion where a system is purchased and installed in segments. The specimen receiving and processing areas of most medium and large operations are very labor-intensive. Front-end robotics, installed to receive, process, store, and retrieve specimens, can improve efficiency and decrease cost (8). The front-end robotic system can be extended to link the automated instruments. A cost/benefit analysis that shows your return on investment can help decide whether or not robotics are feasible.

Testing Site Options

Testing site options include central (main) laboratory, POCT, reference laboratory (send outs), patient home testing, and in vivo testing. When considering what testing options to utilize within a medical facility, one needs to consider the following:

- Quality—the accuracy, sensitivity, specificity, and clinical importance of the procedures
- Turnaround time requirements
- Service—who will maintain and support instrumentation, to include calibration, quality control, and proficiency testing
- Cost—the total cost to provide specific testing options

Usually a centralized automated laboratory operation provides the lowest cost per test (17). However, a centralized laboratory may not always deliver the fastest turnaround time. Sometimes it is more cost-effective to send certain procedures to an outside reference laboratory rather than incur the cost to set up and perform low-volume procedures in-house (21).

POCT may be the only test option that can provide the turnaround time clinically needed for certain procedures (Fig. 4.3). Convenience to the physician and the patient drive POCT demand in both an inpatient and outpatient setting (25, 33). Some POCT may be categorized as waived testing under CLIA. The regulations governing waived tests are substantially less stringent than those for nonwaived testing. The list of waived tests changes rapidly, and the latest information can be obtained from the CMS website at http://cms.hhs.gov/clia/waivetblopdf (accessed 5 January 2003).

Table 4.7 lists a few procedures approved by the Food and Drug Administration (FDA) for over-the-counter purchase and home use by the public without a prescription. These tests automatically are categorized under CLIA '88 as "waived." This test option does not require a physician's prescription. This list will most likely increase over time (FDA website, http://fda.gov/cdrh/ode/otclist.html [accessed 5 January 2003]).

Research efforts to develop noninvasive laboratory procedures, such as bilirubin and glucose testing, are ongoing. This may replace some of the POCT procedures at the patient's bedside (20).

Doing More with Less

Systematic Approaches to Managing Change

The healthcare environment today is one of constant change. The challenge in many facilities is to keep a positive financial bottom line. With reimbursement for healthcare services decreasing and operational costs increasing, a positive bottom line is difficult to achieve. Maintaining the status quo is not an option today, since the changing environment requires changes in our laboratory operations in order to maintain financial stability. Those laboratories that have not made incremental operational changes in the last 15 years may now face the reality of having to make revolutionary changes to survive. These necessary changes may be highly disruptive for a period. Laboratories need to take a systematic approach to managing their

Table 4.7 Tests approved by the FDA for home testing

Human immunodeficiency virus

Pregnancy test

Glucose

Occult blood

Tests for drugs of abuse (cannabinoids, cocaine, amphetamines, opiates, phencyclidine)

Hemoglobin A1c

Ketones

Cholesterol

Prothrombin time

operations (16, 32). Managing the clinical laboratory should integrate all specialty sections. Open laboratory designs facilitate the ability to function as an integrated system (13). Instrument manufacturers are designing instruments that integrate the testing of traditionally separate areas of the laboratories (for example, chemistry, immunochemistry, toxicology, and immunology) into one analytical platform.

A systematic approach allows changes that result in efficiency and economic savings. Cross training of personnel and consolidation of separate sections into one operational area help laboratories meet the demands of the present healthcare environment. But there is a cost to change. Many people are not comfortable with change. With a good strategic plan, good communication, and involvement of the staff, positive change can result.

Rightsizing

Personnel represent as much as 50% or more of the direct operating costs of a laboratory. When the operating budget needs to be significantly reduced, the labor component is one of the first considerations. How does one determine the correct number of staff?

Benchmarking tools such as the Laboratory Management Index Program (College of American Pathologists [CAP] Northfield, Ill.) and Healthcare Benchmarking System International (Soclucient, Evanston, Ill.) can be helpful in evaluating your laboratory's productivity. When using benchmarking tools it is very important that you compare "apples to apples." You should benchmark against peer laboratories. The items for count (such as "test" or "FTE") must be precisely defined. The way procedures are counted must be defined. Are profiles counted as one procedure or broken out into separate components? Labor costs per procedure, worked hours or paid hours per procedure, procedures per FTE, laboratory costs per discharge, and laboratory cost per patient day are a few of the productivity indices that can be used for comparison. For larger laboratories, section-specific benchmarking may be helpful once you have documented the need to rightsize.

There are several ways to approach labor reduction if it becomes necessary. Every time a position comes open, carefully review the need for filling the position. Can the position be eliminated (attrition) or can it be moved to another area of the department where there is a greater need? Consolidation of two or more areas of the laboratory can improve cross coverage ability and decrease the overall need for personnel (for example, consolidation of chemistry and toxicology sections or microbiology and immunology sections). Front-end robotics and new automation may result in labor savings (23). Attrition is less traumatic than layoffs to decrease the workforce.

A review of current laboratory services may reveal some labor-saving opportunities. Can some procedures be performed less often (for example, twice a week versus daily)? Can night coverage in microbiology be eliminated? Can some procedures be sent to outside reference laboratories in place of being performed in-house?

Working with the medical staff to change the way they utilize laboratory services may also save money. Are more procedures coming into the laboratory on the night shift than necessary? Are some tests being ordered too often? Are standing laboratory orders not being reviewed soon enough to discontinue unnecessary testing?

Shrinking Reimbursement

Gross versus Net Revenue

The bill a medical facility sends a patient or a patient's insurance company lists what is termed the "gross billing" charges. Rarely are these gross billing charges paid in full. There are adjustments that are made (discounts) from the original charges based on the contractual payment agreements set up with various insurance payors. The original patient charge represents the gross revenue that is billed. The adjustments lower the gross revenue and determine the amount the medical facility should receive. This is the net revenue or expected dollars received. The difference between the gross revenue and the net revenue can be as much as 50 to 60% or more. A medical facility could bill a total of $100,000,000 for patient services but actually receive only $40,000,000 to $50,000,000. What are some of these adjustments that lower the payments?

Medicare

The federal government initiated the Medicare program in 1966. This program provided healthcare for the elderly. Initially hospitals were paid based on their actual expenses for inpatient care for Medicare patients. In 1983 this all changed when the government instituted the prospective payment system that reimburses hospitals based on DRGs for hospital inpatient services (Medicare Part A) (3). This system was based on reimbursing hospitals after Medicare patients were discharged and paying a set amount based on the discharge diagnosis. The government has developed over 500 DRGs that are specific for a disease or procedure. If a hospital could treat a patient with a specific DRG for less than they were reimbursed, then they made money; if it cost them more than the DRG reimbursed, they lost money. The government is now instituting a similar program for outpatients with ambulatory payment classification (APC) (5). Both the DRG and APC system have shifted the financial risk from the government to the provider.

Physician services and most nonphysician outpatient services are paid by the Medicare Part B program based on a fee schedule. Over the years the Medicare Part B fee schedule for laboratory services has not kept pace with the medical price index, so the reimbursement for laboratory services by Medicare Part B has been decreasing in constant dollars (1).

Managed Care

Managed-care organizations are constantly negotiating with healthcare providers regarding reimbursement. They may pay a set fee for each day a patient is in the hospital (per diem). They may pay on a per-case basis. They may pay a set fee per month per member for any healthcare needed (capitated payment).

The net effect of the prospective payment system is a significant decrease in reimbursement and cash flow for providers. It does not appear that this trend will change soon. The payment for laboratory services reflects this trend, and reimbursements are usually less than half of the gross laboratory charges. There is very little "profit margin" left for providers of laboratory services (30, 31).

Billing

Another factor causing decreased reimbursement for hospitals and clinical laboratories is the billing system itself. Hospital billing systems struggle to keep up with the complexity of the healthcare environment. The need for correct diagnosis codes (International Classification of Disease, 9th Revision), billing codes (Current Procedural Terminology, 4th edition), demographic information, and current insurance information can easily result in missing or wrong information in the billing system. This results in lost charges or payment denials. Hospitals have identified such lost income, and the emphasis has shifted from cutting operating expenses to fixing billing systems to recover dollars "left on the table" (14).

Regulations and Unfunded Mandates

Regulations

There has been a steady increase in regulatory control by both federal and state government of the healthcare industry (4). This increase in regulation extends to all clinical laboratories supporting both inpatients and outpatients. All clinical laboratories must be certified as fulfilling the requirements of CLIA '88. Those requirements include personnel qualifications, quality control, quality assurance, laboratory procedures, proficiency testing, and laboratory safety (2).

The certification of a clinical laboratory performing moderate- or high-complexity testing as defined by CLIA '88 is accomplished through an onsite biannual inspection process (2). This inspection can be performed by the federal government, state government, or a voluntary organization such as the Joint Commission on Accreditation of Healthcare Organizations (JCAHO) or the CAP. The voluntary inspecting organization must be granted "deemed status" by CMS, which ensures that the standards of voluntary organizations are equivalent to their own. Other agencies granted deemed status include the Commission on Office Laboratory Accreditation (COLA), which inspects and accredits physician office laboratories, and the American Association of Blood Banks (AABB), which inspects and accredits blood banks.

Once a laboratory successfully passes its inspection, CMS issues the appropriate certificate of compliance (if inspected by government agency) or certificate of accreditation (if inspected by a "deemed" organization).

Unfunded Mandates

Many of the government regulations imposed on clinical laboratories come with a price tag. There is a cost to laboratories to obtain a CLIA certificate as well as to keep it current. There is a cost to have an inspection by JCAHO, CAP, AABB, or COLA as well as the required proficiency testing programs. New government compliance regulations as well as the new Health Insurance Portability and Accountability Act of 1996 (HIPAA) rules have resulted in unplanned expenses for clinical laboratories and hospitals to modify existing computer systems and even add personnel to help meet the regulations (HIPAA Complete, available at http://www.hipaacomplete.com/history.asp [accessed 5 January 2003]). The FDA has recommended that blood banks have their own quality assurance coordinator. This may result in adding a new position to the payroll. All of these expenses incurred by clinical laboratories to meet mandated regulations represent additional costs for which there is no additional revenue.

Summary

We live in very exciting and challenging times and must constantly utilize new ideas and changes to obtain the resources, both personnel and nonpersonnel, to move ahead. Automation, computerization, POCT, and robotics will allow a more integrated, system-wide approach to providing high-quality laboratory services in support of patient care. Laboratory networks and multihospital systems may achieve economics of scale. The status quo is not a viable option.

The economics of healthcare have changed, decreasing the flow of dollars into diagnostic laboratories. It is imperative today that every laboratorian have a basic understanding of laboratory and healthcare finances (9). This financial knowledge will help the laboratory team work toward those changes that create a more efficient and cost-effective operation.

KEY POINTS

- Since 1983 more than 57% of CLS programs have closed or become inactive.

- As many as 60% of laboratories in this country report understaffing.

- The next 5 to 10 years will bring a shortage of CLS and MLT personnel up to 5,000 nationally.

- CLS and MLT on-the-job training programs must be approved by the medical director of the laboratory.

- It is not unusual to see a cost of $10,000 or more to recruit and retain new hires.

- The cost of one FTE to staff satellite laboratories 7 days a week and 24 h a day can easily exceed $130,000 a year.

- Four critical tools that help the clinical laboratory industry meet the economic challenges of today are automation, computerization, POCT, and robotics.

- Three criteria that should be considered before the addition of new technology to any laboratory are quality, service, and cost.

- Usually a centralized automated laboratory operation provides the lowest cost per test.

- The difference between gross revenue and net revenue can be as much as 50 to 60% or more.

- The prospective payment systems have shifted the financial risk from the payor to the provider.

GLOSSARY

Ambulatory Payment Classification (APC) An outpatient prospective payment system similar to the inpatient DRG system.

American Association of Blood Banks (AABB) A professional organization that provides a voluntary inspection and accreditation program for blood banks and transfusion services.

Centers for Medicare and Medicaid Services (CMS) Formerly known as the Health Care Financing Administration (HCFA), CMS administers the Medicare program and enforces the CLIA '88 regulations by conducting laboratory inspections, determining test reimbursements, auditing billing for medical necessity, and contracting with carriers and fiscal intermediaries to provide reimbursement.

Clinical Laboratory Improvement Amendments of 1988 (CLIA '88) The primary government rules that govern clinical laboratory operations. The final rules were first published in *The Federal Register* on February 28, 1992.

Clinical laboratory scientist (CLS) Term generally used to refer to a person that has completed a four-year college-level program that requires specific training in the clinical laboratory sciences. In recent years, CLS has replaced the older term medical technologist (MT). The designation of MT also indicates a specific level of professional certification by the American Society for Clinical Pathology. A CLS can perform a full range of laboratory tests.

College of American Pathologists (CAP) A professional organization that provides a voluntary laboratory inspection and accreditation program. It places a major focus on peer review and education.

Commission on Office Laboratory Accreditation (COLA) An organization granted deemed status by CMS to inspect physician office laboratories for accreditation.

Core laboratory This term may have several meanings. It may refer to a main (central) laboratory within a multiple laboratory system, or it may refer to a dedicated section within a single laboratory that does the majority of routine and stat testing.

Diagnostic related groups (DRGs) Based on the discharge diagnosis, DRGs are a system developed by the federal government for prospective payment of Medicare inpatient services to providers.

Food and Drug Administration (FDA) One of the administrative components of the Department of Health and Human Services of the federal government. The FDA regulates the laboratory instruments, reagents, and systems provided by the medical device industry. The FDA also regulates blood and blood products and can inspect laboratory blood banks and donor centers.

Full-time equivalent (FTE) A person working 40 hours in a week (full-time position).

Healthcare Benchmarking System International HBSI is a benchmarking tool used by many healthcare facilities to compare specific departmental operations, including the laboratory, to other similar healthcare facilities.

Hospital information system (HIS) This term usually refers to a hospital computer system and its support personnel.

Joint Commission on Accreditation of Healthcare Organizations (JCAHO) A professional organization that provides a high-level peer review, on-site survey, and accreditation program for healthcare facilities, including laboratories.

Laboratory information services (or system) (LIS) This term usually refers to a laboratory computer system and its support personnel.

Laboratory Management Index Program The LMIP is a benchmarking tool managed by the CAP. It allows a clinical laboratory to compare its operational effectiveness to that of other similar laboratories using ratios from operational management data.

Laboratory network A system (formal or informal) of clinical laboratories spread over a geographical area to provide laboratory services in a coordinated, integrated manner. A laboratory network can include commercial laboratories.

Managed-care organization (MCO) An organization that provides medical insurance to beneficiaries within a framework that manages patients' access to certain healthcare services with the goal of providing care at a lower cost. The amount of healthcare coverage varies from one MCO to another depending on the program and fee paid by the client (patient).

Medical laboratory technician (MLT) An MLT can perform general tests under the supervision of a CLS.

National Accrediting Agency for Clinical Laboratory Sciences (NAACLS) An international agency responsible for accrediting educational programs in the clinical laboratory sciences and related healthcare fields.

Point-of-care testing (POCT) Usually refers to tests performed near the patient. Often performed by a nonlaboratorian. POCT is often managed or overseen by clinical laboratory personnel.

Physician office laboratory (POL) A laboratory run by a physician who performs laboratory tests on his or her own patients.

Robotics Computerized, mechanical equipment that automates specimen handling and delivery to automated laboratory analyzers.

Return on investment (ROI) ROI analysis shows how much profit (or loss) will be made on an investment (usually capital dollars) for laboratory equipment, projects, or programs.

Satellite laboratory A laboratory separated from the main laboratory, usually with a limited test menu, that is dedicated to a specific set of patients and locations in a medical facility.

Waived testing Certain simple laboratory tests meet requirements for waived testing as outlined in CLIA '88. Waived testing may be performed without concern for personnel standards or written procedures. Some of these tests are approved by the FDA for home use, such as blood glucose monitoring, are simple, and supposedly have little chance for error or major effect on the patients if an error occurs. (CMS, available at http://cms.hhs.gov/clia/waivetblopdf [accessed 5 January 2003]).

REFERENCES

1. **Barrow, B.** 2000. CLMA spearheads fee schedule updates. *Vantage Point* **4**:8–9.

2. **Clark, G. B.** 1998. Laboratory regulation certification and accreditation, p. 369–393. *In* J. R. Snyder, and D. S. Wilkinson (ed.), *Management in Laboratory Medicine*, 3rd ed. Lippincott-Raven, Philadelphia, Pa.

3. **Crolla, L. J., and P. W. Stiffler.** 2000. Reimbursements and finance, p. 97–103. *In* A. S. Kurec, S. Schofield, and M. Wattens (ed.), *The CLMA Guide to Managing a Clinical Laboratory.* Clinical Laboratory Management Association, Inc., Wayne, Pa.

4. **Curren, D. J.** 2000. HCFA proposes rule on lab test coverage, payment. *Nat. Intell. Rep.* **21**:3.

5. **Curren, D. J.** 2000. Outpatient reimbursement—final countdown to July 1 prospective payment launch. *Nat. Intell. Rep.* **21**:3–6.

6. **Dadoun, R.** 2000. Automation strategies to improve personnel utilization. *Adv. Adm. Lab.* **9**:58–62.

7. **Dilts, T. J.** 1998. Point of care testing: a step to the future. *Lab Notes—A Newsletter from Becton Dickinson* **8**:1–7.

8. **Eggert, A. A., K. A. Emmerich, E. R. Quam, and K. L. Bowers.** 2000. The LIS as process manager. Save money and reduce tech fatigue. *MLO Med. Lab. Obs.* **32**:32–33, 36–38, 40 passim.

9. **Falcone, D. M.** 2000. Basic financial management for laboratorians. *MLO Med. Lab. Obs.* **32**:30–34, 36–37.

10. **Felder, R. A.** 1997. Automation: innovative and inevitable. *Clin. Lab. Manag. Rev.* **11**:365–367.

11. **Forsman, R. W.** 2001. Joint venture versus outreach: a financial analysis of case studies. *Clin. Leadersh. Manag. Rev.* **15**:217–221.

12. **Foster, K., G. Dispotis, and M. G. Scott.** 2001. Point-of-care-testing: cost issues are impact on hospital operations, p. 269–284. *In* K. Lewandrowski (ed.), *Clinics in Laboratory Medicine: Point of Care Testing.* W. B. Saunders Company, Philadelphia, Pa.

13. **Garikes, R. W., and S. Maxwell.** 2001. Flexible and functional: a case study in efficient laboratory design. *MLO Med. Lab. Obs.* **33**:28–33.

14. **Grider, M., and K. Boles.** 2002. Managing your revenue pipeline. *Clin. Leadersh. Manag. Rev.* **16**:211–214.

15. **Ho, D. K. H.** 2000. Mission (almost) impossible: merge 2 hospital labs in 6 months. *MLO Med. Lab. Obs.* **32**:46–52.

16. **Hunter, L., J. Lien, J. R. Snyder, and R. Teixeira.** 2000. Competencies in clinical systems management. *Clin. Leadersh. Manag. Rev.* **14**:166–172.

17. **Kilgore, M. L., S. J. Steindel, and J. A. Smith.** 1999. Cost analysis for decision support: the case of comparing centralized versus distributed methods for blood gas testing. *J. Healthcare Manag.* **44**:207–215.

18. **Klipp, J.** 2000. Who wants to work in the lab? *MLO Med. Lab. Obs.* **32**:25–29.

19. **Klipp, J.** 2000. Personnel turnover, shortages cited as biggest challenge for labs today. *Lab. Ind. Rep.* **9**:1–4.

20. **Kost, J. G., and H. Clifford.** 1996. In vitro, ex vivo, and in vivo biosensor systems, p.717–722. *In* J. G. Kost (ed.), *Handbook of Clinical Automation, Robotics, and Optimization.* John Wiley and Sons, Inc., New York, N.Y.

21. **Labeau, K. M., M. Simon, and S. J. Steindel.** 2001. Clinical laboratory test menu changes in the Pacific Northwest: an evaluation of the dynamics of change. *Clin. Leadersh. Manag. Rev.* **15**:16–22.

22. **Lehmann, C., and A. M. Leiken.** 2000. Diagnostic technology for laboratories in an integrated delivery system. *Clin. Leadersh. Manag. Rev.* **14**:118–123.

23. **McPherson, R. A.** 1998. Robotics, automation, and the new role of process control. *Clin. Lab. Manag. Rev.* **12**:339–346.

24. **Mooney, B.** 2000. Staffing problems top concerns plaguing phlebotomy supervisors. *Adv. Med. Lab. Prof.* **12**:14–17.

25. **O'Brien, J. A.** 2000. Point-of-care-testing. *MLO Med Lab. Obs.* **12**:38–43.

26. **Pearlman, E. S., L. Bilello, J. Stauffer, A. Kamarinos, R. Miele, and M. S. Wolfert.** 2002. Implications of autoverification for the clinical laboratory. *Clin. Leadersh. Manag. Rev.* **16**:237–239.

27. **Root, J. M.** 1996. Competitive strategies for regional laboratory systems, p. 21–27. *In* J. W. Steiner, J. M. Root, and D. K. Watt (ed.), *Road Map for Laboratory Restructuring.* Washington G-2 Reports, Washington, D.C.

28. **Smythe, M. H.** 1997. Automation: triumph or trap? *Clin. Lab. Manag. Rev.* **11**:360–364.

29. **Steiner, J.** 1995. Regionalization of laboratory services to consolidate? to network? to do both? p. 7–9. *In* J. W. Steiner, R. L. Michel, and D. K. Watt (ed.), *Case Studies for Laboratory Reconstructing.* Washington G-2 Reports, Washington, D.C.

30. **Watson, K., and J. F. Boothe.** 2001. Government study calls for change in Medicare reimbursement. *Vantage Point* **5**:1–5.

31. **Weissman, D. W.** 2000. Hospital profits continue to fall. *Lab. Ind. Rep.* **IX**:1, 5–7.

32. **Wilkinson, D. S., and T. J. Dilts.** 1999. Role of medical, technical, and administrative leadership in the human resource management life cycle: a team approach to laboratory management. *Clin. Lab. Manag. Rev.* **13**:301–309.

33. **Wright, J. H. U.** 1998. Rethinking point-of-care-testing. *Adv. Adm. Lab.* **7**:23–20.

APPENDIX 4.1 Websites

http://cms.hhs.gov/clia/waivetblopdf: Since the list of waived tests tends to change frequently, the latest information can be obtained from CMS.

http://fda.gov/cdrh/ode/otclist.html: Procedures approved by the FDA for over-the-counter purchase and home use by the public without a prescription can be found at this website.

These tests automatically are categorized under CLIA '88 as "waived." The list tends to change with time, so you may wish to check the list content periodically.

http://www.hipaacomplete.com/history.asp: the complete HIPAA can be found at this website.

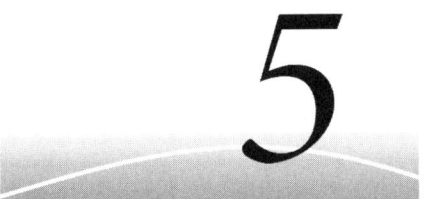

5

The Impact of Regulatory Requirements

Susan D. Roseff, Ann L. Harris, and Carol H. Rodgers

OBJECTIVES

To give readers a basic understanding of the regulatory requirements facing laboratories

To discuss the basics of laboratory inspection and accreditation

To present an overview of Clinical Laboratory Improvement Amendments of 1988

To describe the impact of increasing scrutiny on the practice of transfusion medicine

To evaluate model compliance plans and review the intent and impact on patients, physician providers, hospital and laboratory providers, employers, and payors

To review medical necessity, local medical review policies, advance beneficiary notification, and Medicare secondary-payor requirements

Law and regulation are man's product. The sum of their content is of less importance than the manner in which they are applied.

J. M. SOLOMON (125)

Introduction

Brief History

Prior to the passage in 1970 of the Occupational Health and Safety Act, providing a safe workplace was left to the ethics and knowledge of each employer. Before this law was passed, laboratory safety took a backseat to other priorities like profits, productivity, automation, unions, and other concerns (65). In recent years laboratories have seen an ever-increasing plethora of rules, regulations, and laws governing their operations (109). The many laws emanating from the federal and state governments and their details, interrelationships, and complexities are too much for most individuals to understand. In a large institution, there should be an office with environmental health and safety professionals to act as a resource. Smaller institutions should assign an individual responsible for seeking advice from professionals at other institutions, the regulatory agencies themselves, or private consultants (109).

Overview of the Current State of Laboratory Regulations

Clinical laboratories operate in a constantly changing environment. Much of that change is driven by rules, regulations, and laws, as well as voluntary standards affecting the operation of every clinical laboratory in the United States. Today's laboratory manager and laboratory director must spend considerable time and effort ensuring that their laboratory maintains compliance with what sometimes seems like a constantly moving target.

In an effort to protect laboratory workers from work-related diseases and injury, laws and regulations are enacted by the federal government through its various agencies. The health and safety of employees, their fair and equitable treatment, management of pathogens and chemicals, shipping of specimens, and accreditation of clinical laboratories are a few of the aspects of laboratory medicine regulated by law or standard. The federal agencies and voluntary organizations that set these regulations and standards form a veritable alphabet soup of acronyms.

Through the use of increasingly restrictive donor criteria, screening of donor blood for pathogens, and increased oversight, the federal government seeks to protect the safety of the blood supply. Donor units are screened for a large variety of pathogens prior to transfusion. Because there is a short period after exposure when an infected unit might test negative, extensive records are maintained and a lookback (LB) program identifies recipients of those units. The blood supply has never been safer, but the cost of achieving that safety continues to rise.

Laboratory business practices do not escape the scrutiny of the federal lawmakers. As the single largest payor of healthcare services, the Centers for Medicare and Medicaid Services (CMS) drives much of laboratory business practice. Hospitals should have a system in place to develop and administer programs to ensure regulatory compliance. Laboratory employees should have a basic understanding of laws prohibiting self-referral, fraud and abuse, and ethics and standards of conduct. Failure to comply with federal laws and regulations can lead to institutional, as well as individual, fines and penalties.

The Health Insurance Portability and Accountability Act of 1996 (HIPAA) is a progressive, patient-friendly law which has two sections. Title I deals with protecting health insurance and coverage for people who lose or change jobs. Title II includes language that mandates healthcare providers to establish safeguards that guarantee the privacy of patient information, requiring extensive changes in the way business is conducted. Section II has the greatest impact on clinical laboratory operations. HIPAA codifies institutional security measures to protect the confidentiality of any information that specifically identifies patients.

Regulation of Workplace Safety and Human Resource Management

OSHA

The Occupational Safety and Health Administration (OSHA) was created as a result of the passage of the Williams-Steiger Act of 1970, commonly known as the Occupational Safety and Health Act (129), in keeping with its mission to "save lives, prevent injuries and protect the health of America's workers." (More information about the OSHA's mission and a link to the Occupational Health and Safety Act of 1970 are available at OSHA's website, http://www.osha.gov/oshinfo/mission.html [accessed 10 July 2003].) OSHA establishes and enforces legally enforceable protective standards. Most of the standards applicable to the clinical laboratory fall under *Code of Federal Regulations* 29CFR1910.

ANSI

The American National Standards Institute (ANSI) was founded in 1918. ANSI is comprised of over 1,000 companies and organizations, both public and private (129). A private, nonprofit organization, ANSI "administers and coordinates the U.S. voluntary standardization and conformity assessment systems" (ANSI website, available at http://www. ansi.org [accessed 10 July 2003]). ANSI publishes safety standards developed by its accredited standards committees and publishes specifications for safety equipment, including eyewash and emergency shower facilities and protective eye equipment (safety glasses and goggles). ANSI, through its membership in the International Standards Organization (ISO), coordinates internationally adopted safety standards (129).

NIOSH

In addition to creating OSHA, the Occupational Health and Safety Act of 1970 created the National Institute of Occupational Safety and Health (NIOSH). NIOSH is an agency of the Department of Health and Human Services (DHHS) and functions as a research agency charged with conducting research, providing technical assistance, and recommending standards adoption. (More information about NIOSH is available at http://www.cdc.gov/niosh/about.html [accessed 10 July 2003].) NIOSH recommends safety hazard controls, is a leader in assessment and documentation of hazard control technology, and conducts classes throughout the country, but it possesses no enforcement authority (129). NIOSH works to reduce the enormous toll of workplace injury and disease in the United States. Every day about 9,000 workers incur a disabling injury, 16 die from a work-related injury, and 137 die from a work-related disease. (Additional information about the toll and cost of workplace injury and disease is available at http://www.cdc. gov/niosh/about.html [accessed 10 July 2003].)

ANSI and NIOSH work closely with OSHA in setting laboratory standards. On 19 January 2001, OSHA issued "Memorandums of Understanding: ANSI and OSHA working together to enhance and strengthen the national voluntary consensus standard system of the United States."

This agreement recognizes OSHA's authority in the development and enforcement of health and safety standards while at the same time recognizing the important role that national consensus standard-producing organizations play in the development of occupational health and safety standards. The memorandum states that ANSI will continue working to develop national consensus standards for OSHA's use and that OSHA will cooperate with ANSI and assist in its mission. The agreement calls for close cooperation in the areas of technical support, consultation in planning of standards development activities, sharing of reports, and other areas. This cooperative effort is intended to assist OSHA in carrying out its responsibilities through the use of ANSI's technical support and resources.

NCCLS

Formerly known as the National Committee for Clinical Laboratory Standards and now known by its acronym, NCCLS is a voluntary global organization that develops consensus standards and guidelines for clinical laboratories and other audiences. Over 2,000 member organizations drawn from government, industry, and the professions propose, review, comment on, and approve standards and guidelines. (Information about NCCLS can be found at http://www.nccls.org [accessed 10 July 2003].)

CDC

The Centers for Disease Control and Prevention (CDC) is an agency of the federal government. The CDC tracks, monitors, and researches disease. Of interest to laboratories is the CDC publication *Morbidity and Mortality Weekly Report*. This weekly report provides information on blood-borne pathogens and infectious-waste disposal recommendations, among other topics. Guidelines published by the CDC are published in the *Federal Register* and may be incorporated into OSHA standards. The blood-borne pathogen exposure control guidelines set forth by CDC became the OSHA blood-borne pathogen standard published as 29 CFR 1910.1030 (129).

FDA

The Food and Drug Administration (FDA), an agency of the DHHS, is charged with regulating laboratory instruments, reagents, and blood banks. The focus of the regulations is to ensure that good manufacturing practices are followed and that instruments, blood, and blood products are safe and effective (43). The categorization of diagnostic laboratory tests according to their complexity also falls to the FDA. Tests are classified according to the level of potential public health risk in one of three categories: waived, moderate complexity, or high complexity (Table 5.1). Tests that have been approved by the FDA for home use are automatically classified as waived. However, versions of those tests marketed for professional use are not automatically granted waived status. Such tests qualify for an expedited review, as any differences in the two versions are all that must be reviewed. (Information on categorization criteria, Clinical Laboratory Improvement Amendments [CLIA] waiver information, and a searchable database are located at the website http://www.fda.gov/cdrh/clia/index.html [accessed 10 July 2003].)

EEOC

The Equal Employment Opportunity Commission (EEOC) was formed in 1965 as the federal agency charged with enforcing the Civil Rights Act of 1964 (135). Title VII of the Civil Rights Act of 1964 put into place guarantees of equal treatment for all persons. The emphasis of Title VII was on protecting individuals from employment discrimination through enforcement of individual rights (124). Since the 1960s the emphasis has shifted to addressing and correcting past deficiencies through affirmative action programs (Table 5.2).

Table 5.1 CLIA categorization criteria for test systems, assays, and examinations[a]

Knowledge (required to perform the test)

Training and experience (required of personnel in preanalytic, analytic, and postanalytic steps)

Reagent and material preparation (evaluates stability, reliability, handling and storage conditions, and preparation steps)

Characteristics of operational steps (evaluates steps in the testing process—pipetting, timing, calculations, etc.)

Calibration, quality control, and proficiency testing materials (evaluates the availability and stability of calibration materials and of quality control and proficiency testing materials)

Test system troubleshooting and equipment maintenance (evaluates degree of test operator troubleshooting and maintenance required as well as the decision making and special skills or knowledge required to perform the test)

Interpretation and judgment (evaluates the degree of interpretation and judgment required to resolve problems in preanalytic, analytic, and postanalytic processes)

[a]CLIA categorizes laboratory tests as waived or moderate or high complexity. Each test system (test plus instrument), assay, or examination is graded. A grading system using the seven criteria listed and scores of 1, 2, and 3 is employed. A score of 1 is the lowest, 3 is the highest, and 2 is intermediate. Scores are totaled. A test system, assay, or examination with a score equal to or less than 12 is assigned to the moderate-complexity category; those with scores of greater than 12 are assigned to the high-complexity category. The FDA website, at http://www.fda.gov (accessed 11 July 2003), provides additional information on grading of test complexity.

Table 5.2 Federal laws prohibiting job discrimination (EEOC)[a]

Civil Rights Act of 1964 (Title VII). Prohibits employment discrimination based on race, color, religion, sex, or national origin.

Equal Pay Act of 1963. Protects men and women doing substantially the same job in the same establishment from wage discrimination based on sex.

Age Discrimination in Employment Act of 1967. Protects workers over 40 years old.

ADA of 1990 (Titles I and V). Protects qualified individuals from employment discrimination.

Rehabilitation Act of 1973 (Sections 501 and 505). Prohibits discrimination against disabled federal government employees who qualify.

Civil Rights Act of 1991. Provides monetary damages in cases of intentional employment discrimination.

[a] The website of the EEOC, at http://www.eeoc.gov (accessed 10 July 2003), provides details regarding the various laws prohibiting employment discrimination.

DOT and IATA

The Department of Transportation (DOT) is responsible for coordinating the safety program for shipment of hazardous goods within the United States. Of particular interest to laboratories, biohazardous materials, infectious materials, and dry ice are classified as hazardous goods (Table 5.3). The Office of Hazardous Materials Safety, which is located in the Research and Special Programs Administration Office of the DOT, develops and administers the Hazardous Materials Regulations (HMR). The DOT HMR can be found in the *Code of Federal Regulations* (49 CFR Parts 100 to 185).

Both the DOT's HMR and the International Air Transport Association (IATA) regulate shipment of hazardous goods sent by air. Air carriers worldwide have a major interest in ensuring the safe shipment of dangerous goods. The IATA functions as their international trade association. The DOT and IATA both base their regulations on the recommendations of the United Nations Committee of Experts. However, IATA's adds additional restrictions. The IATA regulations, updated frequently and published annually, are published in the *IATA Dangerous Goods Regulations*. Laboratories adhering to the IATA regulations for shipping infectious or biohazardous materials can be assured of also complying with the DOT's HMR (55).

HAZCOM

The OSHA standard 29 CFR Part 1910.1200, also known as the hazard communication (HAZCOM) standard, was originally published in 1983. Intended to protect workers from hazardous chemicals in the workplace (81), this version of the standard specifically included employees and employers in specific industries. Laboratories in academic institutions and in other industries were not included. Following court challenges, OSHA was required to extend the standard to all employees who work with, or are exposed to, chemicals. The final HAZCOM standard was published in 1987 and became effective on 23 May 1988 (72).

As a result of comments and concerns from the laboratory community that OSHA standards designed for industrial-scale operations were not appropriate for laboratories, an effort to craft a separate regulation for laboratories began. The result was OSHA Standard 29 CFR Part 1910.1450, "Occupational exposure to hazardous chemicals in laboratories," also known as the laboratory standard, which became effective in 1990 (109). In most cases laboratories are held to the laboratory standard rather than the HAZCOM standard (73).

Although the laboratory standard and the HAZCOM standard are very similar, they do have some differences. Key differences are that the laboratory standard adds requirements for development of a chemical hygiene plan and appointment of a chemical hygiene officer and a requirement that there be available standard operating procedures (SOP) (73). The OSHA laboratory standard is not intended to supercede *all* OSHA standards. OSHA rules and standards on areas not mentioned in the standard are

Table 5.3 Hazard classes and definitions[a]

Class	Definition
1	Explosives
2	Gases (flammable, nonflammable, and poison)
3	Flammable Liquids
4	Flammable Solids, Spontaneously Combustible Material, Dangerous When Wet
5	Oxidizers, Organic Peroxide
6	Poisonous Materials, Infectious Substances (6.2)
7	Radioactive Materials
8	Corrosive Materials
9	Miscellaneous Hazardous Materials (includes dry ice)
Other Regulated Materials	

[a] See reference 52.

still in effect. For instance, the Occupational Health and Safety Act contains a "general duty" clause which requires employers to provide a workplace free from recognized hazards that may cause death or serious harm and an employee to comply with all OSHA rules and health standards. Because the requirements of the HAZCOM and laboratory standards are similar, many institutions have chosen to institute programs that meet the requirements of the HAZCOM standard while adding the requirements for a chemical hygiene plan (109).

Blood-Borne Pathogens

Over time, and with increasing knowledge, laboratories have seen changes in the precautions used in handling laboratory specimens. Laboratories have moved from procedures that employed special handling of known or suspected infectious specimens to those requiring the handling of virtually all human specimens as if they were infectious. Over the years, handling of human specimens has progressed from labeling known infectious specimens as "blood and body fluid precautions" to following the recommendations from the CDC and advisories from the DHHS and the Department of Labor on ways to protect healthcare workers from occupational exposure, warnings from OSHA that healthcare institutions not following the guidelines were subject to fines and prosecution (84), and federal requirements as promulgated in the OSHA blood-borne pathogen standard.

OSHA's blood-borne pathogen standard (29 CFR 1910.1030) and its companion compliance directive, OSHA Instruction CPL2-2.44C, became effective 6 March 1992 (33). The standard protects employees who work with blood, body fluids, or other potentially infectious materials by requiring that employers provide certain safeguards. Recognizing that carriers of blood-borne pathogens are not always identified and that contaminated materials are not consistently labeled, the standard fundamentally changed previous practices. Standard precautions, the practice of assuming that all human blood and body fluid specimens are potentially infectious, are the basis of the standard (45).

The standard requires employers to do the following:

- Develop a written exposure control plan. The plan must include an exposure determination (made without regard to use of personal protective equipment [PPE]). This determination must contain a list of job classifications where all employees are exposed, a list of job classifications where some employees may have exposure, and a list of tasks and procedures where occupational exposure might occur.

- Provide a schedule and method of implementing methods of compliance, hepatitis B virus (HBV) vaccinations and postexposure follow-up, communication of hazards to employees, and record keeping.

- Create a procedure for evaluating any exposure incidents.

Reference to the blood-borne pathogen standard (45) will provide detailed information on methods of compliance, including engineering and work practice controls, PPE, laboratory hygiene, management of sharps, precautions while transporting specimens, warning labels, and waste disposal.

On 5 November 1999, OSHA released an updated compliance directive, "Enforcement Procedures for the Occupational Exposure to Blood-borne Pathogens" (CPL 2-2.44D) (112). The directive provides clarification to OSHA inspectors and sets policy for use in conducting inspections to enforce the occupational blood-borne pathogen standard. Some of the clarifications include the following:

- All employees (part time, temporary, and per diem) are covered. OSHA jurisdiction does not include students.

- An exposure control plan must be a "cohesive entity," or a guiding document must be provided stating what separate policies make up the plan.

- The plan must be updated on an annual basis at a minimum. Updates should include changes in technology, changed or new tasks that present exposure, and changed or new job classifications presenting exposure. The plan must include provisions for reviewing exposures and the circumstances under which they occurred.

- Because HBV is easily transmitted by environmental contamination, contaminated work surfaces must be cleaned with an "appropriate disinfectant." Dilute bleach is an effective disinfectant. A 1:10 dilution of stock household bleach (0.5% sodium hypochlorite) is considered to be effective in the time it takes to dry. For commercial products, users must follow the instructions. Gross contamination must be cleaned first with a soap-and-water solution to ensure a disinfectant's effectiveness. Other Environmental Protection Agency-registered products may be obtained from the Environmental Protection Agency Hotline at 703-308-0127.

- Sharps containers must not be overfilled. OSHA notes that the Exposure Prevention Information Network study *Uniform Needlestick and Sharp Object Injury Report*, including data from 77 hospitals in 1993 to 1995, found 717 injuries that occurred during disposal into a sharps container.

- Potable-eyewash facilities are not acceptable unless they contain at least a 15-min supply of free-flowing water and both hands are free to hold the lids open.

- OSHA notes changes in treatment of HBV. Employers are required to use the most current CDC guidelines. (Current guidelines may be located on the CDC website, located at http://www.cdc.gov [accessed 17 May 2003].)

- Exposure documentation, to be useful in creating recommendations to prevent future accidents, must contain useful information, including the circumstances of the exposure, route of exposure, engineering and work practices in use, what device was in use, and PPE in use at the time.

- Training must include description of blood-borne pathogens in addition to human immunodeficiency virus (HIV) and HBV. OSHA notes that hepatitis C virus (HCV) is now the "most common chronic blood-borne infection in the United States." Training need not include a discussion of the transmission and symptoms of less common diseases.

- Training may not be accomplished solely using a film or video. Trainees must have the opportunity to ask questions of the trainer.

- Accurate training records must be maintained for 3 years. Such records should include the names and job titles of the attendees.

Ergonomics

Work-related ergonomic injuries, also referred to as repetitive-motion injuries or cumulative trauma disorders, constitute 65% of reported injuries (118) and are the fastest-growing category of work-related injuries according to NIOSH (89). OSHA has been working toward creating an ergonomics standard since it hired its first ergonomist in March 1979. In 1990 OSHA created the Office of Ergonomics Support. The following decade saw proposed rule making and publishing of a proposed ergonomics standard culminating in November 2000 with President Clinton signing the first ergonomics rule. The OSHA ergonomics standard went into effect in January 2001 (57). Court challenges and politics (56) resulted in Congress repealing the standard in March 2001, thus marking the first time a rule as been successfully overturned through use of the Congressional Review Act (57).

OSHA's interest in ergonomics was not diminished by the congressional action. On 5 April 2002, OSHA announced a "Comprehensive Plan to Reduce Ergonomic Injuries." This comprehensive plan calls for guidelines targeted at specific industries combined with enforcement, assistance with compliance, Hispanic outreach, and ergonomics research (132).

Although the OSHA standard is at least temporarily stopped, employers should continue to be concerned about ergonomic injuries. Not only is OSHA likely to implement ergonomics reviews under OSHA's "general duty" clause (57), but also with an estimated 90 million work days lost each year to ergonomic illness (118), employers cannot afford to ignore ergonomics issues.

Ergonomics has been defined as "the science of fitting jobs to people" (56). Some laboratory tasks posing a particular risk of ergonomic injury include conventional microtomy, microscope use, manual pipetting, phlebotomy, sitting for long periods, and long periods of computer entry (89). Managers can work to reduce ergonomic injuries by studying, e.g., the amount of time spent at a particular task, how long people are in the same position, how long people engage in repetitive motion or are in awkward positions, etc. (Some ergonomics guidelines are listed in Table 5.4.)

TB

Increases in nosocomial tuberculosis (TB) over the past few decades have prompted the CDC to issue guidelines and OSHA to propose a new health standard. Alarmed over the increases in nosocomial infections seen in the 1980s and early 1990s, the CDC issued guidelines in 1990 that were further expanded and revised in 1994 (97). In 1993 OSHA was petitioned by several labor unions requesting a

Table 5.4 Computer workstation and general ergonomic guidelines (not a comprehensive list)

Hold head, neck, and body upright and facing forward.

Forearms, wrists, hands, and thighs should be parallel to the floor.

Feet should rest on the floor or on a footrest.

Top of the monitor screen should be at or below eye level and directly in front of the employee.

The mouse or trackball should be next to the keyboard and be easy to activate.

Wrists and hands should not rest on sharp or hard edges. Wrist rests, if used, should be padded, with no sharp or square edges.

Chairs should provide lumbar support and have armrests and a seat size appropriate for the employee.

Chair seats should be cushioned; the front edge of the seat should not be sharp or push against the back of the employee's lower legs or knees.

Avoid repetitive motions.

Limit microscope use to a total of 5 h a day, preferably spread over the day.

Position the microscope so the operator sits as straight as possible.

Use armrests to support the forearms while using adjustment knobs.

Use an antifatigue mat if long periods of standing are required.

Take frequent short breaks to stretch.

[a] OSHA provides an "e-tool" on hospital ergonomics, with specifics for laboratories, on its website at http://www.osha.gov/SLTC/hospital_etool/mainpage.html (accessed 24 April 2003). The CDC provides more detailed information on laboratory ergonomics, including a checklist, at the website http://www.cdc.gov/od/ohs/ergonomics/labergo.htm (accessed 24 April 2003).

permanent standard for occupational exposure to TB. In their petition the labor unions noted the recent increase in the number of active TB cases and their contention that the 1990 CDC guidelines were not being implemented (130). On 16 October 1997, OSHA released its proposed TB standard. According to OSHA, more than 130 lives can be saved annually under the new proposed standard and implementation of the standard will prevent 70 to 90% of occupationally acquired TB. Noting increased concern due to the emergence of multidrug resistance and new and often deadly forms of the disease, OSHA projected an expected prevention of 21,000 to 25,000 new infections per year with implementation of the standard.

The basics of the proposed standard are very similar to the 1994 revised CDC recommendations for healthcare facilities and include the following (130):

- *Exposure control.* Employers will be required to identify employees who have occupational exposure to TB and to develop a written exposure control plan reviewed at least annually and available to all employees.

- *Work practice and engineering controls.* Employers will be required to identify individuals with TB (suspected or confirmed) and to segregate them, use negative-pressure rooms, and inform contractors of any potential occupational exposure.

- *Respiratory protection.* Employees who enter TB isolation rooms, work in or enter an area where an individual known or suspected to have TB has been segregated, or may be otherwise exposed to aerosolized *Mycobacterium tuberculosis* (such as work on air-handling systems) must be provided with respirators that meet NIOSH guidelines.

- *Medical surveillance.* All employees will be required to have medical surveillance before assignment to a job with occupational exposure and then annually after known exposure, when displaying signs and symptoms of TB, following a skin test conversion, and within 30 days of termination of employment.

- *Hazard communication and training.* Employers will be required to post signs at the entrance to laboratories where *M. tuberculosis* is present, label exhaust systems noting that aerosolized *M. tuberculosis* may be present and that respiratory protection is required, and require employees to attend a training program.

- *Record keeping.* Medical and training records, OSHA logs, and other records have specific retention requirements (130).

Latex

Latex allergy has become a major healthcare concern. While the reasons are uncertain, the number of healthcare workers exhibiting sensitivity to latex has increased markedly over the last 10 to 15 years. The increase is most likely attributable to the increased use of latex gloves to prevent the spread of blood-borne pathogens following implementation of OSHA's blood-borne pathogen standard and its requirement that employees use gloves when working with blood and body fluids. Struggling to keep up with the increased demand, manufacturers made changes in their manufacturing processes and materials that may have contributed to the increased level of extractable latex proteins in the gloves. Latex proteins are the cause of sensitization and allergic reaction. When these proteins become attached to the powder used in the gloves, the proteins are more easily spread throughout the environment (107). The FDA has concluded that the powder commonly used on latex gloves poses a hazard. While not banning its use outright, the FDA intends to develop a rule that will recommend restrictions on the powder (61).

Workers exposed to latex may exhibit three types of reactions:

- Irritant contact dermatitis, though not a true allergy, is the most common reaction. It is caused by skin irritation resulting in skin rash, inflammation, or itchy areas on the skin.

- Allergic contact dermatitis or chemical sensitivity dermatitis results from a reaction to the chemicals used in the manufacturing and harvesting processes. It can cause a delayed skin reaction (usually 24 to 48 h after exposure).

- True latex allergy can be a much more serious reaction to latex. Reaction is usually much more immediate, often occurring within minutes of exposure, and may vary in severity from mild reactions such as hives or itching to respiratory symptoms, and rarely, shock (107).

NIOSH recommends that employers adopt policies to protect workers from undue latex exposure in the workplace. Some strategies to consider include the following: provide nonlatex gloves where appropriate (minimal contact with infectious materials); when latex gloves are used, use reduced-protein, powder-free gloves; ensure good housekeeping practices to minimize latex-containing dust; educate workers about latex allergy; periodically screen high-risk workers for latex allergy; and evaluate your program whenever a worker is diagnosed with latex allergy (107).

Sharps

As a result of the efforts of healthcare worker advocates, the Federal Needlestick Safety and Prevention Act (HR5178) was signed into law on 6 November 2000. The bill mandated that OSHA revise and enforce the existing blood-borne pathogen standard (29 CFR 1930.1030). Specifically, the law required that OSHA revise the blood-borne pathogen standard by strengthening employer requirements for "identification, evaluation, documentation and use of safety engineered sharp devices" (96). In a news release on 9 May 2001, Secretary of Labor Elaine Chao was quoted as saying, "Prevention is the best medicine. The more emphasis we place up front on education and prevention, the better able we are to protect workers. By revising this standard, OSHA is giving employers a stronger tool to help reduce serious injuries and illnesses caused by needles and sharps" (131). Highlights of the revised standard include the following: employers must maintain a sharps injury log that contains, at a minimum, the type and brand of device involved, where the incident occurred, and a description of the incident; exposure control plans must be reviewed annually and include documentation that consideration of available safety devices reflective of technological advances has been made; input must be solicited from frontline employees for the "identification, evaluation and selection of effective engineering controls, including safer medical devices." Other revisions include amendment of the term "engineering controls" and the addition of definitions for "needleless" systems and "sharps with engineered sharps injury protection" (131).

General Laboratory Safety

Laboratory safety is one of the most important responsibilities of a manager. A complete laboratory safety program includes all aspects of laboratory safety, from identification of hazards and procedures for training, maintaining records, and reporting accidents to comprehensive biohazard, microbiological, microbiological, chemical, and waste disposal policies and procedures. Laboratory safety programs should include these components:

- Provision for maintenance and inspection of the laboratory, including appointment of a laboratory safety officer, training policies, and provisions for proper reporting of incidents and illnesses

- Requirements for general hygiene and personal safety. Smoking, eating, drinking, and applying cosmetics (anything that brings the hand to the mouth) should be prohibited in areas where there are biohazards or chemicals. Proper PPE must be described and provided. Emergency showers and eyewashes must be provided where hazards exist.

- Warning signs and labels should be used to alert employees and visitors to particular hazards such as flammables, combustibles, biohazards, and hazardous chemicals. Where applicable, OSHA-specified signage should be used.

- Fire prevention procedures, including requirements for handling flammable liquids, smoke detection and alarm systems, fire prevention and control equipment, and evacuation procedures

- Electrical safety, including provisions for electrical safety checks of instruments and outlets and proper repair and maintenance

- Proper handling of compressed gases, including provisions for proper storage, labeling, transport, maintenance, and pressure regulators and valves, of both flammable and nonflammable gases

- Proper handling of chemicals, including procedures for proper classification of chemicals, material safety data sheets, labels, storage, transportation, PPE, spills, cleanup procedures, and hoods. OSHA requires that laboratories have a chemical hygiene plan which includes specified information (Table 5.5).

- Proper handling of carcinogens, including special precautions, labeling, disposal, medical exams, storage, and transport

- Microbiological hazards may be broken down into three categories: blood-borne pathogens (HBV, HIV, and HCV), pathogens commonly encountered in the clinical laboratory, and specimens and procedures involving highly virulent agents.

- Radiation safety

- Reporting of accidents, illnesses, and incidents

- Hazardous-waste disposal (111)

Chemicals

Four basic principles should underlie all work with chemicals: plan ahead, minimize exposure, don't underestimate risks, and be prepared for accidents (107). Planning ahead allows the worker to prepare for possible mishaps. Material safety data sheets should be reviewed, especially for unfamiliar chemicals, to understand the hazards associated with the chemical. General safety procedures should be observed when working with or around chemicals. Exposure via the skin, eyes, mucous membranes, lungs, or ingestion should be avoided. Eye protection should be required. Gloves should be chosen for their resistance to the chemical in use. Long hair, jewelry, and loose clothing should be confined. Sandals and open-toed shoes should be prohibited. Work areas should be uncluttered and clean, with exits and emergency equipment unobstructed. Minimum quantities of chemicals should be purchased.

Table 5.5 Elements of a chemical hygiene plan[a]

Basic rules and procedures
Chemical procurement, distribution, and storage
Environmental monitoring
Housekeeping, maintenance, and inspections
Medical program
Protective apparel and equipment
Records
Signs and labels
Plan for handling spills and accidents
Information and training program
Waste disposal program

[a] See reference 47.

Chemicals should be labeled properly, with special hazards noted on the label, and stored with attention to incompatibilities. A plan for disposal of waste should be in place before an activity begins. Equipment should be maintained in good condition through a program of regular inspection and maintenance. All employees should be familiar with emergency procedures and the location and use of emergency equipment (Table 5.6) (110).

Transportation of Clinical Specimens

Shippers of hazardous materials are required not only to follow the regulations but also to have documented training. The individual signing the shipping documents as the "certified shipper" is assuming responsibility for the complete shipping process. According to law he or she is the one person deemed fully responsible for the condition of the packaging of the specimen. He or she is responsible for determining whether the specimen is a regulated substance, the regulations governing that substance, the appropriate packaging to use, accurate completion of all required documentation and shipping papers, correct marking and labeling, and notifying the recipient of the shipment. Fines for improper shipping or lack of training are substantial. The Federal Aviation Administration employs lawyers and cargo security specialists to conduct preventative measures ensuring safety. One of the Federal Aviation Administration's recent initiatives is to send "strike teams" to airports, where they spend 1 week checking every package coming through (85).

The DOT document "How to Use The Hazardous Material Regulations CFR 49 Parts 100 to 185" provides information useful in reading and interpreting the regulations governing shipping and transportation of hazardous materials. (The document can be located on the website of the Research and Special Programs Administration Office of Hazardous Materials Safety, located at http://hazmat.dot.gov [accessed 10 July 2003].)

Employment Discrimination

The American Disabilities Act (ADA) of 1990 (Titles I and V) prohibits employment discrimination based on disability in qualified individuals. Disabilities are defined as mental or physical impairments limiting at least one major life activity. Major life activities are defined as walking, breathing, seeing, hearing, speaking, learning, and working. It is important to understand that the act protects "qualified individuals." Qualified individuals are those who possess the necessary skills, job requirements, education, and experience for a particular position and who can perform the functions of the position. While not required to lower production standards, an employer is required to make reasonable accommodation(s) for such a qualified individual. Reasonable accommodations may include such things as altered job schedules, restructuring a job, acquiring or modifying equipment, or providing readers or interpreters. Applying for a job, performing a job, or enjoying the benefits of employment may also require reasonable accommodation. (A more detailed explanation of required accommodations can be found on the website of the EEOC, located at http://www.eeoc.gov [accessed 10 July 2003].)

Perhaps the disabled employee most likely to require accommodation is the mobility-impaired employee who requires use of a wheelchair. Wheelchair use is relatively easy to accommodate by providing wider aisles, space to turn the wheelchair, and variable-height workbenches with access to the equipment on the bench (72).

Reasonable accommodations are required unless they create an undue hardship. An undue hardship is defined as one that imposes significant difficulty or expense in relation to the size, resources, and nature of the business. Employers may inquire about an applicant's ability to perform the job, but not about specifics of any disability. A job offer may be conditional based on a medical examination only if the same examination is required of all applicants in the same job category. The ADA does not protect employees or applicants currently using illegal drugs when an employer acts on the basis of the drug use. (Additional information about reasonable accommodations may be found on the website for the EEOC, located at http://www.eeoc.gov [accessed 10 July 2003].)

Since its passage in 1990, many employers have been concerned about the implications of the law. It is the inclusion of psychiatric and mental, along with physical, disabilities that most concerns employers. Unfortunately, EEOC guidelines do nothing to relieve their anxiety, as the guidelines state that "credible testimony from family members and coworkers may be sufficient notice to the employer that a psychiatric disability exists" (93). The Job Accommodation Network notes that most ADA accommodations cost relatively little. Data from a survey of employers using Job Accommodation Network's services showed that 70% of accommodations cost $500 or less (with 21% costing nothing) (93). Accommodations for people with psychiatric or mental disabilities tend to be no more difficult or expensive than other types of accommodation. Such accommodations may include to-do lists, tape-recorded instructions, and division of large tasks into smaller components (93).

Table 5.6 Safe handling of chemicals[a]

Review the material safety data sheet.

Plan ahead.

Observe general safety procedures.

Wear eye protection or face protection.

Use the proper gloves.

Purchase minimum quantities of chemicals.

Properly label and store chemicals.

Leave exits and emergency equipment unobstructed.

Know emergency procedures and use of emergency equipment.

[a] See reference 110.

While the ADA regulations strive for voluntary compliance, it is important to note that the act does include legal remedies for noncompliance. Employers should ensure that employees involved in any part of the process of interviewing, hiring, promoting, or firing are well versed in the law. Lack of such knowledge could result in a legal challenge where no intention of discrimination was intended.

Accreditation and Licensure

Brief History

Laboratory standards and testing have been evolving for centuries. The evolution has progressed from urine testing done before 400 B.C. to diagnose boils by observing whether insects were attracted to urine poured on the ground (19) to today's modern laboratories. As testing sophistication grew and hospitals began to appreciate the skills of laboratory professionals, self-regulating groups emerged to ensure laboratory quality. The first inspection of laboratories occurred in 1918, when the American College of Surgeons inspected hospitals utilizing standards that required an adequately staffed and equipped laboratory. The year 1918 also saw the first call for a national method to certify technologists and a Pennsylvania state law requiring that hospitals install and equip a laboratory staffed with a full-time technician (20).

Regulation of clinical laboratories began in earnest soon after the Medicare and Medicaid laws went into effect in 1966. The Clinical Laboratory Act of 1967 (CLIA '67) established minimum quality standards for Medicare participating laboratories engaged in interstate commerce, a relatively small portion of clinical laboratories. Lawmakers soon saw the need to regulate all laboratories engaged in testing human specimens. Thus began the effort to amend CLIA '67 in order to establish minimum standards for personnel, accuracy, and quality control and to mandate inspections. When the CLIA '67 final rule was enacted in 1978, it included rules for quality control, proficiency testing, and personnel competency. Personnel working in laboratories receiving Medicare reimbursement were required to be medical technologists with a bachelor's degree or equivalent or to demonstrate satisfactory performance on a proficiency exam administered by the Department of Health, Education and Welfare, the precursor to the DHHS.

In the years following the implementation of CLIA '67 there were repeated attempts to update the act to include all laboratories. The breakthrough came in 1988, when President Reagan signed the Clinical Laboratory Improvement Amendments of 1988 (CLIA '88) into law. Practical problems delayed implementation until 1992. This more comprehensive law requires all laboratories doing human clinical testing to have a certificate issued by the DHHS (21). CMS, a division of the DHHS, carries out the CLIA program.

The enactment of CLIA '88 brought virtually all laboratories doing clinical testing for diagnosis or disease management on human specimens under the umbrella of federal regulation. Laboratories are classified according to their level of testing complexity, with tests classified as waived, moderate complexity (including provider performed microscopy procedures [PPMP]), or high complexity. Laboratories registering for a certificate of waiver or PPMP may apply directly, as they are not subject to routine inspections. Waived laboratories must pay the applicable fee and follow manufacturers' instructions. Laboratories performing moderate- or high-complexity testing must be surveyed (inspected) routinely. To enroll, these laboratories must register, pay fees, and be surveyed before being granted a certificate. Moderate- and high-complexity laboratories have the option of choosing to be surveyed by CMS or by a private accrediting organization that has been granted "deemed status" (Table 5.7). (An excellent overview of the CLIA program is located on the CMS website at http://www.cms.hhs.gov/clia/progdesc. asp [accessed 14 January 2004].)

The final CLIA regulations published on 28 February 1992 set forth standards for proficiency testing, quality control, patient test management, personnel requirements, and quality assurance (QA) in moderate- and high-complexity laboratories.

Laboratory Inspection and Accreditation

The type of CLIA certificate held by a laboratory determines whether routine inspections are required. Routine inspections are not required for laboratories registered with a certificate of waiver or a certificate for PPMP. Over time the number of waived laboratories has increased to 56% of the total laboratories enrolled. Combined with the 22% of enrolled laboratories that hold a PPMP certificate, 78% of all laboratories do not have routine inspections or oversight. Random inspections are conducted at a small percentage of waived and PPMP laboratories each year. These inspections are focused on ensuring that the laboratories are not performing testing at a higher level than their certificate warrants and that they are following other CLIA regulations. Laboratories holding certificates of waiver may only perform waived tests. They must enroll in the CLIA program, pay applicable fees, and follow manufacturers' test instructions. Laboratories holding a certificate for PPMP must enroll in the CLIA program, pay applicable fees, and meet specified quality and administrative requirements. Pilot studies conducted during 1999 to 2001 in 10 states found significant problems with quality and certification (laboratories testing beyond their certificate). As a result, in April 2002, CMS began on-site educational and information-gathering visits to approximately 2% of waived laboratories.

Laboratories performing moderate- or high-complexity testing are required to have an inspection every 2 years. The

Table 5.7 Accrediting organizations having deemed status under CMS

American Association of Blood Banks (AABB)
8101 Glenbrook Rd.
Bethesda, MD 20814-2749
General number: 301-907-6977

American Osteopathic Association (AOA)
142 East Ontario St.
Chicago, IL 60611
312-202-8070

American Society of Histocompatibility and Immunogenetics (ASHI)
1700 Commerce Pkwy.
Mt. Laurel, NJ 08054
856-642-4415

College of American Pathologists (CAP)
325 Waukegan Rd.
Northfield, IL 60093-2750
1-800-323-4040

COLA
9881 Broken Land Pkwy., Suite 200
Columbia, MD 21046-1195
410-381-6581

Joint Commission on Accreditation of Healthcare Organizations (JCAHO)
One Renaissance Blvd.
Oakbrook Terrace, IL 60181
630-792-5000

[a]CMS maintains a current list of accrediting organizations having deemed status at its website, http://www.cms.hhs.gov/clia (accessed 10 July 2003).

Table 5.8 Types of laboratory CLIA certificates

Certificate of waiver. Issued to a laboratory to perform only waived tests.

Certificate for PPMP. Issued to a laboratory in which a physician, mid-level practitioner, or dentist performs no tests other than the microscopy procedures. Permits the laboratory to also perform waived tests.

Certificate of registration. Issued to a laboratory that enables the entity to conduct moderate- or high-complexity laboratory testing or both until the entity is determined by survey to be in compliance with the CLIA regulations.

Certificate of compliance. Issued to a laboratory after an inspection that finds the laboratory to be in compliance with all applicable CLIA requirements.

Certificate of accreditation. Issued to a laboratory on the basis of the laboratory's accreditation by an accreditation organization approved by CMS.

[a]Information about the various types of CLIA certificates is available at the CMS website, http://www.cms.hhs.gov/clia (accessed 14 January 2004).

laboratory may opt to be inspected by CMS or by an organization that has been approved by CMS (granted deemed status) as having program requirements at least as stringent as those of CLIA. CMS awards a certificate of compliance to laboratories that are successfully inspected by CMS and a certificate of accreditation to laboratories based on a successful inspection by an organization having deemed status with CMS (Table 5.8). A provision of CLIA '88 exempts from CLIA requirements "all State licensed or approved laboratories in a state that has a State licensure program established by law" if the state licensure requirements are at least as stringent as the CLIA requirements. Two states, Washington and New York, are currently exempt. (CMS maintains a list of exempt states on its website at http://www.cms.hhs.gov/clia/exemstat.asp [accessed 10 July 2003].)

As noted above, before CMS grants an organization's laboratory inspection program deemed status, the organization must show that its inspection criteria are at least as stringent as those of the CLIA program. Thus, the basic focus of all accredited inspection programs is to ensure compliance with the CLIA standards. However, organizations having deemed status use different approaches to achieve that goal.

CMS. Laboratories inspected under the CMS program experience an outcome-oriented survey process. CMS inspections utilize a QA focus combined with an educational approach to assess and ensure compliance. (General information about the CLIA program can be found on the CMS website at http://www.cms.hhs.gov/clia/progdesc [accessed 14 January 2004].)

JCAHO. Experienced in surveying laboratories since 1979, the Joint Commission for Accreditation of Healthcare Organizations (JCAHO) gained deemed status under CLIA '88 in 1995. JCAHO surveys are conducted by experienced medical technologists who provide consultation on performance improvement throughout the survey process. (The JCAHO survey process is further explained on the organization's website at http://www.jcaho.org [accessed 10 July 2003].)

CAP. The College of American Pathologists (CAP) laboratory inspection and accreditation program encompasses all of the laboratory disciplines. It provides the most comprehensive offerings of any of the accrediting bodies. Conducted as a peer review process, inspections are performed by experienced working professionals. The peer review process provides the opportunity for laboratories to learn both from their own inspection and from the experience of inspecting other laboratories. CAP has deemed status with both CLIA '88 and JCAHO. (Detailed information about the CAP inspection program is available on the CAP website at http://www.cap.org [accessed 10 July 2003].)

AABB. The American Association of Blood Banks (AABB) has been developing voluntary compliance standards for blood banking since 1957. AABB inspections have deemed status under CLIA '88. The inspections are based on compliance with federal regulations and documents as well as AABB standards. (More information about the AABB accreditation programs is available at the association's website at http://www.aabb.org [accessed 10 July 2003].)

COLA. Formerly known as the Commission of Office Laboratory Accreditation, but now known by its acronym, COLA is a nonprofit, physician-directed organization. COLA was founded in 1988 to provide a private alternative for complying with CLIA '88. Originally established to inspect physician office laboratories (POLs), COLA's accreditation program now covers many types of laboratories, from POLs to community hospitals and industrial laboratories. COLA inspections are conducted in an educational and friendly peer review process. COLA has had deemed status with CLIA '88 since 1993 and with JCAHO since 1997. (Laboratories interested in COLA accreditation can find more information at the organization's website at http://www.cola.org [accessed 10 July 2003].)

ASHI. The American Society of Histocompatibility and Immunogenetics (ASHI) conducts a voluntary inspection program encompassing over 200 histocompatibility laboratories. ASHI's laboratory accreditation program has been evolving since 1976. Deemed status with CLIA '88 was granted in 1995 and with JCAHO and the states of Florida, Oregon, and Washington in 1997. ASHI's accreditation program evaluates facilities to ensure compliance with ASHI standards. Laboratory procedures, staff, and facilities are surveyed with emphasis on education and assistance with correcting deficiencies. (The ASHI website, located at http://www.ashi-hla.org [accessed 10 July 2003], provides more information about the ASHI accreditation process.)

AOA. The American Osteopathic Association (AOA) has deemed status under CLIA '88 to accredit laboratories that are in AOA-accredited hospitals. (Laboratories in hospitals accredited by AOA can find information about the laboratory accreditation program at the association's website, located at http://www.aoa-net.org [accessed 10 July 2003].)

FACT. The Foundation for the Accreditation of Cellular Therapy (FACT), while not granted deemed status under CLIA '88, does set voluntary standards and accredit laboratories in the field of cellular therapy. Previously known as the Foundation for the Accreditation of Hematopoietic Cell Therapy, FACT is a nonprofit corporation which establishes standards covering all phases of cellular therapy. FACT accredits programs and laboratories voluntarily meeting these standards. (Information about FACT and its parent organization, the International Society for Cellular Therapy, can be located at http://www.celltherapy.org [accessed 10 July 2003].)

Laboratories exempt from CLIA '88. The CLIA '88 law states that laboratories will be cited as out of compliance unless they have a "current, unrevoked or unsuspended certificate of waiver, registration certificate, certificate of compliance, certificate for PPM procedures, or a certificate of accreditation..." or are CLIA exempt. Laboratories falling under the exempt category include the following:

- Laboratories performing forensic testing only
- Research laboratories testing human specimens but not using patient-specific results in the diagnosis, prevention, treatment, or assessment of disease or health of individuals
- Laboratories certified by the Substance Abuse and Mental Health Services Administration (SAMHSA). This exemption applies only to drug testing meeting SAMHSA guidelines and regulation (all other testing is subject to CLIA regulations).
- Federal laboratories under the jurisdiction of an agency of the federal government are subject to CLIA regulations unless the application is modified by the Secretary.
- Laboratories licensed in states that have their own inspection programs that are exempt under CLIA. These states have inspection programs that CLIA has deemed at least as rigorous as a CLIA inspection. Washington and New York are the only two states currently in this category. (Information regarding laboratories exempt from CLIA regulations may be found in 42 CFR 493.3, which is available at http://www.phppo.cdc.gov/clia [accessed 10 July 2003].)

Personnel Certification and Licensure

Certification is a voluntary program, usually administered by a professional association or governmental agency, recognizing an individual for having met predetermined criteria as set by that organization (122). Certification programs began as a voluntary method of demonstrating competence and enhancing competitiveness in the job market. Current CLIA '88 regulations emphasize specific education and experience, rather than certification, for the various levels of testing complexity. In general, the requirements of certifying organizations are more stringent than those of CLIA '88 (43).

Licensure is the process of a governmental authority granting an individual legal permission to engage in a specific practice. Typically, licenses are granted after examination or proof of specific education. The public is protected from incompetent practitioners by defining regulated practices and making unlicensed practice illegal (122).

Table 5.9 Summary of personnel responsibilities under CLIA '88[a]

Laboratories performing PPMP

   (Note: The moderate-complexity procedures defined as PPMP are only considered as such when performed personally by a physician, dentist, or mid-level practitioner during the patient's visit.)

   Laboratory director. Responsible for the overall operation and administration of the laboratory, including the prompt, accurate, and proficient reporting of test results.

   Testing personnel. Responsible for specimen processing, test performance, and reporting of test results.

Laboratories performing moderate-complexity procedures

   Laboratory director. Responsible for the overall operation and administration of the laboratory, including the employment of personnel who are competent to perform test procedures and record and report test results promptly, accurately, and proficiently, and for ensuring compliance with the applicable regulations.

   Technical consultant. Responsible for the technical and scientific oversight of the laboratory. The technical consultant is not required to be on-site whenever testing is performed but must be available to the laboratory on an as-needed basis.

   Clinical consultant. Provides consultation regarding the appropriateness of testing ordered and interpretation of test results.

   Testing personnel. Responsible for specimen processing, test performance, and reporting of test results.

Laboratories performing high-complexity procedures

   Laboratory director. Responsible for the overall operation and administration of the laboratory, including the employment of personnel who are competent to perform test procedures and record and report test results promptly, accurately, and proficiently, and for ensuring compliance with the applicable regulations.

   Technical supervisor. Responsible for the technical and scientific oversight of the laboratory. The technical supervisor is not required to be on-site whenever testing is performed but must be available to the laboratory on an as-needed basis.

   General supervisor. Responsible for day-to-day supervision or oversight of the laboratory operation and personnel performing testing and reporting test results.

   Testing personnel. Responsible for specimen processing, test performance, and reporting of test results.

[a]A more detailed description of personnel responsibilities under CLIA '88 is available on the CDC website at http://www.phppo.cdc.gov/clia (accessed 24 April 2003).

Personnel requirements under CLIA '88. The personnel regulations under CLIA '88 do not rely on either certification or licensure, although some states may require either or both. CLIA '88's personnel requirements are determined by the level of testing complexity. There are no personnel requirements for waived testing. For PPMP and moderate- or high-complexity testing, CLIA '88 personnel regulations define specific job titles and associated qualifications and responsibilities (Table 5.9). The regulations spell out several ways an individual may qualify for each of the job titles, with the qualifications growing slightly more stringent as complexity increases. Only laboratory directors are limited in the number of lab affiliations. Each director may direct no more than five laboratories.

Qualifications and responsibilities are delineated for the laboratory director and testing personnel at each testing level. For moderate-complexity certificates, the titles of technical consultant and clinical consultant are added. In addition to the laboratory director and testing personnel, high-complexity laboratories must also have a technical supervisor, clinical consultant, and general supervisor.

Specialty boards. CMS is tightening the qualification for directors of high-complexity laboratories who hold a doctoral degree. Until 31 December 2002, they were required to have 2 years of laboratory experience or training and 2 years of experience directing or supervising high-complexity testing. On 31 December 2002, the requirement for certification by a specialty board was added. As of that date, in addition to having a doctoral degree in a chemical, physical, biological, or clinical laboratory science and two 2 years of experience, such individuals must also be board certified (Table 5.10). This additional requirement does not apply to laboratory directors who are already serving and prior to 28 February 1992, qualified under the law of the state in which the laboratory is located, were previously qualified or could have qualified as a laboratory director under the CLIA regulations published in 14 March 1990, or for the subspecialty of oral pathology, or are certified by one of several pathology boards. (More detailed information can be found in 42CFR493. 1443, which is available at http://www.phppo.cdc.gov/clia [accessed 10 July 2003].)

Table 5.10 CMS-approved certification boards, doctoral degree clinical consultants, and directors of high-complexity testing[a]

American Board of Bioanalysis

American Board of Clinical Chemistry

American Board of Forensic Toxicology

American Board of Histocompatibility and Immunogenetics

American Board of Medical Genetics

American Board of Medical Laboratory Immunology

American Board of Medical Microbiology

National Registry of Certified Chemists

[a] The most current list of approved certification boards may be found at the CMS website at http://www.cms.hhs.gov/clia (accessed 10 July 2003).

National certifying organizations. Certification by a professional agency is valued (and in many cases required) by employers because it is a demonstration of basic competence in the area of examination. There are several options for certification as a laboratory professional. The majority of graduates of programs accredited by the National Accrediting Agency for Clinical Laboratory Sciences choose to take a certification examination. Successful completion of a certifying examination demonstrates basic competency in laboratory science. Two national organizations offer the most widely recognized certifying examinations. The exams to certify medical technologists (MT) and medical laboratory technicians (MLT) offered by the American Society for Clinical Pathology (ASCP) are most popular. Also offering certification, the National Credentialing Agency for Laboratory Personnel (NCA) administers exams for laboratory personnel but uses the terms clinical laboratory scientist (CLS) and clinical laboratory technician (CLT) (10).

The ASCP, an organization of pathologists and other clinical laboratory personnel, was the first organization to offer a certifying examination. Responding to a need for programs that would allow documentation of the basic competence of laboratory workers, the ASCP established the Board of Registry in 1928 to certify nonphysician laboratory personnel. Certification by the ASCP does not require recertification or mandate continuing education. The ASCP does, however, recognize the importance of continuing documented competence. The ASCP Board of Registry offers a voluntary program to recognize competence based on documentation of 60 h of continuing education, obtaining a higher level of certification (specialist or diplomate), or an on-site assessment completed by a supervisor. The ASCP Board of Registry certification program has expanded from its initial offering of the MT exam to its current offering of 21 different certifications (10).

In 1978, NCA offered its first credentialing examinations (10). A voluntary, not-for-profit organization, NCA offers the "only peer-developed and peer-administered examination for medical laboratory personnel." NCA's website, http://www.nca-info.org (accessed 10 July 2003), is an excellent resource for information about NCA's certification programs. A major difference between certification by ASCP's Board of Registry and NCA is NCA's emphasis on continuing education. NCA requires 36 h of continuing education every 3 years to maintain certification. Ten different certifications are currently available from NCA (10).

Other organizations offering certification include the American Medical Technologists (AMT) and the American Association of Bioanalysts (AAB). AMT offers certification in eight areas of practice. Individuals with an appropriate bachelor's degree and 1 year of laboratory experience are eligible to sit for the MT certification exam. The AMT MT certification may be awarded in some circumstances without taking the examination. (Information about the certification criteria of many organizations may be found at the website http://www.nssb.org [accessed 10 July 2003].) The AAB Board of Registry requires the applicant to pass an examination that AAB deems acceptable and to meet one of several education and/or or experience requirements. (Information about the AAB certification process can be found at the website http://www.aab.org [accessed 10 July 2003].)

States requiring licensure and certification. While certification demonstrates a basic level of competence that may make it easier to get a job, 10 states and one territory also require that laboratory personnel obtain state licensure. Requirements for obtaining a state license vary by state but usually include a licensing fee, documentation of certification, some evidence of continuing education, and demonstration of education and competency as defined by the state. Most states accept certification from a recognized certifying organization. The exception is California, which administers its own examinations and does not recognize any certification or grant reciprocity for any other state's license. Requirements for state licensure may change. (The most current information is available at the American Society for Clinical Laboratory Science website, http://www.ascls.org/jobs/grads [accessed 10 July 2003].) (Table 5.11).

Some states and U.S. territories require that laboratories operating in their borders, and in many cases performing testing on samples from that state, obtain a license from that state or territory. CMS maintains a list on the Web at http://www.cms.hhs.gov/clia (accessed 10 July 2003) of state and territory laboratory licensure programs. However, because the number of states requiring laboratory licensure is fluid, an individual laboratory is advised to contact the appropriate state survey agency for the most current information.

Regulations Impacting Transfusion Medicine

Overview of Changes in Transfusion Medicine That Have Resulted in Increased Scrutiny

One of the greatest defining moments in the recent history of transfusion medicine was the realization that HIV, the virus that causes AIDS, could be transmitted by transfusion. With all eyes on transfusion safety, blood banking and transfusion medicine went through dramatic changes. Blood banking evolved from a laboratory discipline into transfusion medicine, focusing on patient care through clinical consultation, and then into a blood manufacturing industry (126). Blood donors, previously seen as the altruistic givers of life, were increasingly seen as sources of infection and risk (25).

In 1991, hearings in the U.S. House of Representatives, chaired by John Dingell (D-Mich.), clearly expressed the lack of faith that our elected officials, echoing the sentiments of their constituencies, had in the safety of the blood supply. By referring to blood banking as an indus-

Table 5.11 States and territories requiring licensure of laboratory personnel

State or territory	Licensing entity
California	Department of Health Services Laboratory Field Services 510-873-6327
Florida	Department of Health Division of Medical Quality Assurance 850-488-0595
Hawaii	Hawaii Department of Health State Laboratory Division 808-453-6653
Louisiana	Clinical Laboratory Personnel Committee Louisiana State Board of Medical Examiners 504-524-6763, ext. 261
Montana	Montana Department of Commerce Board of Clinical Lab Science Practitioners 406-841-2386
Nevada	Nevada Bureau of Licensure and Certification 702-687-4475
North Dakota	North Dakota Department of Health Division of Microbiology 701-328-5262
Puerto Rico	Puerto Rico Medical Technology Board of Medical Examiners 809-792-6400
Rhode Island	Rhode Island Department of Health Division of Health Services Regulation 401-222-2827
Tennessee	Lynda England, MT (ASCP), Administrator Tennessee Medical Laboratory Personnel Board 615-532-5128
West Virginia	Marilyn Richards WV Office of Laboratory Science Department of HHS 304-558-3530

[a]The American Society for Clinical Laboratory Science maintains a list of states requiring licensure of laboratory personnel at http://www.ascls.org (accessed 25 April 2003).

try, an important paradigm had shifted (104). The generalized concern was apparent when looking at the changes in blood usage that began in the 1980s: decreases in the use of volunteer allogeneic blood, against the backdrop of an aging and sicker population, and more use of autologous blood and directed donor blood (11, 76, 98).

This climate served as a catalyst for a variety of changes, from purely medical to regulatory and legal. The lay public, concerned about exposure to known and unknown pathogens, sought ways to decrease their risk. The medical community responded, using pharmacological alternatives and blood salvage techniques (collecting and reinfusing blood from the operative field) and adopting more conservative transfusion guidelines. On the production side of the equation, more sensitive tests were added to screen donor blood, more restrictive donor criteria were applied, and more regulations were added to blood banking to increase oversight and scrutiny (76). The complex process of supplying blood to patients was also taking place in a more litigious and cost-conscious environment (98). With infectious complications on the decline, concerns about adequacy are on the rise (5, 105). The public seeks zero risk, and the industry strives to move closer to that ideal.

Safety

HIV and HCV. As a result of changes in blood donor screening implemented in response to concerns about transmissible disease, the United States' blood supply has never been safer. In 1993, in order to prepare for future threats to the blood supply, The Institute of Medicine established a committee to retrospectively study the spread of HIV in the American blood supply. Their report, published in 1995, and two reports published by the U.S. General Accounting Office in 1997 acknowledged the current high level of blood safety while recommending continued enhancements in specific manufacturing practices and in FDA oversight (88, 133, 134). (These reports are available on the U.S. General Accounting Office website at http://www.gao.gov [accessed 10 July 2003].) To gain perspective into the vast improvement, it is helpful to compare the risk of acquiring HIV in the early 1980s to the current risk. Using a mathematical model, Busch et al. estimated that the overall risk of posttransfusion HIV infection was 1.1% per transfused unit in San Francisco between 1978 and 1984, prior to implementation of HIV testing (36). This is in contrast to the current risk of receiving a unit infected with HIV that is negative for all markers (including nucleic acid testing [NAT]), which is 1 in 1.93 million (59).

Despite all the attention paid to HIV, other pathogens that currently pose greater risks are now drawing attention (76). While the risk of acquiring HIV through transfusion was being greatly diminished, the risk of HCV transmission was actually two to four times higher than the risk of HIV transmission in 1996 (121). With the implementation of NAT, the risk of receiving a unit of blood from a donor during their infectious window period has gone from 1 in 103,000 (121) to 1 in 1.543 million (59). Bacterial pathogens are now recognized as a major threat to the blood supply, far greater than that of hepatitis and HIV (76).

LB. It is important to remember that both HIV and HCV were present in the blood supply prior to the availability of screening methods. In addition, early HCV testing was neither sensitive nor specific (1). To address the risk of window period transmission to blood recipients transfused prior to testing, a variety of processes known as lookback (LB) were initiated, essentially looking back at patients with a risk of acquiring a pathogen through transfusion. Targeted LB, triggered when a blood donor is found to be positive for HIV and/or HCV, is the process of identifying and informing transfusion recipients that they might have been exposed to an infectious agent from individuals who previously donated blood during a clinically serosilent window period. In other words, donations from an infected individual with disease are looked back upon. The recipient can then be notified of their risk, tested, counseled, and referred for proper medical care. This can also prevent secondary transmission of disease, which was especially important prior to testing (34).

LB programs have been fraught with limitations. For LB to be successful, it means that the recipient is found, has the disease, and was previously unaware of the infection. Targeted LB requires that high-risk individuals come

back and donate again, so that recipients of the products donated *prior* to their seroconversion can be alerted. By asking high-risk individuals to refrain from donating, this trigger is removed. In fact, through an education program aimed at high-risk individuals, it was calculated that about 90% of infected donors either self-deferred or were deferred during the donation process in San Francisco prior to implementation of HIV screening. In contrast, only about 6% of transfusion recipients were identified through early donor-targeted HIV LB programs in the same area (34).

Other factors also contribute to the lack of success of LB programs, with success being defined as finding people unaware of their risk. One of the major problems, finding the recipient of the blood product, is the result of limitations of early record keeping. Assuming the blood center can track the product to its destination and then the hospital can trace a unit back to a recipient, the mobility of our society makes it likely that the recipient has moved and cannot be found. In addition, even when the recipient is located, he or she may have already learned of the infection through other means or may have already died of underlying disease. In more stable, less mobile populations, there may be greater success (34, 42, 75).

In contrast to HCV LB, HIV LB was initiated voluntarily, as a means to trace infected donors back to their blood recipients. In the heated climate of blood safety concerns, it served as one of the few ways to do something to stop the spread of disease in the early years of the epidemic. By 1984, the general blood banking community endorsed the process, which began in earnest as targeted LB in 1986, the year following implementation of HIV screening. In high-risk metropolitan areas, the process was expanded by using additional means, such as reports from health departments, to trigger LB. In an attempt to find individuals at risk more rapidly, the CDC recommended a broader alert to the public and medical community known as universal or general LB. Through wide-range communication and a public health campaign, transfusion recipients were advised to get tested for HIV. Some hospitals in high-risk areas also sent out letters to all transfusion recipients to alert them of the risk (34).

Due to the low yield and high cost of HIV LB, there was a great deal of debate regarding HCV LB in the early 1990s, with the availability of the first serologic assay. It was estimated that the yield might be even lower, recognizing that HCV had been present in the general population for decades and in a larger proportion than HIV. In addition, most people with HCV infection have less clinically significant and serious disease than those with HIV. The prevention of secondary infection was not as great a concern, either, since the sexual transmission of HCV is not very effective. The current state of knowledge suggested that the task should not be initiated (34). Implementation of HCV LB was ultimately deferred due to concerns that informing blood recipients without complete information might create more harm than good (13, 34).

In January 1998, Donna E. Shalala, the Secretary of the Department of Health and Human Services, endorsed the August 1997 recommendations of its Advisory Committee on Blood Safety and Availability regarding HCV LB. With more sensitive and specific testing for HCV available, a greater understanding of the virus, and new treatment options, it was felt that the time for HCV LB was upon us (2, 70). This intervention could improve the patient's prognosis by preventing further liver damage and disease progression (12). HCV LB was initiated in 1998 under guidance from the FDA (70).

As predicted, HCV LB has yielded poor results. When 85.5% of the initial phases of LB were complete, the CDC reported that only 1.5% of recipients targeted for notification found out about their HCV infections in this manner. It was concluded that targeted LB was of limited value and that other means needed to be used to identify the majority of people with disease acquired due to lifestyle (58). The yield in Quebec, Canada, was only slightly better, at about 3% (95).

Proponents of LB argue that it is the legal and ethical responsibility of the blood banking community to provide transfusion recipients any and all knowledge related to their health. Against the backdrop of previous concerns about blood safety, the public believes that it is their right to have all relevant information. Furthermore, this might renew the public's trust in the blood banking industry, by fully disclosing such information (12). Table 5.12 summarizes the pros and cons of LB.

PDI. Another method to prevent the transmission of disease during the infectious window period relies on donors reporting postdonation information (PDI). PDI is collected when a donor presents for donation and reports information putting previous donations at risk. As an example, a donor successfully donated 4 months ago. During a subsequent attempt to donate, the donor reveals that he got a tattoo 5 months ago, which requires a 12-month deferral. The donor is deferred, but there is concern about the status of recipients of the blood donated 4 months ago, 1 month after the tattoo. If the donor had been in a serosilent infectious window period, the product, though testing

negative, may have been capable of transmitting infection. To handle such situations, the FDA issued PDI guidance, through a memorandum in 1993, describing the process for blood manufacturing facilities to retrieve products and to notify the hospital of the possibility of the increased risk of that donation (68). The guidance does not address the process by which the transfusion facility evaluates the information and/or the process of recipient notification. Therefore, each transfusion service is able to develop its own policies and procedures.

Increases in testing and screening leading to decreases in supply. As mentioned earlier, there is increasing emphasis on regulatory compliance and safety. Due to heightened concerns, theoretical risks are being monitored and proactively addressed. New variant Creutzfeldt-Jakob disease provides an example of the response to an emerging pathogen with possible transfusion transmissibility. In November 2002, FDA guidance required the deferral of all donors who had been in the United Kingdom for 3 months from 1980 to 1996 and Europe for 5 years from 1980 to the present. This defers approximately 5% of current blood donors (67). Since 17 September 2001, the American Red Cross (ARC) has been deferring all donors who have been in the United Kingdom for 3 months and Europe for 6 months from 1980 to the present, estimated to cause the deferral of 8% of donors (7). New York, a state that imports 25% of its red blood cells from Europe, is bracing itself to face severe shortages (8, 128). Of interest, an article from the *Wall Street Journal* in August of 1999 entitled "Mad Regulatory Disease" focused on concerns of imposing new regulations on the ever-diminishing blood supply, without concrete evidence of transmissibility (137). The balance between safeguarding the blood supply from pathogens versus adequacy of supply is an ever-present theme as blood shortages in the United States are more common and last longer.

Shift to a pharmaceutical manufacturing model. In the 1960s and early 1970s, blood establishments were monitored by the National Institutes of Health, an arm of the Public Health Service. Their focus was on public health and research through a collegial relationship, not one of legal enforcement. It wasn't until 1973 that the FDA an-

Table 5.12 Pros and cons of LB

Pros	Cons
Public health initiative	Unnecessary anxiety for recipients
Inform people of their health	Low yield
Change people's lifestyles	High-risk people must donate again
Bring to medical attention	Record keeping dependent
Ethical and moral obligation to inform	Recipient died of underlying illness
Renew public's trust	Disease not acquired by transfusion

nounced that all blood banks, including hospital transfusion services, were required to register as drug manufacturers. The FDA began writing new regulations specifically applicable to blood establishments. Regulations used by the FDA are published in the *Code of Federal Regulations* (CFR) (98, 126).

In the middle to late 1980s, in response to the nightmare of HIV, the public and elected officials raised concerns about the processes and scrutiny being used to ensure a safe blood supply (126). The FDA, charged with the responsibility to monitor blood establishments and enforce regulations related to the production of blood and blood products, was also under the magnifying glass. Whereas the relationship between the FDA and blood banking community had been professional, it too changed, since the FDA was also being criticized for its role in the spread of HIV through the blood supply. As a result, the FDA in the late 1980s and early 1990s focused on enforcement. Inspections were conducted annually, and they were more thorough. The FDA began frequently citing blood manufacturers for their lack of process control and for QA deficiencies (101, 104, 126).

By 1992, the FDA's direction was clear. Previously, blood products were governed by 21 CFR 600, which classifies blood products as biologics, and 21 CFR 606, specifically outlining good manufacturing practices for blood and blood components. Suddenly, 21 CFR 210 and 211 were also enforced. Regulations that had previously been reserved for pharmaceutical manufacturers with details of QA requirements now applied to blood products. Blood was therefore classified as both a biologic and a drug (66). Since the FDA was finding problems in the areas of process control and QA, it felt that applying current good manufacturing practices (CGMP) from 21 CFR 210 and 211 would be the best way for blood manufacturers to improve their operations. This was especially important since blood manufacturing had become increasingly complex with the addition of new tests, computerization, and automated operations (48, 49, 50, 51, 104).

Pharmaceutical manufacturing facilities have been adhering to CGMP in compliance with 21 CFR 210 and 211. The most important aspect of CGMP is process control, which results from strict and consistent adherence to standard operating procedures (SOP). The elements of CGMP ensure that products are made the same way every time, resulting in safe, pure, potent, efficacious products (50, 51). A QA function is defined as being outside of technical operations, reporting independently and directly to management. This gives QA staff the ability and authority to report serious infractions outside of the operational chain of command and to shut down production and/or product release when deemed necessary (69). The QA group must make sure that personnel follow CGMP. The QA group monitors all aspects of SOP development, training, and education, competency and proficiency training, validation, audits, error and accident reporting (as is discussed in greater detail below), and product release. The QA group audits manufacturing operations and defines critical control points (4, 69, 104, 120).

Manufacturers also have product specifications with manufacturing pathways that identify and clearly define the critical steps, or critical control points, of the process. Documentation is an essential part of CGMP, so that each step of the process can be recreated as necessary. An individual designated the responsible head is identified. This individual is responsible for ensuring compliance with the CFR and enforcing discipline and proper performance of all individuals engaged in manufacturing. The responsible head must understand the principles and techniques of the manufacturing process and serve as the establishment's representative to the FDA (104).

By adopting CGMP, many pharmaceutical manufacturers have been able to perform complex operations while providing safe, pure, potent, and efficacious products. It was theorized that using the same principles for blood manufacturing should produce the same results. It is essential to have control of the manufacturing process to provide the highest-quality, safest blood products (25, 101, 104, 120).

Defining blood manufacturing as equivalent to pharmaceutical manufacturing was not straightforward and was consequently met with resistance (25, 101, 104, 126). The most apparent incongruity was trying to apply the regulations that outlined requirements for product release of manufactured goods. Usually in a pharmaceutical operation, these relate to groupings of goods coming off a production line. In blood manufacturing, since the source material is an individual blood donor, the same processes are hard to apply. Since each unit of blood comes from a different donor, the units aren't uniform and cannot be "manufactured" in a consistent process each time (126).

There was also concern that by placing so much emphasis on conformity and process control, other important aspects of transfusion medicine would be overlooked. Instead of spending time working on new and innovative therapies, practitioners would be sidelined into regulatory concerns, leading to stagnation. Furthermore, the innovative and creative technologists and physicians would be attracted by the greater intellectual freedom of other disciplines and turned away by the mundane, bureaucratic field of transfusion medicine (101).

Opponents to this reclassification also feared that creating a manufacturing arm, with a mission different from that of the patient-oriented hospital transfusion service, would create a rift. The two "sides" of the profession would be no longer colleagues but different sides of a supply-demand relationship. Another consequence might be that clinical colleagues would rely less on the consultative services of transfusion medicine specialists, who would be viewed as "product oriented," nonclinical decision makers (25, 101).

The not-for-profit status of the majority of blood collection facilities also sets them apart from their pharmaceutical counterparts. Concern has been voiced that regulatory actions due to violations of procedures that are not truly related to patient safety could have serious effects on the already tenuous blood supply (126). This is in addition to the added cost of implementing CGMP (101).

Regulatory Organizations That Specifically Impact Transfusion Medicine

AABB. The AABB was established in 1947 as an international association of blood banks whose mission is "to establish and promote the highest standard of care for patients and donors in all aspects of blood banking; transfusion medicine; hematopoietic, cellular and gene therapies; and tissue transplantation." Its membership boasts more than 2,200 institutions (community and hospital blood banks, hospital transfusion services, and laboratories) and 8,500 individuals comprising physicians, scientists, administrators, medical technologists, blood donor recruiters, and public relations personnel. It supports voluntary donation of blood and tissue and supports high standards of medical, technical, and administrative performance, scientific investigation, clinical application, and education. The committees and board of directors are comprised of volunteer members, as described in the Association's website, http://www.aabb.org (accessed 10 July 2003).

The AABB publishes the "Standards for Blood Banks and Transfusion Services," which are updated every 18 months. The standards are written by experts in blood banking and transfusion medicine and are consistent with FDA regulations. The AABB maintains a voluntary accreditation program, based on its standards, with voluntary compliance activities that began in 1957. The Association is currently working on a different set of standards that can be used for International Organization for Standardization (ISO) certification. ISO certification is being granted to various blood establishments (103).

The AABB Accreditation Program "strives to improve the quality and safety of collecting, processing, testing, distributing and administering blood and blood products." This voluntary inspection program serves as an independent assessment of the facility's compliance with Standards, CFR, and other federal regulations. The AABB's program has deemed status for CLIA '88. In addition, the AABB conducts proficiency testing programs in coordination with CAP, provides a variety of educational venues, and publishes textbooks as well as the journal *Transfusion*. Additional information about these programs is available at http://www.aabb.org (accessed 20 January 2003).

The AABB Standards require that blood banks and transfusion services establish and maintain a quality system (78). The responsibility for the supervision of the quality system must be given to a specific individual who reports to upper-level management. The program must contain essential elements as listed in Table 5.13. Full implementation of a quality program was required of all AABB-accredited facilities by 1 January 1998. The focus of full implementation was to change the approach from one of detection of errors to one of prevention of errors, in accordance with requirements put forth by the FDA in 1995. The essentials required were consistent with both the AABB Quality Program and the FDA's QA requirements (4, 69). In distinction from the FDA's 1995 requirements, the AABB required transfusion service members, not just manufacturers of blood and blood components, to develop their own quality programs. It's also interesting that the AABB voluntary standards were written in 1957, 18 years before federal CGMP for blood and blood components were published by the FDA. Also, some parts of the CFR refer to AABB Standards (120).

Despite the voluntary nature of its activities, the AABB is legally responsible for its standard-setting activities, according to one recent court ruling. In 1996 the New Jersey Supreme Court upheld a lower court ruling and found that the AABB breached its duty when providing care to a man who was infected with HIV following transfusion in 1984. Since the AABB was a standard-setting organization and did not require certain surrogate tests that *might* have detected HIV in 1984, it was found to be negligent and liable for 30% of the patient's injury. The AABB has expressed concerns about the impact of this decision on its role in protecting the nation's blood supply (9). (A case summary is available at the website for the Rutgers School of Law, http://lawlibrary.Rutgers.edu [accessed 20 January 2003].)

Table 5.13 Essential elements of a quality system[a]

Organization. The facility must be organized so the quality system can be implemented.

Resources. Personnel, training, and competency assessment process.

Equipment. Process of management and installation qualification.

Supplier and customer issues. Qualifications, contracts, and inventory control.

Process control, final inspection, and handling. To include change control and validation of key processes.

Documents and records. Creation, approval, and management process.

Incident, error, and accident management. Procedures and processes to manage.

Internal and external assessment programs. Audits, quality monitoring, and how to respond to external assessments.

Process improvement. Correction as well as preventative action.

Facilities and safety. Disaster preparedness program and employee safety.

[a]See reference 32.

FDA. In stark contrast to the role of the AABB, the FDA has enforcement power over blood establishments. The FDA has been a part of the DHHS since 1979 and is authorized by Congress to enforce the Federal Food, Drug and Cosmetic Act. The FDA's mission is to "promote and protect the public health by helping safe and effective products reach the market in a timely way, and monitoring products for continued safety after they are in use." On its website, it describes its work as a "blending of law and science aimed at protecting consumers" (http://www.fda.gov [accessed 20 January 2003]).

The Center for Biologics Evaluation and Research (CBER) is a center of the FDA whose mission is to "protect and enhance the public health through regulation of biological products including blood, vaccines, therapeutics and related drugs and devices according to statutory authorities. The regulation of these products is founded on science and law to ensure their purity, potency, safety, efficacy, and availability." As such, CBER can be viewed as the "blood arm" of the FDA. Its role is to ensure compliance with laws and regulations through review, education, surveillance, and enforcement. (The website for CBER is available at http://www.fda.gov/cber [accessed 20 January 2003].) CBER regulates biological products under the authority of the Public Health Service Act and specific sections of the Federal Food, Drug and Cosmetic Act. The safety of this nation's entire blood supply and the products derived from it falls into the realm of CBER's responsibility.

As an example of the FDA's regulatory posture, in the late 1980s, it expressed concern over the ARC's lack of regulatory compliance. In 1988 the ARC entered into a consent agreement with the FDA, promising that it would take steps toward tightening its operations (98, 104). Other blood collection facilities were also under increased scrutiny, but the ARC, representing 45% of the nation's blood supply, was by far the largest (98). The FDA issued additional warnings to the ARC, and the ARC began the process of a major reorganization, separating blood services from the rest of its operations. This reorganization began "transformation," focusing on enhancing their computer system, revamping their training programs, and revising SOP to create both national and local-level compliance with CGMP. The ARC named a responsible head and worked on a QA program. The Council of Community Blood Centers members (now called America's Blood Centers), representing a large number of independent blood centers, also worked on meeting full regulatory compliance (104).

Despite progress, the FDA still felt that the ARC was not meeting the full extent of the law. On 12 May 1993, the FDA turned up the heat and invoked a consent decree on the ARC. A consent decree is a formal, binding enforceable court order requiring full compliance. If violated, a party can be found guilty of contempt of court. The consent decree cited deficiencies in QA, training, computer and database review, record review, record management, error and

accident investigation, adverse-transfusion-reaction investigation, transfusion-transmitted-disease investigations, and LB procedures. It also required that the ARC implement an internal audit system. If the ARC complied with the terms for 5 years, the consent decree would be terminated. As of today, the ARC remains under consent decree. In December 2001, the FDA asked a federal court to hold the ARC in contempt of the 1993 consent decree, citing recent inspections that revealed serious and persistent violations (6). The ARC vigorously refuted the claims made by the FDA, citing its continued progress in all areas of the consent decree and declaring the FDA's actions irresponsible. Though the ARC is the largest and most visible blood manufacturer under consent decree, it is not the only one. As one example, the New York Blood Center entered into a voluntary consent decree with the FDA in 1996 (3).

JCAHO. JCAHO is an independent, not-for-profit organization, formed in 1951, that sets standards for healthcare facilities. JCAHO evaluates and accredits nearly 18,000 healthcare organizations and programs in the United States. Its mission is "to continuously improve the safety and quality of care provided to the public through the provision of healthcare accreditation and related services that support performance improvement in healthcare organizations." An organization must be inspected every 3 years in order to maintain JCAHO accreditation; laboratories are inspected at 2-year intervals in order to maintain compliance with CLIA '88. As with AABB accreditation, JCAHO accreditation is a symbol of an organization's commitment to excellence. Accreditation may also result in secondary benefits such as competitive advantages and greater confidence in the accredited organization by the community. (The JCAHO website is available at http://www.jcaho.org [accessed 10 July 2003].)

Blood and blood products are covered in standards that have broader intent. As an example, JCAHO Standard PI.3.1 requires organizations to collect data to monitor their performance. Within this standard are the requirements to use data to monitor adverse transfusion reactions and identify performance measures related to the use of blood and blood components. Standard MS.8.4 requires peer review of practices in order to improve organization-wide performance (90). To comply with this standard, peer review of blood and blood product usage is usually accomplished through a hospital transfusion committee that monitors the use of blood and blood products against institutional guidelines. Requirements for informed consent are also addressed by JCAHO standards, available at http://www.jcaho.org (accessed 10 July 2003).

Biological Product Deviation Reporting

In the manufacturing facility and transfusion service. Through CGMP the FDA requires all licensed manufacturers of biological products to report errors and accidents affecting the safety, purity, or potency (SPP) of a product to the FDA. (FDA guidance is available at http://www.fda.gov/cber/gdlns/devnbld.htm [accessed 20 January 2003].) On 7 May 2001, the FDA added 21 CFR 606.171 to extend this requirement to unlicensed registered establishments and transfusion services. 21 CFR 606.171 and 21 CFR 600.14 also changed the terminology of errors and accidents to biological product deviations. When a deviation occurs, any blood establishment that has control of a blood product must report such deviations to the FDA within 45 days if the deviation affects the SPP of a distributed product. Distributed products are those that have left the control of the blood establishment. As an example, when a courier comes to pick up a product, and a deviation affecting SPP is discovered before the courier leaves the area but after the product has been released to the courier, this becomes an FDA-reportable occurrence. Control is defined as having responsibility for maintaining a product's continued SPP and compliance with applicable product and establishment standards and CGMP requirements. The events must also represent a deviation from either CGMP, applicable regulations, applicable standards, or established specifications, or must be unforeseen or unexpected occurrences (48, 49, 53, 54).

This highlights the inclusion of the transfusion service as a part of the manufacturing of blood, having responsibility for compatibility testing, processing, packing, labeling, and final distribution of the product (60). When deviations meeting the requirements for reporting are discovered, a biological product deviation report, form FDA-3486, must be completed. Alternately, the deviation can be reported online on the FDA's website. (The form can be found at http://www.fda.gov/cber/biodev/bpdrform.pdf [accessed 20 January 2003].) As part of the reporting process, the initiator assigns a code to characterize the deviation so it can be tracked and trended.

Processing a biological product deviation. For deviations that occur before the product has left control of the blood establishment, the FDA does not need to be informed, but the transfusion service must investigate the deviation. These reports are subject to review during an inspection. The FDA expects a thorough investigation of the cause. In order to have a standardized process, institutional SOP need to be written for this activity. The process should include the mode of documentation of the occurrence, how the cause of the occurrence is investigated, who has responsibility for each step of the process, and how the information is used to prevent future occurrences of the same problem. The steps of the process are summarized in Table 5.14. An algorithm for evaluating each deviation, developed by the FDA, is presented in Figure 5.1. The process of root cause analysis can be used to determine the true underlying or "root cause" of the deviation, not necessarily

Table 5.14 Steps in processing biological product deviations

Identification of deviation—if reportable, must report within 45 days

Documentation of deviation

Immediate corrective action

Investigation of deviation (may involve root cause analysis)

Tracking of deviations

Looking for trends in deviations

Implementing corrective action

Monitoring for effectiveness of corrective action

QA oversight

the most obvious cause. During root cause analysis a group of people delve into the occurrence in a predetermined fashion by asking sequential questions or using standard diagram techniques (99). The AABB's quality program also requires error and accident tracking as well as root cause analysis (32).

The intent of tracking deviations is to improve quality, improve patient outcomes and prevent future deviations (127). The best way to detect these deviations is to encourage employees to report such occurrences in a nonpunitive environment. These principles have been successfully applied outside of medicine, the most well-known forum being the aviation industry. By not just identifying errors but also gaining an understanding of their myriad causes, a true opportunity for process improvement is captured (23).

With a grant from the National Heart, Lung, and Blood Institute, a group of investigators developed a medical event reporting system for transfusion medicine (MERS-TM). (The website for MERS-TM is available at http://www. mers-tm.net [accessed 20 January 2003].) On a Web-based platform, different institutions can anonymously submit their own deviations or events to the database. The information is collected in a standardized fashion, classified using the same categories as the FDA requires and analyzes. The data are then used to study the events reported across organizations in order to "facilitate process improvement efforts." This also enables participants to benchmark their own operations in comparison to others. It is emphasized that only by creating a just culture, where employees can safely report deviations without fear of reprisal, will such a system work effectively. According to the website, "The goal is not to punish people for errors, but rather to prevent the events from recurring." The system has been described in detail elsewhere, and preliminary results have been reported (16, 91).

The Cost of Increasing Regulatory Oversight

Implementation of safety initiatives in conjunction with regulatory requirements is a costly endeavor. Data associating the costs incurred by meeting regulatory compliance are scarce. In this era of cost containment, many employees are asked to add new tasks to their current workload. The true allocation of their time for compliance functions is

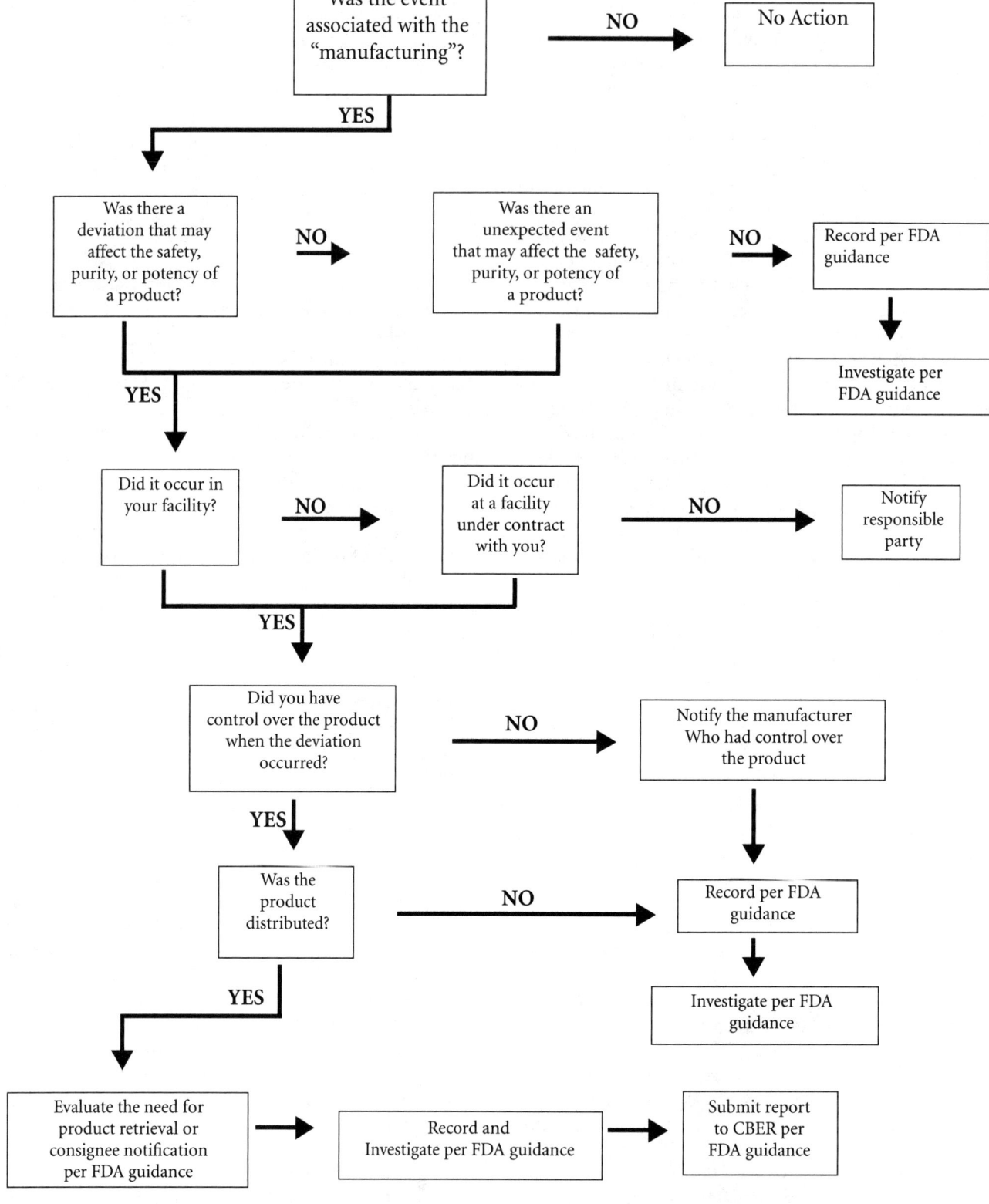

Figure 5.1 Process for evaluating biological product deviations. Available from the FDA, CBER.

hard to capture, since it is "fit" into the rest of their responsibilities. Adding new personnel for compliance functions is more straightforward.

One of the few studies looking at the staff costs associated with implementing a compliance program was performed at a community blood center between 1989 and 1994 (123). In order to maintain compliance and keep the organization on track, the blood center initially hired someone with the sole responsibility of compliance officer. With time, it was necessary to create a separate compliance department. In addition, department heads and other employees within the operational structure devoted increasing time and energy to the effort. A list of activities that comprise "compliance" appears in Table 5.15. During this period, the number of full-time employees dedicated to compliance rose from 7 to 24, with compensation costs rising from $367,000 to $1,298,900. These data focus on personnel cost, but there were additional costs associated with the raw materials necessary for the program. Menitove estimated that on a yearly basis, training in itself might actually occupy about 10% of an employee's time (101).

Of course, there is no alternative to maintaining regulatory compliance. In fact, with the goal of compliance being the maintenance of CGMP, the consequences of poor quality can be quite onerous and costly, from the patient care perspective as well as the blood center perspective. Recalling and withdrawing blood products can incur additional expense (22). Whether or not increasing regulatory compliance leads to an increasingly safe transfusion is unknown (119).

Specific programs aimed at blood safety, as well as their regulatory components, are also cited as increasing the cost of transfusion. As blood gets safer, attempts to further decrease the risks of pathogen transmission come at a higher cost per infection saved (35, 105, 119). In 1999, NAT was introduced to donor blood screening under experimental protocol. Testing is done on samples that are pools of individual donor samples. NAT, as pointed out earlier, has reduced the risk of transmitting HIV and HCV through transfusion (129). NAT for HIV and HCV is now mandated by the FDA. However, using quality-adjusted life year (QALY), expenditures for testing each donation (in contrast to the current pool testing) by NAT will come to about $2 million per QALY gained, far exceeding usually acceptable levels of $50,000 per QALY for most other healthcare initiatives (24, 77, 105).

One of the concerns of the blood industry and the medical system has been that reimbursement for blood and blood products has not kept up with the cost of these new initiatives. In December 2001, the Medicare Payment Advisory Commission (MedPac) released the results of a study to Congress entitled, "Blood Safety in Hospitals and Medicare Inpatient Payment." This report, requested by Congress, looked at the implementation of new safety initiatives such as NAT and leukoreduction. It also accounted for the increasing cost of recruiting donors in the face of a shrinking donor base due to implementation of new safety initiatives, such as deferrals for new variant Creutzfeldt-Jakob disease, and future initiatives, such as pathogen inactivation. The commission unanimously voted to recommend that future Medicare payments "account for blood and blood products by reintroducing a separate component for their prices" (100). (The report is available on MedPac's website at http://www.medpac.gov [accessed 20 January 2003].)

Regulation of Laboratory Business Practices

The federal government's Medicare and Medicaid program is administered by the CMS, a division of the DHHS. Medicare is the single largest payor for healthcare services. CMS maintains the Uniform Bill (UB-92), institutional and professional electronic medical chart format specifications, and other specifications for various certifications and authorizations used by the Medicare and Medicaid programs. CMS also maintains the Healthcare Common Procedural Coding System (HCPCS) medical code set and the Medicare Remittance Advice Remark Codes administrative code set.

Negotiated Rule Making Process

Negotiated rule making describes the process of federal agency representatives and other special interest groups convening to negotiate the text of a proposed rule. A committee, with members from each participating group, develops the language for any proposed regulation before it appears in the *Federal Register* for comment. Congress has

Table 5.15 Typical compliance functions within blood centers and transfusion medicine services

Competency assessment

Documentation of all operational activities

Error and accident reporting

Implementation of new regulatory requirements

Inspections
    Preparation
    Hosting

Internal audits

LB

SOP
    Standardizing
    Writing
    Regular review

Quality control and its documentation

Training: performance and documentation
    Regulatory training
    CGMP training
    Task training

passed three generations of regulatory legislation to offer guidance to healthcare providers:

- Model Compliance Plan in 1984
- Model Compliance Plan for Clinical Laboratories in July 1997 (available at http://oig.hhs.gov/fraud/docs/complianceguidance/cpcl.html [accessed April 2003])
- Model Compliance Plan for Hospitals in February 1998

Copies of the programs are available through professional associations and are published in the United States Code (USC) and the *Federal Register* (CFR).

Corporate Compliance

Corporate compliance has evolved over the last four decades. Starting as a movement to curtail price-fixing and other antitrust violations, it has developed into a quest to solve the national healthcare debt created by fraud and abuse. The Office of the Inspector General (OIG) developed the first Model Compliance Plan after the Reform Act of 1984 was enacted. In February 1998, the Model Compliance Program for Hospitals was released; it included essentially the same elements as the Model Compliance Plan for Clinical Laboratories released in 1997. The Model Compliance Plans for Laboratories and Hospitals are sets of guidelines used to evaluate past behavior and implement policies and procedures for future compliance. The government recognizes that it cannot discover and eliminate every instance of fraud and abuse in healthcare. The intent is for healthcare organizations, laboratories, and providers to police themselves through self-regulation, self-audit, and self-reporting and to proactively practice prevention. Compliance is enterprise-wide attitude, culture, and commitment that support honesty, integrity, and diligence in the workplace.

Key Elements of a Model Compliance Plan for Hospitals

The Compliance Program Guidance for Hospitals developed by the OIG suggests that these key elements be addressed in the compliance plan (63):

- *The chief compliance officer* is typically a high-level individual in the organization authorized to develop, oversee, administer, and monitor any necessary regulatory compliance policies and committees. This individual generally reports directly to the chief executive officer.

  - Other appropriate bodies like the compliance committee consist of representatives from operations, finance, audit, human resources, utilization review, social work, discharge planning, medicine, coding, and legal. Key managers from areas like laboratory and radiology should serve on the compliance committee.

  - The compliance office must have authority to review documents and information that relate to compliance issues.

- *Employee ethics guidelines and standards of conduct.* Human resource policies should include expected behaviors and standards of conduct related to regulations and guidelines for federally funded programs and fraud and abuse. A mission statement that defines the organization's core values and commitment is essential. Hospitals are charged with developing and distributing written policies that identify areas of risk to the hospital and include the following:

  - Written standards of conduct for employees
  - Development of policies addressing areas of risk to regulatory exposure
  - Claim development and submission
  - Medical necessity must be demonstrated by the provider and certified on the claim form.
  - Avoidance of antikickback and self-referral violations created when referrals are made to designated health services in which the physician or an immediate family member may have a financial interest
  - Bad debts
  - Credit balances occur when hospitals fail to refund overpayments by Medicare.
  - Record retention for matters related to compliance is governed by CLIA '88.

- *Education and training programs.* All personnel should be required to attend ethics education and standards-of-conduct training initially. New employees and existing staff must sign a certifying statement following compliance training that indicates thorough understanding of the standards. The compliance office generally maintains these records. Thereafter, managers, supervisors, and employees who interact regularly should receive annual retraining. Annual performance evaluations should include a monitor for measuring adherence, with distinct guidelines for disciplinary actions, including termination when indicated.

- *Compliance communication.* The compliance officer should design a program that ensures each employee's anonymity and guarantees that the lines of communication are open 24 h per day and 7 days per week, without fear of reprisal for any effort to identify or report compliance policy violations or problems. Hospitals should also post in a prominent area the DHHS-OIG hotline telephone number: 1-800-HHS-TIPS (447-8477). Institutions should maintain an anonymous hotline and document all incoming calls in a log. Compliance programs should strictly prohibit the use of termination, demotion, and disciplinary action against employees who report suspected violations.

- *Quality monitors and audits.* An ongoing evaluation process is an essential element of a successful compliance program. Regular, periodic, and random inspections by internal and external auditors should review a random sampling to detect significant variation or deviation from a baseline in each of the areas of risk to exposure as cited above under "Employee Ethics Guidelines and Standards of Conduct." The monitor should include any reserves the hospital may have established for payments that it may owe to Medicare, Medicaid, TRICARE, and other federally funded programs.

- *Disclosure.* Development of a system to respond to allegations of improper activities. Whenever the compliance office becomes aware of any potential employee misconduct or an incorrect claim submission resulting in an erroneous overpayment, it is imperative that a prompt investigation be conducted, in order to make a decision to disclose the misconduct within the 60-day reasonable reporting period allowed by the government. Prompt voluntary unsolicited repayment within 30 days of the finding will eliminate potential exposure to possible fraud and abuse allegations. Repayment is the remedy when the government overpayment is the result of a one-time billing error. If an investigation uncovers a systematic billing problem, you should consult an attorney and consider self-disclosure.

- *Develop policies* to investigate and eliminate systematic problems, including the retention of sanctioned individuals.

Model compliance plan for laboratories. Both the hospital and laboratory must develop and distribute policies that demonstrate a commitment to employee training in areas of marketing, medical necessity, billing, and coding and processing of claims. Key elements include the following:

- Laboratories should design the order screens and requisitions to include approved panels and indicate the need to demonstrate medical necessity when ordering additional individual automated chemistry tests.

- Laboratories should send annual notices to referring physicians that contain the following information:
  - Medicare pays only for medically necessary testing.
  - Lists of Medicare-approved panels and their components
  - HCPCS and Current Procedural Terminology (CPT) codes used to bill for the panels
  - National limitation amount for the tests (also referred to as Medicare expect)
  - How Medicare will be billed for the service

- Physicians who request that laboratories develop custom panels for their patients must acknowledge in writing on an annual basis that they understand the components and billing mechanisms for the profiles.

- Laboratories should monitor the utilization pattern for high-volume testing and investigate shifts in frequency of more than 10% to determine the reason.

- Claims for testing services submitted to Medicare must be correctly coded to avoid charges of false claims.

- Physicians are charged to establish medical necessity and provide the correct diagnosis code (ICD-9 code) for the test order to the laboratory.

- Laboratories must ensure that any claim submitted has a corresponding test order and report.

- Do not bill for both calculations and the underlying tests. The OIG considers this double billing.

Laboratory marketing: compliance issues. Marketing efforts by the laboratory should be honest, clear, correct, straightforward, and informative. Laboratories are prohibited from offering inducements to physicians to gain business. Specifically, laboratories must ensure that physicians are never charged below fair market value for referred testing to avoid the risk of allegations of kickback. Physicians should never be offered lower prices for non-Medicare patients in exchange for obtaining Medicare business that is reimbursed at a higher rate. The laboratory supplies provided to a physician's office should also be scrutinized carefully. Equipment like centrifuges, printers, and faxes must be for the purposes of specimen preparation and result reporting. The laboratory and physician should sign a document that supports the terms and conditions of supplies and equipment provided by the laboratory. The laboratory should have a system to monitor abuse or excessive use of any supply provided.

The Legal Environment

The OIG's position is one of zero tolerance. The office expects a healthcare institution to promote and adhere to compliance at all levels and that noncompliance will not be tolerated.

The government can potentially file charges under the Civil False Claims Act for a period of up to 10 years. The compliance program should synchronize the institution's record retention policies to conform to government regulations. In a 1995 status report (114) issued by the OIG and the Department of Justice joint project, three tiers of penalties were established for hospitals which submit false claims. The tiers are dependent on the extent of the problem in relationship to its size (Table 5.16).

Qui tam provisions of the Civil False Claims Act, which originated during the Civil War, give knowledgeable private citizens the ability to file lawsuits on behalf of the federal government and to share in any recovered damages. From 1987 to 1996, whistle-blower cases filed by current employees, employees with grievances, or competitors alleging individual or corporate healthcare fraud against the federal government increased nearly 1,000%. Federal

Table 5.16 Hospital financial exposure

Tier 1

A hospital's payment or penalty was equal to the potential overpayments plus interest.

Tier 2

Payment or penalty was equal to 100% of potential overpayment plus interest.

Tier 3

Payment or penalty was equal to 300% (treble damage) of potential overpayment plus interest.

prosecutors take advantage of the provisions since they require the lower standard of preponderance of evidence but authorize damages and penalties of $5,000 to $10,000 for each false claim submitted. Over the years, whistle-blowers have received an average of 18% of the total amount recovered by the government in these suits.

The Physician Self-Referral Law, commonly referred to as the Stark Law, originated in 1989. It prohibits doctors from making referrals to an entity for the provision of laboratory services if they or their immediate family have a financial relationship with that entity. Submission of Medicare claims when the ordering physician has a business arrangement with the laboratory is forbidden unless it fits the exception list as defined in the law. The Stark II legislation expanded the law to cover 10 other categories, including physical and occupational therapy, radiology, radiation therapy, durable medical equipment services and supplies, prosthetic devices and supplies, home health services, parenteral and enteral nutrients, outpatient prescription drugs, and inpatient and outpatient hospital services (82). The "Phase I Rules" of Stark II included modification to key terms like referral, indirect financial relationships, indirect referrals, and volume or value of referrals and the definition of group practice. The most significant additions to the Stark I legislation include new exceptions to prohibitions for fair market value, academic medical centers, and nonmonetary compensation.

The antikickback statutes specifically forbid individuals from either seeking, receiving, offering, or paying any compensation (bribe or rebate) in exchange for a referral or for the purpose of purchasing or leasing of goods and services covered by payments from a federally funded program. Inducement is inferred when a laboratory provides anything of value, not paid for at fair market value, to a provider who has a referring relationship with the laboratory. The OIG could consider the following as inducements:

- Provision of phlebotomists who provide other clerical services
- Picking up of biohazard materials unrelated to specimen collection

- Providing medical supplies and equipment not related to testing referred to the lab
- Provision of computers, printers, and faxes unless exclusively used for the outside laboratory's work
- Providing free POL consultation
- Waiving managed-care patient charges in order to retain the client's referral work
- Professional courtesy (free healthcare testing) to the provider and office staff

Violators are subject to criminal penalties and/or exclusion from participating in the federally funded healthcare programs.

Safe-harbor regulations. The Medicare and Medicaid Patient and Program Protection Act directed the agency to give healthcare providers assurance that they would not be prosecuted for engaging in certain practices where they assumed compliance while acting in good faith. Arrangements that may qualify under the regulation include certain investment interests, equipment or space rental agreements, management service contracts, manufacturer's warranty, and gain sharing. Gain sharing results when a hospital agrees to share with a provider a fair market share or percentage of any measurable reduction in costs for patient care where quality and performance criteria were met and said reductions could be directly attributed to the efforts of the provider.

The OIG from time to time issues special fraud alerts to assist contractors and providers who participate in federal programs. (These alerts are also available on the OIG website at http://oig.hhs.gov/fraud/fraudalerts.html [accessed April 2003].)

Legal sanctions. When cited for violations of any of the regulations, sanctions could include denial of payment, refund of monies collected when billed in violation, civil monetary penalties of $15,000/claim and exclusion, civil penalties of $100,000 and exclusion for cross-referral billing schemes, and civil penalties of $10,000/day for failure to report. The *Cumulative Sanction Report* reflects the status of healthcare providers who are excluded from participation in federally funded programs. This report is produced monthly by the OIG and is available on the OIG's website. The General Services Administration also maintains a monthly list of debarred contractors. (The list is posted on the OIG website at http://oig.hhs.gov/fraud/exclusions.html [accessed April 2003].) Hospitals may request information from this data bank as a part of the employee recruitment, screening, and credentialing process.

Settlement agreements. Corporate integrity agreements (CIAs) are executed as a result of a civil settlement between the government and a healthcare provider based on alleged fraud and abuse under the Civil False Claims Act, including qui tam. The most compelling reason for a provider to enter into a CIA is to avoid exclusion from federal programs. Although the government has standard CIA boilerplate agreement, it is in the facility's best interest to work toward developing an agreement that avoids a broad-brush approach using language that closely follows the hospital's existing compliance program, concentrating on the issues prompting the investigation. Over time CIAs have become more rigorous, and they now impose longer terms of duration, investigate a wider span of issues, and include elaborate and expensive provisions and expanded internal and external monitoring of CIA compliance (74).

Impact of compliance on healthcare providers. Facilities should design compliance programs that strive to create a culture that promotes prevention, detection, and resolution of any occurrence that does not comply with federal, state, or private payor healthcare program guidelines (31). The benefits of having an effective program outweigh the managerial costs incurred to establish and administer a compliance program. Healthcare organizations with established compliance plans, that prevent or detect violations and identify employee misconduct prior to an investigation, substantially reduce their exposure to criminal penalties.

Federal sentencing guidelines. Believing that the federal court's sentences for organizations were unfair and unpredictable, under legislation known as the Reform Act of 1984, Congress authorized the creation of a Federal Sentencing Commission to establish guidelines for judges to use in sentencing individuals (first issued in 1987) and organizations (in November 1991). Having a compliance program becomes most valuable when there is a clear understanding of how fines are determined under the sentencing guidelines.

Civil monetary penalties. The complex system of civil monetary penalties enables the government to clearly define the guidelines for an effective compliance plan in the clinical laboratory and the hospital setting (64). After the seriousness of an offense is analyzed, a base fine is determined. Then the organization is scrutinized for the degree of responsibility and degree of involvement of management in the commission of the acts to determine the overall culpability score. These two factors are used to calculate the guideline fine range used by the courts to set the amount of the overall fine. A well-established compliance program shields the healthcare provider from suffering longer sentences or harsher penalties. Under the federal sentencing guidelines, the culpability score for a company being prosecuted for a violation would be reduced by as much as 95% when a corporate compliance program is in effect (62). The challenge is to provide and document evidence of the plan's effectiveness, targeting training as the key.

Laboratory Reimbursement and Medical Necessity

Medicare

In 1999, the DHHS established CMS, formerly known as the Health Care Financing Administration, to provide operational oversight and administer guidance to third-party healthcare contractors.

Medicare contractors: third-party payors. CMS contracts with third-party contractors to administer federally funded programs like Medicare and the Civilian Health and Medical Program of the Uniformed Services (CHAMPUS). The Medicaid program is administered cooperatively between the DHHS and state agencies. The contractors are generally companies whose business is the administration of insurance plans. They must demonstrate financial solvency, adequate infrastructure, and a satisfactory record of service to be awarded a government contract.

- A fiscal intermediary is a primary third-party contractor who administers Part A payments according to policies for hospitals, rehabilitation centers, and skilled-nursing facilities.
- A primary third-party contractor who administers Part B payments according to the policy for physician, ancillary, and commercial laboratory providers is known as a carrier.

Provider designation, responsibilities, and agreements. In order to be designated a Medicare provider, a healthcare facility must first define the types of services being offered as either a hospital, clinical laboratory, rural health clinic, skilled-nursing facility or home health agency. Survey agencies in each state certify that each provider meets the statutory regulations governing the conditions of participation defined by the program (Table 5.17). The Medicare Provider Agreement application is Form 1561. Laboratories as participating suppliers are required to accept the assigned Medicare fee schedule reimbursement as payment in full. The limiting charge covered by Section 1848(g) of the Social Security Act applies to claims submitted by nonparticipating physicians or suppliers who do not accept payment on an assignment-related basis for physician services (30a).

Hospital inpatient services: Medicare Part A. In general, Medicare Part A covers the following services provided to qualified Medicare beneficiaries:

- Services related to a hospital inpatient stay
- Services provided in a skilled-nursing facility
- Home health or hospice services
- End-stage renal disease (ESRD) services

Table 5.17 Medicare provider designation[a]

Provider designation	Certifying agency(ies)	Conditions of participation[a]
Hospital	JCAHO, AOA	Utilization review
		Staffing for psychiatric
		Adhere to DHHS standards or higher
Clinical laboratory	CLIA '88	CLIA certificate current and unrevoked
		No participation agreement needed
		Must accept assignment for negotiated Part B reimbursements
Rural health clinic	Federally qualified healthcare center; 42	Not physician directed
		Located in rural area
		Providers: Participating (Par) and Non-Participating (Non-Par)
Skilled-nursing facility	42 U.S.C. §1395I-3	Participation agreement

[a]See reference 30a.

Medicare excludes, or does not cover, items like most prescription drugs, long-term care, and custodial care in a nursing or private home.

Medicare payments for hospital inpatient stays are reimbursed using the diagnosis related group (DRG), a prospective payment system (PPS). The *Medicare Hospital Manual* contains billing and coding guidelines for Medicare Part A. The Balanced Budget Act of 1997 included a provision to move skilled-nursing facility Medicare payments for Part A and B services to a PPS referred to as consolidated billing (28). In 2000, the Benefits Improvement and Protection Act (BIPA) limited the scope of consolidated billing to the services covered under Part A for skilled bed care, and the payment is referred to as resource utilization group.

Three-day (72-h window) rule. CMS issued the final DRG "72-h window" rule in February 1998; it states that the hospital's inpatient costs are reimbursed by Medicare Part A under the PPS that pays an established rate for all services during the stay, including diagnostic testing. An institution's billing service must ensure that claims are never submitted for any outpatient testing performed by the facility's laboratory within three calendar days of a hospital admission if the services are furnished directly in connection with the admitting diagnosis and are covered by PPS payment (113). Separate payment is not allowed for the following:

- Any nonphysician outpatient service rendered on the day of the admission or during the inpatient stay
- Diagnostic services rendered up to 72 h before the day of admission
- Admission-related nondiagnostic services rendered up to 72 h before the day of admission

Outpatient services: Medicare Part B. Medicare Part B covers physician and other outpatient healthcare services, including the following:

- Physician services and services incident to physician services

- Ancillary services (clinical lab testing, home health services, rehab services, and ambulatory surgical services)

Hospital-based laboratories that perform outpatient and nonpatient testing submit Medicare UB-92 claims as Part A reimbursement to the fiscal intermediary but actually receive payment based on the Medicare Part B fee schedule for the services. The *Medicare Carrier's Manual* contains billing and coding guidelines for independent labs, group practices, and POLs that are useful when filling claims for Part B services.

Outreach (nonpatient) testing. Hospital laboratories provide services to three different patient types: inpatients, outpatients, and nonpatients. Classification of a patient as a hospital inpatient is a straightforward process. Differentiating between an outpatient and a nonpatient is more difficult but very important, since the applicable rules are not the same. The *Medicare Intermediary Manual* describes nonpatient testing as collection of tissue or blood samples or specimens by personnel who are not employed by the hospital who send them to the hospital for testing. Sometimes laboratories are governed by hospital regulations, but there are also instances when the independent laboratory regulations apply.

Tax-exempt hospitals are subject to taxation on their unrelated business income (UBI) for outreach testing activities, because outreach testing activities are not substantially related to the hospital's tax-exempt purposes. UBI is subject to taxation at ordinary corporate rates, and 990-T forms should be filed by the hospital with the Internal Revenue Service. UBI should include outreach testing income minus deductions for expenses directly associated with the program. When hospital employees are used for both patient and nonpatient testing, allocations between the two should be calculated on a reasonable basis. Hospital outreach programs must maintain and retain appropriate records to permit calculation of the outreach testing net contribution to income (71).

COB and coordination of Medicare benefits. The Coordination of Benefits (including coordination of Medicare benefits) program is designed to ensure that a patient's alternative healthcare benefits (workman's compensation and automobile insurance) are identified before a claim is submitted to Medicare. The goal is to eliminate improper payments for services when Medicare should be the secondary rather than the primary payor. CMS maintains a COB page (available at its website at http://www.cms.hhs.gov [accessed April 2003]) to assist providers with their benefit coordination process.

MSP status. Patient registration staff should be familiar with COB and the organization's process to establish Medicare secondary-payor (MSP) status. In certain circumstances another third-party payor, not Medicare, may be the primary insurer for a claim. The claim should always be submitted to the primary payor first and then to Medicare. The MSP regulation requires an MSP questionnaire (Appendix 5.1) be completed that directs providers to other third-party payors first whenever they are primary to Medicare (139). Medicare is considered secondary in the following instances:

- The beneficiary or the beneficiary's spouse is gainfully employed.
- The beneficiary is disabled and under age 65.
- Automobile, no-fault medical, personal injury protection, or third-party liability is involved.
- Pulmonary/respiratory illnesses are associated with mining and benefits are covered by the Black Lung Program.
- The beneficiary is entitled to veteran's benefits.
- The beneficiary's injuries occurred on the job and are covered by workman's compensation.
- An individual entitled to Medicare on the basis of ESRD is covered under an employer group plan.

MSP policies apply in cases where Medicare does not assume the primary obligation to pay for services, as the beneficiary may be covered by other coverage. (MSP policies are available on the United Government Services website at http://www.ugs.com [accessed January 2003].)

A major reason for Medicare claim denials nationwide is the inability to correctly verify a subscriber's eligibility for coverage. CMS Program Memorandum Transmittal AB-00-36 assigns the responsibility for updating the common working files and MSP database to a COB subcontractor (41). Editors of common working files should include prepayment edits, medical-necessity edits, frequency limitations, and postpayment edits. The contractor will not process any claims or handle any mistaken-payment recoveries or claim-specific inquiries (140). CMS intends for the COB contractor to serve as an information-gathering entity to detect and prevent improper payments for MSP by ensuring that the common working files are accurate and current.

Other Federally Funded Programs

Medicare + choice. Medicare + choice is a program administered by Medicare (Part C) and is designed to give beneficiaries freedom to select coverage outside of Medicare Part B (a fee-for-service [FFS] plan) or a Medicare managed-care plan (a prepaid service arrangement). A Medicare + choice organization (coordinated care plan) is a network of providers in a preferred provider organization that have agreed to a contractually specified reimbursement for covered benefits with the organization offering the plan, provides for reimbursement for all covered benefits regardless of whether the benefits are provided with the network of providers, and is offered by an organization that is not licensed or organized under state law as an HMO. The beneficiary and the plan share the expenses under the Medicare + choice arrangement.

Some view Medicare + choice as a failed experiment. The savings that Congress envisioned from the program were based on faulty premises. Since health plans could not cherry-pick the beneficiaries and didn't offer prescription drug benefits, neither the plans nor Medicare subscribers were interested. Moreover, managed care is transforming to resemble preferred provider organizations and fee-for-service models (108).

Medicaid (Title XIX). Medicaid is jointly administered program that is funded by both federal and state government and provides health insurance for certain low-income and needy people. It covers approximately 36 million individuals, including children, the aged, blind, and/or disabled and people who are eligible to receive federally assisted income maintenance payments.

CHAMPUS. CHAMPUS is a program that provides medical and dental care for members and former members of the uniformed services and their dependents. The Department of Defense, DOT, and DHHS administer CHAMPUS. Only authorized providers may participate and must agree to accept the CHAMPUS allowable fee as payment in full, and participating institutions must file claims with the third-party administrator on behalf of the beneficiary. This program is now called TRICARE.

Railroad Retirement Act. The Railroad Retirement Act is a federal insurance program similar to Social Security designed for workers in the railroad industry. The provisions of the Railroad Retirement Act provide for a system of coordination and financial interchange between the Railroad Retirement program and the Social Security program.

NCD and LMRPs

Balanced Budget Act of 1997. The Balanced Budget Act of 1997 mandated the use of a negotiated rule making committee to develop national coverage and administrative policies for clinical diagnostic laboratory services payable under Medicare Part B by 1 January 1999. The bill included provisions for numerous healthcare issues, like civil penalties for fraud and abuse, antikickback violations, guidelines for exclusion from the Medicare program, diagnostic information on medical necessity, coverage for additional screening tests, and prospective payment of Part B services to patients in a skilled bed in a nursing facility.

The provision required that national coverage policies promote program integrity and national uniformity and simplify administrative requirements for clinical diagnostic laboratory services.

NCDs. The national coverage determinations (NCDs) are the national policies that establish whether Medicare will cover certain healthcare services, procedures, or technologies. CMS tracks emerging technologies and patterns of care to determine the application of an NCD and the need for policy change. When an NCD does not specifically exclude an indication or circumstance and does not specify an item or service in an NCD or a Medicare manual, Medicare contractors are responsible for making the coverage decision and publishing and updating the local medical review policies (LMRPs) on a monthly basis. The final rule, published in the *Federal Register* on 23 November 2001 (46), included 23 coverage determinations as listed below. (More detail may be obtained from the publication *Medicare National Coverage Determinations: Clinical Diagnostic Laboratory Services,* available on the CMS website at http://www.cms.gov [accessed January 2003].)

- Culture, bacterial (urine)
- HIV testing (prognosis, including monitoring)
- HIV testing (diagnosis)
- Blood counts
- Partial thromboplastin time
- Prothrombin time
- Serum iron studies
- Collagen cross-links (any method)
- Blood glucose testing
- Glycated hemoglobin or glycated protein
- Thyroid testing
- Lipids
- Digoxin therapeutic drug assay
- Alpha-fetoprotein
- Carcinoembryonic antigen
- Human chorionic gonadotropin
- Tumor antigen by immunoassay (CA 125)
- Tumor antigen by immunoassay (CA 15-3 and CA 27.29)
- Tumor antigen by immunoassay (CA 19-9)
- Prostate specific antigen
- Gamma glutamyltransferase
- Hepatitis panel (acute hepatitis panel)
- Fecal occult blood

Each NCD follows a uniform format that includes policy name, policy number, reason, policy type, bill type, revenue code, a narrative description of the test(s), clinical indications for its use, coverage limitations, HCPCS code, a list of related ICD-9 codes covered by Medicare, a list of ICD codes that will be denied by Medicare, a list of codes that are not generally covered unless certain exceptions are met, national policy, reasons for denial, sources of information, documentation requirements, revision history, and effective dates. The policies include frequency limitations for tests for which Medicare restricts coverage to a specific number of times per year. In some geographic regions, the NCD policies replace the LMRPs. In states where no policies exist, the NCDs become new restrictions (79). Local carriers and fiscal intermediaries can supplement the NCDs with additional requirements before communicating the LMRPs in the form of bulletins to providers, determine eligibility for coverage and reimbursement allowances for services, pay claims, audit, and determine appeals from providers. Medicare requires that providers retain the bulletins for a minimum of 5 years. Medicaid differs from Medicare in that the program is administered jointly by both federal and state agencies. LMRP has a new website at http://www.lmrp.net (accessed January 2003), or the reader may wish to refer to the CMS site at http://www.cms.gov/manuals/108_ pim/pim83c13.asp (accessed January 2003) for easier review of all LMRPs by contractor for a specific area.

Reimbursement Methods

Reimbursement is generally driven by the types of service rendered to a beneficiary and the location in which the service is rendered. Additional information is available in the outpatient prospective payment system patient booklet. (The booklet is located at the website http://www.medicare.gov [accessed April 2003].)

PPS for outpatient services. Congress directed HCFA to develop a PPS for hospital outpatient services in the Omnibus Reconciliation Act (OBRA) of 1986. The Balanced Budget Act established an implementation date of January 2000. Under PPS, hospital services other than those covered under a fee schedule would be included. Excluded services include laboratory, ambulance, occupational therapy, physical therapy, and speech pathology.

APCs. In July 2000, Medicare introduced a new PPS for outpatient services. CMS originally proposed an ambulatory payment group after a study done in 1995. The ambulatory payment groups were mandated by the Balanced Budget Act of 1997. In 2002 the terminology changed to ambulatory payment classifications (APCs) (38, 39). Under APC, there are 451 groups defined by clinical relevance and resource usage (40). In contrast to the Part A DRG approach, which covers a patient's entire inpatient hospital stay, multiple APCs may be assigned to a single encounter. The payment rate for the APC is predetermined and is equal to a national conversion rate multiplied by an APC specific weight and adjusted for local area wage differences. The APC system ensures payment predictability and provides an incentive for efficiency. Clinical laboratory services are excluded from the outpatient PPS and are paid from the Part B clinical laboratory fee schedule (15).

ESRD. ESRD facilities provide services to Medicare beneficiaries who have permanent kidney dysfunction and require dialysis treatment. The facilities have strict medical-necessity guidelines and utilization criteria.

- *MCP or rate.* Reimbursement for physician, supervisory, and direct care services that are routinely rendered in relation to outpatient dialysis (including hemodialysis, continuous ambulatory peritoneal dialysis, continuous cycling peritoneal dialysis, intermittent peritoneal dialysis, or hemofiltration). The costs of certain ESRD laboratory services are included in the composite rate. The three major risks associated with billing for tests included in the composite rate are duplicate billing, failure to document medical necessity for tests not included in the composite rate, and failure to comply with the 50/50 Medicare composite payment (MCP) rule (102).
- The *Medicare MCP 50/50 rule* limits when a multichannel chemistry panel can be included in the composite rate. If 50% or more of the covered tests are included under the composite rate, then the entire panel is to be part of the composite rate paid to the facility and the lab cannot bill for the additional testing separately. On the other hand, if more than 50% of the automated tests are not in the composite rate, then the entire panel may be billed directly to Medicare by the testing laboratory. Laboratories can expect increased scrutiny by the OIG for ESRD claims (92).
- *Medicare fee schedule.* Laboratory testing not included in the composite rate is subject to medical-necessity guidelines and is reimbursed under the Medicare fee schedule when appropriate (18).

Hospice benefits are optional to Medicare beneficiaries whose terminal illness and prognosis are less than 6 months. Payment for treatment and management services is made under the benefit, and all other Part B claims except the professional fees of the attending physician are waived.

Medicare direct billing rules. Medicare pays only the healthcare entity that actually performed or supervised a clinical laboratory test. The exceptions are as follows:

- Laboratory-to-laboratory referrals if the laboratory billing for the service performs at least 70% of the total tests billed within the laboratory
- Laboratory-to-laboratory referrals if the laboratory performing the test is commonly owned by the laboratory billing for the test
- Tests provided under an arrangement with a hospital, critical-care facility, or skilled-nursing facility

Competitive Bidding Demonstration Project. In 1985, the DHHS issued a request for proposals to establish demonstration projects for the provision of clinical laboratory services for Medicare beneficiaries on a competitive bidding basis. The Consolidated Omnibus Budget Reconciliation Act of 1985 prohibited the DHHS from conducting the project until after 1987. Competitive bidding is a method for setting the price of healthcare services through a bidding process to establish payment rates on the lowest price submitted by providers. Although the Balanced Budget Act of 1997 removed the prohibition, the demonstration project remains stalled due to the enormous complexity of the endeavor. The Medicare fee schedule and the system's payment problems are subject to application of different standards in each of the carrier jurisdictions. Competitive bidding would further complicate the system for laboratories that refer tests between jurisdictions while increasing the costs of processing claims. Restricting the ability of physicians to choose the laboratory believed to best serve the needs of their Medicare patients might create access problems. Allowing only a few selected providers might create government-sanctioned monopolies that force necessary providers out of business (44).

Code of Medical Necessity (Reasonable and Necessary Services)

Medical-necessity regulation first originated in the Social Security Act. A test must meet the following criteria to be considered medically necessary:

- The ordered test must be consistent with the signs, symptoms, or diagnosis of the injury or illness being treated and be appropriately documented, both on the test requisition and in the patient's medical record. Medicare does not pay for tests where documentation in the medical record does not support medical-necessity requirements.

- The test must be necessary and consistent with the generally accepted professional medical standards of practice (not investigational or experimental).

- The test must not be ordered for the convenience of the patient or the physician. Medicare generally does not cover routine screening tests even when the healthcare provider ordering the tests considers them to be appropriate for the beneficiary.

- The test must be provided safely and effectively at the appropriate level. Medicare reimburses only for tests that meet the Medicare coverage criteria and are deemed reasonable and necessary to treat or diagnose an individual patient.

The intent of the guidelines was to encourage partnerships between third-party contractors, physicians, and providers in providing appropriate care to patients. The Carrier Advisory Committee was formed to educate and train physicians after analyzing patterns of practice rather than denying claims.

ABN. The Medicare program's purpose for the advance beneficiary notice (ABN) is to ensure that all Medicare beneficiaries are informed in writing prior to receiving a service that the procedure may not be a covered benefit. The ABN serves as a waiver of liability and is intended to assist the patient in making a decision to receive a service and to agree to accept financial responsibility if the claim is not covered. The use of an ABN should be limited to individual instances where the provider feels there is reason to believe reimbursement will be denied. In designing a facility ABN, the correct language to satisfy the CMS requirements is as follows: Medicare will pay only for items and services it determines to be reasonable and necessary. Noncovered services include routine physical exams, screening tests, cosmetic surgery, and experimental or investigational services.

The Balanced Budget Act of 1997 made it a requirement that physicians provide specific diagnostic information when ordering tests for which reimbursement from the Medicare program will be sought. Failure to comply with the medical-necessity regulations could result in the government filing false-claim charges for performing unnecessary tests or services. Tests ordered and performed at a greater frequency than allowed must have medical-necessity documentation.

The most current CMS-approved ABN formats available are as follows:

- *General (CMS-R-131-G).* Can be used by hospital facilities for all general situations, including laboratory, radiology, etc. (Appendix 5.2).

- *Laboratory (CMS-R-131-L).* Specifically for laboratory services (Appendix 5.3).

(Both versions of the ABN form can be obtained and downloaded for replication at http://cms.hhs.gov/medicare/bni [accessed April 2003].) The standard sections of the ABN form must be reproduced in the identical format as the PDF files found on the website, without any alterations. The three areas of the form where the boxes may be customized include the following:

- Header box located above the patient's name
- Test itemization box
- Reason box

CMS recommends that hospitals and laboratories use a legible font, like Arial 10-point font. The ABN can be expanded to an 8.5- by 14-inch format but cannot exceed one page in length.

Authorized representative. The ABN instructions define an authorized representative as a person who does not have a conflict of interest with the beneficiary when the beneficiary is temporarily or permanently unable to act for himself or herself. The representative acts on the beneficiary's behalf, in his or her best interest. This definition differs from the rules on who may sign when the beneficiary is incapable. The following individuals may qualify to serve as an authorized representative:

- A person authorized under state law to make healthcare decisions or exercise power of attorney

- A legal spouse, adult child, parent, adult sibling, or close friend

- A disinterested third party or public appointed guardian

Although the instruction does not define the method of determination of conflict of interest, it does state that an employee of a healthcare provider or supplier of service may have a conflict and therefore be precluded from serving in this capacity (138).

Medical-necessity guide. Laboratories that develop a medical-necessity guide for use by providers and clients who order tests governed by an NCD or a LMRP must avoid code steering, or the appearance that the laboratory is directing or steering the healthcare provider to select a code that will make the claim payable, rather than assigning or selecting the code based on the patient's medical condition. The code choice should always be made before payment issues are considered and should be appropriately documented in the patient's chart (medical record) and the test requisition (141).

Standing orders. A standing order is valid for a limited time as long as it meets medical-necessity guidelines. Regulations require the following criteria for the use of standing orders for any patient type in any type of facility:

- A healthcare provider placed the order.
- The order was specific to the patient and met medical-necessity guidelines.
- An ABN should be executed if the order is for screening or a noncovered service.
- The order must have a start date and indicate the period of time for the standing order (<12 months) and must be documented in the patient's chart.

If testing continues once the order expires or is not necessary, the facility could be liable for fraud and abuse. Laboratory policies related to these orders should include periodic reviews of all standing orders to eliminate the potential risks associated with their performance (27).

Verbal orders. Federal regulations allow laboratories to accept verbal orders or modifications to an existing order and to perform the testing provided the laboratory documents the order within 30 days and maintains the records or the request for authorized signatures for 2 years (17).

Research or investigational testing. Non-FDA-approved testing for research or investigational use could be considered either a noncovered service or not medically necessary. When a third-party payor's LMRP guidelines define a test as a noncovered service, an ABN is not needed. However, if it is deemed not medically necessary, then having a beneficiary sign an ABN informs the beneficiary of his or her financial responsibility.

Reflex testing. The laboratory's test ordering pathway should be based on standards of care developed with physician oversight. When tests include automatic reflex testing (confirmation, sensitivity, antibody elution, or titer), the computer order screen or requisition should clearly indicate that it includes automatic reflex. Billing for reflex testing without a specific order could result in charges of false claims. A laboratory should document a physician's request to automatically reflex certain tests in writing. The agreement should be updated annually. A useful tool for reflex testing is to create a chart or algorithm that maps the sequence or pathway for confirmatory testing (87).

Overview of the Reimbursement Process

The Deficit Reduction Act of 1984 authorized the Medicare clinical laboratory fee schedule and mandated that the laboratory performing the test bill Medicare for the services directly. The ordering physician could only bill if the testing is performed in his office laboratory. In the Balanced Budget Act of 1997, CMS decreased reimbursement to Medicare providers, including the laboratory, by more than $100 billion. BIPA restored some of the reimburse-

ment previously taken away from Medicare providers. BIPA is part of the Consolidated Budget Appropriations Act, which allocated $35 billion over the next 5 years in federal spending, primarily for the hospitals. Pending legislation includes the following:

- *HR 1798/S.1066.* The Medicare Patient Access to Preventive and Diagnostic Tests Act proposes to eliminate the carrier variation and set laboratory fees at the national limitation amount. In addition, tests whose reimbursements were previously set by gap filling at the 74% national limitation amount would be set at 100% of the national median. No action is expected to be taken by the 108th congress.
- *HR 1948.* The Medical Laboratory Personnel Shortage Act of 2001 makes provision for scholarship and loan assistance to attract more people to the profession. The act was reintroduced in 2003 as HR 623.
- *S.416.IS.* Providing Annual Pap Tests to Save Women's Lives Act of 2003 is also pending legislation.

Coverage of new tests. The laboratory environment has witnessed a remarkable growth both in the number of new diagnostic tests and in their complexity. A major problem with the Medicare fee schedule is the method for determining payment amounts for new tests (116). CMS uses either a process called cross-walking to map a new test that is similar to an existing CPT or HCPCS codes or a process called gap filling to establish a baseline reimbursement while assigning a temporary HCPCS code. CMS has not established definitive criteria on how to use the processes, creating many inequities with the fee schedule.

Presently, tests that are similar enough to be cross-walked to an existing code receive the current national limitation amount rate of reimbursement even if the new test's technology is more expensive. In the gap-filling process, CMS and the carriers assess the charge for the new test to determine the median reimbursement and then apply the national limitation amount. The resulting reimbursement is 74% of the median charged by the performing laboratories (28).

Registration and Coding

Institutions have come to understand the need to employ highly trained and qualified coders to assist with the submission of timely and accurate claims, utilization review, and medical record risk management issues. The national accrediting agency that oversees this group of coding and health information management professionals is the American Health Information Management Association (AHIMA). Certified coding specialists convert the healthcare provider's ordering narrative diagnostic description into the corresponding five-digit ICD-9 code (International Classification of Diseases, Ninth Revision) and provide the best CPT code for the service provided. The coding guidelines are disseminated by

CMS, the National Center for Health Statistics, the American Medical Association, and the AHIMA.

Correct-coding initiative. There are five coding systems used by third-party payors (Table 5.18). Each system has coding manuals available to assist coders with filing accurate claims. A facility's correct coding must include the healthcare provider's documentation of the history, examination, and decision-making processes that lead to ordering diagnostic laboratory services that are medically necessary. Coding systems are updated periodically; CPT code changes and updates occur annually. The following practices will ensure that your facility remains in compliance with correct-coding initiatives (117):

- Revise codes and fees in the charge description master (CDM).
- Incorporate edits in CDM into billing systems.
- Modify manual requisitions and electronic order screens if necessary.
- Notify physicians of changes.

CDM. The CDM is the hospital's procedural description for each charge code that cross-references revenue codes and CPT codes to the inpatient and outpatient charges for the services. Other components that can be included in a CDM are productivity values, cost center, and payor billing options (136). Annual review of the hospital's inpatient and outpatient CDM identifies areas for potential compliance risks, such as unbundling of procedural charges and billing for services that are already built into payment rates. Annual changes to the ICD-9, CPT, and HCPCS level II codes should be updated appropriately (106).

Anatomic and surgical pathology. The Omnibus Reconciliation Act of 1989 charged CMS with implementing a reimbursement system for anatomic and surgical pathology services that included both a technical and physician's professional component. The resource-based relative value scale was initiated in January 1992 and included the billing and CPT coding criteria. The suffix modifier TC is added when billing for the technical component, modifier 26 is added when billing for the professional component, and no modifier is needed when one provider is billing for both components. The fee schedule was calculated using relative value units to account for the actual work, any practice expenses, and associated costs of malpractice.

Claim Processing and Submission

Medicare carrier and fiscal-intermediary manuals and communications provide ongoing guidance for providers related to LMRP rules that should be incorporated into the education and training of personnel handling registration, coding, and claim submissions. The billing entity must ensure that all claims submitted accurately reflect the diagnostic information provided by the healthcare professional ordering the test and the most specific code is used for each test ordered for the patient. If the ordering provider uses a narrative description of the diagnosis, the standard practice should be to have only certified coders translate the narrative into an ICD-9 code. Commonly used terms for the more frequent coding errors that might put your facility at risk are found in Table 5.19 (26).

Claim forms. The two claim forms used by healthcare providers when submitting claims are as follows:

- *HCFA 1500 (CMS 1500) (Appendix 5.4).* The current version was created in 1993 to submit Medicare Part B claims for physician services and supplies and is maintained by the National Uniform Claims Committee. Medicare carriers for Part B claims publish instructions for completion of the claim form. The form provides the ability to list ICD-9 and CPT coding on the same line and to use coding modifiers.

- *Uniform bill (UB-92) (Appendix 5.5).* The UB-92 is used by hospital facilities filing claims with a fiscal intermediary. The specification and guidelines for use of the UB-92 are contained in the *National Uniform Bill Committee's Data Specification Manual,* published by

Table 5.18 References for coding systems used for third-party claims

Acronym	Coding descriptive name	Comment(s)[a]
CPT-4 codes	Current Procedural Terminology, 4th edition	7,000 five-digit codes and modifiers used for medical, surgical, and diagnostic service descriptions
HCPCS	Healthcare common procedural coding system	Level I, Level II, Level III
ICD-9-CM	International Classification of Diseases, Ninth Revision, Clinical Modification	Developed by AHA, AHIMA, CMS, and NCHS. Volume 1, disease tabular list; volume 2, alpha index; volume 3, inpatient procedure codes
DRG	Diagnosis-related groups	Over 500 three-digit medical and surgical groupings
		Inpatient stays are split into 25 major diagnostic categories
		DRG for admitting diagnosis paid at an established rate
Revenue code		Code used on UB-92 to identify type of charge

[a] AHA, American Hospital Association; NCHS, National Center for Health Statistics.

Table 5.19 Billing and coding errors: areas of potential risk[a]

Coding term	Definition	Regulation
Simple billing errors	Clerical errors like posting charges to improper account, wrong date of service, misunderstanding about copayments and deductibles, balance billing, etc.	Special fraud alert, November 1994
Insufficient documentation	Billing for items or services that cannot be substantiated by the documentation associated with the claim	
Unqualified personnel	Billing for services provided by unqualified or uncertified personnel	
Lack of system integrity	Must demonstrate computer system integrity; record retention, storage, and retrieval; and an effective backup system	
Up-coding	Term to describe the practice of using a billing code that yields a higher reimbursement than the service actually rendered	42 U.S.C. § 1320a-7a(a)(1)(A)
Reflex testing	Billing for a reflex test performed without a provider's specific order could result in charges of false claims. Carefully design requisitions that clearly indicate that testing includes reflex to confirmation.	
False claim	Intentionally submitting claims for medically unnecessary services not warranted by the patient's condition.	42 U.S.C. § 1395y(a)(1)(A)
	False claims must be reported within 30 days of the discovery to avoid double damages.	31 U.S.C. § 3729(a)
DRG creep	Practice of billing using a DRG code that receives a higher payment than the DRG actually provided	
Duplicate billing	When more than one claim is submitted for the same service, or when the claim is submitted to more than one primary payor at the same time	
Unbundling	Submitting claims for individual tests or procedures rather than together as required to maximize reimbursement	
72 h window	Filing claims for nonphysician outpatient services that are included in the hospital's inpatient payment under PPS	OIG report, *Expansion of DRG Payment Window,* July 1994, A-01-92-00521; OIG report, *Improper Medicare Payments to Hospitals,* May 1996

[a]See reference 26.

the American Hospital Association. A UB-92 (also known as an HCFA 1450) requires the billing entity to specify the revenue code for the accommodation or ancillary service charge, or the type of billing calculation used in field 42 of the claim form. This form does not allow listing of ICD-9 and CPT codes but requires the use of revenue codes with limited use of modifiers.

CPT code billing modifiers. Healthcare providers frequently request the same laboratory testing multiple times within a 24-h period. Payors require use of a two-digit numeric CPT code modifier to ensure payment for this and other special situations (Table 5.20) (94).

Remittance Advice

Third-party payors produce a remittance advice once a claim has been received to advise the billing entity of the status of the claim. The remittance advice permits the laboratory to match the payment received to the actual test and CPT code description as billed. The third-party payors at the same time generate an explanation of benefits

for the covered beneficiary to advise him or her that a claim has been filed and to notify him or her of any impeding financial responsibility to the billing entity.

Audit and Benchmark Monitors

Simple billing errors and misunderstandings can be construed as fraudulent by Medicare beneficiaries and are often reported to the Medicare contractors as fraud. The types of errors reported include posting charges to the wrong account, billing for the incorrect date of service, misunderstandings about deductible or copayment responsibilities, services rendered outside of the outpatient office setting (for example, laboratory), and services rendered by a provider with whom the patient had no encounter (for example, radiologists). An audit is an independent and documented assessment planned to determine if policy requirements are met. Using periodic audits confirms that policies and procedures are being followed and that the monitors selected are effective to analyze coding habits. The audits identify problems, areas of high risk, and the need for training and document and strengthen an effective compli-

Table 5.20 Billing modifiers[a]

CPT code two-digit modifier	Claim form	Description
Modifier 59	UB-92	To identify a separate and distinct procedure performed on the same day
		To report a different or separate patient encounter
		To report tests not usually performed together on the same date of service
Modifier 91	UB-92	Replaced QR (program memorandum AB-97-23)
		Used when the same test is performed more than once on the same date of service
Modifier QW	HCFA 1500	Used for waived tests
Modifier GY	HCFA 1500	Service is not a covered benefit
Modifier GZ	HCFA 1500	Provider expects denial
		No ABN on file
Modifier GA	HCFA 1500	Expects denial. Procedure does not meet LMRP guides
		Provider has an ABN on file
Condition code 20	UB-92	Indicates that a service may be denied for medical necessity
Condition code 21	UB-92	Service is excluded or noncovered
Condition code 32	UB-92	Indicates that an ABN is on file

[a]See reference 94.

ance program. Careful scrutiny of each step in the process from the requisition to coding and claim submission often identifies opportunities to correct patterns of noncompliance or denied payments or lost cash flow (115). The following are useful types of internal or self audits:

- Baseline audits are useful to determine areas of risk. These audits are used at the beginning of a program to identify areas of risk and to establish a baseline for future audits. Keep separate records documenting each issue identified during an audit. Consult counsel prior to initiating audits to ensure protection under attorney-client privilege.

- A chart audit, also referred to as postpayment review, is often used by the facility's compliance officer or legal counsel to determine if a provider's orders were appropriately documented and support the actual services billed on the claim form. Each encounter with the patient should be thoroughly documented in the medical record and should include date of service, reason for visit, physical history and exam, risk factors, review of reports, patient assessment, progress notes and response to treatment, and care and discharge plan as indicated.

- Periodic audits should become a regular routine and ongoing part of any compliance program. Use a checklist to audit problems identified in the baseline audit. Random checks of orders versus billing should be included. Avoid publishing a schedule for audits that is impossible to meet, as it could be viewed as failure to enforce your program.

- *Review of laboratory reports.* An audit of a laboratory report should include a review of the procedural code requested and ordered. The review should check for upcoding, unbundling, and accurate coding to the most specific ICD-9 diagnosis code using a fourth or fifth digit.

The second step should include a review of the CMS 1500 claim and the remittance advice or the explanation of benefits. Periodic audits should review ICD-9 coding to ensure that medical-necessity guidelines are met.

- *Internal audit.* Many hospitals have an internal audit team reporting to risk management and the compliance office that surveys hospital department processes annually. Also referred to as a process audit, an internal audit reviews procedures and forms for their effectiveness. The billing or the laboratory departments can also establish an internal audit process. A charge audit reviews individual charges for accuracy and appropriateness of billing. A denial audit reviews denied claims for system and payor errors. Auditors must have access to all records, resources, and relevant employees and should function independently of the management group. Prompt follow-up and initiation of remedial action on any recommendations demonstrate commitment to compliance.

- *External or special audits.* External audits are used to check the status of a process change. Investigations for Medicare contractor or third-party payor inquiries are privileged and may need to be conducted with advice of counsel. When an outside party requests an audit, hiring an independent third party may be recommended by the compliance/risk management team. Claim submission sampling is a form of prepayment review used by Medicare contractors and third-party payors.

Compliance—the Next Generation: HIPAA

Trust of the consumer is difficult to build and harder to maintain, and it can be lost in the blink of an eye. Healthcare organizations risk losing trust when information is not kept private, confidential, and secure. The rapid growth of e-commerce globally has heightened consumer concerns for privacy. The existing standards for the way health information is transmitted electronically, stored, secured, administered, and utilized, as well as the standards for patient privacy and safety by every healthcare provider and their business partners, are undergoing a dramatic metamorphosis driven by the Health Insurance Portability and Accountability Act of 1996 (HIPAA). HIPAA mandates a set of interdependent regulations that require profound changes in the manner that health information is handled and processed and ultimately in the relationships among patients, healthcare providers, and insurers. CMS has released a number of notices of proposed rule making to implement the HIPAA mandates:

- Transactions and code sets
- National provider identifier number
- National employer identifier number
- Data security and electronic signature
- Data privacy
- Standards for electronic transactions

On 2 July 1999, the DHHS published the final HIPAA national privacy standards in order to regulate how health plans, healthcare clearinghouses, and healthcare providers and their business associates should protect all confidential health information. The final privacy standards were effective 14 April 2003 for most covered entities.

HIPAA allows persons to qualify immediately for comparable health insurance coverage when they change their employment relationships. HIPAA (also known as the Kennedy-Kassebaum bill) gives the DHHS the authority to mandate the use of standards for the electronic exchange of healthcare data; to specify what medical and administrative code sets should be used within those standards; to require the use of national identification systems for healthcare patients, providers, payors (or plans), and employers (or sponsors); and to specify the types of measures required to protect the security and privacy of personally identifiable healthcare information. Organizations must comply with the new privacy rights or standards as set forth by CMS in an interim final rule regarding patient rights and the conditions of participation designed to ensure the emotional and physical health and safety of beneficiaries (29, 30). The purpose of the HIPAA regulation is threefold:

- To protect and enhance the rights of consumers by providing them access to their health information and controlling the inappropriate use of that information
- To improve the quality of healthcare in America by restoring trust in the healthcare system among consumers, healthcare professionals, and the multitude of organizations and individuals committed to the delivery of care
- To improve the efficiency and effectiveness of healthcare delivery by creating a national framework for

health privacy protection that builds on efforts by the states, health systems, and individual organizations and persons (29, 30)

Covered Entities

The HIPAA privacy standards apply to three categories of covered entities:

- Health plans are individual or group plans that provide or pay the cost of medical care, including health insurance companies, managed-care organizations, insured or self-insured employee health plans, and federally funded health plans.
- Healthcare clearinghouses are public or private entities, like billing agencies, repricing companies, and community health information network system companies, that convert health information from nonstandard formats into HIPAA standard formats or vice versa.
- Healthcare providers include institutions, medical professionals, or medical suppliers that bill the Medicare program or receive payment for health services rendered and transmit individually identifiable health information electronically as defined by the HIPAA standard transaction.

Other covered-entity arrangements. An organized healthcare arrangement allows integrated delivery systems to function as a covered entity under the regulations. The arrangement also offers hospital chains composed of legally separate entities the ability to function as a single covered entity operating as an affiliated covered entity (10a). Companies that provide certain covered-entity functions but are primarily engaged in unrelated business activities are considered hybrid entities and must utilize fire walls to prevent unauthorized disclosures to distinguish between the two separate and distinct business activities.

Administrative Simplification

The administrative simplification procedures proposed by HIPAA focus on three elements:

- Privacy standards
- Security standards
- Transaction and code set standards

The regulation requires sweeping changes and ongoing administrative costs to entities covered by the rule. The federal privacy rules preempt all contrary state laws unless the state law is more stringent, provides for reporting of disease, injury, child abuse, birth, death, or public health surveillance, or requires a health plan to report or provide access to information for audits, monitors, or certification.

Privacy Standards: Rules Governing PHI

Health information is any information, whether oral or recorded, in any form or medium, that is created or received and relates to the past, present, or future physical or mental health or condition of a patient. Protected health information (PHI) is individually identifiable information that is transmitted by electronic media, maintained in any medium, and transmitted or maintained in any form or medium. Individually identifiable health information includes 28 types of demographic information that identifies the individual or provides a reasonable basis to believe it will identify the individual, for example, social security number, driver's license number, date of birth, telephone and fax numbers, or patient address.

Minimum necessary. Data privacy standards apply to all health information pertaining to an individual that is electronically transmitted or maintained, while data privacy provisions apply to PHI and individually identifiable health information that are or have been electronically transmitted or maintained in any form. A covered entity must make reasonable efforts to ensure that no more than the minimum necessary PHI is used or disclosed. For example, the patient registration process for signing in at the front desk must limit PHI to the patient's name and appointment or arrival time. Individuals have the right to request records of any disclosure of their PHI for the previous 6 years.

Personnel policies and procedures. Covered entities must categorize personnel consistent with job responsibilities for the purpose of limiting access to PHI to the minimum-necessary standard. Fire walls must be constructed to limit access. Privacy education and training, including password protection and use of the Internet for all employees regardless of their job descriptions, are mandated by the HIPAA final regulation. Human resource policies should be readily accessible and should clearly articulate the penalties for breaches in security or patient privacy.

Patient Informed Rights

A hospital must inform patients of their rights prior to giving care, must have a grievance process, and must identify a representative for the patient to contact. The patient maintains the right to participate in the development of a care plan with the healthcare provider and must be adequately informed to make educated decisions regarding his or her care.

Consent forms and authorization for PHI. Healthcare providers may not use or disclose a patient's health information either verbally, written, or electronically via fax or e-mail in the course of treatment or billing without prior signed consent. Consent allows the use and disclosure of PHI by the covered entity seeking payment, but not by other persons. Consent forms are not needed when the covered entity has an indirect treatment relationship or is providing care to an inmate. The following applies to consent forms:

- It should be a formal written form.
- It should be signed and dated by the individual (patient) at onset of treatment. (Consent remains in effect unless the covered entity changes policies for privacy.)
- It should be used to inform the patient that PHI may be used or disclosed for treatment, payment, or healthcare operations. (The definition of payment includes coverage determinations, billing, claim management, medical-necessity review, and utilization review. Operations includes quality assessment, accreditation, medical review, compliance, business planning, and due-diligence activities.)
- The form should inform the individual of the entity's privacy policies and allow the patient to review before signing.
- The entity may reserve the right to amend, with a procedure to notify the individual.
- The individual may request restriction on disclosure.
- The individual has the right to revoke the consent in writing.

Use and disclosure of PHI for purposes other than treatment, payment, and healthcare operation requires an authorization specific to the purpose and must contain the key elements as cited in the final rule (29, 30). Authorizations are required for preemployment physicals and determination, life insurance, psychotherapy notes, and clinical trials or research and are more detailed than consent forms.

- Information to be disclosed must be specific.
- The person authorized to disclose must be identified.
- The recipient of the information must be named.
- An expiration date is required.
- The patient has the right to revoke disclosure.

Business Associates and Business Associate Agreements

A business associate is defined as a person or business that acts on behalf of the covered entity or organized healthcare arrangement. Associates perform or assist in business activities that are legal, actuarial, accounting, consulting, or data aggregation activities and that involve the use and disclosure of individually identifiable health information. The associate can also provide management, administrative, accreditation, or financial services to or for a covered entity where the PHI is disclosed in the transaction.

After the covered entity obtains satisfactory assurances that the business associate can safeguard PHI according to HIPAA privacy standards for disclosure, a business associate agreement is executed between a covered entity and a business associate that allows for PHI to be created and received. Under the rule, existing contracts are grandfathered until the contract is due for renewal or 14 April 2004. The DHHS has developed a model business associate contract.

Exceptions to business associate arrangements. Healthcare organizations can also ensure confidentiality and security by using confidentiality agreements that are not defined within the scope of business associate agreements for contractors who incidentally encounter individually identifiable health information while in the course of providing a contracted service, like environmental, linen, or dietary services. The decision on the type of agreement used should be made with the advice of counsel (83). Business associate arrangements are not necessary in the following cases:

- The covered entities are disclosing PHI for clinically integrated care and treatment purposes.
- A health plan and another agency are collecting and sharing individual identifiable health information for the performance of authorized functions.
- A financial institution processes consumer-conducted financial transactions for healthcare compensation.

The business associate agreement may not authorize an associate to disclose PHI in a manner that would violate the privacy rules unless proper management, administration, or fulfilling of legal responsibilities of the business associate dictate, or to provide data aggregation services to the covered entity.

Security Standards

The security standard requires covered entities to develop a new standard that integrates every component of security. Procedures must be implemented and certified to ensure the integrity, confidentiality, and accessibility of all PHI data. Formal processes for employee training and termination in order to safeguard controlled access to information and records must be followed. A covered entity's security management must include a contingency plan for backing up data and for disaster.

To comply with PHI security regulations, whenever a healthcare organization submits electronic data for claim submission, COB, referral authorization, or eligibility status to any business partner, a chain of trust agreement should be executed between all business partners (86).

Standards for Electronic Transactions

Healthcare organizations have reduced costs throughout the system in the face of shrinking reimbursements. HIPAA is now mandating standardization and uniformity for claims, eligibility, referral certification, authorization, enrollment data, and premium payments. Using a single format in each of these areas is an untapped basis for further cost savings, estimated to be nearly $30 billion over the next 10 years.

Transactions and code sets. HIPAA mandates that all covered entities and their business associates utilize eight standard transaction and code sets when filing claims. Examples of code sets as defined by the rule include the following:

- CPT codes, used to code provider services
- HCPCS codes, used to code medical equipment, injections, and transportation services
- ICD-9 (Clinical Modification) (ICD-9-CM) codes are diagnosis codes used to classify diagnosis, procedures, signs, and symptoms numerically.

Effective October 2003, all participating Medicare providers are mandated to submit claims electronically. The standards apply only to electronic transactions.

Another by-product of HIPAA-mandated electronic data interface is the opportunity to redesign patient and paper flow from the front door to the back and from information system operations to and through fire walls. Patients, consumers, providers, contractors, and payors will each benefit from HIPAA (80) (Table 5.21).

HIPAA Compliance and Enforcement

Enforcement of the privacy standards rests with the DHHS Office for Civil Rights. Any person, not just the person who is the subject of the allegedly abused PHI, may file a complaint. There are substantial consequences for failure to comply with HIPAA. Civil monetary penalties for an or-

Table 5.21 HIPAA benefits

Stakeholder	Benefit
Patient or consumer	Internal renewal of attention to privacy and security
	System-wide efficiencies reducing costs
Providers	Increased opportunity for work flow redesign
	Improved cash flow by electronic data interfaces
Payor or contractor	Decreased claim inventory
	Improved provider and patient satisfaction
Plan administrators	Utilizing electronic enrollment, eligibility, and authorization processes to reduce time and provide faster coordination of services
Healthcare administration	Reduction in manual processes
	Decreased variation in processes
Customer service	Reduced processing errors
	Shorter claim cycle processing times
	Online claim status reporting

Table 5.22 HIPAA criminal penalties

Tier 1

Up to $50,000 and 1 year in prison for
knowingly obtaining or disclosing PHI

Tier 2

Up to $100,000 and 5 years in prison when
the crime is committed under false pretense

Tier 3

Up to $250,000 and 10 years in prison if
there is intent to sell, transfer, or use PHI
for personal gain or malicious harm

ganization are $100 per violation, or up to $25,000 per standard violated per calendar year. Criminal penalties for individual violations are listed in Table 5.22. However, citizens cannot sue providers for disclosure under the provisions of HIPAA (37).

Summary

Clinical laboratories are governed by federal and state laws. Regulations are promulgated by many agencies. Primary among them are OSHA, the CDC, and the FDA. Other federal agencies and voluntary-standard-setting organizations also regulate and shape the everyday operations of laboratories. A major responsibility of laboratory managers and directors is keeping constantly abreast of new and revised laws and regulations.

In addition to following the laws and regulations governing the operation of clinical laboratories, additional expectations are placed on transfusion medicine services. With increased awareness of transmissible diseases, and the sophisticated methods to detect them in the blood supply, have come mandated programs of donor screening and blood testing. These programs have contributed to the increased cost of blood, but they have also led to a safer blood supply.

In the Model Compliance Plan for Hospitals, the OIG stated that the American healthcare industry continues to evolve. As the number of beneficiaries and the government expenditures grow, there is no time like the present for hospitals to embark on a strong voluntary compliance program. The dynamics of the process enable healthcare providers to police themselves in order to meet the changes and challenges imposed on them by Congress and private insurers. The OIG intended that voluntary participation would allow hospitals to meet their goals, improve the quality of care, and substantially reduce fraud, waste, and abuse and would ultimately reduce the cost of healthcare to federal, state, and private insurers.

HIPAA addresses the five basic principles for the protection of privacy: consumer control, accountability, public responsibility, boundaries, and security. Consumers have the right to see a copy of their medical records, request corrections, and obtain documentation of disclosure of their health information. Health information should only be used for the purposes of treatment and payment. There is a delicate balance among individual rights, public health needs, research, quality of care, and compliance with regulations. Appropriate security measures should protect against deliberate or accidental misuse or disclosure of health information. There are civil and criminal penalties for violations of privacy standards (14).

KEY POINTS

- Federal laws and voluntary standards governing safety and human resource management functions in hospital laboratories are numerous and changing and must be monitored constantly.

- Laboratories performing clinical testing to diagnose, screen for, manage, or treat disease are regulated by the federal government under the provisions of CLIA '88.

- Transfusion medicine has been under increasing regulatory oversight due to concerns about safety of the blood supply in response to the HIV epidemic and risks of HCV.

- Hospital transfusion services and blood manufacturers are inspected by the FDA, with voluntary certification by the AABB and JCAHO for hospitals.

- The FDA requires both hospital transfusion services and blood manufacturers to comply with tracking, trending, and reporting biological product deviations.

- Primary areas of increased compliance risk to exposure include unbundling, up-coding, duplicate billing, billing without appropriate documentation, and failure to maintain confidentiality of records and patient health information.

- The HIPAA administrative simplification standards apply only to the transmission of healthcare data, whereas the security standards apply to all healthcare information maintained electronically or used in an electronic transmission (14).

- Federal regulations preempt all contrary provisions of state law, unless the state law is more stringent, requires the reporting of certain health conditions, or requires a health plan to provide information about covered lives.

GLOSSARY

Advance Beneficiary Notice (ABN) A waiver of liability used by providers to notify Medicare beneficiaries prior to receiving certain services that they may not be covered services and that the beneficiary may incur financial responsibility for the uncovered services.

Allogeneic blood Blood donated by a person other than the recipient.

Ambulatory patient classification (APC) A method of determining payment for outpatient services based on a predetermined rate for outpatient services. Certain services like radiology and blood products have their own APCs; others include supplies bundled into the 345 APCs. Diagnostic laboratory services are paid on a fee schedule and are not assigned an APC.

Americans with Disabilities Act (ADA) A federal law prohibiting discrimination based on disability of qualified individuals.

Authorization Allows the use or disclosure of protected health information for purposes other than patient treatment, payment, or healthcare operations.

Autologous blood Blood donated by a person with the anticipation of its being later transfused back to the donor.

Balanced Budget Act of 1997 A bill which included provisions for numerous healthcare issues like civil penalties for fraud and abuse, antikickback violations, guidelines for exclusion from the Medicare program, diagnostic information on medical necessity, coverage for additional screening tests, and prospective payment of Part B services to patients in a skilled-nursing facility.

Beneficiary Term used for a person who has health insurance through the Medicare or Medicaid program.

Biologics Substances derived from living sources (such as humans, animals, and microorganisms), in contrast to drugs that are chemically synthesized. Most biologics are complex mixtures that are not easily identified or characterized, and many biologics are manufactured using biotechnology. Biological products often represent the cutting edge of biomedical research and, in time, may offer the most effective means to treat a variety of medical illnesses and conditions that presently have no other treatments available. (Additional information is available at the website for the Centers for Biologics Evaluation and Research, http://www.fda.gov/cber [accessed 20 May 2003].)

Blood bank A facility that collects and dispenses blood products, also known as a transfusion medicine service.

Blood center A facility that collects and manufactures blood and blood products.

Business associate A person or organization to whom a covered entity discloses protected health information to perform a function or activity on behalf of a covered entity but who is not part of the covered entity's workforce. A business associate can also be a covered entity in its own right.

Carrier Primary third-party contractors with the Centers for Medicare and Medicaid Services (CMS) who administer Part B payments according to the local medical review policies (LMRP) to physicians, ancillary services, and clinical laboratory providers.

Centers for Medicare and Medicaid Services (CMS) The federal agency that runs the Medicare program. In addition, CMS works with the states to run the Medicaid program. CMS works to make sure that the beneficiaries in these programs have access to high-quality healthcare.

Chain of trust agreement (COT) A pattern of agreements that extends protection of healthcare data by requiring that each covered entity that shares healthcare data with another entity re- quire that entity to provide protections comparable to those provided by the covered entity, and that that entity, in turn, requires any other entities with which it shares the data to satisfy the same requirements.

Civilian Health and Medical Program of the Uniformed Services (CHAMPUS) Administered by the Department of Defense, CHAMPUS provides medical care to active-duty members of the military, military retirees, and their eligible dependents. (This program is now called TRICARE.)

Claim A request for payment for services rendered to beneficiaries by providers.

Clinical Laboratory Improvement Act of 1967 (CLIA '67) First published in 1967 and amended in 1988, CLIA '67 is a statute requiring all laboratories performing clinical testing on human specimens to comply with specific federal certification regulations.

Code set Under the Health Insurance Portability and Accountability Act (HIPAA), a code set is any set of codes used to encode data elements, such as tables of terms, medical concepts, medical diagnostic codes, or medical procedure codes. This includes both the codes and their descriptions. Under HIPAA, the Code Set Maintaining Organization creates and maintains the code sets adopted by the Secretary for use in the transactions for which standards are adopted.

Consent A document signed by an individual that allows the use or disclosure of the individual's protected health information for the purpose of treatment, payment, or healthcare operations.

Coordination of benefits (COB) A program that determines which plan or insurance policy will pay first if two health plans or insurance policies cover the same benefits. If one of the plans is a Medicare health plan, federal law may decide who pays first, in a written statement that states which health plan or insurance policy is primary when two health plans or insurance policies cover the same benefits.

Corporate integrity agreement (CIA) A settlement agreement between a healthcare provider and the Office of the Inspector General (OIG) that sets forth the terms and conditions for continued participation in the Medicare program following investigation and conviction of fraud and abuse.

Cross-walking When a new test is determined to be similar to an existing test, multiple existing test codes, or a portion of an existing test code, the new test code is assigned the related existing local fee schedule amounts and resulting national limitation amount. In some instances, a test may equate only to a portion of a test, and in those instances, payment at an appropriate percentage of the payment for the existing test is assigned.

Current procedural terminology code (CPT code) A code set of medical procedures, maintained and copyrighted by the American Medical Association, selected for use with noninstitutional and nondental professional transactions.

Diagnosis code A descriptive code describing the principal diagnosis or the patient condition established after study to be chiefly responsible for causing the patient to receive medical care.

Diagnosis-related group (DRG) A classification system that groups patients according to diagnosis, type of treatment, age, and other relevant criteria, and is a method of determining payment for hospital services, calculated on a predetermined rate per discharge for inpatient hospital services based on the discharge diagnosis. Under the prospective payment system (PPS), hospitals are paid a set fee for treating patients in a single DRG, regardless of the actual cost of care for the individual.

Directed donor blood   Blood that is donated at the request of a potential recipient by a friend or family member and designated for transfusion to that specific recipient. Many people think that this is safer than volunteer, allogeneic blood, though scientific data do not support this notion.

Disclosure   Release, transfer, provision of access to, or divulgence of information by an entity to persons or organizations outside of that entity.

DRG creep   Use of a DRG code that provides a higher level of reimbursement than the code that accurately reflects the patient's condition.

End-stage renal disease (ESRD)   Terminology used by Medicare to designate beneficiaries having permanent kidney dysfunction and requiring dialysis treatment.

Ergonomics   The science of fitting the job task to the individual in order to reduce exposure to musculoskeletal disorders and repetitive-motion injuries.

Explanation of benefits   A notice that is sent to beneficiaries after a provider files a claim for Part A or B services under the original Medicare plan to explain what the provider billed for, the Medicare-approved amount, how much Medicare paid, and what the beneficiary must pay. This is being replaced by the Medicare Summary Notice, which sums up all the services (Part A and B) that were provided over a certain period of time, generally monthly.

Fiscal intermediary   A primary third-party contractor with the CMS that administers Part A payments according to the LMRP for hospitals and rehabilitation and skilled-care facilities.

Food and Drug Administration   An agency of the Department of Health and Human Services (DHHS) charged (among other things) with regulating clinical laboratory instruments, reagents, and blood banks.

Fraud   The intentional deception or misrepresentation that an individual knows, or should know, to be false, or does not believe to be true, and makes, knowing that the deception could result in some unauthorized benefit to himself or some other person(s).

Fraud and abuse   Fraud is purposely billing for services that were not rendered or billing for a service that has a higher reimbursement than the service actually performed or provided. Abuse occurs when payment is accepted for items or services that are billed by mistake by providers but should not have been paid by Medicare. This is not the same as fraud.

Gap filling   Method used to determine payment for medical services when no comparable existing test code is available. Carrier-specific amounts are used to establish a national limitation amount for the following year.

HCFA-1450   The basic form prescribed by the Medicare program for claim submission for all facility billing, except for the professional component of physician services. Also known as CMS-1450 or UB-92.

HCFA-1500   The basic form prescribed by CMS for the Medicare program for claim submissions by physicians and suppliers. Also known as CMS-1500 or UCF-1500.

Healthcare Common Procedural Coding System (HCPCS)   A medical code set that identifies healthcare procedures, equipment, and supplies for claim submission purposes.

- Level I codes contain numeric CPT codes which are maintained by the American Medical Association.

- Level II codes contain alphanumeric codes used to identify various items and services to supplement services that are not included in the CPT medical code set. These are maintained by CMS, the Blue Cross and Blue Shield Association, and the Hospital Insurance Association of America.

- Level III codes contain alphanumeric codes that are assigned by Medicaid state agencies and local Medicare intermediaries to identify additional items and services not included in level I or II. These are usually called local codes and must have "W," "X," "Y," or "Z" in the first position.

- HCPCS procedure modifier codes can be used with all three levels, with the WA to ZY range used for locally assigned procedure modifiers.

Health Care Financing Administration   Former name of the federal agency within the DHHS established to administer the Medicare, Medicaid, and state children's health insurance programs. The agency is now known as CMS.

Health Information   Any information, whether oral or recorded, in any form or medium, that is created or received, and that relates to the past, present, or future physical or mental health or condition of a patient or the past, present, or future payment for the provision of healthcare to a patient.

Health Insurance Portability and Accountability Act (HIPAA)   Federal privacy standards that regulate how health plans, healthcare clearinghouses, and healthcare providers and their business associates must protect confidential health information.

Individual   The person (adult, emancipated minor, or legal representative) who is the subject of the protected health information.

Individually identifiable health information   Certain health information that identifies the individual or provides a reasonable basis to identify the individual.

International Classification of Diseases, Ninth Revision (ICD-9)   A medical code set maintained by the World Health Organization. ICD-9 classifies morbidity and mortality information for statistical purposes and for the indexing of hospital records by disease and operations for data storage and retrieval.

International Classification of Diseases, Ninth Revision, Clinical Modification (ICD-9-CM)   The American Medical Association's ICD-9-CM is based on the official version of the World Health Organization's ICD-9. The term "clinical" is used to emphasize the modification's intent: to serve as a useful tool to classify morbidity data for indexing medical records, medical care review, and ambulatory and other medical care programs, as well as for basic health statistics. To describe the clinical picture of the patient, the codes must be more precise than those needed only for statistical groupings and trend analysis. ICD-9-CM is totally compatible with ICD-9, thus meeting the need for comparability of morbidity and mortality statistics at the international level.

International Organization for Standardization (ISO) International organization that establishes common voluntary standards for manufacturing, trade, and communications. ISO standards previously applied to manufacturing are now being applied to blood manufacturing (103, 120).

Joint Commission on Accreditation of Healthcare Organizations (JCAHO) A nonprofit voluntary safety and quality evaluation and accrediting organization which accredits nearly 5,000 hospitals and other healthcare facilities.

Leukoreduction The process of reducing the number of leukocytes in a unit of blood to $<5 \times 10^6$. Leukoreduction decreases the risk of febrile, nonhemolytic transfusion reactions, cytomegalovirus transmission, and development of alloantibodies to HLA antigens in transfusion recipients.

Local medical review policies (LMRP) The medical-necessity guidelines established by local Medicare contractors for participating providers.

Medicaid Title XIX is a program administered by state and federal government to provide medical benefits to indigent persons of all ages who meet defined criteria.

Medically necessary Term applied to services or supplies that are proper and needed for the diagnosis or treatment of a medical condition; are provided for the diagnosis, direct care, and treatment of a medical condition; meet the standards of good medical practice in the local area; and are not mainly for the convenience of the beneficiary or the provider.

Medicare Part A Part A is the hospital insurance portion of Medicare. Medicare was established by §1811 of Title XVIII of the Social Security Act of 1965, as amended, and covers inpatient hospital care, skilled-nursing-facility care, some home health agency services, and hospice care.

Medicare Part B Part B is the portion of Medicare insurance that pays for physician services and covered outpatient services, also referred to as supplemental medical insurance. It was established by §1831 of Title XVIII of the Social Security Act of 1965, as amended, and covers services of physicians or other suppliers, outpatient care, medical equipment and supplies, and other medical services not covered by Part A of Medicare.

Medicare Secondary Payor A statutory requirement that private insurers, workman's compensation, and the Veterans Administration, who provide general health insurance coverage to Medicare beneficiaries, pay a beneficiary's claims as primary payors before the claims are submitted to Medicare.

National coverage determination (NCD) National coverage policies developed by CMS that indicate whether and under what circumstances certain services are covered under the Medicare program. It is published in CMS regulations, published in the *Federal Register* as a final notice, contained in a CMS ruling, or issued as a program instruction.

Negotiated rule making The process of federal agency representatives and other special interest groups convening to negotiate the text of a proposed rule.

New variant Creutzfeldt-Jakob disease A disease of the central nervous system, transmitted through a conformational protein change, caused by eating by-products of infected cows.

Noncovered service A service that does not meet the requirements of a Medicare benefit category, is statutorily excluded from coverage on other grounds, or is deemed not reasonable and necessary.

Notice of proposed rule making The document that describes and explains the regulation that the federal government proposes to adopt at some future date and invites interested parties to submit comments related to it. These comments can then be used in developing a final regulation.

Nucleic acid testing (NAT) Amplifying genetic material to detect the smallest amount of a substance. This allows earlier detection of infectious agents.

Office of the Inspector General (OIG) An independent agency of the DHHS established in 1976 to perform audits and investigations of federally funded programs.

Omnibus Reconciliation Act (OBRA) of 1989 Prohibits physicians from referring laboratory testing for Medicare beneficiaries to a laboratory in which the physician has an ownership interest. Also known as the Stark Law.

Omnibus Reconciliation Act of 1990 Denies Medicare reimbursement to a laboratory for a test performed off-site unless at least 70% of the tests for which the laboratory receives requests and submits claims are performed on-site. Also known as the "shell lab" act.

Outpatient prospective payment system (PPS) The method of payment used by Medicare to determine how much Medicare pays and how much the Medicare beneficiary pays for outpatient services at hospitals or community mental health centers under Medicare Part B. Medicare does not pay for all outpatient services under the PPS begun 1 August 2000 (for example, procedures Medicare considers inpatient procedures, such as fixing a fractured hip).

Payor In healthcare, a payor is any entity that assumes the risk of paying for medical treatments for an uninsured patient, a self-insured employer, a health plan, or an HMO.

Personal protective equipment (PPE) Equipment or garments used to protect employees from exposure to workplace hazards.

Preferred provider organization A healthcare organization composed of physicians, hospitals, and other providers which provides healthcare services at a reduced fee. In a preferred provider organization, care is paid for as it is received, rather than as a scheduled fee in advance as with an HMO.

Prospective payment system (PPS) A method of reimbursement in which Medicare payment is made based on a predetermined, fixed amount. The payment amount for a particular service is based on the classification of that service (for example, DRGs for inpatient hospital services.

Protected health information (PHI) Individually identifiable health information, transmitted or maintained in any form or medium, which is held by a covered entity or its business associate, identifies the individual or offers a reasonable basis for identification, is created or received by a covered entity or an employer, and relates to a past, present, or future physical or mental condition, provision of healthcare, or payment for healthcare.

Provider Any entity (for example, hospital, skilled-nursing facility, home health agency, outpatient physical therapy, comprehensive outpatient rehabilitation facility, ESRD facility, hospice, physician, nonphysician provider, laboratory, supplier) providing medical services.

Provider-performed microscopy procedures (PPMP) CLIA '88 term for a limited number of moderate-complexity, microscope-based tests that may be performed by a physician, midwife, or nurse practitioner operating under a PPMP certificate.

Quality-adjusted life year (QALY) Used as a standardized measure of the quality of life. It is a year of life, adjusted for its quality. The measure takes into account both longevity and the quality of life lived (24). One year of perfect health is 1.0 QALY.

Quality assurance The sum of activities planned and performed to provide confidence that all systems and their elements that influence quality of the product are functioning as expected and relied upon (69).

Railroad Retirement Act A federal insurance program similar to Social Security, designed for workers in the railroad industry. The provisions of the Railroad Retirement Act provide for a system of coordination and financial interchange between the Railroad Retirement program and the Social Security program.

Resource-based relative value scale A scale of national uniform relative values for all physicians' services. The relative value of each service must be the sum of **relative value units** representing physicians' work, practice expenses, net of malpractice expenses, and cost of professional liability insurance.

Resource utilization group Payment for services rendered to a Medicare beneficiary in a skilled bed of a nursing home facility; also known as consolidated billing.

Revenue code Uniform Bill 92 (UB-92) requires submission of a "revenue code." This code is used to identify specific accommodation charges, ancillary service charge, or a type of billing calculation. Revenue codes are maintained by the National Uniform Billing Committee.

Risk The chance of suffering a loss.

Risk management A process to identify, reduce, and eliminate exposure to risk that results in financial loss.

Root cause analysis Team-based problem-solving tool used to determine how or why something happened. Asking "why?" five times and using cause-and-effect diagrams are common methods employed (99).

Sanctions Administrative remedies and actions (for example, exclusion, civil monetary penalties) available to the OIG to deal with questionable, improper, or abusive behaviors of providers under Medicare, Medicaid, or any state health programs.

Standard transaction Transmission of any health information in electronic form in connection with a transaction.

Stark I Amendment A federal law prohibiting physicians from referring a Medicare patient to an entity for the furnishing of laboratory services if the physician, or the physician's immediate family member, has a direct or indirect financial interest in the entity providing the laboratory services.

Stark II Amendment An extension of the Stark I Amendment that prohibits physicians from referring Medicare and Medicaid patients for certain types of services known as "designated health services" to entities if the physician, or the physician's immediate family member, has a direct or indirect financial interest in the entity.

Third-party administrator An entity required to make or responsible for making payment on behalf of a group health plan.

Transfusion medicine service Department or laboratory that provides compatibility testing, labeling, and release of blood to patients. Also provides consultative services to clinicians.

TRICARE TRICARE is the healthcare program for active-duty members of the military, military retirees, and their eligible dependents. TRICARE was called CHAMPUS in the past (see "Civilian Health and Medical Program of the Uniformed Services")

Unbundling Submission of bills for various tests in a piecemeal or fragmented fashion. Generally this practice is illegal if done to maximize reimbursement.

Uniform Bill 92 (UB-92) A uniform institutional claim form, developed by the National Uniform Billing Committee, that has been in general use since 1993. The form, also known as HCFA-1450 or CMS-1450, is used by facilities when filing Medicare claims with fiscal intermediaries.

Up-coding Use of a billing code that provides a higher level of reimbursement than the code that accurately reflects the service provided.

Validation Establishing documented evidence which provides a high degree of assurance that a specific process will consistently produce a product meeting its predetermined specifications and quality attributes. A process is validated to evaluate the performance of a system with regard to its effectiveness based on intended use (69).

Window period The period when blood tests are negative for a pathogen though the individual is infected and able to transmit the agent. Lookback and postdonation information are designed to identify recipients of blood who might have been transfused during the window period.

Zero tolerance The OIG's position that a healthcare institution will promote and adhere to compliance at all levels and that noncompliance will not be tolerated.

REFERENCES

1. **Allain, J.-P.** 1998. The status of hepatitis C virus screening. *Transfus. Med. Rev.* 12:46–55.

2. **American Association of Blood Banks.** 1998. Shalala announces support for ACBSA recommendations on HCV. American Associa-

tion of Blood Banks faxnet no. 364. American Association of Blood Banks, Bethesda, Md.

3. **American Association of Blood Banks.** 1996. NYBC and FDA agree to voluntary consent decree. *American Association of Blood Banks Weekly Report,* vol. 2, p. 1–2. American Association of Blood Banks, Bethesda, Md.

4. **American Association of Blood Banks.** Quality program implementation. Association bulletin, 1 August 1997, p. 4. American Association of Blood Banks, Bethesda, Md.

5. **America's Blood Centers.** HHS blood panel says government has role in monitoring blood supply. America's Blood Centers newsletter, 27 April 2001, no. 17, p. 1–6. American Blood Center, Washington, D.C.

6. **America's Blood Centers.** 2001. Judge urges Red Cross and FDA to solve disagreements over consent decree. America's Blood Centers newsletter, 21/28 December 2001, no. 48, p. 4–6. America's Blood Centers, Washington, D.C.

7. **America's Blood Centers.** 2002. New CBER guidance expands vCJD donor deferrals to Europe. America's Blood Centers newsletter, 11 January 2002, no. 2, p. 2–5. America's Blood Centers, Washington, D.C.

8. **America's Blood Centers.** 2001. New York hospitals seek help in mitigating effects of vCJD donor deferrals on blood supply. America's Blood Centers newsletter, 17 August 2001, no. 32, p. 1–2. America's Blood Centers, Washington, D.C.

9. **America's Blood Centers.** 1996. New Jersey Supreme Court jury award holds AABB to ordinary negligence standard. America's Blood Centers newsletter, 6 June 1996, p. 1–3. America's Blood Centers, Washington, D.C.

10. **Appold, K.** 2002. ASCP and NCA highlight their certification options. *Vantage Point* **6**(12/13):8–10.

10a. **Arent Fox Attorneys at Law.** 2001. *The HIPAA Health Information Privacy Standards,* p. 1–9. Alert, February 2001. [Online.] http:// www.arentfox.com (accessed January 2003).

11. **Atlas, S. J., D. E. Singer, and S. J. Skates.** 1994. Changing blood use in the AIDS era: the case of elective hip surgery. *Transfusion* **34**:386–391.

12. **AuBuchon, J. P.** 1999. Public health, public trust, and public decision making: making hepatitis C virus lookback work. *Transfusion* **39**:123–127.

13. **AuBuchon, J. P.** 2000. Paving the road with good intentions: learning from HCV lookback. *Transfusion* **40**:1153–1156.

14. **Ayres, K.** 2000. Be prepared: HIPAA won't go away. *Vantage Point* **4**(7):1, 4.

15. **Ayres, K.** 2000. Hospital outpatient departments soon to face challenge of APCs. *Vantage Point* **4**(6):1, 3–4.

16. **Battles, J. B., H. S. Kaplan, T. W. Van der Schaaf, and C. E. Shea.** 1998. The attributes of medical event-reporting systems; experience with a prototype medical event-reporting system for transfusion medicine. *Arch. Pathol. Lab. Med.* **122**:231–238.

17. **Beasley, D., M. Blanchard, P. Kazon, and C. A. Pontius.** 1999. Use confirmation form to meet oral test order documentation requirements. *Lab. Compliance Insid.,* July, p. 1–3.

18. **Beattie, J., H. M. Casale, and D. Hunt.** 1999. Avoid liability as HCFA targets ESRD billing. *Lab. Compliance Insid.,* August, p. 1–6.

19. **Berger, D.** 1999. A brief history of medical diagnosis and the birth of the clinical laboratory, part 1. *MLO Med. Lab. Obs.* **31**(7):28–40.

20. **Berger, D.** 1999. A brief history of medical diagnosis and the birth of the clinical laboratory, part 2. *MLO Med. Lab. Obs.* **31**(8):32–38.

21. **Berger, D.** 1999. A brief history of medical diagnosis and the birth of the clinical laboratory, part 3. *MLO Med. Lab. Obs.* **31**(10):40–44.

22. **Berte, L. M., and D. E. Nevalainen.** 1997. Quality pays—in every business. *Transfus. Sci.* **18**:589–596.

23. **Billings, C. E.** 1998. Some hopes and concerns regarding medical event-reporting systems; lessons from the NASA Aviation Safety Reporting System. *Arch. Pathol. Lab. Med.* **122**:214–215. (Editorial.)

24. **Birkmeyer, J. D., J. P. AuBuchon, B. Littenbert, G. T. O'Connor, R. F. Nease, W. C. Nugent, and L. T. Goodnough.** 1994. Cost-effectiveness of preoperative autologous donation in coronary artery bypass grafting. *Ann. Thorac. Surg.* **57**:161–169.

25. **Blajchman, M. A., and H. G. Klein.** 1997. Looking back in anger: retrospection in the face of a paradigm shift. *Transfus. Med. Rev.* **11**:1–5.

26. **Boothe, J. F.** 1998. Hospital compliance plan: key elements you need to know. *Vantage Point* **2**(12):1–4.

27. **Boothe, J. F.** 1999. Set standing order review policy to avoid fraud charges. *Lab. Compliance Insid.,* May, p. 6–7.

28. **Boothe, J. F.** 2001. Congressional close brings reimbursement changes, what's ahead for 2001. *Vantage Point* **5**(4):3–4.

29. **Boothe, J. F.** 2001. HIPAA privacy rule issued: the clock is ticking, part 1. *Vantage Point* **5**(7):1–6.

30. **Boothe, J. F.** 2001. HIPAA privacy rule issued: the clock is ticking, part 2. *Vantage Point* **5**(8):1–9.

30a. **Boothe, J., and J. Gayken.** 1997. Chapter 2, Your contract with the Federal Government, p. 27–34. *The CLMA Guide to Medicare Compliance for Laboratories.* CLMA, Wayne, Pa.

31. **Boothe, J. F., and J. A. Gayken.** 1997. Workshop on laboratory compliance, special session. Clinical Laboratory Management Association Annual Conference and Exhibition, Toronto, Ontario, Canada.

32. **Brecher, M. E. (ed.).** 2002. *Technical Manual,* 14th ed. American Association of Blood Banks, Bethesda, Md.

33. **Brown, J. A., and H. Blackwell.** 1992. Compiling employee safety records that will satisfy OSHA. *MLO Med. Lab. Obs.* **24**:45–48.

34. **Busch, M. P.** 1991. Let's look at human immunodeficiency virus look-back before leaping into hepatitis C virus look-back. *Transfusion* **31**:655–661.

35. **Busch, M. P., and R. Y. Dodd.** 2000. NAT and blood safety: what is the paradigm? *Transfusion* **40**:1157–1160. (Editorial.)

36. **Busch, M. P., M. J. Young, S. M. Samson, J. W. Mosley, J. W. Ward, H. A. Perkins, and the Transfusion Safety Study Group.** 1991. Risk of human immunodeficiency virus (HIV) transmission by blood transfusions before the implementation of HIV-1 antibody screening. *Transfusion* **31**:4–11.

37. **Cassidy, B.** 2000. Why comply with HIPAA regulations. *Health Manag. Technol.* **21**(10):12.

38. **Centers for Medicare and Medicaid Services.** 1996. Ambulatory payment classification (APC). Program memorandum A-96-7. Centers for Medicare and Medicaid Services, Baltimore, Md.

39. **Centers for Medicare and Medicaid Services.** 1998. Ambulatory payment classification (APC). Program memorandum A-98-5. Centers for Medicare and Medicaid Services, Baltimore, Md.

40. **Centers for Medicare and Medicaid Services.** 2000. Final outpatient PPS rule. Program memorandum A-00-60. Centers for Medicare and Medicaid Services, Baltimore, Md.

41. **Centers for Medicare and Medicaid Services.** 2000. Transfer of initial Medicare secondary payer (MSP) development activities to the coordination of benefits (COB) contractor. Program memorandum transmittal AB-00-36. Centers for Medicare and Medicaid Services, Baltimore, Md.

42. **Christensen, P. B., K. Groenbaek, and H. B. Krarup.** 1999. Transfusion-acquired hepatitis C: the Danish lookback experience. *Transfusion* **39:**188–193.

43. **Clark, G. B.** 1998. Laboratory regulation, certification, and accreditation, p. 369–394. *In* J. A. Snyder and D. S. Wilkinson (ed.), *Management in Laboratory Medicine,* 3rd ed. Lippincott, Philadelphia, Pa.

44. **Clinical Laboratory Coalition.** 2002. *Competitive bidding.* Laboratory Institute. Washington G-2 Reports, Washington, D.C.

45. **Code of Federal Regulations.** 1991. Occupational exposure to bloodborne pathogens. 29 CFR 1910.1030.

46. **Code of Federal Regulations.** 2001. Medicare program; negotiated rulemaking; coverage and administrative policies for clinical diagnostic laboratory services. 42 CFR 410.

47. **Code of Federal Regulations.** 2001. Occupational exposure to hazardous chemicals in laboratories. 29 CFR 1910.1450.

48. **Code of Federal Regulations.** 2002. Biological products, general. 21 CFR 600.

49. **Code of Federal Regulations.** 2002. Current good manufacturing practice for blood and blood components. 21 CFR 606.

50. **Code of Federal Regulations.** 2002. Current good manufacturing practice for finished pharmaceuticals. 21 CFR 211.

51. **Code of Federal Regulations.** 2002. Current good manufacturing practice in manufacturing, processing, packing, or holding of drugs; general. 21 CFR 210.

52. **Code of Federal Regulations.** 2002. Purpose and use of hazardous materials table. 49 CFR 172.101.

53. **Code of Federal Regulations.** 2002. Reporting of biological product deviations by licensed manufacturers. 21 CFR 600.14.

54. **Code of Federal Regulations.** 2002. Reporting of product deviations by licensed manufacturers, unlicensed registered blood establishments, and transfusion services. 21 CFR 606.171.

55. **Cook, E.** 1999. Specimen transport regulation. *Adv. Admin. Lab.* **8**(3)**:**66–68.

56. **Croce, B.** (ed.). 2001. Are you ready for the impact of OSHA's ergonomics standard? *Brief. Lab. Saf. Accredit.* **7**(1)**:**1–5.

57. **Croce, B.** (ed.). 2001. Congress repeals workplace rules, but ergonomics not dead yet. *Brief. Lab. Saf. Accredit.* **7**(4)**:**1–5.

58. **Culver, D. H., M. J. Alter, R. J. Mullan, and H. S. Margolis.** 2000. Evaluation of the effectiveness of targeted lookback for HCV infection in the United States—interim results. *Transfusion* **40:**1176–1181.

59. **Dodd, R. Y.** 2001. Germs, gels, and genomes: a personal recollection of 30 years in blood safety testing, p. 97–122. *In* S. L. Stramer (ed.), *Blood Safety in the New Millennium.* American Association of Blood Banks, Bethesda, Md.

60. **Downes, K. A.** 2001. FDA tightens rule, targets transfusion services. *CAP Today* **15:**5–8.

61. **Dragon, M.** (ed.). 1998. FDA to regulate powdered latex gloves. *Brief. Lab. Saf. Accredit.* **4**(3)**:**3.

62. **Epstein, Becker, and Green, P.C.** 1996. The National Health Law Practice, January Special Alert. Epstein, Becker, and Green, P.C., Washington, D.C.

63. **Federal Register.** 1998. Publication of the OIG compliance program guidance for hospitals—OIG. Notice. *Fed. Regist.* **63:** 8987–8998.

64. **Federal Register.** 2000. Health care programs: fraud and abuse; revised OIG civil money penalties resulting from public law 104-191. Office of Inspector General (OIG), HHS. Final rule. *Fed. Regist.* **65:**24400–24419.

65. **Flury, P.** 1978. *Environmental Health and Safety in the Hospital Laboratory,* p. 3–26. Charles C Thomas, Springfield, Ill.

66. **Fogle, B.** 1999. Error and accident reporting requirements of regulatory agencies, p. 21–36. *In* J. Rhamy (ed.), *Error Management: an Important Part of Quality Control.* American Association of Blood Banks, Bethesda, Md.

67. **Food and Drug Administration.** 2002. Guidance for industry: revised preventative measures to reduce the possible risk of transmission of Creutzfeldt-Jakob disease (CJD) and variant Creutzfeldt-Jakob disease (vCJD) by blood and blood products. Food and Drug Administration, Rockville, Md.

68. **Food and Drug Administration.** 1993. Memorandum: guidance regarding post donation information reports. Food and Drug Administration, Rockville, Md.

69. **Food and Drug Administration.** 1995. Guideline for quality assurance in blood establishments. Food and Drug Administration, Rockville, Md.

70. **Food and Drug Administration.** 1999. Guideline for industry; current good manufacturing practice for blood and blood components: (1) quarantine and disposition of units from prior collections from donors with repeatedly reactive screening tests for antibody to hepatitis C virus (anti-HCV); (2) supplemental testing, and the notification of consignees and blood recipients of donor test results for anti-HCV. Food and Drug Administration, Rockville, Md.

71. **Foster, H.** 2003. *Key Legal Issues in Laboratory Outreach. Advanced Strategies for Laboratory Outreach.* Washington G-2 Reports and Park City Solutions, Atlanta, Ga.

72. **Furr, A. K.** 2000. *CRC Handbook of Laboratory Safety,* 5th ed., p. 69–197. CRC Press, Boca Raton, Fla.

73. **Furr, A. K.** 2000. *CRC Handbook of Laboratory Safety,* 5th ed., p. 342–352. CRC Press, Boca Raton, Fla.

74. **Gersten, S., C. Anderson, and D. Roach.** 2000. Compliance tip: don't accept boilerplate corporate integrity agreements. *G-2 Compliance Rep.* **2**(5)**:**4.

75. **Gill, M. J., D. Towns, S. Allaire, and G. Meyers.** 1997. Transmission of human immunodeficiency virus through blood transfusion: the use of lookback and traceback approaches to optimize recipient identification in a regional population. *Transfusion* **37:**513–516.

76. **Goodnough, L. T., M. E. Brecher, M. H. Kanter, and J. P. Au-Buchon.** 1999. Transfusion medicine, first of two parts, blood transfusion. *N. Engl. J. Med.* **340:**438–447.

77. **Goodnough, L. T., M. E. Brecher, M. H. Kanter, and J. P. Au-Buchon.** 1999. Transfusion medicine, second of two parts, blood conservation. *N. Engl. J. Med.* **340:**525–533.

78. **Gorlin, J. B. (ed.).** 2002. *Standards for Blood Banks and Transfusion Services,* 21st ed. American Association of Blood Banks, Bethesda, Md.

79. **Graziano, P.** 2002. Capitol scan. *CAP Today* **16**(10):89–90.

80. **Harrington, S.** 2001. HIPAA, HIPAA, hurrah! *Health Manag. Technol.* **22**(4):14.

81. **Hart, P. D.** 1999. HAZCOM, the hazard communication standard. *Facil. Care* **4**(7):19–20.

82. **Hartsfield, S.** 2001. Phasing in Stark II: how the new self-referral rules affect clinical laboratories. *Vantage Point* **5**(6):1–5.

83. **Harty-Golder, B.** 2002. Liability and the lab—defining the business associate provision of HIPAA. *MLO Med. Lab. Obs.* **34**(8):26.

84. **Hicks, R.** 1989. Basics of clinical laboratory safety, p. 325. *In* J. Snyder and D. A. Senhauser (ed.), *Administration and Supervision in Laboratory Medicine,* 2nd ed. J. B. Lippincott Company, Philadelphia, Pa.

85. **Holloway, T.** 2001. Safe specimen packaging begins with you. *Adv. Med. Lab. Prof.* **13**(23):16–19.

86. **Huchenski, J.** 2000. Prepare to make chain of trust agreements with business partners. *Lab. Compliance Insid.,* December, p. 7–9.

87. **Hunt, D., R. E. Mazer, C. A. Pontius, and C. Young.** 1998. How to avoid fraud charges for reflex testing without physician orders. *Lab. Compliance Insid.,* August, p. 1–5.

88. **Institute of Medicine.** 1995. *HIV and the Blood Supply: an Analysis of Crisis Decision Making.* National Academy Press, Washington, D.C.

89. **Johnston, V.** 1997. When pain brings no gain. *Lab. Med.* **28:**380–386.

90. **Joint Commission on Accreditation of Healthcare Organizations.** 2002. *Comprehensive Accreditation Manual for Hospitals,* MS.8.4, PI.3.1. Joint Commission on Accreditation of Healthcare Organizations, Oakbrook Terrace, Ill.

91. **Kaplan, H. S., J. B. Battles, T. W. Van der Schaaf, C. E. Shea, and S. Q. Mercer.** 1998. Identification and classification of the causes of events in transfusion medicine. *Transfusion* **8:**1071–1081.

92. **Kazon, P.** 1997. *Probe,* Module 1. *Medicare Reimbursement,* p. 1–3. CLMA, Wayne, Pa.

93. **Lark, S.** 1998. The Americans with Disabilities Act. *Lab. Med.* **29:**18–24.

94. **Logue, J.** 2002. Modifiers: use correctly and avoid denial of payment. *Vantage Point* **6**(2):6–8.

95. **Long, A., G. Sprull, H. Demers, and M. Goldman.** 1999. Targeted hepatitis C lookback: Quebec, Canada. *Transfusion* **39:**194–200.

96. **Lubbert, P.** 2001. Under OSHA's umbrella. *Adv. Admin. Lab.* **10:**34–39.

97. **Marwick, C.** 2000. Nosocomial TB control guidelines debated: will OSHA's proposed regulations prevail? *JAMA* **284:**1637.

98. **McCullough, J.** 1993. The nation's changing blood supply system. *JAMA* **269:**2239–2245.

99. **McMican, A.** 1999. Sentinel events in hospital performance improvement, p. 11–20. *In* J. Rhamy (ed.), *Error Management: an Important Part of Quality Control.* American Association of Blood Banks, Bethesda, Md.

100. **Medicare Payment Advisory Commission.** December 2001. Report to the Congress: blood safety in hospitals and Medicare inpatient payment. Medicare Payment Advisory Commission, Washington, D.C.

101. **Menitove, J. E.** 1993. Controversies in transfusion medicine: the recent emphasis on good manufacturing practices and the pharmaceutical manufacturing approach damages blood banking and transfusion medicine as medical care activities: con. *Transfusion* **33:**439–442.

102. **Mesaros, F., Jr.** 1999. Laboratory end-stage renal disease testing. *Clin. Lab. Manag. Rev.* **13:**132–136.

103. **Meyers, L. K., N. D. Kalmin, and M. B. Fisk.** 1999. ISO 9002: impact on a blood and tissue center's operations. *Transfus. Med. Rev.* **13:**187–193.

104. **Miller, W. V.** 1993. Controversies in transfusion medicine: blood banks should use good manufacturing practices and the pharmaceutical manufacturing approach: pro. *Transfusion* **33:**435–438.

105. **Mintz, P. D.** 2001. Nishot: on target, but there's no magic bullet. *Am. J. Clin. Pathol.* **116:**802–805.

106. **Mitcheletti, J.** 2000. APC environment poses new compliance risk. *Health Manag. Technol.* **21**(6):54–55.

107. **National Institute for Occupational Safety and Health.** 1997. *Preventing Allergic Reactions to Natural Rubber Latex in the Workplace.* NIOSH alert. NIOSH publication no. 97–135. National Institute for Occupational Safety and Health, Washington, D.C.

108. **National Intelligence Report.** 11 February 2002. Focus on: 2002 Congressional Healthcare Agenda. United against terrorism. Divided over a whole lot more. *Nat. Intell. Rep.* **23**(8):3–6.

109. **National Research Council.** 1995. *Prudent Practices in the Laboratory Handling and Disposal of Chemicals,* p. 197–212. National Academy Press, Washington, D.C.

110. **National Research Council.** 1995. *Prudent Practices in the Laboratory Handling and Disposal of Chemicals,* p. 81–104. National Academy Press, Washington, D.C.

111. **NCCLS.** 1996. *Clinical Laboratory Safety.* Approved guideline GP17-A, vol. 16, no. 6, p. 1–39. NCCLS, Wayne, Pa.

112. **Occupational Safety and Health Administration.** 1999. Enforcement procedures for the occupational exposure to bloodborne pathogens. OSHA compliance directive CPL 2-2.44D.

113. **Office of the Investigator General.** 1994. Expansion of DRG payment window. OIG report A-01-92-000521.

114. **Office of the Investigator General.** 1995. Joint project status report A-03-94-00021.

115. **Padget, D.** 2001. Enhance compliance and reimbursement with chart audits. *Pathol./Lab Coding Alert* **2**(6):41,44–47.

116. **Raab, G., and J. Logue.** 2001. Medicare coverage of new clinical diagnostic laboratory tests: the need for coding and payment reforms. *Clin. Leadersh. Manag. Rev.* **15:**95–105.

117. **Root, J., and D. Voorhees.** 2001. Take four steps to implement CPT codebook changes. *Lab. Compliance Insid.*, February, p. 2–3.

118. **Rorer, M.** 1997. Safety first—a lesson in ergonomics, *Adv. Admin. Lab.* **6**(3):38–45.

119. **Sayers, M. H.** 1995. Cost of compliance: is politics involved? *Transfusion* **35**:625–626.

120. **Sazama, K.** 1996. Current good manufacturing practices for transfusion medicine. *Transfus. Med. Rev.* **10**:286–295.

121. **Schreiber, G. B., M. P. Busch, S. H. Kleinman, and J. J. Korelitz.** 1996. The risk of transfusion-transmitted viral infections. *N. Engl. J. Med.* **334**:1685–1690.

122. **Senhauser, D. A.** 1989. Laboratory accreditation, licensure, and regulation, p. 339–348. *In* J. R. Snyder and D. A. Senhauser (ed.), *Administration and Supervision in Laboratory Medicine*, 2nd ed. J. B. Lippincott Company, Philadelphia, Pa.

123. **Smith, E. N., P. V. Holland, S. M. Holliman, and M. J. Fuller.** 1995. Staff costs associated with the implementation of a comprehensive compliance program in a community blood center. *Transfusion* **35**:679–682.

124. **Snyder, J. R., S. L. Wilson, and L. L. Otis.** 1989. Interviewing and employee selection, p. 177–198. *In* J. R. Snyder and D. A. Senhauser (ed.), *Administration and Supervision in Laboratory Medicine*, 2nd ed. J. B. Lippincott Company, Philadelphia, Pa.

125. **Solomon, J. M.** 1981. Legislation and regulation in blood banking, p. 143–171. *In* M. Schaeffer (ed.), *Federal Legislation and the Clinical Laboratory*. G. K. Hall Medical Publishers, Boston, Mass.

126. **Solomon, J. M.** 1994. The evolution of the current blood banking regulatory climate. *Transfusion* **34**:272–277.

127. **Stanley, L. J.** 1999. Corrective actions for errors and accidents, p. 113–133. *In* J. Rhamy (ed.), *Error Management: an Important Part of Quality Control*. American Association of Blood Banks, Bethesda, Md.

128. **Tagliabue, J.** 16 July 2001. U.S. plan to halt blood imports worries Europe. *New York Times*, New York, N.Y.

129. **Tweedy, J. T.** 1997. *Healthcare Hazard Control and Safety Management*, p. 79–120. HSP Board of Certified Healthcare Safety Management, Bethesda, Md., and Lewis Publishers, Boca Raton, Fla.

130. **U.S. Department of Labor.** 1997. OSHA proposes TB standard to protect 5.3 million workers. OSHA national news release USDL: 97-366. U.S. Department of Labor, Washington, D.C.

131. **U.S. Department of Labor.** 2001. Prevention is the best medicine, OSHA announces outreach effort on needlestick prevention. OSHA national news release USDL: 01-140. U.S. Department of Labor, Washington, D.C.

132. **U.S. Department of Labor.** 2002. OSHA announces comprehensive plan to reduce ergonomic injuries. OSHA national news release USDL: 02-201. U.S. Department of Labor, Washington, D.C.

133. **U.S. General Accounting Office.** 1997. Blood safety: transfusion-associated risks. GAO/PEMD-97-2. U.S. General Accounting Office, Washington, D.C.

134. **U.S. General Accounting Office.** 1997. Blood supply: FDA oversight and remaining issues of safety. GAO/PEMD-97-1. U.S. General Accounting Office, Washington, D.C.

135. **Varnadoe, L. A.** 1996. *Medical Laboratory Management and Supervision*, p. 113–126. F. A. Davis Company, Philadelphia, Pa.

136. **Voorhees, D.** 1999. Perspectives: updating your chargemaster codes for 2000—guidance for compliance management. *Washington G-2 Compliance Rep.* **1**(12):5–6.

137. **The Wall Street Journal.** 25 August 1999. Mad regulatory disease. *The Wall Street Journal*, New York, N.Y.

138. **Waltz, J., and M. A. Allen.** 2002. Perspectives—Using the new ABNs: how to navigate regulatory pitfalls & minimize risks. *Washington G-2 Compliance Rep.*, October, p. 1–4.

139. **Young, C.** 2000. Billing issues: blood smears, claim denials, MSPs. *Vantage Point* **4**(1):4–5.

140. **Young, C.** 2000. MSP questionnaire raises challenging issues for laboratorians. *Vantage Point* **4**(15):9–12.

141. **Young, C.** 2002. Clinical Laboratory Management Association. Compliance 2002 audio conference series. The New ABN: Understanding the Rules/Strategies for Successful Implementation. CLMA, Wayne, Pa.

ADDITIONAL RECOMMENDED RESOURCES

Boothe, J. F. 2000. Negotiated rulemaking: what laboratories need to know. *Vantage Point* **4**(8):1–4.

Boothe, J. F. 2000. HIPAA update. Clinical Laboratory Management Association Audio-Conference, October 2002. CLMA, Wayne, Pa.

Boothe, J. F. 2000. HIPAA data privacy and data security implementation: are you ready? *Vantage Point* **4**(14):1–4.

Brownstone Publishers. 2001. *Health Information Compliance Insider*, February 2001. Brownstone Publishers, New York, N.Y.

Brownstone Publishers. 2001. *Health Information Compliance Insider*, March 2001. HIPAA fact sheet and index to final HIPPA rules. Brownstone Publishers, New York, N.Y.

Brownstone Publishers. October 2000. *Laboratory Compliance Insider*. Brownstone Publishers, New York, N.Y.

Kazon, P. M. 1998. Legal basis and interpretations of medical necessity. *Clin. Lab. Manag. Rev.* **12**(5):375–382.

Keoppel, P. 2001. How to perform a compliance audit of your laboratory. Clinical Laboratory Management Association Annual Conference and Exhibition, St. Louis, Mo.

McCurdy, K., and K. Gregory (ed.). 2000. *Blood Bank Regulations from A to Z*, 3rd ed. American Association of Blood Banks, Bethesda, Md.

Murray, T., and L. Byrne. 1999. To the hill and back: CLMA and the negotiated rule making experience. *Vantage Point* **3**:7.

Young, C. 2001. Crosswalking: the tip of the iceberg. *Vantage Point* **5**(9):1–3.

Young, C. 1999. OIG releases compliance guidance for third party medical billing. *Vantage Point* **3**(2):1–4.

Young, C. 1998. Patient protection from liability: advance beneficiary notices (part 1). *Vantage Point* **2**(9/10):1–6.

Young, C. 1998. Patient protection from liability: advance beneficiary notices (part 2). *Vantage Point* **2**(10):1–3.

APPENDIX 5.1   Medicare Secondary-Payor Questionnaire

Medicare Secondary Payer Questionnaire	
Date of Service:	Physician:
Patient Name:	Location:
Medicare Number:	Phone :
MCVH MRN:	Office Chart #:
PARS Account #:	Interviewer:

MCV LOGO HERE

Part I: Medicare as Secondary Payer to Government Funded Programs	Check Answer	See Instructions
1. Are you receiving Black Lung (BL) benefits and the services being performed are covered by BL? Begin Date: ___/___/___	☐ YES	☐ NO
2. Has the Department of Veteran's Affairs (DVA) authorized and agreed to pay for care at this facility?	☐ YES	☐ NO
3. Are the services to be paid by a government research grant? If yes, list grant number: _____.	☐ YES	☐ NO
4. Is the illness, a work related injury and covered by workman's compensation?	☐ YES	☐ NO, Go to Part II
Part II: Non Work Related Accident /Injury Information		
5. Is the visit or service requested a result of a non-work related accident? Date of Accident: ___/___/___	☐ YES	☐ NO, Go to Part III
6. What type of accident caused the illness/ injury? ☐ Automobile *(Type 02)* ☐ Other than Auto *(Type 05)*	Complete Part III	
7. Was another party responsible for this accident?	☐ YES	☐ NO, Complete Part III
Part III: Medicare Eligibility Information		
8 Do you have Medicare based on Age (A), Disability (D), or E.S.R.D. (E)? *If answer is Age, complete Part IV only. If answer is Disability, Complete Part V only. If answer is ESRD, complete Part VI only.*	☐ Age (A) ___ ☐ Disability (D __ ☐ ESRD (E) ___	Complete Part IV. Complete Part V. Complete Part VI.
Part IV: Employment / Age Related Information		
9. Is the patient currently employed? *If Yes, Provide Employer:* _____ *If No: Provide Date of Retirement:* ___/___/___	☐ YES Continue to #11.	☐ NO Retirement Date
10. Is your spouse currently employed? *If yes, Provide Employer:* _____ *If No, provide Date of Retirement:* ___/___/___.	☐ YES Continue to #11.	☐ NO
11. Is your group health insurance (GHP) coverage based on your own (Yes), or spouse's (No) employment?	☐ YES Continue to #12	☐ NO
12. Does the employer that sponsors your group health (GHP) employ 20 or more employees?	☐ YES Continue to #13	☐ NO Stop! MC =Primary.
Part V: Employment / Disability Related Information		
13. Are you currently employed? List Employer:_____	☐ YES	☐ NO
14. Is a family member (acting as responsible party) currently employed? List Employer: _____.	☐ YES Continue to #15.	☐ NO
15. Do you have group health coverage (GHP) based on their (family) employment? ☐ Self (No) ☐ Spouse (Yes)	☐ YES	☐ NO
16. Does the employer that sponsors the group health plan employ 100 or more employees?	☐ YES	☐ NO Stop! MC =Primary.
Part VI: Employment / End Stage Renal Disease (ESRD) Information		
17. Have you received a kidney transplant? Provide Date: ___/___/___.	☐ YES Continue	☐ NO Stop! MC =Primary.
18. Have you received maintenance dialysis treatment? Date treatment began:___/___/___ Have you participated in a self dialysis training program, Training start date: ___/___/___	☐ YES	☐ NO
19. Do you have group health insurance (GHP) coverage?	☐ YES	☐ NO
20. Are you within the 30 month coordination period?	☐ YES	☐ NO Stop! MC =Primary.
21. Are you entitled to Medicare on the basis of either ESRD & age, or ESRD & disability?.	☐ YES	☐ NO Stop! MC is Secondary.
22. Was your initial entitlement to Medicare based on End Stage Renal Disease (ESRD)?	☐ YES	☐ NO
23. Is the group health insurance (GHP) primary coverage based on age (A) or disability (D)?	☐ YES MC is Secondary	☐ NO MC is Primary

APPENDIX 5.2   Advance Beneficiary Notice CMS-R-131-G

Patient's Name:	Medicare # (HICN):

ADVANCE BENEFICIARY NOTICE (ABN)

NOTE: You need to make a choice about receiving these health care items or services.

We expect that Medicare will not pay for the item(s) or service(s) that are described below. Medicare does not pay for all of your health care costs. Medicare only pays for covered items and services when Medicare rules are met. The fact that Medicare may not pay for a particular item or service does not mean that you should not receive it. There may be a good reason your doctor recommended it. Right now, in your case, **Medicare probably will not pay for –**

Items or Services:

Because:

The purpose of this form is to help you make an informed choice about whether or not you want to receive these items or services, knowing that you might have to pay for them yourself. Before you make a decision about your options, you should **read this entire notice carefully.**

- Ask us to explain, if you don't understand why Medicare probably won't pay.
- Ask us how much these items or services will cost you (**Estimated Cost: $**_____), in case you have to pay for them yourself or through other insurance.

PLEASE CHOOSE **ONE** OPTION. CHECK **ONE** BOX. **SIGN & DATE** YOUR CHOICE.

☐ **Option 1. YES.**   **I want to receive these items or services.**

I understand that Medicare will not decide whether to pay unless I receive these items or services. Please submit my claim to Medicare. I understand that you may bill me for items or services and that I may have to pay the bill while Medicare is making its decision. If Medicare does pay, you will refund to me any payments I made to you that are due to me. If Medicare denies payment, I agree to be personally and fully responsible for payment. That is, I will pay personally, either out of pocket or through any other insurance that I have. I understand I can appeal Medicare's decision.

☐ **Option 2. NO.**   **I have decided not to receive these items or services.**

I will not receive these items or services. I understand that you will not be able to submit a claim to Medicare and that I will not be able to appeal your opinion that Medicare won't pay.

Date	Signature of patient or person acting on patient's behalf

NOTE: Your health information will be kept confidential. Any information that we collect about you on this form will be kept confidential in our offices. If a claim is submitted to Medicare, your health information on this form may be shared with Medicare. Your health information which Medicare sees will be kept confidential by Medicare.

OMB Approval No. 0938-0566   Form No. CMS-R-131-G   (June 2002)

APPENDIX 5.3   Advance Beneficiary Notice CMS-R-131-L

Patient's Name: _____   Medicare # (HICN): _____

ADVANCE BENEFICIARY NOTICE (ABN)

NOTE: You need to make a choice about receiving these laboratory tests.

We expect that Medicare will not pay for the laboratory test(s) that are described below. Medicare does not pay for all of your health care costs. Medicare only pays for covered items and services when Medicare rules are met. The fact that Medicare may not pay for a particular item or service does not mean that you should not receive it. There may be a good reason your doctor recommended it. Right now, in your case, **Medicare probably will not pay for the laboratory test(s) indicated below for the following reasons:**

Medicare does not pay for these tests for your condition	Medicare does not pay for these tests as often as this (denied as too frequent)	Medicare does not pay for experimental or research use tests

The purpose of this form is to help you make an informed choice about whether or not you want to receive these laboratory tests, knowing that you might have to pay for them yourself. Before you make a decision about your options, you should **read this entire notice carefully.**
- Ask us to explain, if you don't understand why Medicare probably won't pay.
- Ask us how much these laboratory tests will cost you (**Estimated Cost: $**_____), in case you have to pay for them yourself or through other insurance.

PLEASE CHOOSE **ONE** OPTION. CHECK **ONE** BOX. **SIGN & DATE** YOUR CHOICE.

☐ **Option 1.   YES.   I want to receive these laboratory tests.**
I understand that Medicare will not decide whether to pay unless I receive these laboratory tests. Please submit my claim to Medicare. I understand that you may bill me for laboratory tests and that I may have to pay the bill while Medicare is making its decision. If Medicare does pay, you will refund to me any payments I made to you that are due to me. If Medicare denies payment, I agree to be personally and fully responsible for payment. That is, I will pay personally, either out of pocket or through any other insurance that I have. I understand I can appeal Medicare's decision.

☐ **Option 2.   NO.   I have decided not to receive these laboratory tests.**
I will not receive these laboratory tests. I understand that you will not be able to submit a claim to Medicare and that I will not be able to appeal your opinion that Medicare won't pay. I will notify my doctor who ordered these laboratory tests that I did not receive them.

_____   _____
Date   Signature of patient or person acting on patient's behalf

NOTE: Your health information will be kept confidential. Any information that we collect about you on this form will be kept confidential in our offices. If a claim is submitted to Medicare, your health information on this form may be shared with Medicare. Your health information which Medicare sees will be kept confidential by Medicare.

OMB Approval No. 0938-0566   Form No. CMS-R-131-L   (June 2002)

APPENDIX 5.4 HCFA (CMS) 1500

PLEASE
DO NOT
STAPLE
IN THIS
AREA

CARRIER →

HEALTH INSURANCE CLAIM FORM

PICA ☐☐   PICA ☐☐

1. MEDICARE   MEDICAID   CHAMPUS   CHAMPVA   GROUP   FECA   OTHER   1a. INSURED'S I.D. NUMBER   (FOR PROGRAM IN ITEM 1)
   ☐ (Medicare #) ☐ (Medicaid #) ☐ (Sponsor's SSN) ☐ (VA File #) ☐ HEALTH PLAN (SSN or ID) ☐ BLK LUNG (SSN) ☐ (ID)

2. PATIENT'S NAME (Last Name, First Name, Middle Initial)   3. PATIENT'S BIRTH DATE MM DD YY   SEX M☐ F☐   4. INSURED'S NAME (Last Name, First Name, Middle Initial)

5. PATIENT'S ADDRESS (No., Street)   6. PATIENT RELATIONSHIP TO INSURED   Self☐ Spouse☐ Child☐ Other☐   7. INSURED'S ADDRESS (No., Street)

CITY   STATE   8. PATIENT STATUS   Single☐ Married☐ Other☐   CITY   STATE

ZIP CODE   TELEPHONE (Include Area Code) ( )   Employed☐ Full-Time Student☐ Part-Time Student☐   ZIP CODE   TELEPHONE (INCLUDE AREA CODE) ( )

9. OTHER INSURED'S NAME (Last Name, First Name, Middle Initial)   10. IS PATIENT'S CONDITION RELATED TO: 11. INSURED'S POLICY GROUP OR FECA NUMBER

a. OTHER INSURED'S POLICY OR GROUP NUMBER   a. EMPLOYMENT? (CURRENT OR PREVIOUS) ☐YES ☐NO   a. INSURED'S DATE OF BIRTH MM DD YY   SEX M☐ F☐

b. OTHER INSURED'S DATE OF BIRTH MM DD YY   SEX M☐ F☐   b. AUTO ACCIDENT?   PLACE (State) ☐YES ☐NO   b. EMPLOYER'S NAME OR SCHOOL NAME

c. EMPLOYER'S NAME OR SCHOOL NAME   c. OTHER ACCIDENT? ☐YES ☐NO   c. INSURANCE PLAN NAME OR PROGRAM NAME

d. INSURANCE PLAN NAME OR PROGRAM NAME   10d. RESERVED FOR LOCAL USE   d. IS THERE ANOTHER HEALTH BENEFIT PLAN? ☐YES ☐NO If yes, return to and complete item 9 a-d.

READ BACK OF FORM BEFORE COMPLETING & SIGNING THIS FORM.

12. PATIENT'S OR AUTHORIZED PERSON'S SIGNATURE I authorize the release of any medical or other information necessary to process this claim. I also request payment of government benefits either to myself or to the party who accepts assignment below.

SIGNED _____   DATE _____

13. INSURED'S OR AUTHORIZED PERSON'S SIGNATURE I authorize payment of medical benefits to the undersigned physician or supplier for services described below.

SIGNED _____

14. DATE OF CURRENT: MM DD YY ◄ ILLNESS (First symptom) OR INJURY (Accident) OR PREGNANCY(LMP)   15. IF PATIENT HAS HAD SAME OR SIMILAR ILLNESS. GIVE FIRST DATE MM DD YY   16. DATES PATIENT UNABLE TO WORK IN CURRENT OCCUPATION MM DD YY FROM TO MM DD YY

17. NAME OF REFERRING PHYSICIAN OR OTHER SOURCE   17a. I.D. NUMBER OF REFERRING PHYSICIAN   18. HOSPITALIZATION DATES RELATED TO CURRENT SERVICES MM DD YY FROM TO MM DD YY

19. RESERVED FOR LOCAL USE   20. OUTSIDE LAB? ☐YES ☐NO $ CHARGES

21. DIAGNOSIS OR NATURE OF ILLNESS OR INJURY. (RELATE ITEMS 1,2,3 OR 4 TO ITEM 24E BY LINE)
1. ⌊___.__   3. ⌊___.__
2. ⌊___.__   4. ⌊___.__

22. MEDICAID RESUBMISSION CODE   ORIGINAL REF. NO.

23. PRIOR AUTHORIZATION NUMBER

24. A DATE(S) OF SERVICE From MM DD YY To MM DD YY	B Place of Service	C Type of Service	D PROCEDURES, SERVICES, OR SUPPLIES (Explain Unusual Circumstances) CPT/HCPCS MODIFIER	E DIAGNOSIS CODE	F $ CHARGES	G DAYS OR UNITS	H EPSDT Family Plan	I EMG	J COB	K RESERVED FOR LOCAL USE
1										
2										
3										
4										
5										
6										

25. FEDERAL TAX I.D. NUMBER SSN☐ EIN☐   26. PATIENT'S ACCOUNT NO.   27. ACCEPT ASSIGNMENT? (For govt. claims, see back) ☐YES ☐NO   28. TOTAL CHARGE $ 29. AMOUNT PAID $ 30. BALANCE DUE $

31. SIGNATURE OF PHYSICIAN OR SUPPLIER INCLUDING DEGREES OR CREDENTIALS (I certify that the statements on the reverse apply to this bill and are made a part thereof.)

SIGNED _____   DATE _____

32. NAME AND ADDRESS OF FACILITY WHERE SERVICES WERE RENDERED (If other than home or office)

33. PHYSICIAN'S, SUPPLIER'S BILLING NAME, ADDRESS, ZIP CODE & PHONE #

PIN#   GRP#

PATIENT AND INSURED INFORMATION →

PHYSICIAN OR SUPPLIER INFORMATION →

(APPROVED BY AMA COUNCIL ON MEDICAL SERVICE 8/88)   **PLEASE PRINT OR TYPE**   APPROVED OMB-0938-0008 FORM CMS-1500 (12-90). FORM RRB-1500.
APPROVED OMB-1215-0055 FORM OWCP-1500. APPROVED OMB-0720-0001 (CHAMPUS)

APPENDIX 5.4 HCFA (CMS) 1500 *(continued)*

BECAUSE THIS FORM IS USED BY VARIOUS GOVERNMENT AND PRIVATE HEALTH PROGRAMS, SEE SEPARATE INSTRUCTIONS ISSUED BY APPLICABLE PROGRAMS.

NOTICE: Any person who knowingly files a statement of claim containing any misrepresentation or any false, incomplete or misleading information may be guilty of a criminal act punishable under law and may be subject to civil penalties.

REFERS TO GOVERNMENT PROGRAMS ONLY

MEDICARE AND CHAMPUS PAYMENTS: A patient's signature requests that payment be made and authorizes release of any information necessary to process the claim and certifies that the information provided in Blocks 1 through 12 is true, accurate and complete. In the case of a Medicare claim, the patient's signature authorizes any entity to release to Medicare medical and nonmedical information, including employment status, and whether the person has employer group health insurance, liability, no-fault, worker's compensation or other insurance which is responsible to pay for the services for which the Medicare claim is made. See 42 CFR 411.24(a). If item 9 is completed, the patient's signature authorizes release of the information to the health plan or agency shown. In Medicare assigned or CHAMPUS participation cases, the physician agrees to accept the charge determination of the Medicare carrier or CHAMPUS fiscal intermediary as the full charge, and the patient is responsible only for the deductible, coinsurance and noncovered services. Coinsurance and the deductible are based upon the charge determination of the Medicare carrier or CHAMPUS fiscal intermediary if this is less than the charge submitted. CHAMPUS is not a health insurance program but makes payment for health benefits provided through certain affiliations with the Uniformed Services. Information on the patient's sponsor should be provided in those items captioned in "Insured"; i.e., items 1a, 4, 6, 7, 9, and 11.

BLACK LUNG AND FECA CLAIMS

The provider agrees to accept the amount paid by the Government as payment in full. See Black Lung and FECA instructions regarding required procedure and diagnosis coding systems.

SIGNATURE OF PHYSICIAN OR SUPPLIER (MEDICARE, CHAMPUS, FECA AND BLACK LUNG)

I certify that the services shown on this form were medically indicated and necessary for the health of the patient and were personally furnished by me or were furnished incident to my professional service by my employee under my immediate personal supervision, except as otherwise expressly permitted by Medicare or CHAMPUS regulations.

For services to be considered as "incident" to a physician's professional service, 1) they must be rendered under the physician's immediate personal supervision by his/her employee, 2) they must be an integral, although incidental part of a covered physician's service, 3) they must be of kinds commonly furnished in physician's offices, and 4) the services of nonphysicians must be included on the physician's bills.

For CHAMPUS claims, I further certify that I (or any employee) who rendered services am not an active duty member of the Uniformed Services or a civilian employee of the United States Government or a contract employee of the United States Government, either civilian or military (refer to 5 USC 5536). For Black-Lung claims, I further certify that the services performed were for a Black Lung-related disorder.

No Part B Medicare benefits may be paid unless this form is received as required by existing law and regulations (42 CFR 424.32).

NOTICE: Any one who misrepresents or falsifies essential information to receive payment from Federal funds requested by this form may upon conviction be subject to fine and imprisonment under applicable Federal laws.

NOTICE TO PATIENT ABOUT THE COLLECTION AND USE OF MEDICARE, CHAMPUS, FECA, AND BLACK LUNG INFORMATION
(PRIVACY ACT STATEMENT)

We are authorized by CMS, CHAMPUS and OWCP to ask you for information needed in the administration of the Medicare, CHAMPUS, FECA, and Black Lung programs. Authority to collect information is in section 205(a), 1862, 1872 and 1874 of the Social Security Act as amended, 42 CFR 411.24(a) and 424.5(a) (6), and 44 USC 3101;41 CFR 101 et seq and 10 USC 1079 and 1086; 5 USC 8101 et seq; and 30 USC 901 et seq; 38 USC 613; E.O. 9397.

The information we obtain to complete claims under these programs is used to identify you and to determine your eligibility. It is also used to decide if the services and supplies you received are covered by these programs and to insure that proper payment is made.

The information may also be given to other providers of services, carriers, intermediaries, medical review boards, health plans, and other organizations or Federal agencies, for the effective administration of Federal provisions that require other third parties payers to pay primary to Federal program, and as otherwise necessary to administer these programs. For example, it may be necessary to disclose information about the benefits you have used to a hospital or doctor. Additional disclosures are made through routine uses for information contained in systems of records.

FOR MEDICARE CLAIMS: See the notice modifying system No. 09-70-0501, titled, 'Carrier Medicare Claims Record,' published in the <u>Federal Register</u>. Vol. 55 No. 177, page 37549. Wed. Sept. 12, 1990, or as updated and republished.

FOR OWCP CLAIMS: Department of Labor, Privacy Act of 1974, "Republication of Notice of Systems of Records," <u>Federal Register</u> Vol. 55 No. 40, Wed Feb. 28, 1990, See ESA-5, ESA-6, ESA-12, ESA-13, ESA-30, or as updated and republished.

FOR CHAMPUS CLAIMS: <u>PRINCIPLE PURPOSE(S):</u> To evaluate eligibility for medical care provided by civilian sources and to issue payment upon establishment of eligibility and determination that the services/supplies received are authorized by law.

<u>ROUTINE USE(S):</u> Information from claims and related documents may be given to the Dept. of Veterans Affairs, the Dept. of Health and Human Services and/or the Dept. of Transportation consistent with their statutory administrative responsibilities under CHAMPUS/CHAMPVA; to the Dept. of Justice for representation of the Secretary of Defense in civil actions; to the Internal Revenue Service, private collection agencies, and consumer reporting agencies in connection with recoupment claims; and to Congressional Offices in response to inquiries made at the request of the person to whom a record pertains. Appropriate disclosures may be made to other federal, state, local, foreign government agencies, private business entities, and individual providers of care, on matters relating to entitlement, claims adjudication, fraud, program abuse, utilization review, quality assurance, peer review, program integrity, third-party liability, coordination of benefits, and civil and criminal litigation related to the operation of CHAMPUS.

<u>DISCLOSURES:</u> Voluntary; however, failure to provide information will result in delay in payment or may result in denial of claim. With the one exception discussed below, there are no penalties under these programs for refusing to supply information. However, failure to furnish information regarding the medical services rendered or the amount charged would prevent payment of claims under these programs. Failure to furnish any other information, such as name or claim number, would delay payment of the claim. Failure to provide medical information under FECA could be deemed an obstruction.

It is mandatory that you tell us if you know that another party is responsible for paying for your treatment. Section 1128B of the Social Security Act and 31 USC 3801-3812 provide penalties for withholding this information.

You should be aware that P.L. 100-503, the "Computer Matching and Privacy Protection Act of 1988", permits the government to verify information by way of computer matches.

MEDICAID PAYMENTS (PROVIDER CERTIFICATION)

I hereby agree to keep such records as are necessary to disclose fully the extent of services provided to individuals under the State's Title XIX plan and to furnish information regarding any payments claimed for providing such services as the State Agency or Dept. of Health and Humans Services may request.

I further agree to accept, as payment in full, the amount paid by the Medicaid program for those claims submitted for payment under that program, with the exception of authorized deductible, coinsurance, co-payment or similar cost-sharing charge.

SIGNATURE OF PHYSICIAN (OR SUPPLIER): I certify that the services listed above were medically indicated and necessary to the health of this patient and were personally furnished by me or my employee under my personal direction.

NOTICE: This is to certify that the foregoing information is true, accurate and complete. I understand that payment and satisfaction of this claim will be from Federal and State funds, and that any false claims, statements, or documents, or concealment of a material fact, may be prosecuted under applicable Federal or State laws.

According to the Paperwork Reduction Act of 1995, no persons are required to respond to a collection of information unless it displays a valid OMB control number. The valid OMB control number for this information collection is 0938-0008. The time required to complete this information collection is estimated to average 10 minutes per response, including the time to review instructions, search existing data resources, gather the data needed, and complete and review the information collection. If you have any comments concerning the accuracy of the time estimate(s) or suggestions for improving this form, please write to: CMS, N2-14-26, 7500 Security Boulevard, Baltimore, Maryland 21244-1850.

APPENDIX 5.5 UB-92

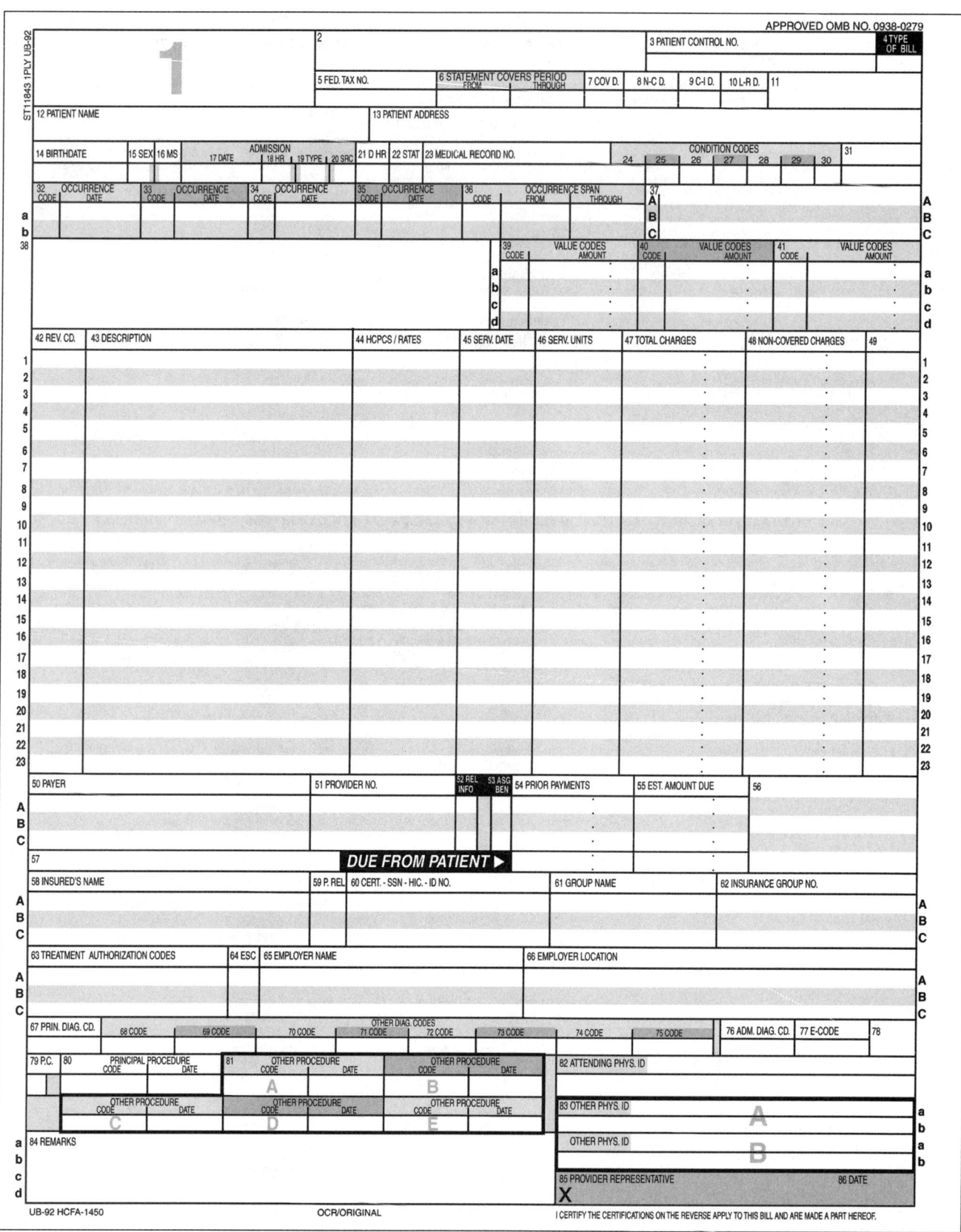

UNIFORM BILL: NOTICE: ANYONE WHO MISREPRESENTS OR FALSIFIES ESSENTIAL INFORMATION REQUESTED BY THIS FORM MAY UPON CONVICTION BE SUBJECT TO FINE AND IMPRISONMENT UNDER FEDERAL AND/OR STATE LAW.

Certifications relevant to the Bill and Information Shown on the Face Hereof: Signatures on the face hereof incorporate the following certifications or verifications where pertinent to this Bill:

1. If third party benefits are indicated as being assigned or in participation status, on the face thereof, appropriate assignments by the insured/beneficiary and signature of patient or parent or legal guardian covering authorization to release information are on file. Determinations as to the release of medical and financial information should be guided by the particular terms of the release forms that were executed by the patient or the patient's legal representative. The hospital agrees to save harmless, indemnify and defend any insurer who makes payment in reliance upon this certification, from and against any claim to the insurance proceeds when in fact no valid assignment of benefits to the hospital was made.

2. If patient occupied a private room or required private nursing for medical necessity, any required certifications are on file.

3. Physician's certifications and re-certifications, if required by contract or Federal regulations, are on file.

4. For Christian Science Sanitoriums, verifications and if necessary re-verifications of the patient's need for sanitorium services are on file.

5. Signature of patient or his/her representative on certifications, authorization to release information, and payment request, as required be Federal law and regulations (42 USC 1935f, 42 CFR 424.36, 10 USC 1071 thru 1086, 32 CFR 199) and, any other applicable contract regulations, is on file.

6. This claim, to the best of my knowledge, is correct and complete and is in conformance with the Civil Rights Act of 1964 as amended. Records adequately disclosing services will be maintained and necessary information will be furnished to such governmental agencies as required by applicable law.

7. For Medicare purposes:

   If the patient has indicated that other health insurance or a state medical assistance agency will pay part of his/her medical expenses and he/she wants information about his/her claim released to them upon their request, necessary authorization is on file. The patient's signature on the provider's request to bill Medicare authorizes any holder of medical and non-medical information, including employment status, and whether the person has employer group health insurance, liability, no-fault, workers' compensation, or other insurance which is responsible to pay for the services for which this Medicare claim is made.

8. For Medicaid purposes:

   This is to certify that the foregoing information is true, accurate, and complete.
   I understand that payment and satisfaction of this claim will be from Federal and State funds, and that any false claims, statements, or documents, or concealment of a material fact, may be prosecuted under applicable Federal or State Laws.

9. For CHAMPUS purposes:

   This is to certify that:

   (a) the information submitted as part of this claim is true, accurate and complete, and, the services shown on this form were medically indicated and necessary for the health of the patient;

   (b) the patient has represented that by a reported residential address outside a military treatment center catchment area he or she does not live within a catchment area of a U.S. military or U.S. Public Health Service medical facility, or if the patient resides within a catchment area of such a facility, a copy of a Non-Availability Statement (DD Form 1251) is on file, or the physician has certified to a medical emergency in any assistance where a copy of a Non-Availability Statement is not on file;

   (c) the patient or the patient's parent or guardian has responded directly to the provider's request to identify all health insurance coverages, and that all such coverages are identified on the face the claim except those that are exclusively supplemental payments to CHAMPUS-determined benefits;

   (d) the amount billed to CHAMPUS has been billed after all such coverages have been billed and paid, excluding Medicaid, and the amount billed to CHAMPUS is that remaining claimed against CHAMPUS benefits;

   (e) the beneficiary's cost share has not been waived by consent or failure to exercise generally accepted billing and collection efforts; and,

   (f) any hospital-based physician under contract, the cost of whose services are allocated in the charges included in this bill, is not an employee or member of the Uniformed Services. For purposes of this certification, an employee of the Uniformed Services is an employee, appointed in civil service (refer to 5 USC 2105), including part-time or intermittent but excluding contract surgeons or other personnel employed by the Uniformed Services through personal service contracts. Similarly, member of the Uniformed Services does not apply to reserve members of the Uniformed Services not on active duty.

   (g) based on the Consolidated Omnibus Budget Reconciliation Act of 1986, all providers participating in Medicare must also participate in CHAMPUS for inpatient hospital services provided pursuant to admissions to hospitals occurring on or after January 1, 1987.

   (h) if CHAMPUS benefits are to be paid in a participating status, I agree to submit this claim to the appropriate CHAMPUS claims processor as a participating provider. I agree to accept the CHAMPUS-determined reasonable charge as the total charge for the medical services or supplies listed on the claim form. I will accept the CHAMPUS-determined reasonable charge even if it is less than the billed amount, and also agree to accept the amount paid by CHAMPUS, combined with the cost-share amount and deductible amount, if any, paid by or on behalf of the patient as full payment for the listed medical services or supplies. I will make no attempt to collect from the patient (or his or her parent or guardian) amounts over the CHAMPUS-determined reasonable charge. CHAMPUS will make any benefits payable directly to me, if I submit this claim as a participating provider.

ESTIMATED CONTRACT BENEFITS

APPENDIX 5.6 Websites

http://www.aab.org: the website for the American Association of Bioanalysts.

http://www.aabb.org: the website for the AABB.

http://www.access.gpo.gov/nara/cfr/index.html: features of this website allow the user to browse the *Code of Federal Regulations* titles and to retrieve specific citations.

http://www.access.gpo.gov/su_docs: Government Printing Office web page. From this page the user can gain access to various federal resources, including the *Federal Register.*

http://www.ansi.org: the website for ANSI.

http://www.aoa-net.org: the website for the AOA.

http://www.arentfox.com: Arent Fox Attorneys at Law, February 2001. Alert. *The HIPAA Health Information Privacy Standards,* p. 1–9.

http://www.ascls.org/jobs/grads: the website of the American Society for Clinical Laboratory Science, a professional organization for clinical laboratory science practiners. This link contains information about certification, licensure, and careers.

http://www.ashi-hla.org: the website for information about the accreditation program of ASHI.

http://www.cap.org: the CAP website. Information about CAP, including the laboratory accreditation program, can be accessed through this website.

http://www.cdc.gov: the website for the CDC. The home page provides links to CDC resources and other websites and has a search function.

http://www.cdc.gov/niosh/about.html: information about the NIOSH. The website has many useful links to health and safety information.

http://www.cdc.gov/od/ohs/ergonomics/labergo.htm: CDC web page giving extensive information on ergonomics and a laboratory self-assessment checklist.

http://www.celltherapy.org: information about the voluntary standards and accreditation program offered by FACT can be accessed at this website for the International Society for Cellular Therapy.

http://www.cms.hhs.gov: the CMS website.

http://www.cms.hhs.gov/clia/progdesc: the portion of the CMS website describing the CLIA program.

http://www.cms.hhs.gov/manuals/108_pim/pim83c13.asp: this website provides a direct link to the Medicare provider manual.

http://www.cms.hhs.gov/medicare/bni: links to CMS information about the Beneficiary Notification Initiative. Copies of beneficiary notices are available for download.

http://www.cola.org: information about accreditation and other programs offered by COLA, a national healthcare accreditation association, can be accessed through the COLA website.

http://www.eeoc.gov: the EEOC website, with links to laws, regulations, and policies as well as other useful information.

http://www.fda.gov: the website for the FDA.

http://www.fda.gov/cber: the website for CBER.

http://www.fda.gov/cber/biodev/bpkrform.pdf: the area of the CBER website where a copy of a biological product deviation report, form FDA-3486, is available.

http://www.fda.gov/cber/gdlns/devnbld.htm: the FDA guidelines that require all licensed manufacturers of biological products to report errors and accidents affecting a product's SPP are available here.

http://www.gao.gov: the website of the U.S. General Accounting Office; it contains copies of its reports.

http://hazmat.dot.gov: the website of the Research and Special Programs Administration Office of Hazardous Materials Safety. Information about transporting hazardous materials by air, rail, highway, or water is located at this website.

http://www.jcaho.org: the website for JCAHO.

http://lawlibrary.Rutgers.edu: the website for the Rutgers University School of Law.

http://www.lmrp.net: LMRP information with links to updates on policy changes and individual contractor websites.

http://www.medicare.gov: the website for use by Medicare beneficiaries.

http://www.medpac.gov: the website of the Medicare Payment Advisory Committee (MedPac), which contain copies of its reports.

http://www.mers-tm.net: the website for a medical event reporting system for transfusion medicine, supported by a grant from the National Heart, Lung, and Blood Institute.

http://www.nccls.org: information about the NCCLS can be found at this website. NCCLS is a global, nonprofit organization that promotes the development and use of voluntary consensus standards and guidelines for use in the healthcare industry.

http://www.nssb.org: the National Skills Standards Board administers certification examinations in many areas including those for AMT.

http://oig.hhs.gov: the OIG of the DHHS website. Information about fraud prevention and detection and compliance guidance as well as the model compliance plan for laboratories is available on this site.

http://www.osha.gov: the website for OSHA contains news, information, and links to laws and regulation topics, safety and health topics, and other related information.

http://www.osha.gov.oshinfo/mission.html: a brief explanation of the OSHA's mission and the services offered by the agency.

http://www.phppo.cdc.gov/clia: this link to the CDC contains links to the CLIA regulations, the *Federal Register, Code of Federal Regulations,* CMS and FDA resources, and more.

http://www.ugsmedicare.com/mspindex.asp: the Medicare secondary-payor index is available at the United Government Services, LLC, website.

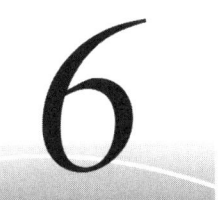

6

The Changing Practice of Medicine

Susan D. Roseff, Brenda G. Nichols, and Margaret M. Grimes

OBJECTIVES

To define changes impacting the practice of medicine over the last two decades of the 20th century

To outline the major cost containment and medico-legal issues faced by physicians and laboratorians

To describe recent advances in medicine and information technology

To describe physician practice and utilization patterns developing in response to societal, reimbursement, and emerging technology

To identify the changes in medical school and residency curricula intended to prepare physicians for medical practice in the 21st century

To change and to change for the better are two different things.

GERMAN PROVERB

SOCIETAL CHANGES, CHANGES IN TECHNOLOGY, and changes in expectations have all come together to create a landscape vastly different for both practitioners and consumers of healthcare over the last two decades. The practice of medicine has changed in response to new discoveries in medicine and science but is being shaped by external pressures such as rising costs, increasing competition, and a new emphasis on customer satisfaction in the information-savvy patient. Patients, looking for zero risk, seem more likely to seek legal avenues when adverse outcomes occur. Due to a focus on the rate of errors in medicine, the medical, regulatory, and legislative communities are interested in ways to deliver consistent, high-quality care. With concomitant concerns about overutilization of certain medical services and investigations revealing fraudulent practices, there is a tremendous amount of attention to and scrutiny of all aspects of healthcare. The training programs that educate future physicians have been restructured to prepare students for the practice environment they will soon enter. The laboratory, always at the forefront of quality issues, is the perfect paradigm of changes going on at a more global level in healthcare.

Overview of Major Changes

Americans are said to enjoy one of the greatest healthcare systems in the world. Improvements in technology coupled with increased demands for greater access are some of the factors responsible for increases in cost. As healthcare costs have risen, there has been pressure to gain control through restructuring, mostly in the form of changes in Medicare and Medicaid regulations as well as the emergence of managed care. Changing the rules of payment and reimbursement has had vast effects on the clinical laboratory (Table 6.1).

Shift from Inpatient to Outpatient Care

Recognizing the high cost of inpatient hospital care has created a shift favoring outpatient treatment, in an attempt to gain control of expenses (70). Insurance companies have decreased the number of days they will provide hospitalization benefits for surgical patients, as care shifts to the less expensive outpatient arena.

Shift from Centralized to Decentralized Testing

The location of laboratory testing has moved, since the hospital's core laboratory may no longer be the best place to perform testing. Though centralization of staff and resources has traditionally been viewed as the most efficient way to perform inpatient testing, as the patient population shifts to outpatient clinics and remote sites closer to residential areas, decentralized laboratory testing has become more common. Within the hospital, other sites, such as the outpatient clinics, the operating suite, or the bedside, may be ideal. Point of care testing (POCT), many times performed by nonlaboratory personnel, has evolved as a means to provide more rapid turnaround times and to

Table 6.1 Themes of change

Financial
    Cost containment
    Managed care
Technological
    Internet-based information
    Automation/robotics
    Miniaturization
    Molecular diagnostics
    Telemedicine
Social
    Client-focused medicine
    Wellness and prevention
    Aging population
    Women's health issues
    Shrinking technical workforce
Legal/regulatory
    Concern regarding errors in medicine
    Concern regarding fraudulent practice
    Increasing malpractice litigation
Training
    Preparation for managed-care environment
    Addressing technological advances in curriculum
    Emphasis on competency

provide a more convenient location for patients. For these same reasons, physicians may also provide limited testing in their offices. The cost of POCT, though, isn't always lower (5, 14).

As the venue for laboratory testing has changed, pathologists and other laboratorians have assumed consultative roles, in lieu of direct management, in order to help nonlaboratorians run operations that maintain compliance and quality. As an example, at the Virginia Commonwealth University Health System (VCUHS) a laboratory located in the surgical suite is being managed jointly by pathology and anesthesia. Such liaisons will become increasingly common as laboratory professionals, specifically trained in these areas, make themselves available to enterprises outside of their exclusive and direct control.

Shift from Specialty to Primary Care

Managed care has evolved to control spiraling healthcare costs. Many insured patients must now go through their primary care provider before seeing a specialist. As a result, primary care providers are seeing and treating patients who would have been referred to a specialist in the past, thus expanding the scope of their practices (79). As the primary care doctor sees a wider variety of patients, one can speculate that more diagnostic testing is done by these physicians to gain a broader picture of their patients' illness. Empirically it seems that this reallocation could affect the use of the laboratory, though such trends are not well documented in the literature.

Independent commercial laboratories have also found a place in the new order (78). As the Clinical Laboratory Improvement Amendments have posed some impediments for physician outpatient laboratories performing more complex testing, outsourcing has become more common. Commercial laboratories have become the centers of esoteric testing, since many hospital laboratories cannot justify the cost of maintaining low-volume esoteric testing.

Technologist Shortages

Echoing the personnel changes in broader aspects of healthcare, the laboratory has also seen changes in the composition of its workers. More generalists staff laboratories than in the past (78). In addition, with shortages of medical technologists, these specialists will assume more supervisory and managerial roles, with testing being performed by personnel not trained in their specific discipline. With many training programs closing, the number of trained technologists diminishes. Some institutions are considering reactivating such programs to fill this void.

Impact of Managed Care on Cost Containment, Quality of Care, and Error Reduction

The government and managed-care organizations would like to see a more efficient, cost-effective practice of medicine, with the provision of high-quality care. The creation of practice guidelines and practice parameters has been encouraged as a means to practice medicine in a consistent manner. Using evidence-based methodologies that lead to the best care should produce the best patient outcomes. Due to such publications as *To Err Is Human,* written by the Institute of Medicine, increasing focus on errors in medicine has also challenged the medical community to improve quality (15). Because of concerns regarding fraud and overuse of testing, laboratories have been required to bundle and unbundle analytes for billing purposes over the last 20 years to maintain compliance with changing regulatory requirements. This may help prevent unnecessary testing and contain cost.

Technological Advances

Technological advances created revolutionary changes in the way medicine and laboratory medicine are practiced. By implementing new technologies, such as nucleic acid testing (NAT), earlier stages of disease and infection can be detected more quickly, leading to earlier treatment. In addition, many instruments have smaller sample volume requirements that make testing safer for neonates and patients requiring frequent testing (47, 87).

Wellness and Prevention

Wellness and prevention are new thrusts of the American healthcare system (78). It seems plausible that by preventing disease and keeping people well, the overall cost of care will decline. Therefore, the use of tests to maintain wellness (e.g., cholesterol) and to prevent disease progression through early screening (e.g., prostate-specific antigen) might increase. If wellness and prevention programs result in improvements in overall health, the rate of reimbursement for wellness testing might also become more favorable.

The Aging Population

The population of the United States continues to live longer, with the elderly representing a larger proportion of patients, as well as a powerful lobbying group. This undoubtedly increases the use of healthcare and laboratory systems. The recognition of diseases that accompany longevity, such as osteoporosis, prostate cancer, and Alzheimer's disease, changes the demands placed on the laboratory. Looking for new ways to diagnose these diseases and monitor treatment in a noninvasive manner is one of the charges of laboratory medicine in the 21st century. It is predicted that this larger group of new healthcare consumers will aggressively manage their own health and take an unprecedented role in the changes to the healthcare delivery system, especially related to "choice" and "service."

Recognition of Women's Health Needs

Recognition that women have healthcare needs distinct from men also shapes American medicine. Men and women have different normal value ranges for many laboratory tests, and they often have different responses to pharmacological agents. Whereas research studies used to preclude women from participation, the inclusion of women is now recognized as essential (85).

The Impact of Technology

The Internet and Information Utilization

New medical discoveries are made at a dizzying pace. Keeping up with these changes has always been challenging for physicians. With the emergence of the Internet, more information is released each day. As healthcare providers try to keep up, patients now have access to more and more information themselves. This has drastically changed the role of patients as consumers of healthcare. There are obviously many advantages to this explosion in information. A more knowledgeable patient can certainly make better and more informed decisions, becoming an integral part of the decision-making process. The notion of the patient as a consumer has now taken on a new and important dimension (4).

Information can also flow more rapidly between practitioners and the medical record (4). Patient records, previously accessible only in a single, poorly legible, paper chart, can now be accessed in many places in the hospital in an easy-to-read, legible format. Laboratory tests and diagnostic tests such as X rays and computed tomography scans can potentially all be accessed at the same time. Managing data information more effectively and efficiently can lead to better coordination of care and faster turnaround times, thus improving patient care (13).

Through teleconferencing, and specifically telepathology, review of problematic clinical presentations or microscopic diagnosis can be accomplished rapidly with minimal cost (13, 26, 87). Commercial laboratories are investigating the use of Web-based technology to allow physicians and patients rapid access to laboratory test results. By using the Internet, two-way communication between the sender and recipient is possible (26). These modalities also provide a mechanism for rural or underserved areas to gain access to healthcare, in particular to specialists who may not be present in each community (41). As information exchange progresses, large databases can be created, affording the opportunity to track individual patient care as well as epidemiological data (13, 55, 65). It is incumbent on all healthcare workers to become proficient with these new modes of information transfer.

Another great promise of the Internet is the use of this technology for training and education. Medical students and residents frequently use Web-based course material in their studies. There are also degree programs for distance learners, who never set foot in a traditional classroom. Continuing medical education can now be easily accomplished through a variety of programs that are entirely Web based.

Unfortunately, a great deal of information on the Internet is neither edited nor controlled for content. There are many reports of incorrect medical information being used by patients leading to inappropriate decisions. Also, more and more prescription medication seems to be available on the Internet, in the absence of medical evaluation. This can cause serious harm. Privacy issues must also be addressed, since not all information transmitted electronically is secure. Concerns have been raised that increasing use of e-mail might damage the doctor-patient relationship (59). Table 6.2 provides a summary of the impact of the Internet on the laboratory.

Advances in Diagnostic Testing

New disease patterns, changing demographics, the aging population, emerging diseases, and the threat of terrorism require innovative testing methods. NAT, as one example, has truly revolutionized the way medicine is practiced. Instead of waiting days or weeks to detect certain viruses in culture, amplifying small amounts of genetic material in a specimen can detect a pathogen within hours. Looking at changes in the genetic material of a tumor may improve the diagnosis of certain malignancies. There is also hope that identifying at the genetic level, disease that is not yet macroscopically evident might lead to earlier treatment (68, 87). Nucleic acid amplification techniques have been introduced to donor blood testing over the last 2 years. Many blood collection facilities use NAT due to its increased sensitivity, though it is not yet required by the Food and Drug Administration (FDA). (Note, FDA guidance is currently being written.)

Miniaturization continues to change the way tests are performed. The use of smaller "micro" components facilitates POCT. As these components become smaller and smaller, the number of analytes in a device can increase, replacing larger analyzers. In some instances, laboratory results are now available while the patient is still in the doctor's office, allowing results to rapidly and directly influence the course of care (65). Using implantable chips as a way to identify patients and their specimens is also on the horizon as a means to ensure proper patient and sample

Table 6.2 Impact of the internet

Increased information available
Information more accessible
Web-based learning
Web-based consultations
Web-based laboratory reporting
More accessible medical record
Results available to patient and physicians
New privacy concerns
Information not always reviewed for accuracy
Improved access to information in rural or remote areas

identification. Developing smaller and faster computers may lead the way to performing noninvasive tests, negating the need for blood specimens (22, 54). The concomitant reduction in sample size is beneficial to the patient (47).

Due to changes and reductions in the laboratory workforce, trying to do more with less is a dominant theme in laboratory medicine. Automation will continue to reduce personnel and laboratory costs (13). The use of robotics can reduce the number of tasks that are currently done manually and thereby reduce the impact of human error (48, 68, 87). By using a system of bar codes that identifies patients and samples throughout the process, misidentified patient samples can theoretically become a thing of the past. This form of process control may have the ability to greatly reduce medical errors (47). Robotics is currently used for the delivery of supplies and blood products in some hospitals.

Introducing new tests, such as troponin levels, can reduce length of stay and decrease the cost of care for certain patients. New treatments for early intervention during myocardial infarction depend on an early, specific marker of myocardial damage, such as troponin. Patients with elevated values can be identified and treated immediately, yielding better outcomes. Conversely, the treatment plan for patients with normal levels can be reassessed and their care redirected to less expensive alternatives (2).

The Emergence of Clinical Practice Guidelines

The Role of Evidence-Based Medicine and Outcome Data

When cost-cutting measures are implemented in response to decreased reimbursement by Medicare, Medicaid, and managed-care companies, quality must be maintained. The use of solid, tangible evidence leads to optimal decision making and the best level of care. Evidence-based medicine is one approach being used to address different aspects of healthcare delivery. Concrete, up-to-the-minute facts are "evidence" that can become a part of the decision-making process. Relying on evidence-based information requires paying close attention to new discoveries and incorporating them into practice. Participating in outcome research provides a mechanism to study the problem and influence future care. Using the Internet to keep abreast of all current changes and to access databases on a daily basis makes the process manageable. Overall, the aim is to objectively evaluate patient management by measuring quality and cost of outcomes. By using evidence-based protocols, variation in practice can be reduced, and this can lead to the validation of practice guidelines, which is discussed later in this chapter (31, 43).

Appropriate utilization (neither over- nor under-) is another central theme in medical and laboratory services. While overutilization might lead to unnecessary expense, underutilization might delay diagnosis and treatment, leading to low quality of care. Outcome assessment or outcome research is an attempt to determine which interventions are necessary. Medical interventions and the use of diagnostic tests must affect the patient outcome in order for them to be considered a necessary part of patient care. Outcomes are diverse and include morbidity, mortality, length of stay (LOS), quality of life, patient satisfaction, length of time to diagnosis, laboratory costs, and rates of laboratory testing, just to mention a few (65, 86). Clinical trials look at similar groups of patients, selected using strict criteria, to assess the impact of changes of single variables. In contrast, outcome research attempts to see what happens after treatment is applied to a more diverse group of patients (51).

As an example, ordering repeated blood cultures for a patient without signs and symptoms of infection would be inappropriate since their use is not supported by scientific facts nor would the culture results (presumably negative) change the outcome for the patient. On the other hand, the use of troponin, as mentioned earlier, has yielded scientific data that support its use and show improvement in patient outcome (2). Therefore, the laboratory has an essential role in fostering both evidence-based medicine and outcome research (65). These principles can be applied to many other services provided by the laboratory, such as POCT and the use of screening tests. To adequately perform such large-scale studies, an integrated information system is essential (43, 86).

Studies evaluating LOS have become common since they measure multiple parameters simultaneously. LOS has financial ramifications since shorter periods of hospitalization are usually associated with a lower cost of care. Extrapolations can also be made on the basis of LOS, with a shorter LOS implying that the patient's care was uncomplicated. A shorter LOS is desirable from the perspectives of the patient, the hospital, and the third-party payor (86).

More complex outcome measures are quality of life and patient satisfaction. These require measures of many subjective parameters, relying on both biological and psychological factors. Finding a way to measure the influence of a patient's underlying perceptions of healthcare, the role of psychological factors in their symptomatology in their functional status, is a challenge (88).

The laboratory can play a major role in studying outcome research by providing objective data that correlate with patient outcomes. Conversely, adverse patient outcomes might be used to screen for laboratory errors. Looking at the outcomes for patients within a critical time frame following the receipt of laboratory data may yield important information related to the performance of the test or the transmission of results. One example would be assessing outcomes for patients on coumadin therapy following recent prothrombin time testing. This process is described as downstream event monitoring (89). Applying outcome research to the clinical laboratory can thereby provide a method to examine quality and prevent errors (51).

Concerns over Utilization and Quality

In 1989, as part of the Omnibus Budget Reconciliation Act, Congress created the Agency for Health Care Policy and Research. Its creation was due to growing anxiety about cost and inappropriate use of medical care. At the same time, there were data pointing toward variations in the use of medical services, questions about the true efficacy of both expensive and commonly used services, and the lack of proven efficacy for many services. Since cost containment measures were not effective, there was a perceived need to study the issues more thoroughly (14).

Through its Forum for Quality and Effectiveness in Healthcare, one of the agency's responsibilities was directly tied to formulating clinical practice guidelines. Its mission, in this regard, was to "sponsor and encourage the development, dissemination, and initial choice of guideline topics" (14). Now the Agency for Healthcare Research and Quality, the agency continues to be the clearinghouse for nationally adopted guidelines (The National Guideline Clearinghouse) in collaboration with the American Medical Association and the American Association of Health Plans. The guidelines are published on their website, available at http://www.guideline.gov (accessed on 12 December 2002). A variety of other parties have worked on practice guidelines, including the American Medical Association, the American College of Physicians, Intermountain Health Care, Kaiser Permanente, and the state of Minnesota (14, 27).

The development of clinical practice guidelines is prioritized based on the prevalence of the clinical problem, burden of illness imposed, cost, variability in practice, potential to improve healthcare outcomes, and potential to reduce cost (14). There have also been suggestions that medical malpractice claims should be used as an additional prioritization for the creation of guidelines to help protect against litigation (8, 72).

The recommendations of the Institute of Medicine's study of errors in medicine, introduced earlier, can also be applied to identify areas needing practice guidelines. Guidelines may be one approach to prevent variations in practice, leading to improved patient safety and outcomes (15).

Clinical Practice Guidelines and Clinical Pathways Defined

The Institute of Medicine defines clinical practice parameters as "systematically defined statements to assist practitioner and patient decisions about appropriate healthcare for specific clinical circumstances." They may provide clinical, ethical, organizational, or other forms of advice and can be presented in a variety of formats, including algorithms, computer-based protocols, and/or policy documents (14). The terms care-maps, care algorithms, clinical pathways, critical pathways, and clinical maps have also been used. The term "clinical pathway" is usually used for prescribed procedures where the patient outcome is more predictable. "Clinical guidelines" refer to situations that have greater variability, such as rehabilitation protocols or complex medical illnesses. When the problem is of even greater complexity or involves chronic disease processes, "case management" may be employed to oversee the overall disease management, usually by nursing personnel under the guidance of a physician. Practice guidelines seem to tie all the trends of healthcare together. They are formulated using evidence-based medicine in an attempt to reduce variation in care, maintain quality, and reduce cost and as a means to influence patient outcomes. Presumptively, when faced with factual evidence, different practitioners will come to the same conclusion. This, in turn, will lead to consistent ways to treat a variety of diseases. It is important to note that the use of these different terms is not standardized and their use may vary in different institutions.

Clinical pathways were traditionally more detailed than initial critical guidelines. Clinical pathways were designed to focus on a multidisciplinary approach to a specific problem, although the line between clinical pathways and clinical guidelines is not distinct. It is important to note, though, that only clinical practice guidelines are defined by the Agency for Healthcare Research and Quality. When working on a project that crosses departments, it is imperative to get the approval and buy-in of hospital administration (39). Looking at it a different way, the use and implementation of practice guidelines can be accomplished through clinical pathways.

Use of Clinical Practice Guidelines

A search of the medical literature as well as a general search on the Internet will identify myriad guidelines. Discussing the specifics of the guidelines available is not within the scope of this chapter, although some examples are listed in the references (35, 37, 38, 40, 45, 55, 66, 77). These papers show the diversity of clinical questions addressed—from psychiatric illness to pediatric transfusion guidelines to the evaluation of unstable angina. Some of these studies have yielded positive outcomes such as decreased LOS, decreased cost of care, increased patient satisfaction, and improved transfusion practice in a pediatric hospital. Others have not been as successful (31).

Legal Implications of Applying Clinical Practice Guidelines

A great deal of concern has been voiced regarding the use of clinical practice guidelines in this increasingly litigious society, especially in the realm of medical malpractice. If one considers these guidelines as actual standards of care, there is speculation that a practitioner who has not followed a practice guideline could be found guilty of malpractice (8, 23, 72).

On the other hand, if a specific guideline has been proven to increase patient safety, adhering to clinical practice guidelines could possibly provide protection from the risk of legal action being brought against a physician. In

some states, adhering to certain guidelines can be used as exculpatory evidence if a physician is sued, thereby ending the lawsuit. It is not surprising, then, that insurance carriers may require their practitioners to follow certain guidelines in order to receive coverage (8, 23, 72).

Pros and Cons

The creation of standard, reproducible algorithms that can be applied to patient treatment offers great promise (Table 6.3). A variety of studies have shown increased efficiency and quality of care with decreased cost and LOS. Some have pointed out that these guidelines may have other uses and serve as a means of education. As stated earlier, they may be used as one means to assess physician competency and proficiency and as a means of conducting peer review, and might also be an integral part of utilization review in the future (14, 30, 73). By having a written, detailed care plan to follow, there is better coordination among the members of the care team. This in itself may lead to the decreased LOS demonstrated. As an example, if a physician is not available, a member of the nursing team or respiratory therapy team may be able to initiate the next step of the protocol in a more timely manner (40).

The introduction of clinical practice guidelines has been met with some resistance, as demonstrated in a survey of members of the American College of Physicians in 1992 (82). Respondents to the questionnaires voiced a variety of concerns. One of their concerns, as discussed earlier, was the fear that implementation would increase their exposure to medical malpractice claims if they didn't strictly adhere to the guidelines. The members were also concerned that they could no longer tailor care to the needs of each individual patient and their autonomy to practice medicine, as it would likely be diminished. This would have a direct influence on their overall satisfaction to practice medicine. In addition, not all studies show improved patient outcomes or decreases in cost.

Table 6.3 Pros and cons of clinical practice guidelines and clinical pathways

Pros	Cons
Increase in efficiency	Too much rigidity
Increase in quality	Decrease in physician autonomy
Increase in patient satisfaction	Decrease in physician satisfaction
Decrease in cost	Increase in cost
Decrease in variations in practice	Increase in variation of practice
Decrease in LOS	Can be used for discipline
Decrease in legal liability	Increase in legal liability
Educational strategy	Outcomes not always favorably affected
Means of peer review	
Means of proficiency/ competency assessment	

Others have voiced concern over the apparent rigidity of guidelines, since very few patients seem to fit the exact mold of the algorithm. This may lead to poor judgment as physicians try to make patients fit into the wrong treatment plan (60). In addition, different practitioners will interpret the "evidence" differently and introduce bias leading to inconsistency and variation in practice (12, 31, 60). An interesting study by Shaneyfelt et al. critically evaluated published practice guidelines and found that between 10 and 25% ignored some of the basic tenets of designing guidelines (76).

In response to charges that clinical practice guidelines may be ambiguous or incomplete, there has been ongoing review of national guidelines. Continual review of existing guidelines is necessary due to the constant changes in the available information (14, 76).

Developing Clinical Pathways

The steps required to develop a clinical pathway are summarized in Table 6.4 and begin with the identification of a problem, where a change in outcome is desired or where there may be a great deal of variation in care. Assembling a team to critically evaluate the areas of concern is also important, especially if the plan will involve a multidisciplinary approach. Enlist the support of hospital administration. The quality improvement team of your institution may be very supportive of efforts to improve patient outcome. A brainstorming session may be the best way to start and to analyze the problem more fully. A full search of all available data and literature should be performed, so that the guidelines are evidence based. Once a list of concerns is raised, it must be prioritized. Specific, desired outcomes should be identified. The methods that will be used to collect and analyze data should be established. A financial analysis should be performed. The pathway should identify patients who may have individual factors not conducive to

Table 6.4 Elements for developing clinical pathways

Identify suitable problem to address.

Identify team members.

Initiate a brainstorming session.

Identify specific outcome objectives.

Search available data and literature.

Assign specific parts of the plan to subteams.

Identify financial impact.

Identify impediments to patient participation (e.g., third-party payor).

Identify data-gathering and analysis tools.

Educate members of team.

Create flow diagram or matrix of process.

Develop method to capture variances.

Develop method to modify plan as it is being used.

Identify individuals to answer questions during process.

Identify individuals to monitor compliance.

Analyze data.

inclusion in the pathway. For example, a patient may be excluded when a pathway requires a specific diagnostic test that the third-party payor will not reimburse (39, 72).

The pathway development team may be broken down into subgroups, each with assignments to address specific parts of the project. All team members should reconvene and a timeline should be created to fit the different pieces of the puzzle together. At this point, the group can work on the specifics of the pathway. Some plans are written in a flow diagram format, while more complex pathways are written in a matrix format. An example of a critical pathway on community-acquired pneumonia from VCUHS is presented in Appendix 6.2. Once the plan is written, the implementation process begins. It is best to develop a comprehensive educational program which includes all staff who will participate. This can occur at a departmental meeting, specific retreat, or grand rounds activity, or one-on-one for specific individuals. Clearly identified individuals should be available throughout the implementation to answer questions as well as to monitor compliance. Variances from the use of the pathway should be recognized, recorded, and analyzed as the process goes forward. Modification of the original plan may occur during the process. Strict record keeping in all aspects of the implementation is required in order to have the necessary information for final analysis (39, 72).

Laboratory Utilization Trends

Medicare pays 29% of laboratory bills in the United States, but this represents only 1.6% of program spending (13). Analyzing a consortium database, Young et al. (90) also found that laboratory expenditures made up only a small proportion of overall costs, with 9% for medical conditions and 6% for surgical conditions. They suggested that shorter LOSs would reduce laboratory costs and overall costs despite the relatively small percentage of the total cost. With the laboratory as a hospital cost center, efforts to reduce unnecessary testing while maintaining quality of care are consistent with global trends in medical care.

Unfortunately, there are little published data linking changes in the practice of medicine directly with changes in specific laboratory utilization. There is also a dearth of data at the national level since there is no single association representing the clinical laboratory industry. As a result, data collected separately by different institutions are not standardized. The laboratory is usually just a small segment of the hospital's business overall and is lumped into other reports. Finally, the laboratory is usually a part of a larger organization that may not keep their laboratory data separated (13).

Changes Due to the Changing Practice of Medicine

One of the greatest changes in medicine that has affected the laboratory is the emergence of managed care. Private insurance carriers often adopt changes in Medicare and

Medicaid legislation; therefore, their impact is universal. The current Medicare clinical laboratory payment structure was developed in the 1980s, and the system has not kept up with all the complex changes (13). As national healthcare expenditures grow, expenditures for laboratory medicine have steadily decreased, with expenditures in 1998 being more than 10% lower than those in 1993. Despite this, the hospital-based market share of laboratory testing continued to grow through the 1990s.

With advancement in POCT, the trend is to perform more testing outside of the main hospital laboratory. A study looking at the laboratory industry found continuing growth of physician office laboratories without any data available to show their profitability. The enhanced efficiency and convenience of the testing might render the financial impact irrelevant (13).

Similarly, growth in outpatient and outreach testing by hospital laboratories has continued. This may be due to attempts by the hospital laboratory to spread fixed costs over a larger volume of service (13). The impact of regulatory agencies on the clinical laboratory is discussed in another chapter.

Laboratory Utilization Management

A variety of factors in today's medical environment impact laboratory utilization. Reimbursement issues dictate which tests are ordered and which ones are reimbursed. The concern about overutilization has stemmed some of the tide. The fear of litigation, though, may drive overutilization in the practice of defensive medicine. In the era of information technology, patients are asking increasingly for certain tests or treatments they have read about on their own. It is easy to speculate that certain test volumes have increased due to our aging population and others have increased due to changing disease patterns as more patients live longer with chronic diseases such as human immunodeficiency virus (HIV) infection and hepatitis C. Unfortunately, there are no direct data to analyze these shifts (61).

With lower reimbursement, the laboratory has a vested interest in decreasing the number of unnecessary tests being ordered. In addition, as the number of tests ordered in a normal population increases, the risk of false-positive results increases. This leads to additional testing and patient anxiety (63). A variety of feedback strategies have been employed with mixed, and sometimes short-lived, results. Usually a combination of passive and active strategies yields the best results. Sending out announcements and educational material by themselves is usually ineffective since not everyone will actually read the material. Changing requisition slips or laboratory ordering screens is a more active intervention. If certain tests that have a high propensity for being overordered are removed from the order list, they are less likely to be ordered unnecessarily. Requiring certain information before a test is performed can also cut down on inappropriate laboratory utilization

(83). A more attractive way to control utilization would be to have the hospital's information system use predetermined acceptance and rejection criteria. The system should also be designed to capture individual data on physician ordering practices as a way to provide feedback (61). Similar systems have been discussed as a means to monitor and decrease inappropriate blood utilization. A combination of both educational and administrative strategies seems to be most effective (63, 83).

Impact of Unbundling

In order to address concerns regarding unnecessary testing and possible fraudulent practices, in late 1996 and early 1997 Medicare and Medicaid required that all tests performed be medically necessary. Therefore, panels of tests previously billed together as a group had to be billed separately, or unbundled. With the exception of certain approved disease panels such as electrolytes, each test must be individually justified as medically necessary (57).

Changes in test utilization patterns based on these rules are not well documented. Of interest, a paper published in the late 1980s found that unbundling actually reduced outpatient laboratory use. Though ordering a panel of 19 chemistry tests was less expensive than ordering each individual test separately, physicians began to order only those analytes that were clinically necessary. There was a 33% decline in the number of tests performed (28).

At VCUHS, there was concern that dismantling panels might have resulted in a temporary increase in the number of orders of thyroglobulin. Formerly, when thyroid panels were available, it was rare to see thyroglobulin ordered by mistake. Due to the alphabetical proximity of this analyte to the other more common thyroid tests, it could easily be ordered in error. This points to the potential importance of test-ordering forms in ordering practices.

Medico-Legal Issues

Increasing Malpractice Litigation

It has been predicted that changes in the healthcare industry over the next 10 to 15 years will far outweigh the changes made over the last 150 years (11). The healthcare industry is already one of the most heavily regulated sectors of commerce. Since the appearance of the professional liability crisis in the 1970s, there has been a proliferation of malpractice litigation. Malpractice premiums continue to spiral upward to amounts higher than in the mid-1980s. A sharp increase began in the year 2000. Insurers raised rates more than 30% after years of price competition that left many insurers unprepared to pay the high cost of claims (81). Many believe that legislation on a national level would help to curb the rising costs of liability insurance, which is driving many healthcare providers away from practice and, in turn, negatively impacting patients' access to healthcare.

The insurance industry blames the increase on the recent trend toward higher jury awards requiring them to pass this cost on as a cost of doing business. The total number of malpractice cases has held steady for many years, but the Jury Verdict Research Group in Horsham, Pa., reports that the average jury award was $3.49 million in 1999, which is up an astonishing 79% from $1.95 million in 1993 (81).

Another factor that may have impacted the severity of claims over the past couple of years is the 1999 Institute of Medicine report on medical errors, *To Err is Human*, discussed earlier (15). This report greatly increased the general public's awareness of medical errors and may have prompted lawsuits by educating consumers to closely examine things they may have previously overlooked. Attention has been focused on the medical community's practice (or the lack of a practice) of disclosing medical errors and injuries to patients. The practice of incomplete disclosure or any perception of withholding of information causes anger. This anger motivates consumers to find answers and may increase litigation.

Without tort reform, the future for liability insurance costs looks very expensive. Increases in life expectancy, the focus on and the ability to maintain good health, and the increase in the population growth will necessitate different approaches to healthcare delivery and payment for those services. These factors, coupled with changes in technology, clearly create challenges and opportunities for all healthcare providers. Future success for healthcare delivery systems will be predicated on their proactive ability to strategically plan to meet the challenges of the future. Comprehensive, proactive risk management strategies that examine insurance coverage and losses over a continuum of operating units will be a key strategy for organizations.

Cost Sharing and Transfer of Liability

As healthcare has changed over the last 30 years, the focus of liability exposure has changed as well. Traditionally, facility risk managers focused primarily on exposures of a professional or general-liability nature. In today's healthcare setting, it is necessary to expand the liability focus to include the following risks: managed care and capitation; merger and acquisition; employment and worker's compensation; electronic data processing and media; automobile, other transportation, and garage; environmental; directors and officers; commercial crime and employee dishonesty; fiduciary; foreign recruitment and foreign travel; research; builders and construction; product liability; and excess liability. An effective laboratory risk management program must examine the exposure for each of the identified and applicable risks and seek the most comprehensive, but also cost-effective, mechanism to manage the risk exposure.

There are some options available to assist with sharing the cost of the exposure. Because there are no national tort reform measures, many of these options will be state specific. Identifying them and determining eligibility to participate will require care. Employing the services of a healthcare consultant firm, while an expense, may prove very beneficial in determining specific exposures and what types of risk-sharing or risk transfer options are available. Some mechanisms, such as birth-related injury funds, may require physician financial contribution, similar to an uninsured-motorist auto fund. When well managed and overseen, specific funding sources have performed well over long periods to meet their intended goals. Others have failed miserably.

Tort Reform

There are no national laws regulating medical malpractice. Many states have specific codes and regulations that have attempted to manage how the legal system handles medical malpractice cases. Currently, a bipartisan coalition of representatives has introduced a national tort reform bill that includes measures from capping noneconomic damages at $250,000 to allowing future economic expenses to be paid over time (1). The Help Efficient, Accessible, Low Cost, Timely Health Care Act of 2002 is currently being reviewed by the U.S. House of Representatives. Highlights of the act are presented in Table 6.5 (34).

Training in Disclosure of Medical Error

In 2001, the National Patient Safety Foundation published a statement of principle titled "Talking To Patients About Health Care Injury" (9). This statement was published under

Table 6.5 Highlights of the Help Efficient, Accessible, Low Cost, Timely Health Care Act of 2002[a]

Lawsuits—with few exceptions—would need to be filed within 3 years of the injury.

A physician would be financially responsible for only his or her share of the liability.

A $250,000 limit on noneconomic damages, such as pain and suffering, would be established.

Economic damages and future medical costs would be limitless.

A higher threshold would be set for juries to award punitive damages, which would be limited to the greater of two times the amount of economic damages awarded or $250,000.

The court could limit the percentage a plaintiff attorney could recover.

Future damages could be paid over time instead of in one lump sum.

A federal law would not supersede state caps already in place.

While this is the seventh time in the last decade that legislation has been considered on this topic, the timing may finally be right for national tort reform (1).

[a] See reference 34.

the premise that patients are entitled to information about the outcomes of diagnostic tests, medical treatment, and surgical intervention. This perspective is the same whether the results are expected or unexpected. The Joint Commission on Accreditation of Healthcare Organizations Patient Safety Standards took effect in July of 2001. The National Patient Safety Foundation, along with the American Society of Health Care Risk Management, has published information and perspectives on how to develop a patient safety policy or position statement for healthcare service entities as well as recommendations for training of staff relative to communication skill development.

There are many situations to consider in framing a policy for disclosure of outcomes, especially those that involve adverse events. There may also be state-specific legal, regulatory, institutional, and cultural considerations. Training should emphasize the importance of effective communication with patients and family members and the need to discuss possible adverse outcomes in the informed-consent process. All healthcare professionals acknowledge that breaking bad news is a difficult, unpleasant, and inescapable part of their role. Although breaking bad news is common in healthcare, there are few known objective facts about how it should be done. The idea of improving one's skills at breaking bad news is viewed as taboo in polite society.

Most clinicians have been taught very little about the techniques of breaking bad news, partially due to the awkwardness of teaching these skills. The goal of training according to Robert Buckman, M.D., is not necessarily to increase an individual's ability to "do it right every time," but to increase the individual's right/wrong ratio, to increase the comfort level and ability to provide support, and to enhance the learning process (9). This learning process should begin in the early days of the healthcare professional's training and should be reinforced in an organizations' new-employee orientation and competency training. The role of breaking bad news, while traditionally thought to be that of the physician, may now be expanded to include other or different members of the healthcare team.

Staffing Shortages

As healthcare organizations respond to changes brought on by managed care, mergers, and acquisitions, they are often faced with the need to do more with less. Elimination of positions and the shortage of many types of healthcare professionals today are creating additional liability exposure. The use of temporary agency staff, or locum tenens, is very expensive but may be necessary to keep operations afloat until recruitment activities can fill vacancies. In some cases, there are no resources to recruit, and services must either be eliminated or added to other areas that already are functioning with tight resources. The development of a strategic staffing plan for both recruitment and retention activities is crucial to controlling the exposures. Oversight

of this function, as well as complete documentation of orientation and training activities of agency staff, is critical to surviving staff shortages. The temporary or permanent transfer of certain functions, as well as outsourcing others, may help an organization to maintain stability.

Insurance

Risk is the possibility of loss. The most common mechanism to transfer or finance risk exposure is to purchase insurance. Insurance alone cannot prevent risk, but it can provide security against loss. Risk transfer and risk sharing are vital elements of an insurance program. Risk is most commonly transferred to an insurance company. By accepting and sharing the risk of many organizations, an insurance company is able to statistically calculate the likelihood that losses will or will not occur. It can also predict the likely severity of the loss and use this calculation to create a premium that it charges back to the organization wishing to transfer the risk. Sound premium calculations allow the insurer to pay the claims that are incurred and still make a profit (11). A comprehensive insurance management program that is carefully monitored can identify exposures and effectively manage them in a timely manner. Insurance requirements can change on a daily basis depending upon the size of the organization and the services it provides.

An organization may be willing to retain a portion of the risk by utilizing a deductible. Virtually every type of insurance can be written with a deductible. Retaining a deductible may cost the organization if the deductible is so large that all of the organization's losses come in at a rate lower than the deductible and have to be paid as operating expenses. In this case, it may cost the organization more than the deductible itself. Careful analysis of losses can determine if the deductible is appropriate for an organization. The insurance provider should provide this service with oversight from the organization's insurance services or legal office staff.

Self-insurance often looks like a commercial insurance policy with a large deductible. In many cases, state regulations must be met for an organization to become a qualified self-insurer. The organization must identify how claims will be administered and who will provide the excess or umbrella coverage. Self-insurance coverage is further complicated by federal reimbursement requirements such as Medicare or Medicaid reimbursement in the case of self-insured programs for medical professional liability.

HIPAA and Patient Confidentiality

The Health Insurance Portability and Accountability Act of 1996 (HIPAA), also known as the Kassebaum-Kennedy bill, is an intricate and far-reaching piece of legislation (Public Law 104-191, 104th Congress, 26 USC Subchapter A) (80). It amends elements of the Employee Retirement Income Security Act, the Public Health Service Act, and the Internal Revenue Code of 1986. The act establishes a variety of health insurance coverage protections, including access to insurance markets for small businesses and the self-employed, access and transferability of coverage for individuals who change jobs, and access by individuals who have preexisting medical conditions. It is important to realize that oral conversations regarding patients are also covered under HIPAA. Discussions that take place on elevators or in hallways must not disclose confidential information if there are individuals present who are not privileged to hear that information.

HIPAA makes the commission of healthcare fraud a federal criminal offense. The act establishes and funds a new healthcare fraud and abuse control program overseen by the Office of the Inspector General of the Department of Health and Human Services (DHHS). The operating capital for the department's enforcement efforts (for example, investigations, audits, inspections, provider and customer education, and prosecutions) comes from the Health Care Fraud and Abuse Control Account, which was created specifically for that purpose (11).

Section 221(a) of this act established a data collection program involving "adverse" actions taken against individual providers, manufacturers, and suppliers, called the Healthcare Integrity and Protection Data Bank. Adverse actions include civil judgments (not including professional liability actions, which fall within the scope of the National Practitioner Data Bank; criminal convictions; actions taken by federal or state agencies responsible for licensing or certifying practitioners, providers, or suppliers; exclusion from federal or state healthcare programs; and any other actions that the DHHS determines are reportable (11). Settlements in which no findings or admissions of liability have been made are excluded from reporting. Mandatory reporting is required only of health plans or when federal or state agencies are involved. Providers, practitioners, suppliers, and manufacturers are not required to self-report but may query the data bank.

The Medicare Integrity Program permits the DHHS to contract with outside entities, known as "intermediaries," to carry out various program oversight functions (11). A list of these functions can be found in Table 6.6. The federal government is serious about its efforts to control fraud in the healthcare setting and imposes fines and jail time for those found guilty of fraud as outlined in Section 242 of the act.

The management of patient-specific data and information is an important responsibility. Over the continuum of care, there are many types of data, including inpatient and outpatient information. Patient records, occurrence reports, committee meeting minutes, healthcare provider performance reviews, quality improvement reports, and similar documents, whether they are provided in an electronic or written format, must be handled in a confidential manner.

Table 6.6 Program oversight functions from the Medicare Integrity Program[a]

To review utilization, fraud prevention, and general program compliance activities or Medicaid ties related to individuals or entities who furnish items or services subject to Medicare reimbursement

To audit cost reports relating to payments made for services provided to program beneficiaries

To determine whether payments made to Medicare secondary payors were appropriate

To provide broad-based education to providers and beneficiaries regarding payment integrity and benefit quality assurance issues

To develop and periodically update a list of safe harbors (permitted activities) and durable medical equipment items that are subject to prior-authorization requirements

[a]See reference 11.

The ability to keep such information confidential is a daunting challenge and a public concern. Centralized databases, e-mail, and computer-based medical record systems link many types of patient facilities, providers, health plans, payors, employers, and vendors. Such technological advances require additional security safeguards to protect the integrity of patient data and to prevent the inappropriate release of confidential patient information. Until recently there were few federal laws protecting confidentiality. State regulations predominated. State protections are often uneven, with large gaps in protection in certain states. Congress recognized the need for minimum national healthcare privacy and security standards through the passage of HIPAA. Congress was given a framework for federal privacy legislation from the Secretary of the DHHS in accordance with HIPAA, which is summarized in Table 6.7.

On 21 August 1999, 3 years after the passage of HIPAA, the authority to promulgate privacy regulations passed to the DHHS, since Congress had failed to pass a privacy statute by that date. On 3 November 1999, in accordance with HIPAA's more limited legislative direction, the DHHS issued proposed regulations in a Notice of Proposed Rule Making on National Medical Records Privacy Rules pertaining to individual identifiable health information privacy and security (80). These regulations are more limited than those proposed in 1997 with regard to entities covered (health plans, healthcare clearinghouses, and healthcare providers) and pertain only to individually identifiable health information maintained or transmitted by these entities in electronic form. According to the DHHS in their introductory statements in the regulations, they are also more limited with regard to strong enforcement provisions and the right to private right of action for individuals. However, despite these limitations and varied opinions about what the final regulations should contain

Table 6.7 Framework for federal privacy legislation (HIPAA)

Allow for the smooth flow of individually identified health information for treatment, payment, and related operations, and for specific additional purposes related to health care that are in the public interest.

Prohibit the flow of individually identified health information for any additional purposes unless specified and voluntary authorization is given by the subject of the information.

Put into place fair information protections that allow individuals to know who is using their health information and how it is to be used.

Establish fair information practices that allow individuals to obtain access to their records and obtain amendments or corrections to them where there is inaccurate or incorrect information.

Require persons who hold individual identifiable health information to safeguard that information from inappropriate use or disclosure.

Hold those who use the individual identifiable health information accountable for their handling of this information and provide legal recourse to persons harmed by misuse.

Allow health information to be disclosed without an individual's authorization for certain national priorities and purposes (such as research, public health, and oversight) but only under defined circumstances.

and whether or not Congress should intervene and pass additional legislation, federal regulations in some form will most likely predominate in the future. They will also preempt state laws that are in conflict with their regulatory requirements and that have less stringent privacy protections.

In the past, the term "medical record" was used almost exclusively in reference to data management. According to the newly proposed federal regulations and some state regulations, the terms health information, healthcare information, and individually identifiable health information are also used in describing types and forms of information associated with confidentiality and privacy protections. The health information referred to in the proposed regulations is related to a person's physical or mental health, the provision of healthcare, or the payment for healthcare. It is information that could identify or be used to identify a person, was created by or received from a covered entity, and has been electronically maintained or transmitted by a covered entity. Typically the medical record is the key document one would be most concerned about protecting. The law of healthcare data management continues to evolve. Healthcare managers need to be alert to the release of the final federal regulations and possible congressional intervention. They should also be aware of its impact on specific state laws to require more precise information to develop the policies and procedures necessary to comply with the confidentiality and security requirements for the protection of health information.

The right to confidentiality and the provider-patient privilege are never absolute. Certain societal interests outweigh the physician's duty to maintain confidentiality of patient records even when there has been no waiver or authorization. Most states have laws mandating that physicians or hospitals report communicable diseases, incidence of cancer, cases of suspected child abuse or neglect, gunshot or knife wounds, physician misconduct, and incidents of adverse patient care. The statute or regulation mandating disclosure usually contains a confidentiality provision restricting the ability of the public to gain access to that information. In the proposed federal regulations, covered entities could use or disclose individual identifiable health information without authorization for treatment, payment, healthcare operations, and national priority activities. With regard to business partners, federal regulations permit covered entities to release protected healthcare information only if satisfactory assurance is obtained that will safeguard this information. A breach by a business partner is deemed a breach by the covered entity.

Special federal rules exist regarding the confidentiality of information on patients treated or referred for treatment for alcohol and drug abuse. In general, the regulations prohibit any disclosure or release of patient information, whether recorded or not, that would identify the patient as a substance abuser. The regulations were amended in 1987 in an attempt to make them clearer and to narrow the application with respect to general-care hospitals. Under the amendments, a general medical facility is not subject to the regulations unless it has either a distinct substance abuse program or specialized personnel whose primary function is treatment, diagnosis, or referral for treatment of substance abuse patients. Information can be released with the patient's consent if the patient gives consent in writing and the request contains certain required elements, listed in Table 6.8. The regulations contain a sample consent form. Each disclosure made with the patient's written consent must be accompanied by a specific written statement, as set forth in the regulations, prohibiting disclosure.

Table 6.8 Requirements of written request for confidential patient information

Name of the program

Name of the proposed recipient of the information

Name of the patient

Purpose or need for the disclosure

Extent and nature of the information to be disclosed

Signature of the patient or of the person authorized to give consent if the patient is a minor, incompetent, or deceased

Date on which the consent is signed

A statement that the consent is subject to revocation at any time

Date, event, or condition on which the consent will expire if not revoked before that time

The regulations permit disclosure without the patient's consent if the disclosure is to medical personnel to meet any individual's bona fide medical emergency or to qualified personnel for research, audit, or program evaluation. They also permit disclosure for certain specific purposes, pursuant to a court order, after the court has made a finding that a "good cause" exists. The information is not otherwise available to the requesting party, and the public interest in disclosure outweighs the potential harm to the patient. The person requesting the court-ordered disclosure has the burden of demonstrating its necessity. A subpoena or other similar court document must be issued in order to compel disclosure.

Because of discrimination against an individual that may result from dissemination of information on his or her HIV status, such information is highly confidential. States have enacted a variety of laws addressing the confidentiality of HIV test results and treatment records. Most states make available anonymous HIV testing but also establish nonanonymous, but confidential, testing programs under which public health officials have access under special circumstances to the names of those testing positive.

It is important to review the laws in your state and to develop written policies that conform to the facility's procedures regarding disclosure. In the absence of a state statute, it may be advisable to model the facility's policy after the federal drug and alcohol rules so that no HIV or AIDS information is released without patient authorization or a court order.

Facilities are also often asked to respond to more informal requests for information by law enforcement officers, district attorneys, and grand juries. In general, without a specific state statute compelling disclosure, law enforcement officers have no authority to examine a patient's medical records. This means that the results (for example, blood alcohol levels on a patient brought into the emergency department) should not be disclosed to the police unless required by statute. Prior to release of privileged information, subpoenas and other legal processes issued by law enforcement agencies should also be carefully scrutinized in consultation with the healthcare facility's general counsel. Within the proposed regulation is a specific provision for its use and disclosure of protected health information for law enforcement purposes without the authorization of the individual. These purposes relate to a legitimate law enforcement inquiry for identifying a suspect or victim as well as for national security activities and healthcare fraud.

With respect to parties to a lawsuit, discovery of documents is initiated by serving a notice specifying, with reasonable particularity, the documents sought to be reviewed, as well as the time, place, and manner of inspection. It is important to understand that despite its official-looking appearance, the court itself rarely issues a subpoena. It may be issued by a clerk or a judge or in some states by an attorney. It is important to carefully scrutinize all subpoenas, including those signed by a judge, and to challenge them in appropriate circumstances when the subpoenas request privileged material.

As custodians of the patient's medical records, healthcare entities often receive subpoenas for records in the context of current litigation not involving allegations of medical malpractice. For example, when an accident victim sues another party to the accident, the facility's medical records contain information necessary to prosecute the suit. One or both of the parties to the lawsuit may subpoena those records.

If privileged medical records are being subpoenaed that the healthcare provider feels are inappropriate, the provider may contact the attorney who requested the subpoena and request that the subpoena be withdrawn or mollified. If this is not successful, an application can be made to the court called a "motion to quash" or a "motion for a protective order" as the appropriate and proper method to test the subpoena (11).

Contracts

Careful contract review protects the assets of the organization. Systematic contract review can minimize problems due to inadequate knowledge of the subject or lack of time to devote to the project. Training and experience will prepare you to focus on areas of liability, insurance, hold-harmless, indemnification, and other risk elements common to many healthcare contracts. This systematic review does not eliminate the need for the general counsel's involvement in major contracts.

To accomplish an efficient review of any healthcare contract, one must understand the type of contract being reviewed, the contractual responsibilities and performance of the various parties, and the negative consequences of a poorly drafted contract. A contract is a legal agreement between two parties that can be enforced through legal channels. It creates an obligation to perform certain actions. Other instruments used like a contract are agreement, letter of intent, memorandum of understanding, lease, purchase agreement, order, or oral contract. A contract contains legally binding obligations between two or more parties and provides one or more of the parties with a legal remedy if another party fails to perform as specified in the document. For a contract to exist, all legal essentials must be included. These are listed in Table 6.9. A well-written contract confirms the understanding between the parties and avoids future disagreements about terms, conditions, and definitions critical to the relationship. Essential contract terms should always be clear and contain adequate detail to avoid subsequent misunderstanding.

Contracting parties can amend contracts, but the amendments should always be in writing and be signed by both parties. There should be a statement in the original contract that amendments should be in writing and

Table 6.9 Essential elements of a legal contract[a]

The parties to the contract must be competent.

The contract represents a "meeting of the minds" between the parties.

There is consideration; a bargained-for exchange of legal value exists between the parties.

The purpose or object of the contract is legal.

The contract is documented in writing if required for law enforcement in that state.

[a]See reference 11.

signed by both parties. The original contract language or provisions that are deleted or changed should be noted in the amendment as well (11). From a practical standpoint, many contractual relationships do not proceed as specified in the contract, and yet, the parties are satisfied with the arrangement. The services may change in scope or focus during the contract term without benefit of a written amendment to the original contract. If the receiving party continues to compensate the other party according to the terms of the contract, a strong argument can be made that the receiving party implied consent to the changes in performance and cannot later plead breach of contract. Contract litigation is expensive and rarely rewarding. Therefore it is important that any changes in the contractual relationship be mutually acknowledged in writing to avoid subsequent problems.

The contract review process should be integrated with the corporate compliance program. In general, federal and state laws prohibit healthcare providers from paying for the referrals of patients or other business, thus requiring careful legal scrutiny of all contractual arrangements between healthcare organizations, physician providers, medical groups, or other potential referral sources. Legal experts are essential to the process of drafting appropriate contracts to ensure compliance with complex federal and state laws.

Many contracts establishing relationships in the healthcare industry have confidentiality or privacy issues contained in the document. As contracts are reviewed, serious consideration should be given to including a confidentiality provision specific to the proprietary nature of business records of the organization, in addition to other protected and sensitive information such as patient information, medical staff records, committee proceedings, personnel file, payroll, and compensation (11). Negligent disclosure of protected information exposes the provider to legal liability. Therefore, access to the organization's protected or sensitive information should be limited to that which the contracting party has a valid "need to know." Any unauthorized disclosure by the contractor and its employees should subject the contractor to the resulting financial liability from the negligent act.

Contracting relationships can include clinical affiliations, sponsorship of educational presentations, tempo-rary staffing agencies, temporary independent contractors of any kind, consulting services, building leases, construction and renovation contracts, equipment purchases, home care, and managed care, to name a few.

Specimens

The laboratory management process presents numerous opportunities for potential liability. Departmental policies should comprehensively address all activities for all hours of operation. These policies should make special reference to exceptional times such as holidays and periods of light staffing or limited service (3, 18).

The two most frequent issues related to specimen collection are mislabeling or misidentification and loss of specimens that are considered to be irretrievable or very difficult and impractical to replace (for example, surgical specimens, samples from interventional procedures, biopsy samples, cerebrospinal fluid). Because of the potential for devastating outcomes related to mislabeling of specimens (leading to misdiagnosis, mistreatment, and the inability to diagnose and treat when specimen is lost), the Commission on Laboratory Accreditation and the College of American Pathologists have developed guidelines and checklists to assist laboratories with effective management of each step within this critical process (3, 18).

Documentation

The healthcare industry is often depicted as drowning in a sea of paper. The paper trail that is required to show compliance with regulations makes documentation a true paradox that is despised for its necessity and cherished for its usefulness. In the medical malpractice arena, documentation is the most reliable indicator of what was or was not done. "If it wasn't documented, it wasn't done. If it wasn't documented, it won't be reimbursed." These statements are repeated daily in the healthcare industry and have become hallmark statements from regulatory bodies. Plaintiff attorneys also use this as a common litigation tactic in the courtroom to argue that if it wasn't documented, it didn't happen (29).

Documentation is viewed in the broadest of senses and includes documents other than the patient's medical record. Critical laboratory documents include policies, protocols, guidelines, position statements, checklists, quality control documents, position descriptions, meeting minutes, personnel schedules, assignments, and any other form of documented information utilized in the management of the laboratory. In the courtroom, documentation carries a great deal of weight, unless something is done to discredit it. Juries will always place more emphasis on the written word versus the memory of events because memories fade over time, and the written word remains. Most documentation is painstakingly maintained with the hope that it will never be needed (16).

When setting up systems to maintain documentation that is accurate, complete, comprehensive, and legible, the biggest challenge is that healthcare providers are altruistic individuals who are more interested in providing care and less interested in capturing the details on paper. Keeping this in mind when creating systems and forms that will quickly and easily capture essential information is crucial to a successful documentation process. Fortunately, laboratory personnel who are more removed from the direct patient care role are generally more detail oriented as required by the nature of their work, making the details of the documentation process less of an obstacle.

With the availability of automation technology in today's world, the challenges of record keeping and storage are somewhat eased. The issue of illegibility of documentation has been eased. However, automation also brings additional challenges such as protection of sensitive and confidential information and recovery of information in the event of technology failure due to natural or other disasters.

By far, the recording and maintenance of information constitute the biggest challenge and biggest headache in the healthcare industry from a medico-legal perspective. All efforts spent on procuring quality technology, training and retraining of healthcare personnel, and maintenance and storage of information will be time, effort, and money well spent, even if the information is never challenged in a courtroom. Proper maintenance and storage of information will enhance patient safety and protect practitioners, the facility, and the community.

Research Liability

The relationships between healthcare organizations and their patients and families are guided by certain basic ethical principles and the morally binding obligations that are derived from those principles. The basic ethical principles that are most relevant to clinical bioethics are presented in Table 6.10. The concepts of doing good (beneficence), avoiding harm (nonmaleficence), privacy, confidentiality, and justice are central to the ethical principles and moral obligations recognized in the Hippocratic oath.

Each healthcare organization that receives federal funding for human research is subject to FDA or Office for Protection from Research Risks (OPRR) regulation and must have one or more institutional review boards (IRBs) with the authority to review, require modification of, approve, or disapprove research proposals. A document assuring compliance with human subject protections must be negotiated between the organization and the DHHS before DHHS-funded research may be conducted. The federal research requirements are founded as well on the respect for the autonomy of the research subject evidenced by stringent informed-consent requirements, the protection of vulnerable populations, the absence of coercion, and the reasonable balance of benefits and burdens of the proposed research for the individual subject, not for society at large. It is the role of the IRB to review and monitor the conduct of research and to educate healthcare personnel about the proper conduct of research (11).

Table 6.10 Ethical principles and moral obligations governing the patient and healthcare organization's relationship[a]

Ethical principles

  Beneficence, which creates an obligation to benefit patients and other persons and to further their welfare and interests

  The principle of respect for patients' autonomy

  Nonmaleficence, which asserts an obligation to prevent harm or, if risks of harm must be taken, to minimize those risks

  Justice, which is relevant to fairness of access to healthcare and to issues of rationing at the bedside

Moral obligations

  To respect the patient's privacy and maintain a process that protects confidentiality

  To communicate honestly about all aspects of the patient's diagnosis, treatment, and prognosis

  To conduct an ethically valid process of informed consent throughout the relationship

[a]See reference 11.

In a time of declining clinical revenue there may be increased pressure from principal investigators and administrators to cut corners and speed up the approval process for sponsored research. Such an approach places the welfare of the researcher and the research institution ahead of the welfare of the subject and is inconsistent with the ethical foundation of biomedical research. As well, the recent compliance activities of the OPRR and the FDA have shown that an approach to research that minimizes the protection of the subject can prove to be very costly, in both revenue and reputation.

OPRR and FDA compliance activities increased significantly in 1999 and are expected to continue at increased intensity, signaling a rise in public interest in the ethical and procedural propriety of biomedical research. Healthcare organizations and their IRBs have the responsibility to educate investigators and monitor the conduct of research as well as the institutional responsibility to provide adequate training to IRB members, which should include periodic didactic or interactive training for IRB members and investigators. The institution is expected to increase IRB infrastructure support to allow for continuous monitoring of research activities. To the extent that any laboratory function or personnel are involved in research activities, the above information related to training, documentation, and monitoring for investigators would apply as well (11).

Infectious Disease Lookback in Blood Transfusion

A lookback process, necessitated by information that is discovered some time after the transfusion has taken place, is a labor-intensive process. Targeted transfusion lookback is a process where blood recipients are notified of possible transmission of HIV or hepatitis C virus by a unit of blood that tested negative at the time of donation. The blood donor, who was negative during the donation, has subsequently tested positive for one of these viruses, creating concern that the unit, though negative by test, could have contained virus not detectable at that time (24). The size of the laboratory operation will impact the size of the lookback process. A key to expediting this costly process lies in timely access to accurate and complete information. Comprehensive and painstakingly detailed documentation will ease both the cost and pain of the process. As well, careful and complete documentation of the plan for the lookback and each step of the process is an absolute necessity. If the laboratory operations include business relationships with other vendors or organizations, it is a good idea to partner with those organizations to complete the process. Including the legal counsel for each entity will be necessary, as will the documentation and sign-off on the plan to accomplish the lookback, with the responsibilities of each entity for each step of the process clearly spelled out in writing. It may also be necessary to consult with your facility's media advisor about how to best communicate the need for the lookback to the public. Engaging the local media in the process in some cases has proven to be a very successful proactive strategy.

Training Physicians for Practice in the 21st Century

The Educational Goal: the Complete Physician

Evolution of medical training in the United States. The sociopolitical and economic currents that are reshaping the practice of medicine in the United States are fostering corresponding reforms in medical education at both the undergraduate and graduate levels. These changes in medical training represent only the most recent phase in the evolution of medical education over the last two centuries. Papa and Harasym (58) describe a series of major shifts in the medical curriculum in North America since 1765, when the prevailing model was that of an apprenticeship with little formalized education. By the second half of the 19th century, the need to improve the quality of medical practice led to a formalized four-year curriculum centered on distinct basic science departments in a university setting similar to the European model. By the turn of the century, emphasis was being placed on active rather than passive learning and on critical thinking skills. In the early 20th century, Flexner's influence further entrenched the separation of basic and clinical science training in medical schools and the importance of scientific reasoning in the practice of medicine (58). By the 1950s, the trend was to develop an integrated cross-departmental approach to teaching medicine based on organ systems and taught by faculty from multiple disciplines. During clinical-training years, students increasingly were exposed to specialists rather than to general practitioners. More recently, problem-based small-group teaching with the goal of developing critical reasoning skills was introduced in some schools. In some institutions the separation of training into "preclinical" and "clinical" years is gradually disappearing as students are being introduced to fundamentals of clinical medicine in their first year in medical school. All of these approaches have both advantages and disadvantages, and elements of each exist in different schools.

The major influences for reform in the current environment may be considered threefold. First, society is demanding increased physician competency and accountability to decrease medical error and to justify rising healthcare costs (21, 44, 67). Efforts to optimize the way in which both the scientific and humanistic aspects of medicine are taught and to develop in physicians the habit of lifelong learning have been ongoing since their introduction in the early 20th century (56). A vigorous attempt is being made to define improved assessment methods to measure training outcomes and the maintenance of competency after completion of training. Second, new knowledge in such areas as molecular biology, gender differences in disease manifestations and responses to therapy, the pathophysiology of aging and of chronic diseases, complementary and alternative medicine, and the applications of advanced technology is rapidly becoming important in the practice of medicine and must be addressed in the curriculum. Finally, medical trainees must be prepared for the practice of medicine in the managed-care environment, in which there is both an emphasis on outpatient care and an increasing recognition of the importance of population-based healthcare, disease prevention, health maintenance, and cost containment.

New paradigms in medical training.

Addressing society's expectations for physician competence. Historically, medical schools design their own curricula. Since 1932, the Association of American Medical Colleges (AAMC) has encouraged the development of learning objectives by medical schools (49). In 1981, the AAMC Project Panel on the General Professional Education of the Physician and College Preparation for Medicine was formed with the purpose of improving educational strategies. The Panel's conclusion was that all medical practitioners should have a "common foundation of knowledge, skills, attributes and values," defined by medical schools and incorporated in the form of specific learning objectives (49). In 1985 the Liaison Committee on Medical Education added defined learning objectives to its requirements for accreditation of medical schools. By the early 1990s, it was evident that despite these efforts, well-defined learning objectives were the exception rather than the rule. In 1996 the AAMC initiated the Medical

School Objectives Project (MSOP), one goal of which was to identify the desired characteristics of graduating medical students. Four attributes were defined: medical graduates should be altruistic, knowledgeable, skillful, and dutiful. For each attribute, 6 to 11 learning objectives were listed. Objectives for the last attribute, "dutiful," include knowledge of epidemiology, of psychosocial and cultural aspects of health, of biomedical information retrieval, and of the organization and financing of healthcare. The MSOP report also emphasized the importance of measuring outcomes of learning objectives and called for the development of improved assessment methods to accomplish this, especially in areas of attitudes and values (46, 49). A second phase of the MSOP report addressed the role of informatics in the practice of medicine and the need to incorporate fundamentals of population health into the curriculum (50). Previously untested aspects of physician training, such as bedside manner, are now being evaluated formally.

The AAMC identified core competency domains, including biomedical ethics, scholarly medical practice, communication in medicine, medical professionalism, and the healthcare system in 2000. These areas of competency cross all disciplines of medicine, and their identification is intended to facilitate development of core curricula to foster the learning required to become competent and independent physicians (62).

In 1999, the Accreditation Council for Graduate Medical Education (ACGME), the accrediting body for graduate medical education (GME) programs in all disciplines of medicine, adopted the General Competencies as part of the Outcome Project, designed to optimize educational outcomes in medical training. (See website for the ACGME. This section describes the rationale, design, and proposed time line for implementation of the General Competency requirements in graduate medical training programs. Available at http://www.acgme.org/outcome/ [accessed 12 December 2002].) Similar to the thrust of efforts being made at the medical school level, the goal of the general competency requirements is to foster the development of training objectives in nontraditional as well as traditional areas of GME to better prepare physicians for the evolving healthcare environment. The competency domains include patient care, medical knowledge, interpersonal and communication skills, professionalism, practice-based learning and improvement, and systems-based practice. As part of accreditation requirements, residency programs must demonstrate training objectives in each area, linked to assessment methods that are designed to provide reliable data documenting resident progress. The program must review assessment methods periodically and use the results to continually improve teaching methods. Ultimately, it is hoped that benchmarks of excellence will emerge.

The American Board of Medical Specialties (ABMS), in a joint initiative with the ACGME, similarly addressed public pressure to improve the caliber of medical care by endorsing the same general competencies and developing requirements for maintenance of competence by board-certified physicians. (See website for the ABMS. This section contains the Web-based version of the organization's newsletter. Available at http://www.abms.org/News.asp; *The ABMS Record*, vol. IX, no. 3, Summer 2000 [accessed 12 December 2002].) Most medical specialty boards now issue time-limited certification with mandatory periodic recertification to demonstrate knowledge of new developments in medicine since the time of the original certification.

Incorporating new knowledge and training techniques into the curriculum. Traditional didactic, largely passive approaches to medical school teaching are gradually giving way to case-based teaching methods, which already have been shown to be valuable in the development of diagnostic competence (19). Some educators citing the complexity of new knowledge and the diversity of the U.S. population have called for a transition from discipline-driven to concept-based education (33). An emphasis on problem-based learning and the development of critical thinking skills are felt to be essential in training students to be lifelong learners (56, 74).

New domains of medical knowledge have emerged over the last two decades and are increasingly being incorporated into medical school curricula. For instance, there is a growing appreciation of women's health needs beyond reproductive medicine; many women's health centers offer comprehensive primary care (85). Women's longevity compared to that of men means that women will comprise the majority of patients in the aging U.S. population and will require medical care that incorporates emerging knowledge of gender differences in disease manifestations and response to therapy (85).

As complementary and alternative medical therapies such as acupuncture, herbal medicine, and homeopathy have become increasingly popular with the public, many schools are recognizing the need to educate medical students about these approaches in order to prepare them to be informed consultants to their patients (25).

While students and graduate medical trainees are encountering rapid technical developments in diagnosis and therapy, technology also plays an increasingly important role in the educational process itself. Paper syllabi are enhanced or replaced by Web-based versions with illustrations, interactive graphics, and self-testing (32). Virtual microscopy is replacing glass slides in Web-based self-study tutorials and is being tested for use in formal examinations. In the near future, computer simulations may be used to train students and to assess their competency in performance of invasive procedures before they encounter patients (36). The accessibility of medical references and drug databases via handheld computers also promises to enhance efficiency and appropriateness of patient care (75).

Training physicians for the managed-care environment. Not surprisingly, medical schools and postgraduate training programs have been relatively slow in adapting to the need to produce physicians prepared for practice in a managed-care environment (6, 7). Medical schools traditionally have emphasized diagnosis and treatment rather than disease prevention and community healthcare. The academic medical center environment, typically a tertiary-care facility with state-of-the-art technology, a faculty rich in subspecialty expertise, and a heavy commitment to research, is inherently not conducive to instructing trainees in a holistic approach to patients, outpatient care, and the practice of cost-effective medicine. Nevertheless, there are areas of overlapping interests in academic health centers and managed care, including high-quality care, customer service, outcome research, and preventive medicine (42).

While in the 1960s approximately 50% of physicians were in primary care, by the mid-1990s the proportion was 30% (20). Over the last few years many medical schools have implemented improved instruction in primary care, ambulatory care, cost-effective healthcare, and disease prevention (10). Increasingly, medical students are exposed to clinical clerkship experience in managed-care settings (84). Some schools have actively addressed the perceived shortage of generalist physicians by committing to a goal of 50% of their graduates entering generalist practice (53).

A national demonstration project, Undergraduate Medical Education for the 21st Century (67), was funded through the Health Resources Services Administration. Over a 3-year period, 18 participating medical schools implemented new educational strategies, including a focus on training in primary care and ambulatory care and the expansion of clerkships or training opportunities to managed-care organizations and community health centers. This triggered curricular changes in 12.5% of medical schools (67).

Provisions of the Balanced Budget Act of 1997 (17), although decreasing GME funding, allow for reimbursement of resident training at certain off-site ambulatory settings. This may facilitate the extension of resident education to these sites, which is becoming an increasingly important aspect of preparing these physicians for practice in today's environment (17).

With the emerging emphasis on health maintenance and disease prevention, there is a growing consensus that medical trainees need to be educated in biostatistics, epidemiology, managerial skills, resource allocation, risk management, medical informatics, social and behavioral sciences, health outcomes, evidence-based medicine, and a population-based approach to healthcare (7, 19, 71, 84). At the same time, there is an appreciation of the need to improve trainees' proficiency in physical diagnosis skills as one way to minimize overuse or inappropriate use of resources (75).

External Forces Affecting Undergraduate and GME

Finding the right mix: how many physicians do we need? During the last 25 years, many questions have been raised regarding overall physician supply, the proportion of generalist or primary-care physicians, and the geographic distribution of physician practices. From the late 1980s through early 1990s, the overall number of trainees in GME programs in the United States increased by more than 15%. This was accompanied by an increase in the proportion of international medical graduates in the system (20). In 1986, Congress authorized the Council on Graduate Medical Education to evaluate physician workforce as well as GME training and financing. The lack of regulation of the numbers and specialist types of physicians being trained, coupled with rising costs and the predicted insolvency of the Medicare trust fund from which most of the funding of GME currently is derived, prompted calls from Congress to establish limits on GME (64). In 1992, Waxman and Rockefeller introduced legislation mandating an allocation system that would limit the number of first-year GME positions to 110% of the number of U.S. medical school graduates and stipulating that half of all these positions be in primary care. The bill also provided for development of an "all-payor pool" to fund GME, essentially placing an assessment on all private payors to contribute to the cost of training physicians (20). The latter concept continues to lack consensus. An independent advisory group, the Medicare Payment Advisory Commission, was established by Congress in the late 1990s to assess physician workforce, funding for international medical graduates, and a possible all-payor system for GME (64). The Balanced Budget Act of 1997, in part addressing the rising costs associated with healthcare, particularly in teaching hospitals, and the perception of an oversupply of physicians, capped the number of residents for purposes of Medicare reimbursement at 1996 levels (17).

Current challenges to academic medical centers. At the same time that curricular changes are being implemented in medical schools, academic medical centers are facing a financial crisis (69). Hospital costs are as much as 20% higher in institutions providing GME (20), largely due to the additional time involved and testing performed in a teaching situation. Teaching hospitals typically serve a greater number of Medicaid patients and the uninsured than do nonteaching hospitals; in addition, increasing numbers of patients are covered by managed-care plans. In addition to placing a cap on the number of residents, the Balanced Budget Act of 1997 decreases both direct (DGME) and indirect (IME) Medicare reimbursements for GME. In addition, the bill stipulates reductions in the disproportionate share payments traditionally made to teaching hospitals because of the relatively large number of uninsured patients treated at these institutions (17). On the positive side, the bill allows for "carving out" of DGME and IME Medicare payments to managed-care organizations and paying them directly to teaching hospitals. Prior to this, managed-care organizations were not required to make payments to teaching hospitals for their enrollees (7). Calls for decreasing the number of medical trainees may be problematic in that non-M.D. physician extenders may be associated with higher costs for academic medical centers (20). The economic duress caused by decreasing reimbursement for clinical service and declining federal support for GME impacts the ability of academic physicians to devote adequate time to training new physicians. Clinicians experience pressure to increase patient care activity in order to improve hospital revenue. (See Web-based version of national weekly newspaper reporting news and information on all aspects of higher education. Available at http://chronicle.com/press/; *The Chronicle of Higher Education:* Daily News: 05/15/2002 [accessed 12 December 2002].)

Responses by academic medical centers to the changing environment have included adaptation to the increased demand for outpatient services, marketing of the sophisticated technology and subspecialty expertise available at teaching hospitals, consolidations or mergers of hospitals for cost cutting and greater efficiency of services, and efforts directed at improving customer service (20, 52).

Summary

The vast changes that have occurred in the practice of medicine over the last few decades reflect the need for cost control within a system that focuses on quality and a low rate of errors. Managed care, which evolved as a means to achieve these goals, has truly changed the face of medical practice in the United States. Along with these trends, American healthcare consumers, equipped with more and more information about their own healthcare, have placed increasing demands on the medical community. The roles of increasing regulatory and legal scrutiny have helped to shape our current healthcare system. In order to prepare future physicians, changes in medical and postgraduate medical education are preeminent.

KEY POINTS

- Major changes in the way medical care is delivered and funded have had a profound impact on the laboratory.
- Technology, including the World Wide Web, improves laboratory turnaround time, communication of laboratory results, disease detection and treatment, availability of information, patient and doctor resources, and all phases of physician training.
- Changes in demographics changed the way medicine and the laboratory function.
- Evidence-based medicine emphasizes cost containment and quality of care.
- Clinical practice guidelines are one approach to standardize medical care.
- Increases in medical malpractice awards impact medical care.
- New regulations and laws change the way medicine is practiced.
- Changes in the practice of medicine impact medical student and resident training.

GLOSSARY

Accreditation Council for Graduate Medical Education (ACGME) Professional organization responsible for accrediting post-medical school training, encompassing more than 7,000 residency programs in 110 specialty and subspecialty areas.

American Board of Medical Specialties (ABMS) Organization of 24 medical specialty boards certifying physicians.

American Society of Health Care Risk Management Organization for healthcare risk management professionals.

Association of American Medical Colleges (AAMC) Association of medical schools, teaching hospitals, and academic societies dedicated to improvements in medical education, research, and healthcare.

Balanced Budget Act of 1997 Package of spending reductions designed to balance the federal budget by 2002. Changes in Medicare financing of graduate medical education (GME) included a cap on number of residents counted for reimbursement and a reduction in indirect graduate medical education payment (IME).

Balanced Budget Refinement Act of 1999 Legislation that offset or revised some of the GME funding provisions of the BBA.

Clinical trial A research study that looks at a similar group of patients selected using strict criteria and assesses the impact of changes of single variables.

College of American Pathologists Association of pathologists dedicated to fostering excellence in pathology and laboratory medicine. Recognized leader in providing laboratory inspection and accreditation programs.

Commission on Laboratory Accreditation Administers the College of American Pathologists Laboratory Accreditation Program, which is approved to inspect laboratories in lieu of the Centers for Medicare and Medicaid Services.

Contract A legal agreement between two parties that can be enforced through legal channels that creates an obligation.

Corporate compliance program The development of effective internal controls that promote adherence to applicable federal and state laws and the program requirements of federal, state, and private health plans. The program is aimed at the prevention of fraud, abuse, and waste in these healthcare plans while at the same time furthering the fundamental mission of all hospitals, which is to provide quality healthcare to patients.

Council on Graduate Medical Education Congressionally authorized body charged with evaluating physician workforce and graduate medical training and financing.

Critical (clinical) pathways Standardized, multidisciplinary approach to a specific problem. Traditionally more detailed than practice guidelines, though the difference may not be distinct.

Direct Graduate Medical Education Payment (DGME) Medicare payment to teaching hospitals for costs directly related to training programs, including residents' stipends, faculty supervision costs, and overhead.

Disproportionate share payment Payment to teaching hospitals to offset costs of treating a relatively large proportion of uninsured patients.

Evidence-based medicine The use and analysis of solid, tangible evidence leading to optimal medical decision making.

General competencies Six domains of competency adopted by the ABMS and ACGME as requisite for physicians: patient care, medical knowledge, interpersonal and communication skills, professionalism, practice-based learning, and systems-based practice.

General Professional Education of the Physician and College Preparation for Medicine AAMC project panel charged with developing improved educational strategies.

Graduate medical education (GME) Specialty or subspecialty training occurring after medical school.

Healthcare Integrity and Protection Data Bank National data collection program mandated by the Health Insurance Portability and Accountability Act of 1996 (HIPAA) to combat fraud and abuse in healthcare delivery. Collects and discloses adverse actions against practitioners, including civil judgments, criminal convictions, injunctions, federal or state licensing and certification actions, and other adjudicated actions.

Health Insurance Portability and Accountability Act of 1996 (HIPAA) Legislation establishing a variety of health insurance coverage protections. Also known as the Kassebaum-Kennedy bill.

Health Resources and Services Administration Agency of the U.S. Department of Health and Human Services charged with ensuring access to quality healthcare for uninsured and low-income populations.

Indirect Graduate Medical Education payment (IME) Medicare payment to teaching hospitals to compensate for higher costs related to severity of patient illness.

Institute of Medicine (IOM) Private, nongovernmental organization, associated with the National Academy of Sciences, whose mission is to advance science and healthcare policy.

Institutional Review Board (IRB) Reviews research proposals and monitors human research conducted in healthcare organizations. Required for healthcare organizations receiving federal funding for such research.

Joint Commission on Accreditation of Healthcare Organizations (JCAHO) Predominant accrediting body for hospitals and other healthcare organizations in the United States.

Length of stay (LOS) The number of days a patient is hospitalized for a specific diagnosis. This metric has been used by managed-care organizations to compare institutions and their utilization of services.

Liaison Committee on Medical Education (LCME) Accrediting authority for U.S. and Canadian medical schools.

Locum tenens A position, usually temporary, for a healthcare professional often in an underserved area.

Lookback A process where blood product recipients are notified of possible transmission of human immunodeficiency virus or hepatitis C virus by a unit that tested negative at the time of donation. The blood donor subsequently tested positive for one of these viruses, creating concern that the unit could have contained virus not detectable by the original test (24).

Medical School Objectives Project (MSOP) AAMC project to examine learning objectives and assessment methods in medical education.

Medicare Payment Advisory Commission Independent advisory group assessing physician workforce and GME funding.

Miniaturization The use of smaller and smaller "micro" components, which allows the number of analytes in a device to increase, replacing larger analyzers. This facilitates point-of-care testing (POCT).

National Patient Safety Foundation Nonprofit organization whose mission is to improve patient safety in the delivery of healthcare.

National Practitioner Data Bank Established through Title IV of Public Law 99-660, the Health Care Quality Improvement Act of 1986, to collect reports regarding medical malpractice payments, adverse licensure actions, clinical privilege actions, and professional society membership actions against healthcare practitioners. Restricts the ability of practitioners to move from state to state without disclosure of adverse actions or incompetent performance.

Nucleic acid testing (NAT) Testing that relies on measuring specific sequences of nucleic acid. This can lead to earlier detection of pathogens and malignancy recurrence.

Office for Protection from Research Risks (OPRR) Section of the Department of Health and Human Services now known as the Office for Human Research Protections.

Outcome Project ACGME initiative emphasizing educational outcomes in the accreditation of resident training programs.

Outcome research Research that looks at diverse patient groups to determine which medical interventions or diagnostic tests have an effect on patients.

Point-of-care testing (POCT) Testing that takes place outside of a centralized or core laboratory setting and closer to the patient encounter. This is also referred to as "near-patient testing."

Practice guidelines Systematically defined statements to assist practitioner and patient decisions about appropriate healthcare for specific clinical circumstances (13).

Risk The chance or possibility of loss.

Tort A legal term for a wrongful act that is done on purpose and causes injury or harm.

Troponin A component of cardiac muscle. Blood levels rise after myocardial damage.

Undergraduate Medical Education for the 21st Century National demonstration project funded by the Health Resources and Services Administration to foster medical school training in primary care and in ambulatory-care settings.

REFERENCES

1. Albert, T. 2002. House bill recognizes crisis, revitalizes tort reform. *AMA Newsl.* **45**(18):1–2.

2. Anderson, F. P., M. L. Fritz, M. C. Kontos, R. A. McPherson, and R. L. Jesse. 1998. Cost-effectiveness of cardiac troponin I in a systematic chest pain evaluation protocol: use of cardiac troponin I lowers length of stay for low-risk cardiac patients. *Clin. Lab. Manag. Rev.* **12**:63–69.

3. Anderson, M., B. Salmon, J. O'Malley, A. Fox, and B. J. Youngberg. 1993. *Legislative, Regulatory and Legal Issues in the Clinical Lab: a Resource Guide,* p. 1–42. University Health System Consortium, Oakbrook, Ill.

4. Berwick, D. 2000. Knowledge always on call: for docs, practicing medicine will mean providing information more than providing care. *Clin. Lab. Manag. Rev.* **14**:250–252.

5. Bickford, G. R. 1994. Decentralized testing in the '90's: a survey of US hospitals. *Clin. Lab. Manag. Rev.* **8**:327–338.

6. Bloom, S. W. 1989. The medical school as a social organization: the sources of resistance to change. *Med. Educ.* **23**:228–241.

7. Blumenthal, D., and S. O. Their. 1996. Managed care and medical education. The new fundamentals. *JAMA* **276**:725–727. (Editorial.)

8. Brennan, T. A. 1995. Methods for setting priorities for guidelines development: medical malpractice, p. 99–110. *In* Committee on Methods for Setting Priorities for Guidelines Development (M. J. Field, ed.), Division of Healthcare Services, Institute of Medicine, *Setting Priorities for Clinical Practice Guidelines.* National Academy Press, Washington, D.C.

9. Buckman, R. 1992. *How To Break Bad News: a Guide for Health Care Professionals.* The Johns Hopkins University Press, Baltimore, Md.

10. Campbell, E. G., J. S. Weissman, J. Ausiello, S. Wyatt, and D. Blumenthal. 2001. Understanding the relationship between market competition and students' ratings of the managed care content of their undergraduate medical education. *Acad. Med.* **76**:51–59.

11. Carroll, R. (ed.). 2001. *Risk Management Handbook for Healthcare Organizations,* 3rd ed. Jossey-Bass, Inc., Publishers, San Francisco, Calif.

12. Clancy, C. M., and D. B. Kamerow. 1996. Evidence-based medicine meets cost-effectiveness analysis. *JAMA* **276**:329–330. (Editorial.)

13. Committee on Medicare Payment Methodology for Clinical Laboratory Services (D. M. Wolman, A. L. Kalfoglou, and L. LeRoy, ed.), Division of Health Care Services, Institute of Medicine. 2000. *Medicare Laboratory Payment Policy: Now and in the Future.* National Academy Press, Washington, D.C.

14. Committee on Methods for Setting Priorities for Guidelines Development (M. J. Field, ed.), Division of Healthcare Services, Institute of Medicine. 1995. *Setting Priorities for Clinical Practice Guidelines.* National Academy Press, Washington, D.C.

15. Committee on Quality of Health Care in America (L. T. Kohn, J. M. Corrigan, and M. S. Donaldson, ed.), 2000 . *To Err Is Human:* *Building a Safer Health System.* National Academy Press, Washington, D.C.

16. Conner, C., and N. Hershey. 2001. *Hospital Law Manual,* vol. 2, p. 1–68. Health Law and Compliance Center. Aspen Publishers, Inc., Gaithersburg, Md.

17. Dickler, R. G., and G. Shaw. 2000. The Balanced Budget Act of 1997: its impact on U.S. teaching hospitals. *Ann. Intern. Med.* **132**:820–824.

18. DiLima, S., N. Frye, and C. Frye (ed.). 1997. *Hospital Risk Management: Forms, Checklists & Guidelines,* vol. II, p. 44:I–44:34. Aspen Publishers, Inc., Gaithersburg, Md.

19. Donoghue, G. D. 2000. Women's health: a catalyst for reform of medical education. *Acad. Med.* **75**:1056–1060.

20. Epstein, A. M. 1995. U.S. teaching hospitals in the evolving health care system. *JAMA* **273**:1203–1207.

21. Epstein, R. M., and E. M. Hundert. 2002. Defining and assessing professional competence. *JAMA* **287**:226–235.

22. Felder, R. A., S. Graves, and T. Mifflin. 1999. Reading the future, the increased relevance of laboratory medicine in the next century. *MLO Med. Lab. Obs.* **31**:20–26.

23. Ferrara, K., S. Mitchell, C. Price, M. Schneider, and B. J. Youngberg. 1995. *Legal Issues Associated with the Use and Development of Practice Guidelines.* UHC Services Corporation, Oakbrook, Ill.

24. Food and Drug Administration. September 1998. Guidance for industry; current good manufacturing practice for blood and blood components: (1) quarantine and disposition of units from prior collections from donors with repeatedly reactive screening tests for antibody to hepatitis C virus (anti-HCV); (2) supplemental testing, and the notification of consignees and blood recipients of donor test results for anti-HCV. Food and Drug Administration, Rockville, Md.

25. Frenkel, M., and E. B. Ayre. 2001. The growing need to teach about complementary and alternative medicine: questions and challenges. *Acad. Med.* **76**:251–254.

26. Friedman, B. A. 1998. Integrating laboratory processes into clinical processes, web-based laboratory reporting and the emergence of the virtual clinical laboratory. *Clin. Lab. Manag. Rev.* **12**:333–338.

27. Glenn, G. C., and Laboratory Testing Strategy Task Force of the College of American Pathologists. 1996. Practice parameter on laboratory panel testing for screening and case finding in asymptomatic adults. *Arch. Pathol. Lab. Med.* **120**:929–943.

28. Golden, W. E., A. A. Pappas, and R. C. Lavendar. 1987. Financial unbundling reduces outpatient laboratory use. *Arch. Intern. Med.* **147**:1045–1048.

29. Goodman, M. L. 19 April 2002. *Medical Malpractice and the Legal Process Goodman.* Allen & Filetti, PLLC, Richmond, Va.

30. Greenfield, S., C. E. Lewis, S. H. Kaplan, and M. B. Davidson. 1975. Peer review by criteria mapping: criteria for diabetes mellitus, the use of decision-making in chart audit. *Ann. Intern. Med.* **83**: 761–770.

31. Grol, R. 2001. Improving the quality of medical care, building bridges among professional pride, payer profit, and patient satisfaction. *JAMA* **286**:2578–2585.

32. Grundman, J. A., R. S. Wigton, and D. Nickol. 2000. A controlled trial of an interactive, web-based virtual reality program for teaching physical diagnosis skills to medical students. *Acad. Med.* **75S**:S47–S49.

33. **Hoffman, E., D. Magrane, and G. D. Donoghue.** 2000. Changing perspectives on sex and gender in medical education. *Acad. Med.* **75**:1051–1055.

34. **H. R. 4600.** 2002. Help Efficient, Accessible, Low Cost, Timely Health Care (HEALTH) Act of 2002 (introduced in House April 25, 2002). 107th Congress, 2nd Session, in U.S. House of Representatives.

35. **Hume, H. A., A. M. Ali, F. Décary, and M. A. Blajchman.** 1991. Evaluation of pediatric transfusion practice using criteria maps. *Transfusion* **31**:52–58.

36. **Iserson, K. V.** 1999. Simulating our future: real changes in medical education. *Acad. Med.* **74**:752–754.

37. **Katon, W., M. Von Korff, E. Lin, E. Walker, G. E. Simon, T. Bush, P. Robinson, and J. Russo.** 1995. Collaborative management to achieve treatment guidelines, impact on depression in primary care. *JAMA* **273**:1026–1031.

38. **Katz, D. A., J. L. Griffith, J. R. Beshansky, and H. P. Selker.** 1996. The use of empiric clinical data in the evaluation of practice guidelines for unstable angina. *JAMA* **276**:1568–1574.

39. **Keiser, J. F., and B. J. Howard.** 1998. Critical pathways: design, implementation, and evaluation. *Clin. Lab. Manag. Rev.* **12**:317–332.

40. **Kelly, C. S., C. L. Anderson, J. P. Pestian, A. D. Wenger, A. B. Finch, G. L. Strope, and E. F. Luckstead.** 2000. Improved outcomes for hospitalized asthmatic children using a clinical pathway. *Ann. Allergy Asthma Immunol.* **84**:509–516.

41. **Kurec, A. S.** 1998. Telemedicine: emerging opportunities and future trends. *Clin. Lab. Manag. Rev.* **12**:364–374.

42. **LaRosa, J. C., P. Whelton, and M. S. Litiwin.** 1999. Academic medicine and managed care: seeking common ground. *Acad. Med.* **74**:488–492.

43. **Larson, D., and L. A. Straub.** 1996. Clinical data repository, a solution for outcomes assessment. *Clin. Lab. Manag. Rev.* **10**:107–114.

44. **Leach, D. C.** 2002. Competence is a habit. *JAMA* **287**:243–244. (Editorial.)

45. **Leibman, B. D., O. Dillioglugil, F. Abbas, S. Tanli, M. W. Kattan, and P. T. Scardino.** 1998. Impact of a clinical pathway for radical retropubic prostatectomy. *Urology* **52**:94–99.

46. **Maudsley, R. F.** 1999. Content in context: medical education and society's needs. *Acad. Med.* **74**:143–145.

47. **McPherson, R. A.** 2001. Blood sample volumes: emerging trends in clinical practice and laboratory medicine. *Clin. Lab. Manag. Rev.* **15**:3–10.

48. **McPherson, R. A.** 1998. Robotics, automation, and the new role of process control. *Clin. Lab. Manag. Rev.* **12**:339–346.

49. **Medical School Objectives Writing Group.** 1999. Learning objectives for medical student education—guidelines for medical schools: report I of the Medical Schools Objectives Project. *Acad. Med.* **74**:13–18.

50. **Medical School Objectives Writing Group.** 1999. The Informatics Panel and the Population Health Perspective Panel. Contemporary issues in medicine—medical informatics and population health: report II of the Medical School Objectives Project. *Acad. Med.* **74**:130–141.

51. **Mennemeyer, S. T.** 1998. Should laboratories be judged by patient outcomes? *Clin. Lab. Manag. Rev.* **12**:57–62.

52. **Meyer, G. S., and D. Blumenthal.** 1996. TennCare and academic medical centers. The lessons from Tennessee. *JAMA* **276**:672–676.

53. **Morse, R. M., G. S. Plungas, D. Duke, L. K. Rollins, V. Barnes, B. K. Brinson, J. R. Martindale, and D. W. Marsland.** 1999. The Virginia Generalist Initiative: lessons learned in a statewide consortium. *Acad. Med.* **74S**:S24–S29.

54. **Narayanan, S.** 2000. Technology and laboratory instrumentation in the next decade. *MLO Med. Lab. Obs.* **32**:24–31.

55. **Nease, R. F., T. Kneeland, G. T. O'Connor, W. Sumner, C. Lumpkins, L. Shaw, D. Pryor, and H. C. Sox.** 1995. Variation in patient utilities for outcomes of the management of chronic stable angina, implications for clinical practice guidelines. *JAMA* **273**:1185–1190.

56. **Neville, A. J., H. I. Reiter, K. W. Eva, and G. R. Norman.** 2000. Critical appraisal turkey shoot: linking critical appraisal to clinical decision making. *Acad. Med.* **75S**:S87–S89.

57. **Office of Inspector General.** 1997. Publication of the OIG model compliance plan for clinical laboratories. *Fed. Regist.* **62**:9435–9441.

58. **Papa, F. J., and P. H. Harasym.** 1999. Medical curriculum reform in North America, 1765 to the present: a cognitive science perspective. *Acad. Med.* **74**:154–164.

59. **Paris, J. J., and J. Ferranti.** 2001. The changing face of medicine: health care on the internet. *J. Perinatol.* **21**:34–39.

60. **Parmley, W. W.** 1994. Clinical practice guidelines, does the cookbook have enough recipes? *JAMA* **272**:1374–1375. (Editorial.)

61. **Pearlman, E. S., M. S. Wolfert, R. Miele, L. Bilello, and J. Stauffer.** 2001. Utilization management and information technology: adapting to the new era. *Clin. Lab. Manag. Rev.* **15**:85–88.

62. **Philibert, I. (ed.).** 2001. AAMC releases report on core competencies. *In* ACGME Bulletin, March 2001.

63. **Plapp, F. V., C. I. Essmyer, A. B. Byrd, and M. L. Zucker.** 2000. How to successfully influence laboratory test utilization. *Clin. Lab. Manag. Rev.* **14**:253–260.

64. **Plaushin, C.** 1997. Microscope on Washington. Federal funding of graduate medical education. *Lab. Med.* **28**:627–628.

65. **Plebani, M.** 1999. The changing face of clinical laboratories. *Clin. Chem. Lab. Med.* **37**:711–717.

66. **Pritts, T. A., M. S. Nussbaum, L. V. Flesch, E. J. Fegelman, A. A. Parikh, and J. E. Fischer.** 1999. Implementation of a clinical pathway decreases length of stay and cost for bowel resection. *Ann. Surg.* **230**:728–733.

67. **Rabinowitz, H. K., D. Babbott, S. Bastacky, J. M. Pascoe, K. K. Patel, K. L. Pye, J. Rodak, Jr., K. J. Veit, and D. L. Wood.** 2001. Innovative approaches to educating medical students for practice in a changing health care environment: the national UME-21 project. *Acad. Med.* **76**:587–597.

68. **Reddick, R. L., and W. W. McLendon.** 1995. Pathology and laboratory medicine. *JAMA* **273**:1707–1708.

69. **Rich, E. C., M. Liebow, M. Srinivasan, D. Parish, J. O. Wolliscroft, O. Fein, and R. Blaser.** 2002. Medicare financing of graduate medical education. *J. Gen. Intern. Med.* **17**:283–292.

70. **Robinson, J. C.** 1996. Decline in hospital utilization and cost inflation under managed care in California. *JAMA* **276**:1060–1064.

71. **Sass, P., and P. Edelsack.** 2001. Teaching community health assessment skills in a problem-based format. *Acad. Med.* **76**:88–91.

72. **Schoenbaum, S. C., and D. N. Sundwall.** 1995. *Using Clinical Practice Guidelines to Evaluate Quality of Care,* vol. 1. *Issues.* U.S. Department of Health and Human Services, Public Health Service, Agency for Health Care Policy and Research, Rockville, Md.

73. **Schoenbaum, S. C., and D. N. Sundwall.** 1995. *Using Clinical Practice Guidelines to Evaluate Quality of Care,* vol. 2. *Methods.* U.S. Department of Health and Human Services, Public Health Service, Agency for Health Care Policy and Research, Rockville, Md.

74. **Schoenfeld, P., D. Cruess, and W. Peterson.** 2000. Effect of an evidence-based medicine seminar on participants' interpretations of clinical trials: a pilot study. *Acad. Med.* **75:**1212–1214.

75. **Shaneyfelt, T. M.** 2001. Building bridges to quality. *JAMA* **286:**2600–2601. (Editorial.)

76. **Shaneyfelt, T. M., M. F. Mayo-Smith, and J. Rothwangl.** 1999. Are guidelines following guidelines? The methodological quality of clinical practice guidelines in the peer-review medical literature. *JAMA* **281:**1900–1905.

77. **Singer, P. A., D. S. Cooper, E. G. Levy, P. W. Ladenson, L. E. Braverman, G. Daniels, F. S. Greenspan, I. R. McDougall, and T. F. Nikolai.** 1995. Treatment guidelines for patients with hyperthyroidism and hypothyroidism. *JAMA* **273:**808–812.

78. **Snyder, J. R., and D. S. Wilkinson.** 1998. The nature of management in laboratory medicine, p. 1–15. *In* J. S. Snyder and D. S. Wilkinson (ed.), *Management in Laboratory Medicine,* 3rd ed. Lippincott, Philadelphia, Pa.

79. **St. Peter, R. F., M. C. Reed, P. Kemper, and D. Blumenthal.** 1999. Changes in the scope of care provided by primary care physicians. *N. Engl. J. Med.* **341:**1980–1985.

80. **Strickland, B. J., and W. O. Quiery.** 17 May 2002. *HIPAA Patient Rights, State Law and You.* Reciprocal of America, Glen Allen, Va.

81. **Trosty, S. R.** 2002. Future looks bleak as malpractice premiums continue upward spiral. *Health. Risk Manag.* **24:**1–12.

82. **Tunis, S. R., R. S. A. Hayward, M. C. Wilson, H. R. Rubin, E. B. Bass, M. Johnston, and E. P. Steinberg.** 1994. Internists' attitudes about clinical practice guidelines. *Ann. Intern. Med.* **120:**956–963.

83. **Van Walraven, C., V. Goel, and B. Chan.** 1998. Effect of population-based interventions on laboratory utilization. *JAMA* **280:**2028–2033.

84. **Veloski, J., B. Barzansky, D. B. Nash, S. Bastacky, and D. P. Stevens.** 1996. Medical student education in managed care settings: beyond HMOs. *JAMA* **276:**667–671.

85. **Weisman, C. S.** 2000. The trends in health care delivery for women: challenges for medical education. *Acad. Med.* **75:**1107–1113.

86. **Wilkinson, D. S.** 2000. Technology assessment: measuring the outcomes of laboratory practice. *Clin. Lab. Manag. Rev.* **14:**267–271.

87. **Wilkinson, D. S.** 1997. The role of technology in the clinical laboratory of the future. *Clin. Lab. Manag. Rev.* **11:**322–330.

88. **Wilson, I. B., and P. D. Cleary.** 1995. Linking clinical variables with health-related quality of life, a conceptual model of patient outcomes. *JAMA* **273:**59–65.

89. **Winkelman, J. W., and S. T. Mennemeyer.** 1996. Using patient outcomes to screen for clinical laboratory errors. *Clin. Lab. Manag. Rev.* **10:**134–142.

90. **Young, D. S., V. S. Sachais, and L. C. Jefferies.** 2000. Laboratory costs in the context of disease. *Clin. Chem.* **46:**967–975.

APPENDIX 6.1   Websites

American Board of Medical Specialties
(http://www.abms.org/News.asp)
This section contains the web-based version of the organization's newsletter.

Accreditation Council for Graduate Medical Education, ACGME Outcome Project
(http://www.acgme.org/outcome/)
This section describes the rationale, design, and proposed timeline for implementation of the General Competency requirements in graduate medical training programs.

National Guideline Clearinghouse (NGC)
(http://www.guideline.gov)
A public resource for evidence-based clinical practice guidelines. The NGC is sponsored by the Agency for Healthcare Research and Quality and provides a catalog of published guidelines.

The Chronicle of Higher Education
(http://chronicle.com/press/)
A web-based version of *The Chronicle of Higher Education,* a national weekly newspaper reporting news and information on all aspects of higher education.

APPENDIX 6.2 Example of a Clinical Pathway: Community-Acquired Pneumonia Clinical Pathway[a]

INITIAL ASSESSMENT

1. Inclusion criteria:

   Infiltrate on chest radiograph ———

   One or more of the following symptoms: ———

      Cough ± sputum production ———

      Malaise ———

      Fever (T > 101.5°F) ———

      Heart rate ≥ 100/min ———

      Respiratory rate ≥ 30/min ———

2. Exclusion criteria:

   No infiltrate on chest radiograph ———

   Age < 18 years old ———

   Suspicion for:

      Aspiration pneumonia ———

      Tuberculosis ———

      Pulmonary emboli ———

      Cystic fibrosis ———

   Depressed immune system:

      HIV ———

      Immunosuppressive medication ———

      Allergy/intolerance to recommended antibiotic ———

3. Stratify by fine criteria:

RISK STRATIFICATION SCORE/CLASS (POINT-SCORING SYSTEM)

Patient characteristics	Points		Patient characteristics	Points	
Demographic factors			Physical examination findings		
Age			Respiratory rate (≥30/min)	+20	
Male Age (in yrs)			Systolic blood pressure (<90 mm Hg)	+20	
Female Age (in yrs)	−10	———			
Admit from nursing home	+10	———	Altered mental status	+20	———
			Temperature (< 95°F or ≥104°F)	+15	
Comorbid illnesses			Pulse (≥125/min)	+10	
Neoplastic disease	+30	———	Laboratory findings		
Liver disease	+20	———	pH (≤7.35)	+30	———
Congestive heart failure	+10	———	BUN (≥30 mg/dl)	+20	———
Cerebrovascular disease	+10	———	Sodium (<130 mq/liter)	+20	———
Renal disease	+10	———	Glucose (≥250 mg/dl)	+10	———
			Hematocrit (<30%)	+10	———
			PO$_2$ <60 mm Hg or O$_2$ Sat <90% on RA	+10	———
			Pleural effusion	+10	———
			Total points		———

A total point score (*risk score*) is obtained by summing the points for each applicable patient characteristic (**M. J. Fine, T. E. Auble, D. M. Yealy, B. H. Hanusa, L. A. Weissfeld, D. E. Singer, C. M. Coley, T. J. Marrie, and W. N. Kapoor.** 1997. A prediction rule to identify low-risk patients with community-acquired pneumonia. *N. Engl. J. Med.* 336:243–250).

Risk: Class I to II: ≤70 points, mortality risk <0.7%   Class III: 71 to 90 points, mortality risk = 0.9 to 2.8%

Class IV: 91 to 130 points, mortality risk = 8.2 to 9.3%   Class V: >130 points, mortality risk = 27.0 to 31.1%

(continued)

APPENDIX 6.2   Example of a Clinical Pathway: Community-Acquired Pneumonia Clinical Pathway[a] *(continued)*

MANAGEMENT OF PATIENT

1. Risk classification I to II:
   - ☐ Manage as OUTPATIENT, unless clinically contraindicated with the following antibiotic regimen:
     - ☐ Doxycycline 100 mg p.o. BID × 10 days
   - *If pregnancy suspected:*
     - ☐ Azithromycin 500 mg p.o. × 1, then 250 mg p.o. QD × 4 days
2. Risk classification III:
   - ☐ Decision for admission based on clinical picture
3. Risk classification IV to V:
   - ☐ Notify General Medicine or ICU team for admission
   - <u>General admission orders</u>
   - ☐ Blood cultures × 2 prior to antibiotic initiation
   - ☐ Sputum culture (if obtainable) prior to antibiotic initiation
   - ☐ Blood (CBC with differential and basic metabolic)
   - ☐ Initiate O_2 therapy if O_2 Sats < 92% on room air
   - ☐ Initiate i.v. fluids at ≥ 75 ml/h, if indicated
   - ☐ Antibiotic therapy:
     - ☐ Initiate oral therapy if:
       - ☐ Tolerating p.o.
       - ☐ Stable hemodynamics
       - ☐ Non-ICU patient
       - ☐ Patient without definite or suspected malabsorption (e.g., decompensated CHF, Crohn's disease, or significant nausea and vomiting)
     - ☐ Initiate i.v. therapy if does not meet above criteria

Caution needs to be exercised when levofloxacin is ordered; oral levofloxacin administration should be separated from antacids (containing aluminum, magnesium, and/or calcium) and other cationic salts (e.g., ferrous sulfate). These medications should not be administered within 4 h before or 2 h after a dose of oral levofloxacin.

On the wards:
When initiating i.v. therapy
Ceftriaxone 1 g i.v. QD
and
Azithromycin 500 mg i.v. QD
OR
Levofloxacin 500 mg i.v. QD
(*If CrCl , 50 ml/min, see dosing schedule below*)

On the wards:
When initiating p.o. therapy
Levofloxacin 500 mg p.o.
QD × 10 days (If CrCl < 50 ml/min, see dosing schedule below)

In the ICU:
When initiating i.v. therapy
Ceftriaxone 1 g i.v. QD
and
Azithromycin 500 mg i.v. QD
OR
Ceftriaxone 1 g i.v. QD
and
Levofloxacin 500 mg i.v. QD
(*If CrCl < 50 ml/min, see dosing schedule below.*)

Dosing adjustment of levofloxacin in renal impairment: (CrCl is creatinine clearance):

–If CrCl = 20 to 49 ml/min:
   Levofloxacin 500 mg (p.o. or i.v.) × day,
     then 250 mg (p.o. or i.v.) QD × 10 days

–If CrCl , < 9 ml/min:
   Levofloxacin 500 mg (p.o. or i.v.) × 1 day,
     then 250 mg (p.o. or i.v.) QOD × 10 days

Generic Name	*Brand Name*	*Dosing*	*No. of pills/prescription*
Doxycycline	Vibramycin	100 mg p.o. BID × 10 days	20
Azithromycin	Zithromax	500 mg p.o. × 1 day, then 250 mg p.o. QD × 4 days	6
Levofloxacin	Levaquin	500 mg p.o. QD × 10 days	10
Azithromycin	Zithromax	500 mg i.v. QD	
Ceftriaxone	Rocephin	1 g i.v. QD	
Levofloxacin	Levaquin	500 mg i.v. QD	

[a]Provided courtesy of Stephen Sigworth, Virginia Commonwealth University Health System.

7

The Changing Healthcare Environment

Ann L. Harris and David S. Wilkinson

OBJECTIVES

To provide a historical overview of reimbursement for laboratory services from 1969 to the present

To present special issues related to contracting for managed care, including prospective payment, capitation, and providing service with payment caps. Discuss the risks related to each of these challenges

To explore the impact of educated and informed consumers, patients, providers, insurers, and employers on the delivery of healthcare

To explore the impact of technological advances, home health devices, and genetic information

To discuss how society is becoming increasingly litigious

To illustrate how consolidation among providers and vendors drives reengineering and restructuring

Nations once measured their national wealth in terms of the gold they were able to hoard. Then came the transition to products, and Gross National Product became the measure of wealth. Now the move is on to information. It's not as if there were no value attached to information in the age of gold. Every university standing today is a testament to the long lasting value of information and knowledge. And gold has not lost its luster in an age of information. It's simply a shift in emphasis. Gold once predominated, then tangible goods, now information. Even if the Internet bubble bursts, this current shift in emphasis is likely to leave the healthcare landscape permanently transformed. Whatever happens with the Internet in healthcare, one truth will remain. It is at the interface between a patient and a caregiver that the greatest opportunity exists for creating value in healthcare. The more technology can contribute to the quality of that interface, the more valuable it will be.

D. BECKHAM (6)

IN THE EARLY 1900s, hospitals performed most of the limited laboratory healthcare testing for the community. By the late 1960s, the volume of laboratory testing increased drastically, and freestanding commercial laboratories emerged to capture much of the physician office and nursing home markets. As the commercial laboratory market matured, laboratories faced declining profits and needed to reinvest in new technology and automation. Local mom-and-pop laboratories became a prime target for acquisition by the larger national commercial laboratories. Their sophisticated, well-financed marketing and service strategies also put the local hospital laboratories at a competitive disadvantage. Physician loyalty to the local hospital laboratory was often undermined by the lure of profit received by marking up their patient's laboratory tests and then sending them out to be performed at low-cost reference laboratories. Before 1984 it was common practice for physicians to sell laboratory testing at retail prices to patients and third-party payors that they purchased from a reference laboratory at wholesale pricing.

The Tax Equity and Fiscal Responsibility Act enacted in 1982 mandated prospective reimbursement for inpatient services rendered to Medicare beneficiaries, subsequently implemented under diagnosis-related groups. The Deficit Reduction Act of 1984 authorized the Medicare clinical laboratory fee schedule and mandated that the laboratory performing the outpatient testing bill Medicare for the services directly, not the physician that ordered the testing. Hospitals were not equipped to measure or account for the decreased revenue. Shifting the Medicare costs to other payors was a temporary remedy. The first Medicare fee schedule, enacted in 1984, set national limitation amounts. National limitation amount payment caps became effective in 1986 and have been lowered repeatedly over the past decade, as demonstrated in Table 7.1.

The Clinical Laboratory Improvement Amendments of 1988 (CLIA '88) further impacted the environment. The costs associated with implementing CLIA performance standards and proficiency testing increased by 67% (40). Then in 1989, the Omnibus Reconciliation Act (OBRA) was passed; it included legislation that prevented physicians from creating "shell laboratories" that contracted out the majority of testing and marked the testing up for direct billing. Laboratories were required to perform at least 70% of all testing on-site to be able to bill for referred testing. The **Stark** legislation prohibited physicians with ownership in a laboratory from referring testing under self-referral legislation. The OBRA of 1993 enacted further reductions in the Medicare fee schedule ceiling amounts (40).

Today, laboratories continue to lobby for the passage of direct-billing legislation to mandate that the laboratory provider universally bill third-party payors for services. Many states have passed such legislation, and some insurers have adopted the ruling using a cost-plus formula based on the Medicare fee schedule. Table 7.2 provides a quick reference and a historical overview of legislation impacting clinical laboratories over the past half century.

The concept of prepaid medical service dates back to the early 1800s. The term managed care, as we know it, didn't gain national attention until coined by a Minnesota physician, Paul Ellwood. The origin of the first health maintenance organization (HMO) traces to the Rural Farmers Cooperative Health Plan in Elk City, Okla. The Ross-Loss Medical Group was founded as a tightly controlled group model on the West Coast as early as 1929. From 1942 to the present, Kaiser of California has been the dominating leader. Following endorsement by the federal government in the HMO Act of 1973, the growth of managed care has not been as rapid as originally predicted. The evolution of managed care has witnessed a change in structure from being nonprofit to for-profit organizations in order to expand access to capital markets. The infusion of federal and private funding and the heightened concern over inflation in healthcare were the early stimuli for growth. Today, the HMO concept has become firmly established and has become a significant segment of the healthcare industry. Future growth of managed care and the response by the stakeholders are dependent on the competitive environment, increased physician supply, and the constraints of the federal budget (43).

A diverse and aging population places increasing demands for long-term care for chronic illnesses in cost-reduced settings. The underinsured and uninsured populations have grown exponentially. In 2002, there were approximately 45 million U.S. citizens without healthcare coverage (50). Refer to Table 7.3.

National health expenditures were projected to reach 14% of the gross domestic product and healthcare spending was projected to increase to $2.8 trillion in 2001, up from $1.3 trillion in 2000 (50). Clinical laboratories account for 3.5% of the nation's total healthcare expenditures, representing $35 billion in revenues annually in 2001 (50) (see Table 7.4). The rising healthcare costs are predictive of the end of a managed-care era that focused on cutting reimbursement and services to achieve lower spending. After consumers experienced a draconian approach to utilization review and utilization management, they responded by increasing demands for less restricted access to providers. Cost containment has slowed, and managed care is returning to the principles of disease

Table 7.1 National limitation amounts

Year	Median payment cap (%)
1986	115
1988	100
1990	93
1991	88
1994	84
1995	80
1996	76
1998	74

"National limitation amounts became effective in 1986. Median payment caps for laboratory services continuously decreased from 1986 to the present. See D. Weissman, *Medicare Reimbursement and Policy Manual for Clinical Laboratory Services,* p. 315–318. (Washington G-2 Reports, Washington, D. C., 2002).

Table 7.2 Legislation and regulation impacting healthcare and clinical laboratories[a]

Year	Legislation title or name of agency	Main feature(s)
1965	Social Security Act	Authorized Medicare and Medicaid programs
1967	Clinical Laboratory Improvement Act	Government assumed licensing and regulatory authority over some clinical laboratories.
1970	Occupational Health and Safety Administration	Agency created to establish and enforce worker safety
1972	Social Security Amendments Office of the Inspector General 42 CFR § 1001.952	Added disability and end-stage renal disease coverage to Medicare program Antikickback Act first enacted Defined elements of safe harbors
1973	HMO Act	Required large employers to offer one federally qualified HMO as alternative to traditional indemnity Migration from FFS reimbursement to capitated payments
1976	Office of the Inspector General	Established to identify and eliminate fraud and abuse in DHHS programs
1977	HCFA	Administers the Medicare program; regulates laboratory testing on humans (except research testing)
1979	NCQA	A private not-for-profit organization that assesses and reports the quality of managed-care providers
1982	Tax Equity and Fiscal Responsibility Act	Mandated the prospective payment system for pathology services covered under Part A
1983		Clinical Laboratory Competitive Bidding Demonstration Project first proposed
1984	Deficit Reduction Act	Enacted direct billing requirement for clinical laboratory tests. Only laboratories that performed testing for Medicare beneficiaries could bill for these services. National laboratory fee schedule implemented
1985	Balanced Budget and Emergency Deficit Control Act	Known as Gramm Rudman Hollins; established limits on federal spending; placed cap on Medicare reduction at 2% per year
1986	OBRA	National limitation amounts established
1986	OBRA Public Law 99-509	Adjustments in prospective payment system and disproportionate share; direct billing for outpatient services
1987	OBRA Public Law 100-203	Physician mandate to accept assignment; $6 billion in Medicare reductions
1989	OBRA Public Law 101-239	Laboratory fee schedule reduced from 100 to 93% of national median payment cap; $2.7 billion in Medicare reductions; prohibited shell laboratories
1990	OBRA Public Law 101-508	Laboratory fee schedule reduced from 93 to 88% of national median payment cap; enacted the 3-day window (72-h rule) eliminating the ability to bill for certain outpatient services within 3 days of a hospital admission
1993	OBRA Public Law 103-606	Laboratory fee schedule reduced from 88 to 76% of national median payment cap
1988	CLIA '88	Established laboratory regulation based on testing complexity (waived, moderate, or high) and extended federal regulatory authority to all laboratories performing clinical laboratory testing for diagnosis and management of human disease
1989	Office of the Inspector General	Issued fraud alert for shell laboratories
1989	Stark I	The original Stark law ("Stark I"), enacted in 1989, prohibited only self-interested referrals for clinical laboratory services.
1990	Shell lab rule adopted	Laboratories billing Medicare for services may not bill for referral testing unless 70% of testing is performed in-house.
1991	Occupational Safety and Health Act	Added regulation on the manner in which laboratories handled and shipped infectious substances and biohazardous wastes
1992		Physician fee schedule moved to relative value units and fully implemented resource-based relative value system by 1996; CLIA '88 final regulations became effective
	HCFA, now the CMS	Established categories for certificate-of-waiver laboratories and provider-performed microscopy procedures
1993	Stark II	Congress broadened the Stark law to include physician self-referrals to an expanded set of "designated health services."
1996	HIPAA Public Law 104-191	Preexisting conditions; established medical savings account; protection of personal health information; mandated administrative simplification for health-care transactions
1997	Office of the Inspector General	Model Compliance Plan for Clinical Laboratories

(continued)

Table 7.2 Legislation and regulation impacting healthcare and clinical laboratories[a] *(continued)*

Year	Legislation title or name of agency	Main feature(s)
1997	Balanced Budget Act	Established Medicare + choice (Medicare Part C); negotiated rule making and national coverage decisions became effective
	Public Law 105-33	Changed reimbursement for skilled nursing beds from prospective payment to consolidated billing and resource utilization groups
	42 USC § 1395 y (a) (1) (A)	Mandated that physicians provide diagnostic information when ordering laboratory tests to be billed by a clinical laboratory; created provisions for Medicare reimbursements for only reasonable and necessary services; administrative simplification required CMS to establish five regional carriers.
1999	Office of the Inspector General Special Advisory Bulletin 42 USC § 1320 a-7a (b)	Gain sharing provisions prohibit hospitals from making payments to physicians as an inducement for patient referrals.
2000	Proposed Balanced Budget Act implementation	346 ambulatory payment classifications
	Benefits Improvement and Protection Act of 2000	42 CFR 410, 411, 414 Pathology Technical Component; proposed coverage for annual pap smear and pelvic exam, colonoscopy, and mammography
2001	Public Law 106-430 Needlestick Safety and Prevention Act	OSHA revised the blood-borne pathogen standard January 2001 to include enforcement procedures and exposure control plans for occupational exposure.
2002	Medicare Policy	Hospital laboratories performing outreach must determine Medicare secondary-payor status every 60 days; two standard advance beneficiary notice forms approved
	Other pending legislation in the 108th Congress:	
	HR 1798 / S 1066	Medicare patient access to testing: methodology for laboratory fee to be revised
	HR 1948	Medical laboratory personnel shortage act
	HR 1201 / S 258	Add Medicare coverage for annual pelvic exam and pap smear to save women's lives.
	HR 1451 / S 730	Physician Pathology Services Fair Treatment Act: grandfather provision for technical component
	HR 3388	Specimen collection fee increased from $3.00 to $5.25
	HR 602 / S 318	Genetic nondiscrimination

[a]HCFA, Health Care Financing Administration; CMS, Centers for Medicare and Medicaid Services.

Table 7.3 Decline of health coverage[a]

Year	Health coverage
1999	17.5% of Americans under age 65 were uninsured; 42.6 million Americans uninsured
2000	39 million Americans uninsured for an entire year
2002	45 million estimated to have no coverage by year's end
2001–2003	86 million estimated to suffer a gap in coverage

[a]From Miller (48a); see also reference 50.

Table 7.4 Percentage of clinical laboratory industry market revenues by segment[a]

Segment	% of market revenue in year			
	1995	1998	2001	% Increase
Hospital laboratories	34	41	62	21
Independent commercial labs	42	36	27	−9
Physician office laboratories	24	23	11	−12

[a]In 2001, the clinical laboratory industry was worth $35 billion. Figures for 1995 and 1998 are from the Centers for Medicare and Medicaid Services Office of the Actuary. According to the SMG Marketing Group, the number of hospitals in integrated networks was 2,060 in 1995, 2,819 in 1998, and >3,100 in 2001, for a 6-year difference of about 1,000. See reference 58.

management for chronic patients to improve outcomes and lower costs (50).

Changing Reimbursement Models

Change from Traditional Indemnity to Managed-Care Insurance

Traditional indemnity insurance pays claims for beneficiaries to healthcare providers (hospital inpatient, outpatient, and provider service claims) on a fee-for-service (FFS) basis. There is little or no control over quality, appropriateness of care, or cost of the services. The goal of managed-care insurance is to keep members healthy by integrating the selected provider arrangements with quality improvement and utilization review using financial incentives to control cost and utilization. Table 7.5 is a comparative summary between traditional indemnity and managed-care insurance.

Managed care, by definition, seeks to enhance value to its customers by lowering overall costs while maintaining or improving the quality of care. Managed-care organizations (MCOs) are under pressure to control cost in uncon-

Table 7.5 Comparison of traditional indemnity and managed-care insurance (27)

Traditional indemnity	Managed care
Patients have few restrictions on choice of providers.	Sets explicit standards for provider participation and restricts patient access to provider's within the network
Reimbursement is FFS based on units of service or may be fee schedule at a percentage of charges.	Pays on contract negotiated rates Per member per month Per diem Contractor's fee schedule
Finance and service delivery function independently of one another.	Integrates finance and access to delivery systems
Role of insurer is limited to paying claim for clinical services.	Role of insurer expanded to provide healthcare management
Plan assumes all financial risk	Shares financial risk with providers
Few incentives to control costs	Offers incentives to control costs
Plan does not measure quality or appropriateness of services.	Participates actively in quality assurance measurements and utilization control

ventional ways. Tools used to achieve their financial goals are as follows:

- Negotiate preferred prices for service (hospital per diems, fees, case rates).

- Limit services rendered to only those that are medically necessary by requiring referrals, preauthorization for inpatient admissions, precertification for costly procedures, adherence to practice guidelines, and active case management.

- Ensure that the services provided are the most cost-effective (least expensive but medically useful alternative).

- Direct patients to an urgent-care setting versus emergency room visits, outpatient surgery center versus hospital inpatient facility, and home care and rehabilitation services versus acute care.

- Provide financial incentives to providers.

- Perform proactive medical management for patient care.

A provision of the HMO Act of 1973 required that federally qualified HMOs charge enrollees an across-the-board community-based rate rather than employer-specific rates that were reflective of the lower utilization in HMOs by the younger healthier patients who typically enrolled in the plan. Both insurers and employers generally perceive federal qualification as a sign of quality. HMOs (as defined under Subpart A 110.102 of the federal HMO regulations) must offer access to certain basic health services, including diagnostic and therapeutic services; inpatient hospital services; short-term rehabilitation; emergency care; short-term outpatient mental health, drug abuse, and addiction services; diagnostic laboratory, radiological, and home health services; and preventative health, such as prescription services, dental care, and vision care (43). Community-based rating creates a global approach to health problems and forces weaker facilities to close. Some argue that community-based rating impeded the HMOs' ability to increase their market share. Using experience rating creates a competitive environment that makes it difficult for small businesses to compete against the stronger players (5).

Four Stages of Managed-Care Market Development

Managed-care markets evolve slowly over time. Purchasers and providers differ in their development stages and the degree of managed-care sophistication according to the actual managed-care market penetration.

Stage 1. During the first stage of managed care, the market is generally an unstructured, traditional environment.

- Purchaser groups (or employers) offer mostly standard indemnity products.

- MCOs that exist are typically preferred provider organizations.

- Maintain satisfied employees with freedom of choice.

- Limited sales to small business

- Low market penetration: 0 to 10% of true managed care

Stage 2. As the market begins to coalesce, HMOs gain endorsements and some consumer acceptance.

- Physicians form loose independent physician associations networks.

- Hospitals develop informal linkage to physicians through physician hospital organizations (PHOs).

- Employers offer little incentive for employees to switch to managed-care plans.

- Increased sales to small business

- Managed-care market penetration is between 10 and 20%.

Stage 3. As the market begins to consolidate, HMOs gain momentum.

- Two or three HMOs dominate the market.

- Managed-care market penetration approaches 20 to 30%.

- Health plans become more sophisticated in tracking and reporting data.

- Group purchasers and employers, concerned over escalating costs per covered life, offer incentives for employees to enroll in managed-care plans.
- PHOs become more formal and sophisticated at credentialing.
- Small business becomes a target segment.

Stage 4. As the market stabilizes and matures, rivalry among HMOs and healthcare providers becomes hypercompetitive.

- Managed-care market penetration is over 30%.
- Purchaser groups and employers become more interested in outcomes for their population.
- PHOs become aggressive and accept full capitated risks.
- Small business becomes a competitive target segment.
- Two or three MCOs dominate the market (13).

Types of MCOs. In order to meet the demands of the stakeholders for geographic service coverage, the large- and small-employer demands for choice, and patient demands for access, MCOs have used several provider network models and healthcare plan options to attract a larger market share. (Refer to Table 7.6.)

Key elements of managed-care contract negotiation. All providers of services within a network must be held accountable for knowing the associated costs to perform the services, to evaluate the risks of capitated payments, and to monitor utilization to maximize efficiencies. You can't manage what you can't measure. Across the continuum of care, providers must accurately forecast revenues against expenses.

- *Price.* Although a major influence in the contract decision, price is not the only determining factor. Other factors that influence the contract award follow.
- *Scope of services.* Providers must be able to provide the scope of services and procedures that meet the needs of the insured population. Demonstrating the capacity to perform and having the necessary infrastructure also influence the contract decision.
- *Service.* Providers must demonstrate a commitment to flexible service strategies.
- *Convenient access.* Providing convenient patient access to services for laboratory, radiology, pharmacy, providers, and procedures drives consumer satisfaction.
- *Geographic coverage.* Healthcare providers should have an established network of physicians, outpatient service centers, and couriers to meet the demands of a defined service area.

Table 7.6 Types of MCOs and services

Acronym	Type of MCO	Definition
ASO	Administrative services only	An insurance carrier or independent organization that handles the administration of claims and benefits for a fee for self-insured group
EPO	Exclusive provider organization	A network contracted with directly by a payor, usually a self-insured employer or third-party administrator
HMO	Health maintenance organization	An MCO that contracts with employers and providers to provide comprehensive health coverage to enrollees
	Group model	The HMO contracts with physician practice groups to provide services. Referred to as a "closed panel," as enrollees are limited to group providers only.
	Network model	The HMO contracts with one or more medical groups for services.
	Staff model	The HMO contracts with a health system's medical staff for services. Providers may be employees of the MCO. Referred to as a "closed panel," as enrollees are limited to staff providers only.
IPA	Independent physician organization	A provider organization that contracts with physicians to provide services to a plan's members at a negotiated cap rate or FFS
ISN	Integrated service network	Specialty networks have developed to provide coverage for a geographic area for care specific to their specialty (e.g., mental health services).
LSO	Laboratory service organization	A laboratory management group that administers contracts for a group of laboratories
MSO	Management service organization	An organization that administers organizational and practice management for physician providers
PHO	Physician hospital organization	An organization acting as a joint venture between a hospital and its medical staff to gain bargaining power with HMOs and PPOs, or directly with EPOs
PPO	Preferred provider organization	An MCO which provides enrollees with freedom of choice. A selective contracting agreement with a specific network of hospital and physician providers at reduced or negotiated rates. Enrollees have financial incentives to use PPO providers in the network.
POS	Point-of-service plan	A managed-care plan that combines the features of prospective prepayment and FFS insurance payments. The enrollees can elect to use the network or opt out of the network, with a sizable copayment as a disincentive.

- *Quality.* Providers must be able to demonstrate quality and consumer satisfaction using surveys, report cards, and utilization management based on developed clinical pathways.

- *Financial stability.* Providers must be able to assess their exposure to risk and sell the MCO on their financial and operational abilities and stability to accept and deliver in such contracts.

- *Informatics.* The enterprise must be able to generate and analyze data in a format that meets the MCO's needs for utilization information required for Health-plan Employer Data and Information Set (HEDIS) reporting by their accrediting agency, the National Committee on Quality Assurance (NCQA).

Reimbursement Strategies in a Managed-Care Market

Payment strategies and associated risk. Managed-care products have become a dominating force in the health-care market over traditional indemnity insurance. As MCOs continue to negotiate contracts that are heavily risk based, the providers are put at increased risk for cost and utilization control. In a risk contract, the payment received is not tied to actual utilization or costs of services. Risk-sharing arrangements should be carefully negotiated and should include safety net and stop-loss provisions.

- Safety net provisions limit the amount of risk assumed. Provisions should include the following:
  - Aggregate payments will be no less than the equivalent discounted FFS payment.
  - Aggregate payments would be subject to a percentage increase when utilization targets are exceeded.
  - Set established thresholds that allow for discounted FFS when thresholds are exceeded for specific services, like extended inpatient stays, costly tests, and costly implants.
- Stop-loss limits are provisions typically used in PHO models where gatekeepers and institutions are at risk for exposure to high-cost procedures (i.e., transplants). The stop-loss limits are defined as dollars per covered member per month or year (14).

Managed-care reimbursement models with low risk. The following are managed-care reimbursement models with low risk:

FFS. The reimbursement method based on payment according to a fee schedule (often as blended fees or MCO's internal fees) for services rendered. It is critical that the fee schedule being used be identified, including geographic and annual adjustments. The Medicare fee or the resource-based relative value system schedule is often used as a reference point in negotiations.

Discounted FFS. The provider agrees to accept a FFS payment that is a percentage of the usual, customary, and reasonable fee schedule.

Cost plus. A method of rating often used to determine a reimbursement rate based on the cost experience plus an administrative markup.

Per diem. The negotiated daily payment rate for delivery of all inpatient hospital services provided regardless of the actual services rendered. These rates are often specific to the type of care for general medical, surgical, and intensive care.

Carve outs. Services and procedures that are defined by contract to be separate and apart from the negotiated capitation rate and that are typically paid on a FFS basis.

Managed-care payment methods with moderate associated financial risk. Capitation is an agreement in which a provider is paid a predetermined amount per member per month in exchange for providing services included in the rate. The rates are typically adjusted by age and sex and are adjusted according to population groups: commercial, industrial, prison, and Medicare. Rates should all differ based on actuarial data. Enrollment guarantees assure the provider that until the targeted membership rates are reached the provider will receive FFS payments. Capitated payments are made prospectively to the provider at the beginning of the month for the total members prior to any utilization or actual services rendered. Adjustments are made the following month based on change in membership. Since the costs for the services rendered may exceed the capitation payment, the provider is at risk.

- To calculate per member per month capitation rate:

$$\frac{\text{Total revenue or expense or utilization units for the period}}{\text{Number of member months for same period}} = \frac{\text{per member}}{\text{per month rate}}$$

- To calculate member months in a given period of time:

(Average number of members for each month in a given period) × (Number of months in period:) = Member months for period

Percentage of premium. An arrangement in which the provider is paid a percentage of the premium billed or collected by the MCO for the services rendered and covered by the rate. Assessing the number of patients, the population type, and the actuarial data is vital. Include a payment minimum in the negotiation.

Fixed rate. Reimbursement agreements that cover all services and costs associated with a specific diagnosis or a procedure. Knowledge of the case mix, average cost per case, and procedures included in the rate is necessary to negotiate the contract rate. The contract defines the payment process based on receipt of a claim (15).

Performance-based risk for service.

Withholds. A payment method that withholds a percentage of a negotiated payment in a reserve fund for specialty provider contracts. Periodically, if negotiated quality and cost criteria have been met, the portion of the fee that was withheld is returned according to the risk-bearing terms of the contract.

HMO reimbursement models with high risk.

Contract capitation is based on experience. There are three types of payments:

- Capitation is paid based on qualifying member types rather than on a random patient population. The provider is at risk only for the costs associated with a referral and not for the number of referrals.
- Global fees are paid for an entire episode of care.
- Monthly fees for a period of time and a specific condition.

Combined health system capitation (hospital and physician)

- Global capitation (caregivers, hospital, ancillary)

Case rate. Per case also bears risk, as the costs of services could exceed the payment per case.

Shared-risk funds. Physician groups, pharmacies, and hospitals share the financial risks and potential profits.

Noncovered services. Services that are not covered need to be identified during contract negotiation, in order to establish the method for billing and payment. In the managed-care environment, patients cannot be billed for services unless defined by the policy. Having the patient sign a waiver of liability prior to services ensures that the patient agrees to accept financial responsibility for the noncovered service.

Laboratory service contract strategies. There are five basic strategies adapted by HMOs. The selected strategy typically generates the most cost savings for the MCO. The five strategies include the following:

- Statewide or regional capitation contracts with a national commercial laboratory
- Inclusion of laboratory services within a global capitation rate (that includes all medical services) and paid to a health system composed of hospitals and physicians
- Inclusion of laboratory services within a physician group capitation

- Capitation paid to a local clinical laboratory, a subcontractor to a national laboratory, or a network of local or regional laboratory providers
- FFS payments based on the HMO's set fee schedule

The advantages of negotiating a statewide contract with an exclusive laboratory provider are compelling.

- The strategy shifts the risk to the national laboratory.
- The data needed for HEDIS reporting and financial analysis reside in a single vendor database.
- The national laboratory promotes consistent quality and correlation of results across the service area.
- National laboratories negotiate on volume, and larger HMOs usually negotiate a lower cap rate.
- Contract administration using a single vendor is more efficient, minimizing claim processing, medical management and customer service issues.

A hospital laboratory that serves as a managed-care contractor or subcontractor for laboratory services should be cautious. Critical knowledge needed to negotiate the contract includes laboratory costs, laboratory utilization patterns, and patient volumes (53). The commodity pricing of healthcare services results in regional competition, volume discount, and intense competition that forces physician groups, hospitals, clinical laboratories, and other healthcare providers to evaluate their ability to compete (73). Managed-care legislation has had a profound impact on the insurance industry. The companies' ability to survive is usually linked to the following:

- Size of the firm and its market share
- Types of product lines and delivery systems offered
- Ability to offer other service lines (workman's compensation and disability)
- Strength of the customer base
- Financial stability in the market

Healthcare Stakeholders in a Managed-Care Market

Plan members. Each patient, beneficiary, or enrollee covered by a managed-care health plan is called a member. The healthcare plan counts them as covered lives. The health plan identifies the enrollees to the providers as the subscriber, or the insured. When the subscriber's policy covers other family members, they are identified as dependents. Both the subscriber and the dependents are considered members. A statement of coverage is issued to the insured under a group contract that outlines the benefits and principal provisions and is called a certificate of insurance or evidence of coverage statement.

Purchasers. Healthcare purchasers include large self-insured employers, coalitions of small employers, associations of trade or professional groups, integrated networks, physician groups, hospital systems, or individuals.

Employers. Escalating costs and changes in healthcare delivery have forced employers to examine their benefit package and role in providing comprehensive healthcare benefits. Employers purchase healthcare for their employees for three reasons: as a form of compensation, to enhance their health status, and to keep them productive at work. Employers (who are classified as large employers under the HMO Act) that offer healthcare coverage are mandated to offer a managed-care plan as an option to traditional indemnity insurance to their employees. Group employers' demands for a wide range of product offering are increasingly more sophisticated.

Providers. Hospitals and physicians have had to change the way they traditionally delivered healthcare in response to the market changes driven by managed-care penetration.

Community organizations or federally qualified healthcare centers. Rural healthcare providers are challenged by the same forces as urban healthcare providers, but they continue to rely heavily on government programs to provide geographic coverage with a shortage of physicians.

Government-sponsored plans. Medicare, Medicaid, Federal Employees Health Benefits Plan, United States Postal Service Employees and Retirees, Department of Defense, Department of Veterans Affairs, Indian Health Services, Department of Justice.

Insurers. Commercial carriers, Medicare contractors, third-party insurance carriers, and third-party administrators who market their indemnity and managed-care products to government, group purchasers, employers, and individuals.

Cost sharing. Patients are generally responsible for paying some portion of their healthcare costs. Cost sharing is a strategy used by MCOs and large employer groups to control utilization of services by the enrollees. Frequency of services accessed is generally inversely proportional to the cost-sharing rate strategy. In a low cost-sharing plan there is generally no deductible and a flat copayment is required for physician and outpatient services. Plans with high cost-sharing strategies have deductibles and copayments similar to those of traditional indemnity insurance products. Point-of-service plans use a combination of the two risks. Low cost sharing applies if the enrollee uses network providers, and high cost sharing applies with a percentage coinsurance when the enrollee goes out of the network (16).

The various types of payments for the patient's financial responsibility are described below (65):

- *Deductible.* A payment defined by the policy that is a percentage of the allowed charges for a procedure or service that must be paid by the member before the insurer will assume liability for the balance. The deductible often varies by contract and group.

- *Copayment.* A specified dollar amount for the medical service that is defined by the policy coverage and is made by the member prior to receiving services.

- *Coinsurance.* In the indemnity market, when a member is covered by a secondary insurance policy, the secondary payor is a coinsurer. To avoid false claim charges, multiple claims for the same service should not be filed with both the primary and secondary insurer (the coinsurer) until denial is received from the subscriber's primary coverage. In the managed-care market, coinsurance is a percentage of the cost of covered services paid by the patient. The coinsurance is calculated after any copayment or deductible is applied. The cost-sharing ratio varies by contract and group.

Another method used by employers to regain control over their healthcare costs is offering a defined contribution plan or medical savings account that shifts control of the healthcare dollars. This forces the employees as subscribers to make decisions about how they spend their healthcare dollars.

Insurance premium pricing cycle. Traditional indemnity and managed-care insurance premiums drive the profits for the companies. If the premiums are too low, even the best healthcare plans will fall short on profits. On the other hand, a plan that has high premiums is not guaranteed profits. The pricing cycle begins when a plan wants to expand its market share and lowers its premiums. Competitive plans respond by matching the premium to maintain market share and position. A premium price war similar to those in petroleum products and airfares ensues. Plans may move toward multiyear contracting. The terms of the multiyear contract make it extremely difficult to solve the problem even when it is apparent. Finally, when the marketplace in general is recording significant losses, an insurer decides to change its pricing strategy, raising the premium, and the competitive players follow the leader. The increases in premium continue until all the insurers are generating profits, and then the cycle starts over again. Additional information can be found in the fact sheets located at Managed Care On Line's website (http://www.MCOL.com [last accessed January 2004]).

Changing Emphasis on Quality

HMO Network Management

NCQA. The government, public health agencies, employers, patients, and purchasers of healthcare coverage and services demand efficiency and demonstrated quality. To that end, MCOs seek accreditation from NCQA, established in 1979. NCQA is a nationally recognized accreditation agency that includes rigorous evaluation of the health plan and the management of the delivery network. Stakeholders use NCQA accreditation as a means to assess managed-care

Table 7.7 HEDIS performance criteria developed by the NCQA for rating MCOs

Effectiveness of care

    Immunizations (child, adolescent, adult)

    Breast and cervical cancer screenings

    Prenatal care (postdelivery care)

    Heart attack treatment

    Eye care for diabetics

    Plan for smokers

    Mental illness follow-up

    Laboratory data reporting: glucose and glycohemoglobin (HgbA1C), cholesterol testing, and pap smears

Access and availability of care

Patient satisfaction

Costs of care

Stability of the health plan

Informed choice for patient healthcare

Utilization of services

Health plan descriptive information

plans. There are 50 standards considered in the NCQA process that evaluate quality improvement, physician credentialing, members' rights and responsibilities, preventative health, utilization management, and medical records.

HEDIS is a set of standard performance measures used to compare the quality of health plans. HEDIS, first published in 1991, requires MCOs to measure and report performance to allow competing plans to be rated on a standard set of criteria. Refer to Table 7.7. NCQA utilizes the accreditation and HEDIS reporting requirement to publish report cards on managed-care health plans (27).

Quality management. Quality management or quality assurance policies ensure that members have access to health services based on established standards of care in the community. Structured care methodologies are tools used to identify best practices, facilitate standardization, and provide a mechanism for variance tracking, outcome measurement, and outcome management. The structured care methodology tools include standards of practice, guidelines, protocols, algorithms, and clinical pathways.

- Standards of practice provide a baseline for the quality of care delivered to the patient and relate care to the operational process.

- Guidelines are systematic statements prepared by professional groups to assist practitioners and patients in making specific clinical decisions about care.

- Protocols are formal guidelines that detail specific clinical therapeutic intervention for health problems within a defined population.

- Algorithms are binary decision trees that combine patient response to intervention with other information to guide stepwise treatment of a specific condition.

- Clinical pathways are written criteria to guide care based on standards of practice by delineating necessary treatment and facilitating appropriate use of resources.

These methods provide an interdisciplinary focus to identify the expected outcomes, the processes for resource management, or the methods that lead to improved quality and cost-effectiveness. Use of the tools should never preclude clinical judgment (19).

Utilization management processes monitor the frequency and utilization of healthcare services to ensure that the care received is efficient and cost-effective, is administered at the correct level, and does not use unnecessary services. Table 7.8 outlines some of the quality management processes used by MCOs.

Table 7.8 Quality management tools used by MCOs

Tool	Management target	Purpose or focus
Quality assurance	Profiling encounter data and claims Chart audits Surveys	Data analysis Health plan, providers, facilities Providers and members for incident reporting and problem resolution
Utilization management	Preauthorization, precertification	Providers must seek approval prior to performing certain procedures or admission.
	Concurrent review Case profiling	Review cases concurrent with ongoing care Analysis of cases as they occur
Outcomes	Record end result	By provider By procedure By clinical guidelines
Demand	Member services	Requests for clinical information Access to MCO triage by nursing Request for patient education resources
Disease (case and outcomes management)	Specific diseases	Claim analysis by procedure Patient and provider education Coordination of care across continuum (hospital, pharmacy, lab, physician)

Medical management. Medical management is the use of organized medical care systems and a routine, preventative care approach to help subscribers avoid health problems rather than treating them after they occur. Plan members select a participating primary-care physician (PCP) or gatekeeper who oversees and approves the medical services for the patient. When a patient requires more technical or specialized treatment, the PCP issues a referral that recommends to the HMO that the patient see another participating HMO provider or specialist for services. Before certain, expensive outpatient procedures are performed, the provider must seek preauthorization (a preservice review) from the health plan to ensure that the services meet the criteria for medical necessity, thereby ensuring that payment will be received for the service provided. If the member needs to be admitted, the health plan may require a preadmission review or precertification to ensure that the service meets criteria for medical necessity and that the services are performed in the most cost-effective setting (66).

Medical management cost control. Medical directors at MCOs evaluate several parameters to help ensure quality: cost, resource utilization, provider profiling, practice guidelines, and outcome studies. Clinical practice guidelines may assist healthcare providers in preventing, diagnosing, and treating medical conditions.

Patient Management

Outcomes. An outcome is defined as a measured change or event that affects the status of a patient during a defined period of time (for example, death, the onset of symptoms, the disappearance of symptoms, discharge, readmission, complications, or diagnosis). "Our reimbursement system focuses on the 'right price' and on volume... We need a system that rewards providers with good outcomes and those that implement safety systems," according to Margaret Amringe of the Joint Commission on Accreditation of Healthcare Organizations.

Outcome research. Outcome research is a formal study into relationships between treatment and effects. It measures the impact of medical management in terms of patient well-being or financial performance. This research in the clinical laboratory requires a systematic collection of data that is best accomplished in conjunction with a broader health service research effort that includes a multidisciplinary team of laboratorians, clinicians, administrators, and statisticians (71).

In the laboratory, test efficacy is measured based on whether a patient's management is influenced by the test result. Test effectiveness is a measure of whether it changes the patient's outcome. The prevalence of disease is affected by the demographics of the patient population (age, socioeconomic status, ethnic background), which in turn influence the predictive value of a given test in a particular population.

$$\text{PV}(+) = \frac{P \times \text{sensitivity}}{[P \times \text{sensitivity} + (1 - P) \times (1 - \text{specificity})]}$$

where PV ($+$) is predictive value of a positive test ($+$), P is the prevalence of disease in the studied population, sensitivity is positivity in disease, and specificity is negativity in health.

The predictive value of the test influences the outcome analysis of cost/benefit ratio. The predictive value of a test performed in the community PCP office varies from the predictive value of the same test performed in an academic tertiary-care medical center, where the patients tend to be at higher risk for disease (71).

The purpose of routine laboratory testing should be not simply to detect abnormalities but also to improve health through diagnosis and treatment of detected conditions. Case finding is an important tool in preventative medicine that screens asymptomatic patients for disease. Screening for possible disease is as much a part of an annual checkup as taking a medical history or giving a physical exam. Outcome research combines studying the actual practice, with the medical exam, and the medical record to uncover the factors (such as the patient's health, demographics, time of last exam, professional experience, gender, reasons for ordering tests, and test expectations) that influence the healthcare provider or the patient during an office visit. The research provides a look at test effectiveness, not just efficacy. The value of a laboratory test is measured by whether it changes the likelihood of disease in conjunction with the clinician's estimate of the probability of disease (M. Silverstein, quoted in reference 49).

In addition to using database repositories, new technology referred to as data mining shows promise for obtaining new knowledge in future research. Outcome research seeks to quantify both the benefits and the costs associated with introducing new technology. Economic pressures to decrease costs of healthcare will impede the introduction of new technology, unless it can be justified by demonstrating improved patient outcomes or financial performance. Laboratory managers will become stewards of both human and capital resources in the future (71).

Outcome management. Outcome management is a proactive concept closely aligned with utilization management and continuous quality improvement. Outcome management applies theory, philosophy, and continuous quality improvement tools to a healthcare treatment or procedure to measure or determine the effectiveness of the treatment or procedure being evaluated. Using multidisciplinary teams, outcome management studies are performed on a specific patient population. The analysis includes both concurrent and aggregate data about specific processes rather than the entire project. The team should have a physician member to champion effective clinical leadership in implementing the finding. Teams must collectively analyze the process, identify the best practice, streamline the process by eliminating variations in practices from provider to provider, and finally educate the physicians, staff, and patients using outside sources as benchmarks. The clinical maps, protocols, guidelines, and algorithms developed by these teams are referred to as multidisciplinary care plans. Focusing on the high cost, high volume, or high-risk populations will yield a bigger impact on future outcomes. The results of the data analysis will be effective only if the data collected can be substantiated and are credible for use in comparative assessments at a later time (67).

Disease Management

Disease management emerged as an MCO management tool in the 1990s with the premise that it would help prevent or better manage disease, reducing the need for expensive medical treatment and hospitalization and ultimately decreasing costs and improving outcomes. When the evaluation process involves the healthcare system or a chronic-disease process, the review is called disease management. Indicators used in this evaluation include length of stay (LOS), turnaround time (TAT), and financial outcomes. Decision support software with algorithms using statistical data are used to identify patients who are at risk for developing severe illness and are more likely to require hospitalization. The ability to rank patients by risk allows the MCO to use case management more efficiently and at the level of care required by the patient. The ability to capture laboratory data electronically and to integrate it with the other data elements enables the health plan to expand the data set used for assigning patient risk and performing gap analysis related to the patient's care. Some of the newest decision support software packages with advanced logic engines combine expert rules with artificial intelligence tools like neural networks that integrate data variables not generally used in traditional clinical models (61). In the past, obtaining provider buy-in has been difficult, as the physician is typically critical of cookbook medicine

and its underlying motives of reduced costs at the expense of quality care. Communication strategies must clearly demonstrate to providers that by individualizing a patient's care plan, the patient's outcome significantly improves. Physician profiling, which compares the individual physician to a group of physicians, helps provider acceptance and stimulates peer pressure.

According to Hewitt Associates, a human resource consulting firm, employers and payors are increasingly using disease management programs. The program growth has doubled since 1997 to 19% in 2002. Hewitt anticipated that employers using disease management programs may have reached ≥30% by 2004. Robert Michel predicts that disease management will drive the next generation of managed care, by focusing on prevention and early detection, and will represent a significant opportunity for clinical laboratories. The ability to provide guidance to physicians and their patients positions the laboratory as a contributing partner in the healthcare continuum (46).

The Educated Consumer

Baby Boomers and Generation Xers: the Educated and Savvy Consumer

The new focus of healthcare will be on the five generations of consumers from the last century. Each generation has distinctively different ethics, values, beliefs, and needs (see Table 7.9). The GI Generation refers to the more than 60 million people born between 1901 and 1924. Known as the can-do generation, they literally lived the American Dream of baseball, hot dogs, apple pie, and Chevrolets. The Silent Generation spanned the years from 1925 to 1942. This generation is full of affluent consumers who are loyal traditionalists that created bureaucracy to maintain control of the world around them. Members of this generation adhere to one basic principle: that if you work hard, you will get ahead. At the same time, they are relatively inflexible and resist change. Then came the Baby Boomers, who represent 76 million births between 1943 and 1960. Baby boomers were flower children, draft dodgers, hippies, and yuppies that benefited from the economic revolution. Also known for regeneration, they have redesigned, redeveloped, reinvented, and reengineered their world. On

Table 7.9 Evolution of the educated consumer[a]

Nickname	Span of years	Description
GI Generation	1901–1924	The "can-do" generation who lived the American Dream
Silent Generation	1925–1942	Affluent and loyal traditionalists with belief that working hard equaled success
Baby Boomers	1943–1960	Flower children, draft dodgers, hippies, and yuppies who redesigned, redeveloped, reinvented, and reengineered the world
Generation Xers	1961–1981	Composed of latchkey, couch potato, and boomerang kids who are extremely savvy with technology but don't read
Millennial Generation	1982–2003	A "get-it-done" generation of achievers who value time and conform with rules

[a]See reference 37.

the one hand, they overindulge in self-gratification; on the other hand, they are type A idealists who are extremely passionate about being successful. Generation Xers are the 44 million people born between 1961 and 1981 who have witnessed everything from human immunodeficiency virus (HIV) to the fall of the Berlin Wall. Known as latchkey kids, couch potatoes, and now as boomerang kids, this generation has a strong need for information and feedback, is typically savvy with both electronics and computers, and generally speaking doesn't like to read. The Millennial Generation, born between 1982 and 2003, represents the newest healthcare consumers just entering the workplace. Generally values, ethics, and needs repeat every fourth generation, so the Millennials should be successful achievers who conform to the rules of society and who will aspire to live the American Dream. They are technologically savvy individuals who dislike wasting time. Like the GIs in the early 1900s, they will be another get-it-done generation (37).

The Increasingly Litigious Environment

In the new millennium, the relationship between the patient and the provider will continue to change. Data, not emotions, will drive the decision-making process. Patients will elect to change providers more frequently during open enrollment. Since the role of litigation is inversely linked to length of relationships, the industry can expect to see an increase in litigation claims. As the population ages, patients' expectations about their rights and access to care will also increase. Patient demand for participation in the decision-making process will increase the need for accuracy and clarity in communications. John Wennberg and his colleagues at Dartmouth developed a new process decades ago known as informed choice, which encouraged patients and their physicians to review all treatment regimens available and then link them to the patients' objectives for treatment. More and more patients may opt for nontraditional, alternative medicine treatments when they become covered services (35).

Changing Technology

Following the onset of managed care, inpatient days decreased as a result of new technology and alternative treatment settings, ultimately reducing routine and inpatient laboratory testing volume. Now, the laboratory's role is expanding to promote prevention. Genetic testing, point-of-care testing (POCT), home testing, and direct public access to preventative testing and screening are increasing (18).

Technological Advances

Fast-occurring changes in microelectronics, chemistry, genomics, imaging software, and miniaturization are converging, integrating, and redefining the landscape of diagnostic testing. The changes include advances in the disciplines of molecular biology and functional genomics, the evolution of technology with high throughput, the escalating costs of healthcare, and the increasing demands of the educated consumer. Information is no longer just a tool but a primary asset used to improve patient management and prevent disease (25).

The information superhighway and the virtualization of healthcare. The funding for the research and development of an experimental, secure data network, now known as the Internet or the World Wide Web, was originally budgeted by the Department of Defense. During the past decade, the Internet has evolved into a powerful new social institution, reaching more than 50 million users in only 5 years. That is roughly one-eighth the time for radio and less than one-half the time for television to reach the same number of consumers. In 1998, consumers spent $8 billion dollars on-line out of roughly $2 trillion in total consumer expenditures (Table 7.10). Although healthcare has not yet totally embraced and adopted it, the Internet is expected to accelerate the development of virtual healthcare. Proponents of the Internet believe that cost savings will ultimately be achieved by eliminating the middlemen, reducing clerical and redundant processes, and decreasing medical errors in the midst of an increased consumer demand. Insurers anticipate cost avoidance through effective disease management supported by Internet-based applications (23). Additional information can be found at the website of Health Futures, Inc. (http://www.healthfutures.net [last accessed Janurary 2004]).

POCT. Microelectronics, microfabrication, and microcomputerization have revolutionized the way that laboratory tests are performed. These technologies allow test results to be obtained in a matter of minutes or even seconds. POCT or near-patient testing has long been touted as the technology that would change patient management in the world of managed care. The most obvious benefit of POCT is decreased TAT. The premise that near-patient testing would radically change patient management in a managed-care environment has not been substantiated (25). Bickford's research concluded that POCT had no significant impact on hospital LOS (76). Receiving rapid results reflects patient status at a given time and improves pharmacological management. However, for physicians to act, they must still wait for a complete manifest of results. As new technologies for POCT evolve, laboratory medicine professionals will continue to question the accuracy and reliability of the instruments and the results. Table 7.11 includes a list of advantages and disadvantages of POCT. Research and development must carefully evaluate instrument limitations, especially for the critical-care setting (43).

Meanwhile, cost minimalization strategies push testing back to the clinical laboratory, where cost-effective testing

Table 7.10 Internet stakeholders: barriers and benefits to healthcare

Stakeholders	Stakeholder barrier(s)	Internet benefits
Physicians	Are skeptical and reluctant to adopt with limitation on time Resent patients with more e-knowledge	Access to consultation is easier. Reduces time spent on phone Access to pharmacy and drug information Online patient access to provider network directory
Administration	Lacks motivation to use and are skeptical	Reduces human resource time Reduces need for clerical support Improves productivity Facilitates needs for outsourcing
Consumers	More aggressive at embracing technology	Consumers seek health information online. Patients are able to discuss conditions more knowledgeably with physician. Consumers seek patient advocates online.
Healthcare institutions	Need system with standardized coding and formats for clinical information Address extensive requirements to protect privacy under HIPAA Security and encryption	Online appointment scheduling and insurance verification Complete preliminary patient history Creation of permanent electronic medical record Paperless transmissions, verification, adjudication, and payment of claims Online marketing to consumers and providers Paperless prescriptions and "mail order" handling reduce time. Access to online outsourcing for administrative management needs (billing, finance, data processing, telecommunications, inventory, and human resources)
Health insurers		Eliminates redundant clerical functions On-line eligibility verifications reduce time on phones. Claim processing and remittance are streamlined. Enables faster electronic fund transfer for payments to providers Assists in outcome and disease management processes Allows for real-time, direct communication with subscribers

and TAT can be maintained. The latest strategy for near-patient testing is the move to specialty centers (for example, chest pain centers), where the focus is on specialized management of the patient for best overall outcome (24). Following the development cycle of personal computers (PCs), inexpensive Internet access, and distributed computing, use of POCT will accelerate in regional care centers, rescue sites, schools, workplaces, rehabilitation centers, law enforcement settings, insurance companies, home health, nursing facilities, and the patient's home. Whole-blood analyzers will be built into stand-alone critical-care monitoring units. The future POCT black boxes will per-

Table 7.11 Advantages and disadvantages of POCT[a]

Advantages	Disadvantages

Shortened therapeutic TAT	Concerns for inaccuracy, lack of precision, and performance
	    Interfering substances
	    Analyte ranges more narrow

Improved patient outcomes	Quality management and assurance practices poorly defined

Reduced preanalytic errors
    Requires smaller sample volume
    Eliminates sample degradation
    Eliminates specimen mislabeling
	Potential for increased clinical errors: test quality is operator dependent
	
	Lack of password security

Self-contained, user-friendly instruments	Lack of connectivity
Shortened critical-care stay	Increased costs over core lab
Handles variety of sample types: whole blood, urine, and saliva	
Potential applications: home health and rescue and military operations	
Convenience for physicians	

[a]See reference 42.

mit ambulatory self-monitoring at home. Patients who take personal responsibility for their healthcare have improved outcomes (36).

POCT and home healthcare. The U.S. population is living longer, and providing care for the elderly has major implications for future healthcare costs. As the population ages, the incidence of disease will increase. In 1997, home healthcare services were provided to approximately 3.5 million Medicare beneficiaries. There are more than 20,000 home health agencies caring for nearly 8 million patients. The cost for home health approached $36 billion in 1999, and home health is anticipated to have substantial growth. Additional statistics about home care can be found at the National Association for Home Care website Homecare Online, at http://www.nahc.org/consumer/hcstats.html (last accessed January 2004). As the number of home care patients increases, it will be important to implement disease management to minimize costs. In the current model, labor costs are high. In order to survive, the home health market will increasing rely on POCT and vital-sign technology in conjunction with patient management and information systems (39).

Telemedicine clinics. Healthcare facilities are now taking a new approach to providing direct access to outpatient services. Telemedicine allows rural communities lacking healthcare professionals to send images to urban medical centers for consultation or a second opinion. Medical instruments such as laryngoscopes and otoscopes, modified to work with a videophone system, are now being placed in suburban malls, major regional referral centers, prisons, and military field offices. The physician located in the medical center miles away makes an interactive diagnosis remotely, using telemedicine technology. The medical information associated with these encounters can be stored in a permanent electronic medical record. The obstacles that limit wider use of telemedicine clinics include the general uneasiness of pathologists in using computers and video instead of traditional slides, lack of standards, and legal issues related to the practice of medicine across state lines (74).

Telemedicine home care. Almost all illnesses were treated in the home setting prior to the 20th century. In the 1900s, the care shifted to institutionally based medicine. Now, 100 years later, healthcare is returning home. The change is fueled by a combination of mounting pressure to reduce costs and emerging telecommunication technologies. A third factor is the sick patient's desire to be treated at home.

Today, nearly 50% of American households have Internet access, and many seek health information on-line. The remaining households that lack Internet access are referred to as the digital divide. The Internet in its present form has limitations. It is not user-friendly to persons with physical and mental limitations and the elderly, and the information available is often incomplete, erroneous, or outdated. Resources to direct patients to reliable and credible sites are limited.

Home telemedicine applications fall into three categories: access to information, transfer of data, and interaction with caregivers. Telemedicine allows for a combination of direct, indirect, and periodic data measurements of blood pressure, heart rate, blood glucose, and pulse oximetry to be transmitted to a central point for storage and analysis and to include immediate patient feedback instructions. In theory, any parameter that can be measured electronically can be transferred, creating ideal conditions for remote patient management via home-based telemedicine. Interaction between the patient and caregiver can be either synchronous (immediate response) or nonsynchronous (delayed response). There are many issues related to patient privacy, quality, and cost that impact the use of telemedicine and need to be addressed. PCs are too complex for ill patients, especially the elderly. Moreover, PCs are too expensive for much of the targeted population. Smaller niche-oriented personal digital assistants are not suitable for patients with visual or orthopedic impairments. Improved technology is needed to support the diverse needs of the home telemedicine market (22).

Although telemedicine and enhanced direct access to care have their advantages, they still have risks and a downside. Consumers armed with a little bit of knowledge may isolate themselves from comprehensive care. Worried about the time or out of fear of the expense, some consumers might even attempt to treat themselves without seeking the benefit of professional guidance (2).

Telepathology. Since the introduction of the PC and the Information Age more than two decades ago, the practice of pathology has been changing. By combining digital imaging, the computer, and high-speed, broadband digital networks, pathologists can now collaborate in real time over great distances. Telepathology capability may be considered a value-added service when marketing reference laboratory services to a pathology practice. The service can be used in the following scenarios:

- Confirm the diagnosis made by a colleague
- Aid in making a diagnosis for a less experienced pathologist just entering practice

Telepathology can also link the pathologists with the surgical suite, where a discussion of relevance takes place and details related to margins are conveyed. Telepathology expands the ability of a pathology practice to provide services to multiple community hospitals and physician office laboratories. Even though there is no additional direct reimbursement for the technology or the overhead costs for the system, the value of the system comes from its potential to break through geographic boundaries (55).

Telecommunication consortia. Major telecommunication, computer hardware, and software manufacturers are working to develop a process to improve the distribution and synchronization of information among electronic devices (computers, personal digital assistants, cellular phones, and other information appliances). The ability to share and update information among devices, sources, and recipients in healthcare should prove useful in the future (72).

Transmitting patient information between business associates over telephone lines and cables is subject to Health Insurance Portability and Accountability Act (HIPAA) security regulations. Integrating security safeguards like passwords and encryption may be necessary depending on system architecture (30).

Direct Consumer Access

The number of people that the Medicare system must manage will soon double as the baby boomers reach the magic age of 66, pushing the financial stability of the healthcare system nearly to its breaking point. Unlike their parents, who were members of the GI and Silent generations, the baby boomers have a much higher expectation for customer-specific services, from paying at the pump for gasoline to managing their portfolios online. Healthcare companies who are progressive recognize that they must meet the needs of this pay-at-the-pump generation to remain competitive in the consumer-savvy marketplace.

Sometimes referred to as a consumer revolution, the desire and expectation for quick, convenient services at the store and the bank have spilled over into the healthcare setting and are more accurately described as consumer demand. Complaints about appointment scheduling and delays, filling out the same form time and time again, and long wait times in a provider's office must drive the changes needed to refocus our energy to the front end to change customer perceptions. Consumers are exposed to self-service technologies in every other industry, why not healthcare?

Focus on the front door. Computer-savvy customers expect to visit a healthcare provider's website from the privacy of their home to schedule a visit, preregister for care, receive patient information instructions, and print out travel and parking directions. Healthcare facilities and their providers whose focus is clearly on the front door have a strong competitive advantage. As a result, physician loyalty is typically increased when patients are no longer required to spend time dealing with the service issues. Healthcare stakeholders all benefit from increased productivity because the physicians have more time for direct patient care. Hospitals that provide the best customer service attract the best physicians, who in turn attract patients (32).

DAT

Direct-access testing (DAT) refers to laboratory testing performed at the request of the patient as the consumer. Over the past 20 years, laboratories offered similar services in the form of health fairs where a designated medical director reviewed the reports prior to providing the patient with the data. Patients who utilize these services are motivated for different reasons:

- Confirm health or wellness as a result of seeing, reading, or family history
- Assess risk from exposure when lifestyle indicates the need
- Monitor the status of their existing conditions
- Ensure confidentiality by avoiding a physician office laboratory visit

Strategically selecting a highly visible location for a personal diagnostic center is critical. The interior should be warm and inviting, versus the sterile appearance typically projected by a laboratory. The employees must be able to support patients in the test selection without giving medical advice, using patient education brochures published by known healthcare associations. Either testing can be performed on-site while the patient waits or results can be directly mailed from the laboratory. The test menu offered can also include other healthcare services from the enterprise like bone density, blood pressure, or electrocardiogram. In most institutions, the personal diagnostic center operations are generally set up as a cash-and-carry service model. A market survey to gather information about the perceived need and revenue projections should be studied along with the state regulatory issues prior to entering the DAT arena (28). The number of states that allow consumers to order DAT has grown from 27 to 34 since 1999. DAT may soon account for up to 10% of the 5.7 billion laboratory tests performed annually in the United States. (20).

Under the DAT model, patients bypass their physician and order tests directly from clinical laboratories or other qualified testing sites. The results are returned directly to the patient. Generally, DAT is not covered by insurance, so the patient pays up front and there is no billing. The DAT model raises important consumer, regulatory, medical practice, medico-legal, economic, and ethical issues.

Consumer perspective. First of all, there are now available a number of diagnostic tests that are Food and Drug Administration (FDA) approved for home use and available over-the-counter. Additional information can be found at Lab Tests Online (http://www.labtestsonline.org [last accessed January 2004]). Some of these are kits that produce results immediately at home. Others are sold as collection kits only, and the collected specimen is mailed to a laboratory for evaluation. Beyond what is sold over-the-counter for home use, the range of DAT available to consumers varies by provider from a very limited menu of simple tests to a virtually unlimited menu of the most sophisticated tests on the market.

DAT increases consumer control of healthcare. The patient may want to save the time and expense of seeing a physician or may want to keep confidential certain aspects of their medical history (illegal drug use or sexually transmitted diseases). The emerging availability of genomic and proteomic testing (for example, BRCA1 and BRCA2 for assessing predisposition to breast cancer) offers a nearly unlimited amount of information potentially interesting to consumers. Much of this testing, at least initially, will not be covered by traditional insurance, and the biotech companies are likely to market directly to consumers (24).

Regulatory and reimbursement issues. All laboratories in the United States that perform clinical tests for the diagnosis or management of human disease are subject to the regulations of CLIA '88. These regulations require that an authorized person order all clinical laboratory tests. However, there are no federal restrictions on who is authorized to order a clinical laboratory test as long as payment is not sought from a government program, such as Medicare, for the self-ordered test. Laboratories that engage in DAT should first investigate state legislation that might restrict the consumer's access to DAT. For hospital laboratories, medical staff policies may restrict who is authorized to order laboratory tests.

Medical practice and medico-legal issues. Test results returned directly to the consumer must be simplified and include some interpretive comments. There must be liability disclaimers that results are provided for informational purposes only, and not for diagnosis or prognosis. The major concern is that the consumer may use DAT in lieu of necessary physician consultation, may not seek medical help appropriately as indicated by the test results, or may react inappropriately to test results taken out of context or without a full understanding of the real medical consequences.

Economic and business issues. Hospital and reference laboratories may see DAT as a promising, cash-based revenue stream that will improve their financial bottom line (60). In some cases, DAT may serve as a hook to get patients attached to a healthcare system or enrolled in long-term chronic disease management programs. Wellness testing, case finding, and disease monitoring through DAT may all be part of a hospital or health system's marketing plan. An insurance company, as one way of avoiding some office visits, might promote DAT.

Internet-based services may facilitate test ordering, result reporting, and patient privacy. Some of the commercial and independent laboratories that offer tests and results reporting through their websites are listed below:

- HealthcheckUSA, an Internet-based company that brokers DAT for participating laboratories (http://healthcheckusa.com [last accessed January 2004])

- Results Direct, a hospital-based company that offers DAT via the Internet (http://results-direct.com [last accessed January 2004])

- QuesTest (http://questest.com), a DAT site offered by Quest Diagnostics, a large national reference laboratory (last accessed January 2004)

Reference laboratories must carefully balance the potential rewards of direct marketing of laboratory tests to consumers against the risks of alienating physicians who are also clients of the reference laboratory and may see DAT as an encroachment on their practice.

Ethical issues. For providers of DAT, the traditional ethical principles should apply. Do no harm. What are the potential risks? Provide a benefit. Will DAT result in better health outcomes? Respect individual autonomy. Is there full disclosure, in understandable language, of the risks and benefits of DAT? Is patient confidentiality protected? Does DAT promote social justice? Will DAT impact overall healthcare costs? Will DAT affect consumer demand for other healthcare services?

Guidelines for providing DAT. Not surprisingly, the College of American Pathologists and much of organized medicine feel that patients' best interests are served when a qualified physician orders laboratory tests. However, if a laboratory decides to offer DAT, the following issues should be considered:

- Is a physician, or other appropriate healthcare provider, available to assist the patient in the proper interpretation of the test results?

- Is there a mechanism to assist the patient with appropriate access to any additional testing, counseling, or therapeutic intervention that may be necessary?

- Does the DAT program comply with state law, informed consent, confidentiality and mandated reporting of certain test results (for example, HIV testing)?

The main financial benefit of offering DAT as a service is the introduction of a new reimbursement stream that is favorable, bringing cash directly to the bottom line. However, there is competition from companies who already are in the business of providing health screening (2).

Over-the-counter testing, self-testing, and self-referral testing. Manufacturers of at-home diagnostics have introduced a wide variety of tests beyond the standard pregnancy and glucose testing in their quest to advance from market potential to profitability. The self-test kit menu has expanded to targeting bladder cancer, HIV and hepatitis C virus, nutrition, fecal occult blood, preterm delivery risks, ovulation cycles, urinary tract infection, cholesterol, anticoagulation therapies, and drugs of abuse, with more in the pipeline. The companies have learned an invaluable lesson during the market's slow evolution. Producing new test kits doesn't come with a guarantee that consumers will purchase them. The market growth is hampered by limitations on direct-to-consumer advertising efforts and third-party reimbursement problems. At-home diagnostic manufacturers may benefit from the growth of e-commerce and the ability to sell kits on-line, coupled with step-by-step directions (64).

California has recently passed legislation that permits state residents to seek laboratory testing for a limited menu of four clinical laboratory services as an alternative to purchasing home testing kits that are not manufactured in the state. As the number of home test kits approved by the FDA increases, consumer access to a broader scope of self-directed testing also increases. The current California legislation (available at http://www.leginfo.ca.gov or http://www.fda.gov [last accessed January 2004]) requires the following:

- The testing must be performed in a clinical laboratory licensed by the state of California.
- The person self-referring assumes full responsibility for the associated costs of the testing to further ensure that healthcare insurance costs are not increased as a result. Third-party payors do not typically cover self-directed testing.
- Tests can be ordered only for oneself and not for dependents or a spouse.
- All results must be reported with reference ranges.
- The report should encourage the person tested to seek a physician for interpretation and follow-up.

Alternative medicine. In the past, alternative medicine was not favored by healthcare providers and insurers, but today, as many as one-third of patients have embraced alternative healthcare treatment. Alternative medicine is generally a noncovered service that patients assume as an out-of-pocket expense. Since therapeutic practices are not well regulated, providers are hesitant to recommend it. Nonetheless, healthcare organizations are integrating new alternative medicine centers dedicated to providing alternative care to capture some of this nontraditional, FFS market (77). Typical services include the following:

- Physical: chiropractic, aromatherapy, and massage
- Psychological: hypnotherapy, meditation, and biofeedback
- Energy: acupuncture and reflexology

Much like self-directed testing, this cash-and-carry model offers convenient access and low cost to the consumer, improving the revenue stream with cash to the bottom line, while eliminating the costs of billing and collections for the visit. Consumers, electing to visit alternative medicine providers for convenience, pay out of pocket nearly 75% of the time.

Costs associated with consumer demand. Consumers increasingly believe that the dollar is more important to

the MCO than is the patient. To regain patient trust, HMOs need to be sensitive to the doctor-patient relationship and put the doctors at arm's length from the direct financial aspects of the patient's care. According to James Sabin of Harvard Pilgrim Healthcare, the American public has shown repeatedly "that it views healthcare as a social good, and even a right, not a commodity." Healthcare organizations spent between $150 and $250 million on consumer-related programs in 1996, and by the year 2000, they pumped nearly $400 million into marketing promotions and customer relations programs (26).

Advances in Genetic Testing and Molecular Pathology

The HGP. Over the past 15 years, the Human Genome Project (HGP), a joint program funded by the Department of Energy and the National Institutes of Health, has completed the sequencing of the total human genome. This project yielded genetic maps and new techniques to further genetic research and clinical testing (79). The HGP significance is vast and has far-reaching implications:

- *Pharmacogenetics.* Designing drugs specifically modified to a person's genetic makeup will be important in the treatment of many genetic diseases.
- *Agricultural genetics.* Engineering genetically modified foods to grow larger, more nutritious, and pest free.
- *Forensic genetics.* DNA-based human identity testing is used to convict or acquit an individual accused of a crime.
- *Evolutional and anthropological genetics.* Genetics is a major source of information about the similarities and differences in humans and other species.
- *Microarray technology.* Research during the HGP has produced one technology, the microarray, with the greatest potential for disease detection and characterization.

The relationships between the DNA sequence and the location in the genome are described by four mapping techniques listed in Table 7.12.

At the forefront of federal and state regulatory activity is ongoing debate about discrimination, quality of testing, informed consent, and storage of DNA samples. Laboratories must carefully weigh the ethical, social, and legal implications associated with genetic testing. The following issues must be considered: patient privacy; patient, professional, and public education; and the application and use of genetic information. The practicality of using genetic testing is hampered by its high costs. The value it adds to medical practice and patient treatment must be carefully weighed against business, political, ethical, and resource-versus-consumption risks (79). To further complicate issues, commercial laboratories commonly license and exclusively offer genetic tests under a patent.

Table 7.12 Genetic mapping techniques[a]

Type of genetic map	Description	Uses of map
Linkage	Assigns a location to a specific landmark in a chromosome	Used statistically to determine if two gene sequences are transferred together in meiosis
Physical (contig)	Continuous gene segments are produced from a chromosome broken into fragments using restriction enzymes.	Gene walking down chromosome to identify genes for specific diseases
Chromosome	Smaller fragments of the contig	Disease genes are often located in regions and not always at specific loci.
Sequence	Contigs are broken down into smaller clones for DNA sequencing to be done.	There are certain regions in the genome that are polymorphic "hot spots."

[a]See reference 79.

Genetic testing. The National Institutes of Health and the Department of Energy task force defines genetic testing as "the analysis of materials derived from the human body, including human DNA, RNA, chromosomes, proteins, and certain metabolites to detect heritable or acquired disease related genotypes, mutations, phenotypes, or karyotypes for clinical purposes. The purposes include predicting the risk of disease, identifying carriers, and establishing prenatal or clinical diagnoses or prognoses in individuals, families, or populations" (52).

Today, there are more than 500 specialized laboratories offering tests with a wide spectrum of application for more than 900 diseases. In 1991, the American College of Medical Genetics was formed to represent providers of genetic services and patients with genetic disorders and to speak for the emerging specialty of medical genetics. The group has issued a number of consensus statements (34) for the following:

- Apolipoprotein E for Alzheimer's disease
- Genetic susceptibility to breast and ovarian cancer
- Laboratory standards for population-based cystic fibrosis carrier screening
- Factor five mutation testing
- Technical and clinical assessment of fluorescence in situ hybridization
- Fragile X syndrome
- Providing samples for DNA testing

In the past, the lack of expertise and the lack of availability of user-friendly test platforms have limited the development of molecular assays for use in academic medical centers, progressive community hospitals, and commercial reference laboratories. The unexpected specificity and sensitivity of PCR analysis have driven the rapid advancement of the molecular diagnostics discipline. The field has moved from the initial ability to isolate DNA and RNA and clone distinct genetic sequences to the present point, where entire sequences of complex genes are routinely analyzed for disease-associated mutations. Future

test offerings for multigenic disorders may be very expensive because of intellectual property rights and the associated royalties. The proprietary protections given to molecular discoveries that offer new value to patients at the same time threaten the very discipline of molecular diagnostics. Another important issue is pending FDA legislation that will require a referring provider to obtain informed consent and will mandate that the laboratory perform reviews of genetic assays for analytic validity and clinical utility before running or charging for the assay (33).

- *Monogenetic diseases.* Using genetic testing to predict and avoid births of children with diseases such as cystic fibrosis or Duchenne muscular dystrophy may have a significant impact on human suffering but may not touch the estimated lifetime costs for the families involved, unless case management and counseling are considered in the equation.

- *Pathogen virulence and drug resistance.* The ability to identify pathogens quickly will eliminate the spread of disease and offer cost savings from avoidance of costly isolation procedures. Selecting the most appropriate drug therapy may shorten LOS or improve mortality rates.

- *Genetic variation in therapeutics.* The cost of genetic variation in therapeutics should not be as great as those observed with monogenetic disease. Genetic variations affecting therapeutic outcomes are 50 to 1,000 times more prevalent in the population. The anticipated cost savings per patient should justify the use of the testing.

The issue is not whether genetic testing will be used as a clinical tool but rather when (70). As pharmacogenetic testing, predictive genetic testing, and gene-specific drug therapies become increasingly available, reimbursement for testing as a covered service will be based on the proven effectiveness of the tests but will probably be subject to frequency limitations. As new genetic test utilization increases, the American Medical Association typically adds genetic specific analyte codes to the Current Procedural

Terminology Code (CPT Code) book to expedite the claim review and payment process (41).

Advances in molecular pathology. A key component in the practice of anatomic and clinical pathology in the future will be molecular pathology. Practice protocols may rely on molecular testing for diagnosis of disease as well as prognosis and treatment in the laboratory disciplines such as hematology, microbiology, histocompatibility, cytogenetics, and surgical pathology.

Common techniques used in molecular diagnostic testing include laser capture microdissection, DNA sequencing, PCR, fluorescent in situ hybridization, micro- and macroarray technology, and proteomics with mass spectrometry. The major obstacles to more rapid advancement in the field of molecular diagnostics include the following:

- Lack of training programs for pathologists, technical directors, and technologists
- Insufficient funding for the costs of development
- Need for well-defined protocols for test utilization (45)

Bioethical issues. The benefits of genetic testing as well as the revolutionary changes and medical, ethical, legal, and socioeconomic issues that the testing raises are recognized by the government and healthcare providers. The Department of Health and Human Services established the Secretary's Advisory Committee on Genetic Testing to evaluate and analyze programs for safety, effectiveness, adequacy, and oversight measures (4). In September 1997, the Task Force on Genetic Testing, created by the National Institutes of Health and the Department of Energy, announced recommendations to ensure the quality of laboratories performing genetic testing. Discrimination, quality of testing, informed consent, and storage of DNA samples are the leading concerns and major focus of state and federal policy issues and activities.

In the future, healthcare will continue to be more regulated, consolidated, and accountable. Consumers will leverage buying power, buying less on price and more on quality. Ethics will influence their decisions. Medical diagnosis and treatment will advance rapidly to the molecular level as it becomes less expensive and less burdensome. Locating single gene mutations and identifying multifactorial conditions whose gene changes have undesirable effects will lead to the study of complex characteristics like obesity, intelligence, and personality disorders. The primary bioethical concern will become what to test for and what to treat (75).

Some believe that pharmacogenetics is the future of laboratory medicine. Advances in gene discovery will lead to increased identification of protein interactions and genetic differences in population responses to drugs. The ability to screen thousands of patients for individual variations in response to drugs enhances the predictive testing and rationale for drug design. Identification of susceptible disease will im-

prove drug utilization, risk factor analysis, and therapeutic management. The opportunities for molecular diagnostic laboratories to partner across the continuum in the industry are unlimited (D. Cooper, personal communication).

Medical records and genetic privacy. The way in which society deals with fundamental issues about health and disease is undergoing profound change in response to advances in electronic information technology and biomedical research in molecular genetics and genomics. At the same time, healthcare delivery has undergone transformation influenced by managed care and the emergence of evidence-based medicine. The very promise of having a greater understanding of diagnosis, treatment, and prevention of human disease and the concept of rationing the delivery of medical services help balance the social burden of human suffering against the costs of medical resources. As a result, there is a widespread and growing concern from the general public related to both the philosophical and ethical consideration of individual autonomy and privacy. At the same time, there are realistic concerns about the security and confidentiality of sensitive, personally identifiable medical information (particularly electronically accessible information) being used inappropriately by an insurer or an employer. The major challenge is to secure all medical information, not just genetic, without impairing appropriate access necessary for medical management (68). In a California-based survey of consumer attitudes regarding ethics and healthcare web services, 75% of the adults indicated concern about sites sharing information without permission. Additional information on ethics and surveys of consumer attitudes about health is available at the California Health Care Foundation and the Internet Coalition website (http://www.chcf.org [last accessed Janurary 2004]).

Ethical guidelines. In any discussion of ethics and medical information, confidentiality should not be the only focus. Quality, medical relevance, and usefulness are also key components (69).

- To provide quality healthcare, physicians need access to accurate, timely, and understandable medical information.
- All available medical information should include any relevant patient decisions.
- Access to the patient's medical information should be limited to those authorized by the patient.
- A onetime patient authorization is no longer sufficient.
- Authorized individuals should not disclose the medical information to unauthorized persons.
- Those entrusted to maintain medical records must safeguard the records to ensure that they are well protected from unauthorized access.

- Laws that require reporting of certain medical information limit a patient's right to confidentiality.

- A patient's right to confidentiality is limited by the provider's responsibility to protect persons from risk and to do no harm.

- Medical information should be provided to patients in a manner that supports the decision-making process.

- Medical information should be objective and educational in nature.

New Regulations To Address Changing Technology: HIPAA

HIPAA regulations, originally proposed as an administrative simplification with an effective date of October 2002, attempt to bring efficiency through standard coding and guidelines for the format of electronic transmissions for enrollment, claims, and authorizations and to further eliminate fraud and abuse, while protecting patient privacy. HIPAA's impact on the costs of providing healthcare for payors and providers is far reaching and will be felt over the next 5 years. Although improved efficiency and financial performance are the goals, maintaining customer satisfaction and loyalty will be achieved only if employee and operation effectiveness can be delivered consistently (38). HIPAA challenges every healthcare organization using e-commerce. Although the technology exists, the cost of compliance may outweigh the benefits.

Push versus pull technology. Using e-mail (a push technology) for laboratory reporting presents many HIPAA issues related to verification of correct address, access, and security. Using a pull technology to access results ensures that only physicians with security clearance can view results out of your system since the results reside in your domain (3).

Consolidation in the Healthcare Industry

Efforts to enact comprehensive national healthcare reform between 1992 and 1994 failed miserably. Driven by powerful economic forces and the fear of the economic consequences, the industry's private sector has undergone radical restructuring over the past 5 years. Those in the healthcare industry turned to mergers, acquisitions, joint ventures, and consolidation to fortify their position and protect their market share. The effects of the consolidation have been felt in every sector of the market.

Laboratories, Hospitals, Physician Practices, and MCOs

Commercial laboratory consolidation seemed to be completed in 1995. However, the dominant players have recently reached across international boundaries to increase their market share. In targeted geographic regions, commercial laboratories will continue to make acquisitions of other independent or esoteric laboratories to solve their need for coverage or complement their test portfolio. According to the CLIA provider files available at http://www.cms.gov (last accessed January 2004), the number of CLIA-licensed independent labs has declined since 1996 from 5,789 to 4,921. The September 2000 *Laboratory Industry Report* indicated that the number of operational hospital laboratories in 2000 was down to 8,563 from 8,888 in 1996 as a result of consolidation to core labs and mergers (38a).

Nationwide, hospitals have joined forces to avoid closings. Independent community hospitals are nearly extinct. In March 2003, Robert Michel noted a steady decline in hospital mergers, acquisitions, joint ventures, and partnerships from more than 700 facilities in 1996 to around 150 facilities in 2002 (48).

Physician practices have merged, becoming group practices and networks, to increase efficiency. Sharing office space in a concept called group practice without walls allows physician groups to expand their service area while eliminating the duplication of leased-space expenses. Solo practitioners are also virtually extinct.

Managed-care companies have been acquired by larger firms to lower expense and increase efficiency through economies of scale. As competition in the market decreases, employers and consumers fear deterioration in the quality of services and price increases more than the reductions anticipated from the efficiencies achieved (31). The maturing of the managed-care market contributed to the consolidation among managed-care plans. Traditionally, managed-care penetration is greatest in large urban areas, and point-of-service plans are more successful in rural communities.

While antitrust laws attempted to promote competition in the marketplace by prohibiting anticompetitive agreements between companies, efforts to enforce antitrust are typically directed at price fixing and geographic market division.

Integrated Delivery Systems

An integrated delivery system is a legal structure formed by hospitals and physicians to share financial risk when collectively negotiating contracts for services with the integrated delivery system health system. Hospitals are encouraged to shift from treating populations in episodes of care to comprehensive health management. Healthcare providers form integrated delivery systems to meet the needs of the payors, purchasers, and consumers. The ability to offer one-stop shopping with convenient access in a defined region allows providers to offer a seamless continuum of care from the PCP to tertiary services. Managed care is suffering from the inflationary costs of healthcare, expected to double to more than $2.7 trillion by 2007 (78). Solutions are focused on changes ranging from industry consolidation and accommodation of the HIPAA regulations to slashing benefits and raising copays. Without an appropriate response, purchasers and employers may move toward direct contracting with purchasers in the future, eliminating the insurer as the middleman and leveraging their buying power.

Irrespective of the national trends, the choice about healthcare is still made at the local level among the stakeholders. In order to provide a continuum of care, integrated delivery systems and regional networks acting as a community-based system must partner with rehabilitation centers, skilled care, home health, and laboratories and must incorporate informatics to be effective (78).

Consolidation in the Laboratory Industry

Change from a Revenue Center to a Cost Center

After decades of profitability based on low incremental cost of testing and favorable FFS reimbursements, the clinical laboratory industry confronted hard times in the 1990s created by the following:

- Severe cuts in Medicare reimbursement levels
- Closed loopholes in federal regulations on unbundling of test panels to increase profits
- Growing influence of managed care

Laboratories watched while as much as one-third of their total sales from Medicare reimbursements disappeared as a result of Medicare reform. Following the shifts from inpatient to outpatient services under managed care, hospital laboratories began to look to outreach to fill excess capacity. Commercial laboratories whose competitive bidding, commodity, and lost-leader pricing strategies had driven their profit margins down to the bottom of the barrel began looking for revenues to offset their losses through joint ventures with hospitals. Since 1992, compliance with CLIA '88 and market dynamics have accelerated the pace of consolidations, mergers, acquisitions, downsizing, and rightsizing in the healthcare industry. Hospital laboratories, independent laboratories, and commercial laboratories came together to form regional laboratory networks. Outreach programs became prevalent in this period to improve the average cost per test by increasing test volume (57).

Internal Consolidation

Consolidation is a strategy whereby several hospital laboratories downsize individual facility laboratories and funnel most specimens into a centralized (also called a core) laboratory. This strategy achieves lower cost per test and improves the competitive position for the consolidated laboratory operation. The primary goals of internal laboratory consolidation include eliminating duplication of services and excess capacity, restructuring work flow, changing staff resources, and centralizing management. Another advantage of internal consolidation is increased test volumes

enabling the laboratory to bring more testing in-house, reducing referrals, lowering costs, and improving TAT. Laboratory consolidation offers the following benefits:

- Integration of clinical information across the healthcare continuum
- Delivering services more economically
- Management of the test cycle/production times
- Electronic links to the providers and consumers
- Providing meaningful and relevant information for improved outcomes

Restructuring trends used in the consolidation process, like downsizing, POCT, internal laboratory consolidation, and interdisciplinary team approaches, paved the way for regional network development and alliances among laboratories. Reengineering efforts of the 1990s that were linked to continuous improvement proved more effective than downsizing or restructuring (62). Reengineering limited to compliance, quality improvement, and cost containment produced some internal financial improvements but had little effect on innovation or long-term growth.

Regional Integrated Laboratory Network

The primary objective for regionalization is to develop a system of laboratories capable of providing services to a larger geographic area and positioning the laboratory system to compete for managed-care contracts (47). Regional networks were formed with core laboratories linked to multiple rapid-response and point-of-service sites. The system enabled the aligned laboratories to market the combined strengths of the collective test menus, keeping more tests within the regional system and eliminating referrals outside of the system.

- Operation and ownership of the laboratories in a regional system remain independent, and internal restructuring is usually not linked to the needs of the system.
- Administration of a regional system is shared among the participants under a separate management group umbrella.

There are many arrangements for this type of system, which may include a combination of independent hospital laboratories, consolidated laboratories, academic medical center laboratories, other independent laboratories, and commercial reference laboratories. Regional laboratories are uniquely positioned to serve their communities. The ability to keep the testing in the local community benefits the internal customers (laboratory employees), doctors (with shorter TAT), and patients (better continuity of care). Outreach sales and marketing for the system are not a part of this model. Each individual laboratory would continue to market their services independent of the regional system, established primarily for managed-care opportunities (47). (See Fig. 7.1.) In a network model, independent laboratories affiliate under a network organization without any consolidation. In a consolidation model, two or more laboratories consolidate core operations to one primary site operating rapid-access operations in remote sites. In a regional laboratory system, a hybrid operation is formed with participants from academic medical center laboratories, a commercial laboratory partner, and participating consolidated hospital laboratory models. According to Michel, even though regional laboratory systems did not develop as rapidly as originally anticipated, several successful models (like Detroit and PacLab) continue to operate effectively in their markets.

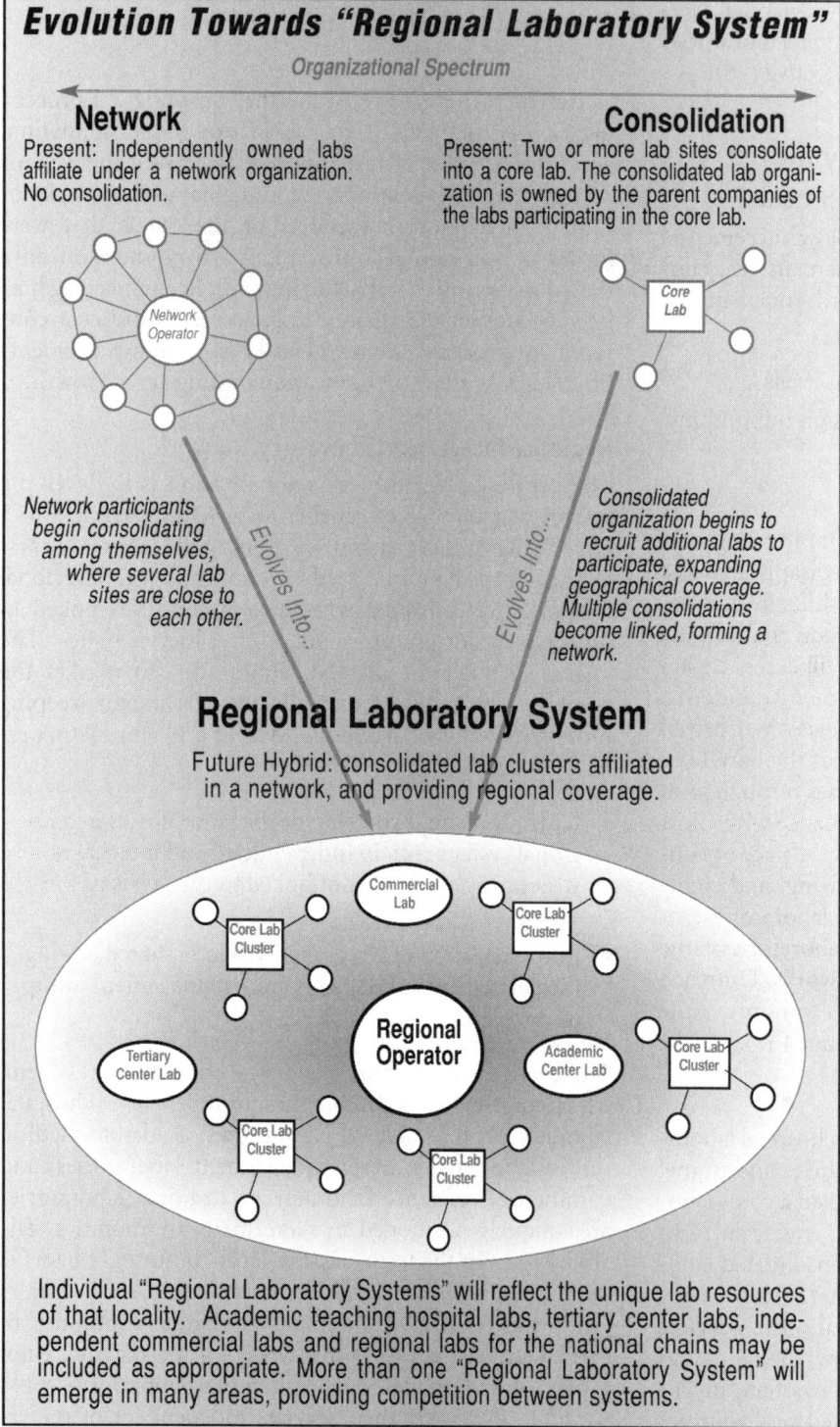

Evolution Towards "Regional Laboratory System"

Organizational Spectrum

Network
Present: Independently owned labs affiliate under a network organization. No consolidation.

Network Operator

Consolidation
Present: Two or more lab sites consolidate into a core lab. The consolidated lab organization is owned by the parent companies of the labs participating in the core lab.

Core Lab

Network participants begin consolidating among themselves, where several lab sites are close to each other.

Evolves Into...

Evolves Into...

Consolidated organization begins to recruit additional labs to participate, expanding geographical coverage. Multiple consolidations become linked, forming a network.

Regional Laboratory System

Future Hybrid: consolidated lab clusters affiliated in a network, and providing regional coverage.

Commercial Lab

Core Lab Cluster

Core Lab Cluster

Tertiary Center Lab

Regional Operator

Academic Center Lab

Core Lab Cluster

Core Lab Cluster

Core Lab Cluster

Individual "Regional Laboratory Systems" will reflect the unique lab resources of that locality. Academic teaching hospital labs, tertiary center labs, independent commercial labs and regional labs for the national chains may be included as appropriate. More than one "Regional Laboratory System" will emerge in many areas, providing competition between systems.

Figure 7.1 Evolution towards regional laboratory system. In a network model, independent laboratories affiliate under a network organization without any consolidation. In a consolidation model, two or more laboratories consolidate core operations to one primary site operating rapid-access operations in remote sites. In a regional laboratory system, a hybrid operation is formed with participants from academic medical center laboratories, a commercial laboratory partner, and participating consolidated hospital laboratory models. (Reprinted with permission from reference 47.)

A virtual laboratory concept is an organization or network of separate companies strategically aligned to develop and market products giving the appearance of a larger organization but does not include merger of assets.

During the past decade, healthcare facilities have implemented various strategies to address the impact of the shrinking healthcare dollar on laboratory operations. The trend has shifted to the creation of integrated delivery systems. In this model, hospitals eliminate redundancy by sharing services and moving the patient to a more cost-effective setting. Successful managers working in an integrated laboratory system will need additional knowledge and new skills akin to industrial and systems engineering combined with an ability to blend them with healthcare economics, fundamental business principles, human resource management, and information technology. Successful consolidated and regional networks will be the winners, leveraging their strengths, surpassing the competition, and using exceptional customer services to create value, adding buying power in contract negotiations (57).

Strategies for Success in the 21st Century

Strategic Redesign

Strategic redesign is emerging as the tactical strategy of the new decade. First, an organization must decide to differentiate its products or services from the competition by adding value. Then, it must develop a structured process to add value and create an environment that welcomes change by empowering the employees. To accomplish the mission, the organization needs a clear vision, a change leader to communicate the vision, and a management team that consistently walks the talk.

Next, the organization must review and redesign each of the necessary support processes to eliminate steps that don't add value. According to Michael Hammer and James Champy in *Re-engineering the Corporation: a Manifesto for Business Revolution* (28a), process redesign involves the fundamental rethinking and radical redesign of business practices to achieve dramatic improvements in key performance measures like quality, service, and timeliness. In strategic redesign, the quality indicators chosen for measurement should never be revenue oriented but should include process cycle times, process costs, costs of servicing the customer, and patient outcomes. Leaders must celebrate milestones of improvement with employees throughout the process and not just during implementation.

There are enormous gaps between what we know and what we do. Typically, the time lapse from recognizing the need for process change to making the change happen is unacceptably long. Ohno, a Japanese engineer at Toyota, developed the kanban system, which encompasses just-in-time inventory and assembly line production with no waiting, to ensure continuity in the process flow. By study-ing Ohno's work, healthcare systems of the future should be able to accurately predict consumer demand and allocate resources by anticipating the needs for care rather than reacting to them, virtually delivering healthcare kanban style (8).

Develop System-Wide Thinking and a Common Culture

Healthcare is suffering from internal turmoil and conflict resulting from the effects of restructuring, mergers, and acquisitions. To succeed in the future, hospital administration, employees, and physicians must develop an appreciation for each other's culture, values, beliefs, language, and goals. Once these things are understood, a new system-wide culture can be agreed upon. By redefining the symbolic barriers of authority, tasks, and politics, the new system should incorporate business, clinical, and ethical dimensions. If not identified early in the process, differences in ethical values will be the crux of ongoing conflict. In order to achieve the mutual goals, the following components are essential (63):

- Mutual understanding and agreement on system goals
- Enhanced communication between administration and physicians
- Greater physician involvement in decision making and governance
- Treatment based on evidence beyond controlling costs
- Emphasis on prevention, self-care, and outpatient services
- Focus on quality patient outcomes

Developing a new culture is a difficult and time-consuming task. A common culture must be flexible and based on shared values and constant learning. A rigid culture is more focused on form. Trust is a perception and an attitude that influences how people will accept change. Truthfulness, keeping promises, treating all employees fairly and equally, and respecting employees as individuals build trust within the organization (51).

Organizational climate. Employees' perceptions about their working environment impact their ability to do a good job. Creating a desirable climate is key to employee retention. The environment must include the following:

- *Flexibility.* With minimal red tape.
- *Rewards.* With performance feedback.
- *Responsibility.* Employees empowered to make independent judgment.
- *Clarity.* Goals and expectations must be clear.
- *Standards.* Hold each employee accountable to the same standards.
- *Team commitment.* Lead by example; create pride.

The trust factor. Organizations that create a culture with an atmosphere of trust among employees and customers maximize their intellectual assets and maintain a competitive advantage in the marketplace. Developing professional relationships and networks, forming strong lines of communication, promoting teamwork, and having a common mind-set are key (29).

Differentiating a Competitive Advantage

As laboratories enter the 21st century and market pressures continue to increase, service industries, knowledge management, and virtual partnerships will lead the way to future survival. The strategies used to differentiate a competitive advantage will move away from a primary focus on cost containment to new strategies that include the following:

- Optimization of new and innovative products
- Flexibility of services
- Forming strong partnerships with stakeholders (suppliers, customers, employees)

The short-term survival mechanisms of cost cutting, whether by restructuring, downsizing, or reengineering strategies, have not always resulted in increased productivity. Instead, they may actually decrease morale, increase anxiety, and ultimately decrease productivity and innovation.

Loyalty-based management. The last and most critical step in achieving a competitive advantage is to create a business environment that sustains customer loyalty. Developing a system-wide culture for understanding the economic effects of customer and employee retention on revenues and costs begins with management. Reinvesting cash flow from knowledgeable decisions attracts and retains loyal employees and loyal customers. When employees are satisfied and happy with their work, they are more productive, which ultimately leads to increased customer satisfaction.

To evaluate the cost per benefit of the business decision, customer, product, and employee needs must all be synchronous. Loyalty-based management systems thrive on effective feedback measurements. Customers are an invaluable resource. Long-term employees are more familiar with the business and the needs of the customer. The ability to constantly deliver value in an ever-changing healthcare environment can be cultivated only through effective listening and learning. In the final analysis, loyalty-based management puts creating customer loyalty ahead of revenue. The only losers in this environment are the competitors who get the leftover customers and leftover employees (56).

Move from Top-Down Management to Bottom-Up Customer Focus

Quality is one of the most talked-about and least understood concepts in healthcare. It is a chameleon phrase that means different things to different stakeholders depending on their needs, beliefs, and motives. Informatics firms offer software tools that capture and measure quality without being able to demonstrate the impact and usefulness to their customers. Employers, insurers, and accreditation organizations demand provider commitment to quality improvement processes but have articulated only minimal standards for measuring and evaluating their effectiveness.

Collaboration is process driven and result oriented. Collaboration commits each side of the business relationship to fulfill their responsibilities and becomes the vehicle to implement quality strategies. The business needs of each stakeholder must be met in order for quality management to become a core competency rather than a tactical business strategy. Business trust, cooperation, a realistic commitment to change, and collaboration are critical to achieving quality management (10). Everyone in managed healthcare that is involved in care delivery is a customer who depends on someone else for information or cooperation to get the job done. Recognizing the interdependence with one another and establishing performance expectations develop trust and buy-in among members of the partnership (11). Placing the patient in the driver's seat ensures that we are listening to and addressing patient needs (Fig. 7.2). More reliable communication systems should decrease errors, prevent miscommunications, and avoid costly delays in the processes, thereby streamlining the encounter. Evidence-based medicine will encourage decision making based on reliable data. Donald Berwick believes that the practice of medicine will migrate from being an enterprise that provides personal service to being one that provides information by the year 2020 (8).

Evidence-Based Medicine

Science and technology have advanced at a rapid pace over the last four decades, but the healthcare delivery system has fallen short in providing consistent, high-quality serv-

Figure 7.2 Bottom-up customer focus: the inverted paradigm. In the new business paradigm, the customer as king maintains the position of influence at the top of the chart. Employees are empowered and trained to provide exceptional customer service, exceeding the customer's expectation. The management teams within the organization must lead by example, building trust among the staff.

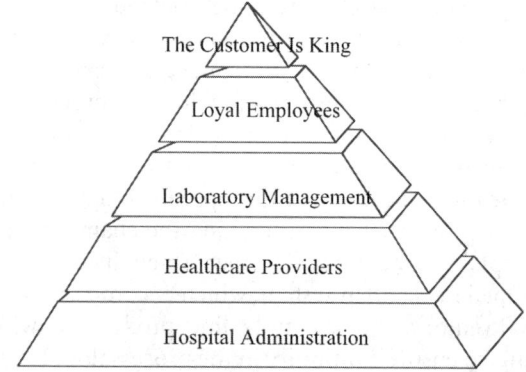

ices to transfer its knowledge into practice. The practice of evidence-based medicine allows for the judicious integration of literature, clinical experience, and patient understanding. Clinical guidelines, based on scientific evidence, and tools for measuring outcomes and patient compliance effectively bridge the gap between knowledge and practice.

In traditional medicine, the physician depends primarily on his memory, opinions formed without data, and anecdotal experience to prescribe treatment. The patient's participation is minimal. In evidenced-based medicine, the physician incorporates current literature and data with memory and experience. The patient participates in actively making joint decisions about treatment modalities. The physician is monitored for adherence to guidelines, and the patient is monitored for compliance. Evidence-based medicine is gaining support from many groups as the foundation for healthcare reform and the future of medicine. Obtaining physician support in this quality-of-care movement is critical. Defining the appropriateness of care for patients, the appropriate practice for providers, and the appropriate payment from payors for future generations will all depend on evidence-based medical practices (21).

Meaningful and Relevant Information

Managed care was not originally formed to focus on utilization control. The purpose was to keep track of the patient's medical record and steer the direction of care from treatment to prevention. This was next to impossible, since the HMOs primarily handled claims and billing data. Integrated delivery networks evolved on the provider side in an attempt to gather more complete information about the patient. In response, hospitals and providers formed community health information networks to build a centralized database that would contain all the medical records for every patient in the community network. This thinking was correct because the goal was connectivity. Other attempts at data collection include data warehousing and development of an electronic medical record. Ultimately the ability to assemble the complete patient treatment experience in one single electronic medical record will decrease medical errors, improve patient care, and fundamentally change the way healthcare is delivered (12).

Healthcare is changing throughout the world, with screening, diagnosis, and chronic disease management being redirected from the hospital environment to the physician providers. Demand for faster responses in patient triage, critical-care medicine, and high-technology and rapid-response diagnostics in the tertiary-care environment reinforces the premise that time is money. C. Price from the Royal London School of Medicine has commented that the potential to provide more value for the money lies in the evolving new culture that is founded on evidence-based medicine, which focuses on outcomes and is manifested in the laboratory as new technologies, competitive advantage, ethical promotion, and distribution of information.

The laboratory's role in informatics. Laboratory test results are of limited use in the absence of supporting clinical information. Descriptive elements of clinical information include gender, race, age, occupation, health status, signs and symptoms, patient status, family and medical history, and social behavior. Fueled by a complex healthcare environment and an ever-expanding array of diagnostic procedures, there is a growing need for increased integration between clinical information and laboratory data during the decade ahead. Genetic testing in particular requires that the test be performed as an adjunct to patient management and used in conjunction with the patient's clinical information. The trend toward evidence-based patient care while focusing on the patient will be challenging. The role of the laboratory in response to these challenges and opportunities will be to contribute medically relevant and value-added information to the future multidisciplinary approach to the management of the patient (44).

To determine value, laboratory information must be differentiated from laboratory data. If we only consider data, laboratories simply perform the right test on the right patient, in the right time and format at the right price. The element that brings value to information is the ability to provide the right result referenced to the right ranges, with the right interpretations and consideration of the test limitations. The information may also include the right advice on how to use the test information with the right knowledge of the clinical context of the testing. For laboratory information to be of value, it must convey results in a manner that assists the provider in estimating the probability of disease and affect subsequent patient management decisions toward improving patient outcome (9).

Impact of bioinformatics on pathology. Pathologists have long suspected that bioinformatics would turn their world upside down. As test results and clinical patient data merge, the previously clear distinction between the roles of the anatomic and clinical pathologists blurs. The recent technology explosion requires that pathologists understand how molecular diagnostics bridges the gap between the worlds of research and clinical care. Pathology will witness a gradual shift from cell morphology to the molecular structure and function of cells as an adjunct to the diagnostic process, including genomic and proteomic testing. As bioinformatics becomes a significant driving force in pathology, result reporting will steadily demand a larger share of the pathologist's daily routine. At the same time, bioinformatics is raising difficult questions about the nature of disease. The concept behind boinformatics is to study significant patterns in large data sets, not in individual biological entities. Pathologists must understand the stewardship of the resource that will become the foundation for bioinformatics research, the development of a comprehensive, well-organized clinical biorepository. The clinical laboratory must have expertise in biochemistry and handling of large data sets, while the anatomic laboratory must have a keen perspective and understanding of cellular biology (59).

Summary

During the first half of the 20th century, hospital-based laboratories almost exclusively delivered a limited menu of anatomic and clinical test procedures. Then in the 1950s, advances in technology paved the way for rapid growth in the areas of automation, instrumentation, quality assurance, and quality control. The improvements in precision and accuracy led to more efficient analytical processes. Computerization was introduced to the laboratory in the 1960s, opening the door for the laboratory to become a repository of clinical information and knowledge about wellness and disease. Concepts of sensitivity, specificity, efficacy, effectiveness, predictive values, and analytical variability emerged. The capital development of the 1960s shifted the testing to remote independent laboratories, where large test volumes were performed in a factory-like setting. The 1980s witnessed the evolution of more sophisticated laboratory equipment and computers that supported bar coding and instant patient identification. During the last decade, visionaries predicted that molecular biology had the potential to change the industry. Since its inception, the laboratory has provided physicians with valuable information that supports the diagnosis and treatment of disease. In the new millennium, the laboratory is strategically positioned for success, providing more information about the human condition faster and more accurately than ever before (7).

During the golden age of healthcare, clinical laboratories focused on increasing on-site test menus, reducing TAT, and acquiring the latest technology. Costs were essentially passed through, and laboratorians and pathologists became specialists in a discipline. Hospitals ignored the service demands of the non-hospital patient market, allowing the independent commercial laboratories to get a stronghold. The reference laboratories were profitable due to the economies of scale from automation and the favorable reimbursement environment. The prospective payment system for inpatient reimbursement and managed-care capitation in the outpatient market led to a commodity pricing strategy, with commercial laboratories using loss leaders to gain managed-care contracts. The industry responded with attempts at consolidation, regionalization, acquisitions, and mergers to offset the losses.

The future of the healthcare industry is being driven by these five market forces (1):

- *Marketization.* The force of marketization means that the stakeholders demand a higher level of performance and accountability for demonstrated efficiency.
- *Consumerization.* During the golden age, patients didn't act like consumers. Today, patients demand choice, access, quality of care, service, and price. The consumer is driving the healthcare paradigm toward prevention and wellness. New metrics for quality and performance in the laboratory hinge on the following four general approaches to outcome evaluation: cost minimization, cost-effectiveness, cost utility, and cost/benefit analysis.
- *Mass customization.* In an efficient healthcare market, competitors must create value for customers by differentiating their products and services. Healthcare is becoming a business of managing relationships rather than events. A complete and longitudinal medical record will become a metric in the future.
- *Value chain optimization.* Stakeholders in the industry are restructuring their internal and external customer focus.
- *Digitalization.* The information revolution and digitization are driving the next wave of technological restructuring in healthcare and information-intensive industries. Information is knowledge, and knowledge is power. Educated consumers are becoming more responsible and involved in their healthcare. Laboratories that embrace change through information technology are positioned for success in the future.

KEY POINTS

- The current healthcare reimbursement system focuses on the right price and volume. The healthcare system of the future should reward providers who demonstrate good outcomes and implement safety systems in the course of treatment.
- The value of a laboratory test is measured by whether it changes the likelihood of disease in conjunction with the clinician's estimate of the probability of disease.
- Patients who take personal responsibility for their healthcare have improved outcomes.
- DAT may soon account for up to 10% of the 5.7 billion laboratory tests performed annually in the United States.
- Consumers electing to visit alternative medicine providers for convenience pay out-of-pocket nearly 75% of the time.
- Consumer demands are forcing change. Consumers want accurate, legible bills and simplified eligibility determination and registration. Their focus on prevention and wellness means that diagnostic testing must identify early and monitor individuals at high risk.
- Hospitals that provide the best customer service attract the best physicians, who in turn attract patients.
- Healthcare is becoming a business of managing relationships rather than events.
- Disease management will drive the next generation of managed care, by focusing on prevention and early de-

tection, and will represent a significant opportunity for clinical laboratories.

- DNA testing used to adjust dose and to select specific cancer treatments will allow treatment regimens to be tailored to the patient, reducing side effects, as specific genes often control the metabolism of drugs (34).

- Evidence-based medicine is gaining support from many groups as the foundation for healthcare reform and the future of medicine.

GLOSSARY

Actuarial data Information used by an actuary to make projections regarding service utilization in order to determine the financial risk of providing the service.

Age/sex rating A method of structuring capitation payments based on membership enrollee age and sex.

Algorithm A binary decision tree using patient response to intervention and other information to guide stepwise treatment of a specific problem.

Bioinformatics The science of developing computer databases and algorithms for the purpose of speeding up and enhancing biological research.

Capitation A predetermined, fixed amount paid to providers in return for rendering a specified set of health services. The payment is usually on a per-member-per-month basis related to the number of patients enrolled in the health plan.

Carve out Services and procedures that are defined by contract to be separate and apart from the negotiated capitation rate that are typically paid on a fee-for-service (FFS) basis.

Catchment/market/service area A specific service area defined by geographic boundaries targeted by health plans, providers, and service networks to market products and services.

Clinical pathways Practice guidelines for patient care that have been adapted to local conditions to standardize treatment.

Coinsurance The percentage split of the agreed-upon cost sharing ratio between a health plan participant and the insurer or employer. Usually the employer assumes 80% and the employee assumes 20%.

Community-based rating A method of calculating insurance premiums based on the combined experience of multiple groups within a geographic region adjusted for age, sex, and high risk.

Composite rate A uniform premium that applies to all eligible members in a subscriber group regardless of the number of dependents covered. Commonly used with labor unions and large employer groups.

Consolidation An internal laboratory system strategy to reduce cost by eliminating the duplication of services and excess capacity, restructuring of the work flow, implementing changes in staff resources, and centralizing operation management.

Consumer In healthcare, the consumer is the patient. The patient is sometimes also an employee, a subscriber, or a beneficiary.

Contract mix The distribution of enrollees by number of dependents (single, double, family).

Copayment (copay) A fixed dollar amount paid by the subscriber to the provider at the time of services.

Critical pathways Written criteria to guide care based on standards of practice, delineating necessary treatment and facilitating appropriate use of resources (also referred to as clinical pathway).

Data mining Sorting through data to identify patterns and establish relationships. Data mining parameters include the following:

- **Association.** Looking for patterns where one event is connected to another event.

- **Sequence or path analysis.** Looking for patterns where one event leads to another later event.

- **Classification.** Looking for new patterns (may result in a change in the way the data are organized, but that's okay).

- **Clustering.** Finding and visually documenting groups of facts not previously known.

- **Forecasting.** Discovering patterns in data that can lead to reasonable predictions about the future.

Deductible The amount of medical expense that the insured must pay before the insurer assumes liability for all or part of the remaining cost of the covered service.

Deficit Reduction Act of 1984 Public law that authorized the Medicare clinical laboratory fee schedule and mandated that the laboratory actually performing the testing, not the physician who ordered the testing, bill Medicare for the services directly (direct billing requirement).

Diagnosis-related group Classification system developed at Yale University that defines 467 major diagnostic categories and places patients into case types based on the International Classification Disease (ICD-9-CM) code classifications (54).

Direct billing Medicare mandate that claims for laboratory services be submitted by the laboratory rendering the service and not billed by the provider that ordered the test.

DNA sequencing A method used to determine the order of base pairs along a stretch of DNA.

Economy of scale Whenever output is increased without increasing the cost of production, economy of scale is achieved.

Electronic medical record Documentation of the patient care treatment experience in an electronic format.

Evidence-based medicine The application of current best evidence from clinical research to the management of patient care, taking into account patient preferences and the physician's experienced judgment. The practice of evidence-based medicine allows for the judicious integration of literature, clinical experience, and the patient's understanding and needs.

Experience rating A method of calculating insurance premiums based on the experience of one group in terms of claims submitted.

Fee for service (FFS) The method of reimbursing providers a fee for each unit of service provided rather than by capitation, case rate, or per-diem payment. Payment may be based on a percentage of charges or an agreed-upon fee schedule.

Fixed rate The negotiated payment rate for a service or group of services linked to a diagnosis code or procedure that is paid either prospectively or retrospectively.

Gap analysis A study of the differences between systems, procedures, or applications, often for the purpose of determining how to get from the current state to a new state. The analysis defines the space between where we are and where we want to be, bridging the gap.

Gatekeeper The primary care provider (PCP) responsible for managing the healthcare of a health maintenance organization (HMO) enrollee.

Gene therapy The introduction of therapeutic genes into cells to treat or cure disease.

Genotype All or part of the genetic constitution of an individual.

Group practice without walls When two or more physician groups share the costs of a lease for an office space. Each group has assigned days of the week for use of the space. This time-sharing business arrangement enables physician groups to expand their service area and eliminates the duplication of lease expenses for the entire month.

Healthplan Employer Data and Information Set (HEDIS) A survey methodology developed by the National Committee for Quality Assurance (NCQA) that standardizes the quality performance data the managed-care organizations provide to NCQA. HEDIS allows NCQA to compare managed-care organizations and issue report cards on the quality of services they offer.

Kanban A Japanese system that monitors production line, inventory, consumer demand, and feedback to deliver goods and services just in time (8).

Ligase chain reaction A DNA sequence amplification reaction using thermostable DNA ligase.

Mapping The method used to determine the chromosomal location of a gene.

Outcome An outcome is a measured change or event that reflects the status of a patient during a defined period (for example, death, the onset of symptoms, the disappearance of symptoms, discharge, readmission, complications, or diagnosis).

Payor Any third-party insurance company that sells traditional indemnity and managed-care products to group purchasers, large and small employers, and private individuals for healthcare coverage.

PCR A technique for amplifying millions of times a single target DNA sequence using thermostable DNA polymerase so it can be detected and studied more easily.

Per diem The negotiated daily reimbursement rate for services provided for inpatient hospital services. The rates are negotiated specific to the type of service rendered (for example, general medical, surgical, or intensive care).

Point of Service A managed-care plan with reduced benefits that allows the enrollee to select services and benefits at the point of service for a network, prepaid plan and an out-of-network,

FFS plan. The out-of-network plan usually carries a copayment that is a percentage of the FFS charges to the health plan.

Progressive rates A method used by some HMOs in which they implement new rates monthly, quarterly, or semiannually when contracting with large employer subscriber groups.

Prospective payment system A method for payment by Medicare for hospital inpatient services, in which the payment is according to the diagnosis-related group classification of the discharge, that was enacted by the Social Security Amendments of 1983 (Public Law 98-21).

Purchasers Buying groups, employers, or individuals who purchase healthcare policies from third-party payors (insurers).

Referral A recommendation by the primary-care physician that a member receive services from another network provider. It is a notification process and not a review to establish medical necessity.

Regionalization A system of laboratories capable of providing services to a larger geographic area. Regional systems allow the aligned laboratories to market the combined strengths of the collective testing menus to keep more tests within the regional system and eliminate referrals outside of the system, positioning the regional laboratory system to compete for managed-care contracts.

Resource-based relative value system A system of reimbursement that reimburses providers for the true cost or value of the services they provide. True cost and value are determined using a formula that multiplies a relative value unit by a monetary conversion factor. The relative value unit rates the value of the actual cost of the service based on a physician cost component (work), a practice cost component (overhead), and a malpractice cost component. The cost-based approach more closely approximates a normal, competitive market than charge-based systems.

Restructuring Tactical measures used in laboratory consolidation include downsizing, point-of-care testing, consolidating work at benches, and interdisciplinary teams on utilization.

Risk pool A portion of provider fees or capitation payments that are withheld as financial reserves to cover unanticipated utilization of services.

Risk sharing The process of establishing financial arrangements, utilization controls, and other mechanisms to share the financial risks of providing care among providers, payors, and users.

Stop-loss A provision within a health plan that limits the members' or providers' out-of-pocket expense to a maximum allowance.

Tax Equity and Fiscal Responsibility Act of 1982 Public Law 97-248, which established payment for inpatient stays for Medicare beneficiaries based on diagnosis-related groups and introduced the clinical laboratory competitive bidding demonstration project.

Telecommunication Voice, video, or data information is transmitted from one location to another using integrated services digital networks, phone lines, T1 (fiber optic) lines, or digital subscriber lines or various forms of wireless communication (74).

Telemedicine The practice of medicine using telecommunication technology to transmit data, sound, and images between two or more distant sites.

Telepathology The practice of pathology using telecommunication technology to link patients with pathologists and other healthcare providers.

Universal access The concept that all persons, regardless of health or economic status, have access to a minimal, standard package of healthcare benefits that provides quality healthcare.

Usual, customary, and reasonable fees Fees paid to a physician under one of the following conditions:

- If the charge does not exceed the "usual" charge from his office
- If the charge does not exceed the amount "customarily" charged by other physicians in the area
- If the charge is otherwise "reasonable" (17)

Utilization management The concurrent or prospective process of monitoring, assessing, and controlling the utilization of healthcare services to promote efficiency and quality. The process includes review of length of stay, admission rates, coordination of physician and nonphysician services, and use of services like emergency room, laboratory, pharmacy, and radiology.

Utilization review A retrospective healthcare assessment tool used by managed-care organizations to ensure that their members have received appropriate quality services. Admissions, length of stay, and utilization of services are included.

Withhold A payment method that withholds a percentage of a negotiated payment in a reserve fund for specialty provider contracts. Annually, if the negotiated quality and cost criteria have been met, the portion of the fee that was withheld is returned according to the risk-bearing terms of the contract.

REFERENCES

1. **Allawi, S. J., B. T. Hill, and N. R. Shah.** 1998. New frontiers for diagnostic testing: taking advantage of force changing healthcare. *Clin. Lab. Manag. Rev.* **12:**3–7.

2. **Appold, K.** 2002. Legislative update: law permits more self-referral tests in California. *Vantage Point* **6**(9):1–3.

3. **Appold, K.** 2002. Laboratorians find the future on the information superhighway. *Vantage Point* **6**(3):1–4.

4. **Ayres, K.** 2000. Genetic testing in the new millennium: government agencies and the public working together. *Vantage Point* **4**(9):1–7.

5. **Baldwin, M.** 1986. HMOs' special status an impediment to modernizing the industry, execs say. *Mod. Healthc.* **1986**(1):26.

6. **Beckham, D.** 2001. What to watch for in the next three years as the Internet transforms the health-care landscape. *Clin. Lab. Manag. Rev.* **15:**107–111.

7. **Berger, D.** 1999. A brief history of medical diagnosis and the birth of the clinical laboratory. Part 4—Fraud and abuse, managed care, and lab consolidation. *MLO Med. Lab. Obs.* **31:**38–42.

8. **Berwick, D.** 2000. Knowledge always on-call: for docs, practicing medicine will be providing information more than providing care. *Clin. Lab. Manag. Rev.* **14:**250–252.

9. **Bissell, M.** 1996. Defining laboratory related outcomes measures—establishing a link to patient focused care. *Clin. Lab. Manag. Rev.* **10:**95–97.

10. **Boland, P.** 1993. Quality prerequisites for providers, purchasers, and payors. *Manag. Care Q.* **1**(2):1–3. Aspen Publishers Inc., Gaithersburg, Md.

11. **Boland, P.** 1993. Role and purpose of performance standards. *Manag. Care Q.* **1**(1):1.

12. **Brailer, D.** 2001. Peer-to-peer technology: connection tops collection. *Health Manag. Technol.* **22**(8):28–29.

13. **Combs, K.** 1995. Regional progress toward managed care. *Va. Med. Q.* **1995**(3):159–160.

14. **Cooper, R., and McDonald, Hopkins, Burks and Haber Co., LPA.** 1995. Principal elements of risk arrangements, p. 27–35. *In* Washington G-2 Reports and CLMA's *The Laboratory Guide to Negotiating Managed Care Contracts*. Managed care series. Washington G-2 Reports in association with CLMA, Washington, D.C.

15. **Coopers & Lybrand.** 1993. Health care reform: new choices, new decisions, section II, p. 9. Presented at the Richmond Area Business Group on Health, Inc., 1993 Annual Health Care Conference and Exhibition, Health Care Reform: Adapting to Change, Richmond, Va.

16. **Coopers & Lybrand.** 1993. Health care reform: new choices, new decisions, section II, p. 11. Presented at the Richmond Area Business Group on Health, Inc., 1993 Annual Health Care Conference and Exhibition, Health Care Reform: Adapting to Change, Richmond, Va.

17. **Coopers & Lybrand.** 1993. Health care reform: new choices, new decisions, section IX, p. 76–79. Presented at the Richmond Area Business Group on Health, Inc., 1993 Annual Health Care Conference and Exhibition, Health Care Reform: Adapting to Change, Richmond, Va.

18. **Counts, J. M.** 2001. Washington clinical laboratory initiative: a vision for collaboration and strategic planning for an integrated laboratory system. *Clin. Lab. Manag. Rev.* **15:**97.

19. **Davis, D., L. Connelly, and V. Fuldauer.** 1998. The total package for laboratorians: resource management, clinical guidelines, process improvement, outcomes management. Presented at the Clinical Laboratory Management Association Annual Conference, Philadelphia, Pa.

20. **Dollemore, D.** 2003. Secrets in your blood—skip the doc, order your own tests. *Prevention* **2003**(4):42.

21. **Ellrodt, G., and P. Keckley.** 2001. Evidence based medicine, where medicine and technology meet. *Health Manag. Technol.* **22**(8):44–46.

22. **Friedewald, V. E., Jr., and R. J. Pion.** 2001. Telemedicine: home care returning home. *Health Manag. Technol.* **22**(9):22–26.

23. **Goldsmith, J.** 2000. How will the Internet change our health system? *Health Tracking* **19**(1):148–156.

24. **Gollust, S. E., S. C. Hull, and B. S. Wilfond.** 2002. Limitations of direct-to-consumer advertising for clinical genetic testing. *JAMA* **288:**1762–1767.

25. **Gorman, E.** 2000. The new futures of diagnostic testing. *Clin. Lab. Manag. Rev.* **14:**26–29.

26. **Greene, J.** 1997. Has managed care lost its soul? *Hosp. Health Netw.* **5:**36–42.

27. **Haller, C.** 1997. Managed care contracting from the insurer's perspective, Finger Lakes Blue Cross Blue Shield. Presented at the Executive War College 1997, New Orleans, La.

28. **Halsey, J.** 2000. Direct access testing in the clinical laboratory: should laboratories offer testing services directly to the consumer? *Clin. Leadersh. Manag. Rev.* **14:**261–265.

28a. **Hammer, M., and J. Champy.** 2001. *Re-engineering the Corporation: a Manifesto for Business Revolution.* Harper Business, New York, N.Y.

29. **Harari, O.** 1999. The trust factor. *Clin. Lab. Manag. Rev.* **13:**28–31.

30. **Harty-Golder, B.** 2003. Telemedicine: look before you leap. *MLO Med. Lab. Obs.* **35:**40.

31. **Hirschman, S.** 1994. Merger mania strikes MCOs, but is bigger better, or will it be harmful to market competition? *Manag. Healthc.* **1994:**5.

32. **Holton, J.** 2002. Viewpoint: meeting the needs of the pay-at-the-pump generation. *Health Manag. Technol.* **23**(1)**:**78–79.

33. **Kant, J.** 2001. Molecular diagnostics: promise, pain for labs. *Adv. Admin. Lab.* **10:**14.

34. **Katz, F.** 2002. Genetic testing in mainstream medicine. *Lab. Med.* **33:**501–504.

35. **Kennedy, M., and R. Pickett.** 1997. Will your laboratory be ready for the future? *Clin. Lab. Manag. Rev.* **11:**233.

36. **Kost, G.** 1998. Optimizing point of care testing in clinical systems management. *Clin. Lab. Manag. Rev.* **12:**361–362.

37. **Kraft, C.** 2001. Who's managing whom? The silent generation, boomers, Xers, and the newly evolving millennials. *Vantage Point* **5**(2)**:**1–7.

38. **Kuriyan, J.** 2001. HIPAA and MCOs: administrative simplification or IT modernization? *Health Manag. Technol.* **22**(10)**:**40–41.

38a. **Laboratory Industry Report.** 2000. **9**(9)**:**7. Washington G-2 Reports, Washington, D.C.

39. **Lehmann, C.** 2002. Management of point-of-care testing in home health care. *Clin. Leadersh. Manag. Rev.* **16:**27–30.

40. **Lips, Bradley and Harris, Geoffrey, CFA.** 1995. The clinical laboratory industry. New opportunities from a changing competitive environment, no. 12, p. 14. SmithBarney, Traveler's Group, New York, N.Y.

41. **Logue, J.** 2002. Pharmacogenetic testing, coverage, and coding. *Vantage Point* **6**(10/11)**:**1, 6–8.

42. **Louie, R. F., Z. Tang, and G. J. Kost.** 2001. Trends in POCT—a glimpse into the future of this new paradigm of distributed testing. *Adv. Admin. Lab.* **10:**26–32.

43. **Lovic, R., and J. Gentry.** 1984. *Dimensions in Healthcare*, p. 1–5. Peat, Marwick, Mitchell & Co., Philadelphia, Pa.

44. **Marques, M., and J. McDonald.** 2000. Defining, measuring the value of clinical information. *Clin. Lab. Manag. Rev.* **14:**275–278.

45. **McClatchey, K.** 2002. Perspectives in pathology—advances in molecular pathology. *Adv. Admin. Lab.* **11:**14.

46. **Michel, R.** 2002. Disease management relies on lab testing. *Dark Rep.* **9**(15)**:**16–17.

47. **Michel, R.** 1997. Regional lab systems beginning to emerge. *Dark Rep.* **4**(7)**:**5–14.

48. **Michel, R.** 2003. Hospital mergers down for fourth straight year. *Dark Rep.* **10**(3)**:**10–11.

48a. **Miller, J. E.** 2001. A Perfect Storm: the Confluence of Forces Affecting Health Care Coverage. National Coalition on Health Care, Washington, D.C.

49. **Monahan, C.** 1997. Special feature: is disease screening worth it? *Vantage Point* **1**(8)**:**1–3.

50. **National Intelligence Report.** 2002. Focus on: the healthcare crisis. *Nat. Intel. Rep.* **23**(15)**:** 4–6.

51. **Neuhauser, P., and R. Bender.** 1998. Merging, partnering, and restructuring: coping with culture clashes. *Clin. Lab. Manag. Rev.* **12:**405–409.

52. **O'Neal, W.** 1998. Focus on genetic testing—the laboratory's piece of the genetic testing puzzle. *Vantage Point* **2**(15/16)**:**1–3.

53. **Parrot, J.** 1998. Proactive management in the managed care era. *Clin. Lab. Manag. Rev.* **12:**310–312.

54. **Professional and Economic Affairs Committee.** 1999. *Professional Relations Manual*, 11th ed., p. 254-263. College of American Pathologists, Northfield, Ill.

55. **Rainer, R.** 2000. Is telepathology right for your lab? *Adv. Admin. Lab.* **9:**53–57.

56. **Reichheld, F.** 1993. Loyalty-based management. *Harv. Bus. Rev.* **1993**(3)**:**64–73.

57. **Salk, J., and F. Ray.** 1997. The buoyancy of laboratory networks. *Adv. Admin. Lab.* **6:**76–80.

58. **Salomon, Smith Barney.** 2002. Industry overview, Fig. 22. *Salomon, Smith Barney Equity Research Report.* Reprinted with permission for Lab Institute 2002 in Washington, D.C.

59. **Skjei, E.** 2002. Getting ready for the bioinformatics shakeup. *CAP Today* **16**(8)**:**1–6.

60. **Soloway, H. B.** 1995. Establishing a direct laboratory access program. *Clin. Chem.* **41:**809–812.

61. **Solz, H.** 2001. Disease management: getting better all the time. *Health Manag. Technol.* **22**(9)**:**42–44.

62. **South, S.** 1999. Seeking the competitive advantage: it's more than cost reduction. *Clin. Lab. Manag. Rev.* **13:**173–177.

63. **Swisher, K., J. Begun, and D. Ulmer.** 1999. Hospital-physician relationships in the integrated delivery system: an ethical analysis. *Clin. Lab. Manag. Rev.* **13:**3–11.

64. **Titus, K.** 1999. Future of self-test market not in the bag. *CAP Today* **13**(6)**:**1–10.

65. **Trigon Blue Cross and Blue Shield.** 1996. *Trigon Blue Cross and Blue Shield Professional Provider Manual*, p. 39–41. Trigon Blue Cross and Blue Shield, Richmond, Va.

66. **Trigon Blue Cross and Blue Shield.** 1996. *Trigon Blue Cross and Blue Shield Professional Provider Manual*, p. 74–75. Trigon Blue Cross and Blue Shield, Richmond, Va.

67. **Walker, A., and B. Ziegler.** 1997. Quality and outcomes management: what is the laboratory's role. *Probe*, Module 9: *Outcomes Management*, p. 1–8. CLMA, Wayne, Pa.

68. **Weber, L. J., and Bissell, M. G.** 1998. Case studies in ethics—consent and confidentiality in genetic research. *Clin. Lab. Manag. Rev.* **12:**435–436.

69. **Weber, L. J.** 2000. Access to medical information: 10 ethical guidelines. *Clin. Leadersh. Manag. Rev.* **14:**280–283.

70. **Wedlund, P.** 2001. The cost of genetic testing. *Adv. Admin. Lab.* **10:**20.

71. **Wilkinson, D. S.** 2000. Technology assessment: measuring the outcomes of laboratory practice. *Clin. Lab. Manag. Rev.* **14:**267–271.

72. **Wills, S.** 2000. The 21st century laboratory: information technology and healthcare. *Clin. Lab. Manag. Rev.* **14:**289–291.

73. **Wilson, M. J.** 1998. Enhancing managed care opportunities of group practices. *Health Care Finance* **24:**65–77.

74. **Yablonsky, T.** 2000. Bringing healthcare and education within reach—distance learning, telepathology transform laboratory medicine. *Lab. Med.* **31:**198–205.

75. **Zeiger, B.** 1997. Ethics: genes, clones, and other "neat stuff." Special interview with Arthur Caplan. *Vantage Point* **1**(14):1–6.

76. **Zeiger, B.** 1998. At the wheel of a point-of-care program. *Probe,* Module 14: *Point of Care Testing,* p. 1–6. CLMA, Wayne, Pa.

77. **Zeiger, B.** 1998. A closer look at alternative medicine: considering the alternative. *Vantage Point* **2**(15/16):4–6.

78. **Zeiger, B.** 1998. Say hello to the future. *Probe,* Module 24: *Laboratory Trends for 1999—A Look Ahead,* p. 2–10. CLMA, Wayne, Pa.

79. **Zneimer, S.** 2002. The Human Genome Project: exploring its progress and successes and the ethical, legal, and social implications. *Clin. Leadersh. Manag. Rev.* **16:**151–157.

ADDITIONAL SUGGESTED READING AND RESOURCES

Beazley, D. 1998. Designing an outpatient laboratory requisition to reduce suspended claims. *Clin. Lab. Manag. Rev.* **12:**438–449.

Bernstein, L. H., and F. I. Scott, Jr. 1997. Strategic considerations in clinical laboratory management: a laboratory leadership role in clinical pathways—establishing the laboratory's direct contribution to the institution's performance. *Clin. Lab. Manag. Rev.* **11:**116–124.

Blanchard, M. R. 1997. High impact process redesign: the art of leading radical change. Presented at the Clinical Laboratory Management Association Annual Conference and Exhibition, Toronto, Ontario, Canada.

Braley, G. 1997. What's the Internet and how can I use it? Presented at the Clinical Laboratory Management Association Annual Conference and Exhibition, Toronto, Ontario, Canada.

Cooper, R. S., and J. P. Wood. 1997. The art of contract negotiation. *Adv. Admin. Lab.* **6:**100–106.

Dress, A. 2002. Lab-on-a-chip: platform in development. *Adv. Admin. Lab.* **11:**54–58.

Eisenberg, D. 2002. The coming job boom: the help wanted ads may look thin—but thanks to aging baby boomers, that's about to change. *Insights* **2002**(8):41–44. (Reprinted with permission from Time Inc.)

Elevitch, F. R. 1998. CE update—laboratory economics I. Impact of managed care on laboratory economics. *Lab. Med.* **29:**747–752.

Jahn, M. 1995. The managed care era strikes the lab. Part I. *MLO Med. Lab. Obs.* **27:**35–43.

Jahn, M. 1995. Dying for care: capitation and it discontents. Part II. *MLO Med. Lab. Obs* **27:**57–60.

Keiser, J. F., and B. J. Howard. 1998. Critical pathways: design, implementation, and evaluation. *Clin. Lab. Manag. Rev.* **12:**317–331.

Kimball, M. C. 1993. Future is now for healthcare reform. *CAP Today* **7**(1):1–4.

Kisner, H. 1999. "Home brew" laboratory tests. *Clin. Lab. Manag. Rev.* **13:**104–106.

Kurec, A. S. 1998. Telemedicine: emerging opportunities and future trends. *Clin. Lab. Manag. Rev.* **12:**364–371.

Lehmann, C., and A. M. Leiken. 2000. Diagnostic technology for laboratories in an integrated delivery system. *Clin. Leadersh. Manag. Rev.* **14:**118–123.

Lewis, M., J. Quinn, and P. Goldstein. 2002. Mapping your HIPAA compliance itinerary. Analysis & perspective. *BNA's Health Care Policy Rep.* **2002**(9):35.

Lieder, K. W. 1999. Excitement builds in molecular biology. *Adv. Admin. Lab.* **8:**50–52.

McGlennen, R. 1999. Microminiaturization: technology in the palm of your hand. *Adv. Admin. Lab.* **8:**31–33.

Michel, R., and R. J. Carlson. 2002. Newsmaker interviewer: laboratories sit squarely between new genetics and today's medicine. *Dark Rep.* **9**(18):3–21.

Poeggel, J. 2000. The lab on the Internet: is it safe? *Vantage Point* **4**(17):1–3.

Sandrick, K. 2000. For HEDIS to succeed, MCOs must get a read on lab's needs. *CAP Today* **14**(7):30–38.

Sodeman, T. 1997. The integrated delivery system: opportunities for leadership. *Clin. Lab. Manag. Rev.* **11:**310–317.

Strazzella, M. P., and A. J. Walsh. 1998. Microscope on Washington: Congress and states delve into genetic concerns. *Lab. Med.* **29:**140–142.

Venner, A. 1997. A method for capitation rate calculation using financial data readily available to the laboratory manager. *Clin. Lab. Manag. Rev.* **11:**382–387.

Walker, A., and B. Zeiger. 1997. Roundtable—ethical dilemmas in genetic testing. *Lab. Med.* **28:**311–315.

Weber, L. J., and M. G. Bissell. 1996. Case studies in ethics: the ethics of billing. *Clin. Lab. Manag. Rev.* **10:**409–411.

Wisecarver, J. 1997. The ABCs of DNA. *Lab. Med.* **28:**48–51.

Yablonsky, T. 1997. Genetic testing helps patients and researchers predict the future. *Lab. Med.* **28:**316–322.

Zeiger, B. 1997. A crystal ball for healthcare. *Vantage Point* **1**(11):4–6.

APPENDIX 7.1 WEBSITES

http://www.ascls.org: American Society of Clinical Laboratory Science. Site last accessed January 2004.

http://www.ascp.org: American Society of Clinical Pathology. Site last accessed January 2004.

http://www.atmeda.org: American Telehealth Association. Site last accessed January 2004.

http://www.atsp.org: Association of Telehealth Service Providers, in Portland, Oreg. Site last accessed January 2004.

http://www.cap.org: College of American Pathology. Site last accessed January 2004.

http://www.phppo.cdc.gov/dls/genetics/: CDC—Division of Laboratory Systems Laboratory Genomics Branch. Site last accessed January 2004.

http://healthcheckusa.com: Healthcheck USA, an Internet-based company that brokers DAT for participating laboratories. Site last accessed January 2004.

http://www.healthfutures.net: The website for Health Futures, Inc., and health futurist Jeff Goldsmith, President. Site last accessed January 2004.

http://www.hl7.org: Health Level Seven. Site last accessed January 2004.

http://labtestsonline.org: Lab Tests Online, a public resource on clinical lab testing. Site last accessed January 2004.

http://www.labautomation.org: Association of Laboratory Automation. Site last accessed January 2004.

http://www.mcol.com/ at http://mcareol.com/factshts/mcolfact.htm: Managed Care On Line. Site last accessed January 2004.

http://www.mot.com/bluetooth: Motorola Wireless. Site last accessed January 2004.

http://questest.com: Quest Diagnostics, a large national reference laboratory that offers DAT. Site last accessed January 2004.

http://results-direct.com: Results Direct, a hospital-based company that offers DAT via the Internet. Site last accessed January 2004.

http://www.webmd.com: Web MD. Site last accessed January 2004.

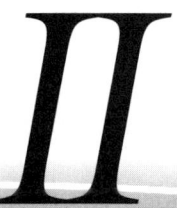

Managerial Leadership

(Section Editor, *John C. H. Steele, Jr.*)

Leadership Styles

Riley M. Sinder and Dean Williams

OBJECTIVES

To help managers identify their personal leadership strengths and opportunities

To help the reader assess when leadership is lacking from either management or the exercise of authority

To provide a better sense for when to exercise authority and when to delegate authority

To enable the reader to discern whether a delegation of authority is sufficient to support an assignment of responsibility

To help the reader improve in his or her ability to change leadership style without taking events too personally

---

All style is gesture, the gesture of the mind and of the soul. Mind we have in common, inasmuch as the laws of right reason are not different for different minds. Therefore clearness and arrangement can be taught, sheer incompetence in the art of expression can be partly remedied. But who shall impose laws upon the soul?

WALTER RALEIGH, STYLE, 1896

W**E BEGIN WITH THE IDEA** that you can change your style of leadership much like you can change your wardrobe. Furthermore, you might alter your leadership style depending on the occasion. Leadership style would include the method, approach, personal details, and mannerisms that affect group problem-solving processes and the accomplishment of tasks in an organization.

But let's be practical. Before you change your leadership style, you need a chance to try the nuance. You need to see how people react to it. If you change your wardrobe, you need at least a mirror. And if you are making a big change, you need to see how it comes across in a real-enough situation before you would try it at work.

How could you get a view of what a change in your leadership style might be? What would serve as a "mirror" for you when you think about changing your leadership style? And where would you practice the new moves and nuances of changing your leadership style?

It would be nice if each of you could attend one of the leadership courses that we give. These leadership courses provide a series of safe experimental situations in which you could "try out" various leadership styles. Since that is not feasible, we will do what we can do with words to build for you a metaphor for planning and evaluating changes in your leadership style.

Imagine that we could provide you with a leadership simulator, like a flight simulator, so that you could practice different leadership maneuvers. By our estimation, current technology could not manufacture the leadership simulation device we describe below. But, we suggest, the reflection you will do as you follow the metaphor can exercise your ability to do leadership diagnosis and evaluate alternatives for your own leadership style.

If the leadership simulator would construct accurately for you the sights, sounds, and reactions of your current workplace, then you could experiment with such leadership techniques as pushing people more than you do, comforting people more than you do, or jolting people more than you do to remind them of their own ideals. And to the extent that the leadership simulator would model accurately the responses of the people in your organization, then you could get a practical feeling for the different results you could get from different leadership styles.

How would a leadership simulator work? The leadership simulator might consist of a helmet, gloves, and body armor connected to a computer. We provide a few details to make the metaphor more real for you.

Imagine you are standing in front of the people who look to you for "leadership" in your organization. To begin the simulation, you put on the helmet, and the computer projects a three-dimensional picture to the inside of the faceplate so that you see the people in your organization exactly as they appear when they stand in front of you. The computer even removes the shadow from the inside of the helmet so that you have your natural peripheral vision in the scene. And the computer generates the sounds of your organization and sends them to the earphones in the helmet so that you hear the individual voices that you recognize.

Most importantly, the computer simulates the individuals in your organization with exactly the conflicting values, priorities, and interests that they have. So, you can expect the experience of leadership in the simulation of your organization to be exactly what you experience in your real-world attempts to exercise leadership.

Do you see the advantage of the simulator? You can run the scenario over and over as you plan and do different things to get better results from your organization. When you want to try out a different leadership style, you can press the reset button at the top of the helmet. And in the more difficult leadership quagmires of a simulation, you can save at any time and replay that section. You have the option of being more flexible when your coworkers try to convince you, and you can compare the organizational results with the outcome when you play the scene with a rigid or domineering leadership style.

When you consider getting better results from your organization, you might consider changing your leadership style. And we will use the metaphor of the leadership simulator to assist you in reflecting on which changes in your leadership style might trigger the greatest improvements in the results in your organization.

Patterns of Leadership Style

We present the leadership simulations that follow to illustrate some of the ways that the leadership style of the senior managers can affect the quality of performance in the organization. You will first play the role of a senior manager, and then you will play the role of a junior manager to get a sense of how your leadership style as senior manager can coordinate with your junior manager's decisions to shape the performance and quality in your organization.

The first leadership simulation is titled "You Hire an Inexperienced Manager." As the simulation begins, you are preparing for an initial meeting with Emily New, a group leader you have selected recently for your hematology unit. You are looking through Emily's personnel folder again and making notes on the points you want to discuss with Emily. You notice that Emily has been a star performer with innovative ideas, high productivity, and a very professional attitude. But apparently this is her first chance to manage a team.

You have a unique opportunity to influence Emily's leadership style. You might focus on your relationship with Emily, you might focus on the job that has to be done, or you might focus on job history. These three different focuses might be characterized, respectively, as a relationship, task, or expertise orientation. And you might consider the likely different effects that would result from your different choices for emphasis.

As Emily comes into your office, you have further options for personal detail that you might add to your role of boss. You might congratulate her, you might welcome her to the management team, or you might begin by asking her what her family did over the weekend. Some people use talk about family as a deliberate technique of leadership style to get on friendly terms. Each of those options might be part of a number of different leadership styles, just as a particular blazer might be part of a number of different ensembles in a wardrobe. You might do all three options, in different orders.

What should be your approach to choosing your options? We suggest that you need to watch for real-time clues to the effects that you are having.

Suppose you choose to begin with a brief exchange of what your families did over the weekend. Then you tell her briefly what you will value highly in what she does. You have several options at this point. You might stress the performance of her team; you might emphasize that your door is always open. Or you might explain that you will give her a gold star if she does a job well, but that you give her *two* gold stars if the people that work for her get your praise. You might do each of those in that order.

Why might you explain to a new manager that you will rate her extra high when a person that works for her gets your praise? To develop an answer to that question, think about playing that same leadership simulation from the role of the new manager. This simulation is titled "You Take the Leadership Style of Your Boss Seriously." As the simulation begins, this time you are Emily New, and you have just had your first meeting with your new boss.

On your way back to your new office, an ambitious young man on your team congratulates you but then adds as if it is a joke, "The boss should have picked *me*, but I know the boss wants to promote women." You both laugh, but you wish he had not said that. During the following weeks, you notice that he tells several jokes making fun of women, and some women on your team object. You have several options. You can try to ignore the troubling jokes. Alternatively, you could ask the ambitious young man to your office and, in private, tell him in very certain but friendly terms that you will insist that he not tell jokes that offend women during work hours in the lab. Suppose you choose to do nothing about the troubling jokes. (If you replay this portion of the simulation several times, you may see that, to the extent that you had power to make some change in the situation, both your use and your nonuse of that power are interventions that change the outcome in the organization.)

As the simulation proceeds, your team encounters several emergencies, including a growing backlog of samples to be tested. The routine processes and emergencies have overworked you and your team. One day, the ambitious young man comes to your office and offers to stay after hours to see if he can figure out how to set up a computerized procedure that could cut the analysis time by half. Since computerized procedures are your particular area of expertise, and since you are quite sure that you can do a better job than the ambitious young man, you were tempted to do it yourself, perhaps with his help. You feel that you should supervise him, and you know that he would resent it.

But suppose you have taken seriously your boss's statement that management will rate you more highly if the people that work for you get management's praise. You might delegate to the ambitious young man the entire task of implementing the computerized procedure.

Surely, you would praise the ambitious young man when he is successful. His success would cut the work effort required by your whole team. But, when your boss actually lavishes praise on the successful and ambitious young man, check your own feelings. Your specialty is the technical area that the ambitious young man improved. And your boss is praising the man who works for you. You might feel left out, but for your boss's promise.

Right after the session where your boss lavished praise on the ambitious young man, the boss asks you to come to her office. (You might notice in real time the effect of reading "her office." We will touch on the phenomenon of surprise, if any, in the next chapter on employee needs compared to expectations and "hungers.")

On your way to the boss's office, a colleague in another unit stops you in the hall and says, "Are you okay? I hear that your boss was upset with that new computerized procedure." You try to keep a straight face, but you might feel a little like you are in quicksand. You might not know whom you can trust. Maybe your boss has some very bad news for you?

When you enter, your boss says, "Emily, I want to tell you what a good job you did with that ambitious young man." You both laugh. You feel great relief. Then your boss continues, "I want you to know that there are pits out there waiting to catch you. And I don't expect you to know yet when it is that you should come by my office. So I would like to set up weekly meetings with you for a while so that you begin to know how to use my office as a resource. Does that make sense?"

You tell the truth and say, "I'm not sure what you mean. But I sure am glad you called me to talk to you just now. There is a series of puzzling events that I would appreciate your helping me to clarify."

The simulation ends there. And now it is time for reflection.

You may ask at this point, "How can a senior manager have the time to assist all the inexperienced managers?"

We propose the following standard. Anyone who has power in an organization is responsible for the results that the use or nonuse of that power produces in the organization. In particular, the senior manager must manage the calendar to make time for advising inexperienced managers—with a realistic view of the trade-offs for the performance of the organization.

And we know that it might be easy to postpone the vague work with the inexperienced managers. All the technical problem solving that crosses the desks of upper management is mesmerizing and consuming.

But, we suggest, the leadership style of the inexperienced managers has an enormous effect on the quality of work in the organization. And, if the senior managers do not shape the leadership style of the inexperienced managers, then who will, we ask (7)?

Two Contrasting Styles of Leadership and Many Between

What management style gets quality results? We suggest that the good answer to that question depends on the situation in your organization. We might contrast (i) a directive style with (ii) "requiring the employees to manage themselves." At times a directive style is the most efficient means of getting quality results. Think of various situations in an emergency room of an urban hospital. In the moment of action, there is usually one physician that makes the decisions. The rest of the team is there to provide sufficient information to the decision maker and to carry out the decisions of the decision maker.

Notice that there is a vast repertoire of tested procedures for dealing with the situations that arise in emergency rooms. There exist solid data and knowledge about the probable quality of outcome of the various decisions that the autocrat of the emergency room can make. To use our metaphor of the leadership simulator, people all over the world have played the "emergency room" scenario so many times that there are published strategies that a novice can learn to repeat to get similar results of quality.

So we will call the emergency room situations technical problems because the existing repertoire of tested procedures can resolve those problems to the satisfaction of the current values in the society. Accordingly, a directive style may get high-quality work from a team that faces only technical problems, the kinds of problems that the current repertoire of tested procedures can solve. And we note that the quality of effort required of the team is technical work characterized by conscientiousness and diligence in implementing the tested procedures; that is, the team does not go through an upheaval of reexamining its fundamental values and deciding which values it can sacrifice to get some progress.

But we suggest that the tested procedures in the current repertoire fail to resolve many problems. And some of these unsolved problems become an issue in the organization when enough individuals hold values that insist that the organization should address the unsolved problems.

We make an analogy with the problem-solving processes of evolution. Every species has a repertoire of tested procedures for dealing with the threats of a particular environment, namely, the environment that honed the problem-solving skills of the species. And as long as the environment is stable and offers the same set of threats, the species survives. That is, the technical solutions of the existing repertoire deliver sufficient quality to satisfy the values that forced the species to develop its current structure, tendencies, and responses.

However, changes in the environment can contract the territory of a species to a mere niche, unless the species evolves a new set of responses that take into consideration the changes in the environment. For example, the rising of antibiotics in the 1950s threatened to reduce some bacteria to a mere niche, but several bacterial species evolved new responses to resist antibiotics. That is, the introduction of antibiotics required an adaptation, not just a mere enforcement of inherited procedures for dealing with the environment. Furthermore, as in the case of evolving bacteria, an effective adaptation is not merely a change, but rather a change that actually resolves the threat and takes advantage of what the environment offers.

We note that in evolution, adaptive change introduces a much greater degree of trial and error than does mere routine problem solving. In adaptive change, each shift is an experiment that generates the data on whether or not the shift is effective.

Below we associate leadership with experimenting by trial and error to see what actually gets employees to tackle tough problems. At times, an autocratic style might get employees to tackle tough problems. But, we suggest, when the existing repertoire of tested procedures cannot solve the problem, then an autocratic style can be detrimental.

As an extreme comparison to an autocratic style, we might consider "letting the employees manage themselves," a laissez-faire style—from the French term that economists use to express a trust that unregulated individual decisions can accumulate to maximize results for the society as a whole. But, as we consider further in the next chapter, employees who work together in the same physical environment may need at least the symbol of a strong "boss" to coordinate their work even though the "boss" may give the employees considerable freedom in making choices.

Elements of Leadership Style that You Can Learn To Command

As we will see in the scenario that follows, the manager who takes the quality of the organization seriously must consider the autocratic style to be but a trial that must be abandoned if it turns out to be an error. This leadership simulation is titled, "Change the Style to Get the Results." When you put on the helmet of the leadership simulator, the simulation begins.

You are Greg Jefe, the supervisor of a team of five technical experts that run special analyses on a variety of advanced equipment. In addition, your team develops advanced procedures for the rest of the laboratory. Technology is always changing. New processes are reported weekly in your journals. The job is exciting, and you are the hero of your team. Your team is very professional and tight-knit, generously offering to help others in the laboratory when the computers or measurement devices do not work as expected. In a very real way, you and your team are the brains of the whole laboratory. So your span of influence extends far beyond your job description. You love it.

Nevertheless, you have decided to make the big move to upper management. You have accepted an offer to be the Director of Specimen Analysis for a referral laboratory which does the specimen testing under contract for several hospitals nearby. At first, you assume that the new job will be very similar to your old job. Instead of having only 5 people under your control, you will now have 80. But you know what it will be like, you think, because in your old job you took care of troubleshooting the equipment and processes for 80 people.

However, you find at the new job that the people are different, the culture is different, and the business is different. Your boss is negotiating a deal to expand from the one laboratory site to four additional sites by acquisition.

The immediate problems are low productivity and high error rates. You schedule a meeting with your supervisors. You have several options for that meeting. You might walk into the meeting with an agenda that you try to sell to them. Or you might throw the problem on the table and make your supervisors come up with an answer. You decide that you will lead by example.

Your supervisors like your idea; they all vote for trying first the style of leading by example. You and your supervisors organize "pep sessions" with the employees to address low productivity. And you and your supervisors stay at work until the job gets done. You are giving good examples for the troops. Nonsupervisory employees get generous overtime.

But you and your supervisors end up doing too much of the work yourselves. Productivity and error rates do not improve. You have several options. A consultant tells you that you should be more forceful.

You decide that you will try an autocratic style. You get your supervisors in the mood by being autocratic with *them.* You will punish offenders. You produce reports of productivity and error rate by person. You and your supervisors have meetings with underperformers and error makers. And you try to issue the punishment with a bit of humor; you issue "traffic tickets." The error rate does not go down. Unfortunately, productivity actually decreases because, people tell you, they are too afraid they will make an "error." Furthermore, unplanned absences increase. People say that, when it came time to go to work, they were "too stressed out and couldn't face it."

You have several options. Suppose you decide that you will try a different style.

If you can't win them by vinegar, maybe you can win them with sugar. So you and your supervisors get approval from upper management to offer $500 to anybody who can make their production, attendance, and error rate goals for the month. You call it "leadership by incentive." Dollar incentives may work with some people in some situations, but suppose you find after a year that productivity and error rates are unchanged. So what do you do next?

We suggest a time-out from the scenario to reflect on what has happened to you. You have experienced the frustration of an adaptive challenge—because the problem does not resolve to satisfy the current values in the organization even when management applies the best-known methods and procedures. And at the root of an adaptive challenge, there is often a conflict of values.

You have several options. You might continue to invent technical solutions—intervention plans that (i) assume a fixed statement of the problem and (ii) measure success by fixed criteria defined before the intervention was made. If you look back on the three approaches explored so far in the above scenario, you might find that each of the three variations in leadership style assumed a fixed statement of the problem and measured success by the fixed criteria of whether or not performance and error rates improved. We suggest that these three technical approaches manifest the old style of leadership in which the manager attempts to build sufficient power, expertise, and reputation so that people will see the wisdom in the manager's decision.

We suggest a different approach, an adaptive approach: you might intervene for the purpose of learning what parts of the system need fixing, with the understanding that the "system" that needs fixing will include your own style, priorities, and values. When you (i) intervene to learn what the problem is and (ii) measure success by what you have learned for the next intervention, then you have begun an adaptive approach. If you take an adaptive approach, you should have an idea of the turmoil you are likely to cause. People are likely to be upset, because you are insisting that they do adaptive work; you are challenging their values and pointing to areas where they do not live up to their own values.

Suppose you take seriously the possibility that the problems in productivity and error rate manifest an underlying conflict in values, with the understanding that likely your own values hinder the success of the organization in some way.

The Ethical Dimension of Leadership

Because leadership often involves processes that shift the values of employees, you may want to explore your feelings of responsibility for the shifts in values that you make. We suggest for your consideration a practical standard of ethics: managers and employees are better off if they are able to solve to their satisfaction a greater set of problems in their life.

Let us explore the dynamics of how shifts of values among managers and employees occur. After you put on the helmet of the leadership simulator and release the pause button, the simulation continues. Suppose you and your supervisors look again at the conflicting values in the organization. How might you assemble a diagram of the various value sets in your organization?

You might poll each of the employees by questionnaire and by structured interview to get a sense of the values that each individual in your organization protects. You might find that each employee and manager is a representative of a family, cultural, and peer group with a corresponding set of family, cultural, and peer group values. And you might find that the values that the employees import into your organization are in conflict with the values of your workplace.

For example, you might find that over half of your employees are under 35, and you might find that your employees under 35 protect the set of values generally ascribed to their peer group, Generation X. That is, you might find that your employees under 35 generally want to take time off from work on the spur of the moment. In contrast, you might find that your employees over 35 generally want to plan their time off from work far ahead. Perhaps, if you set standards for attendance that will not accommodate the Generation X value of "spontaneity" to the satisfaction of your employees under 35, then you have ignored the real underlying problem, which is a conflict in values.

In a similar fashion, you might consider the cultural and family values of the various ethnic groups of Latinos, Native Americans, African-Americans, Slavs, and others among your employees. You may find that the very production schedule in your laboratory, requiring that over 70% of the work be done on second shift from 5 p.m. to 1 a.m., may conflict with parents wanting to be home for their children.

You have several options. You might attempt to refine the various programs for enforcement of standards that you have already tried. Or you might consider an intervention to learn how to fix the system, keeping in mind that your management style and the design of the workplace may be parts of the system that need fixing.

Suppose your boss actually completes the acquisition of the four other laboratory sites. When you see that the new laboratory sites have similar production and error rate problems, you see that you have a huge system to consider fixing.

If your approach is an adaptive approach—to learn how to fix the system—then you would not want to implement a change to all five laboratory sites at once. You might make an intervention at one site or one module of a site so that you could iterate the following cycle: (i) plan the intervention, (ii) make the intervention, (iii) hold steady to analyze the effect of the intervention, and (iv) plan the next cycle of intervention.

You select one smaller laboratory to generate your learning; your personal learning, your supervisors' learning, and your employees' learning—even learning within the organization, because what you learn will stay behind as corporate "memory" even when you move to your next job. You might first get an overview of the conflicting values of the employees at this particular site. You might find that your employees at this site say that they get little professional or personal reward from their job, other than their paycheck. So you attempt a few experiments to see how you might restructure the workplace and work culture to raise the employees' sense of professional and personal reward from their job. You decide that you will explore low-cost restructuring first.

You have several options. You might devise a system of monetary rewards. Or you might restructure the job descriptions and flow of promotions to give more of an appearance of professional achievement. Suppose you decide to restructure the job descriptions and redesign the pro-

motion system with a view to satisfying the values that your employees bring from their family, cultural, and peer groups. You and your supervisors draw up a plan for a regular 6-month cycle of promotion review. After all, over half of your employees are Generation Xers that put a high value on quick reward for little effort. And you may notice that Generation Xers value highly inserting new technologies into their resumes. So you build in a lot of possible movement between technologies, with enough training, thus redirecting your training budget to accommodate parallel shifts between technologies. Furthermore, you make explicit concessions for attendance to allow for "spontaneous" time off and for family emergencies.

You decide that you must give salary increases with each promotion; otherwise your scheme will have no credibility. However, you design with your payroll department an overall compensation plan that you hope does not increase your overall payroll; you will cut the pay of those with the lowest performance and worst error rate scores. You tie the promotions to performance and error rates, but you design the semiannual award ceremony to be a cultural celebration with an ethnic theme: a fiesta, a cookout, a luau, or an Academy Awards-type ceremony. These might not be what you would sit down and plan yourself, but this is your attempt to satisfy many of the family, cultural, and peer group values that your employees bring to the workplace.

So you try it; then you hold steady to get your employees to generate the data and knowledge you need; then you analyze the situation to see what you can learn about shifting the underlying conflict of values, your own values, and the values of the employees; and then you plan the next intervention. We call this attitude the new style of leadership, attending to the real-time effects that you have on the quality in an organization.

In the simulation, after 1 year of iteratively restructuring the work environment to honor the family, cultural, and peer group values that your employees bring to the workplace, you find surprising improvements in both productivity and error rate. You find that the per-employee productivity has risen by 30% and the average error rate has dropped by 10%. In addition, the annualized turnover rate has dropped by half, reflecting the general impression that "the place has become a better place." Furthermore, the productivity increase results in a 20% drop in labor costs for overtime and temporary contract help. The payroll department informs you that your rapid-advancement program has increased your wage and benefit costs no more than the average annual increases for the last two years.

At the end of the year, you and your supervisors look at the charts, and you look for what it was that made the difference. You decide that what made the difference was management involving the employees in a process wherein management and employees learned to own their fair share of the job to be done. The final design of job descriptions and promotion gimmicks may not matter much.

You have managed a learning process: your own learning process, the learning process of your supervisors, and the learning process of the employees, and the process has generated mutual shifts in values such that the underlying conflicts have decreased.

As the scenario comes to a close, you may pull off the helmet of the leadership simulator and say, "But *that* was just a simulation!"

"Yes," we say, "but there are documented cases very similar to what you just experienced. And they got numbers in real life that were better than what *you* did (2). What we have tried to do is to provide a real-enough simulation so that you get a sense of flying the plane by the seat of your pants; that is what a flight simulator is for. If you did exactly in the simulation what the managers did in the real-life case, you should get the same numbers *they* did—if the situation in the organization was the same as the situation in the simulation."

Let us reflect on this experience. The power that you have in an organization is a resource, for good or evil. But you may not realize the effects that your use or nonuse of your power will create. Hypothetically, if you had a leadership simulator, you could try out different choices in the situations of your organization. Sometimes you might find that there is nothing you can do that will improve the quality in your organization. At other times, you might find that even small gestures make a big difference in the final outcome. Since the small gestures of your leadership style that make a difference to others might not be important to *you*, you may not think of them—unless you practice reflecting with your coworkers to uncover the effects that follow from your actions. We suggest that reflecting with your coworkers on recent events can serve the important functions of a leadership simulator, namely, (i) to give you a chance to consider options other than what you did, (ii) to remind you of the impact of even small gestures that you did not consider to be important, and (iii) to provide you with a wide-angle view of how your actions coordinate with the actions of others to create the organizational outcome.

Evaluating Leadership

How might you organize your managers and employees to improve the leadership in your organization? To explore answers to that question, we offer the following simulation, titled "Organizing Your Allies." As the simulation begins, you are Emily New, now 3 weeks into your new position as group leader in the hematology unit. It is time for your weekly meeting with your boss. Your boss has made it clear to you that she expects you to come prepared to discuss some important issue, a leadership puzzle on your team. You have notes on a new robotics idea that might make it possible to handle the projected increases in number of specimens to be analyzed without increasing staff.

You are looking for ways to cut costs. You think your boss will find that commendable.

After you tell your boss your new idea, she nods and asks you, "Why do you think there is a leadership problem there?"

You say, "Because, how can I convince them? To work right, the whole laboratory and our customer hospitals would have to convert to the new test tubes with the serial numbers integrated into the glass. That way nobody would have to fuss with the labels on the samples—and make errors. The machines would read the serial number in the glass accurately. They would read the serial number at the hospital. And we would read the serial number here. The computers would connect the data, accurately."

"You may be right," she smiles. "But look. I want you to think of this as a leadership challenge. And if you take it as a leadership challenge, your job is not to convince people. Your job is to get people to own the problem and along the way consider your idea together with other ideas for the solution."

"Okay," you say; after all, you are new at this. "I'm game. How could I do that?"

"I suggest you organize allies in the other units. And what I mean by an ally is someone that is not in your chain of command but is someone in your meetings and is someone that you can trust to tell you the truth. You get your ally to debrief you on how you come across in getting other people to own what you think is the problem."

You discuss some other staff issues with your boss, and then you part. You go to your office and think about whom you might get to be a truthful ally in telling you how you come across in trying to get people to own this robotics opportunity that you see.

You consider several people. You consider Jim Tug. He is a tough guy, very critical, and very demanding. He even looks like a wrestler. You are not sure that he would tell you when you do something right.

Then you think of George Balans. You remember a time before your promotion when you and he conspired to organize a sports team, as a means of getting to know the people around you at work personally. When he came up with a plan for a softball team to rival your idea for a bowling team, he told you privately that he thought "they need a little competition to get their interest." So you worked together putting on a "good show" of competition that captured the interest of your coworkers. He did not seem to mind that your idea of a bowling team won in the end; he was one of the first to sign up. Maybe you could work with him on your boss's idea of an "ally," you wonder.

You stop by your boss's office; she is free. "I thought I would talk to George Balans about being my ally."

"Good idea," your boss says. "Just make sure from the beginning that he will tell you what you most need to know. Tell him that you need to know when you do something *well*. You may not notice the times that you electrify your audience for a moment and make them think hard. It would be easy for George to tell you what you did wrong; he has so much experience. Tell him that what you need to know most importantly and first of all is what you did *right*."

George agrees when you ask him to be an ally. And shortly thereafter, at a meeting on integration of services, you bring up your robotics idea. George is there, and you and he have your first discussion session. You have coffee and George has a diet soda in a corner of the employee lounge.

"What do you think?" you ask.

"I think you should have sent around a memo first outlining your idea so that everybody could be prepared."

"Wait! Please, George. I need to know what I did right first."

"Sure. I was amazed at that time in the meeting when you raised your hand, your left hand as I recall, and everybody in the room fell silent."

"Really?" you ask.

"Didn't you notice? It was like even your opponents didn't know why they stopped talking."

George has several other positive comments about your tone of voice, your speaking slowly, and your pausing without reacting when someone cracked a joke in the middle of your sentence. Then you ask George if he will look over a short written summary of your robotics idea that you would like to send out to everybody who was at the meeting. He agrees.

After several meetings and debriefings with George, you notice that you can sometimes glance at him as you are speaking and, in wondering what he has noticed, you find that you are more aware of your own tone of voice, your gestures, and your posture. As time goes on, you pay more attention to the faces of your audience than you did before.

This is the end of that simulation scenario. Let us reflect on occurrences.

We might have started this discussion with a definition for "leadership." But we have reserved the time for stating a formal definition. We first developed some "firsthand data" about "leadership" using the metaphor of a leadership simulator. How would you evaluate your performance in a leadership simulator?

We suggest that, from the many possibilities, you might consider some standard for evaluating your personal leadership in real time. How can you tell at the time of your intervention whether your attempt to exercise leadership scores a 1 or a 10? The moments immediately following your intervention are critical, because you can make corrections then, immediately. But you don't want to shift directions too quickly. Following an intervention, you might impose upon yourself a few minutes of holding steady on the intervention you just made.

Some situations in "leadership" might be like driving a car on ice; you may need to do something, but you don't want to do too much. You cannot lay down the detailed rules beforehand for what you should do, but with experience, you can develop an interactive "feel" for what might work. That is, with practice, you can develop an interactive feel for balance between too little and too much.

To give you an interactive feel for what works in leadership, we suggest that you develop allies in your organization. Your allies can give you important data on what works in your leadership style. And, we suggest, when you focus your attention on what works in your leadership style, you may find that you have less tendency to fall back on the flawed parts of your leadership style. For example, suppose your allies have pointed out to you that people listen more attentively when you speak more slowly and use the lower tones of your voice. If you focus more of your attention on speaking in slower and lower tones, then you will have less tendency to revert to a more frenetic and higher-pitched voice.

Suppose you have willing allies. Must your allies have the same definition of leadership as the one that you use? We suggest that it does not matter as long as your allies will give you their raw data. However, it might be good if you have your own definition of "leadership" that is true for you.

A Manager May Master Many Areas and Fail Leadership

Let us examine what might be the elements of your own definition of "leadership." First, we suggest that you may have an idea of something in your organization that needs fixing. Perhaps there is a new opportunity, such as a new technology that your organization does not use properly. Or there may be a chronic problem that is so tough that your organization has never found a satisfactory response.

Think for a moment about some specific tough problem in your organization. And we ask you the following: Wouldn't it take exceptional "leadership" to mobilize your organization to resolve that tough problem?

Admittedly, you might use your leadership style for purposes other than getting people to fix the organizational flaws that cause the tough problems. But within your current standards for exceptional leadership, would you not agree that the highest score for leadership should go to the person who triggered a process that caused the organization to resolve some tough problem that has caused great distress, among other costs?

If you take seriously the task of getting your organization to fix a problem, it matters greatly whether you have the authority to fix the problem. Greg Jefe in the example above had authority to fix the problems of low productivity and high error rate in the referral hospitals that were under him. In contrast, Emily New in the example above did not have authority to fix the system to take advantage of robotics in her laboratory. So Greg and Emily might have to diagnose the responses of their organizations quite differently. And they might have to apply different leadership strategies to influence the outcome of events. Nevertheless, each might have to mobilize a similar learning process in their organization if they are to fix what needs to be fixed in the organization.

Many people who have little authority to fix the problem in their organization will postpone doing something about it until they have some authority to fix the problem. Many people wait for the coach to give them the call to get onto the field and do something about the problem. In the next chapter, we examine why people wait for authority.

But if you think of yourself in a leadership simulator, having authority means merely that you have more influence over people, and you might expect less flak from people who because of their current values would resist your attempts to fix the problem. That is, within a leadership simulator, you can act with the same mannerisms and inflections of a given leadership style whether you are playing the Greg Jefe scenario with great authority or the Emily New scenario with little authority, but people likely would respond to you differently. That is, to get a similar advance in quality in the organization, you likely must do different things and assess events differently if you have less authority in the organization.

"But can't people respond just to the ideas that I present to them?" you might ask.

"Not likely," we would reply. That is, in many situations, someone like Emily with an inventive technical idea cannot convince her colleagues even when she is right. If the problem is endemic, then it's likely that some people, in light of their current values, will resist even the obvious solutions to the problem. Emily might have to mobilize a learning process in which many of the people involved, including Emily, can learn their way to a new understanding of how their organization should work. Likely, a successful learning process would involve a shift in values and priorities of the people in the organization, including Emily.

Even being a master manager may give Emily merely more power to influence people without making her more effective at getting the organization to solve the problem at hand. She still might have to mobilize a trial-and-error learning process for the people in the organization, including herself. With greater authority, she may have more tools to mobilize the trial-and-error learning process. But Greg Jefe's case illustrates the likelihood that a tough problem will involve a conflict of values that will resist even brilliant technical solutions.

If you are a manager, you have authority to supervise and control what people do within your span of authority. But supervision and control imply that the values of management will dominate. So a manager can be a master at supervision and control without ever addressing the conflict of values that may underlie the tough problems in the organization. We suggest that leadership, different from supervision and control, is required to get progress on tough problems. For example, Greg Jefe found that getting

progress on productivity and error rates followed from leadership that mobilized a learning process for both management and employees.

An Authority May Fail Leadership

Suppose you set yourself the goal of fixing the flaw in your organization that causes some serious problem. For example, your organization may be under a severe budget crunch: revenues may be down and costs may be rising. People in organizations tend to lay the blame for problems elsewhere, somewhere out of their own office.

How can you use the power that you have to trigger action that addresses the problem realistically? As we suggested above, you can make the same intervention with the same style whether or not you have authority to make the intervention. But people likely oppose your ideas more if you have little authority in the organization.

If people respond to your intervention by following your proposal, then you have exercised your authority, your "power to enforce laws, exact obedience, command, determine, or judge" (3). Perhaps some of your authority derives from a well-reasoned argument that people follow. Or perhaps people view you as having the power to punish them if they ignore your "recommendation." Either way, people have let your proposal determine the way that they will go.

We suggest that you view your authority in terms of the source of your authority rather than merely as your "power to exact obedience." That is, you should be concerned over whether your intervention likely will diminish your authority in your organization. We suggest that your authority is your power granted to perform a service. That is, if you want more authority, then you must make yourself perceived as performing a greater service.

But in a situation where a problem persists in the organization, when you trigger a process that starts shifting the values that hold the problem in place, people likely will see your action as a disservice. Hence, you may find that your authority diminishes if you insist that people work the more threatening problems in the organization.

Generally, we suggest, authority dynamics in our culture do not reward or promote individuals for mobilizing people to solve the tough problems in the organization. As a result, brilliant technical wizards often give up on fixing the organization because they get burned by "dirty office politics." So, in a very real way, we encourage brilliant technical people to reexamine their experiences of failed leadership with the understanding that authority dynamics in our culture do not reward or promote individuals for mobilizing employees to solve the tough problems in the organization.

So what is a brilliant technical mind to do? We suggest that you set up your own system to collect the data and knowledge you need; we suggest that you find allies across the boundaries of authority in your organization, that you need feedback on what parts of your presentation actually get people to examine their own values that contribute to the problem in your organization. For example, we suggest that Greg Jefe in the scenario above finally got both management and employees to examine their own values that contributed to the problems in productivity and error rates.

Accordingly, when you intervene in an organization, one possible reaction of your colleagues might be to follow your "recommendation," and that following of your edict would make a score in your authority bucket. In a separate tabulation bucket, you might score only if there is a discovery in the organization. For example, when Greg Jefe intervened with his autocratic style, the employees submitted to his "traffic citations," so that intervention would make a series of scores to the authority bucket. But Greg's autocratic intervention triggered zero discoveries about how to improve productivity and error rates. Greg may have made discoveries about what did *not* work to improve productivity and error rates. So to be generous, perhaps Greg's autocratic intervention deserves one or two scores in the discovery bucket.

In contrast, Greg's intervention to recreate the workplace environment and promotion system scored *many* useful discoveries. In particular, Greg's intervention to honor the values that his employees imported from their family, cultural, and peer groups resulted in discoveries about actually improving productivity and error rates. Notice that he found the discoveries surprising, but that is the nature of discovery, is it not? Though you might plan to maximize the possibility of discovery, when you actually make a discovery, it will be surprising or unexpected in some way.

You may suspect that we will attribute discovery to "leadership"—as something scored independent of "authority," your power to get people to do what you say. And so we will, by starting with the standard dictionary definition of the verb *lead*: "to show the way to by going in advance" (3). We note that you have not shown the way to something if people already know it, and we note that what you show people the way to need not be what you told them about. Hence, there can be a discovery in the process both by the one who leads and by the one who is led. For example, if Emily New is able to trigger a process wherein the various teams in the laboratory devise a successful method to increase efficiency, we would score that intervention as leadership even if Emily had no authority across the organizational boundaries and even if her colleagues did not adopt any variation of her ideas, such as her idea to tie the data in the laboratory's computer with the data in the client hospital's computer using the serial number read from the etching on the specimen tube.

We would score your intervention as leadership if you mobilize the employees in your organization to tackle tough problems—even if you have little authority and develop no following (4). And we hasten to add that you should not be surprised if resolution of the tough problems in your organization requires an evolution of values of both management and employees.

Assessing Whether There Is "Progress"

If you are a senior manager, one of your concerns might be the design of the system within which the managers under you operate. Should you change the authority dynamics in the organization to reward leadership—the mobilization of employees to tackle tough problems? We suggest not and provide some of the reasons in the next chapter.

We suggest that you should continue to reward progress, the achievement of actual improvements, as did Emily New's boss above. However, also like Emily's boss, you might consider what you could do to protect and encourage leadership among your managers.

Let us remember that leadership is a trial-and-error process. So you might reward an actual improvement that resulted from the trial-and-error process even while you might not give a specific reward for the trials that were just errors. At the same time, you might consider how valuable it is for the organization if you have a mechanism for encouraging those who organize worthy but unsuccessful trials to try, try again. And you might provide some leadership coaching, including guidance on mobilization of allies across organizational boundaries, as in the Emily New scenario above.

How might you protect and encourage leadership in your organization? We suggest that leadership is an entrepreneurial activity in your organization, and as an entrepreneurial activity looking for discoveries, leadership must compete with the other forms of problem-solving activities in the organization. If you could play several versions of the Emily New scenario above in the leadership simulator, you might find that you, as Emily, have many innovative ideas, and you might find repeatedly that there seems to be no appropriate time to insert your innovative ideas in a way that they are actually considered.

We suggest that Emily's boss might have about the right mix of encouragement and caution in advising Emily so as to protect leadership and the progress that leadership brings. First, Emily's boss encouraged her to foster and promote the innovative ideas from her team. That is, Emily in managing her team must ensure that her competitive impulses do not squelch the useful innovative ideas from those that she manages. Second, Emily's boss cautioned her that she should consider the leadership challenge in introducing innovative ideas. That is, the leadership challenge is more than merely convincing others. Rather, developing an innovative idea might be a leadership challenge of getting her colleagues to take a good look at the problem, come up with their own approaches, and consider her ideas along with others in getting a resolution. Third, Emily's boss has committed a considerable amount of her time to coaching Emily in leadership and in assisting Emily to set up a network of leadership allies among her colleagues.

Delegation of Authority

We suggest that if leadership is an entrepreneurial activity, then leadership cannot be delegated. The boss might encourage and protect leadership, but leadership is not a power that can be delegated.

Leadership is a style, a whole host of personal details and mannerisms that an actor adds to the text and stage directions. As a senior manager, you might delegate a role of manager, but you cannot delegate the effective style. For what makes a particular leadership style click with the audience cannot be predicted.

From our experience in teaching leadership, we suggest that each person does have some personal style that will click with the audience of colleagues to get colleagues to consider the work they must do to resolve the tough problems in the organization. And we suggest that Emily New's boss had the right idea in organizing a network of allies that will notice the elements of leadership style that make a particular person effective.

Though a boss may not be able to delegate leadership, the boss *can* delegate to a manager the job of protecting and encouraging leadership within the manager's team. And the boss can assign a manager the task of resolving a particular problem in the organization.

You Want an Employee To Be Responsible

If you are a senior manager, the junior managers under you are your on-the-spot troubleshooters. Your junior managers add the detailed decisions that give your vision real life. And of course, your junior managers have to invent the details of their decisions to fit the situation they see.

So how should you prepare a junior manager in the proper use of your office? To get a clearer view of the quandary of the junior manager, consider the following leadership simulation titled "Own the Standard." You put on the helmet of the leadership simulator, and you are Jorg Junior, the manager of the toxicology unit of the laboratory.

As the simulation begins, you are in a meeting where your boss is laying down the law on tardiness and error rates. Your boss writes on the flip chart, "Zero Tolerance," and then she looks at you and says, "What does that mean to *you*, Jorg?"

Your colleagues in the room look straight ahead, very serious. You almost start to laugh, but you know that *that* would be a bad idea. "It means zero tolerance," you say in a level voice.

When you take the message to your teams, you have several options. You might tell them that making exceptions has taken too much of your time. Or you might try to give the message a voice of authority by saying that "this

came straight from the executive vice president herself." And there are other possibilities (6).

Suppose you decide to roll down the edict as a message straight from the desk of top management. You summarize what your boss told you, and you even imitate her style of delivery. To close your presentation you say, "This is a top priority of our management, and there will be no exceptions." After a pause, you ask, "Are there any questions?" No one has a question.

Two days later, your boss asks you to come to her office. She holds up some papers and says, "I have five e-mails from people on your team complaining about *my* policy of zero tolerance." She pauses and looks at you piercingly, "Why *is* that?"

You explain that some people on your teams are very skilled at inventing excuses.

"No," your boss says, "I mean why are these people writing to *me*, instead of you."

You decide to ask your boss something that has bothered you: "Might I ask why you singled me out at your presentation?"

She gives you a surly look. "I thought *you* of all people would have something useful to say about zero tolerance. Doesn't the error rate problem bother *you*?"

"Sure. But I am not sure that zero tolerance is the way to go."

"That's fine. My policy is zero tolerance. Now what does that mean to *you*? How can you make that work for you?"

You feel like you are supposed to give in, to bow, and accept zero tolerance, even if it is unreasonable.

Your boss continues, "I suggest that you and I look at this as *our*, notice that I say 'our,' leadership challenge. The people on your teams apparently protect some values that trump the values that you and I honor most, accuracy and precision."

"So, are you upset by the e-mails from my people?"

"No. Your people are great to give us data to work from. But let's figure out some way that you can own this idea of zero tolerance. There is something in these error rates that you would not tolerate in yourself. Isn't that true?"

"But they are just people."

"Maybe, but let's not tolerate the current situation. It seems to me that the people in these e-mails represent some values that conflict with good professional standards. But let's not target these people. I suggest you look at these e-mails they sent me. And come back with some plan to figure out what the conflict of values is. These e-mails are just representative of the rest of your teams. Maybe we can accommodate their values. Find out what their values *are*. We can shift how we do things. But I will keep up my zero tolerance message until something gets done about the problem, because the situation is intolerable. Help me figure out how to fix the system, and let's remind ourselves that our management attitudes may be part of what needs fixing."

But You May Want To Retain Authority

As we discuss in the next chapter, there can be dysfunctional uses of authority. However, one functional use of authority in the modern organization is the enforcement of standards. Apparently, for genetic and cultural reasons, people in modern organizations look to an authority figure to keep them from abusing their freedoms of choice. And sometimes employees have the idea that their freedoms of choice include whether or not they will get to work on time and whether or not they will focus their attention intently enough to prevent errors.

We suggest that generally people in an organization do not spontaneously volunteer the behavior that benefits either themselves or the organization as a whole. Accordingly, the organization grants power to certain authority figures specifically in exchange for the service of enforcing necessary standards to constrain freedoms of choice.

However, as the Greg Jefe scenario illustrates, many styles for attempting to enforce the standards do not actually enforce the standards, particularly when a conflict of values gives rise to the problem that the standards attempt to resolve. What can a senior manager do?

As the Jorg Junior scenario illustrates, the boss can delegate the job of developing the data and knowledge on a problem even while the boss retains authority for deciding what to do about the problem. That is, when a problem manifests as a difficulty in enforcement of a standard, we suggest that management might take an adaptive approach of iteratively developing more data and more knowledge, to learn by trial and error what values of management and employees can shift to make the solution to the problem possible.

Maintaining Standards

The Jorg Junior scenario illustrates several issues for an authority figure facing a problem that looks like a difficulty in enforcing standards. First, the authority figure can intervene for purposes of mobilizing management and employees in tackling the real issue underlying the difficulty in enforcing standards. In imposing the "zero tolerance" standard, Jorg's boss at least started a dialogue among management and employees about the problems of attendance and error rates.

Second, by analyzing the organization's response to the last intervention, the authority figure might get clues to what next intervention could be effective for mobilizing management and employees to tackle the real issue. For example, the boss tasked Jorg to develop a plan to determine the possible conflict of values within his teams. Though there may be similar conflicts in the teams of other managers, apparently Jorg's teams are so anxious to "volunteer" crucial data that they wrote to the boss herself with their issues and complaints. That is, within an adaptive approach, the rebels have "volunteered" to engage in a dialogue to discover how to shift values to resolve the un-

derlying problem. So, to a certain degree the rebels should be protected, not punished, as long as they are engaged in a dialogue about shifting values.

Third, ideally the junior manager would own the standard in a way that the employees would not see the junior manager as merely the puppet of upper management. For example, Jorg's preference for presenting the standards as coming "straight from the desk of the Executive Vice President herself" is but another clue among many to the underlying conflict of values among management and employees. Perhaps, at some stage, the boss might coach Jorg further in how he should use the boss's office. We suggest that the boss might begin that coaching session with Jorg by giving him some exercises in distinguishing his own person from his role as manager. For example, if he had personal enthusiasm for the zero tolerance policy, likely he would have provided his own justifications for the policy when he presented it to his teams. But, we suggest, a manager should consider the duties of his role as manager separate from his personal inclinations. At times, leadership may require the assumed style of an actor to be effective at mobilizing management and employees to tackle the priority tough problems in the organization.

Distinguishing Self from Role

There are some great stories about Shakespearean actors in times of personal pain shaking off their feelings, saying, "The show must go on," and striding forth on the stage to become the monarch, to play the role with such humanity that the audience felt like they and their values were part of the drama on stage. And after the play was over, the actors removed their costumes and took on again the personal pains that they had postponed for a brief time. Similarly distinguishing self from role, the actor can leave the monarch's problems on the stage and not carry them home (5).

We suggest that in your role as manager, you may have opportunities and problems that are not your personal concerns but rather the concerns of the organization. So distinguishing your self from your role can be important for diagnosing what must be fixed in the system. Surely, you would not like to work on your self when the problem is in the organization. Likely, the difficulties you encounter in your role you will feel personally. But you might find it easier to fix the problem when you develop an objective view of which of your personal feelings derive from the forces in your role and which feelings derive from weaknesses in your self, the actor that takes on the role of the manager.

When You Take Off the Mantle of Your Office, Who Are You?

Think back on the scenario when the ambitious young man said to Emily New, "The boss should have picked *me*, but I know the boss wants to promote women." The young man made two attacks on Emily's role, her role as a manager and her role as a woman.

"Her *role* as a woman!" you may exclaim. "Is a man or a woman just a role?"

In real life, people may not get a chance to experience firsthand that man, woman, and manager are just roles. But consider for a moment the metaphor of playing in succession the leadership simulation of Emily New and then the simulation of Greg Jefe above. If you are a man in the Emily New simulation, the computer would alter your voice to be that of Emily, and when you looked in the mirror, you would see that you looked like Emily, in a dress and medium heels.

And most importantly, the computer would generate the reactions of your coworkers and bosses in your organization to be the reactions to a woman, Emily. There is substantial empirical evidence that, in some settings, generally both women and men react negatively to a woman being just as assertive as a man, while both men and women generally approve of a man being as assertive as a woman (1). This may not be fair. But any accurate simulation of your organization would simulate the prejudices that the women and men in your organization have against women.

We do not imply that women should refrain from being assertive. Rather, a woman may get a negative reaction from women and men when she is effective—especially if the effectiveness has derived from the woman's assertive style.

Hence, we suggest that the player of Emily's role in the leadership simulator would have a better chance at fixing what needs to be fixed in the organization if the player interpreted the young man's insult as an attack on her role, not on her person. For example, that ambitious young man likely is but one representative of family, cultural, and peer group values that have a long history of views on women. And we suggest that a process like Greg Jefe's learning process for both management and employees may produce more progress than an autocratic style of laying down the law on comments like the young man made to Emily.

Of course, the manager must lay down the law on sexual harassment to the extent that the law in the outer society enforces the law. But a comment like the young man's comment may manifest a problem in the organization even if the comment does not amount to sexual harassment. That is, if women make significant contributions to the success of the organization, then likely it harms the organization when comments hinder women doing the important work of the organization.

If you are a woman, consider taking the role of Greg Jefe in the leadership simulation above. The computer would project your voice into the scene as a low gruff voice even when you tried to soften it. And your body would take up more space. Your elbows would reach further. And the computer would generate the reactions of the men and women in your workplace as if you were Greg, the medium-height man in black wingtips that you could see in any mirror in the simulation.

In particular when playing the role of Greg, you might find that your associates would rally to your point of view more readily if you hogged the meeting time and talked down objections with an assertiveness that your associates, both women and men, would criticize you for showing when you played the role of Emily. Does this mean that when playing the role of Greg, you should hog the meeting time and talk down objections? Not necessarily; you may find that your associates might give you a great following when you act with a competitive style, but you may find that the organization still cannot improve the productivity and error rates on the lab floor.

That is, we suggest that you should assess the effectiveness of your leadership style independent of whether you get praise, criticism, or a following—particularly in the tough stages of progress when there seems to be little to show for the pain and tribulation that you put people through. People may find it easy to praise you as a manager if you can give them an easy life, but they likely find it difficult to find praise for you when you insist that they do tough work to improve themselves.

When People Attack or Praise, to Whom Are They Speaking?

If you are a manager now, think back on your first days of becoming a manager. Were you not surprised at how differently friends treated you now that you were their manager? Perhaps your friends were more guarded. Or perhaps your friends now stopped talking and looked at you when you entered the room. Your friends now saw you as the role of manager.

You may have experienced the role change when a friend and peer of yours became your manager. Perhaps you felt a change in how open your friend would be with you. Or perhaps you found that your friend had a different reaction to jokes about the incompetence of management. You may have seen the onset of the boundary that distinguishes the role of manager from the role of subordinate. And the boundary between manager and subordinate likely generated new personal feelings for you and for your friend on the other side of the boundary of the role.

If you can distinguish the feelings that derive from your role and the feelings that derive from your self, your person that plays the role like an actor, you might respect your own managers more. And you might have more compassion for yourself in the role of manager.

We suggest that you may find that both manager and subordinate have an opportunity for leadership, that is, opportunity for mobilizing the employees to tackle the tough problems of the organization. But we suggest that because people in the organization respond differently to the roles of manager and subordinate, you likely will find that effectiveness in the manager role will require a quite different leadership style, where style includes the whole range of personal details and mannerisms that you can add to the role of manager that your organization expects from you. In the next chapter, we discuss the "authority" elements that people may expect you to add to your leadership style when you are a manager.

Summary

Different leadership styles may call forth different results from a group of people. Thus, to the extent that a leader can assume different styles for different contexts, a leader can expand the possibilities for the organization. In this chapter, we have explored some ranges of leadership style and have suggested the elements of leadership style that a leader can learn to command. The different effects of different leadership styles arise from the complex of needs and potentials of people. Accordingly, in the next chapter, we consider the needs of employees, first from the standpoint of what they think they need and second from the standpoint of what you may find they actually need in order to get the job done in a modern complex organization, such as a clinical laboratory.

KEY POINTS

- A small change in a manager's leadership style can make a big difference in the ability of clinical laboratory staff to solve tough problems such as productivity, attendance, and error rate. For example, at times an autocratic style can exact obedience even while that autocratic style discourages leadership, the mobilization of employees to tackle the tough problems in the organization.

- In some cases, even nonmanagement employees can exercise leadership, that is, mobilize employees to tackle tough problems. And, in those situations, the manager can exercise leadership by encouraging and protecting the employees' leadership, mobilizing the employees to tackle tough problems.

- Several observational techniques can assist the manager in assembling the data and knowledge on what leadership style actually mobilizes employees to tackle tough problems.

  - First, a manager can organize a network of allies, peers that notice particularly the elements of a manager's style that actually mobilize employees even for a brief time to tackle the tough problems in the organization.

  - Second, the metaphor of a leadership simulator, like a flight simulator, may assist the manager in noticing the different constraints and pressures on the different organizational roles, such as middle managers, upper managers, and subordinate employees.

- A conflict in values often underlies tough problems such as low productivity and high error rate. Accordingly, managers sometimes can improve productivity and error rate by engaging management and employees in adaptive work, an iterative process to learn shifts of values that accommodate what is most important for management and most important for employees.

- For situations where both managers and subordinates can contribute to mobilizing employees to tackle tough problems, the distinction between leadership and authority serves to highlight the different roles of subordinates and managers in improving the organization.

- Generally, authority is power granted for performing a service, such as providing direction, keeping order, and enforcing standards. But in many situations, such as some low-productivity and high-error rate situations, management cannot fix what is wrong in the organization by merely exercising authority. We call these problems adaptive challenges.

- Some adaptive challenges can be resolved by engaging the subordinates in a creative process in which either the subordinates or the manager may provide leadership. The duty of managers in such a process still is to provide direction, keep order, and enforce standards—but in a way that protects and encourages whoever in the organization actually exercises leadership by mobilizing employees to tackle tough problems.

- People in an organization take on roles, such as the role of manager or the role of subordinate. Though the actor playing various roles may be the same, the different roles in an organization give the actor in the different roles different powers of persuasion and influence. Hence, altering your leadership style to accommodate your role rather than your self-image may make you more effective.

- Distinguishing self from role amounts to noticing which attacks, praise, or frustrations are associated with the role and not with the self, the actor that takes on the role. For example, if you can notice which of your frustrations derive from your role of manager and not from your personal relationships, you might leave more of your problems at work and you might be more compassionate with the people in the various organizational roles around you. Furthermore, you might be able to enforce standards more vigorously if you understood which resistances derived from the roles in the organization and not from your personal relationships.

GLOSSARY

Actor The self; the one doing the acting, the speaking, and the gesturing.

Adaptive approach An intervention that seeks to learn how to fix the system, with the understanding that the system for fixing includes the intervenor's own style, priorities, and values. Generally, an adaptive approach consists of an iterative cycle as follows: (i) plan the intervention, (ii) make the intervention, (iii) hold steady to analyze the effect of the intervention, and (iv) plan the next cycle of intervention.

Adaptive challenge A problem that does *not* subside to satisfy the current values in the organization even when management applies the best-known methods and procedures. Generally, the resolution of an adaptive challenge requires a shift in values. For example, at least two competing values might shift to resolve a budget crisis. On the one hand, the "problem" would be resolved if the employees shifted their values to take less pay and still be satisfied. On the other hand, the "problem" might be resolved if management shifted the values in the organization to direct the business to new profitable markets, perhaps global markets.

Adaptive work Effort that produces the organizational learning required to tackle tough problems, the problems that often require an evolution of values. The learning in adaptive work often requires (i) addressing the conflicts in the values that people hold or (ii) diminishing the gap between the values people espouse and the reality they face. For example, dealing with reduced budgets may require (i) addressing the conflict between "We are doing a good job" and "We could do better" together with (ii) diminishing the gap between "We are doing the best that is possible" and current reality, which may be "The public will not pay for quality service."

Authority Power granted to perform a service. The exchange of power for a service may be informal. Formal authority arises when the officeholder promises to meet a set of explicit expectations, such as a job description or professional standards. Informal authority arises where employees confer power on a person based on implicit expectations; for example, "If Sally were here, she would know what to do."

Delegate Appoint someone to act in a particular role. A principle delegates to an agent portions of the principal's authority, the power to perform a service.

Leadership The activity of mobilizing employees to tackle tough problems, the problems that often require an evolution of values. Generally, any employee in the organization can exercise leadership, the activity of mobilizing employees to tackle tough problems. But the actions of those with authority in the organization inadvertently can discourage employees from exercising leadership. Alternatively, those with authority can exercise leadership by mobilizing employees generally to exercise leadership, the activity of mobilizing employees to tackle tough problems.

Management The act or practice of supervision and control.

New style of leadership Noticing in real time the effects that you have on the quality in an organization. From this view, anyone in the organization can exercise "leadership" by mobilizing employees to tackle tough problems. But the actions and words of those with authority and power can discourage the "leadership" of others without intending that result.

Old style of leadership Expecting to build sufficient power, expertise, and reputation so that people will see the wisdom in your decisions.

Reflection The actor's careful consideration of the effects that follow from the actor's words and deeds. Reflection is like an instant replay in which the actor can watch from a wide-angle camera view the coordination of the actor's deeds with the deeds of others to create the organizational outcome.

Repertoire The collection of tested problem-solving procedures that the organization is prepared and competent to perform.

Responsibility The state or fact of being accountable. Generally, people exercise leadership when they have a feeling of personal responsibility for improving quality in the organization.

Role The character or part played by an actor. Each adult person has experienced at least playing the role of child. In addition, many adults have experienced playing the role of mother or father.

Self The actor that can take on many different roles, including mother, father, child, manager, or employee.

Style The personal details and mannerisms that an actor adds to the text and stage directions. Within a modern organization, the actor must invent even the text and stage directions for doing the job. Furthermore, for anyone who attempts leadership—mobilizing employees to tackle the tough problems in the organization—there may be controversies over what the "job" is. Accordingly, leadership is mainly "style," the personal details and mannerisms that a responsible person invents and adds to the routine of the organization.

Technical problem A problem that *does* subside to satisfy the current values in the society when management applies the best-known methods and procedures.

Technical solution An intervention plan that includes (i) a fixed statement of the problem and (ii) fixed standards for success defined before the intervention was made.

Technical work The physical and mental effort that applies known methods for achieving a goal.

Value A desirable standard or quality for which a person will sacrifice what others consider to be of higher importance.

ACKNOWLEDGMENTS

We acknowledge the special role played by Ronald A. Heifetz in helping us understand "leadership" in the terms we use here. Though this chapter expresses the views only of us, significant portions of the text were taken from unpublished drafts and work product that Riley Sinder coauthored with Ron Heifetz going back to the 1970s, as well as concepts further developed by Heifetz in his seminal work, *Leadership Without Easy Answers* (1994, Harvard University Press, Cambridge, Mass.). In addition, Heifetz has read and provided feedback on this chapter.

REFERENCES

1. Butler, D., and F. L. Geis. 1990. Nonverbal affect responses to male and female leaders: implications for leadership evaluations. *J. Pers. Soc. Psychol.* **58:**48–59.

2. Garletts, J. A. 2002. Using career ladders to motivate and retain employees: an implementation success story. *Clin. Leadersh. Manag. Rev.* **16:**380–385.

3. Houghton Mifflin. 1992. *The American Heritage Dictionary of the English Language,* 3rd ed. Houghton Mifflin, Boston, Mass.

4. Pickett, R. B. 2001. What does all of this leadership stuff mean to me? *Clin. Leadersh. Manag. Rev.* **15**:395–400.

5. Redgrave, C. 1996. Michael Redgrave: my father. Trafalgar Square Press, London, United Kingdom.

6. Summers, J., and M. Nowicki. 2002. Management in action: granting exceptions to rules and policies: management issues and ethical guidelines. *Clin. Leadersh. Manag. Rev.* **16**:336–338.

7. Walker, C. A. 2003. Management in action: saving your rookie managers from themselves. *Clin. Leadersh. Manag. Rev.* **17**:115–119.

APPENDIX 8.1 Comparison of Old Style with New Style of Leadership

Emphasis of old style of leadership	Emphasis of new style of leadership
Quality is just fine.	Quality can and must be improved.
Accurate data reporting ensures quality.	Improvement of processes ensures quality, with an emphasis on timely analysis and interactive corrections.
People cause defects and poor quality.	Processes cause defects and poor quality.
Intuition and technology will solve problems.	Resolving conflicts of values, together with solid data and knowledge, will solve problems.
Improvement occurs within one manager's area.	The most valuable improvements arise from integrated changes in several functional areas.
Customers and suppliers are problems.	Customers and suppliers are partners who can benefit mutually from improvements in quality.
There is little time to improve quality.	Improving quality is always on the agenda.

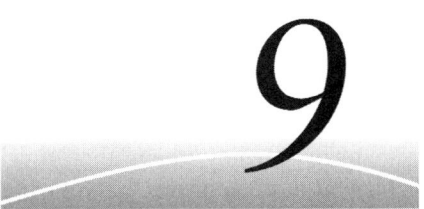

9

Employee Needs

Riley M. Sinder and Dean Williams

OBJECTIVES

To allow the reader to develop techniques for shifting employee and management values to improve the quality of performance in the organization

To distinguish between employee hungers and employee needs for quality performance in the organization

To help the reader develop a results-based view "above the action" to assess the effects of management interventions, such as an autocratic style compared with a laissez-faire style

To guide the reader in altering personal and professional approaches according to actual effects, independent of personal inclinations that may ignore the real problems in the organization

---

But why was it that here most of all he felt that hunger for—for something more?
JOHAN BOJER, *THE GREAT HUNGER*
(TRANSLATED BY W. J. ALEXANDER AND C. ARCHER,
GROSSET AND DUNLAP, NEW YORK, N.Y., 1925).

IN THE PREVIOUS CHAPTER, we presented the leadership simulation of Greg Jefe, who attempted to improve the productivity and error rate scores in his referral laboratory by several traditional methods, including modeling, commanding, and rewarding the desired behavior. When these traditional methods did not improve productivity and error rate, Greg tried reengineering parts of the organizational system that the traditional methods often ignore. In particular, Greg responded seriously to the values that his employees imported into the workplace from their family, cultural, and peer groups outside work.

If you look back on that scenario in the previous chapter, would you say that Greg interpreted the values of his employees as needs? We suggest that he did not. We suggest that Greg, by trial and error, shifted some of his employees' values, in the process making a vital distinction between the needs of his employees and their hungers. Let us examine some of the emotional textures involved in shifting values in the workplace.

Though Greg might want to deal directly with the values of his employees, we suggest that he cannot directly observe or manage "values." What did Greg measure with the questionnaires and interviews? We suggest the metaphor of hungers to characterize the clues that the employees provided Greg in the questionnaires and interviews. That is, Greg's employees expressed various views of their strong desires and cravings, even as they stated what management should do to improve morale.

Distinguishing Needs from Hungers

A manager cannot simply provide what the employee wants. People may not want to work as hard as quality work requires, they may not want to collaborate with other managers or teams, or they might want a lot more recognition than they deserve. We call these "wants" and "don't wants" hungers rather than needs because people seek to satisfy these hungers whether or not the result improves the quality of work. In contrast, what an employee requires for quality work we will term a need. For example, an employee might need appropriate training, motivation, incentive, and up-to-date information. Generally, employee needs represent necessary conditions and not sufficient conditions for quality work.

Using the metaphor of the leadership simulator from the previous chapter, we invite the reader to examine the Greg Jefe case from a different angle—this time from the role of Jeremy Locke, a heavyset smoker and a trivia buff extraordinaire who is also one of Greg Jefe's employees in the cytology lab. This simulation is titled "I want what I want."

As you will remember from the previous chapter, when you put on the helmet of the leadership simulator, the computer projects to your eyes and ears the sights and sounds of your actual clinical laboratory. And the computer simulates perfectly the reactions of your coworkers and managers as they deal with their conflicting values, desires, and dreams in the actual workplace.

In the last chapter, we explained briefly how the armor to the leadership simulator pokes you and presses you to generate the feeling of sitting on simulated chairs and walking up simulated stairs. Now, we draw to your attention that the simulator armor activates your nerve centers to generate the actual hungers and desires of Jeremy Locke. For, as the simulation begins, you find that you want something to eat.

Getting something to eat is a real pain in Jefe's lab. You call your boss "Jefe," with a little contempt because he is a young guy like you, and he walks around like he owns the place. The employee lounge has a few vending machines. But there is nothing for miles around worth the drive. Some poor people bring food from home in plastic, but their concoctions smell up the employee lounge when they put them through Jefe's microwave.

Jefe has announced that a consultant will talk to everybody in the lab. When you receive the preliminary survey questionnaire, you have several options. You could answer the questions with a straight face—but this is not likely, given how much you resent your managers' persistent attitudes of disapproval.

The questionnaire asks all kinds of questions about how to improve morale in the lab. And, as you scan the questions in the survey, you feel it is so unfair how "they" keep telling you to "shape up." You answer every question that you can with some form of telling "them" that "they" make it too difficult for you to do your job. It's your life, not theirs.

To your surprise, when your time with the consultant comes, the consultant looks over your answers to the questionnaire with you and spends the entire time discussing with you how management "should do things different." Maybe they could let you learn some of the other technologies in your lab. You think they should not complain about your taking time off from work unexpectedly—as long as you usually find someone to cover for you. And maybe they could make it easier to get something good to eat. Maybe they could have a caterer come by once in a while; maybe a little lunch surprise, maybe a little atmosphere in the employee lounge.

In a few weeks, Jefe gives a talk to the whole lab saying that he is going to do away with the old job descriptions and design ways to have rapid advancement and to encourage you to move from technology to technology in the laboratory. That sounds good to you. You learn trivia as a hobby. Your job is little more to you than a hobby of medical and lab trivia that pays you some paltry sum of money. You caught on to your current job quickly. And it gets repetitious. You know you are smart. You move fast. You expect to be gone from here to someplace better in a year.

Jefe doesn't say anything about your pet peeve—how the whole place is a desert with nothing to eat. But what Jefe says sounds good. You just don't think he will do what he says.

In the coming weeks, Jefe announces a regular rotation among technologies in your area. You will be responsible for several tasks during the day, so it won't be so boring. And Jefe promises rapid advancement based on productivity and error rate. Seniority will disappear, and job level will be redefined based on quality measures. Some of the long-timers are upset because they lose what they have built up over the years. And that doesn't sound so good to you either because you are sure he is trying to turn the whole lab into a sweatshop. But he says he will throw a "party" for those who get promotions. "Probably not much of a party," you say to one of your smoking buddies. "But that would be *something* anyway," you add.

The new job assignments turn out to be interesting. There is some training, which is a bore, but you like what comes out of it. You move to doing analyses in the neighboring histology lab in addition to some portion of your current assignments. You learn some new technology. Your job gets more interesting, more complex.

One day, when you huff out for your "smoke break," you pass by the employee lounge and, lo and behold, you see that somebody has brought in a caterer—interesting tastes for reasonable prices. There are some strobe lights; there is some new music on a boom box. You try a few dishes, have some conversation, and get back to work. You skipped your "smoke." "Well, I'll be," you say to yourself.

You find it easier and easier to get to work on time. The caterer is not always there, but there is more variety in the vending machines. And you do get a promotion in 6 months. You are not necessarily trying to make fewer mistakes, but your boss tells you that your error rate has dropped. "Isn't that something?" you say to yourself.

And there is a party—somebody's dumb idea of an Academy Awards ceremony. But it's not bad. You win the John Goodman award for "Best Cloud of Smoke." And the "medal of honor" is a full-sized poster of John Goodman, who looks about like you, blowing fire from a trick cigar in a movie you loved, a Steven Spielberg movie about a daredevil firefighter pilot who has a ghost for a buddy for a while.

You feel different about your job. You lose some weight. You think about quitting smoking. You even start calling Jefe "Greg."

The simulation ends, and now it is time for reflection. What did Jefe do that made the difference for Jeremy Locke? In addressing that question, we suggest that you look at the process rather than the exact steps in Jefe's reengineering of the workplace. And maybe the important part of the process was interaction—the kind of trial-and-error interaction that a driver makes on ice. If you drive on ice, you might nudge the system, the car, the wheels, and the ice in a way to use what little power you have, taking advantage of the good things and minimizing the bad things that you sense in the system's response to what you have done. You might make real-time corrections to your interventions based on the effect that you actually have. You might have a firm hand, but you might have at the same time a sensitive hand on the steering wheel so that you *give* in the direction that the car is going when the tires lose traction.

We suggest that there are some pointers for managers in the Jeremy Lock scenario. First, not every person under 35 is the same, but there are some generalities. Many people under 35, the Generation Xers, tend to follow their hungers, their strong desires and cravings, to the detriment of their careers and long-term self-interest. Hence, as Greg Jefe discovered in the scenario of the previous chapter, many of his employees under 35 resisted his initial punishments and incentives even if they would have been much better off if they had followed his direction.

Second, for many people over 35, old-style cultural forces like philosophy, religion, and investing in the future often honor needs while suppressing hungers. However, in many modern situations, the old-style cultural forces are not flexible enough to recognize what is needed for success in the modern workplace. Hence, Greg found that many of his employees over 35 would tolerate his initial punishments and incentives better than the Generation Xers; nevertheless, the mere punishments and incentives did not engage the age and culture groups enough to improve productivity and error rate scores significantly.

Third, by catering judiciously to the various hungers of the various age and culture groups of both management and subordinates, Greg could shift the values of the employees and managers enough to get significant improvements in both the productivity and error rate scores. In actual cases in clinical laboratory workplaces, strategies for catering to employee expressions of what they want in their workplace have cut the annualized employee turnover rate by over 40%, increased productivity by over 30%, and improved quality control measures by over 70% (1).

Analogy with Nutrition

We suggest that catering to the hungers of people is a powerful management tool. But, at the same time, we want to emphasize what you know already—that some human hungers are dysfunctional in modern settings. That is, evolution and culture shaped human hungers not for modern situations, but rather for much simpler times that are long gone—when there were much simpler supply and demand curves. So, for example, someone like Greg Jefe, who caters to the various hungers of his employees and managers in an attempt to solve modern organizational problems in the clinical laboratory, must distinguish between that for which his people (i) hunger and (ii) need for satisfactory performance in the modern setting.

In particular, we suggest that some of your employees even in a modern clinical laboratory setting may crave some great man to solve their problems for them. Furthermore, some of your employees may hunger to take your position away from you. And some of your employees may resent your advice as their manager, especially if they have an inkling that your advice is right for their lives.

Hungers, the strong desires and cravings of people, have both genetic and cultural origins. Some hungers protect important values. For example, without food the body dies. So the human hungers for sugar, salt, and burned fat provide an internal mechanism of incentives to avoid accidental starvation.

But some human hungers are dysfunctional if indulged to the extent of the hungers. For example, indulging your hungers for sugar, salt, and burned fat to the extent of your hungers likely will impair your health. Perhaps the human hungers for sugar, salt, and burned fat provided about the healthiest diet our ancestors could get back in those ancient days in Africa when God and evolution refined our genetic hungers. Sugar, salt, and burned fat were rare and hard to obtain in those days, so the hungers suggested appropriately that you should gorge yourself whenever you could get your hands on some.

In addition to the hardwired hungers for sugar, salt, and burned fat, there are a whole host of latent hungers, such as the addiction to nicotine that family and peer group culture can bring to the fore in the individual. The case of Jeremy Locke above illustrates an employee importing into the modern clinical lab setting hungers that are both an opportunity and a liability for the manager attempting to improve quality in the organization.

The manager might like to instill workplace values—desirable standards and qualities for which the employees will sacrifice some of their personal hungers. But the employees' families, cultures, and peer groups have already instilled a set of values for deciding which of their hungers they will indulge and which they will suppress. Consequently, the employees import into the workplace a set of values that likely compete with the values the manager would like to instill in the workplace.

Nutrition Requires the Determination of Needs

We suggest that by identifying the hungers underneath the employee values that compete with reasonable workplace values, the manager can begin to get a grip on the steering wheel of the car that slides on ice. Your intervention may matter a lot, but to be effective, you might respond interactively with what the organization actually does in response to your intervention. And in the process, you, the manager, might allow your own values to evolve in response to the actual situations that you face as manager.

A first step could be to identify the employee hungers that underlie the employees' rejection of the workplace values that the manager prefers. Likely from Greg Jefe's questionnaire and structured interviews of his employees, he could begin to sketch the employee hungers that interfere with quality work in his lab. A second step might be to determine which of the hungers deserve more attention in a process for fixing what impedes problem solving in the organization.

You may find that "nutrition," a balancing of hungers and needs, can provide a convenient metaphor. Nutrition, we suggest, proceeds on the basis of data and knowledge of what actually proves useful in practice. In contrast, sometimes hungers miss the "vitamins" of what is actually needed, and sometimes hungers produce a craving for what will deter performance. But presumably, nutrition can provide a reasonable means for providing needs in a way to satisfy the hungers well enough.

When Greg Jefe in the previous chapter at first attempted to improve productivity and error rate by traditional punishments and incentives, he appealed to his employees' hungers for reward and freedom from pain. But evidently, the traditional punishments and incentives did not engage the employees' actual hungers enough to change the employees' decisions and actions.

We suggest that traditional punishments and incentives can miss the mark by incorrectly assessing employee needs. To say that the employees need motivation is about as useful as saying that the driver of a car sliding on ice needs to proceed safely to the destination. Anyone in the

midst of the situation likely would say, "I know. I know. Now, how do I actually do it?" And in answering that question, we propose that you engage an interactive trial-and-error process, like unto a leadership simulation. If traditional punishments and incentives fail, then you likely have an adaptive challenge that requires a shift in management and employee values to get some progress toward a solution. And you might begin to shift values by catering to hungers.

Hungers May Give a False Model of Needs

Let us examine the Jeremy Locke case as an illustration of the interactive nature of adaptive work in shifting employee and management values to tackle tough organizational problems. First, when the questionnaire asked about what would improve morale in the laboratory, Jeremy expressed his view of the problem in terms of his own vague hungers for food, for excitement, for freedom from the oppression of management, and for permission to take time off when he pleased. Second, in contrast, management expressed its view of the problem in terms of its own strong desires for improving productivity and cutting error rates.

Third, from some points of view, Jeremy's grumble about wanting management to get off his back was irrelevant to the significant problems in the laboratory. However, if you could play back the Jeremy Locke situation in a leadership simulator and play out the roles of other technicians, you might sample the different grumbles that others had in the laboratory, and you might suspect that the employee grumble expresses some employee value that competes with the management priorities of high productivity and low error rate. That is, Jeremy's grumble about how "boring it is around here" gave management a clue to what might engage Jeremy in a trial-and-error process to shift his values and management's values to improve the quality of work in the laboratory.

However, Jeremy's grumble merely expressed a hunger. And merely catering to the hunger, we suggest, would miss the opportunity of shifting values to improve quality in the organization.

We offer the following as a metaphor for the fault in human hungers. Consider the McDonald's experience in catering to the human hunger for the taste of burned fat. Several food gourmets as well as the fast-food market have asserted that McDonald's fries done in sizzling fat have the best taste. However, several nutritionists complained that all that fat gave people too much cholesterol and fat.

But McDonald's would have a problem switching to pure vegetable oil—because the buyers craved the taste of burned fat. And, we suggest, McDonald's tried a strategy that every manager might adapt to deal with the strong desires and cravings of employees. McDonald's developed a means to deliver just enough of the taste to satisfy the hunger without surrendering to the dysfunction that the hunger creates in the modern setting.

Let us consider the McDonald's strategy as a metaphor for dealing with employee hungers. McDonald's went to a chemist and got the chemist to cook, split, and combine natural products, likely including meat products, to produce a "spice" of which only a few drops in a vat of pure vegetable oil would mimic the intense taste and smell of burned fat so closely that customers thought they were buying fries done in fat. But the "spice" delivered none of the fat and none of the cholesterol that nutrition had found to be dysfunctional in the modern setting (3).

By a similar strategy, Jeremy Locke's management might cater to his vague hungers for management to give him what he wanted even while insisting that he perform to the standards that his job requires in the modern setting. We suggest that the exact mechanisms of your employees' hungers may be unknowable. However, you may find it helpful to consider several metaphors or operational models that you can use in real time to make sense of your employees' reactions to what you do as manager. We offer the following metaphors to assist you in untangling the complexities of office politics so that you see promising options other than what you have tried already for the tough problems in your organization.

Hungers for Authority, the Old Style

When a group of people congregates for a period of hours in close proximity, such as in a clinical laboratory setting, they quickly fall into patterns of competition and hierarchy that might be classed as office politics. If you want to intervene in the system of office politics, you may find it useful to analyze the patterns of behavior in terms of (i) the hungers that maintain the behavior compared to (ii) the hungers that might entice individuals to change their behavior.

The old style of leadership emphasizes the role of the boss. But what are the human dynamics that make the role of boss significant in the organization?

We begin this section with an illustration of the mechanics of the hungers for authority in a normal group of people. We offer you the following leadership simulation titled "The Authority Figure Fails Expectations." When you put on the helmet of the leadership simulator, you are Arthur Spector, a toxicology analyst in the laboratory of a large urban hospital near a high-tech manufacturing corridor.

There have been rumors that your hospital site is for sale to a group of investors from New York—exactly which demeanor of investor they might be changes from day to day. Your colleagues daily have new conjectures and jokes about the transition to whatever is going to happen and about who will stay and who will be kicked out when the new investors start jerking you around in an attempt to "cut costs."

You are not ready to call your feeling "anxiety," but you at least have looked up the symptoms and summary mechanics of anxiety disorder in your *Merck Manual*, home

edition. The chief administrator of your hospital, Joseph Lyon, issues an e-mail under his signature logo of the clasped handshake announcing that he is convening a "staff meeting of the whole to explain matters of interest for all of us in these times."

When the time of the staff meeting of the whole arrives, you get there 15 min early, and you find that the room is already filling. You greet a colleague who manages the rehabilitation team and sit by her. The two of you talk about a recent accident in which several workers were trapped in a safe room and could not get out when a gas main and a solvent line broke. You both have firsthand anecdotes of the emergency room admission of the workers.

When Mr. Lyon strides into the room, everyone falls silent. He walks to the center of the area in front of the first row of chairs, looks at the audience, and does not speak. He stands there, looking like his usual self-assured person. But he does not speak. He scans the room but does not speak.

The tension in the room mounts. There is something wrong; you can feel it. You feel a lump in your throat. There is deathly silence. Someone in the second row, in front of him, asks him quietly, "Are you okay?" He still looks around the room, standing confidently but not speaking. Several people around you stand up. A nurse in the front row walks up to him and feels his pulse. Mr. Lyon does not resist, but allows the nurse to hold his hand limply; he continues to scan the room, looking self-assured, ignoring the nurse.

Someone cracks a joke, "Maybe we've all been gassed." The room breaks into spontaneous laughter. And there is a pocket of applause near the right front of the room near the window.

The simulation ends here. And now let's reflect on what happened. In the situation of crisis and unknown future, the people under Mr. Lyon look to him with several very reasonable strong desires and cravings. And when he does not perform to satisfy those strong desires and cravings, the individuals in the group experience several strong emotions that drive them to (i) get Mr. Lyon to do something else to satisfy their strong desires and cravings, (ii) find out what Mr. Lyon's weakness is, or (iii) do something to divert their attention from the pressing problem that appears to threaten great pain.

Employees Hunger for Someone to Simplify Their Lives

To explore the nature of the hungers that individuals in groups feel for authority, let us consider a variation of Mr. Lyon's presentation. This leadership simulation is titled "Satisfy Their Hunger and Give Them Nothing of Value—Other Than Satisfying Their Hunger." After you put on the helmet of the leadership simulator, you are again Arthur Spector, and the scenario proceeds through the same scene as before until the time of Mr. Lyon's entrance.

You and your coworkers fear that the rumored buyers of your hospital and laboratory facility will interfere with your workplace to cut costs contrary to professional standards of quality and against your personal interests, such as your long personal investments of time to improve quality and performance in the laboratory. You and your coworkers await Mr. Lyon's appearance and speech with a sense of impending doom.

When Mr. Lyon strides into the room, everyone falls silent. He walks to the center of the area in front of the first row of chairs, looks at the audience, and begins with a long description of the history of the hospital, telling many stories about the veterans who can "remember when." He tells a few jokes and gets some applause and laughter.

And even though he talks on for 45 min, he says nothing substantive that has any promise of relieving the employees' real problems in life. But people listen in rapt silence. A few people leave the room without distracting the attention of the audience. But no one says, "Are you okay?" No one walks up to feel his pulse, and no one in your earshot even whispers the joke "Maybe we've all been gassed." For Mr. Lyon has satisfied the hunger for authority that individuals feel in groups.

The leadership simulation ends here. After you remove the helmet of the leadership simulator, you might say, "But Mr. Lyon's talk this time seemed reasonable."

Yes, that is the point! Sometimes you can satisfy your organization's expectations of authority by avoiding the priority work in your organization. For culture and evolution have shaped our human hungers for authority primarily to assess the quality of the boss's posturing while ignoring whether the boss actually mobilizes the employees to tackle the tough problems in the organization. In a similar flaw of hungers for food, many adults crave unhealthy combinations of sugar, salt, and burned fat, even while the craving ignores essential vitamins, minerals, and balanced diet that physical health and performance require.

We suggest that human hungers for authority assess two elements of a candidate's posturing: (i) physical expressions of confidence and (ii) how many people appear to bend to the candidate's will. Hence, for example, if Mr. Lyon can manipulate his posturing so that he (i) comes across as self-confident and (ii) charms a significant coalition in the organization, his performance as boss appears in the interim to be reasonable.

While it is true that human culture may have a great influence on what people want from authority figures, many of our strong desires and cravings for an authority figure may be genetic. For example, among the five species of apes, only chimpanzees and humans organize authority around physical posturing of confidence and coalition building. Orangutans live isolated lives and do not form communities; gorillas form communities but the competition for power goes to the strongest individual; bonobos form coalitions, but the competition among coalitions does not result in a hierarchy of power with only one individual to whom the other individuals in the community defer.

Of the five apes, only humans and chimpanzees typically create communities of individuals that defer to the will of one alpha where the alpha rises to power by competitive posturing in (i) physical displays of confidence and (ii) coalition building. Based on measures of genes in common, the closest species relatives of humans are the chimpanzees. Humans and chimpanzees inherited a common set of genes from the ancestors of the chimpanzees; perhaps 98% of human genes are genes of the chimpanzees. Likely humans inherited from the ancestors of the chimpanzees many of the characteristic strong desires and cravings for authority, including the general deference to the "big boss," the one alpha of the community that wins the competition of physical displays of confidence and coalition building.

Furthermore, apparently the strong desire for gender bias against women in authority comes with those genes that humans inherited from the ancestors of the chimpanzees. A quick survey of modern nations suggests that the industrialized cultures retain an ancient gender bias against women being able to rise to the highest levels of power in the organization. For example, a May 2003 survey of nations shows that Sweden has the highest percentage of women in the legislature, at 43%. And the United States, Andorra, Israel, Sierra Leone, and Ireland are tied for 57th place, with less than 15% of the legislature being women (http://www.ipu.org/wmn-e/classif.htm). Admittedly, those percentages are significantly higher than the occurrence of female chimpanzees becoming alpha of the community, but the trends are similar in manifesting a general gender bias across cultures against females being able to organize coalitions of power in the relevant communities.

That gender bias against females is *not* the natural state among intelligent creatures is illustrated by the general bonobo trend across cultures wherein the females maintain a hierarchy that is physically as powerful as any faction of males—because the males do not form political coalitions. Bonobos presumably inherited from the ancestors of the chimpanzees the same set of genes that humans inherited governing the strong desires and cravings for authority, but bonobos evolved from the chimpanzees about 2 million years later than the humans did and developed very different hungers to take advantage of a very different environment (4).

Notwithstanding natural tendencies, that nature shaped human hungers of strong desire for gender bias against women does not justify gender bias. Similarly, that nature shaped human hungers of strong craving to eat too much sugar, salt, and burned fat does not justify ruining the health of the nation. Facing the hungers and the reality of the dysfunctions that hungers encourage surely suggests that the right thing to do is to manage the hungers to produce the best outcome.

Accordingly, we suggest managing the authority in your organization as an appetite. To a certain extent, authority is an employee need, but indulging the full extent of the appetite for the "boss" form of authority rather than the "responsible citizen" form of authority can be unnecessarily expensive and inefficient. The competitive advantages of a team of "responsible citizens" demonstrate the point, as illustrated by the Orpheus Process described below.

As a complement to controlling the appetite for authority, managing the leadership in your organization might consist of encouraging collaboration and innovative approaches that have promise for improving quality and performance. Similarly, the diet of a world-class athlete requires both (i) curbing the ancient cravings and appetites and (ii) introducing regimen and standards that the ancient cravings and appetites discourage.

In contrast to authority, which caters to the ancient appetite for an alpha "boss," leadership amounts to a "technology," a set of techniques corrected in real time based on data and knowledge of the effects on actual quality and performance. Accordingly, anyone attempting leadership to mobilize employees to be personally responsible for quality and performance, such as in the Orpheus Process described below, must be prepared to manage the distaste, complaints, upset, unreasonableness, and other primitive emotions that express the ancient hungers for the authority of a "boss."

Often, those in authority think that they can afford to ignore the tough and threatening problems in the organization even when the organization is failing. This may be because the human hungers for authority consist of strong cravings for office politics in which the winner of the competition of physical displays of confidence and coalition building becomes the boss whether or not the tough problems in the organization are solved.

Some Employees Hunger To Rise in a Hierarchy

In the above discussion, we have explored the nature of the demand for authority in an organization. Now let us examine the supply side in which some people experience strong desires to be the one to whom people bow. Some people want to give orders, some people want to be adored, some people want to control, and some people want status.

These cravings sometimes lead people to engage in activities that actually impair the quality of performance in the organization. For example, you may be able to rise in the hierarchy by ingratiating yourself to those above you. But that is true even if you impair the quality of performance in the organization. Alternatively, you may be able to rise in the hierarchy by saying yes when, from your best professional data and knowledge, you strongly disagree. Or to rise in the hierarchy you may have to engage in projects that, in your honest and knowledgeable opinion, are a waste of time. That is, your hungers to rise in the hierarchy

and maintain your current status can trump your best professional insights and rational judgment.

In the following section, we explore with you various metaphors for managing the office politics that the hungers for authority produce, both the hungers in the group to have a boss over them and the hungers in individuals that make them strongly desire to become the boss. We first examine the functions of the "boss" that even creative groups without a "boss" must provide within the team.

Dealing with Hungers, the New Style

Notwithstanding the nagging hunger for authority, on the demand side and on the supply side, many creative teams have found that the role of boss costs too much in team performance. That is, in some situations, the maintenance of the boss is too expensive because it either drains the resources of the group as a whole or impedes the creativity within the team, even unintentionally (2). The new style of leadership reduces the role of boss. We offer as an example the Orpheus orchestra, which has performed for over 30 years without a conductor—that is, without a boss—for a team of over 25 members, has drawn discriminating audiences, and has produced over 60 recordings for Deutsche Gramophon in successful competition with the other world-class orchestras with the autocratic or charismatic conductors.

Briefly, rather than an autocratic or charismatic conductor deciding the overall conception of the work and then dictating how each individual is to perform the individual tasks, the Orpheus team generally selects a different "core group" for each piece of music; the core group as a team work out the details of the piece and then present their idea to the whole team; and each member of the whole team then participates in refining the final conception, rehearsal, and product, including checking from various places in the auditorium how the sound is balanced and verifying the quality of the final recording—all without a boss. At times the whole team may follow someone, but whom the team follows rotates from task to task among the members that the team finds capable. The Orpheus team even has developed seminars and training sessions for adapting the Orpheus Process to business (http://www.orpheusnyc.com).

But we warn you. There is a 1997 PBS documentary, "Orpheus in the Real World," of the sometimes painful group dynamics that arise in the Orpheus Process, where there is no boss. Without a boss, each individual in the Orpheus organization must take an extraordinary degree of personal responsibility for ensuring that coworkers engage with the tough problems in the organization. And interestingly, the members of the Orpheus team do ensure that the organization provides the five functional elements of authority in modern settings, which we suggest are (i) prioritizing work efforts among competing goals, (ii) protecting the work from outside influences and distractions, (iii) organizing a division of labor so that necessary tasks are completed, (iv) healing the sometimes painful processes of conflict that surround work, and (v) maintaining standards of quality for work process and final product.

But there is no boss to provide those five functional elements of authority. The team must do it.

The Role of Spices

Why couldn't you do an Orpheus Process in your clinical laboratory? We cannot simulate exactly the scenario for your organization, because we don't know your organization. But we would guess that if you tried to implement an Orpheus Process in your clinical laboratory, office politics would take over. And, as a result, rather than provide the above five functional elements of authority, the authority structure likely would degenerate to the "election" of an alpha in which the candidates for alpha rise in the hierarchy based on a competition in physical displays of confidence and coalition building.

Furthermore, we would argue, an Orpheus Process may not be the most efficient means of providing structure for your organization. To use the analogy with nutrition, the Orpheus Process provides the authority structure that people need without using the "spice" of a boss that caters to the hungers for the alpha that culture and evolution have engrained in people. And many people find the denial of their hungers difficult. Similarly, people may find it difficult to stick to a nutritious diet if they cannot have at least the "spices" to give the tastes of sugar, salt, and burned fat that they crave.

Likely, in your organization, you have many versions of people like Jeremy Locke who do not have the self-discipline to curb their hungers, not even their hungers to be and have a boss. So it may be more efficient to provide the "spice" of a boss, where the boss must take responsibility for making the distinction between what the employees need and what the employees want.

How could you provide the "spice" of a boss? We propose that the Joseph Lyon scenario illustrates the elements of the "spice," namely, (i) projecting confidence and (ii) coalition building. For example, as Mr. Lyon you might use the "spice" of being the boss by opening your talk with the feel-good version, by telling stories of the good old days. Then you might use the "spice" of that diversion to do real work by easing the people into the parts of the real problem that they are ready to engage. Perhaps the people are ready to deal with getting together their resumes; you will help them. But you might at the same time assure people where appropriate that there will be even more promising positions in the future hospital that the organization will become. And, to end the talk, you might make it easier for the people to deal with what the future holds if you tell them that you will be there for them; you will not abandon them. That display of confidence and constancy makes a

"spice" of being the boss. The general structure of a tough talk might be to begin with "spice," ease into as much of the real work as people can handle, and end with "spice."

Basic "Nutritional" Requirements of Authority

In modern settings, the five functional elements of authority might be prioritizing, protecting, organizing, healing, and maintaining standards of quality. However, as the Greg Jefe leadership simulation in the previous chapter suggests, in some situations management's view of those five elements of authority is dysfunctional in going through the motions of those five elements without engaging the tough problems that threaten the organization. For example, when Greg Jefe implemented his "leadership by example," "autocratic style," and "leadership by incentive," he went through the motions of the five elements without tackling the conflict of employee values that created the laboratory problems of low productivity and high error rate.

That is, the five functional elements of authority are necessary for the health of the organization, but they are not sufficient. By analogy, perhaps the five functional elements of authority are like vitamins, necessary but not sufficient for health and functional performance. We suggest that separate from the necessary elements of authority, there must be leadership that provides the energy to mobilize employees to tackle the tough work.

But leadership is not an employee need. Leadership is an organizational need.

Where Employee Needs Likely Differ from Hungers

Possibly, there have been environments where the hungers of people induced them to take advantage of what the environment offered. For example, indulging the human hungers for competitions in coalition building and physical displays of confidence apparently took advantage of what the environment of Africa offered our ancient ancestors a hundred thousand years ago before they left Africa (4). However, the modern situation is quite different.

We suggest that as a modern manager, you face a situation where many employees still engage in the office politics that their hungers crave. Other employees, particularly the bright innovators on your team, in their own way may indulge their own particular hungers by shunning the posturing and coalition building of office politics like a plague. In particular, if you came to management from being a technician, you yourself may resent the posturing and coalition building that seem to come with being a manager.

But for quality work, given their hungers, your employees may need you, their manager, to posture for them in physical displays of confidence and coalition building. "But that is fake," you may protest, especially if your particular hungers do not drive you to rise in the hierarchy.

"Perhaps," we would reply. We don't want to get too philosophical here. But is not all of technology artificial in a similar fashion? That is, given the goal of quality in the organization, the technology for getting people to realize that goal of quality likely is "made up," invented, or artificial in responding to what real problems prevent the quality in the organization.

We close with several analyses to illustrate the variability in the acts of leadership that actually mobilize employees to tackle the tough problems that impede the improvement of quality in the organization. In each situation, we suggest that the manager's job is the supervision and control of (i) leadership and (ii) authority within the organization, taking into account the actual employee needs in the particular situation and considering the full range of leadership styles available, from the autocratic style to the "bossless" style of the Orpheus Process described above.

Case I: Change Management

We assume that the change you want in your organization is the change that improves the quality of performance. Hence, your efforts in change management might provide a means for getting things done more efficiently and more effectively. Leadership-within-change management might involve activities to increase the capability of people in the organization to take on new challenges, solve tough problems, and give up some old practices that give them comfort and stability.

However, a manager's natural inclinations may leave important aspects of change management unattended. For Jorg Junior in the previous chapter, it would have been easy to put off the change management required to improve tardiness and error rates. In addition, he interpreted his boss's insistence on zero tolerance to be an order to which he had to defer rather than a statement of a problem with which he should engage. That is, his natural inclinations reflected the hungers of office politics, such as "not rocking the boat" or "deferring to the boss" rather than "resolving to keep working on the problem until we solve it."

The opportunity for Jorg's boss was to note Jorg's tendency and then to use Jorg's tendency as important data about what needed to be fixed in the organization. That is, perhaps Jorg's tendency was to blame the situation on the boss rather than engage with the problem on his own terms. But, having noted Jorg's tendency, the boss need not correct Jorg's attitude directly. She might go through an iterative process of (i) intervening, (ii) using the data from the employees' e-mail and other reactions to fashion some hypothetical understanding of the underlying problem, and (iii) planning her next intervention based on her best data and knowledge.

We suggest that you as a manager might adopt the leadership style of Jorg's boss; use your authority to intervene forcefully for change management without following your perhaps natural inclinations to impose your answer that the employees must follow. Evidently, Jorg's boss planned to keep up her zero tolerance message until someone came up with an approach that was more promising than zero tolerance. So her intervention was heuristic, to learn clues about possible promising next steps, instead of merely imposing office politics to get her way.

Case II: Encouraging Innovation

Some innovation for improvements can be done only by employees on the front lines. They are closer to the actual problems and work processes. But they may not take responsibility for the politics and processes of innovation because they have been socialized to believe "that's management's job."

For example, an employee with a good idea might be inclined to try to convince the boss so that the boss will use her authority to implement the innovative solution. Emily New, in the previous chapter, exhibited this pattern when she interpreted the leadership problem as convincing others to agree with her idea. A better way to encourage technological innovation might be to say to your managers what Emily's boss said: "Your job is to get people to own the problem and along the way consider your idea together with other ideas for the solution."

A temptation for a senior manager might be to indulge competitive instincts that perpetuate office politics at the expense of genuine collaboration. For example, the senior manager might select a monthly winner of a competition for the Best Innovative Idea. A competition might seem like a reasonable means for getting good ideas to make their way to the top. However, the competitive process may lack the engagement of multidisciplinary perspectives that could provide important design elements to the solution. Emily's boss may have had the right idea in encouraging Emily to develop allies who could work together among the many technical areas to encourage innovation.

Furthermore, within the natural inclinations of office politics, competition may kill innovation. So the senior manager might intervene proactively in the style of Emily New's boss to delegate to the employees with the innovative ideas a little of her power and the encouragement to organize fellow employees to deal with the tough problems rather than just follow their natural inclinations to compete to win the boss's favor.

Where Indulging Hungers May Be Dysfunctional

In case I and case II above, we examined situations where the manager may miss something important if the manager simply follows personal inclinations. By analogy, in nutrition, hungers may not produce appropriate cravings for vitamins even when the person critically needs vitamins.

In the following two cases, we examine situations in which the manager's personal inclinations may indicate that something needs to be done, but the personal inclinations likely cause management interventions that actually hinder the improvement of performance and quality. By analogy, strong cravings to eat repeatedly overpower the dieter's resolve to stick to the regimen that he or she knows will improve health and well-being.

Case III: Crisis

Crisis results when the normal problem-solving processes of the organization fail. Some event or activity happens which the current resources or capacities cannot handle. The fault may be inadequate management planning or incomplete consideration of scenarios. Alternatively, the organization may lack in innovation, such as by failing to give the frontline employees sufficient opportunity to affect management decisions.

The leadership simulations with Joseph Lyon above illustrate the manager's strong inclination at the onset of crisis to step forward and give the employees an easy answer that makes them feel better, whether or not the easy answer has any promise of resolving the problems that caused the crisis. Likely, if there is a crisis, there is no easy answer, so the employees will suffer some loss and maybe substantial loss. Furthermore, during crisis the employees themselves likely must do much of the work of dealing with the problems causing the crisis. Hence, the manager's strong inclination to give an easy answer likely is a dysfunctional hunger—dysfunctional because it lures managers and employees alike into a false sense that the easy answer will keep them from having to sacrifice something that they value highly in order to get on with their lives.

By analogy, a doctor may experience a strong inclination to tell the patient with a badly damaged leg that "everything will be all right." But that strong inclination is dysfunctional if the situation requires amputation of the leg to save the patient's life. Surely it is better for the doctor to tell the patient enough of the situation so that the patient can engage productively with the grieving process that will assist the patient in shifting values, giving up what is lost and learning to take advantage of what life still has to offer.

Accordingly, we suggest that a manager in crisis should display confidence and coalition building to provide some stability in the organization. But the manager in crisis should use the power from that display of confidence and coalition building to assist the employees in mobilizing their own resources for dealing with the tough problem underlying the crisis and with the loss that the crisis will mean. That is, Joseph Lyon in the leadership simulation above should plan for the employees to leave that meeting with enough upset that they are actually dealing with the loss that they must face and with the work that must be done.

Case IV: Enforcement of Standards

People generally acknowledge that standards are necessary for improvement. But, as the Greg Jefe leadership simulation in the previous chapter illustrates, management may try to enforce the wrong standards—wrong because they do not address the real issue in the organization. For example, Greg Jefe at first attempted, in an autocratic style, to enforce clinical laboratory standards for productivity and error rate. But the real issue in the organization was a conflict of values that Greg Jefe untangled eventually by seriously examining what it would take to improve morale in the workplace.

A manager's natural inclination may be to lay down the law: to inform the employees of the standards and then to enforce the standards. And for some simple problem situations, that may work. However, an interactive trial-and-error process, like Greg Jefe's process to improve morale, may get more progress in quality measures than mere enforcement of standards. That is, in some situations, the manager's natural inclination to enforce the standard is dysfunctional because it lures both managers and employees into a competition of wills that prevents managers and employees from seeing opportunities for win-win solutions in which both sides would gain more than they give.

Managing from the View of a "Wide-Angle Zoom Lens"

Let us consider some ways that you might find the metaphor of the leadership simulator useful in untangling the leadership challenges you face as a manager in a clinical laboratory. Imagine that you had your particular organization programmed into a leadership simulator, including your current staff with whatever conflicting values they actually have. We suggest that there are two useful perspectives that you could learn from playing situations over in a leadership simulator: objectivity and choice.

First, you might see the leadership challenges that you face from a wider perspective. Here is a demonstration. Imagine that you have your current moment programmed into the leadership simulator; you are reading this book exactly wherever you are. Then around you are people, perhaps across the room, perhaps on the other sides of walls or partitions. If you had your current moment programmed into a leadership simulator, you could activate the view from a "wide-angle zoom lens" and look down on yourself from the ceiling and then expand the view to include all the people around you in the building where you are reading this book. Then if you watched the scene unfold, you would see how your actions coordinate with the actions of others to generate whatever happens in the scene.

In the view from a wide-angle zoom lens, you could observe what you do without the justifications that your feelings, hungers, and values add to make you different from the other actors in the scene. On the one hand, you might see how your tendency to speak first in a meeting plays into the tendencies of coworkers to let others speak first. On the other hand, you might see how your tendency to wait until you have something important to say plays into the tendencies of coworkers to say in a meeting what is on their mind whether it is important or not.

Second, you might exercise your power of choice. Most people make decisions in their life based on feelings, fears, and desires. However, as a manager, we suggest that your feelings, fears, and desires may tilt your decision-making process repeatedly down the same path without examining alternatives. So we suggest the following exercise in exploring the prerequisites of choice: can you take an alternative route that is different from your natural tendencies or inclinations?

After viewing your general patterns from a wide-angle lens, you might consider the options you actually have. You might insert a moment of choice before you act. For example, if you notice from your examination of the wide-angle view that your tendency is to speak first, then you might consider inserting a moment of choice, a moment of mentally flipping a coin: heads, I will speak; tails, I will wait for five other people to speak first. On the other hand, if you notice that your tendency is to wait until you have something important to say, you similarly might insert a moment of choice: heads, I will speak now; tails, I will wait until I have something important to say. After practice, if you can go the way that the coin says, then you are probably free enough of your natural cravings to go the way that you choose.

If you want to experiment with this technique of acting from the view of a wide-angle zoom lens, consider first trying it in some situation outside your workplace. Maybe the closest thing to a leadership simulator that you can find is your religious community or volunteer organization. In such a safe environment where you can experiment, be polite and courteous, but try pushing people to discover the real and tough problem that impedes quality performance in the meeting.

From a wide-angle zoom lens, you can picture the view looking down from the ceiling in real time. Notice what you do; notice what other people do. After you have noticed your tendency in the moment and have noticed the tendencies of the people around you in the moment, insert a moment of choice; make an intervention. At first, you may make mistakes, but keep going; keep trying to be helpful. And, in assessing your effect and in planning what you might do next, imagine the view looking down from the ceiling in real time. Notice what it is that you do that coordinates with what other people do to determine the outcome of the meeting.

We highly recommend that you discuss your "experimental" meetings with at least one ally, someone who is in your meeting and whom you can trust to tell you the truth. Request that your ally tell you first what you did that

had a beneficial effect on the meeting, even if only for a fleeting moment. If your ally is interested, you might reciprocate with your ally in giving your best and honest opinion of what happened in the meeting, starting first by describing the moments when your ally did something that forwarded progress in the meeting, even if only for a brief moment.

Ultimately, you and your ally might like to discover what the tough problem in your "experimental" organization is and how to tackle it, but that will be a process of discovery, we suggest, because you will be adjusting your point of view at the same time that you are nudging the prevailing points of view in the organization. The discovery process will be an interactive adventure. So you might start noticing the real-time indications of progress, which often snake through moments of despair and then elation in a moment of hope. Perhaps in that moment of hope is an element of an action plan for what might be done to improve the quality of performance in your "experimental" meeting. And all of the evidence of what happened in the meeting will be data for you and your ally to sift through to discover (i) what will make you more effective as a leader and (ii) what will improve the quality in your organization.

Managing from the view of a wide-angle zoom lens provides a real-time technique for noticing the effects that you have while you still have time to make corrections and adjustments. "Looking down on the scene from the ceiling, what can I see that my employees need for them to tackle the tough problems in my organization to improve quality?" From that wide-angle view, you can assess what your employees need independently of your own feelings, hungers, and values.

Summary

If you want quality performance from your employees, you had better give them what they need to do the job. But the manager's determination of employee needs easily pits the values of management against the values of the employees. That is, the employee may respond with some variation of "Who are you to say what I need?"

This chapter has explored the possibility that the employee knows a great deal about what the employee needs. But the manager cannot simply ask the employee to list the employee's needs. For it is likely that the employee will list many strong desires and cravings that have little relation to quality performance.

In this chapter, we have suggested several techniques to assist the manager in determining in a trial-and-error fashion what the employees actually need for quality performance. And along the way, we have explored in a clinical laboratory setting various opportunities for and challenges of leadership: mobilizing the employees to tackle their tough problems.

KEY POINTS

- The natural inclinations of both managers and employees may handicap attempts to improve quality in the organization. For example, employees may lack motivation to provide the extra care that avoiding errors requires. And, if there is a chronic problem of low morale, likely the natural inclinations of managers do not consider approaches that would provide actual motivation for the employees.

- Generally, the natural inclinations of both managers and employees are analogous to the hungers that people have; sometimes natural inclinations are dysfunctional. For example, people who are on a healthful diet may have a strong desire to eat what is unhealthful for them to eat.

  - Analogously, some employees have natural inclinations toward habits detrimental to quality.

  - Nevertheless, managers sometimes have induced a shift in employee values by catering judiciously to the strong desires and cravings of the employees.

- Similarly, managers in certain situations, such as a crisis, have strong inclinations that may be dysfunctional —dysfunctional in avoiding the real problem and chasing a false solution that makes people feel better. For example, in a crisis, a manager may feel compelled to come up with a simple but impractical solution or to find a scapegoat for the crisis.

- Several techniques of observation and analysis may assist the manager in making decisions that do not bend too much to the strong desires that are dysfunctional.

  - If the manager can imagine playing through an event, such as a meeting, in a leadership simulator, perhaps the manager can see options and alternative outcomes that the manager missed in real time. An ally, some peer that was in the meeting, may be able to assist in looking for optional interventions and alternative outcomes.

  - If the manager can imagine in real time looking down on the situation from the view of a wide-angle zoom lens, perhaps the manager can see how his or her actions coordinated with the actions of others to determine the outcome. Looking at the facial expression of an ally in the room may assist the manager in getting an objective snapshot in real time of the manager's effect in a meeting.

GLOSSARY

Adaptive challenge A problem that does *not* subside to satisfy the current values in the organization even when management applies the best-known methods and procedures. Generally, the resolution of an adaptive challenge requires a shift in values. For example, at least two competing values might shift to resolve a budget crisis. On the one hand, the "problem" would be resolved if the employees shifted their values to take less pay and still be satisfied. On the other hand, the "problem" might be resolved if management shifted the values in the organization to direct the business to new profitable markets, perhaps global markets.

Adaptive work Effort that produces the organizational learning required to tackle tough problems, the problems that often require an evolution of values. The learning in adaptive work often requires (i) addressing the conflicts in the values that people hold or (ii) diminishing the gap between the values people espouse and the reality they face. For example, dealing with reduced budgets may require (i) addressing the conflict between "We are doing a good job" and "We could do better" together with (ii) diminishing the gap between "We are doing the best that is possible" and current reality, which may be "The public will not pay for quality service."

Alpha The individual in the community to whom the others defer. Both humans and their nearest species relatives, the chimpanzees, show deference to the alpha of the community by ritualized gestures such as bowing, allowing the alpha to walk first in a procession, or standing aside when the alpha challenges. Furthermore, both humans and chimpanzees select an alpha of the community in a competition of (i) physical displays of confidence and (ii) coalition building. Accordingly, among humans and chimpanzees alike, the alpha of the community often is not the strongest, but rather the one who projects confidence, gives gifts, and strategically curries favor.

Authority Power granted to perform a service. The exchange of power for a service may be formal or informal. Formal authority arises where the officeholder promises to meet a set of explicit expectations, such as a job description or professional standards. Informal authority arises where employees confer power on a person based on implicit expectations; for example, "If Sally were here, she would know what to do."

Hunger Strong desire or craving. Some hungers may be genetic, such as the strong desire to take another breath. Other hungers may have a cultural source, such as the craving for music.

Leadership The activity of mobilizing employees to tackle tough problems, the problems that often require an evolution of values. Generally, any employee in the organization can exercise leadership, the activity of mobilizing employees to tackle tough problems. But the actions of those with authority in the organization inadvertently can discourage employees from exercising leadership. Alternatively, those with authority can exercise leadership by mobilizing employees generally to exercise leadership, the activity of mobilizing employees to tackle tough problems.

Management The act or practice of supervision and control.

Need Something required for performance. Different goals of performance may require different resources, different environments, and different attitudes.

New style of leadership Noticing in real time the effects that you have on the quality in an organization. From this view, anyone in the organization can exercise "leadership" by mobilizing employees to tackle tough problems. But the actions and words of those with authority and power can discourage the "leadership" of others without intending that result.

Nutrition Balancing hungers and needs.

Old style of leadership Expecting to build sufficient power, expertise, and reputation so that people will see the wisdom in your decisions.

Real-time correction An intervention that, based on a comparison of the desired versus actual progress, seeks to cancel the effects of the excessive interventions you have made and to bolster the effects of the interventions you have made that were too weak. One important feature of a real-time correction is holding steady long enough to collect the data and information you need to evaluate actual progress. For example, in driving a car, if you do not hold steady long enough to see what effect you have had, you may oversteer by swinging too much first to the left and then to the right.

Value A desirable standard or quality for which a person will sacrifice what others consider of higher importance.

View from a "wide-angle zoom lens" Metaphorically, a series of snapshots that encompass most of the organization as a whole. The operation of a zoom lens at a sports event illustrates the metaphor. The zoom lens adjusts to provide just enough of the field of action but not too much. In particular, when the player looks up at the instant replay of the view from the wide-angle zoom lens, the player can see more than the player saw when running the play. That is, from the view of the wide-angle zoom lens, the player can see enough of the system to determine how the player's actions coordinated with the actions of others to create the final organizational outcome.

ACKNOWLEDGMENTS

We acknowledge the special role played by Ronald A. Heifetz in helping us understand "leadership" in the terms we use here. Though this chapter expresses the views only of us, significant portions of the text in this chapter were taken from unpublished drafts and work product that Riley Sinder coauthored with Ron Heifetz going back to the 1970s, as well as concepts further developed by Heifetz in his seminal work, *Leadership without Easy Answers* (1994, Harvard University Press, Cambridge, Mass.). In addition, Heifetz has read and provided feedback on this chapter.

REFERENCES

1. Garletts, J. A. 2002. Using career ladders to motivate and retain employees: an implementation success story. *Clin. Leadersh. Manag. Rev.* **16:**380–385.

2. Hackman, J. R. 2002. *Leading Teams: Setting the Stage for Great Performances.* Harvard Business School Press, Boston, Mass.

3. Schlosser, E. 2002. *Fast Food Nation: the Dark Side of the All-American Meal.* Houghton Mifflin, New York, N.Y.

4. Wrangham, R., and D. Peterson. 1996. *Demonic Males: Apes and the Origins of Human Violence.* Mariner Books, New York, N.Y.

APPENDIX 9.1   Sample Suggestions for "Spice"[a]

Group	Possible spice
Generation Xers (people under 35)	Accommodate flexible schedules and approaches.
	Reward independence and self-starting.
	Praise the quality that they like in themselves.
	Provide training and experience in new technology.
Ethnic culture	Celebrate ethnic holidays.
	Produce an award ceremony in a rotating ethnic spirit and decor, such as a fiesta and then a luau.
Parents	Child care
	Family day, designed by parents
New hires	Rapid advancement scheme based on performance and quality
	Special attention to introductions and inclusion in activities
Long-term employees	An appearance of stability
	Encouragement to expand expertise to new technology
Subordinates	Manager displays confidence and ability to organize coalitions
	Opportunities to lead a team in a task

[a]A "spice" may not be an employee need. But a spice may help provide employee motivation by meeting an employee hunger. A survey questionnaire or structured interview process may suggest possible spices for your workplace. Determining whether a spice increases motivation is a trial-and-error process. Probably employee interactivity in designing the spice is more important than the final design of the spice.

APPENDIX 9.2   Suggestions for situations

Situation	Suggestions
A problem resists available approaches for solution.	The problem may require adaptive work rather than mere technical problem solving.
	Likely there is a conflict of values underlying the problem.
You would like to encourage adaptive work on a problem.	Obtain a description, such as by questionnaire, of the values that different managers and different employees represent.
	Cater to values and "hungers" in a way that people can see their own part in creating the situation of the problem.
	Engage managers and employees in an exploration: What would I be willing to give up to get this problem solved?
	Acknowledge progress when there is progress.
You don't have time to do the projects that you have.	Delegate.
	Clarify for yourself the three primary criteria of success for completion of the delegated work.
	Provide the resources required for completion of the delegated work.
Someone attacks you or insults you.	Distinguish your self from your role.
	Ask the following: What aspects of my role threatened my opposition? How could I play my role differently to diminish the threat of my role?
	You may find that the attack had nothing to do with you but rather arose from your opponent's refusal to deal with the problem that you brought into scrutiny.
You would like to practice some change in your leadership style.	Select a volunteer organization. Help them solve their problem.
	Practice different leadership styles in attempting to get the group to tackle the tough problems in the organization.
	Establish a network of allies in your volunteer organization for discussing moments of leadership.
You would like to work with an ally in adjusting your leadership style.	Select for an ally a peer who will tell you the truth.
	Discuss working meetings with your ally, noting the effects that followed different leadership interventions.
	Request that your ally begin each discussion session by noting the times that you were successful in getting the group to work on the tough problems in the organization.

10

Motivation: the Fire Within

Carmen Mariano

OBJECTIVES

To convince every reader that motivation is an internal force that lives in limitless quantities within all human beings

To dispel the myth that some people lack motivation by proving that such people only lack direction

To create a cadre of leaders who, after reading this chapter, will realize that their efforts have no value except through the efforts and accomplishments of those they lead

To encourage every reader to do the following from the day he or she finishes reading

- *Give a daily, written compliment to at least one employee*
- *Use an employee's name at least once in every conversation with that employee*
- *Listen seven times more than he or she talks*
- *Become more powerful by giving more power (and responsibility) to his or her followers*

To help each reader and his or her staff to set a limit of three SMART goals per year for their laboratory, department, or office

To make certain that no one who reads this chapter ever again questions the untold strength of the human spirit or the immeasurable capacity of the human intellect

To ensure that no reader ever again quits a cause unfulfilled or a task unaccomplished

---

The most powerful weapon on earth is the human soul on fire.

FIELD MARSHALL FERDINAND FOCH, COMMANDER
OF ALLIED FORCES IN EUROPE DURING WORLD WAR I

Defining Motivation

MOTIVATION IS A WORD OF WONDER. Many people claim to understand it. Few people do. Denis Waitley describes motivation as "an inner force that causes behavior" (51). Martin Covington calls it "an internal state that impels individuals toward action" (15). Both understand that motivation begins from the inside out, not the other way around. Both understand that motivation is a fire from *within.*

And if the fire comes from within, only the person in whom it burns can light it. Motivation is not something that someone can give or do to someone else. No pressure from a friend, a spouse, a colleague, or a manager is motivation. Pressure is external. Motivation is internal.

There is a myth about motivation that says people can motivate other people. That myth is popular, but not true. People motivate themselves. Their fire comes from within. So the bad news is, people can't be motivated. But the good news is, they don't have to be. All people work hard at something. They are motivated.

That includes healthcare workers. All healthcare workers work hard at something. Most of them work hard at healthcare. Others work hard at asking for a raise, finding ways to leave early, or having weekends off. Still others work hard at bringing up a family, getting through graduate school, breaking 100 in golf, or keeping their grass green.

Some people even work hard at not working hard! I had a friend in graduate school like that. He conducted a nationwide computer search trying to find a research paper on a certain topic so he could copy the paper and submit it for one of his courses. The search took him 2 months and cost $300. It would have been faster and cheaper to write the paper himself, but he was too busy working hard at not working hard.

Everyone works hard at something. Managers must get their staff to work hard on the right things. They must point their staff's inner fire in the right direction.

The Importance of Direction

"Every time you aim nowhere, you get there" (49). People need direction. If you invite someone to your house, the first thing the person would need to know is where you live. He can't go where you want him to go if he doesn't know where that is.

The people you work with are no different. For them to go where you want, they need a map. If you give them a map, they still might get lost, but if you don't, they definitely will get lost! People need to know what you want them to do before they can do it.

"Florence Chadwick was a great swimmer," writes Glenn Van Ekeren (50). "She swam the English Channel many times. Once, Florence tackled the 20-mile swim from Catalina Island to the California coast. But Florence picked a bad day for a swim." The currents were strong. The waves were high. The water was cold. Worst of all, a dense fog made it almost impossible to see. Despite all that, Florence swam for 15 hours. Then, only half a mile from shore, she gave up. Later, when asked why she quit so close to her destination, she replied that it was not the current, or the waves, or the cold. It was the fog. Florence said, "I failed because I couldn't see the shore. I failed because I lost sight of my goal" (33, 50). Florence had inner fire, but she lost direction and failed. Everyone's fire needs direction.

Like Florence, or anyone who's gotten lost in an unfamiliar neighborhood, the lack of a clear direction or goal can leave a person feeling frustrated, helpless, and lost.

Good managers provide directions and goals for their staff. Each person's inner fire needs a goal to work towards.

Setting Goals

Charles Givens tells of a study of university business school graduates who had been out of school for 10 years (23). Eighty-three percent of the graduates had set no goals. This group reported that they were working hard and staying busy but had no specific future plans. Another 14% had goals but hadn't written them down. This 14% was earning on average three times the income of those who had no goals at all. The remaining 3% of the entire graduate group had written goals for themselves. That 3% was earning 10 times more than those with no goals. "The message is clear," concludes Givens. "Goals ... make the difference!"

So, set goals. And make those goals SMART. Make them

- *Specific*
- *Measurable*
- *Attainable*
- *Relevant*
- *Timed*

The purpose of a goal is not to define success or failure but to provide direction. Thus, good goals must be *specific* and *measurable*. You must know if you reach them and if you don't. I had a track coach in high school who told me to "work hard" and "run fast." I never knew if I got there or if I didn't, and neither did my coach. These were not smart goals. I had another coach who told me to "run five quarter miles in under a minute. Then run 5 more faster than that." After every practice, I knew whether I'd succeeded or not, and so did my coach. These goals were specific and measurable.

Take for example the goal "to be all that you can be." Is that goal specific? Is it measurable? Does it define exactly where you are going or exactly when you get there? Where is "all that you can be?" Do you know? Will you know if you get there? What precisely is "all that you can be?" A goal that's not specific or measurable is not much of a guide.

Other goals can be just as vague. Your goal for your laboratory, your office, or yourself may be to "realize your full potential," to "do your best," or to "produce quality work." These sound better, but they're not much help either. What, to be specific, is "your full potential," "your best," or "quality work"? If you don't know what your goals are, you will never reach any of them, and neither will your laboratory or your office.

Goals must also be *attainable*. "If striving for a goal is easy enough to offer 100% probability of success, that goal is of no value. If striving for a goal is difficult enough to offer 100% probability of failure, that goal is of no value either" (12).

Progress is the root of all achievement, and effort is the root of all progress. People will not work toward a goal that they feel cannot be reached. Still, almost all goals can be reached. Something is impossible only until it is accomplished. So reach for the stars. If you fail, you may touch the moon.

To me the biggest danger facing our world, more than nuclear war, overpopulation, acid rain, global warming, or moral decay, is that human beings will stop believing that they can overcome those other dangers. I believe that the world's biggest and only real danger is that people will lose faith in themselves.

Next, the goals of a group must *relate* to the needs of its members. People care about what they own. So make your goals your own. Make your office or laboratory's goals belong to the staff who are involved.

The following story emphasizes this critical point. There were two warring tribes. One lived in the lowlands and the other high in the mountains. The mountain people invaded the lowlanders one day, kidnapped a baby of one of the lowland families, and took it with them into the mountains. The lowlanders did not know how to climb a mountain, but they tried. Their best fighting men made attempt after attempt to climb that mountain and bring the baby home. They finally gave up—and just then they saw the baby's mother walking down toward them with the baby strapped to her back. One man asked her, "How did you climb this mountain when we, the most able men in the village, couldn't do it?" The woman shrugged and said, "It wasn't your baby." That mother climbed that mountain because she owned her direction, her goal. Your staff's goals should relate to them. Sigmund Freud said, "The rider is obliged to guide his horse in the direction in which the horse wants to go" (22). Let staff set and *own* their goals.

W. Edwards Deming was the American industrial engineer who fathered total quality management. Deming brought his beliefs to Japan and turned that country's economy around. Deming believed in excellence. He also believed in people. According to Deming, in the United States, we sell our people short. In Deming's words, "America's greatest mistake lies in its failure to believe in its people." In fact, according to Deming, only about 6% of all organizational performance problems are due to employee error or individual failure. The other 94% are, in his judgment, caused by systems within the organization itself (17, 47).

Those systems separate the employee from the organization and from the organization's goals. This problem can be solved by making an organization's goals belong to its employees.

The philosophical foundation of relating goals to employees looks like this.

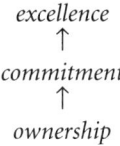

excellence

↑

commitment

↑

ownership

In other words, excellence grows from commitment, and commitment grows from ownership. People care about what is theirs. There is a direct, positive correlation between level of commitment and level of excellence. People can achieve anything if they commit enough of themselves to it, but people will only commit to what is theirs. In the words of Stephen Covey, "Mark it down. Circle it. Underline it. No involvement, no commitment" (13). So, let the goals you set *relate* to your employees.

A minister named Donald Strong, one of my heroes, wrote an essay on leadership called "Letting People Have Your Way" (48). In it he wrote, "Don't force people to do what you want. Help them do what they want." Abide by that advice. Lead people to goals they set and they own.

Last, "a goal is a dream with a deadline." Thus, every goal must have a deadline. Every goal must be *timed*. C. Northcote Parkinson, a professor of history at the University of Malaya in the 1950s and a visiting professor at Harvard and Illinois universities, wrote a book called *Parkinson's Law: The Pursuit of Progress* (41). That "law" asserts that work expands to fill the time available for its completion. So, allocate a specific amount of time to each goal. James K. Polk, the eleventh President of the United States, announced what he called "four great goals" in his 1844 campaign for the presidency (39):

- Acquire California from Mexico.
- Settle the Oregon boundary dispute.
- Lower the tariff.
- Establish an independent treasury system.

To these, Polk added a fifth goal. It was to "serve only one term as President." That goal was the "T" in Polk's SMART! After serving a single term as he promised, and after reaching his other four goals, Polk left office (39). That was a good example for managers: set goals that are *timed*. Set goals that are SMART.

While you are being smart, remember that goals are like children: too many of them will drive you crazy! No individual or organization can achieve excellence in more than three things at the same time. When it comes to goals, less is more. Three is plenty, two is better. When you reach one, add another.

Do you have any goals for your laboratory, your office, or yourself? If you do, write them down right now. Remember to make each goal SMART. Make sure you understand how you will know if you reach it.

Some of you may find it difficult to put your goals into written form. If you have written your goals before, congratulations. You are special. If not, congratulations—you are normal! Only 2 out of every 100 adults in this country have definite written goals related to work, career, life, or their fire within. The other 98% live by what Anthony Robbins calls the "Niagara syndrome" (44). They act as if life is a river. They jump into that river without really deciding where they want to end up. In a short time, they get caught in the currents: current events, current worries, and current problems. When they come to a fork in the river, they don't choose a direction; they just go with the flow of the river. When they finally realize that the river is taking them over Niagara Falls, it's usually too late to do anything about it!

If you and the people you work with have been suffering from the Niagara syndrome, it's okay. You just need to change direction, give your fires direction, and make that direction SMART.

Getting People To Follow Your Direction

People have a fire within, and managers should give that fire direction. They should set SMART goals. However, people don't have to follow that direction or work toward those goals. In every laboratory, hospital, and office, people have the right to do what they want. People can look busy without being busy and can overpromise and underdeliver. They can come late, leave early, or stay home. The people you work with can choose their own direction, and they do! Their time and presence can be purchased, but their commitment must be given and earned. People volunteer to work hard or they don't. They also choose to follow direction or they choose not to.

In America, we are all independent contractors who work for ourselves. We all listen to the same radio station, and it's called WIIFM, otherwise known as "What's in it for me?" Thus, people don't work for anyone else; they work for themselves.

Difficult Employees

Even committed employees at times resort to difficult behaviors. Brinkman and Kirschner (5) put those behaviors on the "Ten Most Unwanted List" as follows:

- The *Tank* is confrontational, pointed, and angry. He or she exhibits the ultimate in pushy and aggressive behavior.

- The *Sniper* uses rude comments, biting sarcasm, or a well-timed roll of the eyes to make you look foolish.

- The *Grenade* explodes (after a brief period of calm) into unfocused ranting and raving about things that have nothing to do with the present circumstances.

- The *Know-It-All* has a low tolerance for correction and contradiction. If something goes wrong, however, the Know-It-All will speak with the same authority about who's to blame—you!

- The *Think-They-Know-It-Alls* can't fool all the people all of the time, but they can fool some of the people enough of the time and enough of the people all of the time, all for the sake of getting some attention.

- The *Yes People* say "yes" without thought, in an effort to please people and avoid confrontation. They react to

the latest demands on their time by forgetting prior commitments, and they overcommit until they have no time for themselves. Then they become resentful.

- The *Maybe Person* vacillates and procrastinates in the hope that a better choice will present itself. Sadly, that choice never comes. Neither does the *Maybe Person's* decision.

- The *Nothing Person* offers no verbal feedback and no nonverbal feedback. The *Nothing Person* offers nothing!

- The *No Person* fights a neverending battle for futility, hopelessness, and despair. Disguised as a mild-mannered normal person, he or she is more deadly to morale than a speeding bullet, more powerful than hope, and able to defeat big ideas with a single syllable.

- Last but not least, the *Whiners* feel helpless and overwhelmed by an unfair world. Their standard is perfection, and no one and nothing measure up to it. But misery loves company, so they bring their problems to you. Offering solutions makes you bad company, so their whining escalates.

Options for Managers

Your staff is no different, in that they don't work for you. They work for themselves, and they will be themselves. They won't follow your direction for you but will follow it for themselves. As a manager, supervisor, and leader, what can you do? Brinkman and Kirschner offer managers four ways to deal with their Ten Most Unwanted (5):

- You can stay in the person's presence and do nothing. That includes silently suffering over it, or complaining to someone who can do nothing.

- You can leave the person's presence, your job, or both.

- You can try to change their behavior. (If you hold your breath as you do this, you will die many times.)

- You can change your behavior.

Choose the fourth option. Some people bring out the best in you, and some people bring out the worst. You can do the same! Never overestimate your ability to change someone else, and never underestimate your ability to change yourself. Leo Tolstoy once wrote, "Everyone thinks of changing the world, but no one thinks of changing himself" (43). When faced with any of the Ten Most Unwanted, change yourself! If people exhibit negative or unproductive behavior in response to what you are doing, do something else. To paraphrase Tony Robbins and James Autry, "the definition of insanity is expecting different results from the same action" (3, 44). If you want someone else's behavior to change, your behavior must change first. So, behave in ways that send your employees the same three messages, over and over, day after day. What are those messages?

Three Messages

Send every employee and colleague these three messages as often as you can, as loudly as you can, and in as many ways as you can:

- You are important.
- You can do it.
- Follow me!

Sending those three messages is your best chance of getting people to point their fires in your direction and getting people to want to do what you want them to do.

The Importance of Feeling Important

Say "You are important" to the people you work with. Do all you can to make the people you work with feel important, because they are!

Andrew Carnegie once said, "Take away my people but leave my factories and soon grass will grow on the factory floor. Take away my factories but leave my people and soon we will build new and better factories." Henry Ford said the same thing with different words. He said, "Take my people and leave me my money and I can never recover, but take my money and leave me my people and I can return to success tomorrow." They were both right. If you are a manager, supervisor, leader, or all three, people are your most important resource. Your job has no value without them, so for starters, make people feel important, because they are!

Making people feel important is the best way you have of getting them to point their fire in your direction. If you want people to choose your direction, "You are important" is the most important message you can send!

The Hawthorne Effect

In 1927 the Western Electric Company's plant in Hawthorne, Ill., experimented to see how certain working conditions affected production. They started with lighting. First, the researchers improved the lighting in one of the shops, and they found that the workers in that shop produced more than they had before the improvements. But further studies revealed that workers in a shop that got no change in lighting increased their production, too! Then, the researchers went into a shop and decreased its lighting. In the words of one of the researchers who were there, this is what happened (10).

"The test group is given increased light. Its output goes up. Good, that was to be expected. But the output of the control group—without one candlepower of extra light—goes up too! This was not expected. It is contrary to common sense—indeed, it is completely screwy. But screwier results are to follow. Light for the test group is now decreased below that of the control group. Its output goes up again! What in heaven's name is going on? The research

staff was forced to conclude that intensity of light was not a factor in production. To verify this they put two workers in a locker room with no light at all except what came through a crack under the door. Those workers increased output, even in the dark!"

"Our conclusions," Stuart Chase goes on, after 21,000 interviews, "are as follows: underneath the stop watches and bonus plans of the efficiency experts, the worker is driven by a desperate inner urge to find an environment where he belongs and has a function, where he sees the purpose of his work and where he feels important" (10). In what was later termed the Hawthorne effect, the researchers discovered that it was the attention paid to the workers, and not the amount of lighting, that increased their production. The workers were given attention, were made to feel important, and they responded by working harder.

People hunger to be noticed, to be valued, and to feel important. The people you work with are no different. They deserve and want to feel important, so make them feel important.

Believe that People Are Important

First, learn from the experts! Study the technique of the all-time worldwide authorities on making people feel important. You may have one of these experts at home waiting for you to get there. When you do, he will begin to wag his tail. If you stop and pat him, he will almost jump out of his skin to show you how happy he is to see you. And you know that behind that show of affection, there are no ulterior motives. He doesn't want to sell you any real estate, or get a bigger paycheck from you, or ask for a favor. Dogs are experts at making people feel important, and they make people feel important for free, without conditions!

The first and best thing you can do to make people feel important is to believe that they are important just for being themselves. If you believe that, it will show; if you don't, that will also show. You can't fool people for long, so the only way to be sure you are making people feel important is to believe that they *are* important. Convince yourself once and for all that the people you work with are truly and unconditionally important.

Ego is a word with many definitions. We all want to see ourselves as being important. Feed the egos of the people you work with. Treat them as if they are that important, and believe it, because it's true.

Frederick Hertzberg's Theory

Stuart Chase and his colleagues weren't the only researchers who discovered the importance of feeling important. As detailed by Hersey and Blanchard (26), Frederick Hertzberg interviewed 201 engineers and accountants from 11 industries in the Pittsburgh, Pa., area. He asked what kinds of things on their job made his subjects unhappy or dissatisfied and what things made them happy or

Table 10.1 Hertzberg's factors[a]

Hygiene factor (maintenance)	Motivator
Policies/administrator	Achievement
Working conditions	Recognition
Safety/security benefits	Advancement
Salary	Importance

[a]See reference 28, p. 148.

satisfied. After analyzing the data from these interviews, Hertzberg concluded that people have two categories of needs that are independent of each other and that affect behavior in different ways. Hertzberg called the first category of needs *hygiene factors* or *maintenance factors*. He called the second category of needs *motivators* (Table 10.1).

According to Hertzberg, working conditions, benefits, salary, security, status, and title are hygiene factors. These factors are tangible and environmental. They relate to physical resources and sensory conditions. People feel and see these factors externally. They meet the physiological and safety needs of employees—nothing more. These factors are also preventative. According to Hertzberg's study, having these factors at high enough levels keeps people from being dissatisfied. But, regardless of how high these levels are, they do not make people happy or satisfied. Hygiene factors produce no growth in worker output and only prevent declines in worker performance.

On the other hand, Hertzberg's motivators include feelings of achievement, professional growth, and recognition. These factors are internal and relate to the nature of the job and the ego of the employee. If properly addressed, these factors can increase employee satisfaction and performance. In the words of Hersey and Blanchard, "Hygiene factors, when satisfied, tend to eliminate dissatisfaction, but they do little to effect superior performance or increase capacity. Motivators, on the other hand, will permit an individual to grow and develop; often implementing an increase in willingness and even ability" (26).

Maslow's Hierarchy of Needs

Psychologist Abraham Maslow developed a widely quoted explanation of human motivation (34, 35). According to Maslow, people have an internal hierarchy of needs pushing them from survival, through comfort, to acceptance, and finally toward personal fulfillment. When a person's needs are satisfied at one level, he or she works toward satisfaction at a higher level. Maslow arranged human needs into a five-level pyramid. The groups of needs in ascending order are as follows:

- *Physiological needs* refer to basic bodily needs such as the requirements for nutrition, water, shelter, moderate temperatures, rest, and sleep.

- *Safety needs* include the desire to be safe from both physical and emotional injury.

- *Social needs* refer to needs for love, belonging to a group, and affiliation with people.

- *Esteem needs* reflect the desire to be seen by ourselves and by others as people of worth.

- *Self-actualization needs* refer to the desire to reach one's potential, and they include needs for self-fulfillment and personal development.

Maslow's hierarchy dovetails nicely with Hertzberg's theory. For example, money and benefits are hygiene factors that tend to satisfy needs at the physiological and security levels. Interpersonal relations and supervision are examples of hygiene factors that tend to satisfy social needs. Increased responsibility, challenging work, and professional development are motivators that tend to satisfy needs at the esteem and self-actualization levels (21).

Praise and Criticism

"Raise the Praise; Minimize the Criticize"

According to Hertzberg (26), money does not satisfy people; nor does money motivate people. Recognition does. Praise does. And according to Maslow (34), money satisfies low-level needs only, while praise does more. So recognize and praise people. Praise is always welcome, is never questioned, and does wonders for your credibility. If you praise people, they always believe you. Praise does wonders for a person's sense of hearing, too. If you want your staff to listen to you, say something good about them!

Mary Kay Ash (2) says, "Criticism should be outnumbered by praise at a rate of about eight to one. But in most organizations, it is the other way around or worse. And that is a shame because praise is more productive than criticism!" You probably don't know many people or many employees who can handle criticism. So raise the praise, and minimize the criticize (56)! "Everyone likes a compliment" (43). Those are Abe Lincoln's words. We all like to be praised. It makes us look good in our own eyes, it makes us feel good about ourselves, and no feeling is more important or more powerful. So use praise, and compliment more than you criticize. Rewarded behavior is repeated, and there is no more valuable reward than praise! If an employee does something that is rewarded by praise, that employee will do it again. Praise is like education (28). There is no such thing as too much of it (45). Give your employees as many chances to succeed as you can, and praise them when they do.

If you have been to Sea World in San Diego, Calif., you know that they put on a terrific show. The star of the show is a killer whale named Shamu. In one trick, Shamu jumps from the tank over a rope that is held 22 ft above the surface of the water. Shamu weighs almost 10 tons, and the rope he jumps over is two stories above the water. How did Shamu's trainers get him to perform that trick?

The first thing they did was lower the rope! The trainers placed the rope under the water first. Then, every time Shamu happened to swim over it, the trainers praised him, gave him fish, patted him on the back, and played with him. Every time Shamu succeeded, they complimented him. Then they raised the rope a little. And when Shamu happened to swim over it again, they gave him fish again, and patted him and played with him. They complimented him again.

And what happened when Shamu swam under the rope? Nothing happened. When Shamu succeeded, his trainers complimented him, but when he failed, they did nothing.

Eventually, the rope was raised to the level of the water in the tank. So, for the first time, Shamu had to leave the water to jump over the rope. When he did, he was complimented, but when he didn't, nothing happened. As the rope went higher, the training remained the same. Each success was noticed and complimented, while each failure was ignored. Eventually, the rope rose to 22 ft, and eventually, so did Shamu. Thus, by complimenting his successes and ignoring his failures, Shamu's trainers were able to get him to perform how they wanted.

People are like Shamu. They respond much better to compliments than they do to criticism. So, look for, find, and praise strengths.

Picasso had trouble remembering the alphabet. Beethoven was deaf and notoriously clumsy. Tom Brokaw and Barbara Walters have speech impediments. Da Vinci's writing was atrocious and his spelling was worse. He formed all of his letters backwards, and he constantly made simple mistakes in arithmetic. We all have strengths and weaknesses. Your staff is no different. They all have strengths, so look for those strengths, and when you find them, praise them! Include a positive, true statement in every conversation. Raise the praise, and minimize the criticize.

Does that mean you should never criticize? Dale Carnegie says it does! In his classic book *How To Win Friends and Influence People* (9), Carnegie says that the world's most influential people never criticize, never condemn, and never complain. I disagree.

The Artful Critique

When there is bad news to deliver, you must deliver it. But when you criticize, listen to Daniel Goleman (24) and do the following:

- *Be specific.* Pick a significant incident or a pattern of deficiency. It demoralizes people just to hear that you are generally "displeased with their performance" or that they are "doing something wrong" without knowing what the specifics are so they can change.

- *Offer a solution.* Your identification of a problem should include the suggestion of a solution. Preferably, ask the employee to suggest solutions. Remember, excellence is built on commitment, and commitment is built on ownership. Help the employee own the solutions.

- *Be present.* Always deliver bad news in person and in private. People who are uncomfortable giving criticism often ease the burden on themselves by doing so at a distance, that is, in writing. Employees deserve more than that. They deserve the opportunity to ask questions. They deserve the opportunity to respond. They deserve to be able look into your eyes. They cannot do these things if you are not there.

- *Be sensitive.* Good leaders see the world through the eyes of their followers. They empathize. So, consider the impact of your message on the person receiving it. An old adage says, "Constructive criticism is when I criticize you, and destructive criticism is when you criticize me." It is true. Most criticism is destructive. Your only hope to avoid destruction is to care. Without empathy, the net effect of criticism is destructive. Instead of opening the way for growth, it creates resentment, bitterness, defensiveness, and distance.

Criticize Products, Never People

One more element can be added to Daniel Goleman's description of "the artful critique." Criticize products, never people. As managers, every time we speak to an employee, we send two messages: a product message and a people message. One message evaluates a product, while the other evaluates the people who created the product.

If a laboratory technologist performs a proficiency test and you comment on that test's results, your comment carries a product message about the test and a people message about the technologist who performed it. Each of those messages can be positive or negative. Every product message you give should be honest, accurate, and based on a set of standards. The message you send about the proficiency test should be positive if the results meet your and the accrediting agency's standards and negative if the results don't.

The message you send to the employee should always be positive! If an employee does poor work, tell the employee that he gave you poor work, and tell him why! Give his work a negative product message, but don't give that employee a negative people message. Tell him that he gave you poor work, not that he is a poor employee. Criticize what a person does, not who a person is.

As managers, we should criticize products, not people. However, some people and some managers often do the opposite. They give a negative people message even when the product message is positive! Specific examples can be seen below:

- "Lill, I am going to give you a satisfactory evaluation, even though you don't deserve it."

- "Bill, your cost analysis is good, but if you weren't so lazy, it could have been great!"

- "Phil, your work is good, but your attitude is not!"

- "Mil, you got an 80 on your proficiency test; that is great, for you!"
- Or "Syl, your report was super. I didn't think you had it in you."

If you've ever said anything that resembled those last few comments, it may be time for a change! Give positive people messages with every product message, and compliment more than you criticize. Raise the praise, and minimize the criticize.

Shine Your Light on Your Stars

Have you ever seen a sign like this? **LIMIT 20 COPIES!!!** These signs are generally above the copy machine in your laboratory or office, and they were meant for the three employees who abuse the copy machine. But who takes that sign seriously? It's probably the 30 dedicated, hard-working, "never-a-problem" employees who don't abuse the copy machine! They read the sign and either feel guilty because they ran off two extra copies one day last year or feel mad because they know they don't abuse the copy machine and don't deserve the sign. However, what do the three abusers do? They ignore the sign and continue to abuse the copy machine! So, discard that sign and consider replacing it with this one that raises the praise and minimizes the criticize:

> **This machine can duplicate almost anything, but it can never duplicate you! You cannot be duplicated. You cannot be replaced. No one knows what you know or can do what you do. Most of all, no one is the person you are. We need you and appreciate you just as you are. There is no "US" without "U"!**

I coached high school wrestling for 10 years. When four or five wrestlers didn't show up for practice, I lectured the members who were there on how important it was to show up for practice and how mad I was when wrestlers didn't show up. Unfortunately, these individuals either felt guilty for the one practice they missed all year or were mad at me for lecturing them instead of those who failed to come to practice! I should have waited for the absent ones to return and should have thanked those who came faithfully for doing so, in front of those who missed!

Two years ago, I attended a Clinical Laboratory Management Association conference in St. Louis, Mo. My hotel made a mistake and gave me a $700 suite overlooking the river, the Arch, and Busch Stadium. It was magnificent, until I opened the closet and found 20 theft-proof hangers. I thought, "Here I am in a $700-a-night suite, being treated like a hanger thief!" It made me think of the sign on the copy machine.

Your laboratory, hospital, or office will go only as far as your best employees will take it. So give your time and your attention to your best, and give them the power of your praise. "Raise the praise. Minimize the criticize!" (56)

Names, Notes, and Notice

Use names and notes, and notice often. The most powerful word in any person's vocabulary is his or her name. Nothing attracts attention faster, and nothing says "You are important" louder. In the words of Dale Carnegie, "Even as a boy, Andrew Carnegie discovered the astonishing importance that people place on their names. When he was ten years old, he had a father rabbit and a mother rabbit. He awoke one morning to discover that he had a whole nest full of little rabbits and nothing to feed them. He told half a dozen boys in the neighborhood that if they would go out every day and pull enough dandelions and grass and clover to feed the rabbits, he would name the rabbits in their honor. The plan worked like magic. Andrew Carnegie never forgot that incident, and years later, he made millions of dollars by using the same technique in business. He wanted to sell steel rails to the Pennsylvania Railroad. At the time, J. Edgar Thomson was president of the railroad. Andrew Carnegie, remembering the lesson he had learned from his rabbits, built a huge steel mill in Pittsburgh and called it the J. Edgar Thomson Steel Works. When the Pennsylvania Railroad needed steel rails after that, where do you suppose J. Edgar Thomson bought them?" (8). Be like Andrew Carnegie. Use a person's name at least once in every exchange you have with that individual.

Send at least one written message of "thank you" or "well done" every day. Handwrite them, and make them about something small. Write a note praising or thanking an employee for something that he or she is sure you did not notice. That will astound the employee and will also make him or her feel important.

Listen!

Another way to make people feel important is to listen to them! Pay attention when they talk. We are flattered by other people's attention, and it makes us feel special and important. That is one of the most basic facts of human psychology. So ask people how they feel or what they think, and *listen* when they answer! Oliver Wendell Holmes (27) once said, "It is the province of knowledge to speak, and it is the privilege of wisdom to listen." Be wise and listen!

On the night the *Titanic* sank, it received five clear warnings of icebergs from other ships. All five of those warnings were given to the captain of the unsinkable *Titanic* before it struck the iceberg. However, the captain of the *Titanic* was not a good listener. He heard all of the warnings but listened to none of them. Be a better manager than that man was a captain. Listen to the people you work with, and make them feel important!

A friend who teaches world history once shared an anecdote about Julius Caesar. It seems that Caesar was once riding into Rome on his chariot when an old woman blocked his path. The woman asked him to hear a complaint, but Caesar brushed her aside, saying he was too busy. "If you are too busy to listen, then you are too busy to rule," said the woman. With that, Caesar halted his chariot and listened. As a manager, you are busy, but you can never be too busy to listen to your staff.

If you are a good listener, congratulations—you are special. If you are not a good listener, congratulations—you are normal. Most of us are bad listeners, and on average, we listen only to 20% of what we hear. We communicate in four verbal ways. We speak, we listen, we read, and we write. Of these, we receive the least training in the art of listening (6).

One night, at a White House gala, Theodore Roosevelt grew tired of meeting people who returned his remarks with stiff, mindless pleasantries. So he began to greet people by saying, "Hello, I murdered my grandmother this morning. How are you?" Most of the people he met didn't even respond to what he said. But one diplomat did. Upon hearing Roosevelt's remark, the diplomat leaned over and whispered, "I'm sure she had it coming, Mr. President!" Roosevelt answered, "Thank you! You are the only person that has listened to me all night!" Failure to listen is not surprising because people must do two things to be good listeners, both of which are hard to do! First, before people can listen, they must stop talking. The other thing people must do before they can listen is even harder. To be a good listener, people must stop thinking about themselves.

If someone is talking to you, before you can listen, you must stop thinking of everything except what that person is saying. You must stop thinking about what's for dinner, how tired you are, how many cholesterols you have to check, how you will pay to get your car fixed, and when you will make your next trip to Aruba! Here are some rules that will make it easier to listen:

- *Stop talking!* That's right, you can't listen and talk at the same time. So, good listeners don't talk while they are listening. That isn't easy. Are you still sure you want to be a good listener?

- *Judge the book.* When you listen, judge the book, not the cover, i.e., judge the content, not the delivery. Have you ever heard someone speak or teach and think, "Is that guy alive or dead, and if he is dead, why doesn't someone tell him?" Well, you can even learn from someone like that, if you listen to what he says. So listen. You can learn from anyone.

- *Work at it.* Good listening is no vacation. It takes energy. Good listeners know that, so they work hard: they stay active, they establish eye contact, they lean forward, they nod, and they smile; they forget about what time it is, or who is home to take out the dog, or what's for dinner.

- *Keep an open mind.* Good listeners fight off stereotypes, assumptions, and biases. What? You don't have any of those? Oh really! Tell me, is Carmen Mariano an Italian man, a Spanish woman, or something else?

- *Hear no ego.* We all interpret everything we hear in a way that makes us look innocent, intelligent, and justified. There is nothing wrong with that, as long as it doesn't completely distort what someone else is trying to say. Good listeners know the difference between what they are hearing and what they want to hear. They hear no ego.

- *Ask anyway.* How many times have you heard something that you didn't understand? Did you question it, or did you just let it go because you didn't want to look stupid, or waste time, or hurt the speaker's feelings? Well, good listeners don't fake understanding. They ask any question any time. They take responsibility for getting the right message!

In his book *The Fred Factor*, Mark Sanborn talks about the difference between relational and transactional leaders (46). He explains that transactional leaders focus on process, product, and profit, while relational leaders focus on people. Transactional leaders care about *what* is working, while relational leaders care about *who* is working. However, transactional leaders may not exist. They are an oxymoron or a self-contradiction, like "jumbo shrimp," "loose tights," "guest host," or "old news." Individuals who focus on transactions and not relationships cannot be leaders, because followers require relationships and followers create leaders.

Also, relationships are built with ears and good listening skills. In the words of Dale Carnegie, "The secret of influencing people is not so much in being a good talker; but a good listener" (8). There is an old story about a young man named Johnny who at 16 tells his mother that he has his first girlfriend. "Why does she like you?" asks Johnny's mother. "Because she thinks I am cute and funny and can dance," replies Johnny. "And why do you like her?" Mom continues. "Because she thinks I'm cute and funny and can dance!" replies Johnny. Being interested builds relationships more than being interesting. Be interested in your employees, and listen when they speak.

Give Responsibility

Giving people responsibility can also make them feel important. When given, responsibility is a visible, active expression of trust. When leaders share responsibility with followers, they say "I trust you" to those followers. In his book *Thinking for a Change*, John Maxwell talks about his "10-80-10 principle," which has to do with giving responsibility (36). Maxwell explains that when he delegates a project to a member of his staff, he spends 10% of the time the task will take explaining where he wants the staff to go. Then he gives his staff 80% of the allotted project time to get where he wants them to go. It is in the 80% that Maxwell gives trust to his staff members. He tells them where to go, but not how to get there. He lets them get there themselves. Maxwell then gives the last 10% of the project's time to letting his staff tell him where they went. Be like John Maxwell, and exhibit trust by giving responsibility.

A family of European refugees was driven from their home by invading soldiers during World War II. Their only chance of escape was over the mountains that surrounded their village. But an elderly man was part of that family, and he wasn't sure he could make it over the mountains. "Leave me behind," he told his son and daughter-in-law, but they would not. Finally the old man agreed to try, and the family set out after dark toward the mountains. As they walked, the old man's son and daughter-in-law took turns carrying their 1-year-old baby. After several hours, the old man stopped and hung his head. "I can't make it," he said. "Yes, you can," his son implored him. But the old man refused to move. Finally the son said, "You must come. We need you. It's your turn to carry the baby." With that, the old man's eyes lit up. "Let's go!" he said. He picked up the baby and headed up the mountain, and the rest of the family followed. They all reached safety that night, including the old man and the baby, all because the old man's son gave him responsibility and made him feel important (57).

However, there are some people who can't handle responsibility. I was one of these individuals until I got to the fifth grade, when my teacher put me on the safety patrol! I got a white belt and a badge. My post was on a street that wasn't even paved. No cars ever used that street, no cars, ever. But I made every student stop when they reached my post, and I wouldn't let anyone cross until I checked for cars. Of course, there were no cars, ever. But I really felt important. I wanted to do anything my fifth-grade teacher wanted me to because she gave me responsibility and made me feel important.

The business world uses responsibility to make people feel important, too. The Harley-Davidson Motorcycle Company was about to go bankrupt in 1981. Their motorcycles were poorly made, so people stopped buying them. They bought Japanese bikes instead. Today, new Harleys are so popular that you have to get on a nationwide waiting list before you can buy one. What happened? In 1981, the company gave every employee on the Harley assembly line a button to push; that button stopped the line. Every employee had the right and responsibility to shut down the production of hundreds of motorcycles if that employee saw anything wrong with even one bike on the line. People took that responsibility seriously, and they began finding each other's mistakes, as well as their own mistakes. Those buttons gave people responsibility and made them feel important. Be like Harley Davidson. Make your staff feel important by giving them responsibility.

Hertzberg touches on the issue of responsibility (26). Prior to Hertzberg's work, many other behavioral scientists emphasized what was termed "job enlargement" or "job rotation." The assumption was that workers could gain more satisfaction at work if their jobs were enlarged, that is, if the number or variety of operations in which they engaged was increased. Hertzberg claims that doing a little of this and a little of that does not necessarily result in job satisfaction. For example, washing dishes, then silverware, and then pots and pan does no more to satisfy and provide an opportunity to grow than washing only dishes. Hertzberg suggests that what we really need to do with work is to enrich the job, using deliberate upgrading of responsibility, scope, and challenge.

Attribution Theory

Bernard Weiner et al. (54, 55) bring the power of responsibility to life by expanding on Fritz Heider's attribution theory. Heider (25) began by identifying two factors that partly determine the outcome of an event. He labeled one factor power, which includes such personal characteristics as ability and intelligence and which indicates whether a goal can be attained. Heider called the second factor trying or motivation. He then postulated that both "can" and "try" are necessary to reach a desired goal (25).

The studies of Weiner et al. (54) expanded Heider's approach into a four-part model by defining "can" in terms of effort and task difficulty, defining "try" in terms of effort, and adding the external variable of "chance" (luck). They then introduced a model of attribution theory that proposes that individuals perceive the causes of success and failure to be found in one or more of four elements:

- *Innate ability.* "Innate ability" refers to things we are born with, like intelligence or talent. People who attribute success or failure to innate ability say things like "I was born to sing!" or "I am just no good in math" or "I have two left feet."

- *Task difficulty.* People who attribute success and failure to task difficulty say things like "I tried, but that culture was just too hard to read" or "Trying to make sense out of that cost analysis is impossible" or "The Joint Commission made their regulations so hard to follow, nobody could understand them" or "I just can't spend another day in that job. They want too much from me."

- *Luck.* Some people attribute success or failure to fate. These people say things like "Why me?" or "If it wasn't for bad luck, I'd have no luck at all" or "I don't buy lottery tickets because I never win anything" or "My boss is a jerk. He got where he is by being at the right place at the right time. Those things never happen to me."

- *Effort.* Some people attribute success to hard work and failure to lack of hard work. They say, "I did it the old-fashioned way; I earned it" or "I could have done better if I really tried" or "If I had studied more, that A− would have been an A" or "The harder I work, the luckier I get."

The model (Table 10.2), as developed by Weiner et al. (54), indicates that ability and effort are seen as internal

Table 10.2 Attribution theory

| Stability | Locus of Control | |
	Internal	External
Fixed	Ability	Task difficulty
Variable	Effort	Luck

causes of success and failure, while luck and the difficulty of the task are seen as external determinants of outcome. In addition, while luck and effort can change, innate ability and task difficulty cannot change. So, which of the four elements is internal and changeable? Only effort. This means that effort is the only element of success and failure that people can change and control. According to Bernard Weiner and Andy Kukla (55) and to others, successful people tend to attribute success to internal factors that they can control, like effort. Unsuccessful people attribute failure to task difficulty or to bad luck, with a secret inner fear that they really just don't have enough ability. Other relevant literature (30–32) confirms the existence of a positive relationship between one's level of achievement and one's effort and offers evidence that the degree to which one believes in such a positive relationship affects one's level of achievement and persistence. And that makes sense.

If you attribute failure to luck, why do anything? Just pray and play the lottery! If you attribute failure to innate ability, just sing if you were born to sing, and fail if you were born to fail. If you attribute success and failure to the difficulty of the task, then just spend time trying to find easy things to do. But if you attribute success to hard work, you will probably work hard and succeed!

Thus, research shows that people who succeed don't believe in luck, in being born to succeed, or in finding the easy way out. People who succeed believe in themselves. They believe that the only thing between them and success is effort. They believe that effort relates to success and failure. That is Fritz Heider's theory, as well as Bernard Weiner's theory. Make yourself believe in effort, and help your staff believe in effort. It will give them success and will also give them responsibility.

If your staff believes in the power of effort, they will try. If they fail, they will take the responsibility for that failure. They won't say that they failed because the work was too hard, or because they were born to lose, or because fate made them fail. They will realize that people make fate, not the other way around. This kind of thinking gives them two things. It gives them responsibility for success, and it gives them control over success.

I once saw a teacher on his way to class. "Have a good class," I told him. "If I don't, it's my fault!" he replied. I didn't know that teacher then, but I know him now. From the day I met him, he took responsibility for success in his classroom. Accepting that responsibility gave him the power to make success happen. Responsibility is power.

Give both to your staff. In the words of Denis Waitley, "There should be a Statue of Responsibility in San Francisco harbor to match the Statue of Liberty" (53). Build that statue in your office, laboratory, or hospital.

Effort: Quality versus Quantity

Tell your staff that effort is like calories; it can be measured in quantity and in quality, and both are important. The quantity of our effort is measured in time. The longer one works, the more effort one gives. Quality is not so simple, because it depends on one's focus, commitment, and efficiency.

If you have teenagers and have ever discussed homework with them, you know what I mean. The television is on, books cover the bed, food is being consumed, music blares as earphones are worn, and a cell phone decorates one ear. At evening's end, a conversation takes place. "How much homework did you do?" you ask. "Three hours' worth" comes the proud and exhausted reply. The *quantity* of effort is high, while the *quality* of effort is low. With your help, your staff will do better. Their focus will improve because you will require goals. Their commitment will increase because the goals you require will be their goals. They will set them and own them, and their efficiency will rise because you will teach them what they need to know. As part of an address delivered at a Clinical Laboratory Management Association conference, Mark Sanborn related the story of a director of human resources who once asked his chief executive officer (CEO) to increase their company's professional development budget. The CEO was hesitant. "What if we train them and they leave?" asked the CEO. "What if we don't train them and they stay?" retorted the director. The director got the money; I hope you get the message. Teach your staff, because the only thing better than education is more education. By providing your staff with more education, you will help increase the quality of their effort.

You Started with All There Is

Power Believed Is Power Achieved

So much for your first and longest message to your staff: "You are important. "After you say that, say this: "You can do it!" A visitor to one of Henry Ford's auto plants met Ford after a tour of the factory. The visitor was in awe of what he had seen. "It seems impossible," the visitor told Ford, "that a man who started with nothing could accomplish all this." "You say that I started with nothing," Ford replied, "but you are wrong. I started with all there is. I started with all I needed to do anything. So does everyone."

You have all you need, as do the people with whom you work. Believe that. Believe Henry Ford. As a leader, after you deal in direction and importance, you must deal in faith: faith in yourself and in the people you lead. Faith in yourself comes first. No matter how well you think you can do in leadership or in life, you can do better. Believe that, and believe in yourself.

Think of the most powerful person you know. Can you visualize that person's face? As soon as you could see that face clearly, did you see your own face? Do you think you are the most powerful person you know? How about the second or third most powerful? Are you in the top 10? If not, you are right. If you don't think you are powerful, you are not powerful.

But what if you did see your own face and think you are powerful? Then you are right, too. Yes, if you don't think you are powerful, you are right. And if you do think you are powerful, you are just as right, because power believed is power achieved. Henry Ford once said, "If you think you can't, you are right. And if you think you can, you are just as right!" (7). Power believed is power achieved!

A kindergarten class was having an art lesson one day. The teacher asked one little girl what she was drawing. "I'm drawing a picture of God," the child replied. "But sweetheart," said the teacher, "no one knows what God looks like." "They will in a minute!" said the little girl. Think like that little girl, and have a childlike faith in yourself, no matter what challenges or odds you face.

Do you want to have the most significant educational experience of your life? Try this. Step one: find something you cannot do. Step two: do it. That experience will teach you the most important thing there is to know about the world's most important subject. That most important subject is you. And the most important thing there is to know about you is that you can do much more than you think you can. Believe in yourself and in your power.

In 1998, I read a speech in *Vital Speeches of the Day* (16) which referred to Steven Beering, the president of Purdue University. According to the speaker, President Beering was once asked to name the one book that, if read, would guarantee any college graduate a successful career in any field. He named *The Little Engine That Could!* On its way up that big hill it was trying to climb, the little engine kept saying, "I think I can. I think I can. I think I can." Be like that little engine. Believe in yourself, believe in your power, and after you believe in your power, believe in the power of the people you lead.

Wilma Rudolph was born in Tennessee, one of 22 children. As a child, Rudolph suffered from polio, scarlet fever, and double pneumonia. When she was old enough to go to school, Rudolph had to wear a leg brace to get there. In 1960, at the age of 20, that same Wilma Rudolph ran in the Olympics and won three gold medals, tying a world record in the process. Rudolph was once asked how she overcame such obstacles and became so successful. She answered, "The doctors told me I would never walk again, but my mother told me I would, so I believed my mother" (4, 40). Be like Rudolph's mother and have faith in your employees. Send a message to your employees that says, "you *can* do PTs," "you *can* do PTTs," "you *can* troubleshoot the DAX,"

and "you *can* identify that nonfermenter!" Send a message to the people you work with that says, "You can do more than you think you can!"

Most of us believe that we work with some good people, some of whom deserve our faith. But others just don't. Some people have what it takes, while others just don't. Why should you have faith in the people who don't? You may have some "couch potatoes" working with you, so why should you have faith in them? You might be right, but then again, you could be wrong. If you are wrong, if you are misjudging your couch potatoes, you won't be the first person guilty of selling someone short. Glenn Van Ekeren cites several examples (50). Michael Jordan's coach cut him from his ninth-grade basketball team. Everyone told Renoir to stop painting because he had no talent (52). Dr. Seuss's first children's book was rejected by 23 publishers. In 1902, an editor of the *Atlantic Monthly* returned the works of a young poet with a note that read, "Our magazine has no room for verse like yours." The poet's name was Robert Frost. Katherine Hepburn was fired from several stage roles. She was criticized for talking too fast. She was considered difficult to work with and was evaluated as being too bony, thin, and mannish to be successful on the stage. If you expect the worst from your couch potatoes, that's exactly what you'll get. But if you expect more, you just might get more.

When a man came home from work one night, his wife greeted him with bad news. "My car has water in the carburetor," she said. "What are you talking about?" asked the husband. "You don't even know what the carburetor looks like." "I am telling you, my car has water in the carburetor," insisted the wife. "And I am telling you, you don't know enough about cars to know that," said the husband. "I'll go look at it myself. Where is the car?" "I drove it into the lake," responded the wife. Don't assume people know less than they do. As a leader, have faith: in yourself and in the people with whom you work.

Faith Is Contagious

William James was a great philosopher. He once said, "Faith in ourselves comes from someone else's faith in us" (29). If you believe in your employees, they might believe in themselves. And if your employees believe in themselves, they might accomplish what they can accomplish. Faith, or the lack thereof, can be contagious.

In his book *Failing Forward* (37), Maxwell tells of an experiment that was conducted with a group of monkeys. Four monkeys were placed in a room that had a tall pole in the center. Suspended from the top of that pole was a bunch of bananas. One of the hungry monkeys started climbing the pole to get a banana, but just as he reached out to grab one, he was doused with a torrent of cold water. Squealing, he scampered down the pole and abandoned his attempt to feed himself. Each monkey made a similar attempt, and each one was drenched with cold water. After making several attempts, they gave up. Then researchers removed one of the monkeys from the room and replaced him with a new monkey. As the newcomer began to climb the pole, the other three grabbed him and pulled him down to the ground. After trying to climb the pole several times and being dragged down by the others, he finally gave up and never attempted to climb the pole again. The researchers replaced the original monkeys, one by one, and each time a new monkey was brought in, he would be dragged down by the others before he could reach the bananas. In time, the room was filled with monkeys who *had never received* a cold shower! None of them would climb the pole, but not one of them knew why.

Don't let lack of faith make monkeys out of your employees. Believe in them, because you have no employees who are incapable of performing the tasks you assign to them. In a best-selling book on brain research in education called *The Learning Revolution* by Dryden and Vos (20), this statement is found: "Every human being has a greater learning potential at birth than Leonardo da Vinci ever used." So push your people, and believe in your people.

In the words of Stephen Covey, "The first fundamental transformation of thinking required of American management is to develop new basic attitudes toward the intrinsic dignity and value of people, of their 'intrinsic motivation' to perform to their maximum capabilities. Management must empower its people in the deepest sense and remove the barriers and obstacles it has created that crush and defeat the inherent commitment, creativity, and quality service that people are otherwise prepared to offer" (14). The "barriers and obstacles" of which Covey speaks relate to faith and the lack of faith. Believe in yourself and in the people who work for you.

Example Is Leadership

Motivation is a fire within, and all people have that fire. You can give direction to any person's fire by sending three messages: "You are important," "You can do it," and "Follow me."

Regarding the third message, if you want people to point their fire in your direction, you must point yourself in that direction first. In other words, if you want people to follow, you must lead by example and by action, because actions speak louder than words.

All individuals speak two languages. Your words speak one language, and your actions speak another. People understand the language you speak with your actions much better than the one you speak with your words. People watch you walk before they listen to you talk. Ralph Waldo Emerson once said, "What you do speaks so loudly, I cannot hear what you say." Emerson was right. Actions speak louder than words. Peters and Waterman write, "As it turns out, we can't fool any of the people any of the time" (42). If our words don't match our actions, people will not be fooled and they will not follow.

A mother once asked Gandhi to get her son to stop eating sugar. Gandhi told the child, "Come back in 2 weeks." Two weeks later the mother brought the child before Gandhi, and Gandhi said to the boy, "Stop eating sugar." Puzzled, the woman replied, "Thank you, but I must ask: why didn't you tell him that 2 weeks ago?" Gandhi replied, "Two weeks ago I was eating sugar." Be like Gandhi. Speak with actions and lead by example. As a leader, you can use nouns like support, concern, or loyalty, but until you give those things and your followers feel them, those nouns have no meaning. Verbs speak louder than nouns. Actions speak louder than words.

You spend your days at work and in life full of thoughts, feelings, and values. Those things are always close to you, and you see them clearly. But others don't. Those things are hidden from the world until you share them through your actions. You might truly feel proud, fond, or appreciative of the employees you lead. But if your actions don't show them those feelings, how will they know?

The Ceiling-of-Effort Theory

My "ceiling of effort" theory says that as a leader, you have no right to expect your followers to work harder than you do. Kemmons Wilson founded Holiday Inns of America and understood the ceiling-of-effort theory even if he never heard of it. Wilson was once asked for the secret to his success. "It's really pretty simple," he said. "I just put in a half a day's work every day. It doesn't really matter which half: the first twelve hours or the last twelve" (58). Bill Parcells has coached teams to three Superbowls. Shortly before Christmas one year, a reporter asked Parcells how many days off he planned to give his players for the holidays. Parcells's response was, "What holidays?" Bill Parcells understood the ceiling-of-effort theory, too. It says that managers must work more than harder. They must work hardest.

In the words of Oliver Goldsmith, "You can preach a better sermon with your life than with your lips" (46). Preach well, work hard, lead with action, and lead by example (19).

Give Credit; Take Blame

As a manager, what example should you give? Start with praise, effort, and credit. If you want people to point their fires in your direction, give them the credit for every success, and give yourself responsibility for every failure.

Citizen Kane is considered by many to be the greatest movie ever made. Orson Welles produced it, directed it, and played its title role. His name is not mentioned in the credits as the movie begins. After the final scene, Welles appears on-screen and personally introduces and praises every actor. Then, credits run again to honor casting directors, stage crews, and costume designers. The last name on that list is Orson Welles. The type is small and its movement across the screen is as swift as that of every other name. Welles gave more credit to every other person involved in his movie while taking less for himself.

At 9:30 on the morning of 6 June 1944, General Eisenhower handed his press aide a statement that was broadcast around the world. It read, "Allied naval forces supported by strong air cover began landing allied armies this morning on the Northern Coast of France" (18). The tide of World War II had turned. The free world celebrated. The Liberty Bell rang in Philadelphia, Pa. Few people realize that Eisenhower had written two messages the night before the invasion. The message of success came true and was broadcast. The other was written in case the outcome had been different. That second message read, "Our landing has failed to gain a foothold and I have given the order to withdraw. Our troops did all that bravery and devotion could do. If there is responsibility to be attached to the attempt, it is mine alone" (18).

As leaders, we must take responsibility for the failure of our people while convincing them that they are responsible for their own success. Yes, leadership is hard.

Failing Forward

So far, so good. You have worked harder and given more. Last, but not least, be stronger. Your employees' fire is expensive, and your strength is a part of that price. A leader needs to be strong in the face of many things, particularly in the face of failure.

One of the most important things you will ever do as a manager is define the word "failure" for yourself and for your staff. Webster's *Ninth New Collegiate Dictionary* defines failure as "a state of inability, or a falling short, or a lack of success" (38). However, you may want to consider the definition of "Famous Dave" Anderson (37). He knows about rejection, bankruptcy, alcoholism, and failure because he has experienced them all. Anderson calls failure the "hallmark of success." For him, that success is in the form of 24 restaurants, 3,000 employees, $41.6 million per year in sales, and a $30 million net worth. Lives like Dave Anderson's prove that failure is nothing more than a necessary step on the road to success. Because Anderson failed and failed and failed, if he had defined any of those failures as a state of inability or lack of success, the world would have no Famous Dave's restaurants. And Dave Anderson was not alone!

During his first 3 years in the automobile business, Henry Ford went bankrupt twice. Cyrus Curtis lost over $800,000 on *The Saturday Evening Post* before he realized any profit (50). In 1905, advisors at the University of Bern rejected a Ph.D. dissertation, saying it was irrelevant and fanciful. Albert Einstein wrote that dissertation (50). Everybody fails, and everybody makes mistakes. How we define failure defines our success! In the words of Nelson Boswell, "The difference between average people and achieving people is their perception of and response to failure. Nothing else has the same kind of impact on people's ability to achieve and to accomplish whatever their minds and hearts desire" (37).

Never Give In

Life is nothing more than a series of opportunities to be strong. Every failure is one of those opportunities. "Never give in. Never give in. Never give in. In all things large or small, great or petty, never, never, never give in" (11). Winston Churchill said that to the people of Great Britain in the darkest days of World War II. Churchill knew what he was talking about. It took him 3 years to get through the sixth grade because he had trouble learning English. But he never gave in, and Churchill was not alone.

Richard Bach completed only 1 year of college and then trained to become an Air Force fighter pilot. Less than 2 years after earning his wings, he resigned. He then become the editor of an aviation magazine that went bankrupt. Even when Bach wrote *Jonathan Livingston Seagull*, he failed. Bach could not think of an ending and the manuscript lay dormant for 8 years. Even when finished, the book was rejected by many publishers. But Richard Bach never gave in (50).

Inventor Chester Carlson pounded the pavement for years before he found someone to back his Xerox photocopy process, but he never gave in. Frank Woolworth saw three of his first five chain stores fail, but he never gave in (50). As noted earlier, at 34 years of age, Florence Chadwick tried to swim from Catalina Island to the California coast, but she failed. Two months later, Florence tried that 20-mile swim again. This time she made it. She was the first woman to do so, and she beat the men's record by 2 hours. Be like Florence Chadwick and Winston Churchill. Never, never, never give in (33). Life and leadership are full of problems. However, those problems are nothing but speed bumps on the road to success!

Together Everyone Achieves More

The Meaning of TEAM

A leader must believe in what people can do, and people can do more as a team than as individuals. The letters in the word "team" can be said to stand for "together everyone achieves more." To lead, you must truly believe that people can do much more together than they could ever do alone. The redwood trees of the American Northwest are considered the largest living things and the tallest trees in the world. Some of them are 300 ft high and over 2,500 years old. You would think that trees that large would have a tremendous root system reaching down hundreds of feet under the ground. On the contrary, the redwoods actually have very shallow root systems. But those root systems are unbelievably strong because they are joined to each other. When storms come or winds blow, the redwoods stand tall—because they stand together. Leaders are like redwoods, they know that people stand together much better than they stand alone, and they know that together everyone achieves more.

Knute Rockne once said, "The secret to winning football games is to work more as a team than as individuals. I never play my 11 best. Instead, I play my best 11" (1). Be like Rockne. Know what the word TEAM stands for. As a leader, stick to your dream and stick to your team.

Maslow's Other Theory

"The more influence and power you give to someone else in a team situation, the more you have for yourself" (35). This comment is from the most renowned authority on human behavior our country has ever produced. When it comes to power, you get what you give, so give and share power, authority, and trust with your team because together everyone achieves more.

Summary

A laboratory manager was walking the beach on Cape Cod when a lamp appeared in the sand. After picking it up, the manager rubbed the lamp and a genie appeared. "I am now yours, Master," said the genie. "You may have one wish. What will it be?" After some thought, the manager replied. "My fiancée lives in London. Please build me a bridge from here to there." "But Master," replied the genie, "that is too difficult a task. Please ask for something else." "Fine," said the manager. "I have spent many years trying to figure out how to motivate my staff and I am still confused. Genie, please explain motivation to me." After a moment's thought, the genie replied, "Would you like that bridge to be two lanes, or four?"

This chapter was written for that manager, and for that genie. Motivation is a fire within. And how many people are motivated? All of them. How many people can you motivate? None. What can you do instead? You can give people direction by sending three messages: "You are important," "You can do it," and "Follow me."

KEY POINTS

- Motivation is an individual and internal fire; no outside pressure can create motivation.
- Motivation requires direction.
- True leadership gives more than it gets.
- Set SMART goals for yourself and your employees.
- Together everyone achieves more.

GLOSSARY

Attribution theory The reasons a person assigns to success and failure. Those reasons may be internal or external and either fixed or variable.

Bilingual A term which defines all people because all people speak two languages: one language with their words and another, more loudly, with their actions.

Ceiling-of-effort theory My contention that a leader's perceived level of effort sets a ceiling above which no follower's level of effort can be expected to go.

Effort The only internal and variable cause to which one can attribute success or failure. It is the variable which, if attributed to success or failure, most often leads to success.

Ego The picture of ourselves we want to see.

Example All aspects of a leader's observable behavior. It is the one aspect of a leader which people will follow, or won't.

External locus of control The belief that the requirement for success exists outside people in the form of luck, fate, other people, or task difficulty.

Failure A necessary step on the road to success.

Goals Specific, measurable, attainable, relevant, and timed (SMART) providers of direction.

The Hawthorne effect The proven, positive effect that attention and feelings of importance have on production.

Hygiene factors Tangible, physiological factors whose absence causes employee dissatisfaction but whose presence does not create satisfaction (e.g., salary, working conditions, benefits).

Internal locus of control The belief that the ingredients needed to succeed exist within people in the form of effort, persistence, intelligence, energy, and/or talent.

Intrinsic motivation A redundancy, because all motivation is intrinsic. All motivation is internal. All motivation is a fire within.

Job enrichment The deliberate upgrading of responsibility, scope, and challenge as they apply to a position, title, or employee.

Locus of control The location of the events, traits, circumstances, or people that determine someone's success or failure (32).

Maslow's other theory The theory that the more influence and power you give to someone else, the more you have for yourself.

Motivation An inner force that causes behavior; a fire from within.

Motivators Internal factors that relate to the nature of work and the egos of employees. If properly addressed, these factors can create employee satisfaction (e.g., recognition, appreciation, self-actualization).

Myth of motivation A long-lived, often-believed falsehood that people can motivate other people.

Niagara syndrome The condition affecting all people whose life or work suffers from a lack of direction.

People message A value judgment made by a manager and perceived by staff members as relating to the quality of the staff members themselves.

Product message A value judgment made by a manager that relates to the quality of something produced or accomplished by one or more staff members.

Responsibility When given, responsibility is a visible, active expression of trust. When accepted, it is the true source of power.

Trust The currency of all leadership. Leaders earn followers by earning their trust. Trust is reciprocal; leaders must give it to get it.

REFERENCES

[Note: I have not created this chapter; I have collected it. The following authors, scholars, and teachers have my admiration and appreciation for the contribution they have made to my work and to the wealth of the world's knowledge.]

1. **Anderson, P.** 1997. *Great Quotes from Great Sports Heroes.* Career Press, Franklin Lakes, N.J.

2. **Ash, M. K.** 1984. *People Management.* Warner Books, New York, N.Y.

3. **Autry, J. A.** 1994. *Life and Work: a Manager's Search for Meaning,* p. 72. Avon Books, New York, N.Y.

4. **Biracree, T.** 1988. *Wilma Rudolph.* Chelsea House Publishers, New York, N.Y.

5. **Brinkman, R., and R. Kirschner.** 1994. *Dealing with People You Can't Stand.* McGraw Hill, New York, N.Y.

6. **Brooks, W., and R. Heath.** 1993. *Speech Communication,* 7th ed. W. C. Brown, Dubuque, Iowa.

7. **Canfield, J., and M. V. Hansen.** 1993. *Chicken Soup for the Soul.* Health Communication, Inc., Deerfield Beach, Fla.

8. **Carnegie, D., and Associates.** 1993. *The Leader in You.* Pocket Books, New York, N.Y.

9. **Carnegie, D.** 1937. *How To Win Friends and Influence People.* Simon & Schuster, New York, N.Y.

10. **Chase, S.** 1945. *Men at Work.* Harcourt Brace, New York, N.Y.

11. **Churchill, W.** 1941. Never give up. Speech given at the Harrow School, 29 October 1941.

12. **Connellan, T. K.** 2003. *Bringing Out the Best in Others!* Bard Press, Austin, Tex.

13. **Covey, S. R.** 1990. *The Seven Habits of Highly Effective People,* p. 143. Simon and Schuster, New York, N.Y.

14. **Covey, S. R.** 1992. *Principle-Centered Leadership.* Fireside Books, New York, N.Y.

15. **Covington, M.** 1998. *The Will To Learn.* Cambridge University Press, Cambridge, United Kingdom.

16. **Daly, G.** *Vital Speeches of the Day.* City News Publishing Co., Mount Pleasant, S.C.

17. **Deming, W. E.** 1986. *Out of Crisis.* Summit Books, New York, N.Y.

18. **De Pasquale, S., M. Field, M. Hendricks, D. Keiger, and S. Libowitz.** 1994. Liberating Ike's letters, etc. *Johns Hopkins Magazine* [Online]. http://www.jhu.edu/~jhumag/694web/policy.html.

19. **DePree, M.** 1989. *Leadership Is an Art,* p. 60. Doubleday, New York, N.Y.

20. **Dryden, G., and J. Vos.** 1999. *The Learning Revolution.* The Learning Web, Torrance, Calif.

21. **DuBrin, A.** 1990. *Essentials of Management.* Southwestern Publishing Co., Cincinnati, Ohio.

22. **Freud, S.** 1933. *New Introductory Lectures on Psychoanalysis.* W. W. Norton, New York, N.Y.

23. **Givens, C.** 1993. *Super Self.* Simon & Schuster, New York, N.Y.

24. **Goleman, D.** 1995. *Emotional Intelligence.* Bantam Books, New York, N.Y.

25. **Heider, F.** 1958. *The Psychology of Interpersonal Relations.* John Wiley and Sons, New York, N.Y.

26. **Hersey, P., and K. Blanchard.** 1982. *Management of Organizational Behavior,* 4th ed. Prentice Hall, Englewood Cliffs, N.J.

27. **Holmes, O. W.** 1878. *Poet at the Breakfast Table.* James R. Osgood, Boston, Mass.

28. **Hoy, W. K., and C. G. Miskel.** 1978. *Educational Administration; Theory, Research and Practice,* 2nd ed. Random House, New York, N.Y.

29. **James, W.** 1956. *The Will To Believe.* Dover Publications, New York, N.Y.

30. **Kleiber, D. A., and M. L. Maehr.** 1985. *Advances in Motivation and Achievement,* vol. 4. *Motivation and Adulthood.* JAI Press, Inc., Greenwich, Conn.

31. **Lefcourt, H. M.** 1996. Internal vs. external control of reinforcement: a review. *Psychol. Bull.* **65:**206–220.

32. **Lefcourt, H. M.** 1982. *Locus of Control: Current Trends in Theory and Research.* Lawrence Erlbaum Associates, Hillsdale, N.J.

33. **Lockhart, A.** 1997. *The Portable Pep Talk,* p. 94. Zander Press, Richmond, Va.

34. **Maslow, A. H.** 1954. *Motivation and Personality.* Harper & Row, New York, N.Y.

35. **Maslow, A. H.** 1998. *Maslow on Management.* Wiley & Sons, Inc., New York, N.Y.

36. **Maxwell, J. C.** 2003. *Thinking for a Change.* Warner Books, New York, N.Y.

37. **Maxwell, J. C.** 2000. *Failing Forward.* T. Nelson Publishers, Nashville, Tenn.

38. **Merriam-Webster, Inc.** 1991. *Webster's Ninth New Collegiate Dictionary.* Merriam-Webster, Inc., Springfield, Mass.

39. **Morrel, M. M.** 1949. *Young Hickory: The Life and Times of President James K. Polk.* E. P. Dutton Publishers, New York, N.Y.

40. **Noe, J. R.** 1984. *Peak Performance Principles for High Achievers,* p. 105. Berkley Books, New York, N.Y.

41. **Parkinson, C. N.** 1958. *Parkinson's Law: the Pursuit of Progress.* John Murray, London, England.

42. **Peters, T., and R. H. Waterman.** 1982. *In Search of Excellence,* p. 56. Warner Books, New York, N.Y.

43. **Phillips, D. T.** 1992. *Lincoln on Leadership,* p. 26. Warner Books, New York, N.Y.

44. **Robbins, A.** 1991. *Awaken the Giant Within.* Summit Books, New York, N.Y.

45. **Rotter, J. B.** 1966. Generalized expectancies for internal versus external control of reinforcement. *Psychol. Monogr.* **80**(1)**:**1–27.

46 **Sanborn, M.** 2002. *The Fred Factor.* Executive Books, Mechanicsburg, Pa.

47. **Sashkin, M., and K. J. Kiser.** 1993. *Putting Total Quality Management to Work.* Berrett-Koehler Publishers, San Francisco, Calif.

48. **Strong, D. H.** 1970. *Letting People Have Your Way or Principals of Leadership.* Community action program, Columbia Point, Boston, Mass.

49. **Timm, P. R., and B. D. Peterson.** 1990. *People at Work: Human Relations in Organizations,* 3rd ed. Stevens West Publications, St. Paul, Minn.

50. **Van Ekeren, G.** 1988. *The Speaker's Sourcebook I.* Prentice Hall, Englewood Cliffs, N.J.

51. **Waitley, D.** 1995. *Empires of the Mind.* William Morrow and Company, New York, N.Y.

52. **Waitley, D.** 1983. *The Seeds of Greatness,* p. 43. Pocket Books, New York, N.Y.

53. **Waitley, D.** 1980. *The Winner's Edge,* p. 38. Berkley Books, New York, N.Y.

54. **Weiner, B., H. Heckhausen, W.-U. Meyer, and R. E. Cook.** 1972. Causal ascriptions and achievement behavior: a conceptual analysis of effort and reanalysis of locus of control. *J. Pers. Soc. Psychol.* 21(2):239–248.

55. **Weiner, B., and A. Kukla.** 1970. An attributional analysis of achievement motivation. *J. Pers. Soc. Psychol.* **15**(1):1–20.

56. **Whitaker, T., B. Whitaker, and D. Lumpa.** 2000. *Motivating and Inspiring Teachers: the Educational Leader's Guide for Building Staff Morale.* Bookrights, Raleigh, N.C.

57. **Wickman, F., and T. Sjodin.** 14 August 1997. Mentoring. As quoted by R. Gilbert in *Bits and Pieces.* The Economics Press Inc., Caldwell, N.J.

58. **Wilson, K., and R. Kerr.** 1996. *Half Luck and Half Brains: The Kemmons Wilson Holiday Inn Story.* Hambleton-Hill Publishing Inc., Nashville, Tenn.

11

Successful Communication

Diane C. Turnbull

OBJECTIVES

To describe the process of effective communication

To help the reader to select the communication technique appropriate for a situation based on the advantages and disadvantages

To explain the necessity of using positive language when communicating orally and in written form

To review the necessity of fostering and nurturing a climate that supports effective communication

To discuss how to integrate the six W/H (who, what, when, where, why, and how) points effectively when disseminating information

To describe the types of listeners and explain the benefits of active listening

---

When people talk, listen completely. Most people never listen.

ERNEST HEMINGWAY

COMMUNICATING WITH OTHERS, both professionally and personally, pervades all aspects of everyday life. The root of almost every problem, conflict, mistake, or misunderstanding is a communication problem. Business consultants vouch that communication is the number one problem in most workplaces. Counselors reiterate that communication is the number one problem for interpersonal relationships (15). Communication is defined as an exchange or sharing of thoughts or information between one person and another. Misunderstood communication can be one of the largest problems facing organizations today. Businesses have a multitude of messages being sent, but not all of the information is received or understood. Even though the communication problems experienced may never be completely eliminated, they can be reduced or often avoided entirely.

Managers communicate in all aspects of the daily work environment. Strong leadership cannot be accomplished without communication. For example, communication skills are important when interviewing applicants for a job, delegating responsibility and authority, directing the efforts of others, interpreting policy, and enforcing procedures and regulations. The communication cycle has three points, which consist of the sender conveying the message in a clear and straightforward manner, the receivers accepting the message and confirming that they have comprehended it, and the sender verifying that the message was understood and received in the manner intended. The ability to communicate is essential to leadership and vital to any organization. It is a skill that can be acquired, cultivated, and improved upon. This chapter will help the reader understand how people prefer to communicate and suggests ways to adapt his or her own communication style to enhance understanding and build rapport with others.

Channels of Communication

In every organizational network, there are distinct formal and informal channels of communication. The purpose of both channels is to disseminate information and carry messages from a person or group to others in the organization. This flow of information can be downward, upward, or lateral.

Formal Channels of Communication

Formal channels of communication are typically aligned according to the organizational chart or structure of the facility and usually follow an organizational hierarchy. Typically strict lines of authority are followed, for example, chief operating officer to vice president to administrative director to supervisors to staff.

Downward communication is commonly referred to as flowing from the top down. It is primarily directive in nature and often used extensively by management to state objectives, disseminate policies or policy changes, provide directives, and convey general information to subordinates. One pitfall of downward communication is the possibility of dilution or distortion of information that can occur between the original sender and the ultimate receiver, which may cause the message to be misinterpreted or inaccurate. This is especially true with oral communication when a large number of people are involved, because the more people involved in the downward chain, the greater the chance of error. In supervision, the downward flow is relied upon very heavily for disseminating information.

Upward communication flows through the ranks of staff members to top management. Generally, upward communication is used to report and convey information. Effective managers encourage a free flow of upward communication as a feedback mechanism. This type of communication can serve as a means to determine whether a message has been transmitted and received appropriately and often conveys to management the effects of a message on staff. A manager should encourage upward communication by demonstrating a desire to obtain and use the ideas and information received from one's staff. A manager must also act on information provided by staff; otherwise this channel of communication will eventually close. Lack of an effective upward flow will destroy the staff's desire to communicate, lead to frustration, and eventually cause employees to seek different outlets, such as the grapevine, or ultimately find other employment opportunities.

Lateral communication flows among persons on the same level in an organization. It is important because it allows for the exchange of information among people with similar responsibilities working on common objectives and fosters intralaboratory and interdisciplinary communication.

Informal Channels of Communication

The main type of informal communication is the grapevine, which is the route by which employees spread information to one another. Even if the organization has well-established formal channels, informal channels inevitably develop. Every department has a grapevine. The grapevine is an outgrowth of the social interaction of people and their natural desire to communicate. It is a method of spreading information rapidly and allows employees to keep abreast of the latest information.

The manager should accept the fact that it is impossible to get rid of the grapevine, but with certain skills, a manager can influence it. Managers need to stay attuned to their organization's grapevine by finding a mechanism to keep them aware of what information the grapevine is transmitting. It is unrealistic to believe that rumors can be eliminated since the grapevine flourishes in every organization. Rather, a manager's best approach is to provide the grapevine with facts. This will help to eliminate partial truths and will use the grapevine's energy to the best interest of management; however, this requires effort on the manager's part.

Types (Methods) of Communication

Methods of communication may vary according to the style of the sender, the situation, the audience, and the content of the message itself. These must all be evaluated before deciding the best way to communicate the information. Types of communication include oral, written, and electronic communication; pictures; and body language or other nonverbal signs. Research indicates that managers spend between 50 and 80% of their total time communicating (6). Typically the majority of their time is spent speaking and listening and to a lesser extent writing and reading.

Oral (Face-to-Face) Communication

Speaking is generally superior to written communication in that it usually achieves better understanding because it permits feedback. It can also save time. This type of communication is useful in direct person-to-person communications and group communications. The most important feature of oral communication is that it provides immediate feedback, in that it allows the receiver to ask questions. This type of communication also has some disadvantages. Since nothing is written down, permanence is lost, so the receiver cannot "revisit" the actual words used.

Other potential pitfalls of oral communication include mumbling, speaking too fast or too slowly, mispronouncing words, speaking in a monotone, and using distracting sounds or words such as "err," "uhh," etc.

A spoken message has three elements: verbal, vocal, and visual (3). The verbal elements are the actual words used, the vocal elements include the tone and intensity of one's voice, and the visual elements incorporate everything that the listener can see. The visual is the most powerful element of communication because dynamic visual, nonverbal communication grabs and holds the listener's attention. Once the speaker has the listener's attention through strong visual, nonverbal elements, then powerful vocal and verbal elements can be used to transmit the message. The vocal elements are processed before the actual words are heard and translated, so if vocal sounds detract in any way from the meaning of the words, people will react and understand less of the message intended (3). Because visual and vocal elements are noticed before the actual words, speakers should be sure that their appearance and vocal tones work in harmony with the message. For example, strong messages should not be delivered in weak or soft tones.

Telephone Communication

The telephone is one of the major ways that people use to communicate at work. Because of this, it is important to be aware of how colleagues and customers perceive the caller. On the telephone, there is no visual contact and consequently no nonverbal cues from body language to help the caller better understand and connect with those on the receiving end. Courtesy ranks highest on the telephone etiquette list. The caller should state his or her name and verify the identity of the person on the other end of the line. It is important for the caller to be personable. This develops rapport and trust with those on the receiving end. Be aware that demeanor often affects the tone of voice that comes across on the telephone. Callers should try to begin every call by sounding upbeat to help set a positive tone for the call and make the receiver feel more relaxed. Tone of voice often has more impact than actual words, communicating an important part of the caller's personality to others (11).

Analyze and constructively critique several phone calls by taping your side only of the conversation. Think about volume, speed, rhythm, inflection, resonance, and clarity. Determine what if any vocal qualities need improvement and whether or not you were accurately communicating the emotions you meant to communicate to the caller. Identify areas of improvement, and think about ways to project a positive demeanor and enthusiastic tone of voice. Five aids to developing an assured voice are to (i) project a strong but not overwhelming resonance; (ii) use the mouth and lips to speak clearly and distinctly; (iii) show enthusiasm by using appropriate pitch, volume, and inflection; (iv) avoid speaking in a monotone; and (v) speak naturally and do not attempt to adopt vocal qualities that do not fit your style (4). The telephone can be used as an effective means of communication by following a few simple rules (Table 11.1).

Written Communication

Written communication provides a permanent record to which the receiver can refer to ensure that he has understood the information presented. It provides accuracy of information as well as permanence. However, feedback is limited, and the sender cannot be sure that a written message is actually read. The important ingredients of effective writing are content, style, technique, and format.

Business letters are written contact with people outside the organization. Letters document communication by providing a long-lasting record which can be referred to whenever necessary. Business letters should be clear, courteous, and concise. Good business writing is a combination of clear thinking, good organization, and effective presentation. Correct grammar, spelling, and punctuation are essential elements of all types of written communication and project a professional image. Always reread all types of documents prior to sending to look for errors and ambiguous statements.

Written memoranda are typically used to contact staff and coworkers within the organization. They should be organized, coherent, and not open to multiple interpretations (Table 11.2). Memoranda should be used to facilitate, simplify, and accelerate internal communication. They can be effectively used to give instructions, ask for information or action, and announce or clarify a new policy or procedure. Memos provide a simple method to communicate an identical message to several people. They should be short, complete, and concise. This can be accomplished by the use of headlines, short paragraphs, bullets, bolding of important points, and a modified outline format. Think about key issues before writing the memo. Written and electronic messages can save time and energy, however, they have a tendency to be overused. To ensure quality communication, an organization must define the parameters of these tools and the ways in which they may and may not be used (1).

Table 11.1 Steps for effective telephone communication

Identify yourself and your department or organization.

Converse with patience.

Be aware of your tone of voice.

Do not converse in a monotone. Sound alive.

Tune into the tone of voice of the person you are calling.

Listen carefully. Listen for content and emotion to understand what the speaker is trying to say.

Close the call before you end it.

When leaving a message on voice mail, make the message worth returning.

Table 11.2 Writing guide for memoranda

Take the time to craft clear memoranda that are short, complete, and concise.

Ensure that written messages are organized, coherent, and not open to multiple interpretations.

Anticipate questions the reader might ask.

Include the six W/H (who, what, when, where, why, and how) points. The memo should address who needs to be involved, what action is being conveyed or needs to be accomplished, and when and where the action needs to be completed. The memo should include why the memo is being written and suggestions on how the action is to be completed.

Make memoranda easy to read from a visual-layout point of view.

Avoid sending mixed messages.

Electronic Communication

Electronic communication, specifically e-mail, is being used more and more in the workplace. E-mail borrows the latitude of speech in a format that seems like writing. This type of communication, with the casualness of speech but without the inflections or context, still looks like written communication on the screen (Table 11.3). Fragmented comments and speedy replies compound the potential in e-mail for confusion, offense, and misunderstanding. Speed and spontaneity are the strengths of e-mail but also its downfall. E-mails are easily forwarded to others, therefore, never send something electronically that should not appear publicly. To maximize the use of e-mail and minimize problems, state the reason for the e-mail in the subject line and borrow from standard letter conventions by being sure the e-mail is clear, complete, and concise. Think before e-mailing an important document as an attachment. Incompatible software can leave the document unread, and people in a hurry or worried about viruses do not open attachments. When attachments are sent, be sure to clearly state which files are attached in the body of the email. Everyone has hit Send and then regretted it. To maximize the use of e-mail, follow some basic principles for sending and replying to e-mails (Table 11.4).

Table 11.3 Effective communication in e-mail

Never use e-mail when angry. Wait or talk directly to the person.

Never send anything that cannot be said directly to the other person.

Never send anything that should not be shared in public.

Avoid revealing protected health information.

Recognize that e-mails are permanent and can be used in legal matters.

Maintain professionalism and confidentiality.

Copy others only as necessary and never as an exercise of authority, power, or manipulation.

Avoid using e-mail to discuss a topic that is complex, especially one that people feel strongly about. This is best discussed in a meeting.

E-mail works best as a means of circulating information, providing notice about events, giving someone a message, and communicating quickly and efficiently with a person about a circumscribed issue.

In business, e-mail works best as a means of circulating information, providing notice about events, giving someone a brief message, contacting people with updates, and communicating quickly and efficiently with a person about a circumscribed issue. However, if complicated issues or negotiations need to occur, it is better to do them face-to-face (14). E-mail should not be used to discuss a topic that is complex and requires feedback.

Visual Communication

Photographs, paintings, diagrams, designs, cartoons, and caricatures are examples of types of pictures that are used as visual communication aids. They are important to communication because they are often easier to understand than written explanations. The image being transmitted to the brain is already drawn or formed. Pictures are effective when used with well-chosen words to help the receiver "see" the message. Effective visual aids can also be in the form of videos, charts, posters, models, and digital pictures.

Visual communication is especially valuable in presenting a process or explaining how to do something. This can be used in training employees as well as in educating patients. For example, showing a video about performing venipuncture is much more effective than just providing written instructions. Verbal instructions along with accompanying pictures can be very helpful when asking patients to collect a clean-catch specimen for a urinalysis.

Body Language and Other Nonverbal Communication

Body language and other nonverbal cues reveal much more about attitudes and emotions than words (5). Body language, also known as kinesics, describes human interaction excluding the use of written and spoken words. Studies in the last two decades indicate that more than half of all verbal messages sent have nonverbal components (13). Researchers in the area of nonverbal communications claim that as much as 90% of the meaning transmitted between two people in face-to-face communications

Table 11.4 E-mail tips

Tips for sending

    Keep it short.

    Try to limit the number of important questions or issues presented.

    Include name and contact information in business e-mail.

    Do not type messages in uppercase letters.

    Use the forward function sparingly.

    E-mail works best when one response or no response is required.

Tips for replying

    Reply promptly.

    Reply to all the questions within the message, not just to the last question asked.

    Think twice before hitting Send. Avoid replying without thinking.

    Be especially careful with the "reply to all recipients" option.

can occur via nonverbal channels. Conceivably, only 10% of the meaning derived comes through words alone (5).

Nonverbal cues include posture, gestures, facial expressions, eye contact, and body image or proximity. For example, leaning toward the person speaking conveys attention and interest. In contrast, standing abruptly while talking to a coworker sends the message that the meeting is over. The person being addressed may also feel that the speaker feels superior. Movement made with the eyes, mouth, or forehead conveys a great deal. A scowl usually signifies displeasure. A stern look can mean disapproval, while a smile means approval. Eye contact lends credibility to the spoken message, giving the message much of its meaning and also affecting whether the listener believes and trusts the message.

Barriers to Communication

Many times communication is not as effective as it could be because of communication barriers. Both the speaker and the listener can create communication barriers. A barrier in this context means any behavior that hinders the flow of meaningful, nonjudgmental communication. There are several types of barriers, but basically they fall into these main categories: physical barriers, nonverbal barriers, verbal barriers, and psychological barriers. Once a manager becomes aware of a barrier, his task should be focused on dissolving or controlling it.

Physical Barriers

Barriers that can be detected and removed easily have been identified as physical barriers. Examples of eliminating physical barriers are reducing background noise, moving out of a busy area, removing furniture between the participants, adjusting the physical distance between participants, and ensuring privacy.

Nonverbal Barriers

There are several nonverbal behaviors that should be avoided. These include poor eye contact; unfavorable facial expressions such as frowning, smirking, scowling, and blank looks; poor posture such as slouching; and too much fidgeting and squirming. Ineffective placement not only is a physical barrier but also creates a nonverbal barrier to communication. Speakers and listeners can remain distant from each other by facing away or turning their backs from each other or by being preoccupied with something else. These are all behaviors that should be avoided for effective communication (10).

Verbal Barriers

Verbal modes of delivery causing barriers to communication may be less detectable or correctable. However, once a speaker realizes that there is a problem, steps can be taken to correct it. Examples of verbal barriers to communica-

tion include speaking in an uninviting tone of voice; using condescending, patronizing, harsh, or reactive tones; using biting sarcasm; and speaking in monotone (16).

Psychological Barriers

Psychological barriers develop based on the nature of individuals and their interactions with others. They may consist of preconceived expectations, self-centeredness, lack of self-esteem, and assumptions by either the sender or the receivers. Power and status perceptions or a defensive attitude may also cause psychological barriers (16). Psychological barriers are more difficult to overcome, but managers need to be aware that these types of barriers exist.

The Importance of Listening

Poor listening skills create one of the biggest barriers to effective communication. Listeners inadvertently create barriers, both verbal and nonverbal. Listening is an important element in communication that is often overlooked. It can be defined as the process of receiving a message from a speaker, processing that message to make sense of it, and then responding to it in ways that show that the receiver understands what the speaker means (9). Listening is a powerful means of communication that can increase job effectiveness. It ensures that parties are communicating completely to reach a shared meaning through dialogue (1). Listening is often defined as a manager's most important skill (2).

Effective Listening

Communicating with employees is sometimes considered the hardest aspect of communication, and it cannot occur without effective listening (1). Good communication encourages creative interaction between employees. When managers listen to employees and show understanding, employees will believe that they are valued as a partner. Listening to employees leads to increased trust and credibility and an increased willingness to cooperate. In organizations, this generally means a reduction in turnover and a greater commitment to the organization's goals. Poor listening contributes to low employee morale and increased turnover because employees do not feel that their managers listen to their needs, suggestions, or complaints. Ineffective listening frequently causes misunderstandings, mistakes, jobs done incorrectly, unhappy customers, increased costs, and reduced profits. Listening more effectively enhances the transfer of information, improves teamwork, builds morale, reduces errors, and leads to higher productivity (2).

Ineffective Listening

There are five basic reasons why managers do not listen more effectively (2).

- Listening is hard work. It requires concentrating on the other person rather than on oneself, and as a result, many people just do not do it.

- Competition for attention comes from radio, television, reading material, and more. So many stimuli cause people to screen out information that they deem irrelevant and at times to also screen out important things.

- Managers interrupt and do not take the time required to hear people out.

- The difference between speech speed and thought speed creates a listening gap. The average person speaks at about 135 to 175 words a minute but can listen to 400 to 500 words a minute. That difference between listening speed and speaking speed is time spent jumping to conclusions, daydreaming, planning a reply, or mentally arguing with the speaker.

- There is a lack of training on how to listen. People do more listening than speaking, reading, and writing, yet they receive no formal education in listening. Many people assume that they are good listeners; however, few actually are. Managers must become aware that listening effectively is a skill that can be improved upon by understanding the stages of listening and the types of listeners and by working toward improving listening skills.

Stages of Listening

Listening occurs in three stages: receiving, processing, and responding. Receiving consists of taking in the speaker's message through the senses, usually hearing and seeing. When people are speaking face-to-face, the eyes read the nonverbal cues that play a part in how the speaker expresses the message. After the listener takes in the speaker's message, the internal processing begins. Processing involves analyzing, evaluating, and synthesizing the message. Responding is the third stage in the listening process. In this stage the speaker sees and hears what the listener does. The listener verbally and nonverbally acknowledges that the message has been received and understood (9).

Types of Listening

People typically listen at one of four basic levels of attentiveness: nonlistener, marginal listener, evaluative listener, and active listener (2). These categories are not distinct lines of differences but general groupings into which people fall. Depending on situations or circumstances, listeners may overlap or move from one category to another. The potential for understanding, trust, and effective communication is highest when active listening is used consistently (9).

Nonlistener

The nonlistener does not hear anything the speaker says. Typically the nonlistener is characterized by a blank stare and nervous mannerisms and gestures. Often this type of listener pretends to pay attention while thinking about other unrelated matters. Nonlisteners want to do all or most of the taking, constantly interrupt, and always have

to have the last word. They are perceived as insensitive and nonunderstanding (2).

Marginal Listener

The marginal listener hears the sounds and words but not the meaning and intent. Marginal listeners are often described as superficial listeners, are easily distracted, and prefer to evade difficult or technical presentations or discussions. Marginal listening is hazardous because there is enormous room for misunderstanding since the listener is only superficially concentrating. In the workplace, this type of listening is often a source of low morale, misunderstandings, errors, and problems (2).

Evaluative Listener

The evaluative listener is actively trying to hear what the speaker is saying but is not making an effort to understand the speaker's intent. Evaluative listeners are described as logical listeners and therefore are more concerned about content than feelings. They remain emotionally detached from the conversation and evaluate a message strictly on the basis of the words delivered, totally ignoring that part of the message conveyed by the speaker's tone, body language, and facial expressions (2).

Active Listener

The active listener is the most comprehensive and powerful level of listener. Active listening is also referred to as responsive listening or reflective listening. It requires the deepest level of concentration, attention, and processing effort. The active listener focuses on understanding the speaker's point of view rather than constantly judging the speaker's message. Attention is concentrated on the thought and feeling of the other person as well as what the speaker is saying. Active listeners capture the speaker's whole message, the facts and the feelings. Active listening requires that the listener send verbal and nonverbal feedback to the speaker indicating that what is being said is really being absorbed. Verbal feedback to confirm understanding of a speaker's message, given without being judgmental, makes active listening the most effective form of listening (2, 9). Communication is most effective when both the speaker and the receiver are active listeners.

Elements of Effective Communication

Effective communication begins with developing an active-listening attitude. To develop this type of attitude, the listener must understand that active listening is as powerful as speech and also saves time. Those who listen actively experience fewer mistakes, fewer misunderstandings, fewer dissatisfied customers, and fewer false starts. Managers must also realize that listening is important and worthwhile with everyone with whom they come in contact. Organizations that promote active listening have fewer communication glitches, increased productivity, and increased morale.

Skills for Effective Communication

To develop active-listening skills, it is necessary to develop six separate skills: concentrate, acknowledge, research, exercise emotional control, sense the nonverbal message, and structure (2).

Concentrate. Focus attention only on the speaker, which diminishes environmental noise and aids in receiving the message clearly. It is also helpful to eliminate distractions and physical barriers to create the best possible conditions to allow for a comfortable conversation.

Acknowledge. Acknowledge the speaker to demonstrate interest and attention that encourages and helps the speaker to send a clearer message. This can be done by making eye contract and/or asking questions to clarify points. This gives positive feedback and helps the speaker know that the message is being received. Wait several seconds before replying to indicate that the message was received and evaluated before a response was formulated.

Research. Gather information about the speaker's interests and objectives to help understand the message, ask questions, and respond to the speaker in a way that promotes communication.

Exercise emotional control. Wait until the entire message is received before reacting to the message. It is important to deal with highly charged messages in a thoughtful manner regardless of how provocative the message may be. Concentrate on understanding the message before reacting to it.

Sense the nonverbal message. Pay attention to what the speaker is trying to say, which includes body language and gestures as well as the words being spoken.

Structure. Structure and organize the information as it is received, which improves understanding and retention of the material.

Organizational Climate

In addition to becoming a more active listener, a manager must work on controlling climate and culture. Effective organizational communication requires a climate or culture that supports effective communication. A manager that does not communicate effectively often does not promote a culture where communication within the organization is managed properly. This type of manager not only communicates ineffectively and discourages effective organizational communication but also is unlikely to hear about problems. Poor communication is self-sustaining.

In this type of climate, there is no feedback mechanism. The staff does not communicate their concerns about communication because management is not perceived as receptive (6).

An effective organizational climate involves trust, openness, reinforcement of good communication practices, and shared responsibility for making communication effective. It is up to the manager to be sure that he and the staff have the skills and knowledge necessary to communicate effectively. Effective communication requires attention. It develops as a result of an intentional effort on the part of management and staff. Once the commitment has been made to improve communication, the manager must play a critical role in fostering and nurturing a climate that is characterized by open communication. The manager must bring communication to the forefront of the organization. This can be done by participating in formal training if necessary, providing it for others in the organization, actively soliciting feedback on communication within the organization, defining how communication should occur, and making clear what information will be available and when and how it will be communicated. A communication strategy should support, encourage, and reinforce the mission and culture of the organization (1).

When speaking to a group in a formal setting, a manager must speak assertively and should be an expert on the topic being presented. Generally managers should know 10 times what they think they need to know on a particular subject. The message must contain the six W/H's—who, what, where, when, why, and how (12). This must be done in both oral presentations and written communications by taking the time to clearly anticipate questions a listener or reader might ask (Table 11.5). On a personal level, the manager must be available and approachable. Communication involves more than just the flow of information. In one-on-one conversation or in small groups, the manager can win the attention and confidence of the other person by asking for their views on the subject. This can be done by asking who, what, where, when, why, and how questions. This communicates the manager's interest

Table 11.5 Effective communication at meetings

Listen to others' opinions and value them.

Compliment the work, help, or support of coworkers.

Ensure that there are no surprises. Do not bring something to a meeting that could embarrass or anger another person. Avoid criticizing someone at a meeting.

Avoid confrontation and ill words at a meeting. Nobody wins.

Do not dominate a meeting.

Be clear and open. Avoid cryptic statements.

Use clear, simple, and appropriate language to address the audience.

Include the six W/H (who, what, when, where, why, and how) points.

Do not misrepresent or overdramatize what was said at a meeting to someone who was not present.

in and attention to both the topic of the conversation and the person or persons (8).

Using Body Language

Body language refers to everything done with the body to express the message. The better the manager is able to transmit messages so that they are received by others as they were intended, the more effective the manager. It is very important to be acutely aware of the nonverbal messages being sent. A sensitive, perceptive communicator uses the nonverbal feedback he or she is getting from the other person to structure the content and direction of the message. The ability to project favorable body postures and to read the body language of others is an asset to organizations (5).

Maintain steady eye contact. Look at the person when talking to him or her without staring and glaring, which may be interpreted as aggressive. Sit up and face the receiver. It is sometimes helpful to lean forward occasionally as well. Show life through facial expression by having facial expressions match your voice inflections. Body language pitfalls to avoid include slouching, invading space, hovering over the listener, looking blank or stern, displaying threatening gestures (finger pointing or pounding a fist on the table), folding arms, and distracting habits (picking, scratching, swirling, pulling on jewelry, rattling change).

Body language is an essential part of interpersonal communication. Proficiency with reading and projecting body language is an integral part of communication success. Once managers are aware of the importance of body language, they can become attuned to how others perceive them and to the nonverbal message from the other person.

Using Positive Language

How a manager uses language is an exceedingly powerful tool. Whether communicating orally or in written form, how the message is expressed affects whether the message is received positively or negatively. Negative language creates a negative environment and increased confrontation. A manager who uses negative language frequently criticizes ideas without offering suggestions or alternatives. Negative language usually tells a person that what he or she has done is wrong, without stressing the positive things that can be done to remedy the problem. Positive language stresses positive actions and positive consequences. It suggests alternatives and choices while sounding helpful and encouraging rather than being bureaucratic. If a manager realizes that he uses negative language rather than positive language, he can start improving his communication strategy by incorporating positive language in written material. Once this has been accomplished, it will be much easier to change spoken language to present a more positive tone. This is most helpful in the workplace. Negative language conveys a poor image to coworkers and customers. Positive language projects a helpful, positive image that improves the organizational climate (7).

Leadership Essentials for Improving Communication

A successful communicator must be a catalyst in the workplace. A catalyst in a laboratory setting is defined as a substance that heightens or accelerates a reaction. In the workplace, a catalyst is someone who sparks action in others. Managers must choose to consistently behave in ways that energize and mobilize others. There are several beliefs that are essential to a successful catalyst's behavior. The first is trust, which is an essential ingredient of success. The second is respect. People deserve respect, and there is value in diversity. The third belief is support. A key role of the leader is to support others. By acting on these beliefs, catalyst leaders practice what they preach, make a long-lasting difference in the lives of the people who look to them for guidance and support, and influence people who can make a difference. Successful catalysts are successful communicators. An integral part of this communication includes understanding the interaction process as well as the preferred communication styles of others.

The Interaction Process

When people interact, they generally have two kinds of needs, the practical and the personal. Achieving a productive outcome can satisfy practical needs. Personal needs include feeling valued, understood, involved, and supported.

The interaction process consists of five guidelines that equip the manager with the skills needed to be successful. The five interaction guidelines are open, clarify, develop, agree, and close. When opening a discussion, state the purpose, the importance of the purpose, and the benefits of accomplishing it. Clarify the discussion by collecting facts and figures and then using them to explore issues and concerns. Develop the discussion by involving the person or group by seeking their ideas. Agree on a course of action by specifying what will be done, who will do it, and a date when it will be done. Agree on a tracking process. Close the discussion by confirming that everyone is clear on the subsequent steps and committed to following through with these steps. These guidelines satisfy practical needs by ultimately ensuring that the discussion achieves its purpose. Clarify, develop, and agree are guidelines that can be used multiple times in a discussion. To keep the discussion moving and on target, the manager must remember to check for understanding and make procedural suggestions when appropriate. Using this process provides the framework for the discussion and ensures that the discussion achieves a productive outcome. The interaction process equips a manager with the skills needed to be successful in any type of discussion or communication.

The interaction guidelines should be used in tandem with five key principles. These principles meet personal needs and build trust and stronger working relationships among staff. The principles are maintain or enhance self-esteem; listen and respond with empathy; share thoughts, feelings, and rationales; ask for help and encourage involvement; and provide support without removing responsibility. When the manager communicates using these key principles, it encourages trust by communicating to the staff that the manager supports them. These key principles support the interaction guidelines during discussions. By using the interaction skills and key principles, the manager is able to achieve critical business objectives while enhancing working relationships, which in turn enhances communication.

Meaningful, supportive feedback is also essential to achieving success within an organization. Effective feedback should be timely, balanced, and specific. Timely positive feedback strongly reinforces positive actions and results. Timely developmental feedback provides suggestions soon enough for people to adjust and enhance their performance. Effective feedback balances suggestions for improvement with reinforcement. Specific feedback provides a distinct picture of present performance and clear guidance on actions that will increase the likelihood of success in the future. Staff should be told what they accomplished (or did not accomplish), how they achieved results, and why their actions were effective. This type of feedback is effective because it provides a complete picture of expected performance and enhances communication.

Adapting Communication Styles

One way of improving communication is to modify the communication style of the speaker to match the individual with whom one is communicating. Individuals can be categorized in one of four ways: active doer, methodical plodder, people person, and thinker. Active doers like a minimal amount of discussion and a quick resolution. They prefer bulleted information with an outline of key points. Active doers want things to happen "yesterday." Methodical plodders thrive on extensive facts and data with multiple channels of input. They prefer to mull the situation over extensively before making a decision or a commitment. A people person prefers a personable approach. He does not want to be inundated with facts and data and is more interested in how issues or problems relate to people. The thinker visualizes the finished product but is not interested in the details. She has no idea how to translate needs into a finished plan and becomes bored quickly with facts and figures. A successful communicator

understands these categories, knows her audience, and then adapts her communication method to match the individual (Table 11.6).

There are four case studies in the appendix that illustrate examples of good and bad communication techniques. For each case there is a case scenario, followed by a brief discussion.

Summary

Effective communication is critical in any organization. It is a two-way street that requires both talking and listening. Smart managers realize that they do not have a monopoly on experience and knowledge. They do much more listening than talking because they know that talented individuals can be found in every possible job in an organization—from the very bottom rung of the corporate ladder all the way to the top. By listening, smart managers often hear good ideas. They must evaluate the situation and decide whether they are best served by taking control and directing the conversation or by listening, asking questions, and collecting ideas (15).

To be expert communicators, managers must acquire a variety of skills and learn when to use the appropriate ones. One of the most important skills is active listening. Effective managers learn and use active-listening techniques. This sets the tone and contributes to a positive communication climate (8). Effective managers realize that it is important to avoid communication barriers. Managers can avoid these barriers by preparing, planning, and organizing the environment as well as the time for exchange of communication. Employees are more receptive when the manager acts in a supportive and positive manner. Communication between managers and employees supports performance and work (16). Managers must treat every communication with the care it would receive if it were going to be delivered to a very important customer (Table 11.7).

In every organization, communication from the manager must be considered credible. This must be earned. Credibility means that the staff finds the manager believable, trustworthy, and deserving of respect. A manager

Table 11.6 Adapting communication to specific listening types

Type	Nonproductive communication	Productive communication
Active doer	Long explanations	Bullet points
Methodical plodder	Bullet points	Long explanations
People person	Memos, e-mails	Personalized meeting
Thinker	Details	Big picture

Table 11.7 Communication tips to build strong working relationships

Be positive and upbeat.

Engage and smile at others.

Be up front—no hidden agendas.

Give criticism politely and always privately.

Remember things that are important to others.

Respect others and their opinions.

Do not say something behind someone's back that cannot be justified or said to them.

Listen actively.

earns credibility by taking positive actions after interactions with staff. These actions must match positive words and good intentions. Credibility can be earned by following through, demonstrating expertise, remaining calm under pressure, taking positive approaches to problems, showing sincerity, and listening before acting.

Managers enhance communication by being a catalyst to others in the organization. Communication improves when managers use an interaction process that meets both the practical and personal needs of the staff. Smart managers adapt their communication style to match the individual with whom they are communicating.

Successful managers are successful communicators. Effective communication benefits the entire organization, since communication helps in accomplishing tasks and solving problems. Communication requires several primary ingredients: setting the climate and the tone, removing barriers, listening actively, and achieving and maintaining credibility.

KEY POINTS

- Appreciate that communication is essential to all aspects of the daily work environment. The ability to communicate is essential to leadership and vital to every organization.

- Recognize that while formal channels are the primary means of official communication, the grapevine exists in every organization. Management can often use the information from the grapevine as well as provide the grapevine with facts.

- Evaluate the situation, the audience, and the content of the message to determine the most effective type of communication.

- Identify communication barriers. Work toward eliminating or controlling communication barriers.

- Become an active listener. Learn active-listening techniques and use them consistently.

- Foster an organizational climate that supports effective communication.

- Recognize nonverbal messages, both those you are projecting and those you are receiving.

- Utilize positive language when possible.

- Practice the interaction process and use it to meet the practical and personal needs of the staff.

- Give positive feedback.

- Adapt your communication style to match the individual with whom you are communicating.

GLOSSARY

Active listener One who listens to the whole message, including facts and feelings.

Communication The exchange of thoughts, messages, or information by multiple mechanisms such as speech, signals, or writing.

Communication barriers Any behavior or physical obstruction that hinders or restricts the flow of meaningful communication.

Evaluative listener A listener who hears the words but makes no attempt to understand the feelings of the speaker.

Formal channels of communication Communication networks designed to follow the structure (lines of authority) of the organization.

Informal channels of communication Informal routes that people use to spread information to one another.

Marginal listener One who hears the words but does not comprehend the intent.

Negative language. Words or phrases used to communicate thoughts and feelings by using excessive criticism and confrontation.

Nonlistener A person who does not hear anything that is said.

Organizational culture Social and artistic expression, characteristic of a community or population, that pertains to behavior patterns, arts, beliefs, institutions, and all other products of human work and thought.

Positive language Words or phrases used to communicate thoughts and feelings by using positive actions and consequences.

REFERENCES

1. **Adams, B.** 2001. Information exchange: the art of communication, p. 16–25. *In* B. Adams (ed.), *The Everything Leadership Book.* Adams Media Corporation, Avon, Mass.

2. **Alessandra, T., and P. Hunsaker.** 1993. Active listening, p. 54–68. *In* T. Alessandra and P. Hunsaker (ed.), *Communicating at Work.* Simon & Schuster, Inc., New York, N.Y.

3. **Alessandra, T., and P. Hunsaker.** 1993. Future perfect communication, p.14–16. *In* T. Alessandra and P. Hunsaker (ed.), *Communicating at Work.* Simon & Schuster, Inc., New York, N.Y.

4. **Alessandra, T., and P. Hunsaker.** 1993. It's how you say it, p. 139–141. *In* T. Alessandra and P. Hunsaker (ed.), *Communicating at Work.* Simon & Schuster, Inc., New York, N.Y.

5. **Alessandra, T., and P. Hunsaker.** 1993. The power of nonverbal communication, p. 120–122. *In* T. Alessandra and P. Hunsaker (ed.), *Communicating at Work.* Simon & Schuster, Inc., New York, N.Y.

6. **Bacal, R.** 2004. Improving communication—tips for managers. Work911/Bacal and Associates. [Online.] http://www.work911.com/conflict/carticles/impcom.htm. Accessed 26 February 2004.

7. **Bacal, R.** 2004. Using positive language. Work911/Bacal and Associates. [Online.] http://www.work911.com/conflict/carticles/poslan.htm. Accessed 26 February 2004.

8. **Blair, G. M.** Conversation as communication. [Online.] http://www.ee.ed.ac.uk/~gerard/Management/art7.html. Accessed 26 February 2004.

9. **Brounstein, M.** 2001. Are you really listening? p. 27–38. *In* M. Brounstein (ed.), *Communicating Effectively for Dummies.* Hungry Minds, Inc., New York, N.Y.

10. **Brounstein, M.** 2001. Fixing your radar on the speaker, p. 51–56. *In* M. Brounstein (ed.), *Communicating Effectively for Dummies.* Hungry Minds, Inc., New York, N.Y.

11. **Brounstein, M.** 2001. Ten ideas for effectively handling telephone interactions, p. 323–327. *In* M. Brounstein (ed.), *Communicating Effectively for Dummies.* Hungry Minds, Inc., New York, N.Y.

12. **Lemery, L. D.** 2002. Communications at the 95% confidence level: the impossible dream? *Clin. Leadersh. Manag. Rev.* **16:**127–129.

13. **Martin, B. G.** 1982. Communications, p. 133–158. *In* K. R. Karni, K. R. Viskochil, and P. A. Amos (ed.), *Clinical Laboratory Management.* Little, Brown and Company, Boston, Mass.

14. **McGinty, S. M.** 2001. Electronic communication, p. 120–127. *In* S. M. McGinty (ed.), *Power Talk: Using Language To Build Authority and Influence.* Warner Books, Inc., New York, N.Y.

15. **McGinty, S. M.** 2001. Putting language to work, p. 87. *In* S. M. McGinty (ed.), *Power Talk: Using Language To Build Authority and Influence.* Warner Books, Inc., New York, N.Y.

16. **Wallace, M. A., and D. D. Klosinski.** 1998. Directing: the third management function, p. 238–247. *In* M. A. Wallace and D. D. Klosinski (ed.), *Clinical Laboratory Science Education and Management.* W.B. Saunders Company, Philadelphia, Pa.

APPENDIX 11.1   Case Studies

Case 1

Alvin has been hired as the administrative director of the laboratory in the hospital at a large academic medical center. After a year Alvin has made little effort to get to know his employees. He keeps himself "set apart." For example, he never stops in the hall to chat and makes no attempt to learn the names of his staff. Alvin never eats lunch with his supervisors even though he frequently walks by the table where they are sitting. In laboratory meetings, he makes cryptic statements and tells bad jokes. He seldom asks the supervisors for input and never uses the input he receives. He tells the hospital administrator that he is resigning and has taken a job elsewhere because he can't work with the supervisors.

Discussion: To be an effective manager and communicator at his next hospital, Alvin must learn to develop his interpersonal skills. He must be available and approachable. He should begin to win the confidence of the staff by asking for their views on subjects and following through with some of their suggestions. A few simple changes such as chatting occasionally with the staff and learning names would go a long way toward improving the environment. This will help to establish a better organizational climate, which could be the first step in improving communication.

Case 2

Katherine has recently been appointed interim administrative director in the hospital Alvin just left. Katherine immediately meets with her supervisors. Within her first month, she holds a meeting on all three shifts. She presents information, listens to employee concerns, and answers questions. Katherine makes herself approachable and available. She always has a friendly smile on her face. When Katherine hears of misconceptions through the grapevine, she takes steps to correct the misconceptions.

Discussion: Katherine promotes a climate that supports effective communication. She is an active listener. The staff will communicate their concerns because she is perceived as receptive. She frequently seeks input and acts on that input. Katherine realizes the value of the grapevine in her organization and provides it with facts. She also uses formal channels to disseminate information and give staff the opportunity to ask questions. Communication between the laboratory director and the staff has improved greatly since Alvin left.

Case 3

Alice makes an appointment to see the administrative director. She is very agitated and upset about not being chosen for a promotion. The administrator attempts to communicate with Alice by using a soothing tone of voice, maintaining eye contact, and being an active listener. When the director tries to give feedback to her, Alice constantly interrupts, raises her voice, and speaks in a very accusatory manner.

Discussion: For communication to be effective, both parties must be active listeners. Because Alice is so upset, she is not hearing anything that the director is attempting to say. The discussion is essentially nonproductive. After several attempts at trying to get Alice to remain calm, the director asks Alice to reschedule the meeting when she is in a more positive frame of mind and is able to listen to feedback.

Case 4

Ginny makes an appointment to see her supervisor about some concerns she has in the laboratory data center. When she arrives the radio is blaring. There are multiple projects all over the supervisor's desk. The supervisor has his back turned to Ginny and is working at the computer. He frequently shuffles through the paperwork on his desk looking for the information he needs for the project he is working on. Ginny attempts to ask her questions and state her concerns but does not feel valued by her supervisor.

Discussion: There are many barriers to effective communication in this situation. This supervisor needs to turn off the radio, maintain eye contact, face the speaker, and stack work neatly on the desk prior to the meeting. He should practice active-listening skills, listening to Ginny and then suggesting a course of action. If some crisis at the last minute makes this impossible, the best thing to do would be to apologize to Ginny and reschedule the meeting.

APPENDIX 11.2   Websites

Gerard M. Blair
(http://www.ee.ed.ac.uk/~gerard/Management/art7.html)
"Conversation as communication"; links to other articles by Gerard M. Blair.

The Work911/Bacal and Associates Workplace Supersite
(http://www.work911.com/conflict/carticles/impcom.htm;
http://www.work911.com/conflict/carticles/poslan.htm)
Network of workplace help sites, articles, etc.

12

Effective Meetings*

Christopher S. Frings

OBJECTIVES

To help the reader determine whether or not to have a meeting

To explain how to set up and run an effective meeting

To illustrate how to be an effective meeting participant

To help managers calculate the cost of a meeting

Show me a person who likes to go to meetings, and I'll show you a person who doesn't have enough to do.

JOE GRIFFITH, PROFESSIONAL SPEAKER

HOW MANY TIMES have you been in a meeting thinking, "What a waste of time. I could have accomplished more doing other things instead of being at this meeting?" This information will give you a formula for more effective meetings. The cost of meetings is high. Since middle managers average 11 hours per week in meetings and upper managers average 23 hours per week in meetings, it is important that we master the skill of holding effective meetings (1). Holding an effective meeting is one more way to work smarter, not harder!

Should We Have a Meeting?

The first question to ask when deciding about a meeting is, "Is it necessary that we have a meeting?" The only four reasons to hold a meeting are to:

- Make decisions
- Motivate a team or group
- Coordinate action or exchange information
- Discuss problems or opportunities (1)

---

*Some of the information in this chapter was adapted with permission from C. S. Frings. 1997. *The Hitchhiker's Guide to Effective Time Management*, p. 65–67. AACC Press, Washington, D.C.

A meeting is an investment in time, money, and possible lost productivity in other areas. Here are some points to consider before deciding whether to have a meeting. Would a memo, e-mail, or voice mail message be as effective as a meeting? If the answer is yes, don't have the meeting. If several people can get together informally to discuss and/or act on an issue in a few minutes, don't call a meeting. Don't hold meetings simply out of habit. Assess the continuing need for any regular meeting held more than once a month. What is the worst thing that might happen if a meeting is not held? What is the purpose of the meeting? How can the meeting's success or value be measured? After you have asked these questions and concluded that the answer is, "Yes, we should have a meeting," follow the keys to successful meetings (1) listed below.

Keys to Successful Meetings

Make meetings more effective by holding them only when a conference call, e-mail, voice mail, or memo won't accomplish the goal. When you do hold a meeting, require everyone to be prepared. Have a purpose, written agenda, and time budget for every meeting. See Appendixes 12.1 and 12.2.

Leader Responsibilities

For a successful meeting to happen, the leader must be able to adapt leadership styles to different groups, different members, and different tasks (2). The leader who uses the authoritarian style all of the time will fail! Invite only those who are needed and are essential to the success of the meeting's goals. Ask, Who should participate? Why? What is the best number of participants to reach resolution? Most people will be happy having one less meeting to go to; however, some with easily offended egos may be upset unless you explain the objective criteria for attendance. Have a detailed written agenda in advance with location, time, length of meeting, and any preparation participants need to make. The agenda should include a short description of the goals and expected outcomes and should be distributed to all meeting participants in advance, giving time to review, prepare, and discuss. How far in advance the written agenda is distributed should depend on the amount of preparation required by the participants before the meeting. Preparation prior to a meeting is vital to a successful meeting. The amount of preparation will vary with the topic and the expertise of the attendees. Increase the preparation time and decrease the meeting time!

Start meetings on time and end early or on time. The person chairing the meeting is responsible for (i) leadership, (ii) starting on time, (iii) ending on time or ending early, and (iv) arranging the meeting site. The person chairing the meeting should arrive early and make certain that the meeting room is set up properly. Tell the participants where they can find rest rooms, a coffee machine, a telephone to use at breaks, and whatever else they may need. Review the agenda and reinforce the purpose of the meeting. Modify the agenda as needed to include last-minute developments (2).

Prepared Agenda

Prioritize the agenda. Address A's first, then B's, and finally the C's (A's are the highest-priority issues and C's are the lowest-priority issues). If you should run out of time for the meeting, you will have done the most important things.

Meeting Interruptions

Don't allow interruptions if possible. If the subject is important enough to deserve a meeting, it should not be preempted by distractions. Avoid taking phone calls during meetings. Because you don't know who is calling you, you will give the impression that anyone calling you is more important than the person(s) you are meeting with. Ground rules for participants should include turning off beepers and cell phones before entering the meeting.

Questions and Answers

Plan to end meetings or presentations ahead of schedule. The extra time provides flexibility to expand on a point or answer a question. Questions and answers should be part of almost every meeting. Allow for questions during the discussion of each agenda item. At some point you have to state that the group must move to the next agenda item. If the extra time isn't needed, the audience will be pleasantly surprised by the early conclusion and probably consider it a sign of efficiency and professionalism. Look out for those people with their own agenda who frequently will try to get you to address what they want addressed (not necessarily sticking to the agenda).

Meeting Summary

Recap, summarize, and state conclusions at the end of the meeting. The person chairing the meeting should leave no issues unresolved and should review all decisions and commitments made. Issues not resolved during the meeting due to the need for additional information, absence of a key stakeholder, etc., need to be addressed. This can be included in the action minutes. End the meeting on an upbeat note. An example is summarizing the progress made on the issues.

Meeting Minutes

Provide written action minutes after the meeting. Written minutes do the following: (i) document decisions made at the meeting and (ii) hold those with assignments from the meeting responsible for completing their assignments. After the meeting, prepare the minutes promptly. Distribute them as soon as possible. The minutes should include meeting date, time, place, and purpose; names of atten-

Table 12.1 Hourly cost of a meeting

Annual salary	Cost for indicated no. of attendees						
	2	4	6	8	10	15	20
$150,000	$300	$600	$900	$1,200	$1,500	$2,250	$3,000
$100,000	$200	$400	$600	$800	$1,000	$1,500	$2,000
$80,000	$160	$320	$480	$640	$800	$1,200	$1,600
$60,000	$120	$240	$360	$480	$600	$900	$1,200
$40,000	$80	$160	$240	$320	$400	$600	$800
$20,000	$40	$80	$120	$160	$200	$300	$400

dees, conclusions, agreements, action items; and assignments (2). The minutes should not try to summarize the discussions or point out who said what.

Regularly Scheduled Meetings: Pros and Cons

Try not to hold regularly scheduled meetings. If you hold a regular scheduled meeting, redetermine on a regular basis if the meeting is really needed or not. If you have regular meetings, ask the group periodically, "Do we still need this meeting at this frequency?" Often the answer is no. Listen to what the group says. Exceptions include meetings required by the expectations of accrediting agencies, medical staff bylaws, etc.

Cost of Meetings

The cost of meetings is high, as shown in Table 12.1 (1). This table assumes that all meeting attendees make the same salary, which is rarely the case. The table gives the cost of a meeting based on salary alone and doesn't include meeting room costs and refreshments or any lost time that could have been spent generating income.

The Participant's Role

So far we have looked at skills of the meeting leader. It also takes skills to be an effective meeting participant (3). As a meeting participant you too have responsibilities. You should prepare for the meeting and then have something to offer, be prepared to influence the group, keep on the subject, and help manage conflict if it arises (2). Make certain to ask for an agenda for the meeting if you have not received one in advance. Be a good listener at the meeting. Use good manners at the meeting by following the Golden Rule. Monitor your nonverbal signals such as facial expressions, yawning, and doodling (2).

Summary

Don't hold a meeting if a voice mail, e-mail, or memo will suffice. Hold a meeting for only one or more of the following reasons: (i) to make decisions, (ii) to motivate a team or group, (iii) to coordinate action or exchange information, or (iv) to discuss problems or opportunities. The cost of meetings is high, and meetings use our most priceless resource—time. Use the tips in this chapter to run effective meetings. Specific recommendations to improve your meetings can be seen in Table 12.2.

KEY POINTS

- Make meetings more effective by holding them only when a phone call, conference call, e-mail, voice mail, or memo won't accomplish the goal.
- Have a purpose, written agenda, and time budget for every meeting.
- When you do hold a meeting, require everyone to be prepared.
- Have a prioritized agenda and stick to it.
- Start meetings on time and end early or on time.
- Recap, summarize, and state conclusions at the end of the meeting.
- Provide written action minutes after the meeting.
- As a meeting participant your responsibilities include preparing for the meeting and then having something to offer, being prepared to influence the group, keeping on the subject, and helping manage conflict if it arises.

GLOSSARY

Agenda A list of things to be discussed and acted on at a meeting.

Meeting When two or more people come together to discuss something; usually implies a face-to-face meeting but could be a telephone or electronic meeting. Examples are departmental or staff meeting, committee or task force meeting, and training meeting.

Minutes An official record of the meeting of an organization.

REFERENCES

1. Frings, C. S. 1997. *The Hitchhiker's Guide to Effective Time Management,* p. 65–67. AACC Press, Washington, D.C.

2. Soundview Executive Book Summaries. 1989. *Skills for Success,* p. 99–105. Soundview Executive Book Summaries, Middleburg, Vt.

3. Yeomans, W. N. 1985. *1000 Things You Never Learned in Business School,* p. 133–153. New American Library, Bergenfield, N.J.

Table 12.2 Problems and potential solutions related to more effective meetings

Problem	Recommended solution
No definition of purpose	Schedule meetings only when there is a defined purpose.
Participants don't want to attend or tend to come unprepared for agenda topics	Distribute agenda prior to the meeting (with plenty of lead time), indicate the benefits of attendance, set time that is convenient for the majority, and pay attention to the physical setting.
Overall planning is minimal or missing.	Planning ahead of time will increase the level of productivity and decrease the overall meeting time required to meet objectives.
Inappropriate meeting participants for the discussion topic	Include participants who are relevant to the topics being presented and discussed.
Meeting fails to begin on time	This sends a message that you have no respect for people's time; begin on time, regardless of whether or not everyone is present.
Meeting objectives are unclear	Begin the meeting by clarifying objectives per written agenda (distributed ahead of time).
Participants appear to be disinterested and confused	Make sure correct participants are present (relevant to topics under discussion); continue to clarify throughout the discussion; provide time for questions.
There are interruptions and undercurrent discussions.	Make it very clear that interruptions are not acceptable; talking during any presentation is also unacceptable. Set up the ground rules from the beginning.
One person dominates the discussion (could be the leader or a participant)	It is the leader's responsibility to ensure that everyone has input and to prevent one person from taking over the meeting; be polite but firm.
The overall discussions appears to stray from the original agenda	The leader needs to keep the discussion on track and to follow the written agenda.
There appears to be indecision among the group	Continue to clarify objectives and work toward completion.
The meeting runs over the allotted time	Prior to the meeting, set up realistic time frames; keep the meeting on track and moving forward.
There is no verbal summary at the end of the meeting	Make sure a verbal summary is provided and that all participants understand the decisions that were made.
The participants do not receive a written summary in the form of minutes	A recorder should be identified at the beginning of the meeting (or ahead of time). Record and distribute written minutes within a day of the meeting; this written documentation serves as a reminder of decisions, pending issues, "to-do" responsibilities, etc.
Failure of the leader to follow up on meeting decisions, assignments, etc.	Confirm assignments and due dates, and set up calendar for confirmation of task completion.
Meeting seems to be okay but not super	Assess participant satisfaction and evaluate meeting format for potential improvements.

APPENDIX 12.1 Checklist To Use When Planning a Meeting[a]

Write the purpose of the meeting.

Write the agenda.

Prioritize the agenda.

Decide who needs to attend.

Select the chairperson.

Select the date, time, and place for the meeting.

Reserve the meeting room.

Name a recorder to write the minutes.

[a]See reference 2.

APPENDIX 12.2 Example of a Purpose, Agenda, and Time Budget for a Meeting

Date of meeting: December 1
Time of meeting: 10:00 a.m.–noon
Invited attendees: CF, MB, AS, DA, DM, LY, DC, LS
Purpose: To establish the program for our February management retreat
Homework: Review suggested program. Suggest several keynote speakers. Suggest several in-house speakers.
Agenda:
   Introduction and expectations (10:00–10:05 a.m.)
   Set date, time, and place for management retreat (10:05–10:15 a.m.)
   Review and discuss suggested program; make changes (10:15–11:00 a.m.)

Break (11:00–11:10 a.m.)
Complete—review and discuss suggested program; make changes (11:10–11:20 a.m.)
Select outside keynote speaker (and two alternates to contact if first choice is not available) (11:20–11:35 a.m.)
Select other speakers (in-house) (11:35–11:45 a.m.)
Delegate authority for selecting break menus, lunch menu, and A/V needs (11:45–11:50 a.m.)
Schedule next meeting date and time to finalize management retreat program (11:55 a.m.)
Adjourn (noon)

13

Conflict Management

Jean Egan

> **OBJECTIVES**
>
> *To define and describe conflict*
>
> *To differentiate between constructive and destructive conflict*
>
> *To identify five different strategies for resolving conflict and the pros and cons of each style*
>
> *To describe the role of the manager in resolving conflicts*
>
> *To discuss the seven-step model for resolving conflict*

You cannot shake hands with a clenched fist.

GANDHI

ALTHOUGH CONFLICT IS INEVITABLE, it can be healthy for an organization if it is addressed and resolved in a rational manner. While conflict can be destructive or constructive, managing conflict is a key component to structuring a successful workplace. Success depends on being able to acknowledge, manage, and resolve conflict, and managers need to take the lead in helping staff recognize and manage conflict. Staff training and development along with an organizational climate that values conflict resolution are keys to healthy conflict resolution. Also, open dialogue and creative problem solving are constructive methods to use when dealing with conflict.

The ability to manage and resolve conflict is a universal skill that crosses all life domains, and recognizing and managing conflict is a skill that can be learned. All successful managers must exercise the skills to identify, analyze, and resolve conflict. When conflict is managed and resolved, it can be a source of growth for individuals as well as institutions. Ultimately the success of an organization depends on how well staff members recognize, understand, and resolve conflict, hopefully within a climate and culture where conflicts are expected and not ignored.

Conflict Defined

Conflicts or potential conflicts occur in every life domain and can range from simple disagreements to complex arguments with each person insisting on their version of what is right. Conflict can be defined as the simultaneous arousal of two or more incompatible motives (5). A second common view of conflict is one person blocking another from reaching her goal (2). A conflict is simply a disagreement over goals or how to accomplish them. Two strangers may both want to park their cars but have a conflict over who will get the single open space they have each spotted. Members of a couple may agree that they both want to take a vacation but disagree about where to go or how long to be away. Roommates may agree that sleeping is an important life activity but disagree about the hours during which sleep should occur. Coworkers may want to take time off around a major holiday, discuss it between themselves, and work out an arrangement, but their manager might not want anyone taking vacation at that time of year. Conflict is inevitable; how you deal with it makes all the difference.

Conflict can be resolved at any level in an organization. It does not always involve taking it up the chain of command. In fact, the healthiest organizations are those where employees or members at every level are empowered to resolve conflict. An organization that values conflict resolution will be healthy and has a much better chance of survival in a competitive environment. Organizations that try to ignore or cover up conflicts will be rife with high rates of turnover, unhappy staff, poor communication, lost time spent griping to or about coworkers, rigid adherence to rules, lack of cooperation, and reduced creativity. People are discouraged when they are forced to live or work in situations where conflict goes unresolved. Workplace violence is the worst form of frustration over unresolved conflict. Successful managers in the future will need to know how to recognize, address, resolve, and even encourage conflict. They must train their staff to resolve conflict and reward people for doing so.

What Conflict Is and Is Not

Conflict tends to be viewed through a negative filter. However, it, like stress, is neither good nor bad. In fact, conflict can lead to growth if it is resolved. The disagreement or different views that people bring to a given situation can be helpful and constructive if they lead to open dialogue and creative solutions. The goal of conflict is growth and positive change. What most people refer to when they use the word "conflict" really is what they experience when they are caught in a conflicted situation and either they have no power to improve it or someone else has forced an outcome on them with which they do not agree. This is a classic definition of unresolved conflict. Unresolved conflict is always destructive.

Constructive Conflict

It is important to draw a clear distinction between conflict that is constructive and conflict that is not. Conflict is constructive when the involved parties recognize and acknowledge that they have a disagreement and actively work to resolve it. Constructive conflict resolution results in outcomes that may involve a compromise on both sides,

and the best interests of the organization are served by addressing the conflict (4). Real conflict resolution takes time to work out a creative solution so that both parties are happy with the outcome. Conflict has been resolved if both parties walk away satisfied and neither one harbors the desire to even the score later.

Destructive Conflict

Destructive conflicts occur when people try to ignore a situation and when one person forces a resolution on another that results in a win-lose outcome. The net result is that the organization is harmed (4). People often try to ignore a brewing conflict. They may have learned to keep their mouths shut and keep their heads down. They may have seen a negative outcome for a coworker who tried to bring a conflict to the attention of a supervisor. They may have tried to resolve an issue and felt discouraged and gave up. Managers need to intervene to resolve destructive conflict.

Common Causes of Conflict

Conflict in the workplace differs from conflict in our private lives in one major way—power. Power is not generally evenly distributed at work. The work environment is almost always set up in a stratified hierarchy. That "pecking order" may be established in formal or informal ways (organizational charts versus how things really get done), but power is not evenly distributed to all the staff. Even among members of the same profession, power is not equalized. Among physicians, for example, seniority, specialty, tenure, political connections, grant funding, research projects, gender, race, and a number of other overt and hidden criteria impact who has power and who is expected to yield to it.

Among laboratory technical staff, power differentials can occur based on differences in formal or informal training and statewide or national credentials, as well as years and types of experience. When offices or companies merge, political alliances, seniority, and old reporting relationships have to be renegotiated in combined offices. These and myriad other potential conflicts need to be anticipated, addressed, and resolved. Otherwise, the underlying issues build until they erupt into hostile differences. Common causes of conflict include the following:

- Incompatible goals
- Poor communication
- Style of supervision
- Different ideas about task achievement
- Different perceptions
- Different values and philosophies
- Personality differences
- Work assignments

- Approaches to change
- Competition

Conflict is going to exist. These major categories of conflict must be identified and addressed before they build into major disruptions to the office or laboratory environment.

Internal and External Origins of Conflict

Sources of conflict can be further differentiated by internal or external origins. There are stressful life events that occur both at work and at home. Individuals have different tolerances for managing life stresses. The ability to compartmentalize stress plays a major role in the ability to tolerate, address, or appropriately respond to situations of conflict.

Internal Sources of Conflict

Work-related, or internal, conflict has its origins in the workplace. It can, however, be impacted by nonwork (external) conflicts. Typical examples of internal conflict include the following:

- Work that is not challenging, that has become routine, or that is boring
- Work that is too challenging because of staff shortages, lack of training, or time pressures
- Poor relationships with coworkers
- Poor relationship with the supervisor
- Pay does not seem fair for the work performed.
- Feeling undervalued, devalued, or unappreciated
- Office politics
- Favoritism
- Lack of resources to successfully complete the job, including time, technology, and tools

These types of internal conflicts develop over time. They may result from a lack of attention to employee morale, misunderstandings that are ignored, lack of emphasis on teamwork, lack of staff and management training, or poor management practices. Conflict in the workplace can be managed with good employee relations and setting performance objectives that are uniformly applied and measured for all staff, as well as by providing training in teamwork and conflict management.

External Sources of Conflict

Employees all have stressors in their private lives that can negatively impact their performance at work. These external sources of stress can contribute to conflicts at work. Examples include the following:

- Interpersonal stress at home
- Scheduling conflicts between work and home demands
- Traffic

- Medical problems
- Illness of family members
- Life transitions such as marriage, divorce, becoming a parent, death of a family member, or retirement of a spouse

Frequently, these types of conflict occur simultaneously. An employee may have had a fight with his teenager before work, have encountered two traffic accidents en route, and be debating whether he can afford the time and money to pursue additional college coursework. These issues weigh on the employee before he ever gets to the workplace. A small instance of friction with a coworker on top of the already existing external stressors can combine to create a larger problem. That problem may manifest itself as a negative attitude when it really is a symptom of mounting stress. Stress that continues to build is likely to erupt as workplace conflict. Managers are wise to know their employees and show sensitivity to both the work and nonwork demands all staff face. Managers can take steps to communicate that conflicts are normal, are to be expected, and can be a source of growth in the office when they are addressed and resolved.

Home-related problems are not left at the office door when an employee reports to work. Similarly, work-related problems are carried home. Staff members need to understand how to identify sources of conflict they bring to the work environment, manage their own sources of stress, and work to collaborate with coworkers to resolve conflicts at work. Having an employee assistance plan, providing opportunities to talk formally and informally with managers and coworkers, and training in stress reduction can help. Resolving conflicts improves productivity at work and life satisfaction at home. With proper training, managers can identify multiple sources of stress, spot conflicts that are building, and take action to address them. Employees who learn conflict resolution skills will experience the benefits in both domains of life.

Two Basic Beliefs about Handling a Conflict

Our history with conflict, whether it is resolved or not, and the outcome of a conflict both impact our willingness to engage in trying to address and resolve conflict. Our approach to conflict can take one of two polar positions. Paul and Paul (8) characterize this polarity as two dichotomous choices in looking at a conflict. They state that when faced with a conflict, we can choose to react either with an intent to protect ourselves or with an intent to learn. The choice we make leads to very different outcomes.

The intent to protect themselves leads individuals to defend their position or behaviors and results in negativity and distance between the parties. Approaching conflict with the intent to learn about the other person's views, share your own views, and find a mutually agreeable resolution leads to a healthy outcome and collaboration between the parties. An awareness of whether one is choosing to protect or to learn is the first step toward change. Suspending the pattern of defending one's position, letting go of the need to blame, and adopting a willingness to learn will result in a positive outcome. Conflict can only be resolved when both parties are willing to approach a disagreement with the intent to learn, change, and grow.

Another similar but expansive view of conflict is offered by Kritek (7). She states that in attempting to address conflicts, the parties can choose between staking and winning their "claim" or approaching conflict to create a workable outcome for everyone involved. Kritek's approach to conflict recognizes that people often negotiate at an uneven table. There are different levels of power between parties in a conflict. If one is focused on claiming victory, the outcome is already determined. There is a win-lose certainty. If both want to claim victory, the outcome is the same: win-lose. However, if both parties are interested in creating a mutually agreeable resolution, both can win. A truly collaborative outcome is possible only if neither party needs to be right or to win by making the other person lose.

The desire to reach a mutually agreeable resolution is the core of successful conflict resolution. When all the parties involved want to resolve the issue, are willing to compromise, and seek an outcome that leaves everyone whole, conflict can be resolved. In the absence of this approach, conflict remains unresolved.

Five Conflict Resolution Styles

Five common approaches are forcing, accommodation, collaboration, avoidance, and compromise (5). Most people have a primary style, but it is possible to draw upon more than one approach when faced with a conflict. Two distinct strategies are at play among the use of these five approaches. Each strategy has advantages and disadvantages. At issue is the balance between concern for people and concern for results (3). Figure 13.1 illustrates the dy-

namics of these two polarities and how each of the five conflict resolution styles operates. One primary difference is the degree to which communication between parties is a goal. Collaboration is possible with a strong concern for people and results. Aggression, or forcing, results from a focus on results at the expense of relationship building. Avoidance results when a person determines that an issue is unimportant or the person lacks the skills or drive to address the issues at hand. Accommodation is the end result of a strong desire to please the parties involved, even if task results are delayed or made subordinate. Compromise results from a middle ground with a balance between task results and people, coupled with a strong desire to move ahead. Compromise often sacrifices detail for speed to obtain a "good enough" outcome for all concerned.

A humorous method to understanding conflict resolution styles is to compare the five styles to animals (6), as shown below.

The Teddy Bear. People who use this approach to conflict would rather accommodate your needs than debate, speak up, or ruffle any feathers with their own views. Their approach is "You win—I give in."

The Turtle. People who use this approach to conflict would rather avoid conflict altogether. Like the turtle, they pull into their shells, avoiding, ignoring, stonewalling, or otherwise escaping the entire issue of conflict.

The Owl. People who use this approach to conflict would rather collaborate and work diligently to resolve a conflict no matter how long it takes. The owl shares ideas and works to bring about a win-win outcome. Those with this approach will not settle for anything less than total satisfaction for all sides in the conflict.

The Fox. People who use this approach to conflict would rather compromise. The fox likes to engage in meaningful discussion and move quickly to a resolution that both parties can live with. Each party gets some of what they need but also makes concessions by giving up some of what they wanted.

The Shark. People who use this approach to conflict force others to give in so that the Shark can win. It is a classic "kill or be killed" approach, an "I win, you lose" outcome. Sharks move quickly to vanquish anyone in their way to get what they want—a win at any cost.

Working with Each Style To Resolve Conflict

The Teddy Bear wants to get to agreement and often goes along with the group even when he or she does not want to do so. If you manage a Teddy Bear, get her to state what she really wants and what she is willing to do, and have all parties sign an agreement to preserve the outcome.

The Turtle does not like conflict. Managers need to gently coach the Turtle out of his shell, point out the benefits

Figure 13.1 Conflict resolution styles based on task or people concerns (3).

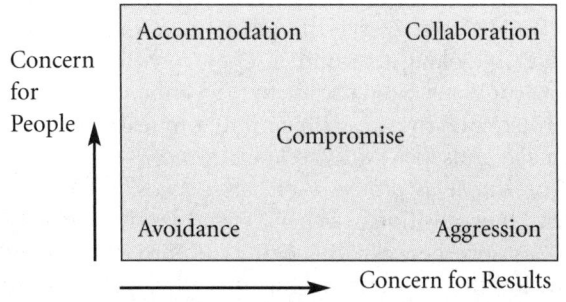

of addressing the conflict, reassure him of his safety, and provide lots of reinforcement for him to engage in the conflict resolution process.

The Owl wants to engage and take as much time as is required to resolve a conflict so that all parties are completely satisfied. In a busy work environment, that is not always possible. Managers need to encourage a deadline, help the Owl focus on the priorities, brainstorm options, find agreement that meets the majority of the priorities, and then move on to the next task.

The Fox wants to compromise and do so quickly. Managers can help the Fox put his cards on the table, set a deadline to explore options fully, find areas of overlap, get agreement, and then move on. Taking time to fully explore the options is a key to success with a Fox.

The Shark is a difficult player to manage. The Shark needs to be managed in ways that encourage her to see the good of the group, not just her own goals. Winning at any cost is not effective for the organization. Requiring her to engage in a 50% win—50% concession approach can contain the Shark. Put any agreements into writing and have the Shark sign off on the document.

Creating an Environment Where Conflict Is Addressed and Resolved

The Role of the Manager

Managers face multiple demands in today's complex working environments. Managing conflict is one of the key skills all managers need to master. Unresolved conflicts result in the staff becoming discouraged and disillusioned and giving up. Problems do not go away when we try to ignore them. Training staff on how to recognize and resolve conflicts empowers them to manage their own experience at work. Establishing an atmosphere of trust and open communication is critical to addressing conflict. Conflicts will occur. However, they can lead to growth and positive change.

The job of every manager involves planning, organizing, directing others, and controlling. The ability to manage conflict runs across each of those skills. Managers who plan well will establish an atmosphere of trust and open communication in the workplace. Those who train staff to recognize and resolve conflicts, who direct staff to manage conflicts successfully, and who organize opportunities for open and constructive communication will control the successful workings of the workplace and the quality of work life for everyone in the laboratory environment.

The Role of the Staff

It is important to create an atmosphere in the laboratory or office environment where telling the truth is rewarded. The biggest problems result when people try to ignore conflict. It is essential to value and reward staff for bringing issues of conflict to the forefront. The key to success is empowering staff members to identify conflicts and to work as a team to resolve them. Staff members need to be encouraged to take steps to identify, analyze, and solve problems at the lowest level possible. Individuals need to be given the power and authority to resolve issues on their own. Managers need to support this process by regularly reminding staff to communicate, collaborate, and resolve problems quickly. The first question a manager or supervisor needs to ask a staff member when she brings a conflict forward is whether she attempted to resolve the issue at a lower level. Taking a conflict to a supervisor should occur only after individuals have attempted to resolve the conflict themselves.

Creating the Right Environment To Resolve Conflict

Every member of the staff plays a role in creating the environment at work. The culture of the organization either supports resolving conflict or supports ignoring it. In today's stressful world, conflicts must be recognized and resolved quickly for the sake of the staff and the organization. Managers need to have simple models to use to resolve conflict.

A Communication Model To Manage and Resolve Conflict

The GGMG Model

Psychologist Robert Carkhuff (1) suggests a model for interpersonal communication that works well when resolving conflicts. In most conflicts, each person wants to be right and communication skills are seldom practiced. The give-get-merge-go (GGMG) model allows all parties to speak, be heard, and negotiate a mutually agreeable resolution and to implement it.

Give ⟷ Get ⟶ Merge ⟹ Go

During a conflict, two individuals frequently give information and expect the other person to simply implement the directive. A common form of this interaction would be "I *give* you instructions—now *go* follow them." If the person on the receiving end does not want to comply, a conflict results. A battle of wits can ensue where each person tries to convince the other to agree with him. No mutual understanding is reached, no merger of ideas is achieved, and progress is stymied.

When the entire GGMG model is implemented, this tug-of-war pattern stops. With the GGMG model, all parties involved need to share information about what bothers them and what their goals are. This is the give and get portion of the model. The parties need to listen and pay attention to what each person wants. In the midst of the interaction, there is an opportunity to find overlap in their goals. This is the merge step. Once overlapping goals are identified, the parties take steps to reach the newly agreed upon goals. The go piece is the final step that leads to conflict resolution.

A Seven-Step Plan for Resolving Conflict

There is a seven-step model for resolving conflict that can be implemented in any organizational setting. It can be used to resolve all types of conflict. The steps are as follows:

1. *Identify the source of the conflict.* What was the source of the conflict? Is it one major issue? Has there been simmering hostility or frustration over time between the parties? Do the parties involved want it resolved? Can it be resolved? What is the goal of each party?
2. *Identify the players.* What are the personalities? What is their history? Did they ever get along? Do you want to keep both people employed? Why? Do they know that?
3. *Have participants state their goals.* What are the areas of agreement or overlap? Have each person paraphrase the other's points. It encourages them to listen to each other and helps avoid a focus on being "right." Focus on what behaviors are getting in the way of effective workplace interaction.
4. *Explore options.* What behaviors need to change? You cannot change an attitude, and it is not essential that you try. What behaviors need to change for the individuals to work effectively with one another? Identify common goals. What steps need to be taken to change those behaviors? Ask the individuals involved to make suggestions of what they are willing to do to improve their part of the problem.
5. *Pick a solution.* After exploring options, select the ideas that are workable and can be immediately implemented. Focus on behavioral steps and the desired outcome. Make sure the outcome is win-win or at least a compromise. Set a reasonable time frame for the employees to implement the solution.
6. *Summarize and seek commitment.* State the ideas to which all parties have agreed. Hold the individuals accountable. You may have all the parties sign an agreement that states what behavioral steps they have committed to implement. Provide support and resources for helping the individuals make the changes they agree to make. Follow up within a day to make sure the parties are implementing the solutions. Follow up on a regular basis with the individuals to ensure that progress continues.
7. *Be open to third-party assistance.* I frequently get called in to resolve conflict in the workplace when individuals reach the breaking point. Employees who throw objects or toss profane comments in open office areas in the general direction of another employee behaviorally characterize the breaking point where the conflict can no longer be ignored. The conflict usually has been brewing for quite a long time before help is requested. If managers and employees were empowered and trained to resolve conflict, it would seldom be necessary to seek outside help. However, do not be afraid to ask for assistance from an internal human resources department if you have one, or from an external consultant trained in conflict resolution.

When Conflict Resolution Fails

There may be extreme cases when parties fail to resolve the conflict. This may be due to employee substance abuse problems, such as drug or alcohol dependency, or employees who refuse to comply with the terms of the conflict resolution agreement. Alternatively, an employee may not have the skills and capabilities to succeed on the job. The conflict between the job performance levels needed and those demonstrated must be resolved by formal personnel actions. Internal progressive disciplinary processes need to be applied. Progressive disciplinary steps generally include an oral warning, a written warning, a final written warning, suspension, and finally termination.

Key Steps in Resolving Conflict

- Listen actively.
- Level with each other about the real issues.
- Avoid sending mixed messages; instead, deal with the identified problem.
- Do not attack.
- Speak for yourself.
- Take responsibility for your role in the problem.
- Focus on ways to resolve the problem.
- Stick to the issue.
- Ask for the change that you want; be willing to compromise.
- Remember that it is not a zero-sum game.

What the Organization Can Do

Whether you are in a management capacity at a hospital, laboratory, or medical office, managing conflict is a critical skill for career success. There are several measures that can be taken by the organization to support an environment where conflict is managed instead of ignored. They include the following:

- Create an organizational culture that supports and tolerates telling the truth. Conflict is inevitable. Resolving it must be, too, in order for productive and meaningful work to occur.
- Provide in-service workshops for staff at all levels to teach conflict resolution skills.
- Provide training to all new employees as a part of new-employee orientation programs. Technical skills

are essential, but if individuals cannot resolve conflict, the technical skills can be overshadowed by interpersonal troubles.

- Have regular "letting off steam" meetings twice a month. Structure lunch meetings where problems can be addressed and resolved. Problems can be submitted anonymously and a team approach to resolving problems can be used.
- Encourage staff at all levels to bring up conflicts with coworkers and empower them to address them to the point of resolution.
- Have managers and supervisors at every level serve as role models in addressing and resolving conflict.
- Provide ongoing support through the human resources department if the organization has one, or outsource the role to a consultant to provide training and guidance for resolving conflict.
- Provide an employee assistance program for employees experiencing job or life stress to resolve issues that contribute to high levels of conflict.
- Provide posters, newsletters, and other visible reminders that resolving conflict is important to the organization.
- Focus on identifying, analyzing, and resolving conflicts so that the quality of life at work is the highest it can be. This enhanced quality of life at work can also serve to attract and retain the best employees.

Summary

Emerson said, "The future belongs to those who prepare for it." Conflict is inevitable and should be expected as a normal part of working with others. It is problematic only when it goes unresolved. Employees at all organizational levels are impacted by events inside and outside of work that cause stresses. Staff members may attempt to avoid conflict or may rely on dysfunctional patterns for dealing with their differences.

Managing conflict is a key component to structuring a successful workplace. Success depends on being able to acknowledge, manage, and resolve conflict. Managers need to take the lead in helping staff manage conflict. Staff training and development along with an organizational climate that values conflict resolution are keys to healthy conflict resolution. Open dialogue and creative problem solving are constructive methods to use when dealing with conflict.

The ability to manage and resolve conflict is a universal skill that crosses all life domains. Recognizing and managing conflict is a skill that can be learned. All successful managers must exercise the skills to identify, analyze, and resolve conflict. When conflict is managed and resolved, it can be a source of growth for individuals and institutions. Ulti-

mately the success of an organization depends on how well staff members recognize, understand, and resolve conflict.

KEY POINTS

- Conflict is inevitable but can be healthy for an organization if it is addressed and resolved.
- Conflict can be constructive or destructive to organizations.
- Individuals have conflict resolution styles and there are pros and cons to each style.
- Both managers and staff members play key roles in identifying and resolving conflict.
- Communication is a key to successful conflict resolution.
- There is a seven-step model to use for conflict resolution.
- The organization needs to create a climate and culture where conflicts are expected and resolved.

GLOSSARY

Conflict A disagreement over the goals or methods to achieve them.

Conflict resolution The process of identifying, analyzing, and eliminating conflict.

Conflict resolution styles Five approaches to resolving conflict.

Constructive conflict Disagreements that are acknowledged and lead to resolution.

Destructive conflict Disagreements that are not addressed or resolved.

External sources of conflict Issues and concerns in the environment.

Give-get-merge-go (GGMG) model A communication model used to resolve conflict.

Internal sources of conflict Issues and concerns within the individual.

Win-win outcome A resolution that works well for all parties.

Zero-sum game When one person wins by making the other person lose.

REFERENCES

1. Carkhuff, R. R. 1983. *The Art of Helping*, p. 14–27. Human Resource Development Press, Amherst, Mass.

2. Catt, S. E., and D. S. Miller. 1991. *Supervision: Working with People*, p. 398–414. Irwin, Boston, Mass.

3. Cloke, K., and J. Goldsmith. 2000. *Resolving Conflicts at Work*, p. 39–40. Jossey-Bass, San Francisco, Calif.

4. DuBrin, A. J. 2000. *Fundamentals of Organizational Behavior*, p. 133–159. South-Western, Cincinnati, Ohio.

5. DuBrin, A. J. 2000. *Essentials of Management*, p. 390–401. South-Western, Cincinnati, Ohio.

6. Egan, J. 2003. *Conflict Resolution Workbook.* Jean Egan Associates, LLC, Suffield, Conn.

7. Kritek, P. B. 1996. *Negotiating at an Uneven Table: Developing*

Moral Courage in Resolving Our Conflicts, p. 17–19, 71–72, 241–244. Jossey-Bass, San Francisco, Calif.

8. Paul, J., and M. Paul. 2002. *Do I Have to Give up Me to be Loved by You?* p. 47–52. Hazeldon Information Education, Center City, Minn.

APPENDIX 13.1   Case Studies

Conflict management requires three major steps: Identify, analyze, and resolve the conflict. While viable solutions always include the option to do nothing or fire the person you perceive is causing the problem, there are better approaches. It is helpful to consider the following questions to resolve conflict. Apply them to the case studies.

1. What is the background to this conflict?
2. What are the major issues that are contributing to the conflict?
3. How would you identify the conflict in this case?
4. What are possible strategies for managing this conflict?
5. What could go wrong with your resolution strategy and how will you handle that problem if it occurs?
6. How will your conflict management solution solve the problem?
7. What is your implementation strategy and timetable?
8. How will you know if your solution worked?

Case Study 1

Donna has been working as a laboratory technician for 6 years. She joined the hospital laboratory 3 months ago. She has good technical skills and impressive credentials. She seemed a little formal during the interview, but you suspected that it was due to nerves. Now that she has been hired, she talks to the older staff in a way that others have described as "superior" because of her national credentials. Most of your staff have been to at least some college, but there is a mix of credentials and on-the-job training among laboratory staff. Donna works well alone and often ignores the requests of coworkers to help with the backlog of work in the laboratory. She gets her own work assignments done on time and well, but when she needs to interact with other staff members, she is abrupt, impatient, and often rude. Several of the other staff members have complained to you to do something about Donna. You see the value of her technical skills in the laboratory environment but need to step in to manage the situation.

Case Study 2

Jennifer is a happy, productive, effective team player. She shows up for work on time, works overtime if needed, and even asks coworkers if they need assistance. On her last performance appraisal, she earned high marks for her rate of production and her ability to get along with coworkers. The hospital has just installed new software for processing orders and returning laboratory results. You have tried several times to schedule Jennifer for the training to update her skills, but she seems to be making one excuse after another. You overheard Jennifer telling a coworker that she was not interested in learning any new software because it took a long time to learn the system currently in use. You need everyone in the department to be up to date on the new software and procedures for using it. You need to take action as the manager of the entire laboratory.

Case Study 3

You have just merged your practice with another group and have moved your staff into their office. The office staff from the original group seemed friendly enough during the initial stages of the merger, but you note some friction developing. There seem to be cliques forming between the staff of the two former offices. You had hoped that everyone would just merge their desks and operating procedures and get along well. Your office manager, Daniel, is having difficulty adjusting to being under the direction of the group office manager. He had systems and processes set up and ran the office efficiently. You do not know if his trouble is the result of the recent changes or caused by now reporting to a younger female supervisor, Amanda. Daniel seems to be lining up the old staff to challenge Amanda at every turn. You are busy with your own issues as a result of the merger and really had hoped that the staffs would be operating as one big happy family by this point. You have been ignoring the small disagreements that you have witnessed between the two groups of staff members but are not sure if more action is needed.

14

Managing Change*

Christopher S. Frings

OBJECTIVES

To help the reader understand the changes and trends occurring in the healthcare arena

To clarify the paradigm shifts occurring in the healthcare arena

To explore why people resist change

To instruct the reader on how to become a change agent

To discuss survival and winning strategies for workplace changes

To identify the skills needed for the future to succeed in the healthcare arena

---

It is not the strongest of species that survive, nor the most intelligent, but the one who is most responsive to change.

CHARLES DARWIN

My theory is that the dinosaur doesn't exist today because it couldn't change and it couldn't adapt. Therefore, the dinosaur became extinct. We will become extinct in the 21st century if we are not able to change and adapt!

CHRISTOPHER S. FRINGS

THE HEALTHCARE INDUSTRY continues to sail in a turbulent environment through a period of dramatic change. With the varied pressures of cost containment, little ability of the consumer to judge quality, Medicare funding problems, and the powerful for-profit healthcare companies and insurers with the actuarial smarts to seek out and insure only the healthy and wealthy among us, you may not recognize your healthcare system in 10 years. To survive and thrive you will have to change some of the things you are doing. The best supervisors, managers, and leaders are masters of change. A manager's most important survival skill is the ability to anticipate change and identify new opportunities (2). We must all become receptive to change.

My prediction for the future for clinical laboratory scientists is unprecedented opportunity with keen competition. There will be more opportunities for clinical laboratory scientists than we ever imagined several years ago, but with more competition for each opportunity than ever before. This means that the good news is that your services will be needed in the future. The bad

---

*Some of the information in this chapter was adapted with permission from C. S. Frings. 1998. *The Hitchhiker's Guide to Self-Management & Leadership Strategies for Success*, p. 29–46. AACC Press, Washington, D.C.

news for some of us is that new skills will be required for these opportunities. This means sharpening the tools in your toolbox and developing new tools now. If the only tool you have in your toolbox is a hammer, then every problem looks like a nail!

Healthcare reform is not over. It will continue, with additional changes for clinical laboratory scientists.

Understanding the Changing Workplace and the Information Age

Three things catalyze all change in this country: (i) cost, (ii) technology, and (iii) politics (or legislative issues). As of the writing of this chapter, the forces driving healthcare are cost and legislative issues. In the future, technology hopefully will play a larger role in healthcare changes than it has in recent years.

We are in the middle of a true revolution in how work gets done, the third one to hit us in the history of civilization. First came the Agricultural Revolution, which totally changed society. Instead of hunting food, we started growing food. This revolution lasted from about 8,000 B.C. to the late 1600s. It was ended by the Industrial Revolution. We started to depend on machines to get things done. Pulling levers and pushing buttons replaced much of the heavy lifting. The third revolution is in progress right now. Beginning about 1950 with the development of the computer and improvements in telecommunications, we entered the Information Age. Now horsepower is being replaced by brainpower. Work is again being completely transformed. The situation is confusing lots of people, and many are upset with the way the Information Age is affecting their careers. The information age requires keeping up with information technology, including informatics, computers, software, digitalization, and communications systems.

We cause progress because we are demanding customers. When companies restructure, outsource, merge, downsize, or go out of business for good, ordinary people like you and me often have a hand in it. As customers, we cause change. That's the American way. We demand better customer service and quicker turnaround time for services than before. We require more user-friendly reports such as bank statements and brokerage statements.

Work is becoming less physical and more mental in the Information Age. Knowledge is needed more than muscles. Concepts, information-type ideas, formulas, concepts, and other data are replacing things. Things are being made by other things, rather than by people. Computers are running assembly lines, and robots are making automobiles. Modern telecommunications and computers are reshaping the work environment. With a laptop computer, modem, cellular phone, pager, and other technologies you can work at home, in your car, or in other places as easily as in your office. This ability to work remotely means we can enjoy much more job freedom, but it also means that companies can go almost anywhere in the world to employ people with the best skills at the lowest salaries.

World War II ended the Depression. The postwar years brought a period of renewed confidence. The economy boomed and people displayed optimism and pride in the American way. For the next 30 years, politicians and businesses acted and talked like we could create the perfect society. The United States became extremely generous with its own people, and government programs grew much larger, with more free spending. Corporate America followed suit with high profits.

We gradually programmed ourselves to believe that big business and big government would protect us. We convinced ourselves that we deserved all of this and that it was our right. The ethic of personal responsibility grew weaker and weaker as we shifted toward an "entitlement" mind-set. We actually started depending on corporate America to protect our careers. We started expecting "our fair share" from our employer and the government.

In the 1970s productivity growth was not happening. Spending by the private sector and the government had grown like wildfire. Corporate profits dropped below what they had been in the 1950s and 1960s. Then in the 1980s businesses reacted by reengineering, restructuring and downsizing. Many jobs disappeared, and the government decided that it also needed to get smaller. The money was no longer there, so companies had to change their spending habits.

So today we are in a situation in which corporate America cannot guarantee our job future and government cannot deliver on what the politicians have promised. Welfare is being drastically reformed. We are in the paradigm shift from entitlement to earning and from rights to responsibilities. Globally we are seeing a greater equality of opportunity. This historical thumbnail sketch explains why we are in these turbulent times of change and can expect more changes in the 21st century (1).

Product life cycles are getting shorter, as shown by the following examples. (i) In 1990 automobiles took 6 years from concept to production. Today they take 2 years. (ii) Most of Hewlett-Packard's revenues come from products that didn't exist 1 year ago. Businesses have changed the way they want to do business. In response, workers are changing the way they work. Workers are substituting flexible scheduling and telecommuting for the 8-to-5 grind of working in the same place for the same boss. Employers have finally recognized that a leaner, more efficient staff leads to a better bottom line. I predict that by the year 2020, 85% of people will be employed by small businesses, and 50% of workers will be in nontraditional work arrangements. These arrangements will include temporary employment. Temps have become one of the fastest-growing segments in the workforce. Outsourcing using temporary employees will be a major trend.

Start figuring out now how your job and profession are changing and how tomorrow's tools and methods will alter the way you work. Don't try to defend old methods of doing things. Resisting change is a no-win battle for us. The new tools that we will use will cause further change. The corporate ladder is about gone with today's leaner, team-based organizations. It is critical that we reinvest our own money and time in skill development for the future. The new source of power in the Information Age is knowledge. The biggest challenge today is not getting an education, it's keeping one! I predict that at least 50% of our skills will be outdated in 3 years.

The good news is that information has never been more available and knowledge has never been so easy to acquire. Technology gets user-friendlier every day. While the Industrial Age was about powerful organizations, the Information Age is more about powerful individuals with knowledge as their power. The days of maintaining job security by just doing your job, "keeping your nose clean," and "holding the fort" are over for the most part. We must do more! We are responsible for our own success. We must make the company work and succeed. Part of our new job is to make our own services and products obsolete before our competitor does. We must be innovators in the Information Age.

Change Is Not Easy

When someone complains about changes, tell this story. Some changes are hard to accept. In 1829 Martin Van Buren, then the governor of New York, wrote this to the President (1): "The canal system of this country is being threatened by the spread of a new form of transportation known as railroads. As you may well know, railroad carriages are pulled at the enormous speed of 15 miles per hour by engines, which, in addition to endangering life and limbs of passengers, roar and snort their way through the countryside. The Almighty certainly never intended that people should travel at such breakneck speed."

When was the last time you did anything to change your behavior? You can't win tomorrow's game with today's score. There is an old saying: if you do what you have always done, you will always get what you have always gotten. This is no longer a valid statement. Today if you *do only* what you have done in the past you will get left out! To survive and thrive, you will have to change some of the things you are doing. The best supervisors, managers, and leaders are masters of change. A manager's most important survival skill is the ability to anticipate change and identify new opportunities. We must all become receptive to change! I have a plastic dinosaur on my desk to remind me that if I don't change and adapt, I will become extinct in the near future.

When a new idea is presented, at first it's not the content of the change that matters; it's peoples' attitudes toward it. To illustrate this point, do the following. Write the word "attitude" on a piece of paper with your nondominant hand (not your usual writing hand). When you look at the word "attitude" written by the non-dominant hand, you see a picture of the kind of attitude we often have when we try something new, especially if the change was imposed on us! A first-time experience threatens our security. We feel awkward and incompetent, and we are out of our comfort zone. Therefore, since we feel this way, when implementing change we must support our team until they get through the initial change period.

Suggestion: Remember the difference between writing with your dominant hand and the other hand when asking someone to make a change or to learn something new.

You can change yourself if you can change what goes into your mind. While it is true that every improvement is the result of change, not every change is an improvement. The past has value and it will continue to have value. At the same time you should not let the past have a veto. Take the best from the past and the best from the future to forge yourself into a success in the future. That means turmoil!

Why People Resist Change

To cope with resistance to change it is important to understand the five reasons why such resistance occurs.

Self-Interest

People often fear that they will lose something that they once had. For example, when the new senior vice president decided to create a new manager position, the existing supervisors resisted because they feared losing their right to approve decisions that affected the company.

Misunderstanding and Lack of Trust

If people don't trust the person who has the new idea, they will suspect that he or she has a hidden agenda and/or harmful motives for proposing the change. For example, the staff opposed the proposal of flexible scheduling because they did not trust the personnel manager who suggested it.

Differing Viewpoints

Different people will view the change differently. People frequently like their own ideas better than ideas of others. They would rather try their ideas than try the ideas of others.

Fear of Failure

People sometimes resist change because they fear that they will be unable to handle the new conditions competently. They may also resist breaking up comfortable social and work relationships with coworkers.

Fear of Uncertainty

Some people resist change just because it is change. They fear change because they know it will alter their comfortable routine.

Forms of Resistance to Change

The following are different ways people resist change: (i) the negative view ("It won't work! We already tried that"), (ii) apathy and indifference ("I just work here"), (iii) pet project attitude ("Are you criticizing my plan?"), (iv) unconscious dissension ("Whatever the boss says . . . but it won't work"), (v) free translation ("We'll implement my variation . . . it's better anyway"), and (vi) authoritarian approach ("You are not to reason why. . . .").

Changes that Are Common Today

The following are changes that are common today: change in the name of your professional organization, change in the name of your company or business, technology changes, reengineering, merger, acquisition, divestiture, layoffs, downsizing, start-up of new company, division or department changes, changes in top management, culture change (new policies, values, and/or expectations), deregulation, reorganization, serious new competitors, changes in your company benefits, reporting to a different manager or a different reporting structure, and promotion to a "higher" position in the organization. Which of these changes have you already experienced? Are you ready for the other changes listed?

Looking Ahead

The following are some of the changes you might expect to see in many organizations in the future: more employee involvement in all levels of decision making; increased emphasis on meaningful work; more responsibility for individual employees; fewer managers; a focus on human intellectual capital as demonstrated by an investment in training, retraining, and new skill development; an atmosphere that encourages more mutual respect and trust; an increase in the protection of employee rights; a continuing need for workers with good communication skills; programs (for example, flextime) that support both work and family; better recognition of and reward for superior performance; greater diversity in the workplace, with more women and minorities; a continuing need for workers with specialized skills; emergence of multiskilled, cross-trained professionals (generalist) with specialized skills; smaller workspace area per employee (smaller cubicles); and use of surveillance tools to maximize productivity and security and to minimize loss. How many have you already noticed in your organization?

Steps to Managing Change

We all go through the following four stages in responding to change, whether it's major or minor.

Denial

It doesn't sink in right away that the change is occurring and that it will affect us. A typical response might be, "They can't be merging our laboratory with that reference clinical laboratory across town." When in the denial stage we are in withdrawal and tend to focus on the past.

Resistance

Here strong feelings about the change emerge, such as anger, blame, depression, anxiety, uncertainty, frustration, and self-doubt. Change is frequently resisted, just because it is change. Often change is resisted because it is someone else's idea.

Acceptance

During the acceptance phase we draw upon internal resources and creativity to figure out new responsibilities and to visualize our future. This can be an exciting time if we take on change as a new adventure and a new opportunity. In this stage we have concern about details, confusion, new ideas, and lack of focus.

Commitment to Change

At this point we are able to set new goals and make plans to reach our new goals. Here we are cooperative, and focused and anticipate our next challenge.

The longer we stay in the denial and resistance stages, the harder and more painful the change will be. Try to get through the denial and resistance stages quickly and go on to a commitment to change. Exchanging the familiar for the new, even if it's better, means the "death" of something familiar. We need to make certain that we allow for mourning and recovery.

How to Become an Agent of Change

The following are things you can do to become receptive to change. When you do these things, you are no longer part of the problem but are part of the solution.

- Keep a positive mental attitude. A positive mental attitude will help you do everything better than a negative attitude.
- Make managing change part of your job description (5).
- Don't fight losing battles.
- Be tolerant of management mistakes by supporting upper management. Management is not trying to make mistakes. They are frequently in uncharted waters in the healthcare arena.
- Keep a sense of humor. Humor is healing!
- Don't let your strengths turn into weaknesses. Refocus rapidly.
- Practice good stress management. Worry is the misuse of imagination!
- Invent the future instead of trying to redesign the past.

The key to implementing change is to give clear and direct communication (3, 4).

Paradigm Shifts in Today's Healthcare Industry

Paradigm shifts that are occurring in the healthcare arena are listed in Table 14.1. Many of these are occurring in other industries. Each industry has its unique set of paradigm shifts; however, many share some of the same changes.

Trends and Changes

Expect the expected and the unexpected. Changes you can expect in the future in the healthcare industry and many other industries are discussed in this section. Many are already happening. Which changes are you ready for? What skills do you need to develop to get ready for the others?

Trends are rapidly changing and so are attitudes, expectations, and roles. More changes are occurring, and this will continue for years to come. Due to the failed proposed healthcare reform by the Clinton administration, healthcare professionals are forming more alliances with those previously looked upon as enemies. Healthcare professionals are reforming themselves before mandatory change is

Table 14.1 Paradigm shifts in today's healthcare industry

From	To
Illness care	Healthcare
Treating mental illness	Mental health
Illness care	Outcomes management
Competition	Partnerships
Quality control	Continuous quality improvement
Quality assurance	Service excellence
Fragmented services	Integrated care
Department focus	Interdisciplinary focus
New technology	Appropriate technology
Fee for service	Managed care
Downsizing	Rightsizing
Boss	Mentor, facilitator, or coach
Turf protective values	Group productive values
Revenue from services	Revenue from covered lives
Competition based on price	Competition based on quality
Economics of scale	Economics of coordination
Activity orientation	Outcome orientation
Task focus	Customer focus
Manager	Leader
Individual	Teamwork
Individuals and groups	Teams committed to common mission
Low trust and guardedness	High trust, openness
Revenue	Cost
Providing services	Providing outcomes
Reacting to change	Initiating change
Controlling others	Empowering others
Periodic improvement	Continuous improvement
Fixing the blame	Fixing the problem
Resisting change	Viewing change as an opportunity

imposed. This affects all healthcare professionals in some way. This results in the rate of change increasing, while expectations at all levels are rising, there are fewer managers, and costs (a very important issue) are being reduced. Most workers are expected to increase their personal productivity and their team's productivity.

Medical care is being managed, which results in reduced test volume, cost containment, right sizing, capitated reimbursement, reduced reimbursement, and appropriateness of laboratory test selection. Healthcare professionals must become better managers of budget, personnel, self, and business. Opportunities are different and thus different skills are required. Changes are technology driven in addition to cost driven and driven by legislative issues. Our environment is not going to change to please us. Some of us are only rearranging the chairs on the deck of the *Titanic*!

There will be an unprecedented demand for "alternative" therapies; this reflects a trend from institutionalized managed care to self-managed care. More and more consumers will turn to alternative therapies, such as biofeedback, herbs, prayer, and chiropractic, whose holistic approaches often seem more natural and less intimidating. More than one-third of Americans spend $14 billion a year on alternative care, most of it out-of-pocket. Demand will accelerate for alternative remedies, fueled mostly by aging baby boomers' openness to new concepts. This will not be a threat to conventional medicine but will be a complement to traditional medicine.

Moore's (Gordon Moore) law says that the number of components that can be packed on a computer chip doubles every 24 months while the price remains the same. This law has amazingly held true for more than 30 years. This means that computer power per dollar doubles every 24 months. Moore's law will probably not hold true forever. The lesson to be learned from this is that personal computers become obsolete about every 3 years due to improved computer technology. I treat my personal computer as a 3-year disposable (only the CPU; not the screen, keyboard, mouse, printer, etc.). I plan to replace my computer and software about every 3 years (± 1 year).

Competing in the Future in the Healthcare Arena

The following are things you can do to become a master of change and your destiny in the healthcare arena and in other arenas:

- Get involved.
- Be part of the solution, not part of the problem.
- Demonstrate your worth.
- Develop positive relationships.
- Expect and get ready for the expected.
- Expect and get ready for the unexpected.

- Lead the technology revolution.
- Keep a positive mental attitude.
- Make managing change part of your job description.
- Don't fight losing battles.
- Be tolerant of management mistakes.
- Keep (or develop) a sense of humor. Humor is healing.
- Don't let your strengths turn into weaknesses. Refocus rapidly.
- Practice effective stress management. Worry is the misuse of imagination.
- Support upper management.
- Initiate or join cross-functional teams.
- Invent the future rather than trying to rediscover the past.
- Look 3 to 5 years into the future.
- Don't be constantly reacting to each new competitive threat as it comes. Be proactive, not just reactive.
- Become different.
- Shape the future of your industry.
- Anticipate the evolution of the healthcare industry, and build capabilities now to win in the future.
- Build skills you'll need for the future. These include the following:
  - Financial management
    - Cost analysis
    - Budgeting
    - Return on investment
    - Break-even analysis
  - Outcome assessment and outcome analysis
  - Continuous quality improvement and total quality improvement
  - Resource management and utilization allocation
    - Personnel
    - Materials
  - Self-management and personal development skills
    - Setting and reaching goals
    - Time management
    - Managing change and making change work
    - Stress management
    - Team building
    - Negotiation skills
    - Presentation skills
- Informatics (systems, reporting, and telecommunications)
- Risk assessment and risk management
- Regulatory issues and laws affecting your industry

Suggestion: When you are resisting change, use a rubber band to snap out of it! Some of those attending my seminars and workshops on managing change wear a rubber band around their wrists as a self-motivator. When they are resisting change, they snap out of it by snapping the rubber band. The snap of the rubber band serves as a self-motivator to remind them to take action toward getting out of the denial and resistance stages so they can make the change happen in a positive way.

Summary

Not all change is good. However, all good comes from change.

KEY POINTS

- The reasons we resist change are (i) self-interest, (ii) misunderstanding and lack of trust, (iii) differing viewpoints, (iv) fear of failure, and (v) fear of uncertainty.
- The different ways people resist change include (i) the negative view ("It won't work! We already tried that"), (ii) apathy and indifference ("I just work here"), (iii) pet project attitude ("Are you criticizing my plan?"), (iv) unconscious dissension ("Whatever the boss says . . . but it won't work"), (v) free translation ("We'll implement my variation . . . it's better anyway"), and (vi) authoritarian approach ("You are not to reason why . . .").
- We all go through the following four stages in responding to change, whether it is a major or a minor change: (i) denial, (ii) resistance, (iii) acceptance, and (iv) commitment to change.
- Track trends by identifying major new trends that affect your workplace and its environment.

GLOSSARY

Change   The process of transforming the way in which an organization or individual acts from one set of behaviors to another.

Paradigm shift   A change from one way of doing things to another; often encompasses a change in an entire concept, model, or standard.

Resistance to change   A force active in groups and individuals that limits the amount of change that occurs.

REFERENCES

1. **Frings, C. S.** 1998. *The Hitchhiker's Guide to Self-Management & Leadership Strategies for Success,* p. 29–46. AACC Press, Washington, D.C.

2. **Montana, P. J., and B. H. Charnov.** 1993. *Management,* 2nd ed. Barron's Educational Services, Hauppauge, N.Y.

3. **Nigon, D. L.** 2000. *Clinical Laboratory Management,* p. 293–307. McGraw Hill, New York, N.Y.

4. **Wilkinson, I.** 1998. *Managing ME Incorporated,* p. 23–28. Clinical Laboratory Management Association, Wayne, Pa.

5. **Yeomans, W. N.** 1985. *1000 Things You Never Learned In Business School.* New American Library, Bergenfield, N.J.

APPENDIX 14.1   Case Studies of How to Overcome Resistance to Change

One example is given below for each change situation. These examples are not meant as the best or only way to deal with the situation. The examples are included to give you one way to handle each change situation.

Change Situation A

Situation: Employees do not understand or have little or inaccurate information about the problem.

Response: Provide in advance as much information as possible about the change and why you are making the change.

Example: A new branch reference laboratory located 61 miles from the central laboratory was opened. Initially the laboratory was open from 8:00 a.m. until 5:30 p.m. Some of the laboratorians worked from 8:00 a.m. to 5:00 p.m., and some worked from 8:30 a.m. to 5:30 p.m. The laboratory has been open for 6 months; the flow of work has changed due to new clients, and there is a need for the laboratory to be open until 6:30 p.m. There is a need for only one laboratorian to arrive at 8:00 a.m. The work schedule must be changed to meet the needs of the physicians and their patients. The laboratory manager meets with all of the employees as soon as possible after the decision is made. He informs everyone that the working hours must be changed to meet the needs of the clients and gives specific information. He gives everyone a 30-day notice of the change in hours to allow affected employees time to make appropriate transportation and child care arrangements.

Change Situation B

Situation: You do not have all of the information needed to implement the change and others have considerable power to resist.

Response: Allow the people who will be affected by the change to participate in the decision as to what needs to be done and how to implement the change. This could be a great team-building opportunity.

Example: An HMO recently purchased two hospitals in the medical center of a large metropolitan area. The chief executive officer and chief operating officer of the HMO don't want to duplicate nonessential laboratory services. There are a lot of talk and rumors as to when and how the duplicate services will be eliminated. You appoint a team with a team leader that consists of two individuals from each lab, an assistant administrator from each hospital, and the medical director of both hospitals to work out the details during the next 14 days. They are to present a written and oral proposal of how to implement the change.

Change Situation C

Situation: Speed is essential and you have considerable power to enforce your ideas.

Response: Announce the change and enforce the change with authority, certainty, and firmness.

Example: The hospital chief executive officer, chief operating officer, and laboratory director have decided to offer point-of-care (POC) testing in the hospital effective in 2 weeks. One laboratorian will have to act as a troubleshooter, problem solver, and quality control and quality assurance coordinator for the nurses who are performing the POC testing under the central laboratory's Clinical Laboratory Improvement Amendments license. This position will be rotated weekly among four laboratorians. Several of the laboratorians are upset about the change because they will not be able to have the same off days as before. After hearing complaints, the laboratory director called the four laboratorians together and stated that the decision has already been made and that it will take place in 2 weeks.

Change Situation D

Situation: Someone will clearly lose out in the change and they have lots of resisting power.

Response: Negotiate for a win-win situation.

Example: Organizational changes are necessary due to the merger of two large reference laboratories to form one central laboratory. There were two laboratory managers (Jim Bob and Georgia Lou), and now only one laboratory manager is needed. Both laboratory managers have been productive, key employees with positive attitudes and great team-building skills. The chief operating officer talks to Jim Bob and Georgia Lou together and separately. He lets both laboratory managers know how important they are to the newly combined reference laboratory. Georgia Lou is given the new laboratory manager position. Jim Bob is given the job of coordinating laboratory operations between all six satellite laboratories and the central laboratory. Each is given a 6% raise effective immediately to let them know that the reorganization is not a demotion for either person. This results in a win-win situation for everyone.

Change Situation E

Situation: People resist change because they are unconvinced by the change.

Response: Help them adjust by making the change as easy and as comfortable as possible.

Example: Refer to the example in change situation C above. One of the laboratorians is extremely upset by the change because it will cause hardships for her and her son. By changing her off day she will have a problem getting her son with cystic fibrosis to the clinic each Wednesday for therapy. The lab manager explains the situation and repeats that POC testing is needed and the nurses will do some of the test volume previously performed in the laboratory. The laboratorian states that her parents will be moving to this city in 2 months and can take her son to the clinic on Wednesdays. The lab manager makes an exception and will give this employee 2 months to make the adjustment due to the special situation.

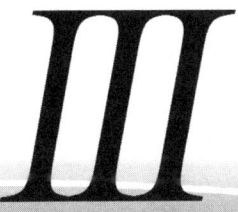

Personnel Management

(Section Editor, *John C. H. Steele, Jr.*)

15

Employee Selection

Anthony S. Kurec

OBJECTIVES

To describe the differences in attitudes attributable to generational group

To discuss the desirable elements of a job description

To distinguish the appropriate search process for a supervisory position from that for a technical position in the clinical laboratory

To list, then critique, various approaches to the interview process

To give examples of appropriate and inappropriate interview questions

To describe the ideal orientation process

To address potentially useful retention techniques available to managers

To describe the steps of progressive discipline

In every human heart there is a tiger, a pig, an ass, and a nightingale. Diversity of character is due to their unequal activity.

AMBROSE BIERCE

LABORATORY PERSONNEL HAVE EXPERIENCED SIGNIFICANT CHANGES over the past decade in how they are managed. The function of the clinical laboratory is critical to good patient care; it is estimated that 85% of medical decision making by a physician is based on laboratory results. The need for trained laboratory personnel will increase over the next few years. However, concern is growing regarding the decrease in the number of training programs and the decreasing number of graduates from the remaining programs. These changes have resulted in vacancy rates ranging between 9 and 20% (15, 27). Also, the laboratory profession is aging; in one survey the average age was 46 years, with less than 5% of the respondents being under the age of 29 (15). The projected number of individuals needed to fill these vacancies is about 9,000, yet only about 5,000 graduates are anticipated to be available from the existing programs.

Supply and demand will result in intense competition for qualified candidates. Predictions indicate that 2-year Medical Laboratory Technician (MLT) graduates will be performing the majority of laboratory tests, while 4-year Medical Technology (MT) graduates will be more involved in data gathering, analysis, monitoring, information dispersal, and consultation (11). As molecular-based testing increases, it is clear that managers will need the best and brightest to meet the challenges of these advanced technologies. To attract and keep these key people, a collective effort between employer and employee will be required so both reap the benefits of this relationship.

Diversity in the Workplace

If human nature were consistent and everyone had the same characteristics, there would be no need for supervisors, policies and procedures, kings or queens. This is particularly true with today's globalized world and the respective diversity of the workforce. Because of this diversity, leaders, through learned or innate skills, must take charge in identifying and selecting those individuals who can accomplish the tasks at hand. For today's administrators, 75% of the population is "different" from themselves (in race, gender, ethnicity, language, culture, age, or social, psychological, or personal attributes); thus, administrators must be aware of these differences when hiring new employees (2). Stereotyping, based on the "like me syndrome" (a clone of you), can lead to a stifled workforce (19). You cannot judge a potential new employee on the basis of technical- and knowledge-based skills alone but must be aware of other potential characteristics that are critical in selecting the right person for the job. Table 15.1 lists some of these characteristics (7).

Over the past 7 to 8 decades, various distinctions in attitudes that influence the workforce have been identified by generational differences. Five age-based groups of workers have been identified based on birth year, each with characteristics common to that group (12). They are Preboomer (1934 to 1945), Boomer (1946 to 1959), Cusper (1960 to 1968), Buster (1969 to 1978), and Netster (1979 to today). Others describe these groupings as "generation X" (roughly 1961 to 1980), "generation Y" (1980 to 2000), and "millenniums" (present) (1, 8). Specific identities for each stage are reflected through each group's lifestyle, social activities, and motivational characteristics. Administrators must be aware of these differences to ensure that they are not unduly influenced to select the wrong candidate. Listed in Table 15.2 are some characteristics that have been identified for each generational work group. While many are unique to an age group, some overlap.

There is a considerable range of cultural and ethnic differences that managers must consider when hiring new

Table 15.1 Performance-based characteristics[a]

Common characteristics to look for in potential employees	
Ambition	Communication
Creativity	Energy
Enthusiasm	Independence
Interpersonal skills	Initiative or motivation
Leadership	Professional skills
Organizational skills	Persuasiveness (sales ability)
Resilience	Work standards
Teamwork	Tenacity

[a]From reference 7.

Table 15.2 Age-related differences[a]

Age group	Characteristics
Preboomer	Work first, loyal to employer, work hard, save money, family first, exercise if forced to, community service, quality first, must vote, motivated by money and responsibility
Boomer	Work first, care about what others think, work hard, play hard, spend hard, family and friends first, some exercise is good, community service and vote if convenient, want even more money and recognition, loyal to self
Cusper	Driven somewhat by money but also by principle, work hard, play hard, worry about money, exercise is a duty, the "Gap" generation, looks for bonuses and stock options
Buster	Principle/satisfaction, don't care what others think, prefer to work alone, individual first, exercise for mental health, will vote but privately, friends are family, cheap, wants time off, concerned about own goals
Netster	Lifestyle first, like small groups, state-of-the art, individual first, live with parents, community service is punishment, Abercrombie's generation, wants time off, portable skills, self-employment

[a]From reference 12.

employees (4, 13, 14). Modern technologies have enhanced opportunities to identify a greater pool of potential applicants, thus requiring a process that allows for the selection of the best-qualified and capable individuals. Lost opportunities for both employer and employee may occur if cultural, ethnic, and gender-related traits are not well understood or accepted. Misunderstandings based on cultural, religious, or ethnic differences may inadvertently cause a missed opportunity for an otherwise excellent employee. Administrators who find themselves managing in a multicultural environment must take the time to learn and understand some of the fundamental differences encountered with each group. Failure to do so may mean the loss of a hardworking, loyal employee. Table 15.3 identifies four cultural dimensions that may be helpful in the pursuit of understanding cultural differences. These differences may be the basis of how an individual responds to questions or situations that come up in the workplace and need to be recognized in order to sustain communication.

Job Description and Requirements

Selecting the right person for the job is not easy. Finding qualified candidates starts with establishing the right criteria needed to meet the goals of the organization. Identifying a candidate's ability to be the "right fit" with education, specific technical skills, and experience is generally not difficult. Often, the more difficult part is identifying those personality traits that are conducive to being a team

Table 15.3 Cultural differences

Four dimensions of cultural value	Definitions	Examples	
		High	**Low**
Power distance	Power distance addresses the distribution of "power." A culture that reflects low power distance views power as being distributed rather equally. Cultures with high power distance define the workplace as "the haves" and the "have nots," where there is a clear distinction between employer and staff.	Malaysia, Philippines, Mexico, Arab countries, Indonesia, India	Austria, Sweden, England, Australia, The Netherlands, Canada
Individualism-collectivism	Individualism is found in those social structures that promote the individual and encourage people to take care of themselves and their immediate families. Collectivism focuses on the extended family and loyalty to that clan. The clan will take care of the individual.	United States, Australia, England, Canada, The Netherlands	Colombia, Indonesia, Pakistan, Taiwan, Korea
Masculinity-femininity	Cultures that rank high are aggressive, competitive, and focused on material things. "Machismo" is a common characteristic. A culture that ranks low tends to be more nurturing and focuses on the quality of life. One works in order to live.	Japan, Austria, Mexico, Jamaica, England	Sweden, The Netherlands, Thailand, Korea, Taiwan
Uncertainty avoidance	This is a more intuitive dimension of social behavior. It reflects how a culture generally reacts in unstructured, ambiguous situations. Those ranked low are more tolerant of differing opinions. Those ranked high tend to be more structured so as to avoid the uncertainty.	Greece, Japan, Argentina, Korea, Mexico	Singapore, Jamaica, Hong Kong, Sweden, England

[a]From references 13 and 14.

player. Traits such as honesty, initiative, ethics, loyalty, and attitude toward the job and to people are subjective and are not quantifiable or tangible. While there is no one scheme available to select the perfect employee, there are some guidelines that might assist in maximizing the chance of making the right choice. As you learn how to hire employees, the experience must be retained and built on so it may be applied to future hiring practices.

Needs Assessment

To hire the best person for the job, it is necessary to clearly define what the job entails. A needs assessment for the desired position is appropriate. This not only includes delineation of duties, skills, and education but also justification of whether the position is truly needed. This is a good time to determine if the position should be eliminated, redefined, downgraded, or upgraded. Most laboratories use some form of productivity measurement to determine the need for replacing or adding staff (16, 25).

Job Description Review

As part of the needs assessment, the job description should be reviewed for accuracy because it potentially sets the foundation for the scope of the job for many years to come. This will ensure that job duties listed are really needed,

have not changed, or could be improved. Pay particular attention to the minimum requirements. While there are some legal guidelines that have to be followed, employers do have some flexibility in establishing job requirements. Those that are too loose may invite applicants who are not qualified, thus deterring recruitment efforts. Conversely, requirements that are too confined may discourage good candidates from submitting their applications.

Minimal Personnel Requirements

For the laboratory, minimum personnel requirements are addressed in the Clinical Laboratory Improvement Amendments of 1988 (CLIA) (6). These requirements have reduced traditional laboratory titles to the following, which are described in detail elsewhere: Director, Technical Consultant, Clinical Consultant, Technical or General Supervisor, Testing Personnel, and Cytotechnologist (22). In addition, all of healthcare has faced financial constraints that have forced laboratories to reconsider their operations, including staff organization. Laboratories have downsized, combined sections into core facilities, and outsourced laboratory tests. In some laboratories, compression of traditional laboratory sections has resulted in adding or eliminating certain duties or levels of authority and in reducing the number of staff and supervisors required, thus affecting the job description when refilling vacant positions.

Criterion-Based Job Description

In the laboratory a criterion-based job description offers a clear and complete format that addresses the expectations of the employer and the employee. A typical job description might include the information presented in Table 15.4 (16). It is based on legal regulations, certification needs, educational essentials, critical tasks related to the job, and work environment needs (Table 15.5) (21). Within the job description, each job duty may be classified as a core task, a basic or advanced technical duty, or a management or administrative responsibility. Some examples are listed in

Table 15.4 Job description

Job title: Official title of the job to be offered.

Education requirements: List minimum requirements, not desired characteristics.

License or certification: Identify what specific statutory required license and certification category are needed to fill the position.

Experience requirements: State the minimum number of years of experience required by law or by established policy.

Duties

General: What duties are required of all or most employees regardless of job title? These may include safety, confidentiality, customer service, and/or time and attendance responsibilities.

Technical: What technical duties are specific to the job title?

Administrative

Supervisory: Does this position require direct supervision, work under general supervision, or provide direct supervision?

Accountability: Are tasks well defined, requiring little interpretation? Do tasks require limited to moderate knowledge of departmental/institutional policies and procedures? Does incumbent develop and implement policies and procedures?

Fiduciary: At what level is this position responsible for budgetary expenditures: none, recommends, or approves?

Teaching responsibilities: Does this job require training or teaching of staff, students, or the public?

Research responsibilities: Does this job require research activities such as research and development of new techniques, instrumentation, etc? Will the incumbent have to provide on-the-job training of staff?

Professional development: What are the regulatory requirements for professional development and continuing education?

Organizational

Table of organization: How does this position fit into the departmental or institutional table of organization?

Direct reports: To whom or to which position(s) does the incumbent report? Which positions report to the incumbent?

Table 15.5 Job description criteria

Criteria	Attributes
Regulatory	State or federal laws mandate qualifications and may require licensure of some laboratory personnel. Often denotes specific scope of practice
Certification	Voluntary action that declares that the individual has taken an examination indicating that they possess at least an entry-level knowledge of the job
Education	Educational requirements related to academic degrees and/or specific course work
Training	On-the-job training that is directly related to the position
Experience	The number of years of experience that is preferred and/or required
Physical demands	Any specific physical requirements (such as color recognition, standing, walking, etc.) related to the job
Skills, abilities, knowledge	Special individual skills such as speaking a second language, writing skills, communication or presentation skills
Work environment	Where the major amount of work is to be performed (clinical lab, nursing home, satellite labs, home draws, etc.)

Table 15.6 (26). This is not an all-inclusive list, and each position will include some or all of these tasks.

Job Description Sections

There are five key sections common to most job descriptions: job title, qualifications and worker traits, job duties, responsibilities and accountability, and job relationships (16). Job titles should be consistent throughout the laboratory with consideration of local and national nomenclature that may be used in describing laboratory job titles. Inconsistency in title usage can result in confusion internally as well as externally, especially with the public. Only minimum qualifications (education, experience, etc.) should be listed in the job description. Other desired worker or personal traits that reflect a humanistic picture of the kind of individual you wish to hire (e.g., honesty, reliability, ambition, personality, etc.) should also be considered. Specific job duties must be identified to ensure that the incumbent understands what he or she is to do. Other attributes to be noted include levels of responsibility and accountability that identify how much authority the individual has in making decisions. It is useful to list job relationships so the incumbent knows to whom to report, who reports to him or her, and what other internal/external relationships may be required of the position.

Table 15.6 Core job tasks

Function	Task
Core	Specimen collection
	Test performance
	Quality control
	Data entry
	Troubleshooting
	Preventive maintenance
	Reporting results
	Continuing education
	Training staff
Advanced technical	Quality assurance
	New test implementation
	Instrument evaluation
	Developing standard operating procedures
	Laboratory safety
Management	Purchasing responsibilities
	Quality assurance-utilization studies
	General personnel supervision
	Financial responsibilities
	Billing activities
	Laboratory inspections, compliance, CLIA

Search Process

Search Committee

The search process can be simple or complex, depending on the level of the position. When hiring at the supervisory level or above, it is advisable to assemble a formal search committee consisting of an appropriate mix of individuals. While the committee should remain small (five to seven people), the mix should reflect the desired diversity of the department. Consider including a physician or pathologist, another supervisor(s), or a staff person. In adding a front line staff member to the group, subtle nuances of the job may be made evident. This also creates a type of ownership within the work environment and offers training opportunities for individuals who wish to learn interviewing skills. Also consider an appropriate gender, ethnic, and age mix, as well as other characteristics that may influence the decision of identifying the "ideal" candidate (28). This is consistent with affirmative action and equal opportunity guidelines. If a committee is not formed, ensure that at least two individuals review résumés, interview candidates, and provide some level of input to the final decision.

It is important to have a written policy that prevents discrimination in the workplace and provides guidance in appropriate hiring practices. Table 15.7 lists a few laws that address these issues. These laws were designed to prevent discrimination in hiring and retention of employees based on gender, age, race, religion, sexual orientation, or other non-work-related characteristics. Through these laws, the Equal Employment Opportunity Commission (EEOC) was created to provide oversight and address violations. President Lyndon Johnson created affirmative action programs by the Civil Rights Act in 1964 and Executive Order 11246 in 1965. Employers were required to establish plans to ensure that hiring and promotion practices paid particular attention to the number of minorities employed (29).

Advertising

An employer must ensure that there are equal opportunities for all qualified candidates to become aware of the open position; thus, the position must be advertised correctly. The advertisement should be concise, stating the job title, the minimum educational requirements, and any appropriate licensure or certification requirements (where applicable), and giving a one- or two-sentence job description. The salary range should not be stated as it might deter good candidates or encourage less qualified candidates. It also may create internal conflicts for those already employed, especially if the salary advertised is higher than for current equivalent employees or is perceived as inappropriate (10). (Salary ranges may be discussed as part of the interview process, but they are often best addressed as part of the final negotiations.) Consider also where to advertise. Internal postings in consideration for hiring from within should not

Table 15.7 Equal opportunity employment regulations

Regulation	Purpose
Civil Rights Act of 1964 (amended 1972 and 1991)	Prohibits discrimination based on color, race, religion, gender, or national origin; established EEOC
Age Discrimination in Employment Act of 1967	Prohibits employment discrimination based on age
Equal Pay Act of 1963	Prohibits discrimination in compensation based on gender
Vocational Rehabilitation Act of 1973	Prohibits discrimination in employment based on physical or mental disability
Guidelines on Sexual Harassment (1980)	Defines sexual harassment and establishes standards
Americans with Disabilities Act of 1990	Prevents discrimination on the basis of a disability

be overlooked. The advantages of hiring from within include portraying the opportunity for internal advancement and placing an individual in the position who already has institutional experience or knowledge. An internal hire is also less costly then hiring from the outside (no travel expenses, minimal advertising expenses, and possibly a salary less than might be commanded by an external candidate). The major disadvantage of hiring from within is the lost opportunity to bring in "new blood." This can be particularly important when hiring for senior-level positions, for which leadership and innovation are often desired.

If you have access to potentially good internal candidates, a limited search could be completed, thereby reducing the time to hire for that position and related costs often incurred with a national search. The placement of an advertisement in the classified section of the local newspaper is inexpensive and often leads to a quick response. Other popular advertising venues are your hospital's web site, professional associations' web sites (such as the American Society for Clinical Pathology [http://www.ascp.org] or the Clinical Laboratory Management Association [http://www.clma.org]), or a general employment web site (http://www.monster.com). Also consider advertising with organizations affiliated with underrepresented populations, such as the NAACP, the Urban League, or other appropriate associations. For a national search, advertising can cost thousands of dollars, and it may be several months before the advertisement is placed. Such a search also generates a greater number of resumes that will have to be reviewed and processed, creating additional work for the search committee. An alternative is to use a job search service that handles the overall process, thus significantly minimizing the time commitment of the search committee. A fixed fee or a certain percentage of the incumbent's annual salary (about 15 to 20%) is charged for this service.

Interview Process

Screening Résumés

Depending on the number of résumés received, screening for the appropriate qualifications can be very time-consuming and should not be taken lightly. While there is no one great technique for screening résumés, a common one is to divide them into three groups. Group 1 consists of those individuals who have outstanding qualifications and are strong candidates for the job. Group 2 includes those who just meet the minimum qualifications. If none of the group 1 candidates is available or accepts a job offer, group 2 becomes viable. Group 3 includes those individuals who do not meet one or more of the qualifications.

Interview Formats

Once several viable candidates are identified, you should decide which of the three types of interviews you will use: structured interview (questions are prepared in advance); unstructured interview (questions are not prepared); and semistructured (a combination of both structured and unstructured) (19). The semistructured approach tends to work well in most situations. The use of prewritten questions can serve as a guide during the interview process, offering consistency in questioning and avoiding inappropriate queries. This format also offers the flexibility of asking questions not on the list as follow-up to information presented by the candidate during the interview.

Another consideration is use of the group interview technique. In some instances it may be appropriate to have two to four individuals interview a candidate at one time. The advantages are that a greater number of individuals can be involved in the process, questions and answers are heard by all at one time, time commitments and scheduling difficulties are minimized, and the candidate can observe interactions among potential new coworkers. The disadvantages include potentially overwhelming the candidate, lessening the chance for making a personal connection with the candidate, and requiring a coordinating effort on the interviewers' part.

Interview Questions

There are various kinds of questions you might ask during the interview process; in general, these fall into five categories (17, 29):

- *Leading questions* are easy and often not very informative questions with obvious answers. An example might be: "Are you a hard worker?" These types of questions should be avoided.

- *Direct questions* require short or simple answers, usually yes or no or another one-word answer. Again, a limited amount of information is obtained, but these can be helpful in gaining specific information. An example is: "Are you a certified technologist?"

- *Open-ended questions* are more difficult for the interviewer to construct and require the interviewee to provide a more complex answer. A significant amount of information can be obtained from these types of questions. You may learn from the specific answer to the question asked, but also the interviewer can observe the candidate's manner, style, affect, and level of articulation presented in the response. The candidate must think about the response and articulate an acceptable answer. An example is: "What are your long-term goals?"

- *Probing questions* are often follow-up questions. Once a candidate comments on a question, a specific point can be probed with another question that reveals even more information. An example is a follow-up question to a query about the level of training/education a candidate professes to have, such as, "How does your training apply to the job offered?"

- *Hypothetical questions* can be useful and are often asked towards the end of the interview as an opportunity to determine how candidates think on their feet. These are problem-solving questions that require the candidates to utilize their training and/or experience to properly answer the question. A question such as "If you had to reduce your budget by 20%, how would you go about it?" gives interviewees the opportunity to demonstrate their knowledge of budgeting, staffing, finances, and other related operational skills. Questions unrelated to the job duties that may be construed as "psychological" or "stress-situation" questions are not appropriate.

Interview "Do's and Don'ts"

You should prepare for the interview by reviewing the job description, résumé, and questions to be asked in advance of the actual interview (see Appendix 15.1). Table 15.8 offers some tips to consider when interviewing. You should put the candidate at ease by asking a question not related to the job—about the weather, the commute to the interview, or some other light topic ("developing rapport"). You should avoid any personal comments about the candidate's dress, suit, haircut, hair color, the "2-carat diamond earrings," or any other personal feature, as well as questions about marital status, age, nationality, family, sexual orientation, religion, or affiliations (17). During the interview process, you should keep in mind the Americans with Disabilities Act and avoid any questions that may appear to be discriminatory to those with physical or mental disabilities. You may ask the candidate if there are any tasks listed in the job description that he or she could not do, but you cannot discriminate based on the *perception* of a candidate's being unable to accomplish job-related requirements. Those individuals who appear to have a disability may be able to accomplish assigned tasks with the use of technological aids. It is appropriate to ask about

Table 15.8 Ten interview tips[a]

- Prepare before the interview; do not use the interview time to look at the candidate's résumé for the first time.
- Allow an adequate amount of time for the interview.
- Avoid interruptions. Schedule the interview in a quiet area.
- Welcome each candidate warmly and make the candidate feel at ease.
- Explain the interview process and what follow-up the candidate might expect.
- Avoid utilizing "stress" interviews.
- Avoid controversial issues. Do not ask illegal questions (see text).
- Do not make promises to the candidate that you cannot keep.
- If you do not know the answer to a question, don't guess.
- Don't do all the talking.

[a]From reference 17. (This information was originally printed in the September/October 1999 issue of Clinical Leadership & Management Review, published by the Clinical Laboratory Management Association. For more information, visit www.clma.org.)

gaps in work experience, about a lack of job progression or responsibilities as noted in the résumé, or about the candidate's time and attendance history (29).

Hiring Process

Candidates interviewed should be evaluated based on their qualifications, education, abilities, experience, and responses to the interview questions. A fixed ranking system can be developed to assist each member of the search committee in presenting an objective evaluation of the candidates. Before any job offer is made, it is essential that each reference be checked. References that do not include an immediate supervisor or some other higher-level individual should be scrutinized carefully unless the candidate has specifically addressed this issue during the interview. Given America's litigious society, most employers are very discreet in what information they release (generally, confirmation of employment, dates employed, and job title) unless the candidate has given them specific permission to be a reference. While you may learn much in what is said about the candidate from the reference, listen carefully to what is *not* said. A reference will offer high accolades for an exceptional employee with little or no prompting, while only basic information (confirmation of employment, dates of employment, duties) will be offered for a marginal or poor employee.

Orientation

Proper orientation is critical to the initial success once a candidate is hired (5). Implementing an organized orientation program provides needed guidance that will minimize confusion and frustration for the new employee, yet maximize the feeling of being part of the team. This also protects the employer from future problems that may arise when critical information has not been shared from the beginning and results in an undesired incident at a later date. Some key points that should be covered during orientation are listed in Table 15.9. Current staff should also be informed that a new employee is joining them and that they should make him or her feel welcome. This sets an impression for the employee as to the tone of the work environment.

The more the new employee knows about operations, expectations, and the general atmosphere of the workplace, the better the assimilation into the team. A prepared orientation checklist that can be signed by the new employee and the trainer documents what has been covered, thus preventing any misunderstandings about responsibilities. Reviewing the job description and initiating a performance program during this orientation process will establish a foundation for what will be expected from the employee and, conversely, what will be expected from the employer. The immediate supervisor should provide ori-

Table 15.9 Employee orientation program check list

Item		Done
Table of organization		
Historical overview of the organization		
Laboratory tour and meet the staff		
Mission and vision statements (departmental, hospital, or other)		
Share/review job description		
Laboratory safety; fire safety; Universal Precautions; environmental safety; hospital security; ID cards		
Health Insurance Portability and Accountability Act of 1996/confidentiality		
Laboratory compliance plan		
Customer service; telephone etiquette; fax machine usage; personal phone calls; dress code/appearance		
Time and attendance expectations		
Vacation, sick leave, overtime accruals, and requests for time off		
Quality assurance, quality control, total quality management and continuous quality improvement programs		
Continuing education policies		
Laboratory information system training		
Purchasing requests: supplies, equipment, etc.		
Performance evaluation; progressive discipline; continuing competence training; continuing education; promotion/raises		
Policies	Right to know	
	Material Safety Data Sheets (MSDS)	
	Sexual harassment policy	
	Patient Bill of Rights	
	Total quality management	
	Advance directives	
Miscellaneous issues	Educational opportunities (personal development, continuing education)	
	Lunch/break area	
	Pay day	
	Parking	
Signatures		**Date**
Employee signature:		
Supervisor signature:		

entation; however, other designated staff who would best be able to educate the new employee can also be involved. The duration of orientation depends on the nature of the job; it should last as long as deemed appropriate to convey the needed information and ensure a successful start to the job. This will also give the employer a basis for evaluation of the employee at a future date (usually 6 weeks after the start date). With a clear path forward, both employer and employee will start off knowing there is an established line of communication and accountability. However, any problems that arise before the formal evaluation should be dealt with immediately and must be appropriately documented.

Documentation

It is important to generate documentation throughout the search, hiring, and orientation process. This ensures that the process is consistent, addresses any legal requirements, and demonstrates fairness in hiring practices. Examples of the kind of documentation to be retained include a description of job duties, résumés of those applying for the position, a copy of the advertisement(s) and where posted, a sample of interview questions asked, the ethnicity of candidates (when possible), and responses from references. These records must be retained for a minimum of 4 years, but in practice, most employers keep documentation for 10 years. This offers protection for the employer for any one individual hired, in addition to providing a track record that demonstrates a consistent and fair hiring process.

Retention

The cost of hiring and training new employees can be very expensive in terms of real dollars and in loss of productivity. Thousands of dollars are spent in advertising, overtime, training, processing, and other recruitment or startup expenses (18). Losing an experienced employee can be particularly costly in terms of lost productivity, institutional knowledge, and experience. Thus, when an employee asks for a pay raise, the administrator must consider replacement costs versus the raise. If the vacancy is unavoidable, another consideration is the opportunity for promotion from within, if appropriate. Maintaining high staff morale is very difficult. One way to show employer support is to recognize existing staff talents by promoting a qualified individual. This is also a good time to consider how responsibilities related to this vacancy might be shared with existing staff, and if the position actually needs to be refilled.

People leave their jobs for many reasons. Some are personal (marriage, pregnancy, illness, self-esteem, burnout), others are work related (hate boss, want more money, poor work conditions, poor work hours, no recognition), and

others relate to professional development (returning to school or military, further education, promotional opportunity) (17). Whatever the reason(s), a good leader will listen to his or her employees and establish avenues of bidirectional communication. Employers need to be sensitive to employee needs, stress levels, multicultural differences, and general morale. Some options, such as implementing pay raises, enhancing benefits, offering continuing education opportunities, or providing promotional options, may be beyond the control of the immediate supervisor. However, acknowledgment by an employer shows a level of sensitivity that is appreciated by staff. Recognizing what can and cannot be done and sharing that with employees often demonstrates to them that you, as the representative of the employer, are not indifferent to their concerns and may serve as encouragement. Table 15.10 offers some suggestions that may help in employee retention (3, 20).

Table 15.10 Suggested retention options

Practice	Option
Good hiring practices	Hire the right people to do the job.
	Have realistic goals and expectations.
	Perform a thorough job search.
	Check references.
Communication	Bidirectional communication.
	Have frequent staff meetings.
	Manage by walking about.
Training	Develop an orientation process.
	Adequately train staff and supervisors in job duties, interpersonal skills, communication, etc.
	Encourage teamwork.
	Encourage continuing education.
Recognition	Find people doing something right.
	Praise people often.
	Foster a positive work environment.
	Encourage ideas, positive attitudes, and innovative thinking.
	Allow more employee participation in decision making.
	Celebrate successes.
Work environment	Maintain a safe work environment.
	Provide adequate tools to do the job.
	Establish a workable infrastructure.
Surveys/feedback	Measure outcomes as part of quality assurance.
	Monitor attitudes.
	Be aware of workplace stress inducers.
	Know employee problems and how they relate to the workplace.
	Communicate.

Resignation and Termination

One goal of all good managers is to ensure that they make the best attempt in hiring what they hope will be long-term and productive employees. Loss of an employee may be due to voluntary or involuntary discharge. The former may be due to a number of issues, as suggested above. In some cases, voluntary resignation may be averted through better channels of communication or through other adjustments (remuneration, promotion, change in job duties, etc.).

Yet, there are circumstances that may lead to the involuntary termination of the employee due to reduction in the force, failure in communicating expectations, or poor job performance. The first is generally a function of fiduciary responsibilities of the employer that may be necessary to keep laboratory expenses within budget. Often, a decision to terminate an employee based on financial need is not a reflection of the employee's performance or job ability but is a bottom-line decision. There are other times when the selection of an employee has not been a good fit for either the employer or employee and thus may require involuntary termination. While it is incumbent on the employer to make every reasonable attempt to correct a problem situation and help the employee to understand where the lack of communication exists, there are times when it is best for both to seek other options. Involuntary termination must be free from any discriminatory actions based on race, age, sex, or disability (23). Over the years, a number of laws and court cases have addressed wrongful termination issues; thus an employer must use care in proceeding to terminate an employee. Table 15.11 lists a few of the more common reasons for termination with good cause (24). You must also be aware of employee situations that may fall under the Americans with Disabilities Act, such as alcoholism, substance abuse, job stress, mental illness, or cumulative trauma disorders such as carpal tunnel syndrome (9).

The process of progressive discipline gives the employee ample opportunity to address the employer's concerns and take necessary corrective actions. Conversely, it also provides the employer with an opportunity to review and adjust any unreasonable expectations that set the employee up for failure. How far the counseling is taken depends on the severity of the problem and the employee's history and status. If initial discussions between the supervisor and the employee do not result in the desired outcome, a more aggressive approach is required that progresses in an established manner. This progressive process will end either with a mutually acceptable resolution or with employee termination. This process is rigidly adhered to for state or federal government employees and in those facilities that have union representation. In the private sector, the rules may be less stringent. The main steps in progressive counseling are:

- *Verbal counseling.* This is an important communication between the employer and employee in a manner that specifically addresses the concerns. This is the first "official" recognition of the problem and is documented for the record only. Depending on the degree of severity, several episodes of verbal counseling may be appropriate.

- *Written counseling.* If there is no performance improvement on behalf of the employee after verbal counseling, additional counseling occurs with preparation of a formal written memorandum. The memorandum must be specific, noting the circumstances, times, dates, and individuals involved. Copies may be circulated to the evaluator's supervisor, the director of human resources, and the employee's personnel file.

- *Penalty stage.* If unacceptable employee actions continue after the written counseling, penalties may be imposed, such as a fine, leave without pay, demotion, or a decrease in pay. Documentation of the additional improprieties and a written memorandum are required. When discipline reaches this level, the relationship between employee and employer is very strained and can create additional problems. Attitudes, a loss of productivity, and inefficiencies may be evident. Other employees may also be directly or indirectly affected when working in a tense environment. Termination may be the only option at this point.

- *Discharge.* The final stage, when no other options or corrective actions are apparent, is termination of employment. This part of the process should be under the direction of the human resources department to ensure that all legal procedures are followed, thus minimizing any basis for legal recourse by the dismissed employee.

A good manager creates the kind of work environment that offers opportunities for employees to be the most productive and efficient in their jobs. The goal is to maximize use of available resources, whether human, financial, physical, or other, to ensure that the workforce is fruitful, content, loyal, and proud of what they do. Employees who know what is expected from them, what to expect from their employer, work in a clean and safe environment, and have the right training, tools, and materials to do the job

Table 15.11 Common dischargeable circumstances

Job incompetence

Insubordination

Excessive tardiness or absences

Verbal abuse

Physical violence

Falsification of records

Theft

Impairment on the job

Criminal charges

are satisfied employees who will provide a long-term service to the institution.

Summary

There are about 171,000 CLIA-certified laboratories performing more than 7.25 billion tests a year in the United States. It is undeniably evident that the function of the clinical laboratory is critical to good patient care. About 85% of medical decision making by physicians is based on laboratory results. It is anticipated that the need for trained laboratory personnel will increase over the next few years. Yet, there is a growing concern regarding the 61% decrease in the number of relevant training programs and the decreasing number of graduates from the remaining programs. This has resulted in vacancy rates ranging between 9 and 20% (15, 27). Also, laboratory professionals are aging. In one survey, the average age was 46 years; less than 5% of the respondents were under the age of 29 (15). The projected number of individuals needed to fill these vacancies is about 9,000, yet only about 5,000 graduates are anticipated to be available within the existing programs.

As in any business, supply and demand will predominate resulting in competition for qualified candidates. It is predicted that 2-year medical laboratory technician graduates will soon be performing most lab tests, while 4-year medical technology graduates will be more involved in data gathering, analysis, monitoring, and dispersal of information (11). As more of the Human Genome Project succeeds and becomes the basis for new technology-based testing, it is clear that managers will need the best and brightest to meet the challenges of these new technologies. Attracting and keeping these key people will take a collective effort between employer and employee so both reap the benefits of this relationship and are able to provide quality patient care.

KEY POINTS

- Every vacancy should prompt a reconsideration of the necessity, qualifications, and requirements for the position.

- The job description, advertising method, interview process, and selection criteria should be carefully analyzed before attempting to fill a job vacancy.

- Those responsible for these processes must be aware of local policies and legal requirements governing the selection and hiring process and of the progressive discipline process.

- Managers must constantly work to retain valued employees by using a variety of techniques.

GLOSSARY

Job description Written delineation of the title, duties, responsibilities, and reporting relationships of a position and the requisite qualifications needed to meet these.

Equal Employment Opportunity Commission (EEOC) Established to prevent discrimination in hiring and retention of employees based on non-work-related characteristics.

Executive Order 11246 of 1965 Created affirmative action programs requiring employers to establish plans to address racial disparities in hiring and promotion, in conjunction with the Civil Rights Act (1964).

Structured interview An applicant interview in which all of the interviewer's questions are prepared in advance.

Unstructured interview An applicant interview in which no interview questions are prepared in advance.

Semistructured interview An applicant interview using both prepared and "spur-of-the-moment" questions.

Americans with Disabilities Act Federal act that precludes discrimination in hiring and retention based on non-job-related characteristics.

Progressive discipline Stepwise process to address deficiencies in job-related activities or attitudes.

REFERENCES

1. **Blackmon, R. K.** 2001. Bridging the laboratory generation gap. *Lab. Med.* **32**(6):299–302.

2. **Cameron, M., and J. R. Snyder.** 1999. Strategic human resource management: redefining the role of the manager and worker. *Clin. Lab. Manage. Rev.* **13**(5):242–250.

3. **Dressler, G.** 1994. Employee safety and health, p. 617–655. *In* G. Dressler (ed.), *Human Resources Management*, 6th ed. Prentice-Hall, Englewood Cliffs, N.J.

4. **Dressler, G.** 1994. Global HRM: Managing intercountry differences in human resource management, p. 687–692. *In* G. Dressler (ed.), *Human Resources Management*, 6th ed. Prentice-Hall, Englewood Cliffs, N.J.

5. **Ehrhardt, P.** 1999. The new employee: proper orientation and training go a long way toward job success. *Clin. Lab. Manage. Rev.* **13**(5):262–265.

6. **Federal Register.** 1992. CLIA '88. *Fed. Reg.* **57**:7001–7288.

7. **Gober, M.** 1999. As we see it: finding Mr. (or Ms.) Right. *Clin. Lab. Manage. Rev.* **13**(5):320–327.

8. **Gross, L.** 2001. Educating and employing gen X & Y. *Adv. Health Inform. Profess.* **11**(21):10–12.

9. **Henry, J. B., and A. S. Kurec.** 2001. The clinical laboratory: organization, purposes, and practices, p. 3–49. *In* J. B. Henry (ed.), *Clinical Diagnosis and Management by Laboratory Methods*, 20th ed. W. B. Saunders, Philadelphia, Pa.

10. **Johnson, C. M.** 2001. Best hiring practices to keep your laboratory running smoothly. *Vantage Point* **5**:1–4.

11. **Katz, F.** 2001. Medical technologists prepare for change. *Lab Med.* **32**(9):502–505.

12. **Kennedy, M. M.** 1999. Understanding the demographics of evolving workforce. *Clin. Lab. Manage. Rev.* **13**(5):310–316.

13. **Ketchum, S. M.** 1992. Managing the multi-cultural laboratory, part I: tools for understanding cultural differences. *Clin. Lab. Manage. Rev.* **6**(4):287–307.

14. **Ketchum, S. M.** 1992. Managing the multi-cultural laboratory, part II: tools for understanding cultural differences. *Clin. Lab. Manage. Rev.* **6**(4):521–536.

15. **Kinjo, M.** 2000. Professional prospectives: the future of medical technologists-through survey and statistics. *Lab Med.* **31**(10):539–540.

16. **Kurec, A. S.** 1998. Staffing and scheduling of laboratory personnel, p. 221–243. *In* J. R. Snyder and D. S. Wilkinson (ed.), *Management in Laboratory Medicine,* 3rd ed. Lippincott, Philadelphia, Pa.

17. **Kurec, A. S.** 1999. Recruiting, interviewing, and hiring the right person. *Clin. Lab. Manage. Rev.* **13**(5):251–261.

18. **Kurec, A. S.** 2000. The role and function of the clinical laboratory, p. 1–20. *In* A. S. Kurec, S. Schofield, and M. C. Watters (ed.), *The CLMA Guide to Managing a Clinical Laboratory,* 3rd ed. Clinical Laboratory Management Association, Wayne, Pa.

19. **Lussier, R. N.** 1995. Selecting qualified candidates through effective interviewing. *Clin. Lab. Manage. Rev.* **9**(4):267–275.

20. **Mass, D.** 1999. Staff retention: a major key to management's success. *Clin. Lab. Manage. Rev.* **13**(5):266–275.

21. **Nigon, D. L.** 2000. Managing people, p. 63–106. *In* D. L. Nigon, (ed.), *Clinical Laboratory Management: Leadership Principles for the 21st Century.* McGraw-Hill, New York, N.Y.

22. **Passey, R. B.** 1998. The Clinical Laboratory Improvement Amendments (CLIA), p. 17–34. *In* J. R. Snyder and D. S. Wilkinson (ed.), *Management in Laboratory Medicine,* 3rd ed. Lippincott, Philadelphia, Pa.

23. **Sams, P. S.** 1999. Involuntary termination of employment: legal and practical considerations. *Clin. Lab. Manage. Rev.* **13**(5):291–300.

24. **Schuler, R. S.** 1981. Employee rights, p. 507–535. *In* R. S. Schuler (ed.), *Personnel and Human Resource Management,* 3rd ed. West Publishing Co., St. Paul, Minn.

25. **Snyder, J. R.** 2000. Staffing: managing the human resource, p. 43–58. *In* A. S. Kurec, S. Schofield, and M. C. Watters (ed.), *The CLMA Guide to Managing a Clinical Laboratory,* 3rd ed. Clinical Laboratory Management Association, Wayne, Pa.

26. **Ward-Cook, K., D. S. Tatum, and G. Jones.** 2000. Medical technologist core job tasks still reign. *Lab Med.* **31**(7):375–379.

27. **Ward-Cook, K., M. G. Daniels, and C. Brito.** 2001. ASCP Board of Registry 2000 annual survey of medical laboratory science programs. *Lab Med.* **32**(11):655–660.

28. **Wilkinson, D. S., and T. J. Dilts.** 1999. Role of medical, technical, and administrative leadership in the human resource management cycle: a team approach to laboratory management. *Clin. Lab. Manage. Rev.* **13**(5):301–309.

29. **Wilson, S. L., and J. R. Snyder.** 1998. Interviewing and employee selection, p. 195–220. *In* J. R. Snyder and D. S. Wilkinson (ed.), *Management in Laboratory Medicine,* 3rd ed. Lippincott, Philadelphia, Pa.

APPENDIX 15.1   Internet Addresses

American Association of Blood Banks
http://www.aabb.org

American Association for Clinical Chemistry
http://www.aacc.org

American Society for Clinical Laboratory Science
http://www.ascls.org

American Society for Clinical Pathology
http://www.ascp.org

American Society for Microbiology
http://asm.org

Clinical Laboratory Management Association
http://www.clma.org

Job search tools and guidelines
http://www.monster.com

National Association for the Advancement of Colored People
http://www.naacp.org

Detailed job descriptions and qualification factors for U.S. Army enlisted jobs (blood banking, clinical laboratory testing)
usmilitary.about.com/library/milinfo/arjobs/bl91k.htm

APPENDIX 15.2   Example of a Search Committee Interview Process and Evaluation[a]

Position: _____

The search committee consists of (*names of individuals*). The Committee met on the following dates: (*insert dates*). The purpose of the committee is to interview and set the agenda for the interviewee. It was explained that committee members may take notes for better accuracy in remembering some details. Specific duties of the job description will be shared at the end of the interview process. A consensus of the committee will be obtained and the incumbent selected based on educational background, technical experience, and personal attributes. The following questions were used as general guidelines in the evaluation process.

Please rate applicant on a scale of 1 (low) to 5 (high) for each item (circle rating).

I. Personal:

1 2 3 4 5   How would a person who knows you well describe you to us?

1 2 3 4 5   What are your career goals?

1 2 3 4 5   What continuing education have you been involved with in the last two years?

1 2 3 4 5   Briefly explain your current position to us.

1 2 3 4 5   What are your two most important achievements in your current job?

1 2 3 4 5   What is your level of computer expertise, including spreadsheets and word processing?

1 2 3 4 5   How do you best communicate with staff? Employer? Non-lab personnel?

1 2 3 4 5   Describe a stressful situation you encountered and how you resolved it.

II. Supervisory:

1 2 3 4 5   Describe your supervisory experience. How long? Number supervised?

1 2 3 4 5   Describe your experience in preparing employee evaluations, counseling sessions, recruiting, and interviewing.

1 2 3 4 5   Describe your involvement in quality assurance practices.

1 2 3 4 5   How would you handle an increased workload that exceeds the normal capabilities of your staff?

1 2 3 4 5   Knowledge of medico-legal issues and procedures.

1 2 3 4 5   Marketing experience in developing proposals and client interaction.

1 2 3 4 5   What is your experience in providing customer service?

III. Clinical or professional experience:

1 2 3 4 5   Where did you do your training? Under whose supervision?

1 2 3 4 5   What is your background experience?

1 2 3 4 5   What is your technical experience in? [*specific task or function*]

1 2 3 4 5   What other specific skills do you bring that would be an asset to this job?

IV. Teaching/training experience

1 2 3 4 5   What is your teaching experience?

1 2 3 4 5   What is your area of interest in [*specific area*] teaching?

1 2 3 4 5   Give an example of your teaching/training experience.

1 2 3 4 5   Describe your experience in training new employees.

1 2 3 4 5   Describe your involvement in continuing education programs.

V. Research:

1 2 3 4 5   Describe your research experience.

1 2 3 4 5   Are there any specific interests you would like to pursue?

1 2 3 4 5   Do you have any publications? Presentations?

(*continued*)

APPENDIX 15.2   Example of a Search Committee Interview Process and Evaluation[a] *(continued)*

Rating

Item	Score	Comments	
Personal			
Supervisory			
Clinical/professional experience			
Teaching/training experience			
Research experience			
		Hire:	
		Hold:	
Total points:		Not acceptable:	

Final comments: _____

_____

Evaluator: _____   Date: _____

Title/position: _____

[a]From reference 17. (This information was originally printed in the September/October 1999 issue of *Clinical Leadership & Management Review,* published by the Clinical Laboratory Management Association. For more information, visit www.clma.org.)

16

Introduction
Performance Appraisals

Competency Assessment

Summary
KEY POINTS
GLOSSARY
REFERENCES
APPENDIXES

Performance Appraisals and Competency Assessment

Diane C. Halstead and Donna L. Oblack

OBJECTIVES

To understand the purpose of performance appraisals

To define the key elements in developing a meaningful performance appraisal

To identify methods to measure employee performance

To describe the steps that may be taken in conducting a successful appraisal interview

To list three accreditation agencies that issue competency standards

To specify three intervals or events that require competency assessment

To describe four competency assessment methods

The quality of a person's life is in direct proportion to their commitment to excellence, regardless of their chosen field of endeavor.

VINCENT T. LOMBARDI

T HE GOAL OF THIS CHAPTER is to provide you with tools that will allow you to develop and execute a successful formal performance appraisal process and competency assessment program. Specific examples of documentation are provided in the appendixes to this chapter.

Performance Appraisals

Definition of Performance Appraisals

The word "appraisal" is derived from the Latin word *appratiare,* to set a price or value (35). In this context, employees work for compensation. Does this mean that the appraisal process was developed solely for the purpose of financial rewards? Certainly not, but the concept of performance appraisals was introduced in the mid-twentieth century as a result of the recession years when companies found it necessary to decrease costs and increase efficiencies. It was not until the 1980s that performance appraisals gained a foothold due to a need for an equitable means of determining pay for performance.

A formal performance appraisal, also known as a merit review, performance evaluation, interview, or rating (28), is a planned, periodic management activity to evaluate an employee's on-the-job behavior, competency, work skill improvement, need for training, progress towards completing goals, and salary and promotion (28, 46, 50). It is a key human resource function that is closely integrated not only with compensation and training but also career planning.

Purpose of Performance Appraisals

Some leading management authorities, such as W. Edwards Deming, renowned for his transformation of Japanese business philosophy, believe that performance appraisals are unnecessary and, in fact, may destroy initiative and encourage competitiveness rather than teamwork, process performance, and a concern for organizational success (28, 37). Others contend that formal performance appraisal programs cost billions of dollars annually (35) for questionable benefits (5, 29, 35, 37). Stress associated with the appraisal process is another reason cited for not conducting performance appraisals (35). In contrast, many human resource experts believe that by implementing a well-designed performance appraisal program, the competitive aspect can be minimized and the motivational aspect can be emphasized (44).

Disadvantages to performance appraisals:

- Destroy initiative
- Encourage competitiveness
- Produce stress
- Require large financial investment

Some managers and employees dislike and even dread performance appraisals (40). They go through the motions, albeit halfheartedly, because senior management requires them to participate in a formal appraisal process. Unfortunately, they do not realize the potential benefits that can be derived from performance appraisals, nor have they developed the skills necessary to conduct or participate in a productive performance appraisal process. An objective of this chapter is to provide you with an appreciation for the performance appraisal as a powerful motivating tool.

Benefits of Performance Appraisals

Appraisals can be challenging as well as productive, rewarding, and energizing (36). Positive feedback provides employees with the opportunity to learn their strengths and weaknesses (2). Employees can be empowered to control their growth and development, as well as the outcomes of the performance appraisal (18). If carefully performed, the appraisal process can enhance relationships with employees and open doors to communication. Managers and their employees can set realistic goals that reflect and support the mission and goals of the organization as well as the employees. Finally, the performance appraisal system and the performance standards specifically are objective tools to use as a basis for merit pay increases, promotions, and termination.

A successful performance appraisal promotes good communication and constructive feedback between managers and their staff. It provides an opportunity to clarify job requirements and performance expectations. When used as an evaluation tool, the appraisal becomes a critical component of reinforcing appropriate behaviors and providing a fair and consistent foundation for promotions, transfers, demotions, terminations, and salary adjustments. An effective appraisal process can be used as a recruitment tool to attract candidates for employment into a program that recognizes employee accomplishments. Employers may highlight how their organization provides opportunities for skill development and promotion. Retention in today's market is important, given the dwindling work force that the laboratory is now facing. When employees feel valued, they tend to remain on the job as loyal employees. In summary, performance appraisals can be used as a tool to recognize outstanding employee achievements and to provide desirable work-related experiences and career opportunities.

Advantages to performance appraisals:

- Foster good communication
- Provide constructive feedback
- Clarify job requirements
- Provide an opportunity to refine job skills
- Define performance expectations
- Promote behavioral modification
- Identify educational needs
- Provide documentation for promotion, compensation, and termination decisions
- Promote recruitment and retention
- Protect organization from discrimination lawsuits
- Provide an opportunity to share departmental and organizational visions
- Encourage teams to improve the way their organization operates

Appraisal Types: Formal and Informal Appraisals

An effective appraisal system should include formal as well as informal ongoing performance feedback. A formal performance appraisal generally occurs at least annually on a specific date and time, such as the anniversary of the employee's hire date (28, 50). Performance appraisals can also be given at a set time of the year identified by the Human Resources department for larger groups of employees within an organization. Appraising everyone during the same time period is generally viewed as most fair because the same guidelines can be applied to all employees evaluated (28, 35). A performance appraisal form is generally completed during the interview, and this written documentation is placed in the employee's file as part of the permanent record. In contrast, informal performance feedback appraisals are useful for monitoring behavior modification, recognizing accomplishments, identifying stumbling blocks in achieving set goals, giving support where applicable, and fostering ongoing communication between formal appraisals. Informal appraisals also ensure that the formal appraisal does not come as a surprise to employees. They know what is expected and can work at fulfilling those expectations.

Benefits of informal performance appraisals:

- Provide an opportunity to monitor behavioral modifications
- Allow for timely recognition of accomplishments
- Identify stumbling blocks to achieving goals
- Provide ongoing support
- Foster good communication

Responsibility for Developing a Performance Appraisal Program

The organizational philosophy and purpose for having performance appraisals should be clear to those who are designing a performance appraisal system. The performance appraisal program is frequently developed by one or more members of upper management and supervisory level employees, including the chief executive officer, managers, human resource professionals, and staff employees, particularly those who are strong performers or who welcome new opportunities. There are several reasons for including staff employees in the planning process. First, they are intimately acquainted with all of the tasks that make up their jobs and with the factors that affect their ability to get the job done. By valuing their input, they will feel that their opinions matter and that they are an important part of the decision-making body of the organization. In turn, their involvement is likely to engender support for the program and loyalty to the organization. Finally, they will feel that they are being given a new opportunity to learn and advance in their career (28).

Who is responsible for developing a performance appraisal program?

- Upper management
- Supervisors/managers
- Human Resources staff
- Staff employees

Legal Aspects of a Performance Appraisal Program

The form itself that is used to document the performance appraisal may be a standardized form or it may be created by Human Resources and/or organizational managers and staff (35). Performance appraisals are discoverable in a court of law. In other words, the information may be considered evidence in a legal case, so it is important to always apply the performance appraisal process fairly and equitably (32, 45). Discriminatory policies can and will get you in trouble. Clearly defined standards, feedback, and documentation are key factors in defending your program and appraisals (32, 50).

Evaluating employees and awarding pay increases consistently is paramount to keeping your program defensible. Performance appraisals are confidential and should be shared with individuals only on an as-needed basis, except by subpoena (28). The following factors help to ensure that you are using a legally defensible performance appraisal system:

- Appraisers should receive written instructions and specific training on how to utilize the appraisals correctly.
- Job descriptions should be used to determine what is evaluated.
- Performance expectations should be reviewed in advance with the employee.
- Appraisals should be designed to evaluate behavior, not personality traits.
- The content of a completed appraisal form should be discussed with the employee, and the employee in turn should have a chance to add his or her own comments.
- Everyone should be evaluated fairly and consistently.

Legal considerations:

- Train appraisers
- Review job descriptions and performance expectations prior to interview
- Evaluate behavior, not personality
- Provide employees with an opportunity to respond to appraisal
- Evaluate fairly and consistently
- Document appraisal

Elements of a Meaningful Formal Performance Appraisal

An effective program is based on an honest and sincere discussion of expectations, job performance, and plans for improvement and follow-up between appraisers and their employees. Performance appraisals must be clearly developed to meet the requirements of specific positions. It takes a concerted effort and up-front expense to develop and maintain an effective performance appraisal system. Time must be devoted to analyzing and preparing job descriptions for each job title within an organization; designing performance appraisal forms; executing a successful performance interview, including preinterview planning; follow-up (21, 32); ongoing monitoring; documenting; training; and compensation. An effective program requires total management commitment of time and money (35).

Elements of a formal appraisal:

- Clear expectations: mission statement, job description, performance standards
- Valid and fair performance assessment

- Plan for improvement
- Follow-up

Mission statement. A meaningful performance appraisal should begin with a current organizational mission statement. The organizational philosophy should be incorporated into the mission statement of each performance appraisal. Understanding organizational goals and values is paramount to setting goals for the employees and ultimately to ensuring organizational productivity and success. As a manager, it is important that you convey the goals and values of the organization and department to your employees.

Job description. A job description is a written document that generally includes the title of the position; department; job code or number, if applicable; Federal Labor Standards Act Status as to whether the position is exempt (salaried) or nonexempt (hourly), full-time, part-time, or temporary; job summary; four to six essential functions or tasks; level of authority; reporting relationship; essential skills or traits required to perform the tasks; qualifications; physical requirements; and effective date of the job description (28) (Appendix 16.1). All employees in an organization should have an up-to-date job description so they know what is expected of them (35).

A job description is a valuable tool when terminating an employee for failing to do the job. It provides documentation that the employee knew what was expected of him or her. "Essential functions" are those duties and responsibilities that are an inherent part of a particular job. The term is included to protect the rights of disabled workers under the 1990 Americans with Disabilities Act (ADA) and is applicable to organizations with at least 15 employees. The ADA is enforced by the Equal Employment Opportunity Commission (28). To meet legal requirements, a skill must be shown to be a valid, true, and necessary requirement of the job. The two controlling principles in developing written job descriptions and standards are job-relatedness and fairness (28).

Performance standards. Evaluations based on performance standards were introduced in the 1990s and are commonly used in the laboratory setting. Standards are formal requirements that outline expectations of job performance, i.e., how well a job should be performed (Appendixes 16.2 and 16.3). Performance appraisals must contain specific, measurable, and realistic standards of performance (40, 50). In other words, the job description defines the job responsibilities and the standards quantify your expectations, e.g., how many cultures are read per day and percent of errors tolerated. Standards can be used to compare the quality of work among staff members. Different types of jobs may call for demonstrable skills or behaviors rather than numerically quantifiable units of production. For example, a stan-

dard of performance in the laboratory may be to demonstrate familiarity with safety regulations in order to provide a safe work environment. Another method of measure is to include percent timeliness, e.g., technologist will finalize 75% of the 48-h cultures on time. Established and specific performance standards allow employees to know how they are doing compared to expectations (17, 18). It makes them accountable (35).

Criteria. A criterion is a standard for judging task performance. Three to four specific, detailed, and realistic written criteria should be developed, understood, and agreed upon by employee and supervisor for each key task (18, 50). These need to be objective, observable, and measurable (40).

Norms. Norms (36) are informal behaviors that are generally accepted in the workplace. For example, treating coworkers with respect is an organizational norm. Norms are more difficult to identify and more subjective than standards. The problem with using norms to measure employee performance is that they are situational. A behavior may be considered acceptable to one manager and unacceptable to another. Alternatively, a behavior may be considered acceptable by a manager when exhibited by one individual and unacceptable when exhibited by another individual. Norms are not less important than standards because violations of an organization's norms can have as much impact as violations of its standards. For example, one of your employees may exceed all standards but frequently offends or insults other coworkers. As a manager, you may find yourself repeatedly calming the other coworkers from the ongoing violation of the laboratory's norms. In this case, when the violation of a norm interferes with the performance of other employees, the individual violating the norm needs to be counseled.

Characteristics of performance standards:

- Specific
- Measurable
- Realistic

Competency-Based Appraisals

Appraisals are often position-specific and competency-based using observable and measurable standards. The Joint Commission on Accreditation of Healthcare Organizations (JCAHO) initially required employers to use criteria-based performance appraisals and later replaced the requirements with competency-based appraisals. In other words, performance appraisals must ensure that all healthcare workers are competent in all areas necessary to perform their jobs. Competency is the state of having the correct or needed skills for the position. In a competency-based performance appraisal, each required competency should be evaluated in some quantitative format. Appraisal forms that use a rating system with a structured scale generally are easy to complete. The disadvantage of a rating system is that it tends to set up a competitive feeling among employees. It is important that the appraiser qualify a rating with behavioral examples. For example, if you score an employee above or below what is considered the minimally acceptable score, you should provide written detail.

Rating Methods

The validity of a rating system depends on such things as rater training and observable and quantifiable behaviors. Employees should have a current, detailed job description and know performance standards and criteria used for assessing performance. Appraising an employee's performance means that you are rating actual performance, not ability. A person may have the ability but may not be performing up to the standards set for that job. Characteristics commonly assessed are competency, accuracy, communication, creativity, productivity, problem solving, decision making, delegating, and administrative effectiveness. You must be able to consistently observe the employee performing the assigned tasks, and your rating criteria must be the same for all employees doing the same job. Performance must be described accurately and must be based on documentation. Be careful when rating subjective qualities such as attitude, cooperation, enthusiasm, and initiative. A qualitative characteristic such as interpersonal skills may be appraised, e.g., unsatisfactory, fails to meet acceptable standards in relationships with others; average, gets along well with others; and outstanding, excels in developing relationships of trust and respect with supervisors and peers (35). Quantifiable performance measures, such as the number of times stat turnaround times were within acceptable limits, specimens were processed, critical values were called, errors were made, and percent of time within budget, are productive measurements that are easier to defend.

Results-based evaluations (RBEs) are performed by managers who focus on attainment of specific measurable results. RBEs may be used in intangible areas such as attaining specific goals in management development, reaching personal goals, and collaborative efforts. Key results areas and expectations are agreed upon at the beginning of a period and measured regularly by staff submittal of monthly progress reports. This type of evaluation allows a manager and employee to set and prioritize reasonable goals.

A rating system may be used to compare the performance of employees through a set of criteria that produces a numerical value. There are four factors to consider when designing a written performance appraisal and selecting a rating system: the purpose of the appraisal, your work environment (e.g., self-directed teams), verbal and analytical skills of employees being evaluated, and the manager's management style (50). Rating requires clear definitions of

the terms "exceeds standards," "meets standards," and "does not meet standards." Absolute methods include graphic rating scale, critical incident evaluation, behaviorally anchored rating scale, and use of a checklist.

Factors to consider when selecting a rating system:

- Purpose of appraisal
- Work environment
- Skills of employees
- Manager's management style

A graphic rating scale provides a ranking scale (usually 1 to 5) for unsatisfactory to outstanding performance (50). An overall rating can be calculated by averaging the individual rankings. This is one of the most popular methods. It is easy to use and understand. The forms are easy to revise and the method is not usually time-consuming.

Free-form or narrative rating (50) is generally an adjunct to other methods (2, 28, 32, 35). A variation of this rating is the critical incident evaluation—documenting written notations of exceptional performance, good or bad, that is then summarized in the written performance evaluation (32). A disadvantage is the lack of reference to the day-to-day, noncritical performance that makes up the greatest portion of an employee's on-the-job behavior.

A behaviorally anchored rating scale (BARS) entails writing a competency statement for each aspect of the job. The BARS (9) focuses on employee behaviors and avoids any evaluation of attitudes. A numerical rating scale is used with a description of behaviors that correspond to each of the ratings (32). It is based on critical incidents or actual examples of how employees behaved in a given situation. This type of rating is generally more expensive and time-consuming to implement. It is also more difficult to develop because it must identify all work behaviors of a job with a specific description of each behavior, ranging from unsatisfactory to outstanding.

Checklist adjectives evaluation is based on the use of descriptive phrases to describe a laboratory worker's most outstanding personal characteristics (50). Checklists include statements describing positive and negative behaviors that may be exhibited on the job. If the employee exhibits one of the described behaviors, the item is checked off, otherwise the item is left blank. When using a weighted checklist, each behavior is weighted differently rather than considering them of equal importance. Points are assigned based on the organizational value placed on that behavior.

Forced choice rating is not commonly used. A rater chooses the most applicable of several unrelated descriptions of performance. The choices are purposefully difficult, with the intent of improving the reliability of the rating (35).

Comparative methods used in the 1980s included forced distribution, ranking employees, and paired comparison. Forced distribution (18, 36, 50) requires the rater to distribute a certain percentage of employees in each ranking category, e.g., 5% outstanding, 10% above average, etc. (18). This helps an organization control and forecast salary budgets.

In a ranking, employees are compared and ranked numerically from best to worst among their peers. Because it is not possible for all employees to be ranked as excellent even if they are, a ranking system (36, 50) does not provide feedback about the employees' performance and generally is neither reliable nor valid.

Paired comparison means that employees are compared two at a time (50). Ranking occurs on the basis of the number of times a given employee is deemed to be the better performer of a pair.

Person-to-person comparison is similar to paired comparison. Employees are ranked below average, average, above average, or outstanding on the basis of comparison of employee performance with that of peers who are currently performing similar tasks (50).

Absolute methods of ratings and ranking:

- Graphic rating scale
- Free-form
- Critical incident evaluation
- Behaviorally anchored rating scale
- Forced choice
- Forced distribution
- Paired comparison
- Person-to-person comparison

Other Types of Performance Appraisals

Self-appraisal. Self-appraisal forms are generally distributed approximately 2 weeks prior to a formal appraisal and are not meant to take the place of a manager's appraisal. They give a different perspective of an employee's performance and possibly a better understanding of the potential obstacles that may impede performance. Employees may be provided with a copy of the same form used by the manager so that they can use the same criteria for evaluation of their performance. Ratings and scores can then be easily compared. Interestingly, most employees tend to appraise themselves at the same level or lower than their manager does (28). As an alternative, some laboratories design a form with a different format that elicits additional information by asking open-ended questions (28). The self-appraisal generates active participation by employees. It provides an opportunity for employees to reflect on their own performance and achievements (18, 38). They may identify additional accomplishments that the manager may not have identified. The self-appraisal also promotes a two-way conversation regarding the need for additional training and development (32, 35).

Peer-to-peer appraisal. Peer-to-peer appraisals require trust among employees working together. Coworkers are asked to evaluate each other. This approach may engender fears among staff members, some without foundation, that need to be addressed. The provision of a comprehensive training program on how to give feedback is required to successfully implement this type of appraisal (28). The technique may be risky when conflict exists among employees, thus preventing an objective evaluation. Conversely, if you are working with an experienced and mature group of employees, the process may be very educational. If performed honestly and sincerely, employees may gain great insight into their work relationships and performance. If you are using a team approach to accomplish institutional goals, you may want to consider a variation of this concept. One team of employees may be asked to evaluate another team, rather than appraising individual coworkers.

360-Degree evaluation. 360-degree evaluations are designed to obtain well-rounded appraisals that tend to be reserved for individuals in management-level positions (36). As with peer-to-peer evaluations, both trust and a comprehensive training program are required to successfully implement this technique (28). The evaluation is often performed anonymously and invites open, constructive in-depth feedback (8) from all levels, i.e., peers, subordinates, supervisors, customers, and self (35, 40). Raters are frequently asked to complete a series of open-ended questions. Solicited evaluations with rater identity removed may be given to the employee being appraised, or they may be summarized to obtain an overall feedback appraisal. This type of evaluation is used for developmental purposes, not for salary adjustments.

Who Should Perform the Appraisal?

The appraiser should be a direct observer of work performance in order to give a credible appraisal (28). He or she should have a firm foundation in what needs to be accomplished to get the job done successfully. Some managers will ask for input from other individuals who interact with the employee being evaluated to ensure an unbiased appraisal. Just remember that sincerity and honesty are the keys to a successful performance appraisal.

Preappraisal Preparation

Appraiser. Approximately two weeks before the performance appraisal, appraisers should schedule the appraisal in a comfortable, nonthreatening, neutral location where there will be no interruptions (43). Prepare for the meeting by reviewing your documentation and the employee's self-appraisal and/or list of accomplishments (32, 35, 43, 47, 50). Make the appraisal a priority and start on time. It is advisable to sit next to the employee rather than across a desk to encourage open conversation. Refrain from taking phone calls during the interview. Allow enough time (at least 1 h) to complete a formal appraisal (28, 36).

Preparation by appraiser:

- Schedule meeting
- Select neutral location
- Prepare/review documentation
- Start on time
- Hold phone calls
- Allow enough time

Employees. Employees should be on time for the meeting. Self-appraisals should be submitted to the manager, preferably before the formal appraisal meeting. Employees should review their job description, the standards for the position, the organizational mission statement, and their goals and accomplishments (40, 47). They should connect their goals with the organizational goals (28). Employees should prepare a list of goals for the coming year and should discuss any obstacles that might impede the accomplishment of those goals. They should be prepared to suggest a solution to a problem. Goals should be established that stretch the employees' capabilities. Employees should be forthright, positive, and honest and provide feedback to their managers. Employees should listen and be open to suggestions. They should ask for specifics and clarification if they believe the appraisal is not reflective of their performance. When given the opportunity to provide written comments, they should document any specific disagreements on their performance appraisal form (35, 47).

Preparation by employee:

- Complete self-appraisal
- Review job description, performance standards, mission statement, goals, and accomplishments
- Relate personal goals with organizational goals
- Prepare list of future goals
- Identify obstacles
- Provide feedback
- Listen and be open to suggestions
- Ask for specifics and clarification

Steps to a Successful Performance Appraisal Interview

Preliminary meeting with employee. The purpose of the meeting is to explore ways to achieve personal and organizational goals and make improvements. Begin the interview by initiating friendly conversation to put the employee (and yourself) at ease. Explain the purpose of the performance appraisal and review the organizational and departmental mission statements, the job description, the performance standards, the goals of the organization and those previously set with the employee, and the self-appraisal before

beginning the formal interview. Remember that performance appraisals should hold no surprises and should not be punitive. Reinforce that the overall intent is for feedback to be motivational (28). Instead of covering every point on the form, be more conversational because the employee will receive a copy of the form to read later.

Formal meeting. Approach the performance appraisal in a positive and respectful manner. The performance appraisal process should motivate employees and should encourage their feedback, so don't do all of the talking and don't answer your own questions. Ask open-ended questions to stimulate discussion and obtain employee responses (28). For example, you may ask questions (47) such as, "What is your understanding of the performance expectations?" "Do you need more training?" "What kind of support can I provide for you to help you accomplish your goals?" Listen actively and intently, do not interrupt, and give feedback. Summarize comments made by the employee during the discussion to ensure that you understand what the employee is conveying to you. Be forthright and constructive in your evaluation, but not critical. Now is not the time to be timid. Most employees have some room for improvement. Using the halo effect (28, 35, 36, 40, 43), whereby you give positive performance appraisals even when undeserved, does nothing to stimulate behavioral modification (35). Likewise, avoid the pitchfork effect (36, 40), by which a single instance of poor performance adversely affects your overall assessment.

If you point out deficiencies without a plan for improvement, the employee may leave the meeting not knowing how to change the situation (40). The end result is that you will not see behavioral modification. Even if behavior modification is needed, focus on how you and your employee can work together to create a positive outcome. Set goals (generally at least four) for the coming year and help the employee specify the behaviors that must be changed to meet these goals. Make sure the goals are realistic, but at least one of them should be a stretch (28, 40, 43, 44). It is important that you communicate with your staff on a daily basis and keep them informed. Listen to them and share your vision and the organization's vision. Celebrate small and large victories and be generous with your praise. Finally, treat others with respect.

At the beginning of the meeting, inform the employee that you may refer to your notes, and that you may take notes during the discussion that will become part of the personnel file. Let the employee know that he or she will have an opportunity to review your written summary, add statements to the document, sign it, and receive a copy before you place it in the personnel file (28). If the employee refuses to sign the performance appraisal, document this and sign the form along with a witness. Also include the date of the meeting and a summary of the agreements you have made. Set follow-up dates and make sure you keep the appointments (21, 32). Disciplinary sessions should be scheduled separately from the performance appraisal. The "do's" and "don'ts" of a performance appraisal (28) are summarized in Table 16.1.

Steps to be taken by appraiser during formal appraisal:

- Observe directly
- Rate behavior
- Measure productivity
- Determine if specific goals have been accomplished
- Establish organizational initiatives
- Identify incidents
- State impact or consequences of behavior
- List additional training received
- Identify future goals

If managers lack the skills necessary to execute an appraisal, they should receive training in how to effectively give feedback to staff members (28). Training should include a review of the organizational philosophy, the purpose of the program, and how to complete the forms and score the evaluation (50), give feedback in a positive man-

Table 16.1 Do's and don'ts when conducting a performance appraisal[a]

Do's

Prepare ahead.

Explain the purpose of the appraisal.

Review the mission statement, job description, standards, and goals.

Focus on performance.

Provide specific performance examples and offer actions.

State impact or consequences of behavior.

Communicate sincerely.

Ask open-ended questions.

Listen to employees.

Summarize to ensure understanding.

Encourage feedback.

Be objective and use objective language.

Be as clear and concise as possible.

Use examples of behaviors you observed.

Set new goals and standards.

Develop an action plan.

Document the appraisal.

Follow up.

Don'ts

Do not use the appraisal to discipline for past negative performance.

Do not focus on personality issues.

Do not make gender-based statements.

Do not generalize.

Do not use subjective language.

Do not interrupt.

Do not discuss salary until after the appraisal.

[a]From reference 27.

ner, focus on performance and not personality, coach for improvement (5, 29, 35, 46), make wage and promotional decisions using performance data, and discover weak spots and correct them. Establish a list of words or phrases to be used for coaching and appraisal discussions (34, 35). Some organizations provide this training at orientation for new managers and annually thereafter.

Appraiser training:

- Review organizational philosophy
- Understand purpose of performance appraisals
- Know how to complete the form and score the evaluation
- Provide feedback in a positive manner
- Focus on performance, not personality
- Coach for improvement
- Understand how to make wage and promotional decisions based on performance appraisals

Benefits of Becoming a Mentor

The appraisal process can be a forum for career development by focusing on employee development, coaching, and training needs. You may, in fact, take on the role of a mentor or trusted advisor to your employees. A mentor typically shares information, experiences, and lessons in leadership. You must believe in your employees, encourage, support, and coach them to aspire to higher goals. Proudly represent your employees to others, lead by example, and exhibit a positive attitude. Mentors tend to take a big-picture approach, getting involved only when help is requested. Mentors thus become a positive force in employee career development (28).

Mentor responsibilities:

- Share information and experiences
- Believe in your employees
- Encourage, support, and coach your employees
- Proudly represent your employees to others
- Lead by example
- Exhibit a positive attitude

Salary Adjustments

Merit increases usually are the end product of formal performance appraisals that connect levels of performance with varying levels of salary increase. It is better to have separate meetings for the performance appraisal and salary increase so that you do not run the risk of feeling pressured to start the conversation by announcing a salary adjustment and then justifying your decision (36, 43).

Strategies To Reinforce Appropriate Behaviors

According to the law of effect, behaviors that are followed by positive consequences are more likely to be repeated. Providing positive consequences or rewards increases the probability that an appropriate behavior will be repeated (35). To be effective, however, positive reinforcement should be applied as soon as possible following the behavior and must be contingent on the desired behavior. This is one reason why informal appraisals are crucial to the success of the appraisal process; the employee does not have to wait a year to learn which behaviors are appropriate and which are inappropriate.

Guidelines for Appraising Poor Performers

Ensure that the employee has a current copy of his or her job description and performance standards. During the interview, give examples of poor performance to support your assessment and the consequences of the behavior (2). This can best be done by providing documentation of how the employee's work does not meet standards and by reviewing previous discussions you may have had with the employee regarding the problem. Prepare a list of specific changes you would like him or her to make and the time frame in which to correct the behavior. Present the information in a manner that shows confidence in the employee's ability to improve. Set measurable standards for improvement and plan together how this can be accomplished. It is important that you plan on meeting in the interim to review the improvement and assess and encourage the employee.

Dealing with Emotional Outbursts during Performance Appraisals

If the employee engages in an emotional outburst or demonstrates signs of aggression, the manager should deal cautiously with the individual. You may want to encourage the employee to seek assistance from the employee assistance program (EAP) (28), if your organization has one. If you anticipate an interview with a negative employee, spend extra time preparing for the meeting. This may require consultation with Human Resources on how to deal with out-of-control employees. It is important that you do not respond emotionally to an employee who is out of control (32). Results of performance appraisals can incite emotions that sometimes are difficult to deal with. For example, crying or shouting may call for a time-out so the employee can regain composure and the appraisal can be productive. Employees can disengage either due to the appraisal or for personal reasons. You will need to conduct an intervention as soon as possible, particularly if you are interested in retaining the employee.

Completed Performance Appraisal Documents

A fully executed written appraisal is a complete and confidential original document, with any changes, added comments, and signatures in place (28) (Appendix 16.4). The original document should be placed in the employee's personnel file and kept in a secure place for the number of years that is specified by organizational policy. Employees should be given a completed copy for their records. Finally, the manager should keep a copy in his or her files.

Requirements for performance appraisal documents:

- Maintain confidentiality
- Complete original, sign, and date
- Place original in personnel file
- Keep documents according to policy
- Provide a copy to employee
- Place copy in manager's file

Improvement Plan

One of the most important points of the appraisal form is to document feedback and improvements (32, 35). An improvement plan may be added to the performance appraisal form to identify ways to help an employee improve or attain a higher level of performance. Courts tend to rule more favorably when an organization assists poor performers in improving their performance. Examples of ways to improve performance may include working side-by-side with a more experienced technologist, attending continuing educational programs, and working in another section of the laboratory in order to understand how each section is related to other sections.

Web-Based Software Products and Websites

Software can be purchased to automate the performance appraisal process (Appendix 16.5). A software program may provide action plans for an employee who is rated below average for a task. Although software programs may make it easier to execute appraisals, the downside is that they tend to decrease interpersonal communication, one of the key factors in a successful appraisal program.

Competency Assessment

Even though laboratories regularly evaluate the performance of their employees for salary increase and job promotion, a regulatory requirement to have an objective system to document employee competency did not exist prior to 1988. Although external proficiency testing is a measurement of the ability to achieve a desired outcome for a particular analyte in question, it is not synonymous with competency. What is competency? JCAHO defines competency as a determination of an individual's capability to perform up to defined expectations (24). Another helpful definition of competency is the ability to do a job correctly and safely and to recognize and solve minor problems without needing assistance (41).

Regulatory Foundation for Competency Assessment

Assessment of personnel competency is mandated by federal statute and is a component of the accreditation programs of the College of American Pathologists (CAP), JCAHO, and COLA. This section reviews the specific regulations.

A federal statute resulted from passage by Congress of the Clinical Laboratory Improvement Amendments (CLIA)

Table 16.2 Responsibilities for competency assessment mandated by CLIA[a]

Moderate-complexity testing	High-complexity testing
42 CFR Sec. 493.1407	42 CFR Sec. 493.1445
"The laboratory director must ensure that policies and procedures are established for monitoring individuals who conduct preanalytical, analytical, and postanalytical phases of testing to assure that they are competent and maintain their competency to process specimens, perform test procedures and report test results promptly and proficiently, and whenever necessary, identify needs for remedial training or continuing education to improve skills. . . ."	"The laboratory director must ensure that policies and procedures are established for monitoring individuals who conduct preanalytical, analytical, and postanalytical phases of testing to assure that they are competent and maintain their competency to process specimens, perform test procedures and report test results promptly and proficiently, and whenever necessary, identify needs for remedial training or continuing education to improve skills. . . ."
42 CFR Sec. 493.1413	42 CFR Sec. 493.1451
"The technical consultant is responsible for evaluating the competency of all testing personnel and assuring that the staff maintain their competency to perform test procedures and report test results promptly, accurately, and proficiently."	"The technical supervisor is responsible for evaluating the competency of all testing personnel and assuring that the staff maintain their competency to perform test procedures and report test results promptly, accurately, and proficiently."

[a]Available at http://www.phppo.cdc.gov/clia/default.asp.

of 1988 and subsequent signature by the president of Public Law 100-578 (3). CLIA '88 (4) classifies commercially marketed in vitro diagnostic tests into three levels of complexity (waived, moderate, and high) and defines qualifications for personnel performing testing across the spectrum of sites in which testing is performed (i.e., qualifications are site-neutral). The CLIA '88 personnel standards provide a number of routes for individuals with diverse educational and training backgrounds to meet the federal regulations. To provide quality assurance of personnel within this framework, the laboratory must have an ongoing mechanism to evaluate the effectiveness of its policies and procedures for assuring employee competence (42 CFR Sec. 493.1713).

CLIA '88 charges both the laboratory director and the technical consultant or technical supervisor with specific responsibilities for the competency assessment program of the laboratory. Policies and procedures should address the entire testing process, including preanalytical, analytical, and postanalytical phases (Table 16.2).

Through the Laboratory Accreditation Program, CAP provides inspection checklist guidelines (6) that address employee training and experience, performance reviews, and competency assessment (Table 16.3). In 1996, JCAHO initiated a standard to be used by hospitals to assess, document, and improve the competency of all employees. The standards focus on job-specific, measurable, demonstrated, age-specific competency statements (11). In addition, JCAHO standards specify the responsibilities of laboratory management pertaining to the assessment and maintenance of employee competency and ongoing learning and development (24). For office-based laboratories, COLA re-

quires that the laboratory director or technical consultant periodically evaluate personnel performance (7).

Regulatory agencies specifying competency requirements:

- CAP
- JCAHO
- COLA

Table 16.3 CAP checklist questions pertaining to competency[a]

GEN.54400 Phase II

Do technical personnel records include all of the following mandatory items?:

1. Summary of training and experience,
2. Formal certification or license, if required by state,
3. Description of duties (may be generic to a position),
4. Records of continuing education.

GEN.54750 Phase II

For laboratories subject to US federal regulation, do all testing personnel meet CLIA-88 requirements?

GEN.55200 Phase II

Are there annual reviews of the performance of existing employees and an initial review of new employees within the first six months?

GEN.55500 Phase II

Has the competency of each person to perform his/her assigned duties been assessed?

[a]From reference 6. Reprinted by permission.

Timing of Competency Assessment

CLIA '88 mandates that the technical consultant of a laboratory performing moderate-complexity testing (42 CFR Sec. 493.1413) or the technical supervisor of a laboratory performing high-complexity testing (42 CFR Sec. 493.1451) be responsible for evaluating and documenting employee performance at least semiannually during the first year of employment. Subsequent evaluations are to be performed annually unless test methodology or instrumentation changes have occurred, in which case, prior to reporting patient test results, the individual's performance using the new test methodology or instrumentation must be evaluated.

Upon employment, all new hires should participate in a laboratory orientation program to ensure that patient test results will not be reported until the desired skill level has been demonstrated. An orientation checklist (Appendixes 16.6, 16.7, and 16.8) may facilitate this process and may help to ensure standardization when multiple trainers are involved. Orientation may encompass a variety of activities such as reviewing laboratory procedure and policy manuals, observing the procedure being performed, performing the procedure under supervision, and completing a posttest examination. A guideline from NCCLS provides a framework by which the laboratory may develop a program for training verification (33). The length of time required for orientation will vary depending upon the employee's formal training and work experience and the number of test procedures to be mastered. CLIA '88 (42 CFR Sec. 493.1425 and 42 CFR Sec. 493.1489) specifies that training (Table 16.4) of testing personnel

> must ensure: 1) The skills required for proper specimen collection, including patient preparation, if applicable, labelling, handling, preservation or fixation, processing or preparation, transportation and storage of specimens; 2) The skills required for implementing all standard laboratory procedures; 3) The skills required for performing each test method and for proper instrument use; 4) The skills required for performing preventive maintenance, troubleshooting and calibration procedures related to each test performed; 5) A working knowledge of reagent stability and storage; 6) The skills required to implement the

Table 16.4 Employee skills required for competency[a]

Collect, label, process, transport, and store specimens.

Implement all standard laboratory procedures.

Perform each test method.

Perform preventive maintenance, trouble-shooting, and calibration procedures.

Understand reagent stability and storage.

Implement the quality control policies and procedures of the laboratory.

Understand factors that influence test results.

Assess quality control sample values prior to reporting patient test results.

[a]Available at http://www.phppo.cdc.gov/clia/default.asp.

quality control policies and procedures of the laboratory; 7) An awareness of the factors that influence test results; and 8) The skills required to assess and verify the validity of patient test results through the evaluation of quality control sample values prior to reporting patient test results.

Both the employee and the trainer must sign the documentation showing the specific training performed and the skill level attained. This documentation is maintained in the employee's file.

Both CLIA '88 and JCAHO require that competency of testing personnel be maintained on an ongoing basis. In addition to changes brought about by technological advances that may affect specific laboratory procedures or instrumentation, changes may also occur in the mission of an organization as delivery of healthcare evolves. To meet these challenges, ongoing education may be offered through a variety of formats, such as in-service educational programs, on-the-job training, audioconferences or teleconferences, self-instructional materials, local or national workshops, and local or national professional meetings. Documentation of the educational event, including the topic, date of presentation or participation, name of the presenter or trainer, and the individual participating, should be maintained in the employee's file as supporting evidence of ongoing competency.

Timing of competency assessment:

- Semiannually during first year for new employees
- Annually for all employees
- Preceding implementation of new methods or instrumentation

Methods for Assessment of Competency

CLIA '88 standards for assessment of personnel competency are the same for laboratories performing moderate- or high-complexity testing (42 CFR Sec. 493.1413 and 42 CFR Sec. 493.1451). The procedures (Table 16.5) for evaluation of competency

> must include, but are not limited to: 1) Direct observations of routine patient test performance, including patient preparation, if applicable, specimen handling, processing and testing; 2) Monitoring the recording and reporting of test results; 3) Review of intermediate test

Table 16.5 Methods to assess competency[a]

Directly observe specimen collection, handling, processing, and testing.

Monitor recording and reporting of test results.

Review preliminary/interim test results or worksheets, quality control records, proficiency test results, and preventive maintenance checks.

Directly observe performance of instrument maintenance and function checks.

Assess test performance through testing previously analyzed specimens, internal blind testing samples, or external proficiency testing samples.

Assess problem-solving skills.

[a]Available at http://www.phppo.cdc.gov/clia/default.asp.

results or worksheets, quality control records, proficiency test results, and preventive maintenance records; 4) Direct observation of performance of instrument maintenance and function checks; 5) Assessment of test performance through testing previously analyzed specimens, internal blind testing samples or external proficiency testing samples; and 6) Assessment of problem-solving skills.

There is no requirement that each method must be used for all tests that are being assessed (25).

CLIA '88 does not specify in detail how competency assessment should be accomplished to preserve flexibility for laboratory managers to design programs that will meet their own unique needs. Examining, documenting, and continually expanding the competency of staff is essential for maintaining test quality, particularly in an environment in which allied health training programs are closing and the workforce is downsizing. When designing a competency assessment program, laboratory managers must determine which assessment method(s) will best suit their needs (13, 30). Assessment may be targeted at functions identified as problem-prone or at critical functions in which errors are likely to go unnoticed (16). It is the intent of CLIA '88 and JCAHO that competency assessment programs be grounded in staff development (24) and efforts towards quality improvement (12). The assessment plan should be designed to give objective measurements (27). The assessment plan should also delineate who will conduct the assessments. Senior technologists proficient in a subspecialty area may be recruited to perform subspecialty evaluations (31), or experienced staff members may be trained in performing and documenting competency assessment (48).

Direct observation of technical skills is especially useful for those procedures that are manually performed, such as primary plating of cultures and venipuncture procedures. A checklist of predetermined skills (Appendixes 16.9 and 16.10) will enable systematic documentation of the critical procedural steps under review (1, 42). Direct observation is also indicated for monitoring performance of instrument maintenance and function checks.

Review of preliminary and final result work sheets, reported patient results (either via on-line or hard-copy format), quality control records, proficiency test results, and instrument preventive maintenance records should be occurring as part of the quality assurance program of the laboratory. Documentation of the review is the essential component that will satisfy the competency regulations. For example, in the competency program of one laboratory, three patient reports for three to six analytes were monitored and documented (39).

Assessment of test performance may be accomplished using previously analyzed specimens, internal blind testing samples, or external proficiency testing samples. Given the limited amount or number of samples provided in external proficiency testing programs, a laboratory with many employees may need to utilize a combination of several methods to assess test performance. In one hematology laboratory, an exam based on microscope slides proved to be better than one based on color transparencies for improving daily practice skills (20). Another laboratory used a computer-assisted chi-square calculation on a 100-cell differential as an effective competency assessment tool (49). In the microbiology laboratory, retention of challenging Gram-stained smears (e.g., unusual organisms, gram-negative diplococci in blood cultures, cerebrospinal fluid, or other body fluid with occasional organisms present) can be used for a microscope slide-based competency evaluation.

A JCAHO standard requires assessment of age-related competencies of those staff providing direct patient care (23, 24). This standard is therefore applicable to laboratory phlebotomists whose practices vary with the patient age group. A continuing education exercise pertaining to age-specific phlebotomy techniques has been published (26). Demonstration of problem-solving skills may be assessed through self-reports of problem resolutions submitted by the employee. For example, if the quality control of an assay is outside expected limits, an employee can report the corrective action taken to achieve quality control results within range. Documentation of the steps taken to resolve receipt of unlabeled or mislabeled specimens is another example of problem-solving skills. Alternatively, an employee may complete a written exercise indicating how he or she would resolve an issue (14). This documentation should be maintained in the employee's file to support ongoing competency.

The laboratory's competency assessment plan should include procedures to address employees who fail the assessment. These procedures should include the time for retraining, reassessment, and expected outcomes (15, 19, 24, 43a).

Current Practices

Current practices of employee competency assessment are reflected in data from a recent interlaboratory survey (22). In this study, employee competency was evaluated through the use of test and quality control results (77.4%), direct observations (87.5%), instrument preventive maintenance (60.0%), and written testing (52.2%). In 77 to 95% of laboratories surveyed, the supervisors/managers performed the competency evaluation of employees, whereas in 19 to 31% of laboratories, the evaluations were performed by peers. Delegation of competency assessment may be necessary to execute the plan. If the employee failed the competency evaluation, in 52% of laboratories, the employee was retested within 4 weeks, while in 8.6% of laboratories, the policy was to disallow the employee from continuing usual work. Adherence to the plan was inversely related to the number of full-time equivalents, the total number of employees, and the number of supervisors in the laboratory. There was less compliance with the plan in teaching hospitals compared to nonteaching hospitals. These data indicate that difficulties may occur in completing the assessment of each employee each year as the size and complexity of the laboratory increases.

JCAHO requires that hospitals provide annual competency evaluation of employees in fire safety, infection control, and blood-borne pathogens. Beyond traditional lectures or written self-study modules, computer-based programs can be a cost-effective and efficient method of providing and documenting this assessment (51). This modality offers uniform presentation and 24-hour availability, features that are particularly helpful in healthcare organizations that must assess staff on three different work shifts.

Personnel Excellence

In addition to specific competencies reflected in job skills and knowledge, managers and executives should encourage professionalism, accountability, and self-esteem as competencies required to ensure customer service (10). These three competencies form the foundation of a hierarchy of all other generic competencies (10). In the 21st century, the quality and success of your laboratory depends on selecting, developing, and retaining competent staff.

Summary

In summary, always remember that a successful appraisal recognizes people as the most valuable resource of an organization. The most important reason for doing appraisals is to motivate your employees positively, not to punish. Recognizing accomplishments is a powerful way to motivate. Providing performance appraisals will show employees that you and the organization are interested in their work and in their development. An integral part of assessing employee performance is a well-designed competency program. Documentation of each individual's job-related competency is one way that a laboratory can not only ensure quality results, but also fulfill federal and accrediting agency requirements.

KEY POINTS

- Performance appraisals are powerful motivating tools that are closely integrated with compensation, training, and career planning.
- An effective appraisal system includes formal and informal ongoing performance feedback.
- A well-designed appraisal program requires clearly defined standards, feedback, and documentation that are applied consistently among all employees.
- Job expectations must be clearly stated.
- Elements of a formal appraisal should be based on an organization's mission statement, the job description, and the performance standards.
- Performance standards should be specific, measurable, and realistic.

- An employee's performance, not his or her ability, should be rated.
- Selection of a rating method depends on the purpose of the appraisal, the work environment, the skills of the employee, and the management style of the manager(s).
- Self-appraisals give a different perspective of the employee's performance and a better understanding of obstacles that may impede performance.
- Peer-to-peer and 360-degree evaluations, if performed honestly, sincerely, and anonymously, may provide the employee with insight into his or her work relationships and performance.
- Preappraisal preparation by employees and managers is essential for a successful performance appraisal interview.
- Performance appraisals should hold no surprises and should not be punitive.
- The performance appraisal process should be motivating and should encourage feedback.
- If behavior modification is needed, focus on how you and your employee can work together to create a positive outcome.
- The employee should set at least four realistic goals for the coming year.
- Individuals performing appraisals should be given training and review the do's and don'ts of conducting appraisals to sharpen their skills in executing a successful interview.
- The appraisal process can and should be a form of career development.
- A manager can become a mentor and a positive force in an employee's career development.
- Appropriate behaviors may be reinforced with positive consequences.
- Recognizing accomplishments is a powerful way to motivate.
- A manager should provide examples of poor performance, if applicable, and the consequences of an unsatisfactory behavior.
- A manager should not overreact if an employee has an emotional outburst during an interview. Encourage the employee to seek assistance from the EAP, if available.
- Documentation and confidentiality are essential components of any performance appraisal program.
- A manager should identify ways to help an employee attain a higher level of performance.
- A successful appraisal program recognizes employees as the most valuable resource of an organization.
- Employee competency should be assessed semiannually the first year of employment and annually thereafter.

- Employee competency should be assessed whenever a change in test method or instrumentation occurs.

- Ongoing training and education are necessary to maintain and enhance employee competency.

- Thorough documentation of employee competency must be maintained for inspection by accreditation agencies.

- Competent employees are the foundation for the quality and success of any laboratory.

GLOSSARY

360-degree evaluations Multilevel assessment adopted by AT&T, IBM, and other Fortune 500 corporations. May be used to identify how a manager is viewed by his or her supervisor, peers, subordinates, and customers. Full-circle feedback.

Americans with Disabilities Act (ADA) Prohibits discrimination against qualified disabled individuals. Applies to institutions with 15 or more employees.

Appraisal type Formal and informal appraisals, self-appraisals, peer-to-peer appraisals, 360-degree appraisals.

Behaviorally anchored rating scale (BARS) Assessment of performance requiring input from other observers based on how employees behaved in a given situation.

Checklist adjectives evaluation At least three adjectives (e.g., aggressive, articulate, meticulous) from a checklist are selected to describe desirable as well as undesirable characteristics of an employee.

Clinical Laboratory Improvement Amendments (CLIA) '88 An act passed by Congress in 1988 that required an objective system to document competency of employees performing testing on patient specimens.

COLA (formerly the Commission on Office Laboratory Accreditation) A national nonprofit physician-directed organization that provides continuing medical education programs, accreditation standards, and accreditation of physician office laboratories.

College of American Pathologists (CAP) A medical society of board-certified pathologists that provides proficiency testing samples, continuing medical education programs, accreditation standards and accreditation of pathology and laboratory services.

Competency Ability to do a job correctly and safely and to recognize and solve minor problems without needing assistance.

Criterion Standard of judging task performance.

Critical incident evaluation Written notations of exceptional performance are summarized in the performance appraisal.

Employee Assistance Program (EAP) Psychological assessment and brief treatment; considered an employee benefit.

Equal Employment Opportunity Commission of 1972 Enforces ADA.

Forced distribution Rater distributes a certain percent of employees in each category (e.g., outstanding, above average, average, below average, unsatisfactory).

Graphic rating scales A quality or characteristic rated by choosing a point along a horizontal axis. The scale may be discrete (1-2-3-4-5, excellent-good-fair-poor-unacceptable) or continuous.

Halo effect Appraiser gives all employees an acceptable rating, regardless of their performance. When an employee is outstanding in one area, an evaluator ignores performance problems in other areas. Opposite of the "pitchfork effect."

Interview A two-way discussion between employee and manager about employee's performance (inter "between," view "look").

Joint Commission on Accreditation of Healthcare Organizations (JCAHO) An independent, not-for-profit organization that develops accreditation standards and accredits healthcare organizations.

Key results area An aspect of a job on which employees must concentrate time and attention to ensure that they achieve the goal for that job. Forces manager to focus only on those activities that add value. Although motivational, staff may be slow to accept.

Narrative rating Includes concise, specific illustrations. Easy to construct, but subjective and difficult to compare employee's ratings.

NCCLS (formerly the National Committee for Clinical Laboratory Standards) A voluntary national organization that issues guidelines for laboratory practices.

Norms Informal behaviors that are generally acceptable in a workplace.

Performance appraisal A planned, formal, and periodic management activity in which an employee's on-the-job behavior is evaluated to enable salary and promotion decisions, change an employee's behavior, determine competence, improve work skills, identify training needs, and determine progress toward goals and career development.

Performance standards Defined performance expectations that are specific and measurable.

Pitchfork effect Poor performance in an isolated instance that adversely affects an employee's assessment.

Ranking system Evaluates employees based on comparison with their peers (e.g., paired comparison, person-to-person comparison). This system does not allow all employees to be ranked as excellent, even if all employees have an excellent work performance.

Rating system Compares employee performance to some set of criteria and produces either a number or a letter grade that represents the employee's level of performance (e.g., graphic scale, free form, critical incident, behaviorally anchored scale, checklist of adjectives, forced choice, or distribution). Allows everyone to be rated highly, if they deserve it.

Results-based evaluations (RBE) Evaluations performed by managers who focus on attainment of specific, measurable results.

Standard Operating Procedure (SOP) Organizational approved protocol that defines step-by-step instructions for all staff to follow when performing a particular test or activity to ensure a consistent and accurate result or outcome.

REFERENCES

1. Baer, D. M. 1997. An operational approach to competency assessment. *MLO Med. Lab. Obs.* **29**(2):55–58.

2. Buhler, P. 1992. *Human Resources Management,* p. 5–103. Amacon, New York, N.Y.

3. Clinical Laboratory Improvement Amendments, Public Law 100-578, 102 Stat. 2903-2915. October 31, 1988. 42 U.S.C. 263a.

4. Code of Federal Regulations. 1992. Clinical Laboratory Improvement Amendments of 1988, final rule. *Fed. Regist.* 42 CFR 493.

5. Coens, T., and M. Jenkins. 2000. *Abolishing Performance Appraisals: Why They Backfire and What to Do Instead.* Berrett-Koehler Publishers, Inc., San Francisco, Calif.

6. College of American Pathologists. 2002. *Laboratory Accreditation Program Laboratory General Checklist,* rev. August 8. A. Rabinovitch (ed.). College of American Pathologists, Northfield, Ill.

7. Commission on Office Laboratory Accreditation. 2000. *Laboratory Accreditation Manual,* rev. 6. Commission on Office Laboratory Accreditation, Columbia, Md.

8. Constantine, D. 1998. Multisource assessment: rating and compensating employees. *Am. Compens. Assoc. News* **41**(5):30–32.

9. Day, C. M. 1991. A hard look at performance reviews. *MLO Med. Lab. Obs.* **23**(11):61–62.

10. Decker, P. J. 1999. The hidden competencies of healthcare: why self-esteem, accountability, and professionalism may affect hospital customer satisfaction scores. *Hosp. Top.* **77**(1):14–26.

11. Decker, P. J., M. K. Strader, and R. J. Wise. 1997. Beyond JCAHO: using competency models to improve healthcare organizations. Part 1. *Hosp. Top.* **75**(1):23–28.

12. Decker, P. J., M. K. Strader, and R. J. Wise. 1997. Beyond JCAHO: using competency models to change healthcare organizations. Part 2: developing competence assessment systems. *Hosp. Top.* **75**(2):10–17.

13. Elder, B. L., and S. E. Sharp. 2003. *Cumitech 39, Competency Assessment in the Clinical Microbiology Laboratory.* Coordinating ed., S. E. Sharp. ASM Press, Washington, D.C.

14. Ellinger, P. J. 1995. Q & A: Assessing competency of laboratory personnel. *Lab. Med.* **26**(1):19.

15. Ellinger, P. J. 2002. *Tech Sample Management and Education No. MGM-2: Competency Assessment.* American Society for Clinical Pathology, Chicago, Ill.

16. Galel, S. A., and C. A. Richards. 1997. Practical approaches to improve laboratory performance and transfusion safety. *Am. J. Clin. Pathol.* **107**(Suppl. 1):S43–S49.

17. Garcia, L. S. 1989. *Tech Sample Management and Education No. MGM-2: The Development and Use of Performance Standards.* American Society for Clinical Pathology, Chicago, Ill.

18. Garcia, L. S. 1995. *Tech Sample Management and Education No. MGM-6: Employee Performance Evaluations: Past Approaches and New Options.* American Society for Clinical Pathology, Chicago, Ill.

19. Gerbasi, S. 2000. Competency assessment in a team-based laboratory. *MLO Med. Lab. Obs.* **32**(9):46–54.

20. Haun, D. E., A. P. Leach, D. F. Fink, and G. Lipscomb. 2000. A better way to assess WBC differential counting skills. *Lab. Med.* **31**(6):329–333.

21. Heller, R., and T. Hindle. 1998. *Essential Manager's Manual.* D. K. Publishing, Inc., New York, N.Y.

22. Howanitz, P. J., P. N. Valenstein, and G. Fine. 2000. Employee competence and performance-based assessment: a College of American Pathologists Q-Probe study of laboratory personnel in 522 institutions. *Arch. Pathol. Lab. Med.* **124**(2):195–202.

23. Joint Commission on Accreditation of Healthcare Organizations. 1998. *Age-Specific Competence.* Joint Commission on Accreditation of Healthcare Organizations, Oakbrook Terrace, Ill.

24. Joint Commission on Accreditation of Health Care Organizations. 1999. *2000–2001 Comprehensive Accreditation Manual for Pathology and Clinical Laboratory Services.* Joint Commission on Accreditation of Healthcare Organizations, Oakbrook Terrace, Ill.

25. Joint Commission on Accreditation of Healthcare Organizations. 2001. *The Competent Laboratory.* Joint Commission on Accreditation of Healthcare Organizations, Oakbrook Terrace, Ill.

26. Kirven, D. R. 2003. Age-specific techniques in phlebotomy competency: understanding and incorporating age-specific competence in evaluating the phlebotomist's performance. *Adv. Med. Lab. Prof.* **15**(6):11–17.

27. Larison, J. 1993. Laboratory practice: personnel competency assessment. *Clin. Lab. Sci.* **6**(1):13–14.

28. Margrave, A., and R. Gorden. 2001. *The Complete Idiot's Guide to Performance Appraisals.* Alpha Books, Indianapolis, Ind.

29. Markle, G. L. 2000. *Catalytic Coaching: The End of the Performance Review.* Greenwood Publishing Group, Westport, Conn.

30. McCarter, Y. S., and A. Robinson. 1997. Competency assessment in clinical microbiology. *Clin. Microbiol. Newsl.* **19**(13):97–101.

31. McCaskey, L., and M. LaRocco. 1995. Competency testing in clinical microbiology. *Lab. Med.* **26**(5):343–349.

32. McKirchy, K. 1998. *Powerful Performance Appraisals.* Career Press, Franklin Lakes, N.J.

33. NCCLS. 1995. *Training Verification for Laboratory Personnel; Approved Guideline.* NCCLS document GP21-A. NCCLS, Wayne, Pa.

34. Neal, J. E. 1997. *Effective Phrases for Performance Appraisals: A Guide to Successful Evaluations,* 9th ed. Neal Publications, Inc., Perrysburg, Ohio.

35. Neal, J. E. 2001. *The #1 Guide to Performance Appraisals.* Neal Publications, Inc., Perrysburg, Ohio.

36. Nelson, B., and P. Economy. 1996. Performance evaluations: not necessarily a waste of time, p. 153–165. *In* B. Nelson and P. Economy (ed.), *Managing for Dummies.* IDG Books Worldwide, Inc., Foster City, Calif.

37. Nichols, F. 1997. Don't redesign your company's performance appraisal system, scrap it! *Corp. Univ. Rev.* **5**(3):54–59.

38. Nigon, D. L. 2000. Managing people, p. 63–105. *In* D. L. Nigon (ed.), *Clinical Laboratory Management: Leadership Principles for the 21st Century.* McGraw-Hill, New York, N.Y.

39. Nordenson, N. J. 1997. Strategic competency assessment: a plan to minimize extra work in conducting employee reviews. *MLO Med. Lab. Obs.* **29**(10):50–53.

40. Pell, A. R. 1999. Evaluating team members' performance, p. 269–284. *In* A. R. Pell, *The Complete Idiot's Guide to Managing People,* 2nd ed. Alpha Books, Indianapolis, Ind.

41. **Ruthemeyer, M.** 2000. The competency question. *Radiol. Manage.* **22**(5):20–28.

42. **Schiffgens, J.** 2001. A four-part approach to competency assessment. *Lab. Med.* **32**(8):431–435.

43. **Scotto, D.** 1999. Performance appraisals: more than just going through the motions. *MLO Med. Lab. Obs.* **31**(3):38–43, 57.

43a. **Sharp, S.** 2001. Initial training verification and competency assessment in the clinical microbiology laboratory. [Editorial.] *Clin. Microbiol. Newsl.* **23**(10):79–81.

44. **Snyder, J. R.** 1987. *Tech Sample Management and Education No. MGM-4: Refocusing the Employee Performance Appraisal Process.* American Society for Clinical Pathology, Chicago, Ill.

45. **Snyder, J. R.** 1991. Assessing the legality of performance appraisals. *Clin. Lab. Manage. Rev.* **5**(6):483–489.

46. **Swan, W. S.** 1991. *How to Do a Superior Performance Appraisal.* John Wiley and Sons, New York, N.Y.

47. **Umiker, W. O.** 1984. The performance review and planning session, p. 208–215. *In* W. O. Umiker (ed.), *The Effective Laboratory Supervisor.* Medical Economic Books, Oradell, N.J.

48. **Vengelen-Tyler, V.** 2001. *Tech Sample Management and Education No. MGM-6: How to Improve Documentation of Staff Competency.* American Society for Clinical Pathology, Chicago, Ill.

49. **Warner, S.** 2001. Using chi-square and a PC to assess competency. *MLO Med. Lab. Obs.* **33**(7):48–51.

50. **Wolfgang, J. W., and K. E. Wolfgang.** 1998. Standards and appraisals of laboratory performance, p. 245–254. *In* J. R. Snyder and D. W. Wilkinson (ed.), *Management in Laboratory Medicine*, 3rd ed. Lippincott, Philadelphia, Pa.

51. **Wolford, R. A., and L. K. Hughes.** 2001. Using the hospital intranet to meet competency standards for nurses. *J. Nurs. Staff Dev.* **17**(4):182–187.

APPENDIX 16.1 Medical Technologist Job Description

Job code: 4000

Position summary: The medical technologist position performs and interprets specialized laboratory procedures to obtain data for use in the diagnosis, monitoring, and treatment of disease in a timely and cost-effective manner to medical center patients. Essential functions:

(Part A)

1. Behaves in a manner that is ethical, professional, and consistent with the medical center core values.

(Part B)

2. Accepts personal responsibility for self-development as demonstrated by continuing education, licensure, and risk management.

(Part C)

3. Demonstrates good interpersonal skills in communication and collaboration, including team building and teaching.
4. Adapts to changes in technology and in the healthcare environment.
5. Understands and performs the technical and computer skills required for the departmental standard test methods.
6. Complies with policies as described in the departmental standard operating procedures (SOPs) for result reporting, quality control (QC), proficiency testing, occurrence documentation, record keeping, and safety.
7. Demonstrates the ability to organize the work in an efficient and cost-effective manner.

Effective: 12/2002

APPENDIX 16.2   Medical Technologist Performance Standards

Name: _____   Rating Period: _____

	Service excellence standards					
	Consistently exceeds standards	Occasionally exceeds standards	Meets standards	Occasionally meets standards	Rarely meets standards	NA
Care—friendliness, respect, diversity, and commitment						
1. Greets patients with a smile and says "Hello."	4					
2. Makes eye contact, listens, and provides assistance.	4					
3. States name and uses patient's name whenever possible.	4					
4. Knocks on the door before entering patient's room.						X
5. Closes curtains and door during exams and procedures.						X
6. Does not discuss patient information in public areas.		3				
7. Keeps patient information confidential.		3				
8. Works to provide a clean and safe environment.		3				
Professional Appearance						
9. Maintains a professional appearance.	4					
10. Clothing is neat and clean.	4					
11. Wears employee identification badge consistently, in a manner that is easily seen.	4					
12. Hair is clean and well-groomed.	4					
Communication—information, education, call lights, telephone, listening and empathy						
13. Uses easily understood language when interacting with patients or customers.	4					
14. Introduces him- or herself to patients and explains his or her role in the patient's care.						X
15. Answers call lights, addressing patient by name.						X
16. Answers telephone in a pleasant tone, identifying department and giving name.	4					
17. Explains delays and thanks patients for waiting.		3				
18. Concludes interactions by asking, "Is there anything else I can do for you?"		3				

(continued)

APPENDIX 16.2 Medical Technologist Performance Standards *(continued)*

Name: _____   Rating period: _____

Service excellence standards						
	Consistently exceeds standards	Occasionally exceeds standards	Meets standards	Occasionally meets standards	Rarely meets standards	NA
Service—service recovery and teamwork						
19. Recovers service disappointments.		3				
20. If approached for directions, offers to escort patients/customers to their destination.		3				
21. Interacts with coworkers respectfully and professionally.		3				
22. Does not discuss staffing levels or system deficits with customers.		3				
23. Demonstrates teamwork.	4					
Department-specific standards (optional)						
24.						
25.						
Sum	40	27				
Sum of scores for standards:	67					
Number of standards scored:	19					
Score per standard:	3.5263					
Total number of standards:	25					
Total score:	88.16					
Service excellence score	88.16					

(continued)

APPENDIX 16.2 Medical Technologist Performance Standards *(continued)*

Employee mandatory requirements

	Yes	No	NA[a]
Note: By responding yes to the mandatory items, you are indicating that back-up documentation can be provided upon request.			
Licensure is current and appropriate for present job.	X		
Received annual employee health screening in a timely manner.	X		
Meets mandatory educational requirements of regulatory/accrediting agencies by attending training or viewing videos.	X		
Meets mandatory training requirements for the present job. Includes such items as fire safety, etc.	X		
Annually reviews and signs the nondisclosure and appropriate use agreement (Health Insurance Portability and Accountability Act).	X		
Annually attends training or views videos regarding the organizational compliance program.	X		
Attends department-specific compliance testing.	X		
Attends all meetings identified as mandatory.	X		
Meets timekeeping and attendance expectations.	X		
Mandatory score	Met		

[a]NA, Not applicable.

Scoring: 4-consistently exceeds standards, 3-occasionally exceeds standards, 2-meets standards, 1-occasionally meets standards, 0-rarely meets standards

APPENDIX 16.3 Medical Technologist Job-Specific Competencies

Name:		Rating period:	
1. Understands and performs the technical and computer skills required for the departmental standard test methods.	**Weight**[a]	**Rating score**	**Points**

a. Must be able to perform all tests on the check-off lists for which training has been completed as evidenced by initial and/or required competency checks.
 	
May exceed performance expectations by:
 	
  1. Writing and maintaining standard test methods according to the established format.
 	
  2. Developing departmental competency checks.
 	
  3. Being the resource person for a particular instrument or system.
 	
  4. Being database coordinator.
	4.50	3	13.50

b. Identifies and investigates specimen problems utilizing such tools as acceptability criteria and pending lists. Exceeds performance expectations by having no undocumented instances of missed specimens.	1.50	2	3.00

c. Completes and documents scheduled instrument maintenance.
 	
May exceed performance expectations by:
 	
  1. Documenting the review of instrument maintenance logs.
 	
  2. Performing or coordinating special instrument or assay function tests not included in daily, weekly, monthly maintenance, such as spectrophotometric/assay linearity checks, analytical balance checks, centrifuge checks, and pipet checks.
	0.75	3	2.25

d. Demonstrates the ability to identify basic instrument or technical problems and handles troubleshooting and documentation. Notifies manager/resource person of problems when appropriate. Exceeds performance expectations by identifying and resolving difficult problems.	0.75	3	2.25
Total points			21.00
Supporting statements:			

[a]Weight of Standard 1 is 7.5, which represents 30% (25 total) of job-specific competencies.

Scoring: 4-consistently exceeds standards, 3-occasionally exceeds standards, 2-meets standards, 1-occasionally meets standards, 0-rarely meets standards

(continued)

APPENDIX 16.3 Medical Technologist Job-Specific Competencies *(continued)*

Name:		Rating period:	
2. Complies with policies as described in the department (SOP) for result reporting, QC, proficiency testing, occurrence documentation, record keeping, and safety.	**Weight**[b]	**Rating score**	**Points**
a. Accurately performs tests on patient and proficiency specimens. Exceeds performance expectations with no more than one error attributed to carelessness or failure to follow established procedures.	3.375	3	10.125

b. Performs and verifies QC communicating appropriately.
 	
  1. Identifying potential QC problems (i.e., shifts, trends), documenting them, and suggesting solutions to solve them.
  2. Updating ranges and control lot numbers.
  3. Coordinating product evaluations and lot number changes.
  4. Developing and updating QC policy/flow diagrams.
  5. Reviewing monthly Levy-Jennings reports with written explanation/documentation.
  6. Coordinating proficiency testing.
  7. Archiving QC and patient results for storage and retrieval.
	1.500	3	4.500

c. Recognizes when critical or abnormal results must be communicated and documents these communications.
 	
May exceed performance expectations by:
  1. Having no omissions of documentation.
  2. Investigating unusual lab findings through additional testing or information gathering.
	1.125	2	2.250

d. Documents problems/corrections in the quality assurance log. Exceeds performance expectations with no more than one omission of documentation.	0.750	1	0.750

e. Complies with established safety practices so no instances of injury can be attributed to negligence or failure to follow established procedures.
 	
May exceed performance expectations by:
  1. Identifying potential hazards and/or suggesting solutions to them.
  2. Serving as the departmental safety coordinator.
    (a) Actively participates on the laboratory safety committee, reporting to the staff and ensuring that the staff is in compliance with the approved safety practices.
    (b) Maintains the departmental chemicals list and is responsible for labeling chemicals.
  3. Performing yearly instrument electrical safety checks and preparing the report.
  4. Performing the yearly electrical outlet checks.
  5. Being certified in and handling specimens/infectious substances for mailing.
  6. Participating in departmental or hospital disaster programs or events, such as hurricane coverage, mass casualty, or bioterrorism events.
	0.750	4	3.000

Total points			20.625
Supporting statements:			

[b]Weight of Standard 2 is 7.5, which represents 30% (25 total) of job-specific competencies.

Scoring: 4-consistently exceeds standards, 3-occasionally exceeds standards, 2-meets standards, 1-occasionally meets standards, 0-rarely meets standards

(continued)

APPENDIX 16.3 Medical Technologist Job-Specific Competencies *(continued)*

Name:		Rating period:	
3. Demonstrates the ability to organize the work in an efficient and cost-effective manner.	**Weight**[c]	**Rating score**	**Points**

a. Completes work on time, within scheduled shift/work period. Effectively manages work to avoid overtime.
 	
May exceed performance expectations by:
 	
  1. Having no instances of unnecessary or unapproved overtime.
 	
  2. Rearranging personal time to meet staffing needs and thus avoid departmental overtime.
 	
  3. Being responsible for scheduling personnel/workbenches.
	2.0	3	6.0

b. Prioritizes duties, responsibilities, and time to meet turnaround times according to departmental SOPs.
 	
May exceed performance expectations by completing daily assignments and taking on additional duties or responsibilities, such as:
 	
  1. Serving as the departmental United Way campaign coordinator.
 	
  2. Coordinating other charitable projects (Christmas family, cancer/diabetes/heart walks, etc.)
 	
  3. Organizing the National Medical Laboratory Week activities and/or service project.
	1.5	3	4.5

c. Recognizes day-to-day inventory needs and communicates appropriately.
 	
May exceed performance expectations by regularly:
 	
  1. Performing the inventory for a department or a large reagent vendor.
 	
  2. Ordering reagents or supplies for a department or large reagent vendor and updating computerized ordering files.
 	
  3. Receiving and organizing supplies.
 	
  4. Following up on back orders.
	1.0	1	1.0

d. Treats hospital property, equipment, and supplies carefully to avoid damage and rarely makes errors that result in waste of reagents or supplies.
 	
May exceed performance by:
 	
  1. Suggesting and documenting cost-saving ideas.
 	
  2. Preparing, evaluating, and monitoring the departmental budget.
 	
  3. Setting up and maintaining cost-per-test files.
	0.5	3	1.5

Total points			13.0
Supporting statements:			

[c]Weight of Standard 3 is 5.0, which represents 20% (25 total) of job-specific competencies.

Scoring: 4-consistently exceeds standards, 3-occasionally exceeds standards, 2-meets standards, 1-occasionally meets standards, 0-rarely meets standards

(continued)

APPENDIX 16.3   Medical Technologist Job-Specific Competencies *(continued)*

Name:		Rating period:	
4. Demonstrates good interpersonal skills in communication and collaboration, including team building and teaching.	**Weight^d**	**Rating score**	**Points**
a. Provides respectful and effective customer service to nonlaboratory personnel, including proper telephone etiquette. May exceed performance expectations by representing the department in laboratory rounds or lab/nursing liaison committee meetings.	1.500	3	4.500
b. Effectively communicates within the laboratory (changes, problems, special requests, etc.) utilizing the tools (logs, e-mail, etc.) available.	1.125	2	2.250

c. Trains and assists students and coworkers on instrumentation and procedures.
 	
May exceed performance expectations by:
 	
  1. Scheduling training sessions within the department.
 	
  2. Orienting the trainee in the department.
 	
  3. Evaluating the trainee.
 	
  4. Preparing and maintaining training material/protocols.
	0.750	1	0.750

d. Follows through on assignments by completing all projects in a timely manner. Exceeds performance expectations by suggesting projects for performance improvement and enhancement (PIE).	0.375	3	1.125
Total points			8.625
Supporting statements:			

^{c}Weight of Standard 4 is 3.75, which represents 15% (25 total) of job-specific competencies.

Scoring: 4-consistently exceeds standards, 3-occasionally exceeds standards, 2-meets standards, 1-occasionally meets standards, 0-rarely meets standards

Name:		Rating period:	
5. Adapts to changes in technology and in the healthcare environment.	**Weight^e**	**Rating score**	**Points**

a. Stays current with trends and activities as they apply to work processes and uses opportunities for continued learning and growth.
 	
May exceed performance expectations by:
 	
  1. Participating on a CAP inspection team.
 	
  2. Preparing lectures, bulletin board presentations, etc.
	0.625	2	1.250

b. Is receptive to new ideas and flexible to a changing work environment.
 	
May exceed performance expectations by:
 	
  1. Suggesting new ideas or ways to improve work flow and efficiency.
 	
  2. Participating on a PIE team.
	0.625	3	1.875

Total points			3.125
Supporting statements:			

^{e}Weight of Standard 5 is 1.25, which represents 15% (25 total) of job-specific competencies.

Scoring: 4-consistently exceeds standards, 3-occasionally exceeds standards, 2-meets standards, 1-occasionally meets standards, 0-rarely meets standards

(continued)

APPENDIX 16.3 Medical Technologist Job-Specific Competencies *(continued)*

Job-specific	Points
#1	20.000
#2	20.625
#3	13.000
#4	8.625
#5	3.125
Total	66.375

Evaluator's comments:

_____

Supervisor's signature   Date

_____

Employee's signature*   Date

_____

Director/vice president signature   Date

_____

*Employee's signature indicates that the employee has reviewed the completed appraisal form but does not necessarily imply agreement with the appraisal.

APPENDIX 16.4 Annual Performance Evaluation and Planning

Name: _____ Employee number: _____

Job title: medical technologist   Department: _____

Review date: _____

The performance evaluation and planning process is a review of the employee's performance and development advances during the previous 12 months. The evaluator should use the tools provided, plus the current job-specific standards document, to evaluate an employee's total job performance. The employee's performance is evaluated in the following areas: 1) service excellence standards, 2) mandatory requirements, and 3) job-specific standards.

My supervisor has reviewed with me my completed evaluation form to include service excellence standards, mandatory requirements, and job-specific competencies.

*Employee signature _____ Date _____

*Signing this form does not necessarily imply agreement with the evaluation.

Evaluator _____ Title _____ Date _____

Next level leadership _____ Title _____ Date _____

If the evaluator is not a director-level employee, please obtain a second signature (minimally must be a director).

Employee comments:

Scoring summary				
Performance areas	**Points**	**Weight**	**Weighted points**	**Total score**
Service excellence standards	88.160	0.15	13.224	
Mandatory requirements	Met			
Job-specific competencies	66.375	0.85	56.419	70
Total score	**Rating definitions**			
0–24	**Rarely meets** standards—Employee consistently falls below the expected level of job performance.			
25–49	**Occasionally meets** standards—Employee is not consistent about meeting the expected level of job performance.			
50–74	**Meets** standards—Employee consistently meets the expected level of job performance.			
75–89	**Meets** standards and **may occasionally exceed**—Employee consistently meets and may in some circumstances exceed the expected level of job performance.			
90–100	**Consistently exceeds** standards—Employee consistently exceeds the expected level of job performance. Exemplary performance can be demonstrated by exceeding job performance expectations, assuming additional responsibilities/projects, or mentoring other staff members.			

(continued)

APPENDIX 16.4 Annual Performance Evaluation and Planning *(continued)*

Job performance planning (Required if total score is less than 50)
Follow-up review date: Performance goal: Action plan: Follow-up procedure:
Follow-up review date: Performance goal: Action plan: Follow-up procedure:
Follow-up review date: Performance goal: Action plan: Follow-up procedure:
Employee comments:

I have reviewed the performance goals with my manager. I understand that my manager and I will meet regularly to review my progress in achieving these performance goals. I understand that I am on job performance probation.

Employee signature and date: _____

Manager signature and date: _____

APPENDIX 16.5 Web-Based Software Products and Web Sites

Performance Appraisal Software

Performance Impact Enterprise™ (web-based software)

Performance Impact Workplace™ (Windows-based software)

Knowledge Point, 1129 Industrial Avenue
Petaluma, CA 94952
707-762-0333/0375
http://www.knowledgepoint.com

Performance Appraisal Websites
http://www.worldatwork.org
http://www.work911.com

Competency Assessment Websites
http://www.asm.org/Division/c/competency.htm
http://www.medtraining.org/viewlabcomp

APPENDIX 16.6 Training Checklist for Microbiology Medical Technologist

Employee: _____ Employee #: _____

Date: _____ Hire date: _____

Function	Tech initial	Trainer initial	Comp meet	Semi-annual
Communication 1. Calls critical values in accordance with departmental critical value list 2. Calls for additional information as needed 3. Relays results and reports using appropriate laboratory information system (LIS) function to nurse or physicians				
LIS 1. Understands LIS accessioning function for sequencing cultures 2. Uses appropriate computer function to result blood cultures 3. Uses templates to work up cultures and understands how charges are generated in LIS 4. Understands required reports for cultures and knows how to send corrected reports 5. Knows how to order and cancel susceptibilities				
General lab duties 1. Has knowledge of lab safety, including use of the BSC and personal protection equipment 2. Keeps work area clean, stocked, and organized 3. Assists with inventory and QC 4. Completes instrument maintenance as assigned				
Interpretation of cultures 1. Understands purpose of various media for the selection and differentiation of organisms 2. Reports colony count for urine and IC cultures 3. Knows criteria for reporting and working up mixed urine and wound cultures 4. Understands what is normal flora in respiratory, wound, stool, and reproductive specimens				

(continued)

APPENDIX 16.6   Training Checklist for Microbiology Medical Technologist *(continued)*

Function	Tech initial	Trainer initial	Comp meet	Semi-annual
5. Has good colony isolation technique				
6. Understands the principles of isolation and work up of anaerobic organisms				
7. Knows which body sources are normally sterile				
Blood cultures (BC)				
1. Knows how to load and unload bottles, generate reports, and send preliminary and final reports				
2. Prepares, stains, and interprets positive BC				
3. Knows which organisms are considered to be contaminants when isolated in one set of BC				
4. Stocks all isolates				
5. Sends notification form to floor when cultures are contaminated for phlebotomist follow-up				
6. Clears out positive box as cultures are completed				
Biochemical and spot tests				

1. Demonstrates competence in the performance and interpretation of the following tests:
    Catalase
    Oxidase
    Spot indole
    Tube indole
    Staph latex agglutination
    BBL™ coagulase (tube)
    L-Pyrroglutamyl-peptide hydrolase (PYR)
    BBL™ Cefinase™
    Catarrhalis Test Disk™
    Microdase™ disk
    Desoxycholate test
    BBL™ Taxo™ P disk
    Phadebact® pneumococcal reagent
    Strep PathoDx® test
    BE/NACL
    Hippurate Disk™
    Novobiocin test				

2. Understands the frequency and documentation of reagent QC				
Stains				
1. Prepares, stains, and interprets Gram stains on direct specimens and culture isolates				
2. Understands when to perform wet preps				
3. Sets up and reads germ tubes				
4. Prepares and reads India ink smears				
5. Prepares and reads KOH smears				

(continued)

APPENDIX 16.6 Training Checklist for Microbiology Medical Technologist *(continued)*

Function	Tech initial	Trainer initial	Comp meet	Semi-annual
Biochemical identification (ID) systems				
1. Sets up the following ID cards:				
GPI™				
GNI™				
NHI™				
ANI™				
YBC™				
2. Sets up and reads the following ID systems:				
api® 20E				
api® 20 NE				
RapID™ NH				
RapID™ ANA II				
RapID™ STR (Strep)				
Referrals				
1. Refers IDs to SBH when needed				
2. Sends the following isolates to the SBH for serotyping:				
H. influenzae from blood or CSF				
N. meningitidis				
Salmonella (upon request or from blood)				
3. Refers CF isolates as needed for ID and synergy				
Susceptibility testing				
1. Understands colorimeter standardization and maintenance				
2. Demonstrates knowledge of the basic operation and troubleshooting of the Vitek® instrument				
3. Knows how to handle and store Vitek® cards				
4. Knows how to set up GNS™ and GPS™ cards				
5. Understands the Vitek® Expert system				
6. Understands how Etest®s are set up and how they are interpreted, including various types of growth that are seen				
7. Knows how to read Bauer-Kirby disk diffusion				
8. Knows how to read Microscan® or other micro-broth dilution panels				
9. Knows when to set up an anaerobe MIC panel and how to read the results				
10. Understands frequency and documentation of susceptibility QC				
11. Knows how to set up and report experimental antibiotics and how to document QC				

(continued)

APPENDIX 16.6 Training Checklist for Microbiology Medical Technologist *(continued)*

Function	Tech initial	Trainer initial	Comp meet	Semi-annual
Susceptibility reporting				
1. Knows the usual susceptibility pattern for:				
Klebsiella				
Citrobacter				
Enterobacter				
Proteus				
Serratia				
Pseudomonas				
Acinetobacter				
2. Understands the oxacillin screen for *S. aureus*				
3. Knows how to confirm a VRE				
4. Knows when and how to confirm an ESBL				
5. Knows age-dependent rules for the following antibiotics:				
Ampicillin/sulbactam				
Levofloxacin and ciprofloxacin				
Tetracycline				
6. Understands how the following classes of antibiotics cascade:				
Ampicillin/penicillin				
Aminoglycosides				
Quinolones				
Cephalosporins				
Imipenem				
7. Recognizes unusual susceptibility results:				
Vancomycin resistance in *Staphylococcus*				
Imipenem resistance in enteric GNB				
Piperacillin resistance with pip/tazo susceptible				
Levofloxacin resistance in *S. pneumoniae*				
8. Knows which antibiotics are reported in urine, blood, and CSF				
9. Knows where to find antimicrobial susceptibility standards (NCCLS standards) document				

APPENDIX 16.7 Training Checklist for Third-Shift Microbiology

Employee: _____ Employee #: _____

Date: _____ Hire date: _____

Function	Tech date	Trainer	Comp meet	Semi-annual check

Rapid Procedures
1. Interpretation of direct Gram stains
2. Set up and interpretation of:
    India ink
    Wet prep
3. Performs strep A Ag procedure
4. Sets up stool for pus (WBC)				

LIS 1. Understands laboratory information system (LIS) functions for logging in cultures 2. Enters Gram stain results in LIS 3. Results strep Ag and orders beta-strep culture if strep Ag is negative 4. Communicates with day shift through communication log				
Culture set-up 1. Knows how to set up CSF for culture and how to use cytocentrifuge for smear prep 2. Knows how to set up sputum cultures 3. Knows how to set up urine cultures 4. Subcultures GN broths to XLD at 4–6 hours 5. Knows how to store specimens that are not being set up 6. Knows how to use CO_2 bags				
Blood cultures 1. Knows how to enter information in the BC instrument computer 2. Knows how to load bottles into the instrument 3. Knows how to unload positive bottles 4. Knows how to enter the positive BC Gram stain and how to send a preliminary report 5. Orders template to record information 6. Notifies patient's nurse				

APPENDIX 16.8   Training Checklist for Microbiology Medical Laboratory Technician

Employee: _____ Employee #: _____

Date: _____ Hire date: _____

Function	Tech date	Trainer	Comp meet	Semi-annual check
Communication 1. Answers phone courteously and effectively, (giving name and department) 2. Assists floors with ordering tests 3. Calls for additional information as needed 4. Relays results and reports using appropriate laboratory information system (LIS) function to nurses or physicians				
LIS 1. Orders tests through appropriate LIS function 2. Knows proper test for specimen types 3. Aware of all tests that are ordered (specimens may have multiple orders) 4. Knows how to cancel and credit tests 5. Knows how to receive specimens through appropriate LIS function 6. Knows how to receive using appropriate LIS function, BCs with the proper drawn ID 7. Logs cultures into Micro through appropriate LIS function 8. Knows how to change default media 9. Knows how to change the work center 10. Knows how specimens are routed and how to change the routing of specimens				
General lab duties 1. Knows about lab safety, including use of the BSC and personal protective equipment 2. Keeps work area clean, stocked, and organized 3. Assists with inventory control, including putting away supplies and media 4. Knows how to operate the autoclave 5. Works with specimen management to see that specimens are received ASAP				
Specimen setup 1. Knows how to assess the quality and transport time of specimens (specimen rejection policy) 2. Knows appropriate tests for each specimen type, including immunocompromised panel 3. Knows appropriate plates for each culture 4. Knows when to add media to a culture 5. Knows how to prioritize culture set up (i.e., set up anaerobe, surgical, and CSF before other cultures) 6. Sets up cath and cc urine with .001 loop and cysto and suprapubic urine with .01 loop				

(continued)

APPENDIX 16.8   Training Checklist for Microbiology Medical Laboratory Technician *(continued)*

Function	Tech date	Trainer	Comp meet	Semi-annual check
Specimen setup (continued)				
7. Batches stool cultures				
8. Knows how to grind tissue (except for fungus)				
9. Knows which cultures have a Gram stain				
10. Knows how to set up fungus culture on tissue				
11. Knows how to handle AFB cultures				
12. Knows how to set up ANA and Campy jars				
13. Knows what media to set up on fungus cultures				
14. Understands where to incubate plates:				
Peds and all cultures CF, THR, BETA, EAR, CSF				
Pediatric urine				
Adult urine				
Infection control				
Adult cultures				
Fungus cultures				
15. Knows how to handle viral, O&P, and serology specimens				
Blood cultures				
1. Knows how to load and unload bottles				
2. Knows how to process positive BC				
3. Transfers positive cultures to appropriate work card				
Rapid procedures				
1. Prepares smears and performs Gram stains				
2. Knows how to set up				
India ink				
Calcofluor white				
KOH				
Wet prep				
3. Performs strep A Ag procedure				
4. Knows how to set up stool for pus (WBC)				
5. Knows how to set up stool occult blood				
6. Interprets *Helicobacter* screening test				

APPENDIX 16.9   Competency Assessment Form: Microbiology Specimen Processing

Employee name: _____ Evaluation interval: _____

Task - direct observation	Met	Not met[a]	Evaluator	Date
Match order slip with specimen				
Match identification on specimen and order				
Perform laboratory information system (LIS) specimen receipt function				
Utilize specimen rejection criteria				
Select appropriate media for culture				
Place computer labels on media				
Label glass slide for smears				
Operate biological safety cabinet (BSC)				
Wear gloves and protective coat when handling and plating specimens				
Perform plating of specimens inside BSC				
Use aseptic technique handling specimens				
Inoculate and streak plates using method appropriate to body site of specimen				
Use tissue grinder for tissue specimens				
Use centrifugation for fluid specimens				
Place inoculated media in appropriate gaseous/temperature environment				
Achieve well-isolated colonies on cultures				
Smear dried and fixed				
Perform Gram stain on smears				
Interpret Gram-stained smears				
Record Gram stain results on work card				
Call critical Gram stain results				
Enter Gram stain results in LIS				
Complete requisition for reference lab				
Use appropriate packaging materials for referred specimens				
Complete external courier shipping forms				
Store specimens until referred				
QC/instrument function-review records				
Gram stain QC				
Function checks of BSC				
Problem solving - review records				
Mislabeled specimens				
Unlabeled specimens				

[a]Remedial action:

Reassess: [ ] Met [ ] Not met   Date _____ Evaluator _____

Employee name _____ Date _____

Supervisor _____ Date _____

Director _____ Date _____

APPENDIX 16.10   Competency Assessment Form: Blood Culture Procedures - Bactec® 9240

Employee name: _____ Evaluation interval: _____

Task - direct observation	Met	Not met[a]	Evaluator	Date
Use personal protective equipment				
Inspect bottles for fill volume				
Note underfilled bottle on work card				
Note on work card if only one bottle received				
Review order for unusual organisms				
Extend protocol length function				
Use FOS™ for fluid specimens				
Check receipt/collection date/time: if >48 h, perform blind subculture				
Load bottles into instrument				
Resolve anonymous bottles				
Resolve orphan bottles				
Safely dispose of bottles				
Subculture positive bottles in biological safety cabinet				
Perform and interpret Gram stains				
Call Gram stain results				
Results/records review				
Record results on work cards				
Enter results into on-line patient record				
Instrument function - review records				
Perform function checks of Bactec® 9240				
Problem solving - review records				
Resolve failure of tape backup				

[a]Remedial action:

Reassess: [   ] Met [   ] Not met   Date _____ Evaluator _____

Employee name _____   Date _____

Supervisor _____   Date _____

Director _____   Date _____

Staffing and Scheduling

Patti Medvescek

OBJECTIVES

To explain the dynamics of staffing and scheduling laboratory personnel with respect to current labor trends and business requirements

To describe the personnel classifications as determined by governing bodies, accreditation agencies, and specific laboratory needs

To compare and contrast traditional versus alternative staffing plans, using personnel classification and qualification and service requirements

To describe key success factors for laboratory scheduling and metrics for effectiveness and efficiency

Creativity seems to emerge from multiple experiences, coupled with a well-supported development of personal resources, including a sense of freedom to venture beyond the known.

LORIS MALAGUZZI

KATHLEEN MADIGAN WROTE FOR *Business Week Online*: "Labor costs constitute some three-quarters of total (expense) outlays in the corporate sector" (5). The situation is no different in a clinical laboratory, where human resources account for a significant percentage of the laboratory budget. Staff utilization is the key to controlling expenses in the laboratory. The education and experience required of the staff as well as staff scheduling models can optimize laboratory operations. Failure to recognize the impact of staffing and scheduling might diminish services provided and negatively affect the operating budget. Laboratory managers must understand the current and future dynamics that influence staff availability and must be aware of scheduling opportunities to provide efficient and effective laboratory operations.

Laboratory Personnel: Current Dynamics Affecting Staffing

Labor Shortage

Many organizations, including the American Society for Clinical Pathology (ASCP) and HealthOne Alliance, have reported on the shortage of clinical laboratory scientists. The root cause is varied, including fewer people entering the field, resulting in fewer schools for medical technology, combined with decreases in available funds for education and an increase in opportunities outside of the laboratory sector. In February 2003, American Medical Technologists reported, "US hospitals and other healthcare facilities face a critical shortage of clinical laboratory personnel" (1).

HealthOne Alliance reported the national vacancy rate for clinical laboratory scientists at 12% (3). A 1998 Bureau of Labor Statistics report stated that the need for clinical laboratory professionals will increase 10 to 20% over the next decade, while medical technology schools are closing because of the high cost of maintaining quality programs. An online American Medical Technologists news report stated that clinical laboratory science schools may decrease in number due to low enrollment.

The availability of trained individuals to perform laboratory testing is and should be a concern for laboratory managers. Creative staffing and scheduling can reduce staffing requirements, lessening the impact of this shortage.

Business Need

The *Occupational Outlook Handbook* reports, "Technological advances will continue to have two opposing effects on employment [of clinical laboratory technologists and technicians] through 2010. New, increasingly powerful diagnostic tests will encourage additional testing and spur employment. On the other hand, research and development efforts targeted at simplifying routine testing procedures may enhance the ability of nonlaboratory personnel physicians and patients, in particular, to perform tests now done in laboratories". (Bureau of Labor Statistics, http://www.bls.gov/oco/ocos096.htm). As hospitals (and laboratories) continue their evolution from healthcare providers to businesses providing healthcare services, laboratory managers are faced with the challenges of achieving a balance between skill levels of staff and scheduling staff to maintain services while reducing costs. How the laboratory interacts with other ancillary and hospital departments becomes important as cost sharing, cost savings and point-of-care testing are integrated into the hospital.

Increasing Opportunities for Medical Technologists

The Bureau of Labor Statistics, in the *Occupational Outlook Handbook*, lists related fields in chemistry, material sciences, veterinary technologists, technicians, and assistants. Also available to laboratory personnel are positions in manufacturing and industry, including sales, technical support, and research and development positions. Clearly, the labor shortage, the increased need for trained personnel, the availability of jobs in nonhealthcare settings, and the barriers for entry into the field (perceived low salary and schedule demands) mandate the need for effective staffing and scheduling in the clinical laboratory to make best use of available talent.

Personnel Requirements

Education

Medical and clinical laboratory technologists generally have a bachelor's degree in medical technology or one of the life sciences or a combination of formal training and work experience. Technicians generally have either an associate's degree or certification from a hospital vocational or technical school. Several programs provide certifications for technologists and technicians, or training program guidelines, including the ASCP, the American Society of Clinical Laboratory Scientists, the National Credentialing Agency, and NCCLS.

The basic requirements for personnel to perform testing in a clinical laboratory are based on the Clinical Laboratory Improvement Amendments of 1988 (CLIA '88). Tests are grouped by complexity (as defined within the CFR Sec. 493), with specific licensure, education, or experience requirements for each complexity model. The degree required for testing personnel varies and includes doctors of medicine or osteopathy; doctoral, master's or bachelor's degrees; associate degrees; or high school diplomas. The common denominator is documented training for each individual performing laboratory testing, based on the complexity of the tests performed. The credentialing options (for example, Bachelor of Science degree in Medical Technology or chemistry, or high school diploma plus military training, to name a few) provide the laboratory manager with flexibility in hiring decisions and scheduling personnel. This flexibility can be defined in terms of ratios of technologists, technicians, and employees with a high school education plus training. The College of American Pathologists (CAP) and other organizations with deemed status under CLIA '88 to provide accreditation programs for clinical laboratories require that "all testing personnel meet CLIA '88 requirements" (2).

If the overall laboratory staff increases, the ratio of technicians to technologists may change in favor of technicians and those trained on the job. As staffing decreases, more technologists (qualifying as technical supervisors) are needed to ensure that qualified personnel perform all services over all shifts.

Experience

The CAP General Laboratory Checklist (1) addresses inservice training that is adequate to meet the needs of all clinical laboratory personnel. The ASCP, the American Society for Microbiology, the National Credentialing Agency, and the Clinical Laboratory Management Association, among others, provide continuing education opportunities through journal reviews, educational programs, and meeting seminars.

Each technologist or technician must be competent to perform laboratory tests based on the specific policies and procedures for the laboratory. Training and competence must be documented within personnel records. In addition, on-the-job training may be integrated into the laboratory for those with the minimum education required. Consideration should be given to on-the-job training, especially for laboratory assistants or phlebotomy staff, for job improvement and promotion. As the labor pool of skilled employees decreases, developing a pool from within provides the laboratory manager with additional resources to staff the laboratory. Employees who are trained and ready to perform a variety of tests limit the negative impact of staff absence, leaves of absence, or open positions in the laboratory.

Functional Definitions

For purposes of this text, several terms are discussed within the context of staffing and scheduling in the laboratory:

- *Laboratory size* is identified due to the differing needs for the laboratory based on physical limitations (multiple locations, floors, laboratories requiring additional personnel to efficiently perform testing). Small laboratories occupying less square footage may require fewer personnel if a generalist can cover all the areas.

- *Laboratory location*, also a variable, should be considered. For example, for a hospital laboratory, proximity to high-use areas, such as the emergency room (ER) or intensive care unit, will lessen the time required for transportation or personnel services between these areas and the laboratory. Decentralized services will affect staffing requirements. STAT laboratories, outpatient facilities, and nursing unit stations all require additional personnel. The benefit of decentralized services is improved turnaround time for direct services; the cost is trained personnel to staff the areas.

- *Laboratory test menus* are a factor in determining staffing patterns, based on complexity of testing performed. A generalist model may be appropriate for a hospital or physician office laboratory (POL) that refers microbiology identification and susceptibility testing or blood bank antibody identification; the specialist model may be required for laboratories, regardless of size, that provide a tertiary level of service.

- *Laboratory service levels* include activities defined by process or contract. These may include specimen collection on- and off-site, POL support, reporting procedures, and other support provided by the laboratory to one or more facilities.

Generalist versus Specialist

The staffing model widely used 20 years ago was based on specialists for every discipline in the laboratory. Labor-saving instruments and computerization have changed the testing process in the laboratory, allowing ease of test performance. This opens the opportunity to employ a generalist model in the laboratory. Generalists can be cross-trained for all laboratory sections. Cross-training can be defined for staffing purposes as training an individual to perform testing in more than one functional area of the laboratory. Traditionally, medical technologists were assigned to a specific section, e.g., hematology or chemistry, and their competency was assessed only for those tests performed in that area. By training personnel to perform testing in multiple areas of the laboratory,

when multiple areas exist, the laboratory manager has the skill mix available to assign individuals where the need is greatest at the time.

In addition to the generalist versus specialist model, the laboratory manager should review career levels within each job function. Career advancement in medical technology can follow the administrative track (to laboratory supervision) or the technical specialists track, e.g., senior technologists. Having two career tracks does provide options for laboratory employees to stay in the laboratory through job enrichment and job enhancement. When staffing is adequate to accommodate multiple levels of job categories, the potential exists to reduce turnover and provide additional resources for problem resolution, technical consultation, and staff education.

If cost savings are needed in the laboratory and labor accounts for a large percentage of the laboratory budget, then changing the skill mix of the staff is one way to achieve cost savings. However, the optimal mix of assistants, technicians, and technologists (specialists and generalists) should be specific for each facility based on the functional definitions of the laboratory. Once the CLIA '88 requirements are satisfied for testing personnel, it is up to the laboratory manager and director to determine the proper mix. Cost/benefit analysis can assist in determining this mix, as shown in Table 17.1.

Laboratory Staffing

Staffing Requirements

The laboratory manager must assess the needs of the laboratory to determine the number of employees needed as well as the mix of expertise, training, or credentials of technical staff. The following are elements within the laboratory that should be addressed.

Test mix. A large test menu, including moderately and highly complex tests, requires a different group of technical staff than a laboratory performing mostly routine testing on automated analyzers. Specialty areas in microbiology, surgical pathology or cytology, and blood bank also require special consideration.

Table 17.1 Staffing ratio costs and benefits

Staff level	Cost	Benefit
Technologists	Expense and availability	Expertise in testing methods, ability to analyze and solve problems
Technicians	Expertise may be insufficient to review or troubleshoot test results	Less expensive
On-job trained	Training program preparation and implementation	Resource supply, lower labor cost

Hours of operation. For a full-service laboratory supporting an ER or intensive care unit, staffing coverage for 24 h/day, 7 days/week requires a different pattern than an outpatient laboratory or POL providing services Monday to Friday for one shift. The requirements for on-site technical supervision in CLIA '88 mandate the need for technologists in addition to technicians on off shifts, weekends, and holidays.

Service levels. Turnaround time, phlebotomy, results reporting, and sequential testing are all variables to consider when staffing the laboratory. An outpatient laboratory may provide all test results by the next day, allowing for a smaller staff to perform specimen collection during the day with batch testing performed in the early evening. A full-service laboratory performing tests for the ER will require testing personnel 24 h/day to perform a stat test menu with turnaround times within minutes. Computerized result reporting eliminates the need for laboratory assistants to hand-deliver test results. Automatic sequential or cascade testing relieves clerical or technical staff of contacting physicians with results and/or waiting for additional test requests.

Productivity levels. The author has based productivity goals on a "traditional" 80% productivity measure. The key, however, is to know how to define the term "productivity," including the metrics to measure productivity. For example, if the amount of time available to work is used as maximum opportunity, then the 8-h day is actually 6.5 h (assuming 1.5 h for lunch and breaks). Then 80% productivity (based on an 8-h day) is equal to 65% productivity (based on an 8-h day but including 1.5 h/day as unavailable time). Productivity is also a useful indicator to determine optimum staffing in conjunction with minimum staffing. Few laboratories can afford to hire enough personnel to staff the laboratory for maximum workload levels. Similarly, few laboratories can afford the quality issues inherent in minimum staffing levels, so productivity approaches 100% when workload increases. The creative manager will staff for the typical workload day, with additional personnel available to call in when workload exceeds projections. This flexibility is the primary advantage to part-time, flextime, and cross-trained individuals.

Basis for Determination: Workload Recording

Some method should be used to objectively document the amount of "work" performed by the laboratory. The units of work are factored by the hours required to perform the work to determine productivity. The CAP workload recording unit continues to be one benchmark in use today (13). CAP has added management tools, including LMIP, a program that benchmarks management indicators. The workload recording program provides historical information but has not been updated to include newer technologies or instrumentation. It does, however, provide a basic understanding of workload versus hours worked that may be valuable as a learning tool when constructing a staffing model. Other productivity programs are available via Internet search. One website, Health Information Technology Yellow Pages, lists a variety of resources for productivity measures, staffing, and scheduling personnel. Newer workload models may be available and should be investigated for appropriate use in the laboratory. The key to workload recording is to determine the basis for calculation, while reducing the variables that can affect the results and limiting the exceptions that will skew performance.

The laboratory supervisor and director should be informed about projected patient volumes. If inpatient volumes are declining, staff may be downsized, despite an increasing outpatient volume. It is critical to understand the resource requirements for each patient "sector" and to justify staffing requirements via documentation of workload and efficiency.

Staff Scheduling

Once the staffing mix has been developed and implemented, employees must be assigned to their work schedules. To schedule staff effectively, the laboratory manager must understand the needs of the laboratory, hours of operation and the staff required, versus the needs of the employees, for whom work-life balance is becoming more important.

Key Success Factors

The laboratory manager should not only understand the factors that are critical to the success of the laboratory but also be able to demonstrate or document these key areas. For a cost center, two key success factors are financial performance and quality assurance. When reviewing staffing and scheduling, labor costs can target areas of opportunity for improvement. The cost of overtime and turnover will affect overall person-hour and expense budgets. The achievement of targeted performance metrics influences the satisfaction of customers (e.g., physicians, patients).

Metrics for Success

Reporting efficiency. Laboratories have measured their reporting efficiency in terms of percent of tests reported within required or requested time frames. This metric is particularly important to those who take action on the test results, as treatment options and procedures depend on laboratory results. Reporting efficiency also can affect the financial performance of the hospital. When laboratory results are available and patient care is delivered efficiently, the patient length of stay may be decreased. For the reference laboratory, reporting efficiency to their customers is not only an indicator of performance; it may also be included in the contractual agreement, with financial considerations if metrics are not achieved.

Turnaround time. Laboratories with responsibility for collecting patient samples may monitor the percent of tests collected within a time frame around the test request. For example, a hospital laboratory may report the percent of 6 a.m. labs collected between 5:30 a.m. and 6:30 a.m.

Productivity measurements. The productivity of the laboratory is a function of the number of tests performed by the number of personnel working, or workload units per full-time equivalent. Not all tests performed are billed, and there must be a distinction between billed, billable (but not billed for whatever reason), and nonbillable tests when comparing productivity to financial performance. This distinction is also important when contracting for reagent purchases so the correct quantity of reagents for tests performed is used for negotiation and contractual obligation. If the laboratory staff is unable to complete the billable tests within an acceptable percentage of all tests, inventory levels, pricing, and efficiency are all affected.

Impact on staff. The implementation of productivity measurements can affect the laboratory staff. Productivity measures are an objective, quantitative means of reviewing performance but may be perceived as changing the workplace from a laboratory to an assembly line, where productivity is the only indicator or laboratory success. By including quality indicators such as proficiency surveys performance in laboratory metrics, the laboratory supervisor can emphasize the importance of quality as well as productivity.

Scheduling processes. At a minimum, the manual schedule is prepared for the staff in advance. Scheduling software programs are available that include parameters for skills and training. The need for computerized scheduling is dictated in part by the size of the laboratory staff and the time available to devote to maintaining a manual versus a computerized system. Laboratory supervisors should examine the time required to prepare, distribute, post, and amend manual schedules and compare the labor intensity with the cost and implementation of a computerized process. Ultimately, the laboratory must be staffed with sufficient personnel trained for the areas in which testing is provided.

Alternatives

Outsourcing. Reference laboratories have in the past provided esoteric testing not usually done in clinical laboratories. With overnight testing and air couriers, reference laboratories have expanded their menus to include routine testing. The laboratory manager is challenged with deciding which tests to send out versus perform in-house, based on cost per test as well as service levels provided. For some laboratories with minimal test volumes, the ability to bill for tests performed must be also considered. The incremental opportunity for additional tests may justify the additional costs for technologists or equipment.

Opportunity cost and benefit. The laboratory manager should consider the impact of staffing decisions on the facility or physician using the laboratory. The manager should also consider the opportunity to combine job functions across departmental lines when feasible to take full advantage of the benefits provided. For example, locating the phlebotomy staff on nursing units provides efficiency for the laboratory in less travel time to the patient and also provides nursing units with ancillary personnel trained to provide defined levels of patient care. This program can be compared to the option of additional support within the laboratory for the most benefit to the facility and the laboratory.

Creative scheduling. Creative scheduling includes opportunities for job sharing, flextime, part-time, telecommuting, and self-directed teams (Table 17.2). Similarly skilled and trained employees can elect to share a position. This often decreases fringe benefit cost while providing equal hours worked. Flexible scheduling, based on employee need or request, can result in increased employee satisfaction (resulting in reduced turnover). Telecommuting for specific positions such as medical transcription reduces space requirements for the laboratory, may enhance work performance, and provides an additional resource of experienced employees. Using self-directed teams reduces the time demands on the laboratory supervisor while providing job enrichment and satisfaction. Scheduling employees in nontraditional shifts (e.g., 10 a.m. to 6:30 p.m.) or four 10-h days may provide work hours needed by the

Table 17.2 Scheduling alternatives

Alternative	Pros	Cons
Job sharing	Decreases benefits costs	Potential lack of continuity
Flexible schedules	Employee satisfaction	Must be administered consistently and in accordance with human resource policy
Part-time schedules	Increases pool of employees	Lack of continuity
Telecommuting	Reduces overhead requirements; employee satisfaction	Limited to specific jobs; cost to establish and maintain links to the laboratory
Self-directed teams	Improves employee satisfaction; reduces management "hands-on" time	Consistent application of policy

laboratory while meeting personal needs of the staff. Part-time employees can also provide additional resources for staff coverage in emergencies. The author recommended 20-h coverage in one laboratory, from 4 a.m. to midnight, staffed by two 10-h shifts. Testing was limited between midnight and 4 a.m. to the critical test menu, with limited swing shift staffing available to perform routine instrument maintenance and stat testing as needed.

Special Considerations

Inpatient testing requires a 24/7 response for patient testing with more specific criteria for emergency, intensive care, or surgical patients. These requirements may add staff to the laboratory roster. Outpatient testing may still include weekend hours but is more limited in hours of operation. The facility or laboratory may have specific customer satisfaction metrics for outpatient visits, including waiting time. Shared services (inpatient facilities and outpatient testing stations within one department) provide more flexibility for shared staffing and an increase in the pool of trained personnel available for coverage.

The laboratory as a web-based business continues to develop and expand, particularly as national reference laboratories invite web activities. Ellen Hope Kearns et al., in *American Clinical Laboratory*, reported, "Efficiency gains within the healthcare arena have been attributed to the application of information technology and most specifically, the Internet" (4). Innovation in technical support from manufacturers via the Internet, immediate communications to and from physicians, and automatic generation of test reports are changing the requirements for the laboratory. The extent to which the laboratory will utilize the Internet to save time and money and improve services is changing rapidly. The manner in which the public will receive healthcare e-commerce is being explored. The opportunity certainly exists to explore e-business in the future.

Summary

Effective laboratory staffing and scheduling will have a positive impact on the laboratory as a service provider. Changes in the availability of skilled employees, in the way laboratories are operated as businesses (cost center versus revenue center), and in the regulatory environment all create challenges today for laboratory managers hoping to optimize human resource utilization. These challenges can be limited or eliminated by creative scheduling and utilization of available personnel.

KEY POINTS

■ Personnel classification and qualifications for laboratory operations are detailed.

■ Traditional scheduling methods are under review as the laboratory as a service provider evolves (or has evolved) into the laboratory as an integral part of the business of healthcare.

■ A key to understanding the depth of opportunity within a laboratory is to recognize the base requirements and the incremental impact of creative scheduling, labor pool, and services provided.

■ Staffing and scheduling are very dependent on the locale, the availability of technical staff, the practice patterns by physicians, and patient expectations.

■ Scheduling processes are reviewed to provide options and opportunities that meet the key success factors for the laboratory.

GLOSSARY

Contingency workforce Employees not defined as permanent or regular employees, usually assigned jobs based on short-term needs.

Full-time equivalent Forty hours worked per week.

Generalist One trained in multiple areas of the laboratory.

Laboratory supervisor Individual responsible for staffing and scheduling the laboratory.

Medical Technician Also known as Clinical Laboratory Technician; a person with an associate's degree in Medical Laboratory Technology (or equivalent).

Medical Technologist Also known as Clinical Laboratory Technologist; a person with a bachelor's degree in Medical Technology or in a selected health science and who has completed a 1-year practicum.

NCCLS Voluntary consensus standards-developing organization disseminating standards and guidelines to the healthcare community; previously known as the National Committee for Clinical Laboratory Standards.

Outsourcing Contracting with consultants, reference laboratories or other clinical laboratories to provide services.

Productivity measures Raw numbers or calculations that describe work performed relative to hours worked, tests billed, revenue generated, reagents used, etc.

Specialist One trained and experienced in one specific laboratory discipline; formally, one who has a minimum of 5 years' experience in that discipline and has passed a qualifying examination for that discipline by an accepted accrediting organization.

REFERENCES

1. **American Medical Technologists.** 2003. Online news report: February 2003 "Laboratory Staffing Shortages." http://www.amt1.com/site/epage/9836_315.htm (verified 15 May 2003).

2. **College of American Pathologists.** Laboratory general checklist, 2003. #GEN.54750. College of American Pathologists Laboratory Accreditation Program. Northfield, Ill.

3. HealthONE Alliance. 2004. http://www.health1.org/seriousshortage.asp. [Online.]

4. Hope Kearns, E., S. Holmes, and G. Schmidt. 2002. The role of e-commerce in health care. *Am. Clin. Lab.* August–September: 16–19.

5. Madigan, K. 1999. Corporate scoreboard, *Business Week Online,* http://www.businessweek.com/1999/99_20/b3629122.htm (verified 15 May 2003).

APPENDIX 17.1 Further Information

Web Sites

American Medical Technologists
(http://www.amt1.com/site/epage/9836_315.htm)
American Medical Technologists, online news report, February 2003. "Laboratory Staffing Shortages." Includes discussion on the Coordinating Council on the Clinical Laboratory Workforce in a joint effort to identify and define the causes of the personnel shortage and to develop strategies to address this crisis.

Healthcare Information Technology Yellow Pages
(http://www.health-infosys-dir.com)
Lists a variety of resources for productivity measures, staffing, and scheduling personnel.

HealthONE Alliance
(http://www.health1.org/schoolofmedtech.asp)
Description of the Clinical Laboratory Science Education School of Medical Technology, Denver, Colo.

Organizations and businesses

American Medical Technologists
(http://www.amt1.com)
710 Higgins Road
Park Ridge, IL 60068
Phone: 847-823-5169

American Society for Clinical Pathology (ASCP)
(http://www.ascp.org)
2100 West Harrison Street
Chicago, IL 60612-3798
Phone: 312-738-1336

American Society for Clinical Laboratory Sciences (ASCLS)
(http:www.ascls.org)
7910 Woodmont Ave., Suite 530
Bethesda, MD 20814
Phone: 301-657-2768

American Society for Microbiology (ASM)
(http://www.asm.org)
1752 N Street, NW
Washington, DC 20036
Phone: 207-737-3600

College of American Pathologists (CAP)
(http://www.cap.org)
325 Waukegan Road
Northfield, IL 60093-2750
Phone: 800-323-4040

Clinical Laboratory Management Association (CLMA)
(http://www.clma.org)
989 Old Eagle School Road, Suite 815
Wayne, PA 19087
Phone: 610-995-9580

Health Information Technology Yellow Pages
(http://www.health-infosys-dir.com)
911 Douglas Blvd., Suite 85-147
Roseville, CA 95661
Phone: 916-773-2852

HealthOne Alliance
(http://www.health1.org)
600 South Cherry St., Suite 217
Denver, CO 80246
Phone: 303-322-3515

National Credentialing Agency
(http://www.nca-info@goamp.com)
P.O. Box 15945-289
Lenexa, KS 66285
Phone: 913-438-5110

NCCLS
(http://www.nccls.org)
940 West Valley Road, Suite 1400
Wayne, PA 19087-1898
Phone: 610-688-0100

Regulations

Bureau of Labor Statistics, U.S. Department of Labor
(http://www.bls.gov/oco/ocos096.htm)

Occupational Outlook Handbook 2002–03 Edition.
Clinical Laboratory Technologists and Technicians

Clinical Laboratory Improvement Amendment
Public Law 100-578, Section 353
Public Health Service Act (42 U.S.C. 263a), October 31, 1988

18

Teams, Team Process, and Team Building

James W. Bishop and Lei Wang

OBJECTIVES

To define a work team and distinguish it from a work group

To indicate why a precise definition of "team" is important

To explain the concept of group process within teams

To describe the situations in which teams can be productive and those in which they cannot

To define "task interdependence," the types of task interdependence, and their importance. Explain how task interdependence influences choices related to teams

To explain the basic concepts behind selecting team members

To explain the importance of training with respect to teams; distinguish the differences between task-related training and team-related training; and understand the concept of team building

To list the types of leadership associated with teams and the advantages and disadvantages of each

To explain the importance of goals, both individual and team. Explain how team goals can be set and achieved

To explain how to evaluate team and team member performance and emphasize individual performance in terms of contribution to the team

To explain legal issues involved with the use of teams

What sets apart high-performance teams . . . is the degree of commitment, particularly how deeply committed the members are to one another.

JON R. KATZENBACH AND DOUGLAS K. SMITH

THE USE OF WORK TEAMS has become a popular strategy for increasing productivity and worker flexibility in the United States. For example, 82% of companies with 100 or more employees reported that they used teams, 68% of Fortune 1000 companies reported that they used self-directed work teams, and 91% reported that they used employee participation groups in 1993 (12). All 25 finalists for the 1996 America's Best Plants award, sponsored by *Industry Week*, have implemented work teams, and the majority of these companies' production workforces are engaging in self-directed or self-managed teams (56). Organizations have reported a number of benefits derived from the use of work teams. These include increased individual performance, better quality, less absenteeism, reduced employee turnover, leaner plant structures, and substantial improvements in production cycle time (22). In general, teams are considered an important ingredient of organizational success in the modern economy, which is characterized by needs for rapid information exchange and response to customer demands (13).

Definition of a Team

There are multiple definitions of the term "team." These include, but are not limited to

- A small number of people with complementary skills who are committed to a common purpose, performance goals, and approach for which they hold themselves mutually accountable (29).

- A group whose individual efforts result in a performance that is greater than the sum of those individual parts (54).

- Two or more people with different tasks who work together adaptively to achieve specified and shared goals (7).

- A collective of individuals who are interdependent in their tasks, who share responsibility for outcomes, who see themselves and who are seen by others as an intact social entry embedded in one or more larger social systems (for example, business unit or the corporation), and who manage their relationships across organizational boundaries (13).

Teams meet all of the defining characteristics of groups (configurations of more than two interdependent individuals who interact over time), but in addition, teams incorporate skill differentiation in a context where there is a common fate (i.e., success or failure at the team level has consequences for all team members) (25). It should be clear at this point that different authors have different specific definitions of teams. However, in the examples above we can see that there are more similarities than there are differences. Common to each of the definitions above is the idea of blending different skills to accomplish objectives that the individuals, even if their efforts were summed, could not accomplish. Notice that the previous statement indicates that the individuals would not be able to accomplish the team's objectives even if their efforts were summed. The sum of an individual's efforts is devoid of any synergy that may be produced as a result of working together in a concerted, coordinated, or teamlike way. Furthermore, implicit in each definition is the idea of both individual and collective accountability. That is, each individual can be rewarded or taken to task for the results of both the team's efforts and his or her own efforts.

Distinguishing Teams from Work Groups

The words "team" and "group" are often used interchangeably. Nevertheless, some theorists delineate the differences between them. One distinction is that the term "team" is used more in popular management literature, while "group" is used more frequently in the academic literature (13). Another distinction between "team" and "group" is the degree of "groupness" that characterizes the aggregation, that is, the degree to which the group's tasks are interdependent and the members are integrated with each other. "Teams" are aggregations of individuals with a high degree of "groupness" (28).

The difference between "team" and "group" can also be discussed from the perspective of synergy. A "work group" is defined as "a group that interacts primarily to share information and to make decisions to help each member perform within his or her area of responsibility" (54). Thus, a group does not require joint effort. The group's outcomes are just the sum of individual members' contributions. A work team on the other hand, generates positive synergy through the coordinated efforts of its members. Their individual efforts result in a level of performance that is greater than the sum of the individual inputs. Within a work group, members share information, have neutral or even negative synergy, and accountability is at the individual level. Members' skills may or may not complement each other's. By contrast, a team is designed for collective performance, synergy among its members should be positive, and accountability is both individual and mutual. Members' skills are complementary to each other (54).

Differences between groups and teams can be summarized in the following way. Groups tend to have strong, clearly defined leaders, while teams share leadership roles. Members of groups produce individual work products and are held accountable at the individual level. Teams produce collective work products, and accountability is at the individual and group level. That is, team members are responsible for what they do individually, and they are mutually accountable for each other's and the team's production. When groups hold meetings, the emphasis is on efficiency. Decisions are announced, information is disseminated, and assignments are made. When teams meet, these things are also done. But in addition, open-ended discussion is encouraged and problem-solving efforts are made. Following team meetings, members don't just go their separate ways but they perform real work together (29).

Types and Classifications of Teams

There are various ways to categorize teams. Based on how members allocate their time, teams can be full-time or part-time. Teams can be permanent or temporary. From a functional perspective, teams can be classified into three types: teams that recommend things, teams that make or do things, and teams that run things (13).

- Teams that recommend things include task forces, project groups, and audit, quality, or safety groups asked to study and solve particular problems.

- Teams that make or do things include people at or near the front lines who are responsible for doing the basic manufacturing, development, operations, marketing, sales service, and other value-adding activities of a business.
- Teams that run things include groups from the top of the enterprise down through the divisional or functional level.

Other typologies of teams have been identified, some of which overlap in their dimensions. One classification of teams includes work teams, parallel teams, project teams, and management teams (13).

- *Work teams:* continuing work units responsible for producing goods or providing services; memberships are typically stable, well defined, and usually full-time (12).
- *Parallel teams:* teams that pull together people from different work units or jobs to perform functions that the regular organization is not well equipped to perform (36).
- *Project teams:* teams that produce one-time outputs, such as a new product or service to be marketed by the company, a new information system, or a new plant (42).
- *Management teams:* teams that coordinate and provide direction to the subunits under their jurisdiction, laterally integrating interdependent subunits across key business processes (46).

Another classification scheme includes problem-solving teams, self-managed teams, and cross-functional teams (54).

- *Problem-solving teams:* members share ideas or offer suggestions on how work processes and methods can be improved. However, rarely are these teams given the authority to unilaterally implement any of their suggested actions.
- *Self-managed work teams:* groups of employees who take on the responsibilities of collectively planning and scheduling work, controlling the pace of work, making operating decisions, and taking action on problems. Fully self-managed work teams even select their own members and have members evaluate each other's performance.
- *Cross-functional teams:* teams made up of employees from about the same hierarchical level, but from different work areas, who come together to accomplish a specific task.

Based on the degree of autonomy (from low to high), teams and groups can also be classified into traditional work groups, quality circles, high-performance work teams, semiautonomous work groups, self-managing teams, and self-designing teams (3).

- *Traditional work groups:* Workers perform core production activities but have no management responsibility or control.
- *Quality circles:* Members join voluntarily with no financial rewards. The group has the responsibility for making suggestions but does not have the authority to make and implement decisions. The problem-solving domain is limited to quality- and productivity-related issues and cost reduction.
- *Semiautonomous work groups:* Workers manage and execute major production activities.
- *Self-managing teams* (or autonomous work groups): members have control over the management and execution of an entire set of tasks—from the acquisition of raw materials through the transformation process to shipping, including all support activities, such as quality control and maintenance, required to produce a definable product. The product could be a definable part of a production process as well as a completed process.
- *Self-designing teams:* These groups have all the characteristics of self-managing teams. In addition, they have control over the design of the teams themselves and decide such issues as what tasks should be done and who should belong to the teams.

Why Define a "Team" So Precisely?

A precise definition of the term "team" is necessary. By defining the term "team" precisely and paying attention to our own business needs as they relate to team attributes, we can make an informed decision about whether we can or should implement teams. The words of the definition should be a guide for the structure, purpose, and composition of the teams, as well as the decision of whether to implement them. "But wait," one might say. "Isn't the team the 'thing' in business organizations these days?" Well, it's certainly true that teams are quite popular and their implementation has produced good results for many businesses (6). However, that does not mean that every organization or every department in an organization should implement teams or, if they do, that they should expect the same results.

We should recognize that teams are not for every organization. Nor is it always wise to use them. For one thing, teams are expensive to implement and maintain. Hours of training are usually required before employees are comfortable with each other and able to function effectively and efficiently in a team. Trainers and training programs are expensive, and during the time employees are in training, they are not working. This is not to say that training isn't worth it; rather, it should remind us to be sure that the use of teams is necessary and that the possible outcomes are desirable before committing resources for their implementation.

Group Process and Teams

Now that we know what teams are (and are not) we can take a look, in general, at how they go about doing what they do, that is, performing their tasks. Basically, the group process model says that the sum of the individuals' potential plus process gain minus process loss equals group effectiveness (58) (Fig. 18.1). Group processes include communication patterns used by team members when they exchange information and ideas, the techniques and processes they use to arrive at decisions, the interaction with and the behavior of the team leader, the power dynamics in the group, and the way the team resolves conflicts (54). Notice that the use of teams generates process loss as well as process gain. Process loss includes such things as social loafing, that is, a team member who lets others "carry" him or her, and time lost for team meetings, the extra time it takes for a group to come to a decision, and administrative functions required when people work in groups. Process gain can be referred to as synergy. For example, when performing a task that requires diverse skills, such as those found in a laboratory, the quality of the decisions and therefore of the output tends to be better than if the individuals worked alone or independently (54).

The group process model is based on the concept that in order for teams to be worthwhile, process gain must exceed process loss over the long term. The phrase "over the long term" can be illustrated by the following. A number of team-based organizations with which the authors are familiar have weekly team meetings that last approximately 1 h. These weekly meetings are considered important for the teams to achieve important process gains associated with the use of teams in the first place. The hour so used represents part of the process loss that is also associated with the use of teams. For the use of teams to be worthwhile in these cases, the process gain resulting from their use must be such that the workers produce more goods and services in 39 h per week with the team meetings than they would in 40 h without them. That is, in these cases, the process loss part of the equation includes 1 h (times the number of participants) that is lost to the production process. The types of teams that use this procedure of weekly meetings include teams that are both self-directed and non-self-directed; the types of tasks include production, knowledge-based, and service; the types of organizations include manufacturing and service.

Awareness of the time spent for team meetings provokes the following questions: "Are all of these meetings necessary, and are they productive?" and "What would

happen if a weekly meeting was skipped?" The answer to the last question is that if a meeting were skipped one week, production would probably increase by about 2.5% (the percentage increase from 39 to 40 h) during that week. By the same token, if meetings were continually missed and if the meetings were productive to begin with, then their omission would lead to problems not getting resolved, fewer suggestions being made, and no suggestions receiving the benefit of refinement by the group. Furthermore, conflicts would smolder and metastasize. Hence, these meetings are looked upon not only as a corrective mechanism for past issues but also as an investment of time for future efficiency and increased effectiveness. That is, while the time used for meetings represents one component of process loss, the results of the meetings will be in the form of process gain such that the resulting group effectiveness exceeds the sum of the individuals' potential.

It should also be noted and understood that team meetings do not automatically ensure net process gains. There are numerous guides and techniques for conducting effective meetings, and the details will not be repeated here. However, some general guidelines are in order:

- Have an agenda. It should be distributed in advance of the meeting. Be sure that each individual has the opportunity to put items on the agenda.

- The focus of all meetings should pertain to the purpose and objectives of the team. Each agenda item should have a demonstrable relationship to the achievement of the team's purpose and objectives.

  When teams are new, it may be better to be particularly strict with these guidelines. For example, announcements of a general nature that pertain to all employees, and not exclusively to team members, should be made at a different meeting or by other means, if possible. This restriction may be relaxed once the team is fully established and it is felt that extra-team agenda items will not dilute the team's focus or cohesiveness. For some, this suggestion may seem excessive. However, during their formation, teams are very delicate entities. Many people are not used to working in teams, have never worked in teams, and do not know what a team looks and feels like.

  Furthermore, for teams to be effective, team members must at times put the team's objectives ahead of their own. For many, this is not a natural behavior and indeed is contrary to what most people are taught, particularly in the United States. Hence, in some ways, when we ask people to work in teams, we are asking them to do something that is not natural for them. Therefore, anything that would dilute the team in the eyes of the members should be avoided if at all possible, even if it seems trivial.

- All should understand the format of the meetings. Ample opportunity for input from each member should be provided. Input from those who are more reserved, thoughtful, or introverted should be solicited.

Figure 18.1 Group process model.

	Potential team effectiveness
+	Process gains
−	Process loss
=	Actual team effectiveness

- Items that require action should be assigned, resources should be allocated, and action items should be followed up. If this is not done, the message imparted is that the team is not a serious entity and the products and outcomes of the meetings are not important.

Why Have Teams?

Now that we have defined teams and understand their processes, we are in a better position to determine if having them would be in the best interest of our organization. For a situation in which a combination of skills, experiences, and judgments are needed, a team can be expected to outperform a collection of individuals who operate within confined job roles and responsibilities. Superior performance by teams comes from teams:

- Bringing together complementary skills from different individuals.
- Responding to changing events more quickly, more accurately, and more effectively due to communication channels that are built to support real-time problem solving and initiative.
- Being designed and their members being trained to overcome barriers to collective performance. In pursuing this purpose, team members are more likely to develop trust and confidence in each other and to prioritize team objectives ahead of personal objectives. As a result, teams tend to provide unique social dimensions that enhance the economic and social aspects of work.
- Being more fun in which to work for most people. Fun sustains performance and is sustained by team performance. This is not "fun" in the frivolous sense, but in the sense of enjoyment of accomplishing tasks together and enjoying others' company.
- Fostering behavioral changes more readily. This is because (i) teams are less threatened by change because of collective commitment and support; (ii) teams offer more room for growth and change because of their flexibility and willingness to consider a wider range of options and solutions for problems and challenges; (iii) teams, due to their focus on performance, motivate, challenge, reward, and support individuals who are willing to change their ways of doing things (28).

A Cautionary Note

Always keep in mind that teams are not panaceas. Even if it is the right thing to do, even if the teams perform well as independent entities, and even if it appears that the teams' goals are congruent with those of the organization, it does not automatically follow that teams are doing the best for the organization. The example found in case study 1 in Appendix 18.1 illustrates this.

Guidelines for Choosing Whether To Have Teams

Now that we know why an organization would want to have teams, we are in a position to make that determination in our own situation and circumstances.

Common Purpose

Managers can use several guidelines when they are deciding whether to have teams. One precondition that supports the use of teams would be if teams, as units, have a common purpose. "A common, meaningful purpose sets the tone and aspiration . . . inspires both pride and responsibility . . . conveys a rich and varied set of meanings to guide what the team needs to do, particularly in meeting its goals . . . gives teams an identity that reaches beyond the sum of the individuals involved, which keeps conflict constructive by providing a meaningful standard against which to resolve clashes between the interests of the individual and interests of the team (28)." A common purpose is not a nebulous, tautological admonition exhorting people to "work together," nor is it a far removed objective such as "corporate profitability." Common purpose, in the context used here, consists of objectives that can only be reached if all members of the team contribute and the success of a given member's contribution depends upon and is dependent upon the success of other members' contributions. Stated another way, a common purpose is one that is unlikely to be achieved without a meaningful and competent contribution from each team member. Furthermore, this type of common purpose is unlikely to be achieved even if excessive or for that matter heroic contributions are made by some members in an effort to overcome the lack of contributions or poor contributions from others. For example, as we tragically saw in early 2003, a surgeon's skills and the collective skills of a surgical team, no matter how competently applied in performing an organ transplant, cannot offset a botched blood type matching.

A team must not only have a common purpose, members must understand and accept that purpose. Once all members accept and understand it, then attention can be given to how each member will contribute to its achievement. Therefore, an important question is: Can a common purpose be defined in a meaningful way that meets the above criteria? If not, a team approach cannot be used very well and is probably not needed. If so, we can turn our attention to other team-related prerequisites.

Interdependent Tasks

By examining the nature of the tasks that must be performed and the relationships between and among these tasks, we can sometimes reach an understanding of how each member will contribute to the successful achievement of the team's common purpose. This understanding should help answer another important question: Do the individuals who would make up the team really need to have their tasks and responsibilities closely coordinated? In particular, we are interested in the degree of interdependence between and among the tasks. Tasks are interdependent if their progression or completion is influenced by, determined by, or subject to, the progression or completion of one another. Stated another way, task interdependence can be thought of as the degree to which the completion of a given task requires that other tasks are completed, the degree to which the given task must be completed for another task to be completed, or the degree to which the individual performing the given task must interact with others to complete the task.

Task interdependence can be thought of as having three types or forms: (i) pooled interdependence, (ii) sequential interdependence, and (iii) reciprocal interdependence (Fig. 18.2). Pooled interdependence occurs when two individuals function with relative independence but their combined output contributes to the group's or organization's overall goals. An example of pooled interdependence would be an assembly shop that has a number of employees, each working alone to assemble radios. At the end of the day, the completed radios are shipped out together. In this case the workers' efforts are independent but the results of their efforts are pooled, and it could be said that the shop produced x number of radios.

Sequential interdependence occurs when workers depend upon others for their inputs. The dependency is in only one direction, and if those who provide the inputs don't perform their jobs properly, those who are dependent on them will be significantly affected. An example of sequential interdependence is an assembly line. In the above radio shop example, sequential interdependence would exist if each worker installed a component in a partially completed radio and passed the partially assembled unit on to the next worker in the line. That worker would then install a component, and so on. The steps have a specific order, and individuals cannot perform their tasks until the tasks that precede theirs are completed.

Reciprocal interdependence occurs when individuals exchange inputs and outputs. If the performance of any task is compromised, the effect will eventually be visited upon the other tasks. For example, sales people, in contact with customers, acquire information about the customers' future needs. Sales then relays this back to the product development department so they can create new products or alter existing ones to meet customers' needs. By the same token, the product development department would try to anticipate customer needs with their development efforts. By keeping the sales force informed of their innovations, they influence the interactions that the sales reps have with the customers. Another example would be a surgical team in which the actions of one member influence and are influenced by actions of the others (28).

It is possible to make rather objective assessments of the type and degree of task interdependence that exists between and among specific tasks. However, whether the workers who are performing the tasks would agree with the assessment is another matter. Current research indicates that various individuals can perceive the degree of task interdependence of the same set of tasks as different (5). This research also indicates that the level of task interdependence perceived by employees is related to their commitment to the organizations for which they work and, if applicable, their teams. The idea behind this research is that as employees perceive that their efforts are interdependent with the efforts of others, they become more aware of the contributions they are making to the successful attainment of the organization's goals and to the success of those with whom they are working. This heightened awareness, according to the theory, should enhance employees' ego involvement with their jobs and increase their positive affect towards their organizations and their teams (5, 44, 47). The lesson is that it is important for employees to understand how their tasks contribute to (read: "are interdependent with") the success of others' tasks and what the successful performance of these tasks means to the organization.

Summary

In summary, the use of teams should be considered if (i) a common purpose for the *collective* can be identified, (ii) the individuals who would make up the team thoroughly understand this purpose and accept it, and (iii) one or more of the goals that must be met to achieve the common purpose can be achieved only through a collective effort.

Selecting Team Members

Skill requirements for team members can be categorized into three types: (i) technical or functional expertise; (ii) problem-solving and decision-making skills, and (iii) interpersonal skills. While the members can possess these skills when the team is formed or develop them after it is in place, performance by the team cannot happen without them. Thus, it is important that team members are se-

Figure 18.2 Types of task interdependence.

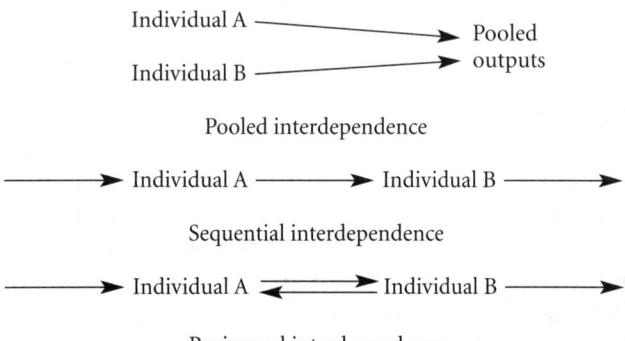

Pooled interdependence

Sequential interdependence

Reciprocal interdependence

Table 18.1 Knowledge, skill, and ability (KSA) requirements for teamwork[a]

I. Interpersonal KSAs
   A. Conflict resolution KSAs
      1. Recognize and encourage desirable, but discourage undesirable, team conflict.
      2. Recognize the type and source of conflict confronting the team and implement an appropriate conflict resolution strategy.
      3. Employ an integrative (win-win) negotiation strategy rather than the traditional distributive (win-lose) strategy.
   B. Collaborative problem solving KSAs
      4. Identify situations requiring participative group problem solving and utilize the proper degree and type of participation.
      5. Recognize the obstacles to collaborative group problem solving and implement appropriate corrective actions.
   C. Communication KSAs
      6. Understand communication networks and utilize decentralized networks to enhance communication where possible.
      7. Communicate openly and supportively, that is, send messages that are: (i) behavior- or event-oriented; (ii) congruent; (iii) validating; (iv) conjunctive; and (v) owned.
      8. Listen without judging and appropriately use active listening techniques.
      9. Maximize consonance between nonverbal and verbal messages and recognize and interpret the nonverbal messages of others.
      10. Engage in ritual greetings and small talk, recognizing their importance.
II. Self-management KSAs
   D. Goal setting and performance management KSAs
      11. Help establish specific, challenging, and accepted team goals.
      12. Monitor, evaluate, and provide feedback on both overall team performance and individual team member performance.
   E. Planning and task coordination KSAs
      13. Coordinate and synchronize activities, information, and task interdependencies among team members.
      14. Help establish task and role expectations of individual team members and ensure proper balancing of workload in the team.

[a]Adapted from reference 59, p. 505.

lected based on either possessing these skills or having a strong aptitude for their development. These three basic skill categories are used to set the criteria for team member selection. In practice, these categories take various forms and degrees, depending on the type of team. For example, one can expect task-related skills for a management team to be drastically different from those for a work team. Similarly, decision-making skills and interpersonal skills in those two contexts are also likely to differ to a large extent (28).

While the technical expertise and decision-making skills may differ across teams depending upon their goals, objectives, and methods, the required team-related skills tend to be common among all types of teams. Team-related skills could be further categorized as shown in Table 18.1. Sample questions from a selection instrument designed to measure these attributes are shown in Table 18.2.

In addition to written tests, other selection tools can be developed to measure such knowledge, skills, and abilities (KSAs). For example, structured interviews can be de-

Table 18.2 Example items from the teamwork-KSA test[a]

1. Suppose that you find yourself in an argument with several coworkers about who should do a very disagreeable but routine task. Which of the following would likely be the most effective way to resolve this situation?
   a) Have your supervisor decide because this would avoid any personal bias.
   b) Arrange for a rotating schedule so everyone shares the chore.*
   c) Let the workers who show up earliest choose on a first-come, first-served basis.
   d) Randomly assign a person to do the task and don't change it.
2. Your team wants to improve the quality and flow of the conversations among its members.
   Your team should
   a) Use comments that build upon and connect to what others have said.*
   b) Set up a specific order for everyone to speak and then follow it.
   c) Let team members with more to say determine the direction and topic of conversation.
   d) Do all of the above.
3. Suppose you are presented with the following types of goals. You are asked to pick one for your team to work on. Which would you choose?
   a) An easy goal. This will ensure that the team reaches it, thus creating a feeling of success.
   b) A goal of average difficulty. The team will be somewhat challenged, but they will be successful without too much effort.
   c) A difficult and challenging goal that will stretch the team to perform at a high level. The goal is attainable so that effort will not be seen as futile.*
   d) A very difficult or even impossible goal. Even if the team falls short, it will at least have a very high target to aim for.

[a]Adapted from ref. 59, p. 519. Asterisks indicate correct answers.

signed to measure whether candidates have adequate levels of these KSAs. Assessment center techniques can be used to measure candidates' leadership and other social skills through group exercises. Biographical data measurement may provide information about candidates' KSAs in dealing with social problems, especially those focusing on experiences candidates had in previous jobs, in school, and in recreational activities involving teams. One can also integrate team-related KSAs into the recruiting process by communicating the importance of these KSAs through such methods as realistic job previews (59).

The following is an example of how individual traits may affect various attributes of teams, including productivity. In a study of work teams conducted at an apparel factory, certain dispositions of team members were found to be negatively related to team performance or quality. For example, team members who possessed a higher degree of aggression and autonomy were less likely to report high levels of team commitment and team cohesion, two factors often regarded as important antecedents of team performance. In addition, teams were found to have more difficulty in controlling quality when members were talkative or valued extraneous communications among team members at the expense of attention to the team's tasks. Teams with more members willing to use cross-training skills tended to have higher productivity, quality, cohesion, and commitment (55).

In teams, as elsewhere, success breeds success. There is evidence that team members' preferences for teamwork are related to the effectiveness of the team (10). Hence, it is important for teams to experience success early; this starts with member selection. For two examples of team self-selection issues, see case study 2 in Appendix 18.1.

Training Team Members

Why is team training such a big deal? Don't people learn teamwork in school? Actually, they don't. More likely they have been admonished to "do your own work." With this type of school experience, most people are *not* well prepared to work in teams. On the contrary, they have been taught to strive for their individual goals and objectives. For a team to be successful, that has to change. Training for teams can be roughly categorized into two basic types: task-related training and team-related training.

Task-Related Training

Task-related training focuses on the actual tasks for which the team is responsible. Because of rapidly changing technology, the associated technical skills and knowledge require continuous upgrading. Hence, task-related training is an ongoing process. Training programs should be designed to satisfy the team's need for particular technical skills. Consequently, the design should consider each individual member's current abilities, interests, and professional direction. Task-related training can be conducted through formal classroom instruction, on-the-job training, and member-to-member mentoring (51).

Team-Related Training

Research indicates that when team members possess the appropriate team-related KSAs (Table 18.1), there will be positive effects on team performance (8, 14, 49, 51, 59, 60, 66). One of the most important of these skills is the ability to communicate well. Teamwork relies on collective actions and decisions. Furthermore, team members achieve these actions and decisions through exchange of opinions, negotiation, persuasion, and compromise. Thus, communication skills are essential for collective creation. Training to enhance communication skills can start before the work teams are formed and should be made available on an ongoing basis as teams develop and mature.

Numerous authors and consultants have also endorsed team awareness training. The purpose of team awareness training is to give employees an overview of what teams are all about, why the organization is adopting them, and how employees can benefit personally from their team membership (51). To the extent that teams are complete operating units, they take over many of the organizational functions that were previously performed by specific organizational departments such as purchasing, payroll, engineering, accounting, human resources and work process analysis (51).

J. R. Hackman has proposed a four-stage process for creating and developing work teams (Table 18.3). A set of questions associated with each stage can be used to guide actions. Once these questions are addressed and all four stages are achieved, team members should get substantial return from their effort in terms of work effectiveness and in the quality of their interactions with teammates (19). For an example of team-related training, see case study 3 in Appendix 18.1.

Table 18.3 Guidelines for team building[a]

Stage 1: Prework
  Q1: What is the task?
  Q2: What are the critical task demands?
  Q3: Will the group be manager-led, self-managing, or self-designing?
  Q4: Overall, how advantageous is it to assign the work to a team? How feasible is it?

Stage 2: Creating performance conditions
  Q5: How should the group be composed and the task be structured?
  Q6: What contextual supports and resources must be provided?

Stage 3: Forming and building the team
  Q7: How can a team be helped to get off to a good start?

Stage 4: Providing ongoing assistance
  Q8: How can opportunities be provided for the group to renegotiate its design and context?
  Q9: What process assistance can be provided to promote positive group synergy?
  Q10: How can the group be helped to learn from its experiences?

[a]From ref. 19, p. 335–337.

Leadership and Teams

General Ideas about Leadership: a Brief Review

Leadership is a process in which one individual exerts influence to structure the behavior of other people within a group (67). Various leadership theories have hypothesized leadership roles and behaviors, their relationship with group performance, and external conditions that moderate such relationships. Two of the earliest behavioral leadership theories are the Ohio State University study and the University of Michigan study. The Ohio State study categorized various leadership behaviors into two basic types, labeled "consideration" and "initiating structure." The Michigan study also identified two basic categories of leadership behaviors, labeled "relationship-oriented behaviors" and "task-oriented behaviors." Both consideration behaviors and relationship-oriented behaviors focus on relationship building and maintenance between leaders and followers. These behaviors have also been referred to as "supportive behaviors" and include acting friendly toward followers, respecting followers' ideas and feelings, appreciating their contributions, recognizing their accomplishments, and showing concern for their welfare and needs. Both initiating structure and task-oriented behaviors are focused on task completion. These include planning, organizing, and scheduling work, planning activities, assigning tasks, coordinating activities, and providing the necessary direction, materials, and support. Initiating structure and task-oriented behaviors have also been termed "directive behaviors" (26). There are numerous other typologies of leadership behaviors, but most tend to be subcategories of the two main categories described above. While there are subtle differences in the definitions of the terms "consideration," "relationship-oriented," and "supportive behavior," as well as the terms "initiating structure," "task-oriented," and "directive behavior," we will not go into that here. For our purposes, we will consider the terms within each category to be synonymous. It turns out that the Ohio State studies have received the most attention by academics and tend to appear in textbooks more often than the others, though in recent years the terms "directive" and "supportive" have appeared more and more. In any event, we will use the Ohio State designations for the rest of this discussion.

One of the most common errors made by students when first confronted with the two categories of leadership behavior is that they tend to think of "consideration" as good and "initiating structure" as bad. Nothing could be further from the truth, and why students tend do this remains a mystery to the authors. We suspect they equate consideration with "being nice" and initiating structure with "bossing people around" in an abrasive manner. Such conclusions are erroneous. Each type of behavior has its place, and employees under the right circumstances appreciate each.

For example, when the employee is new, inexperienced, or lacks knowledge or direction, guidance and direction are needed and usually appreciated. This calls for the leader to initiate structure by providing the needed guidance and direction. Considerate behavior at such a time would likely be seen as ineffective and evidence that the manager does not understand what is going on. Similarly, initiating structure may be called for if the task is very complex, the situation is ambiguous, or the environment uncertain. Some employees lack confidence, are timid, or have an external locus of control. Individuals with these characteristics may respond well to initiating structure. On the other hand, if the employee is experienced, highly skilled, and particularly competent, then initiating structure may not be needed and may even be resented. Such an employee would respond more positively to the behaviors we have labeled "consideration." Likewise, if the task is simple and generates its own feedback—that is, the employee can easily and quickly see how he or she did and corrective action is easily determined—then consideration is likely to be more appropriate. In such cases, initiating structure would be redundant and ineffective.

Even though these examples may be clear, in the workplace we are often confronted with ambiguous and conflicting situations. For example, what about the situation in which the task is simple (suggesting that initiating structure is not needed) but the employee is inexperienced (suggesting that initiating structure is needed)? In such a case, managerial judgment is required. One alternative might be to ask the employee what he or she needs. Those with an internal locus of control may ask for time to figure it out while those with a more external locus of control may ask for instructions. Take the first individual. Suppose time is of the essence and you don't have time for them to "figure it out." Take the second individual. Suppose figuring things out is a skill they must develop. There are two points here. One is that while managerial education may be a fine thing and while management scholars believe that managerial theory and research are important and helpful, they are not immutable dogma. We must realize that theory, research, and education provide important guidelines to help managers make the tough decisions for which, many times, there are no single "right" answers. The second point is that initiating structure and consideration are not mutually exclusive. Managers can engage in both types of behavior as they are required. It is up to managers to apply judgment along with the theories and concepts to the situations they face.

Leadership in a Team Environment

Performing successfully as a team leader requires a number of skills (29). Successful team leaders should know that team performance comes from collective effort and action. Therefore, motivating team members to support collective performance becomes an important focus. To achieve this, team leaders need first to "clarify purpose and goals, build commitment and self-confidence, strengthen the team's collective skills and approach, remove externally imposed obstacles, and create opportunities for others" (29). Depending upon whether the team leader is also a member of the team, he or she may also need to perform team-related tasks within the purview of the team. Second, team leaders should be aware that they do not have to take all the responsibility for decision making by the team. Keeping in mind that team success depends on the combined contributions of all members of the team, team leaders should consciously avoid any action that might threaten the desire of team members to make contributions. Third, team leaders need to confront a number of dilemmas, such as the amount of autonomy given to team members versus giving up control, making tough decisions alone versus letting the team make them or participate in making them, and doing difficult tasks alone versus letting others do them and learn how in the process. The fine line of balancing these decisions varies from team to team, each of which has its own unique characteristics.

Team leaders should take the role of developing and facilitating team members rather than controlling them. They can serve as a liaison between the team and other parts of the organization or even other organizations; they can be resource providers, assisting the team in defining their resource needs and helping to secure those resources; they can be counselors, helping team members develop problem-solving skills; they can be mentors, guiding team members to develop organizational savvy; they can be teachers, passing on technical information to team members; they can challenge the team process of decision making, interpersonal relationships, and progress toward the team's goal (2). Team leaders and members should also be aware that the leader's role changes with growth of the team (11). Team leaders can lead members to lead themselves. To do this, some management scholars suggest the following seven steps:

1. Become an effective self-leader. (For further discussion of self-leadership, see reference 43.)
2. Model self-leadership for team members.
3. Encourage team members to set their own goals.
4. Create positive thought patterns.
5. Reward self-leadership and promote constructive critical feedback.
6. Promote self-leading teamwork.
7. Facilitate a self-leadership culture (43).

Team Leader Selection

There are a number of ways to select a team leader. The leader can be assigned externally, be elected internally, emerge naturally, or be rotated among team members. Different methods of leader selection have different effects on the leader's legitimacy—how followers perceive the leader's source of authority and respond to the leader. Electing the team leader makes it more likely that the followers will identify with the leader, have more sense of responsibility to the

leader, and perceive a greater investment in him or her (23). However, elected leaders will be more likely to face criticism from followers for performance failure (24). Research has shown that teams whose leaders were elected by team members performed better than teams with no leader or teams whose leaders were appointed (17) and that, when compared to appointed leaders, elected leaders received higher ratings from the members on responsiveness to members' needs, interest in the group task, and competence (4).

A naturally emergent leader can be expected to receive similar responses from team members as an elected leader because both kinds of leader selection reflect team members' opinions regarding appropriate qualities of a team leader and the particular person believed to possess such qualities. However, leaders emerge on their own, and depending on the team's timetable, this may not be amenable to the achievement of the organization's and team's goals. There are other dangers in waiting for a team leader to emerge. First, unless the team's production norms are clear and high, an emergent leader may lead the team away from the purpose for which the team was formed. Second, two or more rival leaders may begin to emerge and coalitions may form around them and split the team. Finally, no leader may emerge.

Rotating leaders is another way to generate and maintain team-leading function. In certain self-directed teams, team members rotate the position of team leader. Here, the focus is on the function of the leader position rather than who the team leader is. Rotating leaders tends to work when the task is clearly defined and the direction, vision, and purpose of the team are well understood and do not depend upon who the leader is. It is also an excellent way to give leadership experience to the team members and encourage each member to strongly buy in to the team's purpose.

Another approach for team leader selection is through a process in which both upper management and the team members participate. Participative selection, if properly structured and guided, can have at least four positive results:

- Selection of a high-quality leader;
- A high level of participant satisfaction;
- Facilitating better understanding of the leader's job; and
- Creating positive expectations that can enhance the chances of the leader's success through the process of self-fulfilling prophecy (48).

Motivating Team Performance

Goal Setting and Performance

One of the most viable and successful motivational techniques to appear in the management literature is goal setting. Goal setting theories suggest that goals can improve performance because they generate, direct, and sustain effort (39). In particular, goals should be specific, rather than general or vague; difficult but attainable (also called "stretch goals"), rather than easy; and accepted by the team. Attempts to reach them should be accompanied by feedback (15, 39, 40, 63).

General or vague goals, such as "do your best," do not result in the levels of performance that occur when goals are specific, e.g., "increase production by 10%." The specificity of the goal acts as a guide and stimulus, allowing employees to make reasonable inferences about the effort and resources that will be required. Difficult goals, when met, obviously result in greater performance than corresponding easy goals. However, simply setting difficult goals is not automatically effective. Workers must see the goal as attainable. If the goal is unreasonably high and perceived as unattainable, it could serve to discourage effort rather than motivate it. At the same time, goals, to be effective, must be accepted by those who would strive to attain them. If a goal is not accepted, the individual involved is unlikely to strive very much to reach it.

From this discussion, we might infer that less difficult goals are more likely to be accepted than more difficult ones. However, more difficult goals can be associated with greater rewards, extrinsically as well as intrinsically. Managers who set goals for their employees walk a fine line between setting goals so high as to discourage effort and setting them so low that good performance is not attained. Consequently, managers would do well to ensure that goals are accepted and, to the degree possible, implement a reward structure to support their attainment.

Researchers disagree over the usefulness of having employees set their own goals or participate in setting them versus having goals be assigned by management. One school of thought is that employees will try harder if they have the opportunity to participate in setting their own goals. The other school holds that it doesn't matter. The results of research on this question are mixed (35), with participatively set goals being superior in some cases and assigned goals being superior in others. Regardless of these results, a major advantage of employee participation may be in the acceptance of the goal. That is, as employees consider the resources, effort, and other parameters required to achieve the goals they set, they are likely to conclude that the selected goals are desirable ones to pursue.

The final dimension in goal setting theory is feedback. When people have accepted a goal and are striving for its attainment, they need to know how they are doing. This knowledge helps them identify discrepancies between where they are and where they want to be and what they are doing versus what they should be doing. In effect, feedback acts as a guide for behavior. Research indicates that self-generated feedback is a more powerful motivator than externally generated feedback. In other words, if employees can monitor their own progress, results tend to be better than if they cannot (27).

Goal Setting and Teams

The performance-enhancing effect of goal setting has been found not only at the individual level but also at the group level (9, 31, 39, 50, 52, 53, 64, 65). The results of research with groups parallel those obtained with individuals in terms of goal specificity (50), difficulty (64), attainability (33), and acceptance (59). Conversely, team effectiveness can be lowered because of a lack of unity or clarity about goals (59). Furthermore, improper assessment of goal difficulty leads to team failure (32, 68).

As with individuals, team goals can be assigned or participatively set. Which technique to use depends on the type of team and tasks. Studies show that participatively setting goals is likely to enhance the acceptance of goals by team members (45, 52), increase congruence between individual and team goals (16, 41), lead to better quality goals and satisfaction with the process (37), and increase the likelihood of producing positive outcomes (50). Another possible benefit of team members participating in goal setting is the cohesiveness that can be generated by such interaction. Further, as teams discuss various goal levels, individual members become aware of their teammates' strengths, weaknesses, and overall capabilities. This awareness should assist members in making sound and realistic judgments concerning the team's capabilities as a unit. Frank discussions of member roles in achieving team goals should increase the knowledge of how and to what degree the various tasks are interdependent. As was mentioned before, heightened perceptions of task interdependence are associated with increased organizational and team commitment (5).

Evaluating Teams and Team Members

Performance evaluation gives feedback to the team, which guides the team to make needed adjustments (18). Because of synergy, a team's collective production is not necessarily the simple addition of individual member productions. Therefore, teams need to be evaluated as single units. A team's achievement can be evaluated based on (i) the degree to which the results that a team delivers are acceptable to those who receive them, (ii) the team being able to work effectively together in the future, and (iii) individual members being more satisfied than frustrated in achieving their personal goals (20).

At the time when collective outcome (team performance) is assessed, individual team members' performance must be evaluated as well (61). Different individuals may make disproportionate contributions. In general, this should be avoided. At the same time the nature of a given team may be that one individual (or a subset of individuals) is simply capable of more and the others respond by relieving that individual of some of the administrative or "housekeeping" duties and supporting him or her in other ways. Even so, it is important to monitor individual performance so as to prevent social loafing or free-riding (the tendency to exert less effort in a joint action) (1, 21, 30, 34, 45). Most of the time, a team's visible outcome is the result of a collective effort. Consequently, evaluation of individual team members can be problematic. Some experts suggest creating a behavioral instrument based on the KSAs for teamwork as displayed in Table 1. Honest and constructive peer evaluation is also important.

Rewarding Teams and Team Members

Some managers with whom the authors are familiar have suggested giving rewards to individuals who exhibit outstanding performance. In general, we tend to discourage such action. In fact, there are times when it can be counterproductive. For example, when teams are new and have been recently introduced in an organization, there may be a tendency by individuals to resist sacrificing their own autonomy for the sake of the team. To offer individual rewards during this time would, in our view, undermine the team concept and the idea of subordinating individual goals for team goals. For teams to prosper, especially during the initial stages of their formation, we suggest that all rewards be at the team level and all recognitions be for team results. Later, individual rewards may be appropriate. But this action should be carefully considered and done with extreme caution.

Legal Issues and Teams

Can the use of work teams get you into legal trouble? Yes, actually it can. Here's how. The National Labor Relations Act (NLRA) was passed in the 1930s to define and guide the legal relationships between management and labor (these classes include companies, labor unions, and employees). Section 2(5) of the NLRA defines a labor organization in this way:

> The term "labor organization" means any organization of any kind, or any agency or employee representation committee or plan, in which employees participate and which exists for the purpose, in whole or in part, of dealing with employers concerning grievances, labor disputes, wages, rates of pay, hours of employment, or conditions of work.

By this definition, should an organization's teams discuss with management conditions of work or, as with some gainsharing committees or teams, bonuses, then such a team is, according to law, a labor organization. Therefore, many of the teams in the United States can be classified as labor organizations, just as a union is classified as a labor organization. The NLRA goes on to state in Section 8(a)(2):

> It shall be an unfair labor practice for an employer to dominate or interfere with the formation or administration of any labor organization or contribute financial or other support to it . . .

According to some recent court decisions, the term "other support" can include a computer, office space, or secretarial services. Hence, if your team is a labor organization, as defined by Section 2(5) of the NLRA and you provide support to it as defined by Section 8(a)(2) of the same act and interpreted by the courts, then your organization is guilty of an unfair labor practice. Sound farfetched? See Appendix 18.3 for the wording of a bill before Congress, HR 634. Three days later, the same bill was introduced in the Senate (S 295). The vote on the Bill was along party lines, with the Republicans voting "aye" and the Democrats voting "nay." The bill died when it became clear that there were not enough votes in the Senate to override a veto promised by then-President Clinton. The issue of where teams stand legally is still in limbo.

Summary

The use of teams is not easy, and it is certainly not free. In fact, using teams can have important and salient drawbacks. Such drawbacks must be looked upon as investments in the business before teams are implemented. Organizations should be as sure as they can be that their investment in teams will bring forth worthwhile returns. That is, the use of teams should be evaluated just like any other investment.

KEY POINTS

- Effectiveness of a team can be determined by:
  - the acceptability of its results,
  - the ability of its members to work together in the future,
  - the value of the team experience to each member.
- Conditions that facilitate effective teamwork are:
  - a group structure that promotes competent work on the task,
  - support and reinforcement of excellence by the organization,
  - the availability of expert coaching and process assistance.
- The essence of a team is common commitment leading to specific performance goals.

GLOSSARY

Common purpose A state that is achieved when team members fully understand the team's purpose or reason for existing, and there is significant goal congruence.

Gainsharing A financial plan in which improved group productivity determines the amount of money that is shared among the company, investors, and members of the group.

Goal congruence The degree to which team (or group) members' individual goals coincide with the team's (or group's) goals.

Goal setting The process by which team and/or individual goals are determined, communicated, and agreed upon.

Group effectiveness The sum of the group member's individual capabilities, plus process gain, minus process loss.

Group process The way groups get things done, including communication patterns, decision-making methods and techniques, leader behavior and interaction, power dynamics, conflict resolution methods and techniques, and the way members interact with each other.

Leadership legitimacy The degree to which a team or group leader is accepted by both the team or group members and the employing organization.

Participative selection A process in which team members choose new members of their team based on team-related criteria that were determined and agreed upon prior to candidate identification.

Process loss (gain) The degree to which group processes inhibit (enhance) the successful completion of group objectives.

Task interdependence The degree to which a task's progression or completion is influenced by, determined by, or subject to the progression or completion of one or more other tasks.

Work group Two or more individuals who interact primarily to share information and to make decisions that help each other perform within his or her area of responsibility.

Work team Two or more individuals whose individual efforts result in a performance that is greater than the sum of those individual parts and who have different tasks but work together adaptively to achieve specified and shared goals.

REFERENCES

1. **Albanese, R., and D. D. Van Fleet.** 1985. Rational behavior in groups: the free-riding tendency. *Acad. Manage. Rev.* **10**(2):244–255.

2. **Aranda, E. K., L. Aranda, and K. Conlon.** 1998. *Teams: Structure, Process, Culture, and Politics.* Prentice Hall, Upper Saddle River, N.J.

3. **Banker, R. D., J. M. Field, R. G. Schroeder, and K. K. Sinha.** 1996. Impact of work teams on manufacturing performance: a longitudinal field study. *Acad. Manage. J.* **39**(4):867–890.

4. **Ben-Yoav, O., E. P. Hollander, and P. J. D. Carnevale.** 1983. Leader legitimacy, leader-follower interaction, and followers' ratings of the leader. *J. Social Psychol.* **121**(1):111–115.

5. **Bishop, J. W., and D. J. Scott.** 2000. An examination of organizational and team commitment in a self-directed team environment. *J. Applied Psychol.* **85**(3):439–450.

6. **Bishop, J. W., K. D. Scott, and S. M. Burroughs.** 2000. Support, commitment, and employee outcomes in a team environment. *J. Manage.* **26**(6):1113–1132.

7. **Brannick, M. T., and C. Prince.** 1997. An overview of team performance measurement, p. 3–16. *In* M. T. Brannick, E. Salas, and C. Prince (ed.), *Team Performance Assessment and Measurement.* Lawrence Erlbaum Associates, Publishers, Mahwah, N.J.

8. **Buller, P. F.** 1986. The team building task performance relation: some conceptual and methodological refinements. *Group Organ. Studies* **11**(1):147–168.

9. **Buller, P. F., and C. H. Bell.** 1986. Effects of team building and goal setting on productivity: a field experiment. *Acad. Manage. J.* **29**(2):305–328.

10. **Campion, M. A., G. J. Medsker, and C. Higgs.** 1993. Relations between work group characteristics and efficiency: implications for designing effective work groups. *Personnel Psychol.* **46**(4):823–850.

11. **Carew, D. K., E. Parisi-Carew, and K. H. Blanchard.** 1986. Group development and situational leadership: a model for managing groups. *Training Dev. J.* **40**(6):46–50.

12. **Cohen, S. G.** 1991. New approaches to teams and teamwork, p. 194–226. *In* J. R. Galbraith, E. E. Lawler, and Associates (ed.), *Organization for the Future: the New Logic for Managing Complex Organizations.* Jossey-Bass, San Francisco, Calif.

13. **Cohen, S. G., and D. E. Bailey.** 1997. What makes teams work: group effectiveness research from the shop floor to the executive suite. *J. Manage.* **23**(3):239–290.

14. **De Meuse, K. P., and S. J. Liebowitz.** 1981. An empirical analysis of team-building research. *Group Organ. Studies* **6**(4):357–378.

15. **Earley, P. C., G. B. Northcraft, C. Lee, and T. R. Lituchy.** 1990. Impact of process and outcome feedback on the relation of goal setting to task performance. *Acad. Manage. J.* **33**:87–105.

16. **Erez, M.** 1986. The congruence of goal setting strategies with sociocultural values and its effect on performance. *J. Manage.* **8**(1):83–90.

17. **Goldman, M., and L. A. Fraas.** 1965. The effects of leader selection on group performance. *Sociometry* **28**(1):82–88.

18. **Goodman, P. S. S., R. Devedas, and T. L. C. Hughson.** 1988. Groups and productivity: analyzing the effectiveness of self-managing teams, p. 295–327. *In* J. P. Campbell and R. J. Campbell (ed.), *Productivity in Organizations.* Jossey-Bass, San Francisco, Calif.

19. **Hackman, J. R.** 1987. The design of work teams, p. 315–342. *In* J. W. Lorsch (ed.). *Handbook of Organizational Behavior.* Prentice Hall, Englewood Cliffs, N.J.

20. **Hackman, J. R.** 1990. *Groups That Work (and Those That Don't): Creating Conditions for Effective Teamwork.* Jossey-Bass Publishers, San Francisco, Calif.

21. **Harkins, S. G.** 1987. Social loafing and social facilitation. *J. Exp. Social Psychol.* **23**(1):1–18.

22. **Harris, T. E.** 1992. Toward effective employee involvement: an analysis of parallel and self-managing teams. *J. Allied Bus. Res.* **9**(1):25–33.

23. **Hollander, E. P.** 1993. Legitimacy, power, and influence: a perspective on relational features of leadership, p. 29–47. *In* M. M. Chemers and R. Ayman (ed.), *Leadership Theory and Research: Perspectives and Directions.* Academic Press, San Diego, Calif.

24. **Hollander, E. P., and J. W. Julian.** 1970. Studies in leader legitimacy, influence, and innovation, p. 33–69. *In* L. L. Berkowitz (ed.), *Advances in Experimental Social Psychology,* vol. 5. Academic Press, Inc., New York, N.Y.

25. **Hollenbeck, J. R., D. J. Sego, D. R. Ilgen, D. A. Major, J. Hedlund, and J. Phillips.** 1997. Team decision-making accuracy under difficult conditions: construct validation of potential manipulations using TIDE simulation, p. 111–136. *In* M. T. Brannick, E. Salas, and C. Prince (ed.), *Team Performance Assessment and Measurement: Theory, Methods, and Applications.* Lawrence Erlbaum Associates, Publishers, Mahwah, N.J.

26. **Howell, J. P., and D. L. Costeley.** 2001. *Understanding Behaviors for Effective Leadership.* Prentice Hall, Upper Saddle River, N.J.

27. **Ivancevich, J. M., and J. T. McMahon.** 1982. The effects of goal setting, external feedback, and self-generated feedback on outcome variables: a field experiment. *Acad. Manage. J.* **25**(2):359–372.

28. **Katzenbach, J. R., and D. K. Smith.** 1993. *The Wisdom of Teams: Creating the High-Performance Organization.* Harvard Business School Press, Boston, Mass.

29. **Katzenbach, J. R., and D. K. Smith.** 1993. The discipline of teams. *Harv. Bus. Rev.* **72**(1):111–120.

30. **Kerr, N. L., and S. E. Bruun.** 1983. Dispensability of member effort and group motivation losses: free-rider effects. *J. Pers. Social Psychol.* **44**(1):78–94.

31. **Koch, J. L.** 1979. Effects of goal specificity and performance feedback to work groups on peer leadership, performance, and attitudes. *Human Rela.* **33**(7):819–840.

32. **Kukla, A.** 1975. Preferences among impossibly difficult and trivially easy tasks: a revision of Atkinson's theory of choice. *J. Pers. Social Psychol.* **32**(3):338–345.

33. **Larson, C. E., and F. M. J. LaFasto.** 1989. *Teamwork: What Must Go Right/What Can Go Wrong.* Sage, Newbury Park, Calif.

34. **Latane, B., K. Williams, and S. Harkins.** 1979. Many hands make light the work: the causes and consequences of social loafing. *J. Pers. Social Psychol.* **37**(6):822–832.

35. **Latham, G. P., M. Erez, and E. A. Locke.** 1988. Resolving scientific disputes by the joint design of crucial experiments by the antagonists: application to Erez-Latham dispute regarding participation in goal setting. *J. Appl. Psychol.* **73**(4):753–772.

36. **Ledford, G. E., E. E. Lawler, and S. A. Morhman.** 1988. The quality circle and its variations, p. 255–294. *In* J. P. Campbell, R. J. Campbell and Associates (ed.). *Productivity in Organizations.* Jossey-Bass, San Francisco, Calif.

37. **Levine, J. M., and R. L. Moreland.** 1990. Progress in small group research. *Annu. Rev. Psychol.* **41**:585–634.

38. **Likert, R.** 1961. *New Patterns of Management.* McGraw-Hill, New York.

39. **Locke, E. A., and G. P. Latham.** 1990. *A Theory of Goal Setting and Task Performance.* Prentice Hall, Englewood Cliffs, N.J.

40. **Locke, E. A., K. N. Shaw, L. M. Saari, and G. P. Latham.** 1981. Goal setting and task performance. *Psychol. Bull.* **90**(1):125–152.

41. **Mackie, D. M., and G. R. Goethals.** 1987. Individual and group goals, p. 144–166. *In* C. Hendrick (ed.), *Review of Personality and Social Psychology.* Sage, Beverly Hills, Calif.

42. **Mankin, D., S. G. Cohen, and T. K. Bikson.** 1996. *Teams and Technology: Fulfilling the Promise of the New Organization.* Harvard Business School Press, Boston, Mass.

43. **Manz, C. C., C. P. Neck, J. Mancuso, and K. P. Manz.** 1997. *For Team Members Only: Making Your Workplace Team Productive and Hassle-Free.* American Management Association, New York, N.Y.

44. **Mathieu, J. E., and D. M. Zajac.** 1990. A review and meta-analysis of the antecedents, correlates, and consequences of organizational commitment. *Psychol. Bull.* **108**(1):171–194.

45. **Matsui, T., T. Kakuyama, and M. U. Onglatco.** 1987. Effects of goals and feedback on performance in groups. *J. Appl. Psychol.* **72**(3):407–415.

46. **Morhman, S. A., S. G. Cohen, and A. M. Morhman.** 1995. *Designing Team-Based Organizations: New Forms for Knowledge Work.* Jossey-Bass, San Francisco, Calif.

47. **Morris, J. H., and R. M. Steers.** 1980. Structural influences on organizational commitment. *J. Vocat. Behav.* **17**(1):50–57.

48. **Newstrom, J., M. Lengnick-Hall, and S. Rubenfeld.** 1987. Recruitment: how employees can choose their own bosses. *Personnel J.* **66**(1):121–126.

49. **Nicholas, J. M.** 1982. The comparative impact of organization development interventions on hard criteria measures. *Acad. Manage. Rev.* **7**(3):531–542.

50. **O'Leary-Kelly, A. M., J. J. Martocchio, and D. D. Frink.** 1994. A review of the influence of group goals on group performance. *Acad. Manage. J.* **37**(5):1285–1301.

51. **Orsburn, J. D., L. Moran, E. Musselwhite, and J. H. Zenger.** 1990. *Self-Directed Work Teams.* Business One Irwin, Homewood, Ill.

52. **Pearson, C. A. L.** 1987. Participative goal setting as a strategy for improving performance and job satisfaction: a longitudinal evaluation with railway track maintenance gangs. *Hum. Relat.* **40**(5):473–488.

53. **Pritchard, R. D., S. Jones, P. Roth, K. Steubing, and S. Ekeberg.** 1988. Effects of group feedback, goal setting, and incentives on organizational productivity (monograph). *J. Appl. Psychol.* **73**(2):337–358.

54. **Robbins, S. P.** 1998. *Organizational Behavior,* 8th ed. Prentice Hall, Upper Saddle River, N.J.

55. **Scott, K. D., and A. Townsend.** 1994. Teams: why some succeed and others fail? *HR Mag.* **38**(8):62–67.

56. **Sheridan, J. H.** 1997. Culture-change lessons. *Ind. Week* **246**(2):20–24.

57. **Stein, B. A., and R. M. Kanter.** 1980. Building the parallel organization: creating mechanisms for permanent quality of work life. *J. Appl. Behav. Sci.* **16**:371–386.

58. **Steiner, I. D.** 1972. *Group Process and Productivity.* Academic Press, New York, N.Y.

59. **Stevens, M. J., and M. A. Campion.** 1994. The knowledge, skill, and ability requirements for teamwork: implications for human resource management. *J. Manage.* **20**(2):503–530.

60. **Tannenbaum, S. I., R. L. Beard, and E. Salas.** 1992. Team building and its influence on team effectiveness: an examination of conceptual and empirical developments, p. 117–153. *In* K. Kelley (ed.), *Issues, Theory, and Research in Industrial and Organizational Psychology.* Elsevier, Amsterdam, The Netherlands.

61. **Tesluk, P., J. E. Mathieu, and S. J. Zaccaro.** 1997. Task and aggregation issues in the analysis and assessment of team performance, p. 197–224. *In* M. T. Brannnick, E. Salas, and C. Prince (ed.), *Team Performance Assessment and Measurement.* Lawrence Erlbaum Associates, Publishers, Mahwah, N.J.

62. **Thompson, J. D.** 1967. *Organizations in Action,* p. 54–55. McGraw-Hill, New York, N.Y.

63. **Tubbs, M. E.** 1986. Goal setting: a meta-analytic examination of the empirical evidence. *J. Appl. Psychol.* **71**(3):474–483.

64. **Weingart, L. R.** 1992. Impact of group goals, task component complexity, effort, and planning on group performance. *J. Appl. Psychol.* **77**(5):682–693.

65. Weldon, E., K. A. Jehn, and P. Pradhan. 1991. Processes that mediate the relationship between a group goal and improved group performance. *J. Pers. Social Psychol.* **61**(3):555–569.

66. Woodman, R. W., and J. J. Sherwood. 1980. The role of team development in organizational effectiveness: a critical review. *Psychol. Bull.* **88**(1):166–186.

67. Yukl, G. 1998. *Leadership in Organizations,* 4th ed. Prentice Hall, Upper Saddle River, N.J.

68. Zander, A. F., and T. Newcomb. 1967. Group levels of aspiration in United Fund campaigns. *J. Pers. Social Psychol.* **6**(1):157–162.

APPENDIX 18.1   Case Studies

Case 1: When a Good Team Goes Bad
Team Commitment

(This is a stylized account of an actual situation that occurred in a branch of the armed services in a country that will remain nameless.)

Generally, we think of commitment to one's team and its goals as a precursor to team performance. Certainly team performance is a good thing, isn't it? After all, isn't that what we wish for? However, as the old saying goes, "Be careful what you wish for, you might get it." Consider the following anecdote:

In a branch of the armed services, there was a company of helicopter "flights." Each flight consisted of several helicopters and the company consisted of several flights. Each flight had a maintenance team, or ground crew, that was responsible for keeping the helicopters in their flight up and running.

In one particular company there was an "all-star" ground crew who, it seemed, never had an inoperable helicopter. Their "birds" were always airworthy. Their success was the stuff of legends and was in sharp contrast to the "up-time" achieved by other flight crews. Though competent and hardworking, the other crews seemed to have one or more of their birds down at any given time. Knowing just this, one would be tempted to say, "The 'All-Stars' are really a great team. Clearly their goals and objectives are congruent with the company's goals and objectives. Furthermore, they should serve as a role model for other teams, who should copy their methods."

But do they have goal congruence with the company? Should they serve as a role model for other teams? Let's take a closer look and see.

The Situation

As those familiar with helicopters can attest, because of the nature of the movable wing aircraft design, helicopters are notorious for wearing out parts. Therefore, a good supply of spare parts is absolutely essential to keep a company of helicopters flying. In addition to their skill and motivation, one of the reasons for the success of the All-Stars was that they never experienced a shortage of spare parts. On the other hand, the other crews were constantly short of parts and even resorted to cannibalizing parts from inoperable helicopters, something the All-Stars never had to do. Why was this? Wasn't there a common store of parts from which the flights drew replacements? Yes. Well then, didn't everyone have the same access to parts? Yes, at least officially. But in reality the truth was quite different.

It turned out that the All-Stars had their own parts procurement process to "supplement" company procedures. They went around the chain of command; they established informal relationships with the appropriate quartermaster personnel, and they devised an extra-official parts procurement process and procedure of their own. As if that wasn't enough, they hoarded parts. Because some helicopter parts wear out in a predictable manner, it was known beforehand which parts would likely be needed in greater quantities. It was these parts that the All-Stars hoarded in the greatest quantity. The result was that although the All-Stars had 100% up-time for their helicopters, the company as a whole had a number of helicopters down for want of parts that the All-Star team members possessed in abundance.

The Lesson and What To Do

A major lesson here is that even though the achievement of team goals may appear to coincide with and further organizational goals, the methods of achieving team goals may inhibit or even prevent the achievement of organizational goals.

What should a manager do in such a circumstance? Usually with exercises of this type, students want more information before making a decision. Granted, in such cases it is difficult to know exactly what we would do. Furthermore, we need to keep in mind that this is a military unit and therefore may be subject to military rules and regulations that differ significantly from those in the civilian world.

However, with the information provided we can articulate some reasonable alternative actions that would be appropriate in the civilian sector. First, it is highly unlikely that the All-Star team could be salvaged as an intact unit. The team norms are too strong and run too counter to the objectives of the organization. Second, hoarding parts may be grounds for dismissal. At the very least the team should be broken up and the members dispersed throughout the company, or preferably, across several companies (or units in a civilian organization). Similar action would be required with respect to those in the parts supply chain who enabled the All-Stars shenanigans.

It is easy, though often counterproductive, to point out to people what should have been done. Even so, in this case, what should have been done and what must be done *now* are much the same. In addition to the actions related to the ground crew team and the parts personnel, the organization must reevaluate its team training program and the components that comprise it. Those responsible for training, as well as company management, must ensure that team objectives include knowledge of organizational objectives and techniques for advancing team goals in such a way as to fulfill and not impede these objectives. Care should be taken to ensure that as team norms develop, team members are aware of, concerned with, and take action for the furtherance of organizational goals.

Though our primary purpose in analyzing this case is to consider the issues related to the implementation and use of teams, other aspects of the situation must not be neglected. It is important to do this to avoid a myopic view that would cause us to become one-dimensional in our problem-solving thought processes.

With this in mind we would recommend that a control system for the distribution and use of parts be put in place and its use mandated and supported by management. Particular care must be taken in the design and implementation of such a system. For example, a charge-back scheme has some characteristics that would help prevent situations like the one exemplified by the All-Stars. Charge-backs would require ground crews to have a financial component for which they must be responsible. On the other hand, if the charge-back scheme includes an overly restrictive budget or if rewards for a parts budget surplus are emphasized, then teams may be motivated to skimp on the use of parts

(continued)

and try to stretch the usable life of the parts too far—with disastrous consequences.

Summary

Team goals did coincide with organization goals, but the methods of achieving the team goals inhibited the achievement of organizational goals.

Case 2: Two Examples of How to and How Not to Select Team Members

Example 1: Selecting New Members for Established Teams (an Automotive Outsourcing Plant)

Invariably, the composition of teams will change over time. Members quit or get fired, promoted, or transferred. When a position on a team opens, filling that position presents unique challenges. In addition to the traditional selection criteria involving task-related KSAs, team-related criteria must be considered for a successful match to be made. Some of the additional questions that arise are, "Can the applicant work well in a team environment? Can the applicant work well with the particular team that has the vacancy? Can the team work well with the applicant?"

One organization with which the authors are familiar approached this problem in the following way. First, the human resources department screened the applicants for the traditional KSAs that are required for successful performance on the job in question, checked references, confirmed job history, and performed the appropriate background checks. Following this screening process, three to five candidates whom the company would hire were presented to the team. The team members reviewed the documentation gathered by the human resources department and, considering this information in light of the team's requirements, interviewed the candidates for the purpose of making the final selection. The candidates interviewed with the team members individually and as a group. Team members were trained in structured and unstructured interviews. They were fully aware that their purpose was twofold. One, they were trying to sell their team to the candidate and, two, they were trying to determine if the applicant would make a good teammate.

This system seemed to produce a good amount of initial commitment between the chosen new member and the established team; after all, they chose each other. These initial positive feelings can be enhanced or squandered depending upon subsequent actions by the parties involved. But at least it's a positive start and the system worked well for this organization and its employees.

Example 2: Selecting Members for Newly Formed Teams (a Sewing Plant)

The previous example illustrated a reasonable and effective method of selecting replacement members for existing teams— teams that are up and running. We now turn our attention to an example of a method for selecting team members at the time when teams are first implemented in an organization. In this particular instance, the organization was the owner of more than a dozen sewing plants, both in the United States and overseas.

Management made the decision to go from individual sewing to team sewing. The individual sewing method involved tasks that were characterized by sequential interdependence. Individual sewers performed their tasks on partially completed garments before they were passed on to other stations where other tasks were performed. Each individual was responsible for his or her own task and no other. Compensation was based on piecework.

In the team method the tasks had characteristics of both sequential and reciprocal interdependence. Compensation was still based on piecework but at the team level, that is, everyone on the team was compensated at the same rate for what the team produced. The objectives for implementing teams included cutting costs by reducing work in process inventory, reducing turnaround time between customers' orders and the organization's delivery, improving quality by reducing dirt, oil, grease, and achieving a more flexible workforce by cross-training employees and having them be collectively responsible for results. Employees received task-related and team-related training. The latter included communication skills development, conflict resolution and problem-solving techniques, and other group process training.

Because there were no teams already in place, team member selection meant choosing all members of all teams, not filling an opening on an existing team. This called for the organization to employ a different selection strategy as contrasted with the one described in the previous example. For one thing, the employees were already working for the company. Therefore, initial screening was not required. For another, teams were new in the work environment and required that the employees work in a significantly different way. Consequently, management rightly anticipated some resistance to the change. To reduce resistance, increase employees' acceptance of the team concept, and promote psychological ownership of employees' teams, management concluded that the employees should form their own teams, in their own way, with their own selection criteria. Note that the formation was done after initial training was given in team-related skills.

Management predicted that employees would choose their teams based on friendships and kinship. Management also believed that this initial attempt would most likely fail. Even so, management was willing to accept this initial setback in order to allow employees the decision-making authority management believed would, in the long run, enhance employee buy in to the team concept and obviate some of the initial resistance. Management also felt it was better not to be in the position of forcing people to work together.

Management was right on both of their predictions. First, teams initially consisted of friends and relatives; the employees' selection criteria focused on these attributes and tended to ignore other, more task-related, ones. Second, the teams soon failed. The team strategy was not halted because management's assessment was that the use of teams was not an option but a necessity based on the competitive environment. Hence, the teams were reformed.

When the teams were formed the second time, selection was again left to the employees' discretion. Only this time, on their own, the employees used different selection criteria. This time, the ability to sew at a similar speed as others who would make up the team and the desire to make the same amount of money

(continued)

were the top criteria. This meant that team members shared the same goal and possessed the same means to achieve it. It should be noted that just because the initial teams were composed of friends and family, this was not the problem. In fact, when friends and family members possessed similar skill levels and shared the same monetary goals, their teams worked quite well.

This example illustrates the importance of shared goals and the collective means of achieving them. In no way does this illustration negate the importance of personal compatibility within teams. Rather, it illustrates that while personal compatibility may be important for team success, it does not constitute a sufficient condition. Further, personal compatibility can be enhanced when members possess common goals and the means to achieve them.

Case 3: Team Building Exercises: An Example

A number of exercises are frequently used for team building and to train individuals in group process skills. One of the more popular exercises involves having the trainees rank a list of objects in a survival situation. There are numerous survival scenarios, including being stranded in the Artic, in the desert, on the moon, in a lifeboat, and in the wilderness where it's hot, cold, wet, or excessively dry. Trainees are asked to come up with their rankings of the items based on the situation. First they do so individually and then as a group. The group must reach a consensus and produce a single ranking. Both the individual and group rankings are scored against experts' rankings. Difference scores for the individuals and the group are computed. The individuals' difference scores are averaged; this represents the team potential without considering process gain and process loss. This average is subtracted from the group's score; this difference represents one component of the process gain (positive number) or process loss (negative number). Usually but not always, the team's score is superior to the average of the individuals' scores, indicating a process gain in accuracy by the group over the individuals. In-

variably, the groups take longer than the individuals to complete this task. This added time represents one component of process loss. Changes in members' knowledge about each other and their preference for working together can represent either process gain or process loss, depending upon whether team members perceive the knowledge they gain about each other to be positive or negative and if their preference for working together in the future is increased (process gain) or decreased (process loss).

Such exercises must have several characteristics in order to work. First, the solution to the problem must require knowledge that is not generally known to the trainees. If the solution to the problem is well known, then no problem solving will be required by the group. Hence, group discussion, compromise, give and take, trade-offs, and conflict resolution will not be required. Second, the objects that are on the list should be items with which most people have some familiarity. Third, while the environment described in the exercise can be a place or situation with which the trainees are not intimately familiar, it must at least be recognizable in terms of some of its more unique and salient features. These last two points are important because they move the problem-solving techniques employed by the teams toward the application of logical deductions and away from simple guesswork.

The use of such exercises is designed to show the trainees that teams can make superior decisions when a variety of experiences, viewpoints, and perspectives are brought to bear on a problem. It should also illustrate that team decisions require more time than individual decisions. The trainees should also realize that there are a variety of communication styles and techniques, and the level of communication skills varies from person to person. Trainees should gain insight into their own communication styles as they interact with others to perform a task. These insights should form a base for trainees to evaluate their own and others' styles of working in a team environment and ready them for further training to become productive team members.

National Association for Healthcare Quality
(http://www.nahq.org)
Publications related to quality healthcare, including team building

Training Services On Demand
(http://www.tsod.com/teambuilding_books.htm)
Work teams, team building, and total quality

Viability Group Inc.
(http://www.viabilitygroup.com)
50-Minute Books related to management topics, including team building

BusinessTrainingMedia.com Inc.
(http://Businesstrainingmedia.com/or email sales@business-marketing.com
Videos and training packages, including teams and team building

Clinical Laboratory Management Association
(www.CLMA.org)
Links to relevant government agencies, other organizations, and other resources; excellent resource

[a]Verified 7/24/03.

APPENDIX 18.3   Teamwork for Employees and Managers Act of 1997 (introduced in the House) HR 634 IH

105th CONGRESS
1st Session
H. R. 634

To amend the National Labor Relations Act to allow labor management cooperative efforts that improve economic competitiveness in the United States to continue to thrive, and for other purposes.

IN THE HOUSE OF REPRESENTATIVES

February 6, 1997

Mr. FAWELL (for himself, Mr. GOODLING, Mr. STENHOLM, Mr. DOOLEY of California, Mr. HOEKSTRA, and Mr. HALL of Texas) introduced the following bill; which was referred to the Committee on Education and the Workforce

A BILL

To amend the National Labor Relations Act to allow labor management cooperative efforts that improve economic competitiveness in the United States to continue to thrive, and for other purposes.

Be it enacted by the Senate and House of Representatives of the United States of America in Congress assembled,

SEC. 1. SHORT TITLE.

This Act may be cited as the "Teamwork for Employees and Managers Act of 1997."

SEC. 2. FINDINGS AND PURPOSES.

(a) FINDINGS: Congress finds that—
  (1) the escalating demands of global competition have compelled an increasing number of employers in the United States to make dramatic changes in workplace and employer-employee relationships;
  (2) such changes involve an enhanced role for the employee in workplace decision making, often referred to as "Employee Involvement," which has taken many forms, including self-managed work teams, quality-of-worklife, quality circles, and joint labor-management committees;
  (3) Employee Involvement programs, which operate successfully in both unionized and nonunionized settings, have been established by over 80 percent of the largest employers in the United States and exist in an estimated 30,000 workplaces;
  (4) in addition to enhancing the productivity and competitiveness of businesses in the United States, Employee Involvement programs have had a positive impact on the lives of such employees, better enabling them to reach their potential in the workforce;
  (5) recognizing that foreign competitors have successfully utilized Employee Involvement techniques, the Congress has consistently joined business, labor and academic leaders in encouraging and recognizing successful Employee Involvement programs in the workplace through such incentives as the Malcolm Baldrige National Quality Award;
  (6) employers who have instituted legitimate Employee Involvement programs have not done so to interfere with the collective bargaining rights guaranteed by the labor laws, as was the case in the 1930's when employers established deceptive sham "company unions" to avoid unionization; and
  (7) Employee Involvement is currently threatened by legal interpretations of the prohibition against employer-dominated "company unions."

(b) PURPOSES: The purpose of this Act is—
  (1) to protect legitimate Employee Involvement programs against governmental interference;
  (2) to preserve existing protections against deceptive, coercive employer practices; and
  (3) to allow legitimate Employee Involvement programs, in which workers may discuss issues involving terms and conditions of employment, to continue to evolve and proliferate.

SEC. 3. EMPLOYER EXCEPTION.

Section 8(a)(2) of the National Labor Relations Act is amended by striking the semicolon and inserting the following: ": *Provided further,* That it shall not constitute or be evidence of an unfair labor practice under this paragraph for an employer to establish, assist, maintain, or participate in any organization or entity of any kind, in which employees participate to at least the same extent practicable as representatives of management participate, to address matters of mutual interest, including, but not limited to, issues of quality, productivity, efficiency, and safety and health, and which does not have, claim, or seek authority to be the exclusive bargaining representative of the employees or to negotiate or enter into collective bargaining agreements with the employer or to amend existing collective bargaining agreements between the employer and any labor organization, except that in a case in which a labor organization is the representative of such employees as provided in section 9(a), this proviso shall not apply;".

SEC. 4. LIMITATION ON EFFECT OF ACT.

Nothing in this Act shall affect employee rights and responsibilities contained in provisions other than section 8(a)(2) of the National Labor Relations Act, as amended.

19

Labor Relations

Lynne S. Garcia

OBJECTIVES

To describe the legal framework for labor relations activities

To understand and describe the reasons why employees seek union representation

To discuss the union organizing campaign and the "do's and don'ts" for the union and management

To describe the election process

To discuss the collective bargaining process

Why is it that those who are the quickest to judge are often those in possession of the fewest facts?

JOHN WOODEN

T HE TERM "LABOR RELATIONS" has been defined as the interactions between an employer, represented by management and supervisors, and groups of employees who are in bargaining units represented by a union. These interactions involve the legal rights of employees and unions and the interpretation and application of collective bargaining agreements addressing issues such as wages, hours, and working conditions. Procedures for resolving disputes that may arise over the application and interpretation of the contract are also included (6).

Regardless of whether you support or dislike the concept of unionization, it is mandatory that all parties have a basic understanding of labor relations, including the laws, organizing campaigns, collective bargaining, and contract administration. The topic of labor relations is often discussed within a very emotional atmosphere, and factual information is minimal or absent. It is particularly important that management and supervisory staff understand the ramifications of their actions regarding personnel management within the context of unionization.

There are a number of laws that govern healthcare labor relations within the United States. These laws are generally divided into three categories, those covering federal government employees, state and local government employees, and profit and nonprofit employees in the private sector (Table 19.1). The laws relevant to these three categories undergo constant review and modification, based on changes in the actual laws and regulations and agency or court decisions related to administration of the laws.

Table 19.1 Labor law coverage for healthcare institutions and employees within the United States

Healthcare employees	Coverage
Federal government	1978 Civil Service Reform Act
State and local government	State labor laws
For-profit and nonprofit institutions	1935 National Labor Relations Act, as amended

Labor Law

Current labor law supports two major objectives. First, it supports stability through collective bargaining and defined dispute resolution. Second, it tends to equalize the balance of bargaining power between employees and management. Until the Norris-LaGuardia Act of 1932, unions had very few rights; this act declared a federal policy that employees were free to form unions (4).

National Labor Relations Act (NLRA) (Wagner Act)

Until the NLRA of 1935, employers were not required to collectively bargain with unions. This legislation included some very important provisions: (1) employees have the right to form, join, or assist unions, the freedom to bargain collectively with the employer, and the right to engage in group activity; (2) employers must bargain collectively with the employees' certified bargaining representative and must refrain from employer unfair labor practices (ULPs); and (3) the National Labor Relations Board (NLRB, or Board) became the regulatory body responsible for administration of the NLRA.

Section 8 of the NLRA prohibits certain actions by the employer, which are identified as ULPs. These actions are defined in detail (Table 19.2). Specific examples of employer ULPs include (1) discharging employees for urging other employees to join a union; (2) refusing to reinstate an employee to an open job because the employee participated in a union strike related to a ULP or economics; (3) refusing to hire a qualified applicant for a job because the applicant belongs to a union; and (4) demoting employees for exercising their right to organize (7).

Labor-Management Relations Act (Taft-Hartley Act)

An NLRA amendment, the Labor-Management Relations Act of 1947, addresses four problems that arose after passage of the NLRA in 1935, one of which was ULPs by unions. Union ULPs are also clearly defined (Table 19.3). The Taft-Hartley Act guarantees a broader interpretation of "free speech" for both the union and employer; this provision allows both to express their views, arguments, and opinions. As long as these views are expressed without any threats of reprisal or promise of benefits, no ULP has been committed. The five titles within this act are summarized in Table 19.4.

The requirement for "good faith" bargaining by both the union and employer is also a part of the Taft-Hartley Act; this includes meeting at reasonable times and places and conferring honestly regarding wages, hours, and other working conditions. However, there is nothing in the act that requires either the union or management to agree to concessions or proposals.

The Taft-Hartley Act also set forth notification guidelines in the case that either the union or management wants to terminate or modify a contract upon expiration. Specific requirements include (1) a 60-day written notice prior to the expiration of the contract; (2) an offer to meet

Table 19.2 Employer ULPs that interfere with employee rights (NLRA)

1. Interference with rights to unionize and to bargain collectively
   - Threatening employees with loss of jobs or benefits
   - Withholding customary periodic wage increases
   - Offering increased wages or benefits if and when the union loses the election
   - Threatening to relocate or close the business
   - Questioning employees about their union activities or membership under circumstances that would tend to restrain or coerce employees in their right to organize
   - Spying on union gatherings or pretending to do so
   - Granting wage increases timed to discourage employees from forming or joining a union
2. Domination of or contributing to a union
   - Employer must remain neutral during the organizing process
   - Employer cannot solicit employees to join a particular union or to oppose a competing union
   - Employer cannot contribute financial or other support to the union
3. Discrimination against employees because of their union activities or because they filed charges or testified under the NLRA
4. Refusal to bargain in good faith with the employees' elected representatives

Table 19.3 Union ULPs that interfere with employer rights (NLRA)

- Refusing to bargain in good faith with the employer
- Paying employees for work not actually performed (feather-bedding)
- Charging discriminatory initiation fees or dues
- Interfering with employees' choice of a labor union
- Discriminating against certain employees and/or seeking the employer's discrimination against certain employees or potential employees (e.g., to discourage or encourage membership in a particular union)
- Picketing, striking, and carrying out boycotts against businesses other than the employer involved in the primary labor dispute
- Organizing strikes or boycotts designed to make an employer assign work to a particular group to recognize a union without NLRB certification

Table 19.4 Titles within the Taft-Hartley Act (1947)

Title	Content
I	Amended NLRA (1935)
	Increased size of NLRB from three to five members (adjudicate cases)
	Established the Office of the General Counsel of the NLRB (supervise regional and field offices, investigate and prosecute ULP charges)
	Granted employees right to form, join, or assist formation of union
	Granted employees right to bargain through representative of own choosing
	Granted employees right to engage in other protected activities for purpose of collective bargaining
	Outlined series of employer ULPs that violate employee rights
II	Concerned with prevention of work stoppages (established FMCS)
	Outlined procedures by which president of the United States can obtain federal court injunction when strike or threatened strike endangers national welfare
III	Provided that suits to enforce labor-management contracts be brought in a federal district court
IV	Established a labor-management commission to study labor-management relations in the United States
V	Gave employees the right to refuse to work under abnormally dangerous conditions of employment without such a work stoppage being considered a strike

and confer with the other party; (3) notification to the Federal Mediation and Conciliation Service (FMCS) and any relevant state agency within 30 days of serving notice; and (4) maintaining all terms and conditions of the contract for a period of 60 days after notice has been served or until the expiration date of the contract, whichever is later (1). These notification requirements served as the basis for the 1974 Healthcare Amendments (see below) (Table 19.5).

Labor-Management Reporting and Disclosure Act (Landrum-Griffin Act)

The Labor-Management Reporting and Disclosure Act of 1959 was passed to address some problems with the Taft-Hartley Act and to prevent abuses by union officials. The act prevents unions from restricting members regarding the right of free speech, assembly, or participation in union elections and meetings. Union officers are required to be bonded and accountable for union property and funds. The act also prevents dues from being increased without all members first voting by secret ballot.

Federal regulation for union internal operations is also addressed, including the NLRB's supervision of union officer elections; minimum standards are in place for those wishing to be candidates for office, as well as for voting procedures. These include the following provisions: (1) all union members in good standing must be allowed to vote; (2) elections for local officers must be held at least every 3 years; (3) secret balloting procedures must be followed in local elections, but delegates to a national or international union convention may cast open votes; (4) a reasonable opportunity to nominate candidates must be given to all eligible voting members; and (5) qualifications for candidate eligibility must be reasonable (4).

1974 Amendments to the NLRA

Prior to the NLRA amendments in 1974, nonprofit healthcare institutions were excluded from coverage by the NLRA; after passage of the amendments, these institutions were no longer grouped with employers excluded from coverage under the NLRA. A number of other features of the 1974 amendments involve written notification rules (Table 19.5). In passing these amendments, Congress was very concerned about maintaining the continuity of patient care. Thus, the "ally doctrine" does not apply within certain healthcare settings. This means that if employees in a hospital setting are on strike and patients are transferred to another hospital, the striking employees from the first hospital cannot legally picket the second hospital.

NLRB

Description

The NLRB is an independent federal agency created by Congress in 1935 to administer the NLRA, the primary law governing relations between unions and employers in the private sector. The statute guarantees the right of employees to organize and to bargain collectively with their employers or to refrain from all such activity.

Table 19.5 NLRA notice requirements in the healthcare industry (1974 Healthcare Amendments)

Notice type	Notice to:		
	Other party (days)	FMCS (days)	Appropriate state agency (days)
Modify or terminate contract			
Initial bargaining	30	30	30
Existing contract	90	60	60
Notice of strike or picketing activity			
Initial bargaining	40 (10 days after the initial 30 days seen above)	40 (10 days after the initial 30 days seen above)	40 (10 days after the initial 30 days seen above)
Existing contract	10	10	10

Function

Based on its statutory duties, the NLRB has two main functions: (1) to determine through free-choice, secret-ballot elections whether employees wish to be represented by a union in dealing with their employers, and if so, by which union; and (2) to prevent and remedy unlawful acts (ULPs) by either employers or unions. The agency does not act on its own in either function but processes only those charges of ULPs and petitions for employee elections that are filed with the NLRB in one of its regional, subregional, or resident offices. The NLRB also resolves disputes about what constitutes an appropriate employee bargaining unit—typically defined as a group of employees who have a community of interests, including workplace conditions and concerns. Supervisors and managerial employees, as well as government workers and independent contractors, are not covered by the NLRA.

Structure

The NLRB has two major sections (Fig. 19.1). The Board itself has five members and acts as a quasi-judicial body in deciding cases on the basis of formal records in administrative proceedings. NLRB members are appointed by the President to 5-year terms, with Senate consent; the term of one member expires each year. The General Counsel, appointed by the President to a 4-year term with Senate consent, is independent from the Board members and handles the investigation and prosecution of ULP cases and the supervision of field offices in processing cases.

Processing of Cases

When a ULP charge is filed, the field office investigates the charge to determine if there is reasonable cause to believe the NLRA has been violated. If the charge is determined to lack merit, it is dismissed unless the charging party withdraws the charge. The dismissal of a charge is appealable to the General Counsel's office in Washington, D.C.

If the regional director finds reasonable evidence that the NLRA has been violated, the region seeks a voluntary settlement to remedy the alleged violations. However, if settlement efforts fail, a formal complaint is issued and the case goes to hearing before an NLRB administrative law judge. The judge issues a written decision that may be appealed to the five-member Board in Washington for a final agency ruling. This ruling is subject to review in a U.S. Court of Appeals. Of the approximately 30,000 ULP

Figure 19.1 Structure of the NLRB.

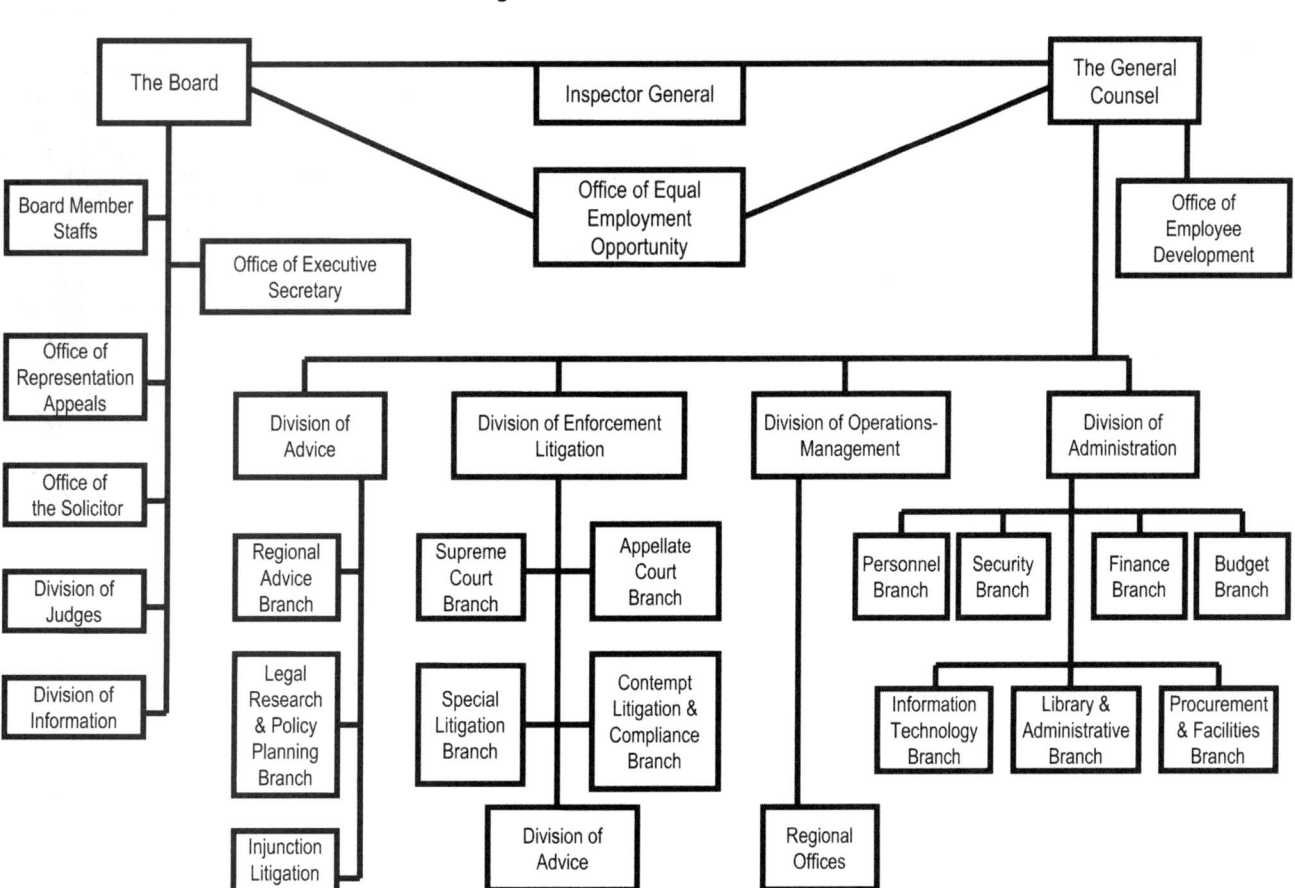

charges filed each year, about one-third are found to have merit, of which more than 90% are settled (9).

Authority To Secure Injunctive Relief from a Court

The NLRB is able to petition a federal district court for an injunction to temporarily prevent ULPs by employers or unions and to restore the status quo, pending the full review of the case by the Board. In determining whether this action is appropriate in a particular case, the main questions are whether injunctive relief is required to preserve the Board's ability to remedy the ULP charge and whether the alleged violator would otherwise benefit from the violation. The act requires the Board to seek a temporary federal court injunction against certain forms of union misconduct, mainly involving "secondary boycotts" and "recognitional picketing."

Union Structure

Formal Structure

The majority of national unions within the United States belong to the voluntary federation, the American Federation of Labor-Congress of Industrial Organizations (AFL-CIO). The AFL-CIO provides research, education, lobbying, and public relations activities for its unions; it does not get involved with the internal affairs of its member unions. The individual unions are autonomous regarding strikes, contract demands, and internal affairs.

Usually, local unions are subunits of a national union. However, in the absence of a national union, a local union may form to bargain with one or more employers. Gener-

ally, local unions vary considerably in size and may range from fewer than 10 members to more than 40,000.

Each union has a constitution on file with the Secretary of Labor; the content specifies the titles and duties of the officers, who are usually elected and may include president, vice president, business manager, treasurer, financial secretary, recording secretary, and grievance committee chair. Some of these positions may be full-time paid officers, but others are volunteers who are reimbursed for out-of-pocket expenses and work time lost while conducting union business.

Union Membership

In 2002, 13.2% of wage and salary workers were union members, down from 13.4% in 2001. This represents a decline of 280,000 over the year to 16.1 million in 2002. Union membership has steadily declined from 20.1% in 1983. Specific data from 2002 are summarized in Table 19.6 (3). Data from the Bureau of Labor Statistics' Healthcare Practitioners and Technical Occupations grouping are summarized in Table 19.7; this table contains labor statistics and does not reflect union representation (2). Unions that have become

Table 19.7 2001 healthcare practitioners and technical occupations (major group)[a]

- This major group comprises the following occupations: Chiropractors; Dentists; Dietitians and Nutritionists; Optometrists; Pharmacists; Anesthesiologists; Family and General Practitioners; Internists, General; Obstetricians and Gynecologists; Pediatricians, General; Psychiatrists; Surgeons; Physician Assistants; Podiatrists; Registered Nurses; Audiologists; Occupational Therapists; Respiratory Therapists; Speech-Language Pathologists; Veterinarians; Medical and Clinical Laboratory Technologists; Medical and Clinical Laboratory Technicians; Dental Hygienists; Cardiovascular Technologists and Technicians; Diagnostic Medical Sonographers; Nuclear Medicine Technologists; Radiologic Technologists and Technicians; Emergency Medical Technicians and Paramedics; Dietetic Technicians; Pharmacy Technicians; Psychiatric Technicians; Respiratory Therapy Technicians; Surgical Technologists; Veterinary Technologists and Technicians; Licensed Practical and Licensed Vocational Nurses; Medical Records and Health Information Technicians; Opticians, Dispensing; Orthotists and Prosthetists; Occupational Health and Safety Specialists and Technicians; Athletic Trainers; and residual "All Other" occupations in this major group.
- Employment: 6,118,970 (4.8% of the total, 127,980,430)
- Mean hourly wage: $24.01
- Mean annual wage: $49,930
- Hourly wage, annual wage, and percentile (median = 50% of workers earn less than the median, 50% earn more than the median):
  a. $10.97, $22,810 (10%)
  b. $15.05, $31,300 (25%)
  c. $20.56, $42,770 (50%, median)
  d. $27.65, $57,520 (75%)
  e. $41.87, $87,090 (90%)

[a]From reference 2.

Table 19.6 2002 Union membership data[a]

- Men (14.7%) were more likely to be union members than women (11.6%).
- Union membership for blacks (16.9%) was unchanged and remained higher than the rates for either whites (12.8%) or Hispanics (10.5%).
- Almost 40% of government workers were union members, but less than 10% of workers were union members in private-sector industries.
- Nearly 40% of workers in protective service occupations, including firefighters and police officers, were union members; this group has had the highest union membership rate of any broad occupation every year since 1983.
- About 1.7 million wage and salary workers were represented by a union, while not being union members themselves.
- Four states had union membership greater than 20% (New York, Hawaii, Alaska, and Michigan).
- The largest numbers of union members live in California (2.5 million), New York (2 million), and Illinois (1.1 million). More than half of the 16.1 million union members within the United States live in six states, although these states accounted for only 35% of wage and salary employment nationally.

[a]From reference 3.

more active within the healthcare environment include the Service Employees International Union; the National Union of Hospital and Health Care Workers; the American Federation of State, County, and Municipal Employees; the International Brotherhood of Teamsters; the Retail Clerks International Association; the American Federation of Government Employees; and the American Nurses Association. Generally, wherever working conditions and salaries are poor, unions will attempt to organize.

Function of the Union Steward

One of the most important positions within any union is the steward; this position is comparable to one of the levels within management (5). The steward listens to grievances by employees within the bargaining unit, counsels them on a course of action, and, depending on the circumstances, intercedes with management on their behalf. Reasons for grievances might include discipline, failure to get a merit increase or promotion, and disagreement with the employee evaluation process. A part of the steward's responsibility is to review all the evidence related to grievances and to obtain a factual account from both the employee and management regarding the issues involved. Generally, a union steward will not defend inappropriate employee behavior, particularly if this approach would result in a loss of credibility with the employer, a situation that would complicate future contract negotiations. In many collective bargaining agreements, the initial grievance must be presented to the employee's immediate supervisor as the first step; employees may ask for assistance from the steward at this beginning step in the process. The Supreme Court has ruled that a member of a bargaining unit has a right to union representation during a management interview if the employee feels that disciplinary action might result from the interview (8).

Unionization Process

Individual, Group, and Union Image: Reasons Why Employees Join Unions

Although there may be a number of reasons why employees decide to join unions, generally these reasons can be categorized as (1) personal, (2) related to the social environment, and (3) related to the image of the union (Table 19.8). One of the main considerations against unionization has been the perception that professionals don't equate being concerned about socioeconomic issues with unionization. However, some groups of professionals have moved beyond this perceived barrier to unionization and are willing to consider collective bargaining as just another component of their "professional activities." In some cases, unions have or have considered establishing a separate professional division within the union in an attempt to make unionization a more attractive alternative. Another approach is to limit the bargaining unit to professional employees, thus fostering the idea that the union and professionals are compatible.

Relevance for Healthcare Workers

For many years, healthcare professionals as a group have been somewhat skeptical and apprehensive about unionization; many always assumed that they would never need to join a union. As professionals, they felt that their concerns could be taken directly to management and they would always have a fair hearing and reasonable outcomes. Employees may question the need for a union if the institution uses a fair system for work assignments, raises, promotions, and corrective action policies and has an appropriate policy for handling employee grievances. However, over the years, some of these perceptions have changed and many healthcare employees are now represented by unions. Often, just the potential of a union entering a healthcare institution may stimulate management to improve salaries and benefits. Generally, if both management and unions are well informed, approach the organizing campaign within specific guidelines, maintain professional attitudes and express appropriate behavior, the outcome of an election may be acceptable to both parties, even if the union receives the required number of "yes" votes. Unfortunately, when either management or the union fails to play by the rules, the outcome can be chaos, inappropriate behavior, anger, and feelings of betrayal and mistrust. How the organizing campaign is handled will affect relations with employees for years to come, regardless of the outcome.

Professional workers are confronting increasing challenges to their careers, brought about by rapidly changing technology, the turbulent world economy, and new work

Table 19.8 Reasons why employees decide to seek union representation

Personal reasons	Social environment	Image of the union

Individual
  Economic benefits (salary, fringe benefits)
  Job security
  Fairness in job conflict resolution
Group
  Unity and togetherness
  Advancement of profession
	Family tradition and history
	Work-category tradition and history
	Unionization within the organization and/or community
	Unionization within the profession, pros/cons
	Based on work group union membership, pressure to conform to the group
		Success in bargaining
		Ability to represent workers
		Goals consistent with individual goals
		Ability to support and advance the profession
		Professional in their approach to labor relations
		Reasonable dues
		No evidence of violence

methods. Like so many other workers, professionals are forming unions to enhance their professional autonomy, to be involved in making the decisions that affect their careers, and for greater professional and personal security. Current information on unions and professionals includes the following:

- The union movement now consists of almost 50% white-collar workers.

- Among the professional occupations, about 22% of workers are union members, a higher proportion than the workforce in general.

- Employment in the professional and technical occupations is growing faster and adding more workers than any other major occupational group. While total U.S. employment is projected to grow 15% between 2000 and 2010, the growth for professional and technical workers is projected to be 26%.

- Eight of the 10 fastest-growing occupations are computer-related.

Organizing Campaign

The first step in the process of gaining union representation is the organizing campaign. Situations may exist in which the employees contact a union representative to initiate discussion regarding union representation. However, union representatives may initiate the contact to determine whether employees want to pursue discussions about possible unionization. The right for employees to seek or aid unionization or to refrain from such activities is guaranteed by the NLRA. More than one union may be involved in an organizing campaign, competing for the employees' interest and eventual votes for union representation.

Authorization Cards

It is highly unlikely that management will voluntarily recognize employees' wishes to be represented by a union for the purposes of collective bargaining. The union must follow set procedures to demonstrate employee interest leading to an election for union representation. The union will ask employees to sign authorization cards, which state that the employee wishes to be represented for purposes of collective bargaining by the union named on the card. The union must have 30% of the employees sign authorization cards before the NLRB will honor a petition for a union-representation election. The union must specify within its petition exactly which occupational groups it seeks to represent; this specification begins the process of defining the bargaining unit.

The Bargaining Unit

Final responsibility for determining the job categories within a bargaining unit resides with the NLRB; often the employer may challenge the union's proposed bargaining unit. Generally, the employer will want to include occupational groups perceived to be unfavorable toward unionization or may want the bargaining unit decreased to eliminate groups perceived to be in favor of unionization. Key factors considered by the NLRB include (1) the history of bargaining within the industry and occupational groups under consideration; (2) the community of interest among employees and common supervision; and (3) the wishes of the employees. Certainly, they will also consider the pros and cons of inclusion and exclusion of various groups as requested by the union and the employer. In general, the NLRB will allow up to six different bargaining units in a healthcare institution: physicians, registered nurses, other professional employees, technical employees, service and maintenance employees, and business office clerical employees. However, recognition of these bargaining units does not mean the NLRB is forced to maintain these categories; several groups can also be combined into a single bargaining unit.

Information Distribution and Solicitation

Information distribution generally refers to distribution of printed materials to employees, the content of which is informational only. Solicitation is directed to a specific individual with the intent to elicit a specific response from that individual; an excellent example is the request for an employee to sign and return an authorization card. Very specific rules govern these activities, both for the union and for the employer (Table 19.9). It is important that a proper balance be achieved between the rights of the employees and the rights of management to guarantee safe and efficient patient care.

Table 19.9 Rulings regarding information distribution and solicitation in the hospital setting

Union	Distribution and solicitation by a nonworking employee (prounion) of other nonworking employees are allowed in nonworking areas on the premises, other than in patient care areas (e.g., patient rooms, operating rooms, treatment rooms).
Union	Solicitation is banned in sitting rooms and corridors adjoining or accessible to patient rooms (crowding issues).
Employer	Cannot ban solicitation in the cafeteria, gift shop, and lobbies on the first floor of the institution; however, employer need only show that solicitation is likely to disrupt patient care or disturb patients in order to enforce a ban on solicitation in nonpatient care areas.
Employer	May allow solicitation in "normal gathering places" for employees but ban certain areas such as lobbies and gift shops.
Employer	If management insists on a very broad "no solicitation rule," it is important that supervisors and managers realize this approach may be judged invalid if challenged by the union.

Election

Once at least 30% of the employees in a proposed bargaining unit have signed and turned in authorization cards, the union may petition the NLRB for a representation election. Certainly, the union would prefer a showing of much more than 30%, particularly because of the time lag between the submission of the petition for election and the election itself. During this interim time, management will campaign vigorously to counteract the union's position and will try to change employees' minds regarding the necessity of unionization. Therefore, some employees may, in fact, change their minds during this time lag between petition submission and the actual election. The NLRB, or in the case of federal workers, the Federal Labor Relations Authority, reviews the petition and makes a number of determinations directly related to approval or rejection of the election proposal (Table 19.10).

If there are no reasons to preclude the election and the bargaining unit is appropriate, agreement is sought regarding "consent" election; there are two types of agreements to consent elections. The first consent-election agreement provides for an election, over which final authority regarding disputes with the NLRB itself resides with the regional director. The second agreement, termed "stipulation for certification," provides for an election, over which the final authority regarding disputes resides with the NLRB itself.

If either the employer or the union(s), or both, fail to agree to a consent election, a formal hearing occurs before a hearing officer appointed by the regional director. Employees, the employer, the union, or any of their representatives may appear at the hearing and may testify and introduce additional evidence. These issues must be relevant to representation and may include the jurisdiction of the NLRA over the employer and the occupational makeup of the bargaining unit. Although the regional director makes the decision either ordering the election to occur or dismissing the petition, a party may appeal the decision to the NLRB.

Table 19.10 NLRB determinations regarding acceptance or rejection of union election petition

1. Confirmation of whether there are any statutory or policy reasons that would preclude an election.
    a. Participation in interstate commerce.
    b. Large enough in size to quality; use of dollar volume amount.
2. Determination of whether the bargaining unit is an appropriate unit.
3. If there are no reasons to preclude the election and the bargaining unit is appropriate, agreement is sought regarding "consent" election.
    a. Consent-election agreement provides for an election; final authority over disputes with the NLRB itself resides with the regional director.
    b. Stipulation for certification provides for an election; final authority over disputes resides with the NLRB itself.

If all parties agree to the consent election based on the filing of the petition, the date is set and normally occurs 60 days after the union files the petition. However, if the parties do not agree and the hearing process is instituted, the election normally occurs between 25 and 30 days following the final decision.

Employees who have been confirmed as being in the bargaining unit at the end of the payroll period immediately preceding the date of the election are eligible to vote. The employer must provide the NLRB and the union a list of names and home addresses of eligible employees within 7 days after the final decision on the consent election. The election is held at a place and time designed to provide maximum participation for all bargaining unit employees to vote for or against union representation; mail ballots may also be used within the election process. The election is by secret ballot, and the union must have a simple majority of the votes cast to win and be certified by the NLRB as the bargaining representative.

All relevant parties may have observers at the polls; an NLRB agent supervises the observers to ensure appropriate behavior during the election process. Ballots may be challenged, and these ballots are impounded. If the number of impounded ballots would make a difference in the election outcome, the regional office investigates these ballots and makes a decision regarding whether or not they will be counted. If the number of impounded ballots will not affect the election outcome, they are not counted. Depending on the ballot count, a runoff election may be required; this occurs if more than one union is involved in the election process and there is no majority vote for one union or for no representation.

Certification

If union representation is rejected, another election within that bargaining unit cannot be held for 12 months. If a union wins the election, the NLRB issues a certification of representative; this certification of representative confirms the union's status as the exclusive bargaining representative for a period of 1 year after the date of certification. During this 1-year period, the employer is required to bargain with the certified union. It is important to remember that although the bargaining unit may be composed of union members and those who choose not to join the union, a negotiated collective bargaining agreement applies to all those within the bargaining unit. All members of the bargaining unit are subject to the contract terms and provisions. Because compulsory union membership is prohibited but all members of the bargaining unit benefit from union representation, some states allow unions to collect some portion of the monthly union dues from nonunion members of the bargaining unit. A review of the organizing, election, and certification phases of the process can be seen in Fig. 19.2.

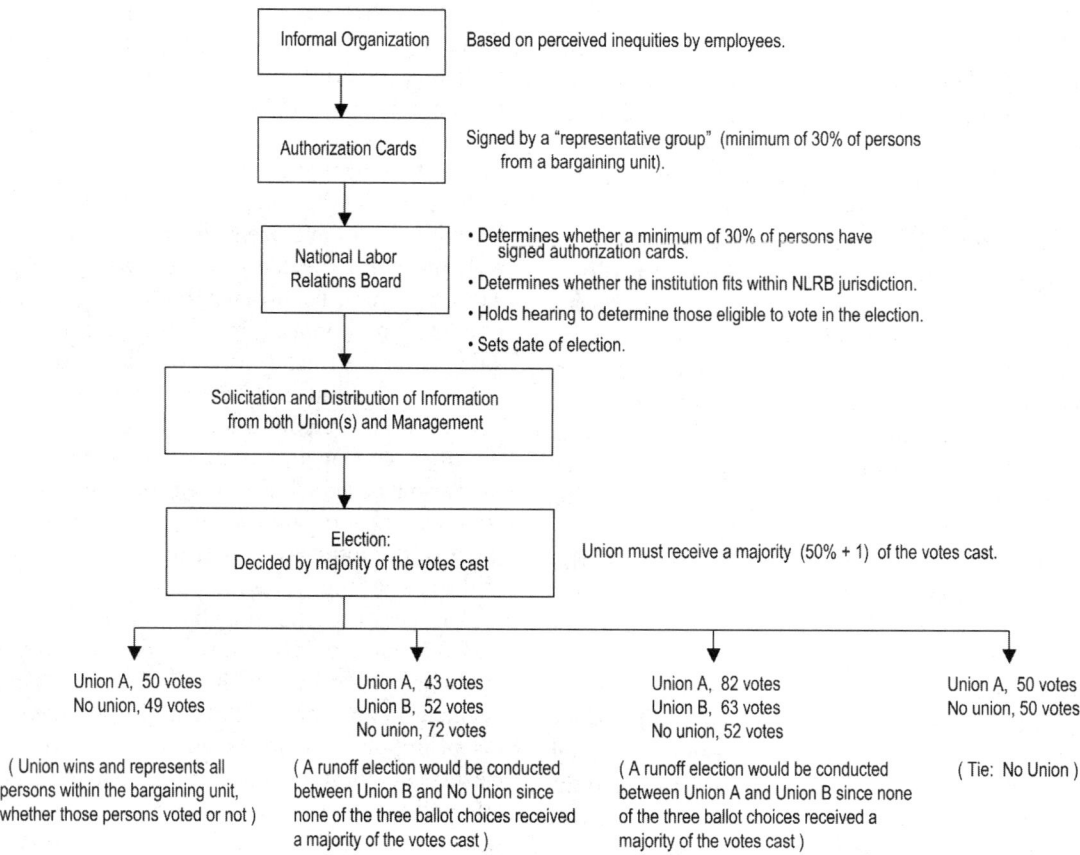

Figure 19.2 Union organizing campaign, from first inquiries to election results.

Collective Bargaining

After a bargaining unit selects a particular union as its representative, the employer and union must bargain in good faith. This negotiating process addresses many issues, such as (1) establishing work rules; (2) selecting the form and mix of employee compensation; (3) providing uniformity among competitors; and (4) setting priorities for both labor and management.

Issues for Bargaining

There are three basic categories of bargaining subjects: mandatory, permissive, and illegal and prohibited (5). Mandatory subjects include wages, hours, and other terms and conditions of employment. Permissive subjects are bargained only if both parties voluntarily agree to do so. However, neither party may refuse to bargain on mandatory subjects to force bargaining on permissive subjects. Illegal or prohibited subjects include those that would cause one or both parties to violate federal or state law, such as bargaining (1) for a closed shop; (2) for a contract clause under which union members could refuse to work with nonunion goods and materials; and (3) for contract language that would permit discrimination as defined by

the Civil Rights Act. Attempts to negotiate these illegal subjects would constitute ULPs. Other ULPs associated with the bargaining process include (1) refusing to bargain collectively; (2) failing to offer meaningful counterproposals; (3) refusing to discuss economic terms until noneconomic issues are resolved; and (4) attempting to delay meetings or move meeting sites. Although the NLRB cannot force an agreement between the parties, as a remedy for a ULP, the Board can order them to bargain or may order a cease and desist order to refrain from bad faith bargaining.

Preparation Phase

The union and employer begin the process of bargaining by selecting negotiating teams. The union team is often led by a full-time paid official, while the management team is led by industrial relations managers and key department managers. Both parties may also include attorneys experienced in labor law and contract negotiations. Depending on the size and complexity of the bargaining units and relevant issues, preparations by both negotiating teams may begin several months prior to actual negotiations or may begin as long as 1 year prior to initiation of the bargaining process.

Negotiation Phase

A representative list of bargaining subjects can be seen in Table 19.11. It is important to remember that almost any topic falling within the context of wages, hours, or work and other terms and conditions of employment is a mandatory bargaining subject. Some issues may be bargained to the point of impasse but not lead to a work stoppage if the union feels they are not issues about which members feel strongly. In these situations, the final contract between the union and employer would just eliminate wording about these particular issues. Some contracts will allow either party to reopen negotiations on any section of the contract by giving the other party a notice of such interest. A change may also be accomplished by amending the contract through a letter of agreement covering a specific issue.

Administration of the Agreement

Unfortunately, there is no such thing as a "perfect" contract. The negotiating teams cannot envision all the potential problems that could arise during the time span of the contract. Different people will interpret the contract differently, especially depending on healthcare environmental changes, economic conditions, and a number of other potential changes. If the union, the employer, or an employee believes that the collective bargaining agreement has been violated, the process for handling such disagreements is contract administration, which uses the agreement's grievance procedure, the final step of which is likely arbitration. The purpose of such a process is to provide a

Table 19.11 Representative topics for contract negotiations

Recognition and representation

Membership requirements

Wage rates (including cost-of-living clause)

Hours and overtime

Flextime options, including 4 days on, 4 days off, etc.

Shift differentials

Seniority

Vacations

Personal leave and provisions for time off

Holiday, overtime, on-call, "incentive," and merit pay

Lunch and rest periods

Employee benefits (e.g., insurance, pensions)

Safety and health

Grievance procedure

Corrective action and discharge procedure

Strikes and lockouts

Effect of agreement and amendments

Use of bulletin boards

Management rights

Union security clause

Dues "checkoff" clause

Terms of the contract

mechanism for handling day-to-day differences among the union, management, and employees.

The grievance procedure includes a series of meetings through which the complaint may move toward resolution. The initial step usually includes a verbal discussion with the opposite party. Each step contains time limits for the appeal and response after the preliminary discussions. Each step in the process also includes the addition of higher levels of decision makers. If resolution is not reached, most collective bargaining agreements provide that either the union or the employer, but not an aggrieved employee, may appeal to arbitration; usually 60 to 120 days must elapse before a grievance reaches arbitration. During arbitration, a neutral third party, or arbitrator, hears the facts and each party's position. The arbitrator then renders a final and binding decision. These arbitrators are selected and agreed upon by both parties prior to the beginning of the arbitration process. The arbitration hearing is similar to a court hearing; witnesses are called and subjected to cross-examination, exhibits are introduced, and the opposing parties present opening and closing arguments. However, there is no jury present. Although a single individual conducts most arbitration hearings, an arbitration panel may be used.

Management Rights Clause

Although the length of the management rights clause in the contract may vary from several paragraphs to several pages, it generally states that management has the sole right and prerogative to unilaterally make decisions concerning the operation of the institution, except as it may be limited by the contract (10). These rights include the right to hire, fire, suspend, and discharge for just cause; to temporarily assign, promote, or discharge employees according to the needs of the business; to determine the methods of work; and other issues. The inclusion of the management rights clause can often eliminate prolonged disagreement over many issues, one of which is the right to suspend and discharge employees for just cause. These policies must be clearly defined and consistently used. Often, the union may challenge a suspension or discharge for lack of just cause. The arbitrator may reinstate an employee who has been improperly terminated. The arbitrator may also decide on remedial action, such as full pay for all time lost and restoration of all benefits that resulted from improper discharge. Because of the potential for lengthy remediation of such issues, many contracts include provisions for an expedited grievance procedure, thus limiting the potential for substantial remedial legal liability.

Summary

Contemporary labor law attempts to balance two goals, the encouragement of stability through collective bargaining and reasonable dispute settlement and the balance of bargaining power between employees and management.

In the past few years, the field of labor relations has become more relevant to the healthcare industry. Therefore, it is critical that all levels of management personnel recognize the importance of understanding labor relations, both as a general concept and as a complex process with many parts. All of the systems inherent in labor relations must be seen as dynamic, changing entities, primarily based on changes in the laws and regulations themselves, decisions of agencies participating in the administration of the laws, and decisions of the federal and state courts.

KEY POINTS

■ Labor laws are relevant for various groups of employees and employers.

■ Specific legal entities support, guide, and confirm appropriate behavior by unions, employers, and employees.

■ The unionization process is very clearly defined, with specific actions that can and cannot be taken by all parties involved.

■ The organizing campaign, election, and certification form a step-by-step process through which a union may or may not be voted in as the exclusive representative of a particular bargaining unit.

■ Collective bargaining includes mandatory, permissive, and illegal topics for negotiation.

■ Although some contracts are very detailed and inclusive, there is no such thing as the "perfect" contract. Therefore, the ability to administer the contract specifications can require a day-to-day working knowledge of the contract and its use.

GLOSSARY

Administrative law judge A member of the NLRB's corps of judges who conduct hearings at which the parties present evidence. These judges work for the NLRB. Decisions of administrative law judges can be appealed to the five-member Board in Washington, D.C.

AFL-CIO American Federation of Labor-Congress of Industrial Organizations: voluntary federation of unions that provides education, lobbying, public relations, and consultation services for unions; currently has 65 member unions representing more than 13 million employees.

Agency shop Requires nonunion members of the bargaining unit to pay a "collective bargaining service fee" to the union; however, non-union members are not required to join the union.

Ally doctrine Acceptance by a neutral employer of work normally performed by striking employees of another company. Thus, the neutral employer becomes an "ally" of the struck employer. The neutral ally employees may be legally picketed by the striking employees of the other employer. "Ally doctrine" does not apply within healthcare settings (e.g., hospital).

Arbitration A process during which a neutral party decides the outcome of a dispute between labor and management, typically regarding a collective bargaining agreement.

Authorization card A card that once signed by the employee, authorizes the union to represent the employee during the collective bargaining process.

Authorization card, required percentage A union must obtain authorization cards from at least 30% of the employees within a bargaining unit as proof of employee interest before the NLRB will allow an election for union representation.

Bargaining unit A group of employees (approved by the NLRB) that shares a community of interest and can vote in a union representation election. They are represented by the union and are covered by the terms of the collective bargaining agreement if the union wins the election and negotiates a contract with the employer.

Bargaining unit, employees Usually composed of workers with a family of closely associated jobs.

Bargaining topics Include wages, hours, and conditions of employment. Neither labor nor management can refuse to bargain on these issues.

Certification election Conducted by the NLRB to determine whether employees want to be represented by the union that wants to represent them.

Certified union Has the exclusive right to bargain on behalf of the employees it represents. Individual employees within the represented group are not allowed to enter into separate agreements with the employer.

Charge An allegation made by an individual, employer, or labor organization of a ULP under the NLRA. Charges are filed at NLRB's regional offices.

Closed shop Illegal; employment site where all employees must join the union prior to employment.

Collective bargaining Contract negotiations between union and employer. Mandatory topics include wages, hours, and conditions of employment.

Complaint If the regional office finds merit in a ULP charge and no settlement is reached, the regional director of the NLRB issues a complaint in the name of the Board, stating the ULP(s) and giving notice of a hearing before an administrative law judge. The complaint does not constitute a finding of wrongdoing, but raises issues to be decided by the judge.

Decertification Election in which bargaining-unit employees vote to rescind the union's certification as their representative.

Decertification requirement Petition for decertification election requires the consent of a minimum of 30% of the employees within the bargaining unit.

Dues Paid by the union members, usually on a monthly basis; with employee authorization, can be paid through automatic payroll deduction.

Feather-bedding Illegal practice by a union of having employees paid for work not actually performed.

Full-time workers Workers who usually work 35 h or more per week at their sole or main job.

Good faith bargaining To bargain collectively is the performance of the mutual obligation of the employer and the representative of the employees to meet at reasonable times and confer in good faith with respect to wages, hours, and other terms and conditions of employment, or the negotiation of an agreement or any question arising thereunder, and the execution of a written contract incorporating any agreement reached if requested by either party, but such obligation does not compel either party to agree to a proposal or require the making of a concession.

Grievance Allegation, typically by union or bargaining-unit employee, that the employer has acted improperly, usually by violating provision(s) of the collective bargaining agreement.

Impasse A deadlock in negotiating between management and union over terms and conditions of employment. According to the NLRB, whether an impasse in bargaining exists "is a matter of judgment" and depends on such factors as "bargaining history, the good faith of the parties in negotiations, the length of the negotiations, the importance of the issue or issues as to which there is disagreement, [and] the contemporaneous understanding of the parties as to the state of negotiations."

Labor laws, agency:

- **1935: National Labor Relations Act (NLRA) (Wagner Act)** Federal law passed in 1935; gave employees the right to organize, select their representative(s), and bargain with the employer regarding wages, hours, and working conditions; established the authority of the NLRB.

- **1947: Labor-Management Relations Act (Taft-Hartley Act)** Federal law passed in 1947; amended NLRA and established the authority of the Federal Mediation and Conciliation Service (FMCS).

- **1954: Labor-Management Reporting and Disclosure Act (Landrum-Griffin Act)** Designed to close loopholes in the Taft-Hartley Act pertaining to internal union affairs; amends the NLRA.

- **1974: Amendments to the NLRA** Provides NLRA notice requirements in the healthcare industry.

- **1978: Civil Service Reform Act** Established the Federal Labor Relations Authority to administer federal-sector labor relations.

- **Federal Mediation and Conciliation Service** Federal agency that provides mediation services to labor and management to resolve bargaining impasse situations or to assist in securing arbitrators.

Lockout Occurs when employer closes the business or dismisses employees to deny current employees access to the workplace.

Management rights clause Contract clause in bargaining agreement that states that anything not covered in the contract remains within the purview of management.

No-solicitation rule Rule instituted by management to prevent solicitation of employees for union membership at the workplace. Rules that are too broad are often found to be invalid by the NLRB and the courts.

No-strike, no-lockout clause Clause in which union agrees not to strike and management agrees not to lock employees out or keep them from reporting to work for the life of the contract.

Part-time workers Workers who usually work less than 35 h per week at their sole or main job.

Professional employees Employees meeting the NLRA (amended) criteria for this category. Generally, professional and nonprofessional employees are not included in the same bargaining unit.

Represented by unions Employees, who may or may not be union members, but whose jobs are part of a bargaining unit represented by a union.

Steward Individual within a union who serves as the union's counterpart of the employer's manager or supervisor.

Union shop Site where all employees must join the union after a short introductory period.

REFERENCES

1. **Bakke, E. W.** 1960. To join or not to join. *In* E. W. Bakke, C. Kerr, and C. W. Anrod (ed.), *Unions, Management and the Public.* Harcourt Brace Jovanovich, New York, N.Y.

2. **Bureau of Labor Statistics.** 2002. *National Occupational Employment and Wage Estimates,* December 23, 2002. [http://www.bls.gov/oes/2001/oes290000.htm].

3. **Bureau of Labor Statistics.** 2003. *Union Members Summary,* February 25, 2003. [http://www.bls.gov/news.release/union2.nr0.htm].

4. **Emerson, R. W., and J. W. Haardwicke.** 1987. *Business Law,* 3rd ed. Barron's Educational Series, Inc., Hauppauge, N.Y.

5. **Fitzgibbon, R. J. (ed.).** 1981. *Legal Guidelines for the Clinical Laboratory,* p. 280–283. Medical Economics Co., Oradell, N.J.

6. **Karni, K. R., K. R. Viskochil, and P. A. Amos (ed.).** 1982. *Clinical Laboratory Management,* p. 519–553. Little, Brown, and Co., Boston, Mass.

7. **National Labor Relations Board.** 1979. NLRB no-solicitation rule guidelines. *Labor Relations Reporter: News and Background Analysis.* Bureau of National Affairs, Washington, D.C. **102:**164.

8. **NLRB v. J. Weingarten Inc.** 1975. 420 US. 251, 35 LRRM 2689.

9. **NLRB.** 2003. *Fact Sheet on the National Labor Relations Board.* [http://nlrb.gov/facts.html].

10. **Snyder, J. R., and A. L. Larsen.** 1983. *Administration and Supervision in Laboratory Medicine,* p. 262–280. Harper & Row, Philadelphia, Pa.

APPENDIX 19.1   Helpful Websites Related to Unions and Collective Bargaining

Workforce Management
(http://www.workforce.com)
Articles on arbitration, employer/employee relations, the NLRA, unions, and nonunion shops.

National Labor Management Association
(http://www.nlma.org)
Power sharing in unionized organizations.
(http://www.nlma.org/f-t/ft-tclmc.htm)
20 commandments of labor-management cooperation.

Federal Mediation & Conciliation Service
(http://www.fmcs.gov/internet/)
Independent agency that promotes sound and stable labor-management relations in such areas as dispute mediation, preventive mediation, and alternative dispute resolution.

Legal Information Institute
(http://www.law.cornell.edu/topics/collective_bargaining.html)
Primer on the law of collective bargaining.

NLRB
(http://www.nlrb.gov/)
NLRB's authority and assigned responsibilities.
(http://www.nlrb.gov/nlrb/shared_files/weekly/2003weekly.asp)
Weekly summary of NLRB cases.

APPENDIX 19.2   Do's and Don'ts for Management Regarding Union Activity

THINGS MANAGEMENT CAN DO REGARDING UNION ACTIVITY (5)

- Tell employees that if a majority of the employees in the bargaining unit select the union, the employer will have to deal with the union on all their daily problems involving wages, hours, and other conditions of employment. Advise the employees that the employer would prefer to continue working with them directly on such issues.

- Emphasize that members of management are always willing to discuss any subject. Remind the employees how earlier problems have been resolved through such discussions.

- Remind employees of the benefits they currently enjoy, all of which have been obtained without union representation; avoid threats or promises, either direct or indirect.

- Point out how wages, benefits, and working conditions compare favorably with other institutions in the area, whether unionized or not; all information must be factual.

- Advise employees of the disadvantages of belonging to a union, such as initiation fees, dues, fines, strike assessments, and membership rules. Quote from the union's constitution and bylaws granting it authority to impose punishment and discipline against its members and giving the international organization power over the local.

- Tell employees there is a possibility that a union will call a strike or work stoppage even though many workers may not want one and the employer is willing to negotiate or has already been bargaining.

- Point out that any strike can cost employees in lost wages.

- Explain that in negotiating with the union, the employer does not have to agree to all of its terms and certainly not to those terms that are not in the economic interest of the institution.

- Relate any experience with unions, especially the ones involving the organizing campaign; be factual.

- Provide employees with information about the union or its officers; identify the source of the information.

- Point out any untrue or misleading statements made by an organizer, in a pamphlet, or through any other medium; management may always give employees the facts.

- Advise employees that signing an authorization card does not mean they have to vote for the union.

- Inform employees of the NLRB election procedures and the importance of voting and emphasize that the vote is by secret ballot.

- Make and enforce rules limiting solicitation of membership or discussion of union affairs to outside working time. However, remember that employees can solicit members and discuss the union on their own time, even on the premises, when it does not interrupt work.

- Prohibit the distribution of union literature in patient care areas.

- Restrict the wearing of union buttons to areas where there is no patient contact.

- Enforce all other institution rules impartially in accordance with established procedures.

THINGS MANAGEMENT CANNOT DO REGARDING UNION ACTIVITY

- Promise employees a pay increase, promotion, benefit, or special favor if they vote against the union.

- Threaten loss of job, reduction of income, or elimination of privileges or benefits.

- Discharge, discipline, or lay off an employee because of union activities (or threaten to do so).

- Spy on union meetings.

- Discriminate against workers actively supporting the union.

- Transfer employees because of union affiliation.

- Show partiality to employees not involved in union activities over those active in union activities.

- Discipline or penalize employees supporting a union for an action permitted to employees not supporting a union.

- Separate prounion employees from other employees through assignments or transfers.

- Ask employees how they intend to vote in a union election.

- Question workers about whether they belong to a union or have signed an authorization card.

- Inquire about internal affairs of the union.

- Ask employees about the union sentiments of their coworkers.

(continued)

APPENDIX 19.2 Do's and Don'ts for Management Regarding Union Activity *(continued)*

- Say that the employer will not deal with the union.
- Urge employees to persuade others to oppose the union.
- Give financial support or assistance to a union, its representatives, or employees; this restriction prevents an employer from favoring one union over another.
- Make speeches to assemblies of employees on institution time within the 24-hour period prior to a representative election.

- Call employees to the office or visit their homes to discuss the union.
- Remember these TIPS; do not do the following:
  - Threaten
  - Intimidate
  - Promise
  - Spy

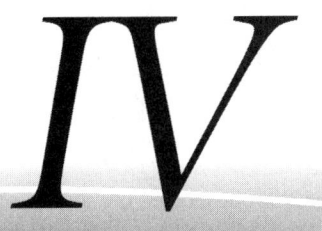

Requirements for Effective Laboratory Management

(Section Editor, *David L. Sewell*)

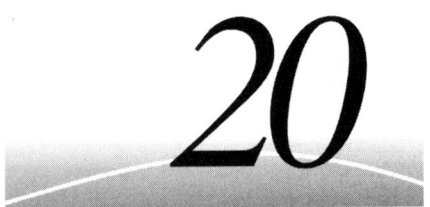

20

Quality Management

Ron B. Schifman, George Cembrowski, and Donna Wolk

OBJECTIVES

To understand the three phases of the total testing process

To understand factors affecting quality of test ordering, specimen collection, and patient satisfaction

To understand basic statistical processes involved in monitoring analytical performance

To understand factors affecting test turnaround time

To understand the role of corrected and incomplete reports in quality management

To understand systems for document control

Quality has to be caused, not controlled.

PHILIP CROSBY, REFLECTIONS ON QUALITY

QUALITY MANAGEMENT IS A SYSTEM for continuously analyzing, improving, and reexamining resources, processes, and services within an organization (5, 68). This is accomplished by defining quality indicators that are measured and analyzed either through time or by comparison to other similar or identical indicators within other departments or organizations (benchmarking) (70). The primary objective is to achieve the best possible outcome. Indicators provide information for improvement, and quality is achieved by reducing variability by standardizing these processes across the organization. Managing the development and implementation of a quality program requires a global understanding of the various resources (structure), processes, and outcomes associated with laboratory medicine as well as healthcare systems in general (23).

The design of a quality management system depends in large part on expected outcomes. For example, processes involving identification of patient specimens in preparation for blood transfusion are much more rigorous than processes for identifying patient specimens for general chemistry testing because the possible risk of a poor outcome from a misidentified specimen is substantially higher for the former (51). Fortunately, poor outcomes from laboratory errors are uncommon. The frequency of laboratory mistakes is estimated to be about 1 per 1,000 patient visits in which laboratory testing is performed. Of these errors, only about a quarter of mistakes are judged to have any impact on patient management, and very few are associated with any significant adverse patient outcome (18, 63).

Developing an effective quality management program is challenging because the goal of the program (good outcomes) is often difficult to quantify and may involve processes that are not directly under the laboratory manager's control (52). In this context, quality assessment of laboratory medicine should be viewed as part of the organization's total quality plan. The "total testing process" is a concept that provides a comprehensive working model for evaluating the components of the laboratory's quality management plan as an interdependent component of the organization's total quality improvement program (38, 61, 73, 74, 95).

The total testing process consists of three phases. The preanalytical phase involves all the various processes and resources that precede the measuring step. This includes proper ordering and test selection by the clinician, patient preparation, specimen collection, identification, transport and/or storage, and premeasurement laboratory processing.

The analytical phase involves managing the reliability of instruments and reagents used for measuring patient specimens and obtaining test results. This phase relies heavily on statistical quality control processes to reduce errors and variation in test measurements. Quality management of this phase of the testing process is the most standardized and regulated and has therefore received the most attention. However, the fewest errors occur during this part of the testing cycle. For example, various studies have shown that only 13 to 32% of laboratory errors are due to analytical problems (7). Howanitz et al. (35) have suggested that the heavy focus on laboratory quality control processes has diverted attention and resources away from other equally important quality objectives associated with the pre- and postanalytical phases of testing.

The postanalytical step involves reporting, interpretation, and clinical use of test results. Application of different quality management processes may involve one or a combination of all three phases. For example, turnaround time and examination of reasons for corrected reports are important quality indicators that may cross over any or all phases of the testing process.

The College of American Pathologists (CAP) (http://www.cap.org) provides numerous management tools to assist laboratories with quality improvement. Two in particular, the Q-Probes and Q-Tracks programs, focus on pre- and postanalytical phases of the testing process (70, 96). Several standardized monitors are provided each year to participants. The Q-Probes program provides a series of cross-sectional quality assurance studies with peer evaluations while the Q-Tracks program provides continuous quality monitors for tracking changes over time. These programs have substantial value for benchmarking performance and tracking improvement. Table 20.1 shows the 2004 Q-Probes and Q-Tracks monitors. A broad range of Q-Probes studies from the last 15 years is available for use by laboratories from the CAP. These predesigned quality

Table 20.1 CAP Q-Tracks and Q-Probes quality assurance program, 2004[a]

Q-Tracks

Patient Identification Accuracy

Assess the incidence of wristband errors within individual institutions and compare performance between participating hospitals.

Blood Culture Contamination

Determine the rate of blood culture contamination using standardized criteria for classifying contaminants.

Laboratory Specimen Acceptability

Identify and characterize unacceptable blood specimens that are submitted to the chemistry and hematology sections of the clinical laboratory for testing.

In-Date Blood Product Wastage

Compare the rates of blood product wastage (i.e., units discarded in-date) in participating hospitals and track rates of improvement over time.

Satisfaction with Outpatient Specimen Collection

Assess patient satisfaction with outpatient phlebotomy services by measuring factors including waiting time, level of discomfort, courteous treatment, and overall satisfaction.

Stat Test Turnaround Time Outliers

Monitor the frequency with which stat test turnaround time intervals exceed institutional stat test turnaround time expectations.

Morning Rounds Inpatient Test Availability

Establish the compliance rate at which laboratories meet morning test reporting deadlines.

Q-Probes

Critical Values Reporting

Evaluate the documentation of successful critical values reporting in the general laboratory for both inpatients and outpatients according to the laboratory's policy.

Type and Screen Completion for Scheduled Surgery

Identify the incidence of avoidable problems associated with the timely obtaining of samples for adequate pre-transfusion testing as well as the practices associated with improved rates of completing testing prior to surgery.

Hospital Nursing Satisfaction with Clinical Laboratory Services

This study will determine and characterize the satisfaction of hospital nursing personnel with clinical laboratory services.

Rate of Peripheral Blood Smear Review

Measure the rate of manual peripheral blood smear (PS) review by laboratory personnel and compare rates of PS review among other institutions. Additionally, determine what institutional factors and practice characteristics influence the rate of manual PS review.

[a]CAP (http://www.cap.org).

assurance studies also come with historical data for benchmarking performance and can be a useful supplement to a laboratory's quality program.

Organizational structure, personnel information, and utilization management as well as laboratory safety are important components of the total quality management plan and are discussed in other chapters. In addition, many of the laboratory's quality management procedures conducted in clinical laboratories today have been mandated by regulatory and accreditation requirements. Participating in on-site laboratory inspections and appropriate external proficiency programs is required to comply with government regulations (see chapter 5).

Quality Management of Preanalytical Processes

Even the most accurate measurement using the most up-to-date technology by a highly trained technologist may cause an untoward clinical outcome if the wrong test is ordered, or the specimen is compromised prior to analysis. The preanalytical phase of the testing cycle is complex and is prone to the most variation and the highest proportion of errors (18, 46, 78). For example, one study uncovered only 0.47% of 40,490 erroneous results from stat tests performed for critical care patients. Of these, 68% were caused during the preanalytical phase of testing, compared to 13% of errors during the analytical phase and 18% in the postanalytical phase. About one-quarter of all erroneous results led to unnecessary additional testing or therapy (65).

Test Selection and Ordering

The first step in the testing process is when a decision is made for a test to be performed. This involves knowledge of the indications for testing, including test sensitivity and specificity for the patient's condition or diagnosis. Many tests are performed for monitoring or screening, so frequency of testing may need to be considered. Many clinical guidelines have been developed that provide expert opinions about clinical indications for testing based on specific signs, symptoms, or suspected disorders (19, 55). However, implementation of these guidelines has proven difficult (9). Some approaches for managing the quality of test selection include monitoring the frequency of testing use by algorithms and instituting test restriction policies (41). For example, some laboratory information systems are capable of notifying the clinician about a potential excess ordering pattern when the number of tests (e.g., two serum cholesterol orders within a week) exceeds a predetermined number (3, 81). Use of algorithms in which indications for ordering a test may depend on the results of another test or other patient parameters can be effective. Examples include deferring serological testing for acute hepatitis A when serum transaminase is normal or defer-

ring ova and parasite examinations in patients who have been hospitalized for more than 3 days (59).

Preanalytical errors associated with ordering tests include inaccuracies or omissions when transcribing from paper requisitions into a laboratory computer system, tests performed but not actually ordered, discrepancies with associating the order with the correct physician, and mistakes with assigning priority status to the order (e.g., stat, routine). Of all tests ordered, about 2% are not completed because of these problems (87). In one study involving 660 laboratories, 4.8% of about 115,000 outpatient orders resulted in mistakes (88). The most common was assignment of the wrong physician with an order and the least common was test priority assignment. High test volume, verbal orders, and lack of laboratory policies and procedures to ensure a quality order entry process were factors associated with higher error rates.

While ordering errors and inappropriate test requests should be tracked and trends should be investigated, major advances in improving the quality of test selection will depend on advances in healthcare information systems that have the ability to assist clinicians based on other information in the patient's electronic record (3, 29, 66). Use of computerized test ordering directly by the physician reduces clerical and transcription errors associated with paper requisitions, reduces costs, and improves utilization (77, 82).

Quality of Specimen Collection

Laboratory test results may be affected by the patient's condition at the time of specimen collection, as well as by the materials and procedures used for specimen collection (57). These types of errors may be easily overlooked and lead to inaccurate test interpretations or incomplete testing due to specimen rejection (e.g., hemolysis), insufficient volume, or incorrect collection container. In one study that examined more than 800,000 outpatient visits among 210 facilities, about 0.4% of phlebotomy procedures were unsuccessful (22). The most common causes in order of frequency were nonfasting patient, missing orders, unsuccessful phlebotomy procedure, patient left collection area, and patient not prepared for test, other than because of nonfasting status. Of the successful blood collections, 0.26% of specimens were unsuitable for testing. In order of decreasing frequency, this was caused by hemolyzed specimen, insufficient specimen volume, clotting of anticoagulated specimen, lost specimen, mislabeling, and rejection based on delta check failure. Other studies have shown that about 0.35% of specimens submitted for chemistry examinations are rejected, hemolysis being the most common reason, and about 0.45% of specimens received for hematology testing are rejected, specimen clotting being the most common reason (39, 40). The quality of coagulation testing depends greatly on good collection technique and full sampling (1, 46).

Well-documented and validated specimen collection procedures used by trained phlebotomy and nursing staff are key factors to prevent these problems from affecting the overall quality of the testing process (4, 6). It is important to provide patients with detailed instructions about preparation prior to collecting the specimen and then to make sure the instructions were followed. For example, one study suggested that up to 25% of toxic serum digoxin levels were likely false positives due to specimen collection too soon after patients ingested their medication (33). False toxicity results can be avoided when phlebotomists are instructed to ask patients when they last took a digoxin pill in order to determine if a specimen should be collected or deferred until a later time. Likewise, phlebotomists should always ask if a patient is fasting prior to collecting a specimen for triglyceride because false elevation of serum triglyceride occurs when a specimen is collected from a nonfasting patient, making this determination meaningless. Measuring total creatinine on 24-h urine specimens helps determine whether a full collection was obtained, and this can be monitored as a quality indicator.

Special attention must be given to collection of specimens for microbiological examinations. Poor quality specimens that are collected improperly or inappropriately will produce useless or even misleading results that may be misinterpreted as having significance to patient care (94). In some cases, specimen quality can be evaluated by smear examinations before cultures are performed, and specimens may be deferred from testing if judged to be of poor quality (60). For example, excessive epithelial cells seen on a Gram stain from a sputum specimen suggest that the specimen contents are from the mouth rather than the lower respiratory tract; this may warrant rejection of the specimen for culture. It may not be possible to eliminate completely contaminated cultures from sterile sources, but they can be reduced with attention to good aseptic collection techniques. Proper sterile preparation of the venipuncture site with the correct materials and careful collection procedures by a professional phlebotomist have been shown to significantly reduce the cost of blood culture contamination, which varies up to fivefold between laboratories (28, 48, 72, 89). This has important implications for costs and outcomes because the average additional patient expense from a preliminary false-positive blood culture result is about $4,000 per episode due to extra hospital days, laboratory tests, and medications (2). Finally, the specimen may be collected properly, but there may be insufficient volume or number of specimens to provide the highest quality result. For example, failure to collect a sufficient number of sputum specimens is the most common cause of delayed diagnosis of tuberculosis in HIV-infected patients (26, 54). Collection of solitary rather than multiple blood cultures makes it difficult to differentiate contamination from true bacteremia when coagulase-negative *Staphylococcus* sp. is isolated (69).

It is critically important that specimens be labeled correctly and properly. The frequency and reasons for incorrect patient identification should be part of the laboratory's quality assessment program. Delta checking (see Use of Patient Data for Quality Control) is a method in which the laboratory manager establishes parameters in the laboratory information system that flag current patient results that differ substantially from previous results (37, 44, 45). Delta checks on some analytes are not very helpful because of large expected changes (e.g., glucose), but others tend to be more sensitive (e.g., red blood cell mean corpuscular volume). Depending on how the parameters are set, only a small proportion of delta check warnings may uncover errors. However, it has been estimated that about 50% of mislabeled specimens can be picked up with delta checking (75). All misidentified specimens should be monitored and contributing factors should be investigated as part of the quality management program (76).

Patient and Client Satisfaction

Typically, the only direct experience patients have with the laboratory is during phlebotomy. Patient satisfaction with this experience is an important preanalytical quality measurement. This is determined by patient surveys as well as objective parameters such as patient waiting times or number of self-reported hematomas (31). Laboratories may also find it useful to conduct nurse and physician satisfaction surveys (58). Typically, turnaround time is found to be the most significant concern expressed by laboratory customers (79). Setting up a hot line through which clients can report potential problems or errors and make inquiries may help large laboratories consolidate customer support services. It is useful to track this information to look for trends or ideas for improving services.

Specimen Transport, Storage, Receipt, and Preanalytical Processing

Specimens may be mishandled through prolonged delays or failure to maintain proper conditions during transport. Some tests are more susceptible than others (e.g., urine culture, coagulation tests) to processing delays. While monitoring transport times is helpful for quality assessment, this is difficult because in situations in which collection is not under the control of the laboratory, it is difficult to accurately determine the time when the specimen was obtained. Specimens that are lost or mishandled in other ways (e.g., broken tube) during transport or preanalytical laboratory processing should be tracked as a quality indicator (see Corrected and Incomplete Reports). Specifications for specimen transport and storage based on stability of analytes should be validated and documented.

Accurate identification of the specimen throughout the testing process is facilitated by the use of bar codes that can be read by laboratory instruments prior to testing (83). This is significantly more reliable than entering patient information manually. It also prevents errors due to misplacement of specimens into instruments or when dividing specimens into secondary containers. Bar code systems work best when integrated into the blood collection process with wristband (inpatient) or identification card (outpatient) positive patient identification schemes. Finally, development of new robotic technology for automated handling of all aspects of within-laboratory preanalytical specimen processing within the laboratory reduces errors (8, 30).

Quality Management of Analytical Processes

Quality management of the analytical phase involves reducing inaccuracy and imprecision (variability) of test methods as much as possible. Attention to standardizing test procedures and monitoring method performance with a well-designed quality control system are the key elements for meeting this management goal. Appropriate method selection and proper training are additional factors that are important for success.

Method Selection and Evaluation

Method selection is laboratory dependent and based on characteristics that best fit goals for cost, timeliness, and reliability (see chapter 25, this volume). These include type of specimen required, sample volume, run size, population to be tested, instrument capacity, analysis time, personnel requirements, existing equipment, safety, utilities (e.g., electrical, water), and space requirements. The complexity of analysis, including calibration, stability of reagents and controls, sensitivity and specificity of the method, linear range of analysis, and interferences, as well as types of internal and external proficiency systems, are factors that may affect method selection decisions. Most laboratory methods are reviewed and approved by the U.S. Food and Drug Administration (FDA) after commercial manufacturers submit data from rigorous premarket evaluations. Validation and implementation of non-FDA-approved methods can be much more complex and labor-intensive and require substantially more development and evaluation. Sometimes, the best decision is to outsource a test when rapid turnaround time is not necessary, test volume is low, or it is difficult to maintain an acceptable quality of proficiency.

Method evaluation and implementation involves assessing the analytical process statistically by the use of control materials, establishing or validating the reference (normal) range of the population being tested, documenting the procedure in writing (both for laboratory use and another document for client use), and training personnel (Table 20.2). When a new method is introduced, it must be compared to the old method before bringing it into use. All procedure changes, training, and analytical perform-

Table 20.2 Method evaluation and implementation

Stage I
Prepare and document procedure
Validate linearity and calibration
Determine within-run imprecision
Evaluate for interferences

Stage II
Determine between-day imprecision
Compare to old method
Evaluate acceptability of imprecision and bias
Perform or validate reference range(s)

Stage III
Establish final quality control ranges, critical values, and delta checks
Train personnel
Complete and sign procedure documents
Notify clients of any significant changes in method

ance data from the previous method should be documented, and clients should be notified of changes affecting interpretation of results.

Quality Control

The term "quality control" describes the approach used to monitor the analytical process to ensure that the test results meet their quality requirements. Quality control includes establishing specifications for the analytical process, monitoring the analytical process to determine conformance to these specifications, and taking any necessary corrective actions to bring the analytical process into conformance (11).

The primary quality characteristic that is monitored during the analytical process is the deviation of an analytical measurement from expected. If the size of this deviation (also known as error) is large, the analytical process may be defective and thus must be investigated. Errors can be classified as systematic (resulting in a shift) or random (resulting in increased imprecision). They may also be classified as persistent or intermittent. Other quality characteristics of the analytical process that are monitored include specific instrument checks that are usually unique to a particular instrument.

The deviation of the analytical measurement from expected is usually monitored by measuring the concentration of analyte contained in quality control specimens. This material is typically a commercially prepared, stabilized surrogate patient specimen. The results of testing these controls are compared to a range of expected values that are obtained by repeated testing over time and calculated as the mean and variance (standard deviation) of these measurements. If the result measured from the quality control specimen deviates significantly as defined by quality control rules (see below), routine analysis is suspended, the analytical run is investigated, and corrective action is taken.

Either two or three different control levels are used. In hematology and hormone (ligand) measurements, it is standard to use three levels; in general chemistry, two levels are standard. As a rule, it is better to have more measurements on fewer control products. Laboratories may also compare these quality control results to others using the same lot of control materials and instrument/reagent systems. This information is provided by most commercial manufacturers of quality control materials and provides a way to assess relative bias and imprecision of the laboratory's methods compared to others' tests performed under similar quality control conditions (Fig. 20.1). Quality control systems for microbiological and serological testing are primarily qualitative in nature. Control testing is performed to check the performance of media, biochemical reactions (positive or negative), immunological reactions, or expected growth in the presence of antibiotics (susceptibility testing).

Quality Control Rules

Quality control rules developed for the clinical laboratory originated in the early 1950s with Levey-Jennings charts. These charts were implemented with three standard deviation (SD) limits, and controls were run just twice per week. By the 1960s, the limits had been reduced to two SD (Figure 20.2). In the next decade, statistical quality control rules started to be used to help reduce the number of false rejections. Table 20.3 shows some of the common quality control rules used to evaluate control measurements today. Westgard et al. have developed a nomenclature for these control rules and devised graphical summaries (power function curves) of their sensitivity and specificity (90, 91). For most applications of clinical laboratory quality control, a combination of the 1-3SD and the 2-2SD control rules is adequate. The 1-3SD rule can detect increases in random error and large systematic errors, while the 2-2SD control rule detects moderate-sized systematic error. This quality control combination is relatively simple to implement and has a relatively low false

Table 20.3 Quality control rules

Rule	Summary	Use
1-2s	Use as a rejection or warning when one control observation exceeds the $x - (\pm 2\text{SD})$ control limits; usually used as a warning.	Use overused. Should only be used with manual assays with low number of analytes/control materials.
1-3s	Reject a run when one control observation exceeds the $x - (\pm 3\text{SD})$ control limits.	Detects random error and large systematic error.
1-3.5s	Reject a run when one control observation exceeds the $x - (\pm 3.5\text{SD})$ control limits.	Detects large random and systematic error. Use only with highly precise assays.
1-4s	Reject a run when one control observation exceeds the $x - (\pm 4\text{SD})$ control limits.	Detects large random and systematic error. Use only with highly precise assays.
2-2s	Reject a run when two consecutive control observations are on the same side of the mean and exceed the $x - (+2\text{SD})$ or $x - (-2\text{SD})$ control limits.	Detects systematic error.
4-1s	Reject a run when four consecutive control observations are on the same side of the mean and exceed either the $x - (+1\text{SD})$ or $x - (-1\text{SD})$ control limits.	Detects small systematic error; very few applications.
10x	Reject a run when ten consecutive control observations are on the same side of the mean.	Detects very small errors; do not use.
R-4s	Reject a run if the range or difference between the maximum and minimum control observation out of the last four to six control observations exceeds 4SD.	Detects random errors; use within run.
x-0.01	Reject a run if the mean of the last N control observations exceeds the control limits that give a 1% frequency of false rejection ($p_{\text{fr}} = 0.01$).	Underutilized.
R-0.01	Reject a run if the range of the last N control observations exceeds the control limits that give a 1% frequency of false rejection ($p_{\text{fr}} = 0.01$).	Underutilized.

Figure 20.1 Examples of interlaboratory quality control reports.

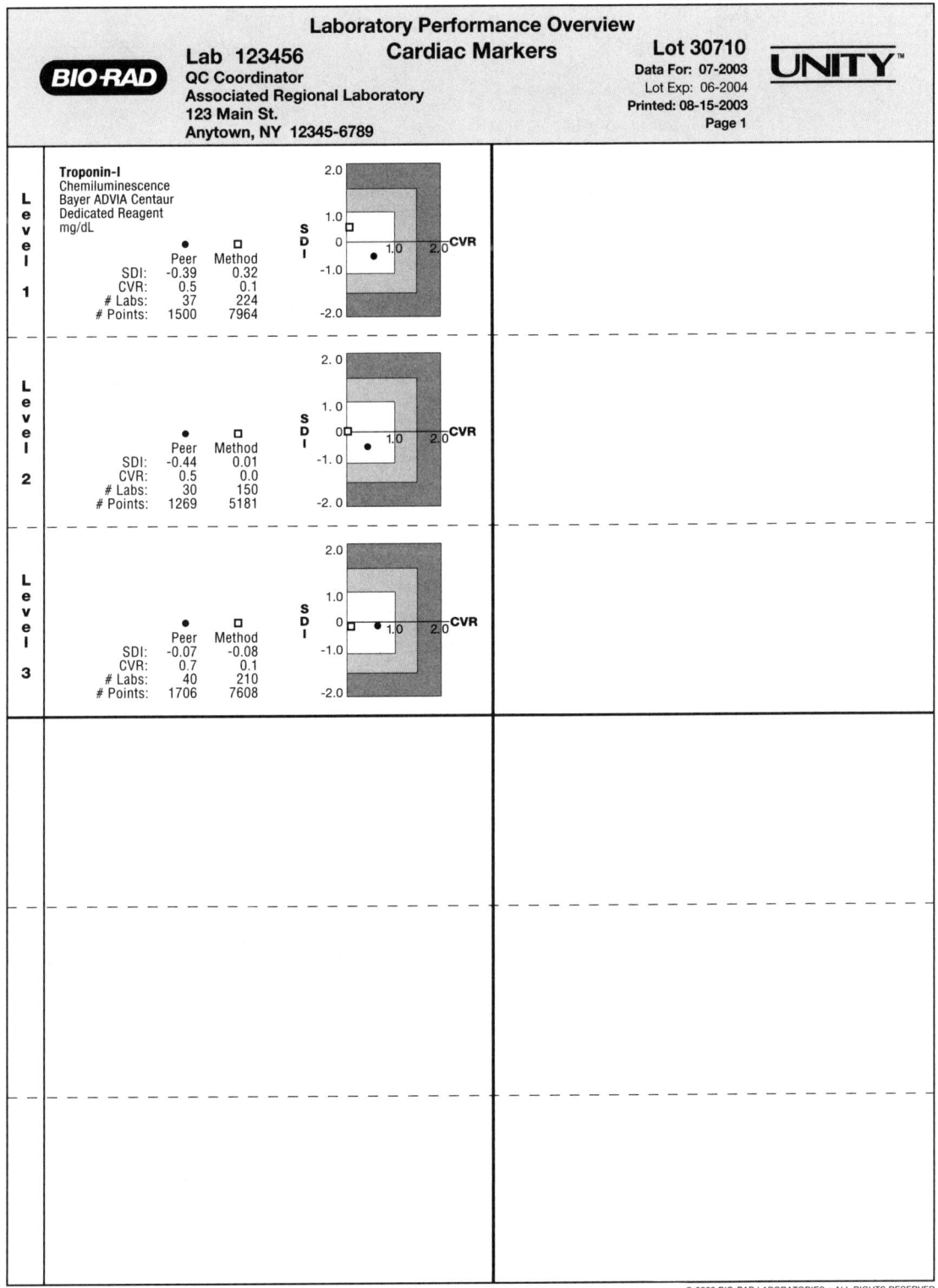

(A) The SDI (a peer-based measure of bias) and CVR (a peer-based estimator of precision) are combined as an *x, y* coordinate within three performance zones: acceptable, acceptable to marginal, and marginal.

(continued)

Figure 20.1 *(continued)*

<table>
<tr><td colspan="7">**Laboratory Comparison Report**
Cardiac Markers</td></tr>
</table>

BIO·RAD

Lab 123456
QC Coordinator
Associated Regional Laboratory
123 Main St.
Anytown, NY 12345-6789

Lot 30710
Data For: 01-2003
Lot Exp: 6-2004
Printed: 08- 5-2003
Page 1

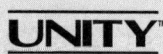

The following statistics are derived from user-supplied data and are provided by Bio-Rad Laboratories as a service to customers. Such action does not imply support of reported analytes and test methods. Refer to the package insert for specific analyte claims and stability information.
Peer group statistics contained in this report may not be used without the express written consent of Bio-Rad Laboratories.

Analyte Method Units Temp Instrument/Kit Reagent		Level 1		Level 2		Level 3	
		Mon	Cum	Mon	Cum	Mon	Cum
Troponin-I							
Chemiluminescence ng/mL							
Bayer ADVIA Centaur							
Dedicated Reagent							
Your Lab	Mean	1.49	1.60	10.78	11.08	38.94	38.17
	SD	0.053	0.074	0.332	0.405	1.60	1.49
	CV	3.6	4.6	3.1	3.7	4.1	3.9
	(Peer) CVR	0.5	0.6	0.5	0.6	0.7	0.7
	(Method) CVR	0.1	0.1	0.0	0.1	0.1	0.1
	(Peer) SDI	-0.39	0.27	-0.44	0.03	-0.07	-0.28
	(Method) SDI	0.32	0.37	0.01	-0.03	-0.08	-0.17
	# Points	4	151	4	151	4	151
Peer Group	Mean	1.53	1.57	11.08	11.06	39.10	38.78
	SD	0.102	0.111	0.677	0.635	2.14	2.20
	CV	6.7	7.1	6.1	5.7	5.5	5.7
	# Points	1500	5889	1269	4917	1706	6900
	# Labs	37	39	30	32	40	41
Group Values by Method	Mean	1.21	1.23	10.70	11.34	40.46	41.98
	SD	.0866	.100	.786	1.023	1.901	2.294
	CV	7.15	8.13	7.35	9.02	4.70	5.46
	# Points	7964	37806	5181	25366	7608	35479
	# Labs	224	254	150	179	210	238

(B) Reports provide monthly and cumulative statistics for the laboratory and between-laboratory comparisons with peer group. Report includes mean, standard deviation, coefficient of variation, CVR, SDI, number of data points, and number of laboratories. CVR, coefficient of variation ratio, a ratio of laboratory imprecision to peer group imprecision. A value less than 1 indicates better than average imprecision; a value greater than 1 indicates more than average imprecision compared to peer group.

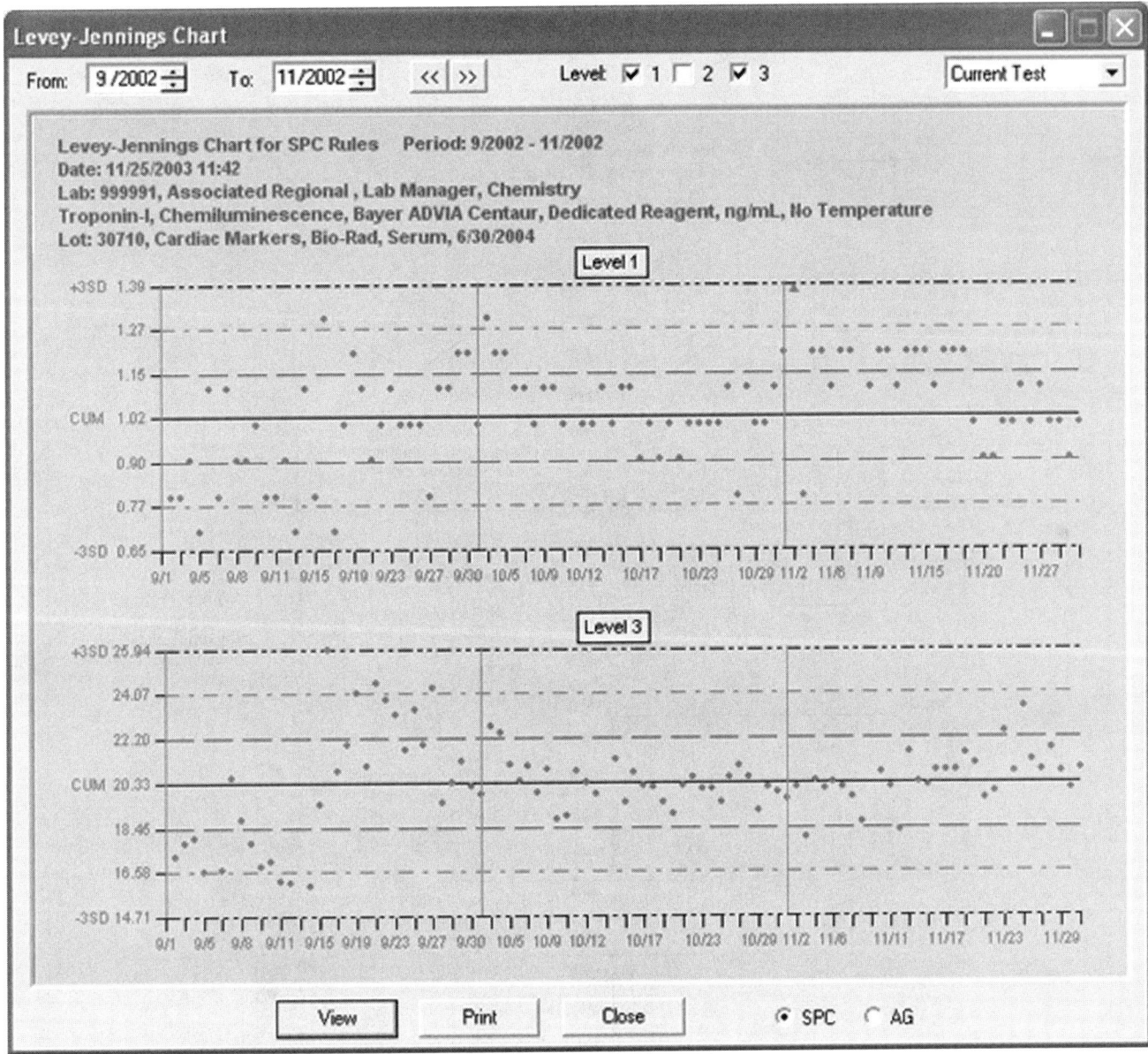

Figure 20.2 Levey-Jennings charts.

rejection probability. Figure 20.3 shows how the 1-3SD and the 2-2SD control rules are applied at one laboratory.

Frequency of Quality Control Analysis

The more frequently that control products are analyzed, the more quickly analytical errors can be detected, investigated, and corrected. For some tests, the longest period over which controls need not be analyzed is specified by government regulations. While many laboratories analyze controls more frequently, the government-mandated period tends to become a de facto standard for control analysis. The average time to detect a persistent error has been shown to be one-half of the period between control analyses (64). Thus, if the period between control analysis is 24 h, an error may impair laboratory testing for an average of 12 h before being detected. It is possible to shorten the interval between control analyses without increasing the numbers of controls analyzed. Rather than analyze several controls together, each can be tested at different times of the day. As a result, the period between control testing is shortened. For example, rather than analyze three blood gas controls every 24 h, one can be tested every 8 h. Using this control analysis schedule, the average time to detect a persistent error will be 4 h.

Some laboratories do not analyze quality control specimens on a periodic basis; rather the number of controls analyzed depends on the number of patient specimens

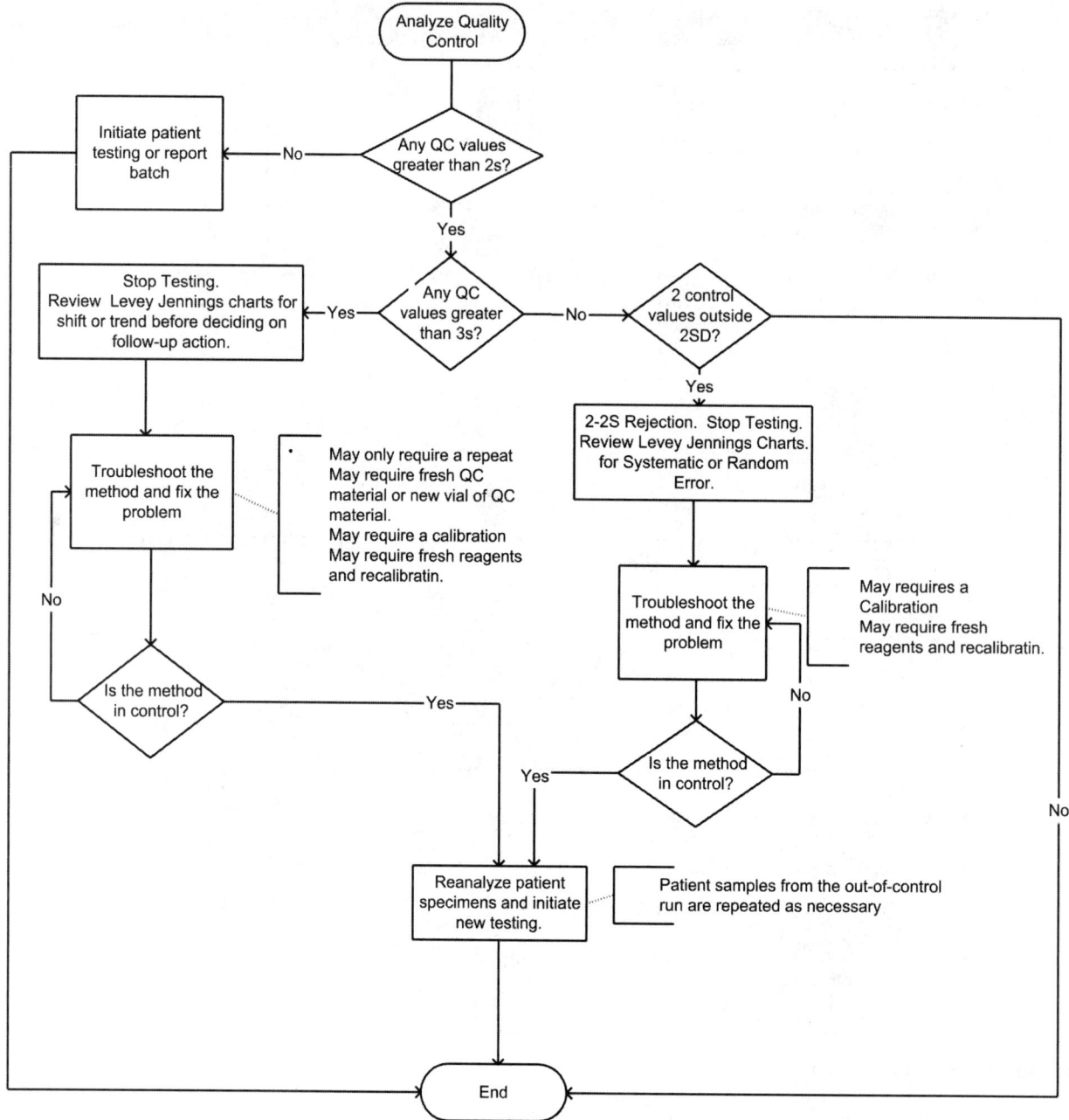

Figure 20.3 Flow chart showing implementation of the 2-2SD / 1-3 SD control procedure. Courtesy Tammy Hofer, BSc (MT), MBA.

run. Because reference laboratories analyze large numbers of specimens over the course of a day, regular but infrequent control analysis may result in large numbers of samples being analyzed with minimal information provided about the run quality. As such, many reference laboratories run their patient samples in batches with a specific number of controls analyzed in each batch. Only when the quality control specimens are within quality control limits is the batch of patient results reported. Some authors have

suggested that for high volume multichannel chemistry analyzers, control specimens be run between every 30 and 100 patient specimens (62).

Specification of MAE

The primary function of quality control is to maintain a stable process. Once the process is stable, then improvements can be made if necessary. Specifications for maximum allowable error (MAE) provide information about how good a test system is for patient care. This is the amount of total error associated with an analytical method that can be tolerated without invalidating the medical usefulness of the result. The analytical quality of a test can be evaluated by comparing its total error to the MAE; this is a method for setting goals for the analytical performance of a laboratory test.

Several different approaches have been used for determining the MAE of laboratory tests. One of the first was offered by Tonks in 1963 (84), who insightfully suggested that the MAE be based on interindividual variation. For most analytes, he suggested that the MAE should be no greater than one-quarter of the analyte's reference range (84). Cotlove et al. proposed the concept that the MAE should be less that one-half of the intraindividual range (20). Ricos et al. have tabulated MAEs for 316 different analytes based on biological variation, associated method biases and imprecisions with estimates of MAE (67).

Table 20.4 compares the MAE for select analytes to maximum imprecisions that are easily achievable by today's clinical analyzers. There is tremendous variation in the MAE among these analytes, ranging from around 1% for serum sodium to 30% for various urine assays. The MAE/imprecision ratio is a very important indicator of analytical quality for the method. It can be thought of as the magnitude of shift, expressed in standard deviations, that will render a test measurement unfit for medical usage. Thus, when MAE is derived from physiological limits for sodium, just a one standard deviation shift in sodium may make the measurement too inaccurate to use. Where a test's MAE/imprecision ratio is less than 2.5, it is attendant on the manufacturer to reduce the method's imprecision. This is a better approach than adding extra quality control samples to more reliably detect smaller analytical errors on a system that has insufficient reproducibility. Whenever possible, instruments with MAE/imprecision ratios that exceed 4 should be used. For analytical systems with such high ratios, it is possible to employ control rules with very low rejection probabilities, such as 1-4SD or 1-5SD (12).

Ideally, each analyte measured in a clinical laboratory should be subject to analyte-specific quality control to prevent the reporting of test results that deviate more than its 99% MAE limits. A computer program is available that

allows the laboratorian to develop more efficient quality control procedures (92). Unfortunately, optimization on an analyte basis is difficult because many analytes are measured together on a single instrument, although some, because of their analytical robustness, may require infrequent testing. It is almost impossible in a busy hospital laboratory to schedule analyte-specific quality control testing and interpretation. At this time, very few instruments can automatically sample and analyze on-board quality control material on a per analyte basis. As a result, most laboratories use the same schedule of control analysis for all of the analytes measured. Some laboratories at least apply analyte-specific quality control rules through the use of a sophisticated laboratory information system or instrument-based quality control systems.

Use of Patient Data for Quality Control

Analytical errors can be detected in other ways. Individual results that are sufficiently outside of their usual physiological limits and that may be incompatible with life (sometimes called critical or alert values) may be followed with reanalysis (42, 43). This kind of a check is sometimes called a limit check. For specimens with large random errors, specimens may be analyzed in duplicate and the average may be reported as long as the difference between duplicates is between certain limits—originally around 15%, but presently around 5%. Some laboratories use duplicate analyses of another type: patient-sample comparisons. These comparisons require the regular analysis of split samples on instruments that measure the same analyte. Differences between instruments that exceed predetermined limits are investigated and corrected (15, 56).

The average of patient (AOP) data is another control procedure that uses patient data. In AOP, an error condition is signaled when the average of consecutive centrally distributed patient data is beyond the control limits established for the average of the patient data. The assumption underlying AOP is that the patient population is stable. Any shift would thus be secondary to a systematic analytical error. The error-detection capabilities of AOP depend on several factors (13). The most important are the number of patient results averaged and the variance in patient population and analytical method. Using averages of patient endocrine data has

Table 20.4 Comparison of MAEs, derived from physiological variation to typical instrument imprecisions

Analyte	MAE (%), 95% limits	Typical imprecision (%)	MAE (%)/imprecision
Serum albumin	3.9	1.5	2.6
Urinary albumin	46.1	8	5.8
Urinary creatinine, 24 h	6.9	2.5	2.8
Activated partial thromboplastin time	4.5	3	1.5
Hemoglobin	4.1	0.8	5.1
Serum sodium	0.9	0.8	1.1
Urinary sodium, 24 h	28.8	4	7.2

demonstrated high error-detection capabilities for thyroid testing (24). However, AOP is not commonly used for clinical chemistry. In contrast, AOP has been used extensively in hematology to monitor patient red blood cell indices and, indirectly, their constituent measurements, hemoglobin and red blood cell count as well as hematocrit (17, 47, 53). The primary limitation of AOP in the hospital laboratory is the lack of randomization in the order of receipt and analysis of patient samples. In hematology, for example, the averaging of a large number of specimens from a neonatal unit or a hematology unit can cause the red blood cell indices to inappropriately indicate an out of control situation. In clinical chemistry, analysis of specimens primarily from renal units will cause large shifts in the AOP of creatinines, glucoses, and urea nitrogens. In reference laboratories, where there is "natural randomization" of patient specimens, AOP is a very powerful tool in guaranteeing acceptable analytical performance (16).

One other quality control approach uses patient data: the delta check, in which the most recent result for a patient is compared to the previous value. The difference between consecutive laboratory values (deltas) is calculated and compared to previously established limits (45, 75). A difference that exceeds these limits is investigated; this difference is either the result of specimen mix-up or real changes in the patients' test results. The difference is usually calculated in two ways: as a numerical difference (current value minus last value) and as a percentage difference (numerical difference times 100 divided by the current value). The percentage of true positives of delta check methods can range from 5 to 29%. While delta checks are used almost universally, there is a high cost in investigating the many false positives, especially in tertiary-care hospital populations in which there are large excursions in laboratory values secondary to disease or therapy (93).

External Quality Control

Proficiency-testing programs provide samples of unknown concentrations of analytes to participating laboratories. The purpose is to determine the ability of laboratory personnel to achieve the correct analysis. Participation in these programs is usually government-mandated with the premise that if performance is acceptable, analysis of patient specimens is proficient. This assumes that proficiency specimens are comparable to and treated the same as patient specimens. Acceptable performance is determined by some form of consensus by peer comparisons using "fixed limits," which are expressed either in measurement units of the analyte (e.g., ±0.5 mmol/liter from the mean for potassium) or as percentages (e.g., ±10% for total cholesterol) (85). Statistically defined limits of acceptability are used for a far smaller number of methods (e.g., thyroid-stimulating hormone) (Table 20.5). The standard deviation index (SDI) is used for this purpose and is calculated as the numerical difference between an individual laboratory's results and the mean of all laboratory results, divided by the standard devi-

ation of all laboratory means. For these analytes, the participant result is acceptable if it falls within ±3 SDI of the group mean.

An alternative multirule system has been proposed for laboratories to evaluate proficiency test results, as illustrated in Fig. 20.4 (10, 14). When significant deviations are detected in a set of five survey results (one or more observations exceeding ±3 SDIs, or the range of the observations exceeding 4 SDIs, or the mean of the five results exceeding ±1.5 SDIs), the laboratory records, including the internal quality-control results, should be reviewed. Mixups of proficiency specimens or of proficiency and clinical specimens should be ruled out.

Whenever possible, aliquots of the survey specimens should be frozen and saved. If the survey results differ significantly from those obtained on peer instruments, these aliquots should be reassayed. Results that still deviate significantly after retesting indicate a long-term bias. If the deviations are variable in magnitude and direction, there may be a problem with imprecision (random error). In the event that repeat analysis yields satisfactory results, the error probably represented a random error or transient bias encountered during the testing period.

Quality Management of Postanalytical Processes

The two most important factors affecting the postanalytical phase of the testing process are test reporting and result interpretation. One source of inaccurate reporting is clerical

Figure 20.4 Flow chart illustrating proficiency test review.

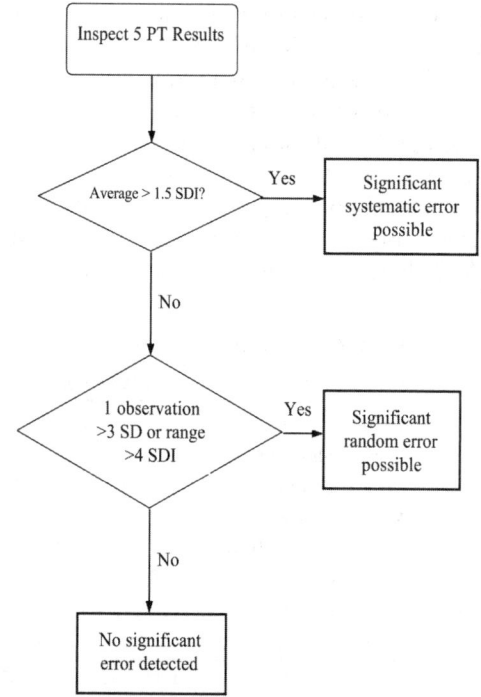

Table 20.5 CLIA testing criteria for acceptable external proficiency testing performance

Test or analyte	Acceptable performance (± target value)
Chemistry, toxicology	
Alanine aminotransferase	20%
Albumin	10%
Alcohol, blood	25%
Alkaline phosphatase	30%
Alpha-1 antitrypsin	3 SD
Alpha-fetoprotein	3 SD
Amylase	30%
Anti-human immunodeficiency virus	Reactive or nonreactive
Antinuclear antibody	2 dilution or positive/negative
Antistreptolysin O	2 dilution or positive/negative
Aspartate aminotransferase	20%
Bilirubin, total	0.4 mg/dl or 20%
Blood lead	10% or 4 μg/dl
Blood gas pO_2	3 SD
Blood gas pCO_2	5 mmHg or 8%
Blood gas pH	0.04
Calcium, total	1.0 mg/dl
Carbamazepine	25%
Chloride	5%
Cholesterol, total	10%
CK isoenzymes	MB present or absent, or 3 SD
Complement C4	3 SD
Complement C3	3 SD
Cortisol	25%
Creatine kinase	30%
Creatinine	0.3 mg/dl or 15%
Digoxin	20% or 0.2 ng/ml
Ethosuximide	20%
Free thyroxine	3 SD
Gentamicin	25%
Glucose	6 mg/dl or 10%
HDL cholesterol	30%
Hepatitis (HBsAg, anti-HBc, HBeAg)	Reactive, positive or nonreactive, negative
Human chorionic gonadotropin (HCG)	3 SD or positive/negative
Immunoglobulin A (IgA)	3 SD
IgE	3 SD
IgG	25%
IgM	3 SD
Infectious mononucleosis	2 dilution or positive/negative
Iron	20%
Lactate dehydrogenase	20%
Lithium	0.3 mEq/liter or 20% (greater)
Magnesium	25%
Phenobarbital	20%
Phenytoin	25%
Potassium	0.5 mEq/liter
Primidone	25%
Procainamide (and metabolite)	25%
Quinidine	25%
Rheumatoid factor	2 dilution or positive/negative
Rubella	2 dilution or positive/negative
Sodium	4 mEq/liter
T3 uptake	3 SD
Theophylline	25%

(continued)

Table 20.5 CLIA testing criteria for acceptable external proficiency testing performance *(continued)*

Test or analyte	Acceptable performance (+ target value)
Chemistry, toxicology *(continued)*	
Thyroid stimulating hormone	3 SD
Thyroxine	20% or 1.0 µg/dl
Tobramycin	25%
Total protein	10%
Triglycerides	25%
Triiodothyronine (T3)	3 SD
Urea nitrogen	2 mg/dl or 9%
Uric acid	17%
Valproic acid	25%
Hematology	
Cell identification	80% or greater consensus on identification
White cell differential	3 SD based on leukocyte percentage
Erythrocyte count	6%
Hematocrit	6%
Hemoglobin	7%
Leukocyte count	15%
Platelet count	25%
Fibrinogen	20%
Partial thromboplastin time	15%
Prothrombin time	15%

errors due to data entry mistakes. Laboratory instrument interfaces with computer reporting capabilities prevent most of these types of errors. Phone reports have a relatively high rate of errors and should be avoided if possible. If computer reporting is unavailable, printed results should be promptly delivered to the patient's chart or physician's office. Whenever possible, calculations should be done by preprogrammed computer systems.

Procedures for defining and reporting critical laboratory test results must be developed and periodically reviewed by the laboratory director in conjunction with the medical staff to ensure that clinicians are immediately notified about abnormal results when necessary (25, 49, 50). Common examples of critical values that require immediate notification include severe hypo- or hyperglycemia, thrombocytopenia, or positive blood cultures. Failure to notify a clinician of a critical test result is a serious quality failure and should be investigated. Quality management of results utilization and proper test interpretation is underdeveloped at this time. For example, improved laboratory communication with physicians of clinically significant bacterial culture results improves appropriateness and timeliness of treatment in patients with serious infections (21, 71).

Turnaround Time

Inadequate laboratory test turnaround time is one of the most common complaints that comes to the laboratory manager. Since clinical evaluations typically require sup-

port from laboratory testing, until results are available, diagnoses are less certain and management decisions are delayed. From an outcome perspective, slow test turnaround times lead to longer waiting times for the patient or incomplete information at the time of a clinical encounter. Pressure to provide test results more rapidly has led, in part, to development of point-of-care devices that enable testing to be done outside of the main clinical laboratory. As a general rule, faster service is associated with higher costs and sometimes lower quality of test results. Therefore, it is the laboratory manager's responsibility to determine the most effective overall testing process and schedules that will provide the most cost effective and reliable results within a time frame that is clinically appropriate.

Evaluation of test turnaround time is an important component of the laboratory's quality assurance program (34, 86). Turnaround time involves all stages of the testing process and is a good way to globally assess performance. Table 20.6 shows the major intervals in the testing process that are potential bottlenecks for delayed testing. Measurement of turnaround time can involve any of these intervals, although the typical measurement is usually specimen collection to result reporting or specimen delivery to result reporting. Typically, the distribution of turnaround times is shifted to the right with a few cases of prolonged times due to various factors such as verification protocols, dilutions, or instrument malfunction. Therefore, simply taking an average of all turnaround time measurements is misleading. A more appropriate measure is to examine the

Table 20.6 Stages in the testing cycle where turnaround time may be measured

Order received and recorded
Patient registration
Specimen collection
Specimen delivery
Specimen processing
Test
Result verification
Result reporting
Interpretation by clinician

percentage of outlier turnaround times (80). These are also the events that will most likely be noticed and be of concern to clinicians. The key to this approach is to establish an appropriate target for turnaround time based on the goals of the clinical staff and the capabilities of the laboratory and facilities infrastructure (32). For example, in one study involving 496 hospitals, about 90% of stat tests from the emergency department were completed in less than 70 min. Test ordering and specimen collection accounted for nearly 60% of all reasons for delays (80).

Corrected and Incomplete Reports

Corrected reports are an important indicator of a failure in one or more laboratory processes. They are analogous to shipping a defective part in the manufacturing industry. Fortunately, only about 4% of these errors have a significant impact on patient care (36). The largest proportion tend to be associated with hematological testing, while the fewest are documented in transfusion medicine. Prior to a result being reported, any number of quality processes may come into play to prevent incorrect results from being reported. However, after the result is verified and reported, it has the potential to affect patient outcome. Incorrect results may be detected in a variety of ways, including input from the physician about a clinical inconsistency, a delta check that uncovers a mislabeled sample that was previously tested, delayed recognition of a significant quality control failure, or a clerical error found during routine supervisory review. All corrected reports should be treated as opportunities to examine processes that can be improved to prevent recurrences of the same problem.

Incomplete reporting of results accounts for about 2% of orders received by laboratories (87). This may occur for a variety of reasons that involve the total testing process, including improper specimen collection, patient unavailable, broken tube, lost specimen, misinterpretation of order, interfering substance in specimen, or failure to document result in patient record. Whenever possible, incomplete testing should be reported as soon as possible to the clinician so that repeat testing can be done, if nec-

essary. As with corrected reports, incomplete tests should be monitored and examined with the goal of changing processes to prevent future occurrences.

Document Control

Clinical laboratories process and handle an enormous amount of information each day. These processes require an organized approach for controlling and organizing this information and making it readily accessible to busy laboratory staff and laboratory inspectors. Document control can be difficult to manage. Nationally, the top three laboratory deficiencies identified during CAP on-site inspections in the years 1998 to 2001 were related to document control items (27). The Joint Commission on Accreditation of Healthcare Organizations (JCAHO) inspection of laboratories yields similar results, especially when off-site or multisite laboratories are involved. A document control policy should state the intent and direction the laboratory takes to document and record the structure it uses for creating, revising, distributing, storing, retrieving, and destroying documents. Processes to be defined in laboratory documents with examples of typical procedures are divided into seven broad document categories that compose the general sum total of documents for most laboratories (Table 20.7).

Table 20.7 Document categories

Manuals
Policies, processes, and standard operating procedures. These are often stratified into sections according to technical specialty

Personnel
Training, competency, qualifications, job/position descriptions

Organization
Organizational charts, definitions, responsibilities and relationships, inspection and accreditation records, provision of service plan, quality plan

Safety
Accident reports, chemical hygiene plan, biohazardous waste disposal plan, shipping and handling of biologicals, infection control plan

Audits
Internal and external

Performance
Quality assurance records, performance improvement records, faults, reporting errors and accidents, root cause analysis records and corrective action plans

Supplies and Equipment
Identification, inventory list, validation records, operation/maintenance checks, and quality control records

Summary

Clinical laboratories are required to have in place a comprehensive quality program. This requires managing the quality of a wide spectrum of resources, procedures, and services by continuously evaluating quality indicators and making adjustments to improve laboratory performance and patient outcomes. The program involves ongoing inspection of the total testing process, from the time a test is ordered until the results are utilized. The quality program is supported by a robust document control system and is conducted by measurement and analysis of indicators to provide information to guide improvement.

KEY POINTS

- Quality management is a system for continuously analyzing, improving, and reexamining resources, processes, and services within an organization.

- The total testing process provides a comprehensive working model for evaluating the components of the laboratory's quality management plan as an interdependent component of the organization's total quality improvement program.

- Well-documented procedures and trained phlebotomy and nursing staff are key factors for ensuring quality of specimen collection.

- Patient satisfaction is an important quality indicator.

- Quality control is a method for establishing specifications for an analytical process, assessing the procedures, monitoring conformance by statistical analysis, and taking corrective actions to bring the procedures into conformance.

- The two most important factors affecting the postanalytical phase of the testing process are test reporting and result interpretation.

- Turnaround time, corrected reports, and incomplete testing are important indicators for monitoring the total testing process.

- A document control policy should state the intent and direction the laboratory takes to document and record the structure it uses for creating, revising, distributing, storing, retrieving, and destroying documents.

GLOSSARY

Accuracy Agreement between the best estimate of a quantity and its true value.

Analyte Sample to be measured.

Analytical error The difference between the result of an analytical method and the true value.

Analytical method Set of written instructions that describe the procedure, materials, and equipment necessary for the analyst to obtain a result.

Analytical range The range of concentration or other quantity in the specimen over which the method is applicable without modification.

Bias Systematic error that describes difference between measured and true or assigned value.

Calibration Process of using standards of known concentration to establish a relationship between measured signal from the instrument and analyte concentration.

Coefficient of variation A measure of variance expressed as a percentage of the mean ([standard deviation/mean] × 100).

Confidence interval Expected range of values within a group with a specified probability.

Constant systematic error An error that is always in the same direction and of the same magnitude even as the concentration of analyte changes.

Control limit A range of expected values that, if exceeded, warns of random and/or systematic error in an analytical process.

Control material Specimen which is repeatedly analyzed and test results are statistically analyzed to monitor method performance.

Delta check Rule-based method to compare patient's current test result to previous measurement to check for unexpected differences that might be due to analytical or nonanalytical errors in the testing process.

Error Deviation of measured concentration from expected or true value.

Gaussian distribution A random distribution of values described by their average and variance (standard deviation); used to described analytical imprecision.

Imprecision Analytical variance, usually expressed as the standard deviation or coefficient of variation ([standard deviation/mean] × 100).

Interference One or more specimen constituents that cause bias by affecting the analytical method.

Matrix Total constituents of the specimen that may affect the analytical process.

Maximum allowable error (MAE) Amount of error associated with an analytical method that can be tolerated without invalidating the medical usefulness of the result.

Mean Arithmetic average of a set of values.

Medical usefulness limits Quality control limits derived from clinical application of results rather than statistical imprecision of the method.

Normal range *See* Reference range.

Proportional systematic error An error that is always in one direction and whose magnitude is a percentage of the concentration of analyte being measured.

Quality assurance A systematic approach to continuously analyzing, improving, and reexamining the total testing process.

Quality control A process for monitoring assay performance to detect deviations from expected outcomes.

Random error A variance from expected that is not reproducible or predictable.

Recovery Amount (usually expressed as percentage) of known quantity of an analyte that is measured when added to a specimen.

Reference range Test results that are within expected parameters for about 95% of all individuals in a defined healthy population. Values outside of the range are classified as abnormal and may be associated with a pathological condition.

Sample Part of specimen that is measured.

Sensitivity, analytical The lowest detection limit of an assay; sometimes measured as the concentration of an analyte that can be differentiated from a blank within a 95% confidence interval.

Specificity, analytical The ability of an analytical method to determine solely the component(s) it purports to measure.

Standard Material of known or assigned concentration used for assay calibration.

Standard deviation A statistic that describes the amount of variance of a set of measurements about the mean value. It is used to describe random error of an analytical method.

Turnaround time The interval between the beginning of one event to the end of another event in the total testing process. Typically measured as the collection to reporting time or as the receipt of specimen in laboratory to reporting time.

Variance Standard deviation squared. Assuming all sources of error are independent of each other, total error is the sum of variances of individual sources of error.

REFERENCES

1. **Adcock, D. M., D. C. Kressin, and R. A. Marlar.** 1998. Minimum specimen volume requirements for routine coagulation testing–dependence on citrate concentration. *Am. J. Clin. Pathol.* **109:**595–599.

2. **Bates, D.W., L. Goldman, and T. H. Lee.** 1991. Contaminant blood cultures and resource utilization. The true consequences of false-positive results. *JAMA* **265:**365–369.

3. **Bates, D. W., G. J. Kuperman, E. Rittenberg, J. M. Teich, J. Fiskio, N. Ma'luf, A. Onderdonk, D. Wybenga, J. Winkelman, T. A. Brennan, A. L. Komaroff, and M. Tanasijevic.** 1999. A randomized trial of a computer-based intervention to reduce utilization of redundant laboratory tests. *Am. J. Med.* **106:**144–150.

4. **Becan-McBride, K.** 1999. Laboratory sampling. Does the process affect the outcome? *J. Intraven. Nurs.* **22:**137–142.

5. **Berwick, D. M.** 1989. Continuous improvement as an ideal in healthcare. *N. Engl. J. Med.* **320:**53–56.

6. **Beto, J. A., V. K. Bansal, T. S. Ing, and J. T. Daugirdas.** 1998. Variation in blood sample collection for determination of hemodialysis adequacy. Council on Renal Nutrition National Research Question Collaborative Study Group. *Am. J. Kidney Dis.* **31:**135–141.

7. **Bonini, P., M. Plebani, F. Ceriotti, and F. Rubboli.** 2002. Errors in laboratory medicine. *Clin. Chem.* **48:**691–698.

8. **Boyd, J. C., and R. A. Felder.** 2003. Preanalytical laboratory automation in the clinical laboratory, p. 107–130. *In* K. M. Ward-Cook, C. A. Lehmann, L. E. Schoeff, and R. H. Williams (ed.), *Clinical Diagnostic Technology. The Total Testing Process,* Vol. 1: The Preanalytical Phase. A.A.C.C. Press, Washington, D.C.

9. **Cabana, M. D., C. S. Rand, N. R. Powe, A. W. Wu, M. H. Wilson, P. A. Abboud, and H. R. Rubin.** 1999. Why don't physicians follow clinical practice guidelines? A framework for improvement. *JAMA* **282:**1458–1465.

10. **Cembrowski, G. S., P. G. Anderson, and C. A. Crampton.** 1996. Pump up your PT IQ. *Med. Lab. Obs.* **28:**46–51.

11. **Cembrowski, G. S., and R. N. Carey.** 1989. Introduction, p. 5. *In* G. S. Cembrowski (ed.), *Laboratory Quality Management: Q.C. Q.A.* American Society of Clinical Pathologists, Chicago, Ill.

12. **Cembrowski, G. S., and P. Champion.** 2003. Simple control rules (1–4s or 1–5s) can be used to quality control the Sysmex XE-2100™ Hematology Analyzer. *Lab. Hematol.* **9:**106–107.

13. **Cembrowski, G. S., E. P. Chandler, and J. Westgard.** 1984. Assessment of "average of normals" quality control procedures and guidelines for implementation. *Am. J. Clin. Pathol.* **81:**492–499.

14. **Cembrowski, G. S., J. R. Hackney, and N. Carey.** 1993. The detection of problem analytes in a single proficiency test challenge in the absence of the Health Care Financing Administration rule violations. *Arch. Pathol. Lab. Med.* **117:**437–443.

15. **Cembrowski, G. S., E. S. Lunetzky, C. C. Patrick, and M. K. Wilson.** 1988. An optimized quality control procedure for hematology analyzers with the use of retained patient specimens. *Am. J. Clin. Pathol.* **89:**203–210.

16. **Cembrowski, G. S., E. Parlapiano, D. O'Bryan, and L. Visnapuu.** 2001. Successful use of patient moving averages (PMA) as an accuracy control for multichannel hematology analyzers in a high volume robotic clinical laboratory: abstract 3. *Lab. Hematol* **7:**35.

17. **Cembrowski, G. S., and J. O. Westgard.** 1985. Quality control of multichannel hematology analyzers: evaluation of Bull's algorithm. *Am. J. Clin. Pathol.* **83:**337–345.

18. **Chambers, A. M., J. Elder, and D. O'Reilly.** 1986. The blunder rate in a clinical biochemistry service. *Ann. Clin. Biochem.* **23:**470–473.

19. **Connelly, D. P.** 2003. Critical pathways, clinical practice guidelines, test selection and ordering, p. 47–63. *In* K. M. Ward-Cook, C. A. Lehmann, L. E. Schoeff, and R. H. Williams (ed.), *Clinical Diagnostic Technology. The Total Testing Process,* Vol. 1: The Preanalytical Phase. A.A.C.C. Press, Washington, D.C.

20. **Cotlove, E., E. K. Harris, and G. Z. Williams.** 1970. Biological and analytic components of variation in long-term studies of serum consitituents in normal subjects. 3. Physiological and medical implications. *Clin. Chem.* **16:**1028–1032.

21. **Cunney, R. J., E. B. McNamara, N. Alansari, B. Loo, and E. G. Smyth.** 1997. The impact of blood culture reporting and clinical liaison on the empiric treatment of bacteraemia. *J. Clin. Pathol.* **50:**1010–1012.

22. **Dale, J. C., and D. A. Novis.** 2002. Outpatient phlebotomy success and reasons for specimen rejection. *Arch. Pathol. Lab. Med.* **126:**416–419.

23. **Donabedian, A.** 1992. Defining and measuring the quality of healthcare, p. 41–64. *In* R. P. Wenzel (ed.), *Assessing Quality Health Care.* Williams & Wilkins, Baltimore, Md.

24. **Douville, P., G. S. Cembrowski, and J. Strauss.** 1987. Evaluation of the average of patients, application to endocrine assays. *Clin. Chim. Acta* **167:**173–185.

25. **Emancipator, K.** 1997. Critical values–ASCP practice parameter. *Am. J. Clin. Pathol.* **108:**247–253.

26. **Finch, D., and C. D. Beaty.** 1997. The utility of a single sputum specimen in the diagnosis of tuberculosis–comparison between HIV-infected and non-HIV-infected patients. *Chest* **111:**1174–1179.

27. **Garcia, F., E. Harrison, C. Wise, and D. Wolk.** 2003. Is your document control out of control? complying with document control regulations. *Clin. Leadersh. Manag. Rev.* **17:**255–262.

28. **Gibb, A. P., B. Hill, B. Chorel, and R. Brant.** 1997. Reduction in blood culture contamination rate by feedback to phlebotomists. *Arch. Pathol. Lab. Med.* **121:**503–507.

29. **Hindmarsh, J. T., and A. W. Lyon.** 1996. Strategies to promote rational clinical chemistry test utilization. *Clin. Biochem.* **29:**291–299.

30. **Holman, J. W., T. E. Mifflin, R. A. Felder, and L. M. Demers.** 2002. Evaluation of an automated preanalytical robotic workstation at two academic health centers. *Clin. Chem.* **48:**540–548.

31. **Howanitz, P. J., G. S. Cembrowski, and P. Bachner.** 1991. Laboratory phlebotomy: College of American Pathologists Q-Probe study of patient satisfaction and complications in 23,783 patients. *Arch. Pathol. Lab. Med.* **115:**867–872.

32. **Howanitz, P.J., G. S. Cembrowski, S. J. Steindel, and T. A. Long.** 1993. Physician goals and laboratory test turnaround times: a College of American Pathologists Q-Probes study of 2,763 clinicians and 722 institutions. *Arch. Pathol. Lab. Med.* **117:**22–28.

33. **Howanitz, P. J., and S. J. Steindel.** 1993. Digoxin therapeutic drug monitoring practices: a College of American Pathologists Q-Probes study of 666 institutions and 18,679 toxic levels. *Arch. Pathol. Lab. Med.* **117:**684–690.

34. **Howanitz, P. J., S. J. Steindel, G. S. Cembrowski, and T. A. Long.** 1992. Emergency department stat test turnaround times: a College of American Pathologists' Q-Probes study for potassium and hemoglobin. *Arch. Pathol. Lab. Med.* **116:**122–128.

35. **Howanitz, P. J., G. A. Tetrault, and S. J. Steindel.** 1997. Clinical laboratory quality control: a costly process now out of control. *Clin. Chim. Acta* **260:**163–174.

36. **Howanitz, P. J., K. Walker, and P. Bachner.** 1992. Quantification of errors in laboratory reports: a quality improvement study of the College of American Pathologists' Q-Probes program. *Arch. Pathol. Lab. Med.* **116:**694–700.

37. **Iizuka, Y., H. Kume, and M. Kitamura.** 1982. Multivariate delta check method for detecting specimen mix-up. *Clin. Chem.* **28:**2244–2248.

38. **Irjala, K. M., and P. E. Gronross.** 1998. Preanalytical and analytical factors affecting laboratory results. *Ann. Med.* **30:**267–272.

39. **Jones, B. A, R. R. Calam, and P. J. Howanitz.** 1997. Chemistry specimen acceptability: a College of American Pathologists Q-Probes study of 453 laboratories. *Arch. Pathol. Lab. Med.* **121:**19–26.

40. **Jones, B. A., F. Meier, and P. J. Howanitz.** 1995. Complete blood count specimen acceptability: a College of American Pathologists Q-Probes study of 703 laboratories. *Arch. Pathol. Lab. Med.* **119:**203–208.

41. **Keffer, J. H.** 2001. Guidelines and algorithms: perception of why and when they are successful and how to improve them. *Clin. Chem.* **47:**1563–1572.

42. **Kost, G. J.** 1990. Critical limits for urgent clinician notification at US medical centers. *JAMA* **263:**704–707.

43. **Kost, G. J.** 1991. Critical limits for emergency clinician notification at United States children's hospitals. *Pediatr.* **88:**597–603.

44. **Lacher, D. A.** 1990. Relationship between delta checks for selected chemistry tests. *Clin. Chem.* **36:**2134–2136.

45. **Ladenson, J. H.** 1975. Patients as their own controls: use of the computer to identify "laboratory error." *Clin. Chem.* **21:**1648–1653.

46. **Lawrence, J. B.** 2003. Preanalytical variable in the coagulation laboratory. *Lab. Med.* **34:**49–57.

47. **Levy, W. C., K. L. Hay, and B. S. Bull.** 1986. Preserved blood versus patient data for quality control—Bull's algorithm revisited. *Am. J. Clin. Pathol.* **85:**719–721.

48. **Little, J. R., P. R. Murray, P. S. Traynor, and E. Spitznagel.** 1999. A randomized trial of povidone-iodine compared with iodine tincture for venipuncture site disinfection: effects on rates of blood culture contamination. *Am. J. Med.* **107:**119–125.

49. **Lum, G.** 1996. Evaluation of a laboratory critical limit (alert value) policy for hypercalcemia. *Arch. Pathol. Lab. Med.* **120:**633–636.

50. **Lum, G.** 1998. Critical limits (alert values) for physician notification: universal or medical center-specific limits. *Ann. Clin. Lab. Sci.* **28:**261–271.

51. **Lumadue, J.A., J. S. Boyd, and P. M. Ness.** 1997. Adherence to a strict specimen-labeling policy decreases the incidence of erroneous blood grouping of blood bank specimens. *Transfusion* **37:**1169–1172.

52. **Lundberg, G. D.** 1998. The need for an outcomes research agenda for clinical laboratory testing. *JAMA* **280:**565–566.

53. **Lunetzky, E. S., and G. S. Cembrowski.** 1987. Performance characteristics of Bull's multirule algorithm for the quality control of multichannel hematology analyzers. *Am. J. Clin. Pathol.* **88:**634–638.

54. **Mathur, P., L. Sacks, G. Auten, R. Sall, C. Levy, and F. Gordin.** 1994. Delayed diagnosis of pulmonary tuberculosis in city hospitals. *Arch. Intern. Med.* **154:**306–310.

55. **McQueen, M. J.** 2001. Overview of evidence-based medicine: challenges for evidence-based laboratory medicine. *Clin. Chem.* **47:**1536–1546.

56. **Metzger, L. F., W. B. Stauffer, A. V. Krupinski, R. P. Millman, and G. S. Cembrowski.** 1987. Detecting errors in blood-gas measurement by analysis with two instruments. *Clin. Chem.* **33:**512–517.

57. **Miller, J. J.** 2003. Specimen collection, handling, preparation and storage, p. 65–90. *In* K. M. Ward-Cook, C. A. Lehmann, L. E. Schoeff, and R. H. Williams (ed.), *Clinical Diagnostic Technology. The Total Testing Process*, Vol. 1: The Preanalytical Phase. A.A.C.C. Press, Washington, D.C.

58. **Morgan, M. S.** 1995. Perceptions of a medical microbiology service: a survey of laboratory users. *J. Clin. Pathol.* **48:**915–918.

59. **Morris, A. J., P. R. Murray, and L. B. Reller.** 1996. Contemporary testing for enteric pathogens: the potential for cost, time, and health care savings. *J. Clin. Microbiol.* **34:**1776–1778.

60. **Morris, A. J., L. K. Smith, S. Mirrett, L. B. Reller.** 1996. Cost and time savings following introduction of rejection criteria for clinical specimens. *J. Clin. Microbiol.* **34:**355–357.

61. **Narajanan, S.** 2000. The preanalytic phase: an important component of laboratory medicine. *Am. J. Clin. Pathol.* **113:**429–452.

62. **Neubauer, A., C. Wolter, C. Falkner, and D. Neumeier.** 1998. Optimizing frequency and number of controls for automatic multichannel analyzers. *Clin. Chem.* **44:**1014–1023.

63. **Nutting, P. A., D. S. Main, P. M. Fischer, T. M. Stull, M. Pontius, M. Seifert, Jr., D. J. Boone, and S. Holcomb.** 1996. Toward optimal laboratory use. Problems in laboratory testing in primary care. *JAMA* **275:**635–639.

64. **Parvin, C. A., and A. M. Gronowski.** 1997. Effect of analytical run length on quality-control (QC) performance and the QC planning process. *Clin. Chem.* **43:**2149–2154.

65. **Peters, M.** 1995. Managing test demand by clinicians: computer assisted guidelines. *J. Clin. Pathol.* **48:**98–100.

66. **Plebania, M., and P. Carraro.** 1997. Mistakes in a stat laboratory: types and frequency. *Clin. Chem.* **43:**1348–1351.

67. **Ricos, C., V. Alvarez, F. Cava, J. V. Garcia-Lario, A. Hernandez, C. V. Jimenez, J. Minchinela, C. Perich, M. Simon.** 1999. Current databases on biological variation: pros, cons and progress. *Scand. J. Clin. Lab. Invest.* **60:**491–500.

68. **Schifman, R. B.** 1990. Quality assurance goals in clinical pathology. *Arch. Pathol. Lab. Med.* **114:**1140–1144.

69. **Schifman, R. B., P. Bachner, and P. J. Howanitz.** 1996. Blood culture quality improvement: a College of American Pathologists Q-Probes study involving 909 institutions and 289,572 blood culture sets. *Arch. Pathol. Lab. Med.* **120:**999–1002.

70. **Schifman, R. B., P. J. Howanitz, R. J. Zarbo.** 1996. Q-Probes: a College of American Pathologists benchmarking program for quality management in pathology and laboratory medicine. *Adv. Pathol.* **9:**83–120.

71. **Schifman, R. B., A. Pindur, and J. A. Bryan.** 1997. Laboratory practices for reporting bacterial susceptibility tests that affect antibiotic therapy. *Arch. Pathol. Lab. Med.* **121:**1168–1170.

72. **Schifman, R. B., C. Strand, F. Meier, and P. Howanitz.** 1998. Blood culture contamination: a College of American Pathologists Q-Probes study involving 640 institutions and 497,134 specimens from adult patients. *Arch. Pathol. Lab. Med.* **122:**216–221.

73. **Schumacher, G. E, and J. T. Barr.** 1998. Total testing process applied to therapeutic drug monitoring: impact on patients' outcomes and economics. *Clin. Chem.* **44:**370–374.

74. **Shahangian, S., R. Cohn, E. E. Gaunt, and J. M. Krolak.** 1999. System to monitor a portion of the total testing process in medical clinics and laboratories: evaluation of a split-specimen design. *Clin. Chem.* **45:**269–280.

75. **Sheiner, L. B., L. A. Wheeler, and J. K. Moore.** 1979. The performance of delta check methods. *Clin. Chem.* **25(12):**2034–2037.

76. **Simpson, J. B.** 2001. A unique approach for reducing specimen labeling errors: combining marketing techniques with performance improvement. *Clin. Leadersh. Manage. Rev.* **15:**401–405.

77. **Smith, B. J., and M. D. McNeely.** 1999. The influence of an expert system for test ordering and interpretation on laboratory investigations. *Clin. Chem.* **45:**1168–1175.

78. **Stahl, M., E. D. Lund, and I. Brrandslund.** 1998. Reasons for a laboratory's inability to report results for requested analytical tests. *Clin. Chem.* **44:**2195–2197.

79. **Steindel, S. J., and P. J. Howanitz.** 2001. Physician satisfaction and emergency department laboratory test turnaround time. *Arch. Pathol. Lab. Med.* **125:**863–871.

80. **Steindel, S. J., and D. A. Novis.** 1999. Using outlier events to monitor test turnaround time—a College of American Pathologists Q-Probes study in 496 laboratories. *Arch. Pathol. Lab. Med.* **123:**607–614.

81. **Studnicki, J., D. D. Bradham, J. Marshburn, P. R. Foulis, and J. V. Straumfjord.** 1993. A feedback system for reducing excessive laboratory tests. *Arch. Pathol. Lab. Med.* **117:**35–39.

82. **Tierney, W. M., M. E. Miller, J. M. Overhage, and C. J. McDonald.** 1993. Physician inpatient order writing on microcomputer workstations. Effects on resource utilization. *JAMA* **269:**379–383.

83. **Tilzer, L. L., and R. W. Jones.** 1988. Use of barcode labels on collection tubes for specimen management in the clinical laboratory. *Arch. Pathol. Lab. Med.* **112:**1200–1202.

84. **Tonks, D. B.** 1963. A study of the accuracy and precision of clinical chemistry determinations in 170 Canadian laboratories. *Clin. Chem.* **9:**217–223.

85. **U.S. Department of Health and Human Services.** 1992. Medicare, Medicaid, and CLIA programs. Regulations implementing the Clinical Laboratory Improvement Amendments of 1988 (CLIA) final rule. *Fed. Regis.* **57:**7002.

86. **Valenstein, P.** 1996. Laboratory turnaround time. *Am. J. Clin. Pathol.* **105:**676–688.

87. **Valenstein, P., and P. J. Howanitz.** 1995. Ordering accuracy: a College of American Pathologists Q-Probes study of 577 institutions. *Arch. Pathol. Lab. Med.* **119:**117–122.

88. **Valenstein, P., and F. Meier.** 1999. Outpatient order accuracy—a College of American Pathologists Q-Probes study of requisition order entry accuracy in 660 institutions. *Arch. Pathol. Lab. Med.* **123:**1145–1150.

89. **Weinbaum, F. I., S. Lavie, M. Danek, D. Sixsmith, G. F. Heinrich, and S. S. Mills.** 1997. Doing it right the first time: quality improvement and the contaminant blood culture. *J. Clin. Microbiol.* **35:**563–565.

90. **Westgard, J. O., and T. Groth.** 1979. Power functions for statistical control rules. *Clin. Chem.* **25:**863–869.

91. **Westgard, J. O., T. Groth, T. Aronsson, H. Falk, and C. H. de Verdier.** 1977. Performance characteristics of rules for internal quality control: probabilities for false rejection and error detection. *Clin. Chem.* **23:**1857–1867.

92. **Westgard, J. O., B. Stein, S. A. Westgard, and R. Kennedy.** 1997. QC Validator 2.0: a computer program for automatic selection of statistical QC procedures for applications in healthcare laboratories. *Comput. Methods Programs Biomed.* **53:**175–186.

93. **Wheeler, L. A., and L. B. Sheiner.** 1981. A clinical evaluation of various delta check methods. *Clin. Chem.* **127:**5–9.

94. **Wilson, M. L.** 1996. General principles of specimen collection and transport. *Clin. Infect. Dis.* **22:**766–777.

95. **Witte, D. L., S. A. VanNess, D. S. Angstadt, and B. J. Pennell.** 1997. Errors, mistakes, blunders, outliers, or unacceptable results: how many? *Clin. Chem.* **43:**1352–1356.

96. **Zarbo, R. J., B. A. Jones, R. C. Friedberg, P. N. Valenstein, S. W. Renner, R. B. Schifman, M. K. Walsh, and P. J. Howanitz.** 2002. Q-Tracks: a College of American Pathologists program of continuous laboratory monitoring and longitudinal tracking. *Arch. Pathol. Lab. Med.* **126:**1036–1044.

APPENDIX 20.1 Regulations, Guidelines, and Information with Application to a Clinical Laboratory

A listing of relevant regulations grouped according to the regulatory agency from which they are issued. Information changes rapidly; the information listed is representative of that available in February 2003.

FDA
21 CFR 11, Electronic Records; Electronic Signatures, Subpart B–Electronic Records
21 CFR 58, Good Laboratory Practice for Nonclinical Laboratory Studies
    58.185 Reporting of nonclinical laboratory study results
    58.190 Storage and retrieval of records and data
    58.195 Retention of records
21 CFR 211, Current Good Manufacturing Practice for Finished Pharmaceuticals
    Subpart J—Records and Reports (211.180–211.198)
21 CFR 600, Biological Products, General
    600.12 Records
21 CFR 606, Current Good Manufacturing Practice for Blood and Blood Components
    606.100 Standard operating procedures
    Subpart I—Records and Reports (606.160–606.171)
21 CFR 640, Additional Standards for Human Blood and Blood Products
    640.72 Records
21 CFR 803, Medical Device Reporting of Adverse Events and Certain Malfunctions
    803.17–803.18 Written MDR procedures, Files
21 CFR 820, Good Manufacturing Practice, Quality System Regulation
    Subpart M—Records (820.180–820.198)

Department of Labor: Occupational Safety and Health Administration (OSHA)
29 CFR 1904, Recording and Reporting Occupational Injuries and Illnesses
    1904.6 Retention of records
    1904.9 Falsification or failure to keep records or reports
29 CFR 1910 Occupational Safety and Health Standards
    Appendix C to 1910.120
        4. Training (records)
        8. Medical surveillance programs (records)

Department of Health and Human Services: Center for Medicare and Medicaid Services (CMS)
42 CFR 493, Laboratory Requirements (CLIA 88)
    493.1107 Test—Records
    493.1201(b) Written quality control procedures
    493.1202(c)(2) Procedure manual, moderate-complexity testing
    493.1211 Procedure manual, high-complexity testing
    493.1221 Quality Control—Records
    493.1721 Quality Assurance—Records

Department of Health and Human Services, Public Health
42 CFR 72, Interstate Shipment of Etiologic Agents

Department of Transportation
49 CFR 171–7 Shipment of Hazardous Materials

Department of Labor
29 CFR 71—Protection of individual privacy and access to records under the Privacy Act of 1974

Miscellaneous sources (specifics not listed)
Multiple Federal Register sources
FDA Guidelines, Guidances, and Memoranda
Various CDC Guidelines
FDA Compliance Program Guidance Manual

Veterans Health Administration
Pathology and Laboratory Medicine Service Procedures—Directive 1106 and Handbook 1106.1 (Feb. 12, 1998)
Chapter 2 Quality Improvement
    2.04 Required elements for quality improvement in major divisions of the laboratory and ancillary testing sites
    2.08 Retention of samples, slides, and records
VA Records Control Schedule (RCS) 10–1, Section VIII, "Laboratory Service" (Feb. 14, 2002)

American Association of Blood Banks
Standards for Blood Banks and Transfusion Services, 21st Ed.
    Std 6.0 and 6.1.1 through 6.1.6—Documents and records; policies, processes and procedures to ensure that documents are identified, reviewed, approved and retained.

College of American Pathologists (CAP)
Standards for Laboratory Accreditation (1999 Edition)
CAP Laboratory Accreditation Program Checklists for Inspection of Laboratories (2002 Edition)
    Requirements under checklists—(too numerous to count)
    Example: GEN.41480 Are laboratory records and materials retained for an appropriate time?

Joint Commission on Accreditation of Healthcare Organizations (JCAHO)
Comprehensive Accreditation Manual for Pathology and Clinical Laboratory Services (2001–2002)
    IM.7 Laboratory—specific data and information; the laboratory develops tools for communication. For example:
        IM.7.1 Written procedures
        IM.7.1.1 Procedure approval
        IM.7.6 Required records and reports are maintained
        IM.7.10 Current descriptions and instructions for all analytical methods and procedures
    LD.2 Directing services—The laboratory director is responsible for developing, implementing, and maintaining policies and procedures.
    IM.8 Aggregate data and information
    IM.10 Comparative data information; defined, collected, analyzed, transmitted, reported and used
    QC.1 Each specialty and subspecialty has a documented quality control program.

National Committee for Clinical Laboratory Standards (NCCLS)
GP2-A4 Clinical Laboratory Technical Procedure Manuals; 4th Edition
GP26A A Quality System Model for Health Care Approved Guidelines (October 1999)
    Part 4.6, Quality system essentials, documents, and records

(continued)

APPENDIX 20.1   Regulations, Guidelines, and Information with Application to a Clinical Laboratory *(continued)*

International Organization for Standardization (ISO)
ISO 9001 (Third edition 12–15–2000)
Section 4. Quality Management System
  4.2 Document requirements
    4.2.1 General; documented procedures to control all documents
    and data

    4.2.2 Quality manual
    4.2.3 Control of documents
    4.2.4 Control of records

APPENDIX 20.2   CAP Laboratory Inspection Checklist Questions Associated with Quality Management

Proficiency testing

GEN.10000 Are the laboratory's procedures for proficiency testing written and sufficient for the extent and complexity of testing done in the laboratory?

GEN.10500 Does the laboratory have an alternative performance assessment system for determining the reliability of analytic results on patient samples for which no external proficiency testing program (e.g., CAP Surveys) is offered?

GEN.10650 Is the above alternative performance assessment system exercised at least semi-annually?

GEN.10710 Has the Laboratory Director or designee reviewed the results from the above alternative performance assessment system?

GEN.11226 Does the laboratory have a procedure for assessing its performance on PT challenges that were not graded because of lack of consensus, or because the laboratory either submitted its results after the cut-off date for receipt, or did not submit results?

GEN.11742 Is there evidence that problems identified by proficiency testing and alternative performance assessment have been recognized and corrected?

GEN.12258 Is there a policy that prohibits interlaboratory communication about proficiency testing samples before submission of data to the proficiency-testing provider?

GEN.13032 For tests performed within the laboratory, is there a policy that prohibits referral of proficiency testing specimens to an outside laboratory?

Quality Improvement

GEN.13806 Does the quality improvement (QI) program follow a documented operational plan?

GEN.16902 Has the QI plan been implemented as designed?

GEN.20100 Does the QI program cover all aspects of the laboratory service?

GEN.20316 Are key indicators of quality monitored and evaluated to detect problems and opportunities for improvement?

GEN.20332 Are appropriate actions taken when opportunities for improvement are identified?

GEN.20348 Do the QI indicators include measures of preanalytic variables?

GEN.20364 Do the QI indicators include measures of postanalytic variables?

GEN.20380 Are graphical tools (charts and graphs) used to communicate quality findings?

GEN.20400 Is there a systematic program to identify and correct problems that may interfere with patient care services?

GEN.20500 Is a physician responsible for ensuring that the QI program is coordinated with others in the facility (medical, surgical, nursing services, etc.)?

GEN.25250 Is the QI program appraised at least annually for effectiveness?

GEN.27625 Is there evidence of improvement in objective measures of the laboratory's quality in the preceding 2 years?

Document Control

GEN.20386 Does the laboratory have a written document control system?

GEN.20392 Are all quality improvement procedures, forms and records managed under document control?

GEN.42950 Are procedure manuals clearly documented, complete and readily available to all authorized users?

Patient Satisfaction

GEN.22875 Have the referring physicians' or patients' satisfaction with the laboratory service been measured within the past 2 years?

Analytical Quality Control

GEN.30000 Is there a written quality control program that clearly defines procedures for monitoring analytic performance, including establishment of tolerance limits, number and frequency of controls, corrective actions based on quality control data, and related information?

GEN.30050 For those tests performed using different methodologies or instruments or at different testing sites, is there a documented mechanism to verify the comparability of patient results throughout the clinically appropriate ranges?

GEN.30200 Are quality control records retained for at least 2 years?

Specimen Collection

GEN.40000 Is there a procedure manual or other source for the complete collection and handling instructions of all laboratory specimens?

GEN.40050 Is the specimen collection manual distributed to all specimen-collecting areas within the hospital (nursing stations, operating room, emergency room, out-patient areas) AND to areas outside the main laboratory (such as physicians' offices or other laboratories)?

(continued)

GEN.40100 Does the specimen collection manual include instructions for all of the following elements, as applicable?

1. preparation of the patient
2. type of collection container and amount of specimen to be collected
3. need for special timing for collection (e.g., creatinine clearance)
4. types and amounts of preservatives or anticoagulants
5. need for special handling between time of collection and time received by the laboratory (e.g., refrigeration, immediate delivery)
6. proper specimen labeling

GEN.40125 For specimens sent to reference laboratories, does the referring laboratory properly follow all requisition, collection and handling specifications of the reference laboratory?

GEN.40535 Is there an adequate process for correcting problems identified in specimen transportation, and improving performance of clients or offices that frequently submit specimens improperly?

GEN.40540 Is there a documented system to monitor the quality of specimens received from remote sites and collection sites not under the control of the laboratory?

Reporting

GEN.41330 Is there documentation of notification of the appropriate clinical individual of all critical values?

Turnaround Time

GEN.41470 Has the laboratory defined turnaround times (i.e., the interval between specimen receipt by laboratory personnel and results reporting) for each of its tests, and does it have a policy for notifying the requester when testing is delayed?

Corrected Reports

GEN.43700 Is there a documented system to ensure that all revised reports for previously reported incorrect (erroneous) patient results are identified as revised, corrected, or amended on all forms of patient reports (paper, video displays, etc.)?

21

Effective Communication in Laboratory Management

Elissa Passiment

OBJECTIVES

To describe the importance of effective communication to laboratory management

To identify the recipients of laboratory communication

To discuss the means and methods of communication

The newest computer can merely compound, at speed, the oldest problem in the relations between human beings, and in the end the communicator will be confronted with the old problem, of what to say and how to say it.

EDWARD R. MURROW

IN THIS ERA OF INFORMATION OVERLOAD, effective communication is one of the most important skills needed in pathology and clinical laboratories. Laboratory services cannot be delivered effectively without a coordinated, intricate system of communication. In many institutions, the laboratory is viewed as a mystery or a black hole, as stated by one hospital administrator, into which money, body fluids, and body parts go, but little comes out. A major contribution to that perception of the laboratory is the necessary practice of sending the laboratory's output—patient test results—directly to the patient's chart or caregiver. However, the mystery of the laboratory is perpetuated by the lack of an organized, systematic, flexible, and bidirectional exchange of information, ideas, standards, and beliefs between the laboratory and its customers, i.e., effective communication.

Communication can be defined a number of ways:

- The exchange of thoughts, messages, or information, as by speech, signals, writing, or behavior (1)

- The art and technique of using words effectively to impart information or ideas (1)

- A system, such as mail, telephone, or television, for sending and receiving messages (1)

- The exchange or transmission of ideas, attitudes, or beliefs between individuals or groups (9)

The importance of communication has been discussed and documented since formal management theories were promulgated. Chester I. Barnard wrote in 1938 in *Functions of the Executive* that the first executive function is to develop and maintain a system of communication (2). Management textbooks

391

throughout the decades have devoted chapters to the need for effective communication. In *The Management of Organizations*, Hicks (6) stated, "Organizational interaction depends on communication. . . . Communication is of prime concern to managers because it makes cooperative action possible." It was his belief that as one moved up any management structure, more time had to be devoted to communication to succeed. Because he taught that "communication is a primary requirement of decision making," it was the only way to achieve any change in direction or activity of the company.

As management theory evolved, the importance of communication grew. Peters and Waterman (10) in *In Search of Excellence*, state, "The nature and uses of communication in excellent companies are remarkably different from those of their nonexcellent peers. The excellent companies are a vast network of informal, open communications." The results of constant communication include getting the right people together and maintaining the continuous transmission of ideas and information. Peters and Waterman (10) say, "The intensity of communications is unmistakable in the excellent companies." If laboratories are to provide excellent service, i.e., function as excellent companies for their clients, communication should still be the first priority of everyone in laboratory management.

Communication within healthcare, or the lack thereof, was a major focus of the Institute of Medicine's (IOM) two reports, *To Err is Human: Building a Safer Healthcare System* (7) and *Crossing the Quality Chasm: A New Health System for the 21st Century* (8) (http://www.iom.edu/; http://www.nap.edu/books/0309072808/html/). The reports discuss the lack of efficient flow of information within healthcare and the misconception in our health system that the need for privacy has been translated into secrecy and has severely compromised the necessary sharing of information. In this era of patient safety concerns, laboratory management must strive to create an "excellent company" to provide the level of care and information every individual hopes to receive.

Many of the concerns that arise surrounding laboratory services are directly attributable to a lack of communication. Communication does not come easy for laboratorians. The traditional scientific personality types attracted to the profession are focused and introverted. Communication skills are not routinely taught in the curricula of nonphysician laboratorians. In fact, communication among members of the healthcare "team" is not taught at all. The IOM study (7) states, "Because medical training is typically isolated from the training of other health professionals, people have not learned to work together to share authority and collaborate in problem solving." The same can be said for the training of all health professionals. It is rare to find an interdisciplinary course on communication and problem solving in any allied health school. The health professions that are visible to the patient and to other members of

the healthcare team can develop their communication skills on the job. But that opportunity doesn't readily present itself to laboratorians.

Communication and information flow or transfer is very complicated. Information must be exchanged between internal departments, external departments, external vendors and regulators, and the laboratory's clients (customers). Any time the flow of information is improved, the efficiency of the laboratory will be improved. For instance, if all of the ordering providers in your client base (hospital, system, network, etc.) know what tests your laboratory offers, when they are performed, and the expected turnaround time (TAT), the service center will field fewer phone calls about these aspects of the operation. The service center will be able to spend more time on the patients, specimens, and reports that are part of their function. If these providers also know when and what tests to order, the laboratory's resources, staff, and materials will be more efficiently utilized. However, most laboratories are reluctant to communicate protocols for the appropriate utilization of laboratory services to divisions.

It is the responsibility of laboratory management to ensure that the information flow is bidirectional. The laboratory should not simply send out information, memos, policies, and procedures but should have a mechanism for receiving information from its clients. Clients (healthcare providers) should be able to retrieve information from the laboratory easily. If the retrieval system is like trying to find a needle in a haystack, these clients will not be happy and their needs will not be met. Those needs include diagnosing and treating patients. For inpatients, the needs include feedback on the effects and efficacy of any medication and/or procedures. For the consumer, that translates to an affable, helpful voice on the phone or a short TAT to an Internet inquiry.

Delivering the Message

Management should have a communication strategy—a plan that is used whenever the laboratory has information that it wants to disseminate (Table 21.1). This plan should first identify the overarching purposes for communication. The purposes should include the education of all clients on:

- the appropriate utilization of laboratory services;
- the extent of services offered; and
- regulations concerning the operation of the laboratory as well as any mandated communication.

Table 21.1 Elements of a communication plan

Define objectives and purpose of the plan.

Identify the structure and format of written communiqués.

List recipients of laboratory communication.

Identify the method(s) of communication.

The plan should also contain the formal structure or format of all written communiqués such as memos, newsletters, and flyers. Once a uniform look and feel of the written word has been adopted, all written notifications from the laboratory will convey an image and eventually establish an identity for the department. The plan should also include the elements of the strategy, i.e., with whom the laboratory believes the information will be shared, the mechanics of communication that the laboratory will use, and the purpose of communication. Communication should be considered a way of marketing the laboratory and its services, and a well-constructed plan will aid in that marketing by focusing the message. Whether the memorandum is about a protocol, a new test, a change in procedure, or a new service, the information should be presented so that the laboratory's expertise and its concern for its customers are obvious. Done properly, effective communication can be a competitive advantage.

Who: Communicating to Diverse Audiences

Laboratories should be communicating with all of their customers: physicians, nursing and allied health professionals, patients, third-party payors, and paying customers. Each of these customers has very different needs and processes information differently. As Hicks (6) states, "A person may not communicate with his supervisor in the same manner that he does with a person of equal standing." Adapting that statement to laboratories means that the laboratory manager may not tell the hospital administrator about federal rules and regulations in the same fashion used to inform the staff of each department. Indeed, the actual information that the hospital administrator needs to know will be different from that required by the staff. It is incumbent on the laboratory manager to tailor the message to each audience so that the message is understood.

Boyett and Boyett (3) implore managers to communicate, communicate, communicate, and communicate some more. There is really no such thing as too much communication. Clients will only perceive that there is too much communication if the information is superficial or not pertinent to their needs.

Visitor encounters in many laboratories are treated as trespassing or interruptions. They should be treated as opportunities to exchange information with other healthcare providers. In my experience as a hospital consultant, the successful laboratories were those in which clinicians could be found looking through microscopes in hematology, microbiology, and pathology and consulting with the staff. These laboratories were highly valued and perceived as very credible sources of important, accurate information. Heller (5) wrote "For successful operations, information must be totally visible." Labora-tories that open their doors to their customers and become visible will be successful and valued.

Laboratories communicate to convey information about policies and procedures (including rules and regulations that determine policies), results of tests ordered, status of testing, and new technology and services that are being added. The job of all managers is to coordinate the human and physical elements of an organization into an efficient and effective working unit. Communication is of prime concern to managers because it makes cooperative action possible (6). The higher one is in the organizational hierarchy, the more likely you are to spend greater time in communication (6).

Means and Mechanics of Effective Communication

Heller (5) wrote, "For effective communication, you must be aware of the means and the channels . . . with which to transmit and exchange information" (Table 21.2). The means of communication are fairly simple: the spoken word, the written word, and visual images. The mechanics include written memoranda, e-mails, reports, notices, newsletters, flyers, telephone service, manuals, and formal presentations, among others. These messages can be delivered by direct mail, the Internet, fax, or video using the hardware of communication such as telephone systems, computer information systems (and their interface with the institution's information system), terminals, fax machines, intercoms, headsets, and beepers. The trick is to match the mechanics to the message so that the message is well received. For instance, many laboratories produce a handbook that describes all of the tests offered (test menus) by the laboratory, with information about the specimen requirements, expected TATs, indications for ordering, and reference ranges. While this is an excellent communication device for anyone needing laboratory services, it isn't always used effectively. In many instances, the reason that this effort does not achieve the intended results is that the book is huge and imposing. The individuals needing the information in this book are the very people who do not have the time to read it. Many laboratories have miniaturized the book; the most successful have made it truly pocket-sized. The real key to communicating all of this information is determining what the ordering providers and nurses use as help aides (e.g., wall charts,

Table 21.2 Methods of communication

Verbal	Written	Visual
Telephone	Memoranda	Videos
Presentations	E-mails	Posters
Intercom	Newsletters	
Face-to-face	Flyers	
	Manuals	
	Personal digital assistants	

the institution's computers, personal digital assistants, the Internet, etc.) and employing that mechanism to transfer this information.

Any type of communication can be misinterpreted or contain errors. That is a risk that must be understood, but it should not impede the flow of information. The IOM's reports remind us that the majority of medical errors occur because of a lack of an open flow of information (7, 8).

Spoken Word

While we may not realize it, communication via the spoken word occurs daily in our laboratories—every time someone answers the phone. This is the most direct means of communication, but it can be the most damaging if words are not chosen carefully and if tone is not modulated. As stated earlier, the professionals practicing in laboratories, at all levels of education and authority, are renowned for being introverted and have traditionally not used the spoken word effectively. However, in our society of instant information, it is necessary to educate laboratorians in the use of the spoken word. Much can be accomplished with a telephone exchange or the clinician-laboratorian encounter in the laboratory if the words are carefully chosen, if body language and facial expressions are positive, and if we state our knowledge clearly without a great deal of laboratory shorthand that may be misunderstood by other members of the health-care team. Staff and management should be encouraged to engage caregivers in a discussion of the tests, the appropriateness of the tests, and the meaning of the results based on their level of knowledge. Each level of staff should be trained in consultation techniques and when to refer the provider to the next level of expertise. The traditional policy that no one other than the physician communicates information to other physicians is no longer workable given the increasing amount of information that needs to be communicated. However, it is necessary that staff are educated constantly and appropriately so that they are capable of expanding the laboratory's consultative services.

It is the responsibility of the laboratory management to provide continuing education opportunities, both in-house and through external meetings, to improve the verbal skills and knowledge level of its personnel. It is not appropriate to rely on self-study modules to improve verbal skills. While self-study continuing education can be very efficient for the transfer of new scientific knowledge, it does nothing to enhance verbal skills because there is no verbalization going on. In this day of personnel shortages, it is difficult to free employees to attend meetings, in-house or externally. However, if one considers the payback when employees become adept at the spoken word and the laboratory's image and usefulness are improved, the sacrifices needed to send them to meetings will be worth it.

Written Word

As Heller (4) states, "the written word is the basis of organizational communication and . . . is relatively permanent and accessible." Laboratory management should learn how to design written communications to optimize readability. The physical design of the piece should be easy to read, with standard fonts and font sizes. The page should not be crowded—the reader will be overwhelmed with the amount of information and either will not read it or will only skim it, potentially missing important information. While clip art has expanded our ability to become artistic, resist the urge when communicating with most clients unless the visual image will really convey the message.

Intradepartmental Communication

Laboratory managers must encourage a routine exchange of thoughts and messages between the laboratory departments, management and staff, and different shifts. The laboratory's organizational structure is based on the disciplines of pathology and laboratory science and is not always conducive to an open flow of information. Many laboratories use established intranets—communication superhighways for internal information exchange.

Without good internal communication, the potential for error increases. It is common for one department or shift to be unaware of new announcements concerning testing or schedules that were disseminated to the laboratory's customers. Laboratory managers may mistakenly assume that because the testing will not occur on that shift or in that department, for instance, that all of the staff don't need to know about the changes. Because your customers (e.g., nurses, physicians, outpatients) read memos at any time of the day and night, you cannot predict when or to whom a query will be addressed. Written intradepartmental communication is very effective because there is documentation that it occurred and it can reach every shift and all staff, whether they were present on the day it was issued or not. However, communication should not be exclusively in the written form. Meetings, informal chats, and impromptu announcements allow the staff to ask questions and exchange ideas immediately. This active communication can improve staff morale, as personnel know that they are being heard.

Interdepartmental Communication

The flow of communication beyond the laboratory includes that between the laboratory and the institution's administration (whether it is the vice president of clinical services or the office manager in a physician's office) and its clients (e.g., patients, physicians, and nonphysician caregivers). Written interdepartmental communication tends to be more formal than intradepartmental and needs to be carefully structured.

Table 21.3 Elements of a formal proposal to change laboratory services

Identify the benefits to the organization.
Project required resources, costs, and revenues.
Specify the responsible individual.
Project completion timelines for implementation of the service.
Describe the final outcome.

Memos, letters, and notices are adequate forms of communication for most announcements and responses to inquiries from other departments of the institution. However, when laboratory management wants to start a new service, change protocols, acquire instrumentation, or reorganize any part of the business, they should communicate through formal proposals (Table 21.3). Structuring a request this way ensures that you will address all of the questions that the reader may have. Before you write the proposal, you need to fully understand the missions and strategies of your institution. Your proposal should always point out how it will fulfill or complement the missions and strategies of the organization. The components of a proposal, or a business plan, should (i) explain why the change or plan is needed and how it will contribute to the strategies of the overall institution/business (e.g., economic benefits, objectives); (ii) estimate the resources required, the cost of the program, revenues from the plan, and the timeline for completion, and identify the individual responsible for completion or the proposal; (iii) produce an outline of a plan of action; and (iv) describe what success will look like. If you cannot verbalize or quantify outcomes, the project will not be noticed and probably will not be approved.

External Communication

Entities external to the organization include insurance companies, the federal government, accrediting agencies, competitors, and others. There are a myriad of regulations that affect a laboratory's operation, such as a license to operate and personnel policies. The federal government requires that every laboratory performing tests for diagnostic purposes be certified by the Centers for Medicare and Medicaid Services under the Clinical Laboratory Improvement Amendments of 1988. Laboratory managers must keep current with these federal rules and regulations and must communicate any changes to their superiors. The changing rules for Medicare reimbursement also require monitoring and reporting up the chain of management. In addition, clinical laboratories are required by the Centers for Medicare and Medicaid Services to have a compliance plan (Health Insurance Portability and Accountability Act) that helps employees avoid actions that might be construed as fraud and abuse. The Office of the Inspector General has outlined what that compliance plan should look like. The human resources department in most institutions dictates personnel policies that must be followed in the laboratory.

The manner in which individuals communicate depends upon the formal organizational structure. In an organization that is rigidly structured, individuals will act and interact differently than in an organization that is very informal. The organizational chart will define how and with whom a manager will communicate.

The most important activity that laboratory managers should undertake is to get out of the office and out of the laboratory. Managers should volunteer to serve on hospital committees and should encourage their staff to do so as appropriate. "Management by walking about" (MBWA) contributes to informal communication. As a manager from Hewlett Packard (identified as an excellent company) states, "We just plain talk to each other a lot without a lot of paper or formal rigmarole" (10). The lesson from all successful companies is that management must be visible. Sitting in the laboratory, monitoring TATs, quality assurance, compliance, and billing, while essential to keeping the laboratory functioning, will not achieve the goals of a good communication system. Laboratory managers should practice MBWA, not just in the laboratory but also in the institution of which the laboratory is a part. The informal communication that occurs will be of immeasurable benefit to the laboratory as a whole. As nurses, physicians, patients, patients' families, and the institution's management begin to recognize the laboratory management, additional impromptu communication will occur. Managers should visit the nursing units (or any departments in which patients/customers are using the laboratory's services) on a routine, predictable basis. The agenda of these visits should include but not be limited to checking on the phlebotomy service, satisfaction with TATs, and the interpretation of laboratory reports.

As care providers come to know that the laboratory is interested in its performance, the department will be increasingly perceived as a member of the team. Some hospital laboratories have assigned personnel to a nursing unit or department so that there is a recognizable liaison with which caregivers can readily communicate.

The laboratory should survey its clients periodically to determine how they get the majority of their information and what information they routinely need. The survey results will also tell management whether the services the laboratory is providing are pertinent and can be used to identify future services. Laboratory management should attend social events to get feedback about their services and the effectiveness of their communication. Managers should encourage staff to join the softball team, the credit union or other similar activities that will increase the visibility of the department. All avenues for communication with people who interact with the laboratory should be explored and exploited to improve laboratory services.

Summary

Communication is the exchange of ideas, attitudes, and information through the spoken word, written word, and visual images. Communication should be targeted to a specific audience and understood by that audience and can be delivered by a myriad of methods (e.g., newsletters, manuals, Internet, videos, etc.). Effective communication is a critical skill that is needed by laboratorians to ensure effective delivery of laboratory services. It must be bidirectional between the laboratory and its customers, clients, and members of the organization's hierarchy.

KEY POINTS

- Effective communication, whether internal or external to the organization, is critical to the management of the laboratory.
- Communication must be tailored to the understanding and needs of its audience.
- Communication occurs by the written word, the spoken word, and visual images.

GLOSSARY

Communication Exchange of thoughts, messages, or information (through speech, signals, writing, or behavior); art and technique of using words effectively to impart information or ideas; system, such as mail, telephone, or television, for sending and receiving messages; exchange or transmission of ideas, attitudes, or beliefs between individuals or groups.

External communication Occurs with entities outside of the organization (e.g., insurance companies, regulatory agencies, accreditation organizations).

Hierarchy A group of individuals organized or classified according to rank or authority.

Interdepartmental communication Occurs between the laboratory and other organizational departments, clients, and healthcare providers. Tends to be structured and formal.

Intradepartmental communication Occurs within the laboratory between management, sections or divisions, and work shifts. Tends to be informal.

Management by walking about (MBWA) A process that promotes informal communication between managers and employees.

Quality assurance A systematic approach to continuously analyzing, improving, and reexamining the total testing process.

Turnaround time (TAT) The interval between the beginning of one event and the end of another event in the total testing process.

REFERENCES

1. American Heritage Dictionary of the English Language, 4th ed. 2000. Houghton Mifflin Company, Boston, Mass.

2. Barnard, C. I. 1938. *Functions of the Executive.* Harvard University Press, Cambridge, Mass.

3. Boyett, J., and J. Boyett. 1998. *The Guru Guide, The Best Ideas of the Top Management Thinkers.* John Wiley & Sons, Inc., New York, N.Y.

4. Heller, R. 1998. *Communicate Clearly,* 1st ed. DK Publishing, Inc., New York, N.Y.

5. Heller, R. 2002. *Manager's Handbook—Everything You Need to Know About How Business and Management Work.* DK Publishing, Inc., New York, N.Y.

6. Hicks, H. 1967. *The Management of Organizations.* McGraw-Hill Book Company, New York, N.Y.

7. Institute of Medicine. 2000. *To Err Is Human: Building a Safer Healthcare System.* National Academy Press, Washington, D.C. [Online: http://www.iom.edu/]

8. Institute of Medicine. 2001. *Crossing the Quality Chasm: A New Health System for the 21st Century.* National Academy Press, Washington, D.C. [Online: http://www.nap.edu/books/0309072808/html/]

9. On-line Medical Dictionary. 1997. Academic Medical Publishing & CancerWEB, Lexico Publishing Group, Los Angeles, Calif.

10. Peters, T. J., and R. H. Waterman, Jr. 1982. *In Search of Excellence: Lessons from America's Best-Run Companies.* Harper & Row Publishers, New York.

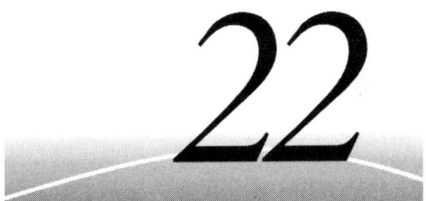

Managing the Laboratory Information System from a Clinical Microbiology Perspective

Joseph M. Campos

OBJECTIVES

To review the principles of laboratory informatics

To review the architecture of information systems

To identify methods to enhance the cost-effectiveness and accuracy of microbiological data through informatics

> What I am going to tell you about is what we teach our physics students in the third or fourth year of graduate school. . . . It is my task to convince you not to turn away because you don't understand it. You see my physics students don't understand it. . . . That is because I don't understand it. Nobody does.
>
> RICHARD P. FEYNMAN, *THE STRANGE THEORY OF LIGHT AND MATTER*

THE MANNER IN WHICH CLINICAL LABORATORIES OPERATE has changed significantly in recent years. For one thing, fewer laboratories exist because of a trend toward consolidating services across institutions to realize cost savings. Such partnerships and mergers generate vexing problems from an information management perspective in that integration of laboratory data stored in disparate information systems can be a major challenge. A second trend has been the "tearing down of walls" that separate the traditional laboratory disciplines of chemistry, hematology, and microbiology and then combining the automated and stat testing services from these disciplines into a multidisciplinary core laboratory. Personnel working in such a laboratory are expected to have competence in all areas of the core laboratory and be able to perform tests as directed by the urgency and volume of test requests received. That can present challenges to the configuration of the laboratory information system (LIS) since poor organization within the LIS will hamper the efficiency of "multitasking" testing personnel. This chapter will focus on the microbiology laboratory; however, the discussion is relevant for all laboratory disciplines.

The responsibilities of the clinical microbiology laboratory leadership team have evolved over the years as well. Along with ensuring that the laboratory produces clinically relevant test results, passes accreditation surveys, and scores well on proficiency tests, the microbiology supervisor, manager, and/or director must have confidence that the LIS is functioning as intended. At least one study in the literature has demonstrated that the preanalytical and postanalytical phases of microbiology testing are more prone to errors than the analytical phase (11). Yet, the preanalytical and postanalytical phases still tend to receive less attention than the analytical phase during test development and implementation. Preanalytical selection of appropriate tests for ordering and postanalytical correct interpretation of test results are quite dependent upon information supplied by the laboratory. That information is frequently furnished to care providers in an on-line format originating from the LIS on a 24-h per day, 7-day per week basis (7). Failure on the part of the laboratory management team to keep that information up-to-date and accurate can lead to serious medical errors.

Most clinical microbiology laboratories today have begun to use the LIS as a management tool, in addition to using it to coordinate the ordering and resulting of laboratory tests (2, 4). The contemporary LIS is able to manage the quality control and quality assurance activities in the laboratory, document the attendance records of laboratory employees, and monitor the inventory levels of laboratory supplies, among other things. In the course of this chapter the principles of laboratory informatics and information system architecture will be reviewed. The potential for the LIS to serve as a tool for enhancing the cost-effectiveness and accuracy of microbiology laboratory testing will also be discussed.

Laboratory Informatics

The primary purpose of the LIS is to manage an abundance of laboratory data, and that activity is the foundation of laboratory informatics (3). In reality, much of the data residing in the LIS are of little concern to the clinical microbiology laboratory. However, ensconced within the data tables of the LIS are the records of microbiology test orders and results. These records are viewable by both laboratory-based and non-laboratory-based users through standard queries of the information system. Results of these queries are usually displayed on video terminals or in printed reports.

Just about all clinical microbiology laboratories interact with at least one information system housed outside of the laboratory, and many laboratories deal with several such systems on a daily basis. Most would agree that tremendous strides have been made in the laboratory over the last 10 years to reap the benefits afforded by important advances in information technology. Nevertheless, changes in the microbiology laboratory resulting from the advent of molecular diagnostics are better understood by most clinical microbiologists than is the impact of information technology. That is probably because most clinical microbiologists lack an understanding of all that happens inside the LIS "black box." On the other hand, they feel a greater incentive to be aware of molecular techniques in order to maintain their laboratory in a competitive stance with others occupying the same marketplace.

A Primer on Information System Terminology

Computer terminology can apply to either hardware or software, and a summary of the various computer components can be seen in Table 22.1; definitions can be found in the Glossary. It is important and very helpful for all personnel levels working within the clinical laboratory to understand the basics of the various computer information systems.

A Primer on Information System Architecture

The information system architecture at many hospitals consists of a patchwork of modular software applications and servers that work in an integrated fashion to meet the information demands of the facility. The centerpiece of the infrastructure is referred to as the hospital or enterprise information system (6). This system is the nexus for patient-related activity, including keeping track of patient admissions, discharges, and transfers. It is the location for the master patient index (MPI), which is a storehouse of information concerning current and past patients who received medical care from the hospital. It is the source of patient demographic data that are provided to other information systems with which it is interfaced. The MPI should be regarded as a precious entity. The manner in which additions, deletions, alterations, and merges of patient records occur in the MPI should be strictly regulated and under constant surveillance. The integrity and accuracy of the MPI should be verified on a frequent and regular basis. User access to MPI editing functions should be restricted to authorized individuals who are thoroughly trained and documented as competent.

Other information systems are also likely to be present in the hospital setting. They may include systems for managing patient care records (electronic medical record), scheduling of patient visits, billing for services rendered

Table 22.1 Information system terminology

Type of system	Term
Hardware	Central processing unit (CPU)
	Client
	Graphical user interface (GUI)
	Hard disk (disk drive, hard drive, hard disk drive)
	Local area network (LAN)
	Random access memory (RAM)
	Server
	Video adapter
	Wide area network
	Workstation
Software	Basic input/output system (BIOS)
	Operating system (OS)

(financial information system), enabling decision support analyses, coordinating physician practice management, aiding in materials management, and operating pharmacy services (pharmacy information system), diagnostic imaging services (radiology information system), and laboratory services. These peripheral information systems may be integrated modules obtained from the same vendor that supplied the HIS, or they may be what are considered "best of breed" systems purchased from other vendors. In the latter case, data transfer interfaces must be built between the HIS and the peripheral information systems to make possible a rapid flow of information between the systems.

To facilitate communication of information across information system interfaces, near-universal adoption of the Health Level 7 (HL-7) standard for healthcare information management is in place. The HL-7 standard's domain is limited to clinical and administrative data. Its specifications identify the appropriate location and sequence of data elements ("segments") in messages between healthcare information systems. Many hospitals elect to install an interface engine at the hub of the information system architecture to manage the flow of data between disparate information systems. A properly functioning interface engine enables hospitals to select HL-7-compatible information systems of their choice from a variety of vendors and link them together to provide systemwide communication.

Each information system in the healthcare enterprise is built around at least one server that houses the operating system and relevant application software. A conservatively designed information system architecture features redundant servers housed in widely separated locations to provide for effective disaster recovery and efficient use of server resources. Locating redundant servers several miles apart minimizes the possibility that all will be destroyed during a single disastrous event (e.g., fire or flooding). The deleterious impact of heavy user activity on system resources during busy periods of the day can be lessened by distributing users across redundant servers (load balancing). Redundant servers are also an important safeguard during system downtime. When one server is not available during scheduled or unscheduled downtime, users can be quickly logged into a different server and remain productive.

One other point regarding information system architecture should be emphasized. There must be a mechanism for engaging in regular system backup. Information stored on each server should be copied to magnetic or optical media on a daily basis. At least one copy of the backed-up system and database files should be stored in a location that is remote from the server location. Should a disaster beset the location where an information system server is located, the stored information within that server can be loaded onto a replacement server using the system backup media as the source.

Transactions that are communicated between the LIS and other information systems are conveyed by one of several interfaces. Typically encountered interfaces include the ones listed below (Table 22.2).

Admission/Discharge/Transfer (ADT) Interface

The LIS depends on the MPI for the most current information regarding patient admissions, discharges, and transfers. Usually, this information is sent to the LIS dynamically via an ADT interface. Such an interface obviates the need for manual entry of patient demographic records in the LIS.

Order-Entry Interface

Direct entry of laboratory orders into information systems by caregivers and other patient care personnel is a definite trend in hospitals today. Although the placing of orders by patient care personnel requires time that might be spent seeing additional patients, this practice is a central strategy in the universal campaign to eliminate medical errors. Because patient care personnel are more familiar with placing orders for nonlaboratory services (e.g., pharmacy and radiology) in clinical information systems, most hospitals have agreed to fund the building of interfaces between the clinical information system and the LIS to allow laboratory orders to be placed in these systems as well. Patient care personnel frequently are confused by the plethora of similar sounding tests on the laboratory menu, thus the likelihood of mistaken orders can be great. Individuals designing the order-entry screens must do their best to simplify the ordering process and eliminate ambiguity from the test name descriptors. Even so, laboratory test orders coming across an order-entry interface should be closely monitored for errors.

Results-Entry Interface

The same clinical information systems used for placing laboratory test orders are often used by patient care personnel for viewing test results. Thus, installation of an

Table 22.2 Interfaces used to communicate between the LIS and other information systems

Interface term	Comments
ADT	LIS depends on MPI for patient updates; information sent to LIS via ADT interface, thus eliminating the need for repeat entry of patient demographic records
Billing interface	Critical to financial success; can be structured so charges are sent across the interface either when tests are ordered or on specimen receipt (pros and cons for either option)
Order-entry interface	Direct entry of laboratory orders into information systems by patient care personnel; system must be carefully monitored for errors
Results-entry interface	Often uses same system as that for order-entry; ongoing system validation critical for accuracy

order-entry interface is often accompanied by installation of a results-entry interface. The microbiology laboratory should play a central role in testing and validating the operation of the results-entry interface to ensure that the test results display is accurate, unambiguous, and clinically helpful. This is especially true for antimicrobial susceptibility results, which should be displayed in a table format.

Billing Interface

From a dollars and cents perspective, the billing interface between the LIS and the financial information system is critical. Laboratory test charges are sent either individually as they are incurred or simultaneously in a daily batch across this interface. A decision must be made by laboratory leadership as to whether charges should be levied upon test ordering or upon specimen receipt by the laboratory. The former choice inevitably means the issuing of many credits for tests on specimens that are not received by the laboratory. An important requirement of financial transactions is that they be precise, complete, and convertible into a format dictated by the payors or denial of reimbursement becomes a real problem.

A Primer on LISs

An LIS consists of one or more servers that provide the services described in the sections above. Of course, the information entered into, housed by, and reported from the LIS is relevant to laboratory testing. The LIS counterpart to the MPI is a living database usually known as the laboratory file (LF). Within the LF resides all of the patient demographic information sent to the LIS across the ADT interface from the MPI, as well as complete information about the laboratory tests ordered and the results for those patients. Laboratory users of the LIS access information via workstations or "dumb terminals" equipped with monitors and one or more data entry devices. Workstations are usually personal computers capable of running software applications other than the LIS (e.g., e-mail, word-processing, spreadsheet, and presentation software). Dumb terminals are devices that generally consist of a monitor and a keyboard, and they serve solely as a client of the LIS server(s).

Peripheral Hardware

Peripheral hardware connected to the LIS server(s) either directly or through a personal computer (PC) workstation includes:

- Data entry devices (e.g., keyboards, light pens, touch screens, barcode wands, scanners, terminal-emulating devices, and digital cameras).
- Printers for preparation of specimen identification labels and reports.
- Laboratory instruments to permit batch or dynamic transfer of patient demographic data and test results. Instrument connections are mediated by interface software, which permits the LIS server and the instruments to communicate in much the same way that an interpreter enables people who speak different languages to understand one another. Interfaces may be unidirectional (instrument to server or server to instrument) or bidirectional (server to instrument to server).

- Interfaces to other information systems (e.g., the clinical information system, the financial information system, the pharmacy information system, the LIS of another organization) or to an interface engine are also common. It is not unusual for the LIS to be part of the enterprise local area network (LAN) or wide area network.

The LIS enhances the utilization of laboratory services by patient care providers and assists in the "back-office" management of testing. Ordering of tests is often performed in an information system other than the LIS and should be streamlined by logically organized, on-line test menus that offer ready access to information concerning specimen requirements. The ordering of medically unnecessary or redundant laboratory tests can be recognized by user-defined, rules-based logic—ideally in real time by the ordering system but as a last resort by the LIS after orders have come across the order-entry interface. Test results should be available in the results viewing system immediately upon the completion of testing. Test result reports may be printed on paper or delivered electronically to patient care personnel by fax, e-mail, alphanumeric pager, or video monitor display. Interpretive comments can be attached to reports to assist clinicians in understanding their significance. Automatic billing for laboratory services can be triggered by transactions sent across the billing interface from the LIS to the financial information system. Complex financial algorithms dictated by contracts with third-party payors, health maintenance organizations, and managed care providers can be handled with tools included in some LISs but are probably better relegated to the province of the financial information system.

Long-term storage and retrieval of laboratory data can be easily accommodated by a suitably configured LIS. The current emphasis by payors and healthcare accrediting agencies on monitoring the outcomes of patient care mandates that utilization of laboratory services be examined on a regular basis. Generation of "canned" or user-defined reports from the LIS can be instrumental to this effort. Reports can be exported electronically to personal computers for analysis by sophisticated software tools.

A Primer on Clinical Microbiology Informatics

Clinical microbiology laboratories should be able to realize the many benefits offered by healthcare information systems. Individuals who are well versed in both clinical microbiology and information system technology enable this to happen. This combination of skills facilitates laboratory participation in patient outcomes studies, detection of unnecessary testing, assistance in practice guidelines development, and participation in hospitalwide performance improvement activities.

To exploit the wealth of information stored within the LIS, individuals who understand the data needs of the microbiology laboratory and who are skilled at using information system tools must be available (5,12). The specialty known as "laboratory informatics" was created several years ago to help achieve this goal (9). The ideal informatics specialist is first and foremost a trained laboratory professional who understands the principles, requirements, and flow of laboratory testing and possesses the knowledge, skill, and desire to participate in the management, use, and continuing improvement of the LIS. Informatics specialists should have a minimal set of hardware and software tools at their disposal, including the following.

Laboratory Data Repository

A laboratory data repository (preferably on-line) should be easily accessible and span a period of at least 3 years. Queries extending over several years make possible meaningful trending of laboratory activity. Given the relatively low cost of LIS memory these days, expense should not be a significant impediment to meeting this requirement. Not to be overlooked, however, is the requirement that the LIS server that will be running these queries be sufficiently robust to conduct searches of large databases within a reasonable period of time and without degrading system performance for other users. Server upgrades can entail a significant financial outlay.

Functionality for Data Repository Query

The functionality for querying the data repository must reside in the LIS. This capability is almost always an extra-cost option purchased from LIS vendors. It may be referred to as an "ad hoc" or user-defined report writer or as a report engine. Whatever it is called, it should be installed on a server that is separate from the server(s) logged onto by regular users so that resource-intensive queries don't degrade the response time for those users. The server housing the report engine must have access to a complete copy of the LF that is kept up-to-date through a dynamic link with the other LIS server(s).

Connectivity

The connectivity to deliver data quickly from the LIS to a PC is a necessity. This may be accomplished in a variety of ways:

- Reports may be "printed" in flat field text format to a file on a PC that is linked to the LIS via a serial connection.
- Report files can be sent directly to a PC from the LIS using file transfer protocol over a network connection.

- The LIS LF can be queried directly with PC-based software, assuming that the LF data are stored in an open database connectivity (ODBC)-compliant relational or relational-like table format and the driver needed to link the querying tool to the LIS is available.
- The screen capture functionality that is part of the terminal emulation software needed to work with the LIS on a PC workstation can be used to capture LIS reports as formatted text files.

Once the data are delivered to a PC, spreadsheet, database, and/or data extraction software can be used to perform sophisticated analyses. The types of analyses that can be carried out are virtually limitless.

Summary

Data analysis tools and skills can be extremely useful to clinical microbiologists. However, they cannot be used to their fullest extent if the information system infrastructure is inadequate. It is the responsibility of the leadership in the laboratory to convince hospital administrators of the wisdom of investing in LIS hardware and software.

Once that is accomplished, all laboratories, including the clinical microbiology laboratory, have the opportunity to benefit fiscally by using these tools to recognize and eliminate unnecessary testing (13). For example, a query of the LF can quickly determine which care providers appear to be overutilizing laboratory services. With the help of PC-based software applications, such data can be stratified and further analyzed by ordering location, patient diagnosis, and other tests ordered simultaneously.

Laboratories can also improve the quality of their testing and eliminate laboratory errors by identifying test performers whose results exhibit questionable characteristics (8). This approach is particularly useful for evaluating qualitative test results that are interpreted by subjective criteria. The very popular lateral flow technology for rapid detection of microbial antigens or antibodies is an excellent example. Test data for the entire laboratory over the course of a year can be extracted from the LF and imported into a PC-based spreadsheet or database application. Then, using either of these tools, test results can be stratified by individual test performer to determine whether any individuals depart significantly from the laboratory mean in the percentage of positive results reported. After taking into account effects caused by potentially confounding factors, such as only working the night shift or only working on weekends, individuals that remain as outliers can have their competency further assessed and be provided with retraining, if necessary.

More than ever, clinical microbiologists are purveyors of information, most of it valuable, but some of it valueless (10). In effect, we have become information brokers as such, and it is one of our jobs to determine what information is clinically important and what is not. The LIS can be a valuable ally in this regard. In the past, they were stand-alone systems that were counted on to streamline the management of laboratory data and capture the billing for laboratory testing. Now they are essential vehicles for communication with laboratory clients. They also must be able to communicate with other information systems and meet the needs of the systems with which they exchange information.

The selection, maintenance, and operation of an LIS have become much more complicated than they used to be. Overseeing these responsibilities has become more than a full-time job in all but the smallest of laboratories. The area of laboratory informatics has become a laboratory specialty for this reason, and there currently is a shortage of knowledgeable personnel. The work is challenging and constantly changing, and carries tremendous potential for job security and career advancement. The combination of clinical microbiology and laboratory informatics is an excellent fit and one that I highly recommend.

The skills addressed in this chapter are easily gained and can be extremely practical for the reasons outlined earlier. Individuals who possess these skills are acknowledged as valuable members of the hospital workforce by laboratory and hospital administrators (1). We presently find ourselves in the midst of a dangerous, change-oriented, healthcare environment in which cost cutting is the order of the day. Clinical microbiologists who have earned the respect of hospital leaders because of the diverse skills they have acquired can expect to be rewarded with continuing employment and promotional opportunities—both within and outside of their workplace.

KEY POINTS

- Failure to keep data stored in the information systems up to date can lead to medical errors.

- The HIS contains the master patient index and is the source of demographic data provided to other interfaced information systems.

- Transactions between the LIS and other information systems occur by four typical interfaces: a) ADT; b) order-entry; c) results-entry; and d) billing.

- The LIS can be used to identify and eliminate unnecessary testing.

GLOSSARY

BIOS (basic input/output system) The program a computer uses to start its operations when it is turned on (booted up). The BIOS also coordinates the flow of data between the OS and peripheral devices such as the hard disk, video adapter, keyboard, mouse, and printer.

Central processing unit (CPU) The main information processor in a computer that interprets and implements instructions.

The CPU performs calculations, makes logical decisions, and stores information transiently.

Client The computer/workstation that requests an action from a server in a client/server relationship.

Dumb terminals Devices that consist of a monitor and a keyboard and serve solely as a client of the LIS.

Graphical user interface (GUI) A "picture-oriented" paradigm for using software applications that depends on use of a pointing device (e.g., a mouse) rather than on key strokes for issuing commands.

Hard disk A peripheral device, also known as a "disk drive," "hard drive," or "hard disk drive," that stores and provides ready access to large amounts of recorded data.

Health level 7 (HL-7) Near-universal standard adopted for healthcare information management. The HL-7 domain is limited to clinical and administrative data; specifications identify the appropriate location and sequence of data elements in messages between healthcare information systems.

Hospital information system (HIS) Total hospital computer system that is often linked to the LIS or a third-party order-entry system.

Instrument interface A hardware and software connection between a server and a laboratory instrument that facilitates communication between the two.

Laboratory file (LF) The LIS counterpart to the MPI; contains patient demographics, information about laboratory tests ordered and results.

Laboratory information system (LIS) The computer system set up for laboratory services.

Local area network (LAN) A group of several computers or workstations that are connected to a server. The server manages client use of software applications and often serves as a repository for the networked client's data. The LAN enables client workstations without storage capabilities to be operational at a much lower cost than for full-fledged, stand-alone workstations.

Master patient index (MPI) Contains data related to current and past patients who receive medical care from the system. Usually contained in the hospital information system.

Operating system (OS) The software that makes a computer operational. The OS prompts users (or peripheral devices) for input and/or commands, takes actions, and then reports back the results of these actions. It stores and manages data and oversees the sequence of software and hardware operations.

Random access memory (RAM) The component of a computer in which the OS, the application software, and the data in current use are stored so that they can be quickly accessed by the CPU. Accessing or storing data in RAM is much faster than accessing or storing it on a hard disk, a floppy disk, or a CD-ROM drive, but the data are present in RAM for only as long as the computer is turned on.

Server A computer that has software applications installed for use by members of a local or wide area network. It also can serve as a repository for data generated by other computers or workstations on the network.

Video adapter An integrated circuit board in a computer that enables digital-to-analog conversion of a video signal so that data can be displayed on a monitor.

Wide area network A group of several personal computers or workstations connected via a geographically dispersed telecommunications network.

Workstation A computer intended for use by an individual for professional purposes rather than for home or recreational purposes. Since processing speed is usually important, it tends to have a fast microprocessor, a large amount of RAM, and a high-speed video adapter.

REFERENCES

1. **Balis, U. J.** 1999. Alternative careers in the laboratory re-engineering paradigm. *Clin. Lab. Med.* **19:**453–461.

2. **Bazzoli, F.** 1999. Laboratory systems evolve to meet data demands. *Health Data Manag.* **7:**66–71.

3. **Block, C.** 1997. Benefits and limitations of computerized laboratory data. *J. Clin. Pathol.* **50:**448–449.

4. **Campos, J. M.** 2003. Laboratory consultation, communication, and information systems, p. 31–43. *In* P. R. Murray, E. J. Baron, J. H. Jorgensen, M. A. Pfaller, and R. H. Yolken (ed.). *Manual of Clinical Microbiology*, 8th ed. ASM Press, Washington, D.C.

5. **Elevitch, F. R.** 1999. Prospecting for gold in the data mine. *Clin. Lab. Med.* **19:**373–384.

6. **Huet, B.** 1998. Hospital information system: reusability, designing, modeling, recommendations for implementing. *Medinfo* **9:**952–956.

7. **Kay, J. D.** 2001. Communicating with clinicians. *Ann. Clin. Biochem.* **38**(Pt 2)**:**103–110.

8. **Kern, D. A., and S. T. Bennett.** 1999. Quality improvement in the information age. *MLO Med. Lab. Obs.* **31:**24–28.

9. **McPherson, R. A.** 1999. Perspective on the clinical laboratory: new uses for informatics. *J. Clin. Lab. Anal.* **13:**53–58.

10. **Miller, W. G.** 2000. The changing role of the medical technologist from technologist to information specialist. *Clin. Leadersh. Manag. Rev.* **14:**285–288.

11. **Nutting, P. A., D. S. Main, P. M. Fischer, T. M. Stull, M. Pontious, M. Seifert, Jr., D. J. Boone, and S. Holcomb.** 1996. Toward optimal laboratory use. Problems in laboratory testing in primary care. *JAMA* **275:**635–639.

12. **Oakley, S.** 1999. Data mining, distributed networks, and the laboratory. *Health Manag. Technol.* **20:**26–31.

13. **Workman, R. D., M. J. Lewis, and B. T. Hill.** 2000. Enhancing the financial performance of a health system laboratory network using an information system. *Am. J. Clin. Pathol.* **114:**9–15.

23

Management of Point-of-Care Testing

Glen L. Hortin

OBJECTIVES

To identify how management of point-of-care testing (POCT) differs from other types of laboratory testing

To describe cost factors in POCT and approaches for analysis of the costs of testing

To provide information about how to operate a POCT program and to assure the quality of testing

To provide an understanding of how technological advances are driving change in the scope of POCT

Ther nys no werkman, whatsoever he be,
That may bothe werke wel and hastily

CHAUCER

POINT-OF-CARE TESTING (POCT) presents some of the most controversial and difficult laboratory management challenges (Table 23.1). There is a commonly held view among laboratory workers that, as expressed in the quote from Chaucer, POCT represents a compromise in test quality in the interest of speed to obtain results. Many of the challenges presented by POCT are substantially different from those of any aspect of centralized laboratory testing. Common challenges include crossing traditional physical and organizational boundaries, performing tests at a large number of locations, training a large number of personnel with limited laboratory experience, using technologies or devices that differ from those in central laboratories, capturing test results and control values into information systems, and difficulty in tracking costs and program activity. In many respects POCT requires management "outside of the box," not only of the physical "box" of laboratory space but also the usual "boxes" of organizational structures, groups of coworkers, testing devices and technologies, laboratory practice, and management information systems. In this chapter, the management challenges of POCT are categorized into organizational, operational, and technological issues as listed in Table 23.1, although some of the issues listed in reality overlap into more than one category.

There is not complete agreement about the definition of POCT, and a variety of other terms such as "near patient," "bedside," or "alternative site" testing have been used as approximate synonyms of POCT. For this chapter, POCT will be defined as testing that is performed outside defined laboratory facilities, including not only central laboratories but also small satellite

Table 23.1 Management challenges of POCT

Organizational challenges
- Historical resistance of laboratories to POCT
- Competition between POCT and central laboratories
- Setting goals
- Cooperation across multiple departments
- Deciding who controls/directs testing
- Developing a management structure
- Assignment of costs and revenue
- Management across usual lines of authority
- Deciding about licensure and accreditation of POCT

Operational challenges
- Determining the scope of POCT services
- Weighing alternatives to POCT
- Analysis of costs
- Performance of POCT at a large number of sites
- Training a large number of staff to perform POCT
- Lack of experience and training of staff in performing laboratory tests
- Lack of centralized records of test results
- Quality assurance
- Inventory management
- Management of information
- Billing

Technological challenges
- Growing menu of tests that can be performed as POCT
- Rapid change in POCT devices
- Rapid changes in testing technology
- Linking POCT data systems
- Lack of equivalence of POCT versus central laboratories
- New monitoring technologies

or special-function laboratories in physician offices, intensive care units, and emergency rooms. This definition is used by the College of American Pathologists (CAP) to define POCT for laboratory inspections (5).

POCT represents one of the most rapidly growing and changing segments of laboratory testing. A recent survey shows that nearly every hospital has some form of POCT (20). Glucose testing is the most widespread component of POCT, but there were substantial increases in the menu of testing in many hospitals between 1999 and 2001 (20). POCT devices are evolving very rapidly, and recent technological advances have made it possible to perform virtually any laboratory test as POCT. The growing scope of POCT has led to the publication of entire books related to this topic which serve as general resources of information about POCT (17, 32, 42, 45). The present chapter concentrates on aspects of the management of POCT that differ from other areas of the laboratory and that are controversial.

Organizational Challenges

Political Challenges

Up until the mid-1990s, laboratory workers often were highly antagonistic to the perceived competition and lower analytical quality provided by POCT. Laboratory directors and managers secured the four walls of the laboratory by building a fortress of organizational boundaries, regulations, and arguments to serve as moats and barriers to prevent outsiders from intruding into the domain of laboratory testing. This management strategy sought the disappearance of POCT. However, the historical resistance of laboratory workers to POCT did not make it disappear. Instead, POCT often developed under separate management from the central laboratory, and testing volume grew rapidly as testing technologies advanced. It was only with recent attention to the licensing of all laboratory testing and efforts to control costs that POCT began to be merged with laboratory management. Nevertheless, the previous independent operation of POCT and the resistance of laboratory workers to POCT serve as political and historical contexts in many organizations that must be overcome in the management of POCT.

Recently, acceptance of POCT among laboratory workers has grown, and laboratories have participated more actively in managing POCT. Input from laboratory professionals in POCT appears to be an important element in promoting the quality of testing based on long-standing problems recognized for POCT (26) and on studies of testing in physician office laboratories (21, 47). Some of the reported problems with testing included inaccuracy of test results, failure to perform quality control (QC) testing and correct test procedures, and inadequate staff training. Despite increased recognition of the importance of teamwork, healthcare organizations are complex political environments. Each department or nursing unit where POCT is performed will have its own experience, expectations, and sense of ownership of POCT performed within its domain. Acceptance of centralized management of POCT requires commitment from central administration and leaders of departments, and the perception from individuals that their needs will be addressed and that there is overall benefit from such a structure.

Setting Goals for POCT Management

One of the key initial steps in the management of POCT is the development of institutional goals. Common motivations for hospital administration and nursing units to seek additional management support for POCT are deficiencies on accreditation surveys; difficulty in meeting accreditation standards; problems with the quality of test results of POCT, resulting in complaints or lawsuits; and requests from nurses who feel the need for assistance to address laboratory regulations. In response to these acute problems, plans to revamp POCT management structure often are made in a crisis mode. Success is viewed narrowly as passing the next inspection or solving the acute problem. However, deciding that the primary goal in managing POCT is to address regulatory requirements is a very limited vision that may lead to overlooking opportunities for improving the quality and efficiency of patient care or potential clinical benefits of POCT. It would be tantamount to saying that the primary goal in the management of a clinical laboratory is to maintain accreditation. Developing a broader vision of the goals of POCT and a commitment from institutional leadership is important for moving beyond a minimal standard of performance and generating a positive sense of mission and purpose. More far-reaching goals in management of POCT are to provide testing that will improve patient care and to improve organizational efficiency (Table 23.2). Meeting regulatory standards is also a necessary goal, but regulations may be of greater value as a means than as an end. Regulations and inspectors provide guidance, incentives, and useful tools for maintaining the quality of testing and meeting more ambitious goals.

Developing Management Structures for POCT

In developing the management structure for POCT, there are political issues that need to be sorted out by central administration and departmental leaders. These include issues such as what department and who will direct testing, institutional priorities for POCT, and how costs and revenues will be assigned. Development of an oversight committee can serve as a useful mechanism to assess evolving needs for POCT. It also provides bidirectional communication with participants in POCT. Considering the diverse range of stakeholders in POCT, it may be useful to have representation of nurses, physicians, laboratory and hospital administrators, information technology specialists, and laboratory directors and technologists. Such a committee can advise about needs for general changes in policy and review requests for changes in the menu of tests or sites of POCT.

Day-to-day operations usually are overseen by testing coordinators and a laboratory director. However, there is much greater variation in organizational structure than there is in other areas of the laboratory. Some POCT programs are organized as extensions of the clinical laboratory with all testing performed by laboratory staff such as phlebotomists or medical technologists. In these circumstances, management of POCT differs little from other sections of the laboratory: All of the staffing, training, employee evaluations, instrument and reagent inventory, analytical and quality assurance processes, reporting of results, data systems, and budgeting are handled within the laboratory. From a management standpoint, this results in the simplest structure. The main practical problems with this model are the need to hire extra staff to perform POCT and to have staff available at the appropriate sites when testing is needed.

A more common organizational structure is that testing is performed by nurses or other nonlaboratory staff, but these are organized under a single POCT management. Problems inherent in the centralized management of a far-flung POCT program are difficulty in training a large number of nonlaboratory staff, maintaining effective communication to and from all units and staff, maintaining accountability, avoiding interdepartmental competition and turf battles, and managing a large number of staff across usual lines of management authority. It is important to identify POCT skills as core competencies and elements of job performance for the staff who perform testing and to have active participation of nursing managers in corrective action. Problems with POCT compete with many other urgent patient care issues on individual units. POCT program managers, then, sometimes need to resort to drastic actions such as withdrawal of testing devices or authorization for testing in order to create the necessary urgency for correcting problems.

A third organizational model, more common in the past, is for POCT in each clinical department or nursing unit to operate as a separate laboratory. This does simplify the management of each unit. However, it has become less common due to the inefficiencies of applying for separate licenses for multiple sites, the lack of standardization of procedures and equipment, and the coordination of testing activities within an institution. This organizational model may apply where POCT or a specific type of POCT is limited to a single unit or at a remote location.

Laboratory Licensure and Accreditation

Decisions about how POCT will be licensed and accredited influence how POCT will be managed and the types of tests that can be performed. Federal licensure is required for all clinical laboratory testing in the United States (8, 10). Specific standards are described for three levels of complexity of testing—high, moderate, and waived. If all testing is in the waived category, laboratory testing can be performed under a certificate of waiver, which has less stringent requirements than other levels of testing. Several agencies including CAP, the Joint Commission on Accreditation of Healthcare Organizations (JCAHO), the American Osteopathic Association, and the Commission on Office Laboratory Accreditation

Table 23.2 Goals of management of POCT

Improve the quality of patient care

Enhance the efficiency of patient care

Increase physician and nursing satisfaction

Improve patient education and satisfaction

Address accreditation standards

Fulfill federal and state laboratory regulations

Decrease liability risk

(COLA) have the authority to accredit laboratories. Some states have specific regulations that must be met.

The initial question to address is how many and what types of licenses to apply for. It is possible to perform POCT under the same license as the central laboratory. However, many laboratory directors have been reluctant to cover POCT under their licenses due to concerns about compliance of POCT with laboratory standards and lack of direct control over how testing is performed. Also, including POCT under the main laboratory license means that the same accreditation standards must be applied for POCT and central laboratory testing. CAP, which does not recognize any relaxation of standards for waived testing, accredits many hospital laboratories (5, 8). Some POCT programs, particularly those including only waived testing, decide to apply for a separate license or certificate of waiver for POCT to simplify requirements. Although CAP may inspect the central laboratory, if POCT is under a different license, it may be inspected by a different accrediting agency, such as JCAHO. POCT can be performed at multiple locations within a facility under the same license. For the sake of efficiency in the application process and avoidance of additional fees, all POCT within a facility often is operated under a single license or certificate of waiver.

Operational Challenges

Determining the Scope of POCT Services

One of the most critical operational challenges is deciding what sites will perform POCT and what menu of tests should be offered. A starting point for this analysis is to inventory the types and testing volumes of ongoing POCT. Obtaining an accurate inventory of POCT can be difficult due to the dispersed nature of testing, the lack of information systems, and, in some cases, the lack of recognition of what represents a laboratory test. Commonly overlooked POCT activities might include occult blood testing, urine dipstick testing, physician-performed microscopy, and whole blood coagulation testing. Many POCT devices are small, portable, and distributed among many sites, so it can be difficult to find or count the devices. Surveys of patient care units often provide incomplete responses. It may be necessary to resort to information from vendors, purchasing departments, or material management departments to determine the number of analyzers and the volume of testing.

The major source of demand for POCT has been from clinicians who desire rapid laboratory results for clinical decision making. A large gap exists between the expectations of clinicians and laboratory targets for turnaround times (25, 48). Surveys of clinicians indicate that they believe that stat test results for analytes such as electrolytes and glucose should be available within about 15 min, while laboratory professionals often have set a goal of stat turnaround times of less than 60 min (25). This gap between clinical expectations and laboratory service delivery has led to the high demand for POCT.

Turnaround time usually is perceived as the key advantage of POCT, but there are a number of other factors that may come into play for specific tests or clinical situations (Table 23.3). Use of a smaller specimen volume for POCT may be an important consideration for care of infants and young children. Lower capital costs of POCT for equipment or facilities may be important advantages for infrequently performed tests. For some tests, such as whole blood coagulation tests, the specimen must be tested immediately, so POCT becomes necessary. For the care of diabetics, POCT of blood glucose can be viewed to have educational value and to address patient expectations.

Some common disadvantages of POCT that must be weighed are lower accuracy and precision of tests, lesser laboratory experience of staff performing tests, lack of comparability with central laboratory results, and the greater difficulty of managing POCT, ensuring quality, and capturing test results into central information systems.

One point that may be overlooked in considering where to perform a test is whether to offer the test at all. Consider, for example, the bleeding time test. A large body of evidence suggests that this test is of questionable clinical value and it should not be performed (37). There must be a clear clinical justification for any test that is performed as well as an assessment of whether increasing the speed of testing will result in significant improvement in the quality or efficiency of patient care.

Weighing Alternatives to POCT

Usually, POCT is not the only option for performing a test. Common choices for delivering a test include performing it in a central laboratory, in a satellite laboratory, or as POCT. A fourth option that has become available recently is a robotic or remotely controlled analyzer. The first option, and in many cases the most efficient, may be to improve central laboratory processes to meet turnaround time goals. This might involve changes in infrastructure such as installation of a pneumatic tube system for rapid specimen delivery, changes in laboratory instrumentation to perform analyses on whole blood rather

Table 23.3 Common advantages and disadvantages of POCT versus central laboratory testing

Advantages	Disadvantages
Faster turnaround time	Lower accuracy and precision
Smaller specimen volume	Less skilled testing personnel
Lower capital cost	Higher supply costs
Testing of labile samples	Lack of comparability with laboratory results
Immediate access to results	Lack of data systems
Patient education/satisfaction	Difficulty in assuring quality
Physician satisfaction	Difficulty in managing testing

than serum or plasma, and improving mechanisms for delivery of test results (17). For tests designed for POCT use, such as fecal occult blood tests, qualitative drugs of abuse tests, urine pregnancy tests, or whole blood cardiac marker tests, sometimes an assumption is made that the tests should be performed as POCT based on history within an organization or the design of a device for POCT use. However, the advantages and disadvantages of performing the test as POCT should be weighed considering factors listed in Table 23.3. As long as the specimens are stable, it may be desirable to perform these tests in the central laboratory even though the test device is acceptable for POCT use. For some tests such as those for drugs of abuse, there may be special considerations such as complicated legal issues and a need to confirm positive results, and this issue must be considered in evaluating whether it is desirable to perform the tests as POCT (13).

An instructive example of the decision to perform a test as POCT or in a laboratory is provided by intraoperative parathyroid hormone (PTH) testing. This test is performed during parathyroid surgery, and test results are needed rapidly (23). The first commercially available analyzer to perform this test was designed to be on a mobile cart that could be moved to the operating room. However, many hospitals that offer this test now perform it in a laboratory setting and set up processes for rapid transport of the specimen in order to use staff and equipment most efficiently (19, 24).

Setting up or maintaining a satellite laboratory represents a major commitment and expense for facilities, equipment, and laboratory staff. Usually, this commitment of resources is justified only when there is an acute clinical need for rapid turnaround time, a high volume of testing, and use of relatively complex testing procedures. Remotely controlled analyzers may represent a new alternative to satellite laboratories. Considerable engineering expertise was required for early application of the approach (11). However, this has become a practical option now that functions such as calibration and QC testing have been automated on some analyzers and operation of the analyzers can be monitored remotely by laboratory workers (see surveys of blood gas analyzers in *CAP Today*, accessible at http://www. cap.org, for current information).

Analyzing Costs and Benefits

Although it would seem that costs of a test would be an objective quantity that could be calculated precisely, the absolute and relative costs of POCT and central laboratory testing are some of the most controversial issues relating to POCT. The majority of older published references conclude that POCT is more expensive than the same test performed in a central laboratory (6, 28, 36). One report went so far as to conclude, "The costs of central laboratory testing are always very much less than that of distributed testing" (55). However, in examining these reports, it is notable

that the major cost identified for POCT is for labor. It turns out to be difficult to account for labor for POCT, which involves small bits of time by a large number of staff. There is a paradox in that if you add up all of the time spent collectively performing POCT, it represents a substantial number of hours that may equal the time of several full-time staff members (full-time equivalents [FTE]). However, POCT usually has no impact on FTEs within the units that perform the testing; usually, the only recognized impact on FTE is one or more positions as central coordinators of POCT.

There are several possible reasons why performing POCT on a clinical unit has no direct impact on FTEs. A time-and-motion study of nurses comparing time spent by nurses to perform a POCT glucose test versus time spent to draw a specimen for central laboratory testing noted that less time was required by nurses to perform a glucose test than to collect a specimen and send it to the laboratory (17) (C. A. Moultrie, G. L. Hortin, and V. R. Randolph, abstract, *Clin. Chem.*, **43:**S162, 1997). The entire POCT process from specimen collection and testing to result retrieval was completed in one brief episode about the length of time required to draw blood. Sending a sample to the laboratory required multiple steps at different locations spread over about 1 h—generating a test requisition and label, performing phlebotomy, transporting the specimen to the nursing station, and retrieval of results from the computer. The timing study points out that there may be an underaccounting of the labor required to send specimens to the laboratory and retrieve results and that there is the potential for POCT to save labor even without accounting for the labor to perform the test within the laboratory. In addition to the greater amount of time directly spent by nurses to send the sample to the laboratory, the delay between testing and receipt of results may lead to indirect inefficiencies and less effective patient care because adjustments of diet and medication wait on receipt of test results.

Based on its higher efficiency and low volume within an individual clinical unit, POCT will rarely result in the need for additional staff or worked hours within the clinical unit. However, the aggregate volume of testing for a large POCT program sometimes reaches hundreds of thousands of tests. This volume of testing can significantly affect laboratory staffing, particularly if there is a demand for stat results at the time of peak demand in the early morning. One published estimate is that each reduction of 100,000 specimens sent to the laboratory would result in the reduction of work by four FTEs (17). This value obviously will vary depending on the levels of automation and efficiency of the laboratory. Coordination of POCT for this volume of testing requires about one FTE, depending on the complexity of testing and the number of testing sites. Analysis of the impact of POCT on FTEs would suggest that at a low testing volume, POCT usually would require an additional

FTE in the form of a test coordinator but would have no impact on staffing within the central laboratory. However, at higher test volume, there is the potential for greater FTE reduction in the laboratory than the additional FTE required for coordinating POCT. One other situation in which POCT may result in an overall reduction of FTEs is in the replacement of a satellite laboratory with POCT. If work is not evenly distributed for a satellite laboratory, often there is a high labor cost for idle time between testing activities. An analysis of the costs of various testing options indicates that POCT may result in direct cost reductions versus satellite laboratories (30).

There are a number of other complicating factors about cost analysis. First, two fundamentally different approaches are applied—a bottom-up or microcost analysis that adds up individual cost elements and a top-down or macrocost analysis that divides budgeted costs. Second is the problem of allocation of overhead or small bits of labor that do not result in changes of FTEs, such as nursing time spent on POCT. Third, most analyses of labor cost do not account for any changes in productivity, e.g., if nursing staff perform an additional task without any increase in worked hours, that represents a change in productivity not a labor cost. Finally, the most important complicating factor is weighing the indirect effects of POCT on the overall cost of patient care (2). Laboratory tests account for a small proportion, perhaps 5%, of healthcare costs (3). If changes in laboratory testing have any impact on factors such as length of stay or changes in clinical outcome, the cost impact potentially could be far greater than the total amount spent on laboratory testing.

A couple of recent studies provide evidence that POCT affects treatment decisions in a substantial proportion of testing episodes, although the net effect on costs was not clear (3, 15). Other interesting examples have been described in which POCT may result in substantial savings by having impacts on processes such as frequency of transfusion (7) or in which rapid intraoperative PTH testing contributes to an overall cost reduction. Although providing intraoperative PTH testing results is an increase in laboratory costs, total costs for patient care appear to be decreased substantially (24, 46, 53). Improvements in the quality and the efficiency of patient care delivery or reduction in transfusion frequency have been considered to result from POCT in a number of other cases, with the potential for overall cost reduction (1, 14, 44). Difficulty in arriving at an exact dollar benefit for a change in clinical process makes these analyses challenging.

In deciding how to analyze the costs of POCT, it is necessary to decide what question is being asked. A common question is: How much is POCT going to cost the organization? That is, what is the overall budgetary impact? Usually, addition of POCT will have little effect on facilities or overhead costs within the organization, so there is negligi-ble effect on these cost factors. In analyzing the budgetary impact of POCT, the labor cost would be represented primarily by any change in FTEs or paid working hours. Management of a POCT program is time-consuming, so it is appropriate to allocate some labor expense for management and medical direction. Depending on the nature of POCT within a facility and the alternatives of POCT versus no POCT, labor costs may be either positive or negative. To these labor costs will be added costs for equipment, supplies, and information systems. Adding all of these expenses together yields an estimate of the annual organizational cost or impact on expense budgets. Dividing these costs by the total number of tests performed will provide an estimate of the average cost to perform a test by POCT.

A second common question is: What charge would be necessary to recover the costs of POCT? In this analysis, there usually would be an allocation of nursing time for performing the analysis and an allocation of a portion of facilities and administrative overhead costs that must be recovered in some manner. These costs would be added to costs for equipment, supplies, etc. In addressing this question, usually there is no accounting for potential savings of expenses for central laboratory testing, changes in worker productivity, or efficiency of clinical care. This type of analysis usually will provide a much higher estimate of per test cost than an analysis of the budgetary impact of POCT.

It is notable that if calculations are performed to address these two questions, very different values usually will result for the average cost of a test. This comparison underlines the importance of understanding exactly how a cost analysis is being performed and what question is being addressed. One of the major problems in many of the published analyses of the costs of POCT (6, 28, 36, 55) is that they use cost allocation approaches that do not directly assess the budgetary impact of a test. Differences in approaches of cost analysis and lack of recognition that there is more than one way to calculate the costs of a test lead to much of the controversy about the economics of POCT. For most purposes, costs of POCT are better represented by an analysis of budgetary impact performed by a macrocost analysis of labor (measured as FTEs) rather than by a microcost analysis of labor (measured as minutes performing tests) because measurement of labor as change in FTEs accounts for changes in productivity and efficiency.

Besides the labor component, there are a number of other ways in which the economics of POCT generally differ from central laboratory testing. Usually, the supply costs are higher for POCT and a higher proportion of tests are used for quality assurance purposes because a much larger number of analyzers need to be checked. The high proportion of tests used for QC and the relatively fixed time required for staff training and management of testing lead to substantial economies of scale for performing a higher volume of testing (36). The significance of this economy of scale for the management of POCT is that efficiency is best served by restricting POCT to sites that perform a high volume of testing. Performing POCT at sites with low volumes of testing leads to higher supply, equipment, and labor costs per test. Due to wide variation in the cost elements of different POCT procedures, there is no fixed threshold value for the volume of testing that reaches a significant economy of scale; each situation must be analyzed with respect to both the direct cost factors and clinical necessity for rapid turnaround time.

Three final potential problem areas in the economics of POCT are in management of reagent wastage, utilization of testing, and duplication of POCT and central laboratory testing. These problems may lead to higher than expected costs for POCT. Checking a small proportion of POCT results with the same test performed in a central laboratory may serve as a useful quality assurance process (29). However, if most POCT is repeated with a duplicate test in the laboratory, this will have a major impact on the analysis of costs, and it may represent a substantial problem either in test-ordering patterns or in clinical confidence in the reliability of the POCT. Keys to managing these sources of increased costs are good systems for inventory management, data systems that allow review of test utilization patterns, agreement with and among clinicians regarding appropriate test ordering practices, and effective training of staff.

Quality Assurance Challenges

POCT has many of the same overall quality assurance requirements as testing in the central laboratory, such as training of staff, confirming competency, equipment maintenance, recording of patient results, inventory control, QC of testing, proficiency testing, documentation of processes to meet regulatory requirements, review of utilization and budgets, and billing for testing activities. Recent reports about patient harm from errors in medical care underscore the importance of developing improved strategies for avoiding error in POCT (31). Although the goals of quality assurance activities are similar to those in the central laboratory, there may be substantial differences in implementation due to the highly distributed nature of testing and the large number of staff involved.

One of the greatest challenges and a key to making POCT work is training and assurance of the competency of staff. Even if test devices are operating perfectly, accurate test results will not be produced if staff personnel are not educated about appropriate specimen collection and operation of test devices. Fecal occult blood testing could be considered one of the least complicated tests to perform. However, without appropriate training a number of breakdowns in test procedure have been noted in the past, such as use of the wrong developer solution, refilling bottles of developer solution with water, incorrect timing of test procedures, and lack of understanding of color changes (16). Completion of training by staff must be an essential component of job-specific competencies. Considering that training is one of the most important functions of the coordinators of POCT, teaching skill should be one of the prime factors in the selection of testing coordinators. It can be difficult to schedule enough training sessions to accommodate a large number of staff, so it may be helpful to have self-instruction videos or web-based instruction as additional options. Vendors of a number of POCT products have recognized the critical role of training and provide assistance with initial training of staff.

Quality assurance of POCT can be a very demanding activity due to the large number of analyzers that need to be tracked. Most POCT devices require limited maintenance such as cleaning and battery replacement, but if this is neglected, devices may fail. Portable devices may be dropped or exposed to vibration, water, extremes of heat or cold, or other environmental challenges that may lead to equipment failure. In part, this is a training issue, but even with appropriate maintenance and use, periodic device failures are likely. The greater potential for equipment damage in an uncontrolled environment emphasizes the need for control processes to detect malfunctions of devices. Usually, failure of POCT devices is handled by replacement of the failed unit rather than attempts at recalibration, service, or repair. This is handled by having one or more devices available as backups or by having a contingency plan for how service will be delivered. Lack of experience of the testing staff with troubleshooting equipment or reagent problems means that there is a need for on-call support by POCT coordinators or other experts. The central laboratory may assist with troubleshooting, particularly with interferences or with systematic changes of analyzers or reagents that may be identified by comparison of test results from POCT and the central laboratory.

Changes in U.S. federal regulation in 2003 affect quality assurance of testing (10). Control processes of POCT ideally should assess equipment, specimens, reagents, and testing personnel. Some POCT equipment has internal checks of electronic components, batteries, photometers, and other components with each use of the device. Mechanisms may exist for detecting specimen problems, such as inadequate specimen volume, clots, or bubbles. Many devices that are interpreted by direct visual inspection, such as tests for fecal occult blood, pregnancy, and other rapid antigen and antibody tests, have internal procedural controls that indicate whether the individual device is operational and whether there are inadequate specimens or interferences with the test. These control processes are highly desirable for POCT and should be sought in the selection of equipment because they check the instrument, specimen, and, in some cases, the reagents with each use.

The primary quality assurance focus of laboratory workers and regulations usually is on external QC testing and proficiency testing. These external controls do serve as additional checks for equipment and reagent failure. However, standard QC processes are designed primarily to detect systematic shifts in performance over time, and these are less of a problem with POCT, where reagents and equipment often are stable for months. A recent standard from NCCLS on unit-use devices has suggested that the frequency of QC testing should be one-tenth of the shelf life of reagents rather than more customary testing per shift or per day (52). Discussion of this standard provides an excellent overview of potential sources of error in POCT (52). Standard QC processes are not well designed to detect sporadic failures of unit-use devices and do not detect specimen problems. Two areas in which QC testing may make a positive contribution in the POCT environment are to evaluate and provide ongoing competency assessment of testing staff and to provide ongoing training of staff who infrequently perform a test. To achieve these benefits, it is important for QC testing to be rotated among all staff.

One controversial issue with respect to QC testing is the suitability of using electronic simulators rather than control materials (9). Advantages of using electronic controls are substantial reduction in the costs for test supplies and control materials. Often, control testing represents as much as one-quarter to one-half of the total volume of testing at a low-volume testing site. Therefore, use of electronic controls could reduce supply cost by as much as 50%. This reduction in cost may be critical to the economic viability of some testing activities in which unit costs of supplies are high. The major argument against use of electronic simulators is that although they check performance of the electronic components of an analyzer, they do not check the performance of the reagents. If electronic simulators are used, there should be some mechanism to periodically check on appropriate function of the reagents. Other drawbacks of the simulators are that they may provide less assistance with ongoing training and competency evaluation of testing staff.

Information Systems and Billing

Extensive record keeping is essential for meeting the regulatory and quality assurance requirements for POCT (31, 32, 39, 42). The only way to prove that appropriate procedures have been followed is to provide documentation of all activities. Historically, this was one of the most onerous aspects of the management of POCT. Most information was recorded manually, and it was a constant struggle to encourage complete recording of necessary data and to collect all of the data sheets. In organizations in which the scope and volume of POCT grew, it became increasingly critical to develop data systems to collect this information. Many POCT analyzers now have data systems that collect information about control testing, patient results, and which operators performed testing. Also, analyzers may have security functions to limit access to authorized users and lockout functions that require control testing at defined intervals before patient testing can be performed. Information from individual analyzers is gathered by periodic uploading of information into a central data station via modem or electronic network or by taking a laptop computer to testing sites.

There is increasing recognition of the value of consolidating all patient test results into central information systems. Entry of POCT results into central laboratory information systems provides many advantages: increased access to the results of POCT for patient care, improved ability to track and manage testing activities, ongoing quality assurance by providing comparison of POCT versus central laboratory results (29), and improved records for liability purposes. A major consideration in the selection of equipment for POCT should be the data-handling capabilities and how it will be interfaced with central information systems.

The decision to bill for POCT and the selection of billing methods are complex issues that have been handled in completely different ways by different organizations (43). Some organizations have decided not to bill for POCT, others have rolled these costs into nursing or room charges, and others have billed for individual tests. To perform billing, it is necessary to have effective information systems that can document ordering of the test, performance of the test, and patient diagnoses suitable for reimbursement. If there is some duplication of POCT and central laboratory testing, this could be identified as double billing. It may be necessary to review the frequency of testing on bills to see that this is within allowable limits. Creating the necessary documentation and reconciling bills with rules for reimbursement is a formidable challenge.

Technological Challenges

Rapid Changes of Menu, Devices, and Technology

Historically, POCT was severely limited by the small menu of tests that could be performed and by the relatively poor analytical quality of tests. However, advances in technology and successful miniaturization of devices have made it technically feasible to perform virtually any test as POCT (31, 42, 45). Ongoing advances in the microfabrication of devices and in nanotechnology provide the promise of substantial future technological change and further reduction in the size of POCT devices. Miniaturization of testing devices alone is not sufficient to make a test suitable for POCT. It is also important to reduce analysis times, to simplify the operation of test devices, and to minimize requirements for specimen preparation. To be suitable for POCT, a test usually must accept an unprocessed sample such as whole blood and the analysis times must be less than about 15 min. If these conditions are not met, it is difficult to perform the procedure as POCT or the advantage in turnaround time of POCT versus central laboratory testing is not sufficient to provide a strong advantage for POCT.

The previously cited example of intraoperative PTH testing provides an interesting example of the interplay between testing technology and the decision to perform a test as POCT. When technological advances reduced the time to perform PTH tests from hours to less than 15 min, it became practical to perform testing during surgical procedures (23). Some organizations decided to perform intraoperative PTH testing as POCT, while other organizations decided to transport specimens rapidly and to perform intraoperative PTH testing in a central laboratory (19). The decision of how to provide this testing appears to be influenced strongly by the characteristics of the testing devices—size, complexity of operation, cost, and testing menu. This test serves as just one example of how technological advances are greatly complicating the management of POCT by expanding the menu of tests that can be performed. In the past, it was easy to make the choice of POCT versus central laboratory when a test such as PTH could not be performed rapidly or no analyzer was available that was suitable for POCT. Now, it is necessary to evaluate critically a much wider range of potential tests and devices for POCT.

The rate of innovation and change of POCT devices has been faster than for high throughput analyzers in the central laboratory. This is possibly due to the lower complexity and much smaller capital investment for manufacturers to design a POCT device than a large laboratory analyzer. As an example, there have been about five generational changes in the fundamental technology applied for POCT glucose measurement over the past 25 years from (i) visually interpreted test strips to (ii) test strips read by optical meters after wiping away blood to (iii) no-wipe test strips read by optical meters to (iv) test strips read electrochemically to (v) microsample testing with electrochemical detection (4, 12, 17, 51). Other further changes in approach allowing testing with minimally invasive or noninvasive technologies are described in the next section; they may be viewed as further generational changes in technology. At the same time as all these changes in POCT devices and testing technology have occurred, there has been little change in the technology applied to glucose testing in central laboratories other than increased automation of analyzers and availability of whole blood glucose testing through expansion of the menu of blood gas analyzers.

The high rate of change and innovation of POCT devices presents a management challenge to stay abreast of information about these products. When advertisements and salespeople tout the latest and greatest new POCT devices and tests, how can your organization evaluate these claims? There are continuous upgrades for existing POCT devices, so a vendor of devices currently in use in your organization is likely to propose or require an upgrade as a change in the product is made and the old product is discontinued. It is difficult for laboratory workers to be knowledgeable about the characteristics of a wide range of new POCT devices, many of which are not used in central laboratory settings. Technologies and performance characteristics may differ from central laboratory analyzers, and extensive track records of clinical use and published evaluations may be lacking. It is difficult to even keep up with the range of test devices that are available, and most published reports become outdated quickly. As a result, the most useful resources for surveying what devices are available are periodically updated surveys such as those in *CAP Today* (accessible at http://www.cap.org). A website of the U.S. Food and Drug Administration includes a list of approved devices and devices that are classified as waived (http://www.fda.gov/cdrh/oivd). For the most current information about individual products, it is necessary to consult with vendors.

At the same time as there has been rapid evolution of the analytical capabilities of POCT devices, there have been major changes in the quality assurance processes, internal data systems, and the ability to transmit data to central information systems. A major problem with POCT devices has been the lack of common standards for internal data systems and for communication between other devices or central information systems. Recent development of standards by the Industry Connectivity Consortium should lead to improved ability to link devices to information systems (41). Consideration of how to link devices to information systems has become an increasingly important consideration in the evaluation of devices.

Lack of Equivalence between POCT and Central Laboratory Tests

In many cases, the specimen type or fundamental measuring principles of POCT devices differ from those used in the central laboratory, and these can be confusing to clinicians who are trying to interpret test results. Thus, it is important to perform careful comparisons of POCT and central laboratory results. Differences in whole blood specimens used for POCT versus serum or plasma samples used for central laboratory testing can lead to systematic differences in results for tests such as glucose (4, 17, 22, 34). Efforts have been made to reach agreement on a common reference standard such as plasma for glucose measurement to reduce the problem with comparison of POCT and laboratory results (22). However, the volume displacement and viscosity effects of hematocrit still can affect the reliability of results for specimens with extremely high or low hematocrits (4, 17). Fundamental problems of comparability of methods often have been experienced for POCT hematocrit measurements by conductivity versus laboratory measurements (49) and for POCT whole blood coagulation tests versus laboratory measurements on plasma specimens (35). Sometimes variation in the site of specimen collection can affect results. The glucose concentration of capillary blood from fingers can differ substantially from the concentration in venous blood (34). Collection of capillary blood from a forearm can yield different results than sampling from a finger (12, 27, 40). Differences in testing technology can lead to differences in the interferences with POCT devices (4, 17, 33), so it is important to become informed about potential limitations of each test device.

Practical consequences when there is nonequivalence between POCT and laboratory methods include a need (i) for careful comparison studies by the laboratory to guide device selection and to provide data about expected differences for clinicians; (ii) for education of clinicians about differences; and (iii) to report values by nonequivalent methods in separate columns in laboratory reports with appropriate reference values. It is desirable to have POCT and laboratory values side-by-side in reports to provide ongoing comparison.

New Monitoring Technologies

One growing source of uncertainty in defining the limits of POCT is the blurring of the boundaries between physiological monitoring—traditionally, measurements such as blood pressure, pulse rate, and temperature—and laboratory testing. It is now possible to perform measurements of analytes such as electrolytes, blood gases, and glucose with new types of devices attached to a patient (18, 38, 50, 54). Electrodes can be inserted into blood vessels or subcutaneously to provide continuous measurements. Specimens can be collected through the skin barrier by micropuncture or iontophoresis and analyzed by devices placed on the skin surface. Measurements can be made photometrically through tissue or by reflectance to measure bilirubin, glucose, hematocrit, or other compounds. The greatest commercial and clinical interest is in noninvasive measurement of glucose for diabetes care. This is a very large and dynamic field for which current information is best obtained through websites such as http://www.diabetesmonitor.com/meters.htm or http://www.childrenwithdiabetes.com.

Federal regulations in the United States (Clinical Laboratory Improvement Amendments of 1988) defined laboratory tests as procedures in which specimens were removed from the body for analysis (8). Procedures that are performed by devices attached to patients such as those described above or that involved the analysis of breath specimens were considered to represent physiological monitoring rather than laboratory testing. This raises the question: Is a glucose measurement performed by a device attached to a patient not a laboratory test while a glucose measurement performed on a specimen physically removed from a patient is a laboratory test? At this point, it is not clear how tests performed by monitoring devices will be classified in the future or whether the same standards will apply to measurements by monitoring devices.

In addition to posing fundamental questions about the limits and regulation of laboratory testing, monitoring technologies pose new challenges in the interpretation of test results. Some of these devices measure concentrations in tissue or interstitial fluids rather than in plasma or blood, and there may be physiological differences in the specimens sampled (27, 40, 50). Accuracy and performance characteristics of these devices may differ substantially from that delivered by usual laboratory tests, and the number of test results may be much greater. These issues will complicate the interpretation of results and the management of a large number of test results. For clinicians to interpret results from these devices, it will be important for any organization using monitoring devices to perform comparisons versus traditional laboratory measurements to generate information about how results from the monitoring device and the laboratory compare. Also, whether these devices are officially classified as laboratory tests or not, there will be a need for mechanisms to assure the quality of the test results. Processes and management structures developed for POCT may be effective mechanisms for supporting monitoring devices even if these are not covered by the same regulations as laboratory testing.

Summary

POCT presents some of the greatest and most controversial political, organizational, operational, and technological challenges for laboratory workers. POCT often crosses traditional organizational boundaries, encompasses testing activities performed at a large number of different sites, and requires training and coordination of a large number of staff with limited experience performing laboratory tests. One of the most controversial issues is whether POCT costs more or leads to lower costs relative to central laboratory testing. Part of this controversy relates to lack of standard approaches for analyzing costs. There is evidence that POCT can reduce total organizational costs in certain circumstances. POCT is also one of the most dynamic and rapidly changing fields of diagnostic testing, driven by rapid technological change as well as evolving clinical demands. There are no simple solutions to the complex issues of POCT that are universally applicable to varying organizational structures, political and historical contexts, laboratory operations, and clinical demands for testing. With all of the organizational and operational hurdles to overcome, perhaps the greatest challenge in POCT is to try to maintain a focus on the goals of using POCT to achieve the greatest organizational efficiency and the best possible patient care.

KEY POINTS

- POCT presents different management challenges than other types of laboratory testing.

- Cost analysis of POCT requires a clear understanding of the question that is being addressed. Analysis of labor costs usually are best addressed by evaluation of impact on FTEs.

- There is evidence that POCT can lower organizational costs in selected circumstances.

- Advances in testing and information technology are driving rapid change in the form and scope of POCT.

GLOSSARY

American Osteopathic Association A professional association of doctors of osteopathy that also provides laboratory accreditation services, primarily for physician office laboratories.

College of American Pathologists (CAP) A professional association of pathologists that provides laboratory proficiency testing and accreditation services.

COLA (formerly Commission on Office Laboratory Accreditation) An organization that provides laboratory accreditation services primarily for physician office laboratories.

Full-time equivalent (FTE) A labor component equivalent to the time worked by one full-time employee on a standard schedule.

Industry Connectivity Consortium A group that has developed engineering standards for electronic communication between POCT devices.

Joint Commission on Accreditation of Healthcare Organizations (JCAHO) An organization that accredits healthcare facilities and components of their services such as laboratory testing.

Macrocost analysis Analysis of costs by breaking down overall budgetary costs.

Microcost analysis Analysis of costs by adding up costs for performing an individual test.

Monitoring devices Devices that are attached directly to a patient and that provide periodic or continuous measurements.

NCCLS (formerly National Committee for Clinical Laboratory Standards) An organization that develops standards for laboratory practice.

Physician-performed microscopy Microscopic examinations such as potassium hydroxide preps and wet preps performed by primary care physicians outside the laboratory setting.

Point-of-care testing (POCT) Testing performed outside of a laboratory facility.

Waived testing Laboratory testing with the lowest level of complexity that can be performed under a certificate of waiver rather than a full laboratory license.

REFERENCES

1. **Alves-Dunkerson, J. A., P. E. Hilsenrath, G. A. Cress, and J. A. Wildness.** 2002. Cost analysis of a neonatal point-of-care monitor. *Am. J. Clin. Pathol.* **117:**809–818.

2. **Asimos, A. W., M. A. Gibbs, J. A. Marx, D. G. Jacobs, R. J. Erwin, J. Norton, and M. Thomason.** 2000. Value of point-of-care blood testing in emergent trauma management. *J. Trauma* **48:**1101–1108.

3. **Boone, D. J., J. W. Hay, J. Aguanno, T. Getzen, and G. Hortin.** 2002. Are the correct economic factors influencing point-of-care testing? *Point of Care* **1:**212–221.

4. **Chmielewski, S. A.** 1995. Advances and strategies for glucose monitoring. *Am. J. Clin. Pathol.* **104**(Suppl. 1):S59–S71.

5. **College of American Pathologists.** 2003. *Point-of-Care Testing Checklist. Laboratory Accreditation Program.* College of American Pathologists, Northfield, Ill.

6. **DeCresce, R. P., D. L. Phillips, and P. J. Howanitz.** 1995. Financial justification of alternate site testing. *Arch. Pathol. Lab. Med.* **119:**898–901.

7. **Despotis, J., J. E. Grishaber, and L. T. Goodnough.** 1994. The effect of an intraoperative treatment algorithm on physicians' transfusion practice in cardiac surgery. *Transfusion* **34:**290–296.

8. **Ehrmeyer, S. S., and R. H. Laessig.** 1995. Regulatory requirements (CLIA '88, JCAHO, CAP) for decentralized testing. *Am. J. Clin. Pathol.* **104**(Suppl. 1):S40–S49.

9. **Ehrmeyer, S. S., and R. H. Laessig.** 2001. Electronic "quality control" (EQC): is it just for unit use devices. *Clin. Chim. Acta* **307:**95–99.

10. **Ehrmeyer, S. S., and R. H. Laessig.** 2003. POCT 2003: testing environment, regulations, and technology. *Adv. Admin. Lab.* **12**(4):28–38.

11. **Felder, R. A., J. Savory, K. S. Margrey, J. W. Holman, and J. C. Boyd.** 1995. Development of a robotic near patient testing laboratory. *Arch. Pathol. Lab. Med.* **119:**948–951.

12. **Fineberg, S. E., R. M. Bergenstal, R. M. Bernstein, L. M. Laffel, and S. L. Schwartz.** 2001. Use of an automated device for alternative site blood glucose monitoring. *Diabetes Care* **24:**1217–1220.

13. **George, S., and R. A. Braithwaite.** 2002. Use of on-site testing for drugs of abuse. *Clin. Chem.* **48:**1639–1646.

14. **Grieve, R., R. Beech, J. Vincent, and J. Mazurkiewicz.** 1999. Near patient testing in diabetes clinics: appraising the costs and outcomes. *Health Technol. Assess.* **3:**1–74.

15. **Gruszecki, A. C., G. Hortin, J. Lam, D. Kahler, D. Smith, T. Daly, C. A. Robinson, and R. Hardy.** 2003. Utilization, reliability, and clinical impact of point-of-care testing during critical care transport—6 years experience. *Clin. Chem.* **49:**(6 Pt. 1):1017–1019.

16. **Hortin, G. L.** 1997. Managing the forgotten bedside test—occult blood testing. *Adv. Admin. Lab.* **6**(7):4–6.

17. **Hortin, G.** 1998. *Handbook of Bedside Glucose Testing.* AACC Press, Washington, D.C.

18. **Hortin, G. L.** 2002. The pursuit of less painful glucose testing. *Adv. Admin. Lab.* **11**(4):10–11.

19. **Hortin, G. L., and A. B. Carter.** 2002. Intraoperative parathyroid hormone testing: survey of testing program characteristics. *Arch. Pathol. Lab. Med.* **126:**104–109.

20. **Hughes, M.** 2002. Market trends in point-of-care testing. *Point of Care* 1:84–94.

21. **Hurst, J., K. Nickel, and L. H. Hilbourne.** 1998. Are physicians' office laboratory results of comparable quality to those produced in other laboratory settings? *JAMA* 279:468–471.

22. **IFCC Working Group on Selective Electrodes.** 2001. IFCC recommendation on reporting results for blood glucose. *Clin. Chim. Acta* 307:205–209.

23. **Irvin, G. L., III, and G. T. DeRiso.** 1994. A new practical intraoperative parathyroid hormone assay. *Am. J. Surg.* 168:466–468.

24. **Johnson, L. R., G. Koherty, T. Lairmore, J. F. Moley, L. M. Brunt, J. Koenig, and M. G. Scott.** 2001. Evaluation of the performance and clinical impact of rapid intraoperative parathyroid hormone assay in conjunction with preoperative imaging and concise parathyroidectomy. *Clin. Chem.* 47:919–925.

25. **Jones, B. A., P. Bachner, and P. J. Howanitz.** 1993. Bedside glucose monitoring: a College of American Pathologists Q-Probes study of the program characteristics and performance in 605 institutions. *Arch. Pathol. Lab. Med.* 117:1080–1087.

26. **Jones, B. A., and P. J. Howanitz.** 1996. Bedside glucose monitoring quality control practices. A College of American Pathologists Q-Probes study of program quality control documentation, program characteristics, and accuracy performance in 544 institutions. *Arch. Pathol. Lab. Med.* 120:339–345.

27. **Jungheim, K., and T. Koschinsky.** 2001. Risky delay of hypoglycemia detection by glucose monitoring at the arm. *Diabetes Care* 24:1303–1304.

28. **Keffer, J. H.** 1995. Economic considerations of point-of-care testing. *Am. J. Clin. Pathol.* 104(Suppl 1):S107–S110.

29. **Kilgore, M. L., S. J. Steindel, and J. A. Smith.** 1999. Continuous quality improvement for point-of-care testing using background monitoring of duplicate specimens. *Arch. Pathol. Lab. Med.* 123:824–828.

30. **Kilgore, M. L., S. J. Steindel, and J. A. Smith.** 1999. Cost analysis for decision support: the case of comparing centralized versus distributed methods for blood gas testing. *J. Healthcare Manag.* 44:207–215.

31. **Kost, G. J.** 2001. Preventing medical errors in point-of-care testing: security, validation, performance, safeguards, and connectivity. *Arch. Pathol. Lab. Med.* 125:1307–1315.

32. **Kost, G. J.** 2002. *Principles and Practice of Point-of-Care Testing.* Lippincott, Philadelphia, Pa.

33. **Kost, G. J., T. H. Nguyen, and Z. Tang.** 2000. Whole-blood glucose and lactate: trilayer biosensors, drug interferences, metabolism, and practice guidelines. *Arch. Pathol. Lab. Med.* 124:1128–1134.

34. **Kuwa, K., T. Nakayama, T. Hoshino, and M. Tominaga.** 2001. Relationships of glucose concentration in capillary whole blood, venous whole blood and venous plasma. *Clin. Chim. Acta* 307:187–192.

35. **Laposata, M.** 2001. Point-of-care coagulation testing: stepping gently forward. *Clin. Chem.* 47:801–802.

36. **Lee-Lewandrowski, E., M. Laposata, K. Eschenbach, C. Camooso, D. M. Nathan, J. E. Godine, K. Hurxthal, J. Goff, and K. Lewandrowski.** 1994. Utilization and cost analysis of bedside capillary glucose testing in a large teaching hospital: implications for managing point of care testing. *Am. J. Med.* 97:222–230.

37. **Lehman, C. M., R. C. Blaylock, D. P. Alexander, and G. M. Rodgers.** 2001. Discontinuation of the bleeding time test without detectable adverse clinical impact. *Clin. Chem.* 47:1204–1211.

38. **Louie, R. F., Z. Tang, and G. J. Kost.** 2001. Emerging technologies for point-of-care testing. *Adv. Admin. Lab.* 10(9):64–68.

39. **Main, R., J. Wright, and F. L. Kiechle.** 1994. Data management programs for bedside glucose testing. *Lab. Med.* 25:784–789.

40. **McGarraugh, G.** 2001. Response to Jungheim and Koschinsky: glucose monitoring at the arm. *Diabetes Care* 24:1304–1306.

41. **NCCLS.** 2001. *Point-of-Care Connectivity; Approved Standard.* NCCLS publication POCT1-A. NCCLS, Wayne, Pa.

42. **Nichols, J. H.** 2003. *Point-of-Care Testing: Performance Improvement and Evidence-Based Outcomes.* Marcel Dekker, New York, N.Y.

43. **Paxton, A.** 2001. Labs waver on whether to bill for POC tests. *CAP Today* 15(8):1.

44. **Price, C. P.** 2001. Point of care testing. *Br. Med. J.* 322:1285–1288.

45. **Price, C. P., and J. M. Hicks.** 1999. *Point-of-Care Testing.* AACC Press, Washington, D.C.

46. **Sokoll, L. J., H. Drew, and R. Udelsman.** 2000. Intraoperative parathyroid hormone analysis: a study of 200 consecutive cases. *Clin. Chem.* 46:1662–1668.

47. **Steindel, S. J., S. Granade, J. Lee, G. Avery, L. M. Clarke, R. W. Jenny, and K. M. LaBeau.** 2002. Practice patterns of testing waived under the Clinical Laboratory Improvement Amendments. *Arch. Pathol. Lab. Med.* 126:1471–1479.

48. **Steindel, S. J., and P. J. Howanitz.** 2001. Physician satisfaction and emergency department laboratory test turnaround time. *Arch. Pathol. Lab. Med.* 125:863–871.

49. **Stott, R. A. W., G. L. Hortin, S. Miller, C. H. Smith, T. R. Wilhite, and M. Landt.** 1995. Analytical artifacts in the measurement of hematocrit by whole blood chemistry analyzers. *Clin. Chem.* 41:306–311.

50. **Tamada, J. A., S. Garg, L. Jovanovic, K. R. Pitzer, S. Fermi, R. O. Potts, and the Cygnus Research Team.** 1999. Noninvasive glucose monitoring: comprehensive clinical results. *JAMA* 282:1839–1844.

51. **Weitgasser, R., B. Gappmayer, and M. Pichler.** 1999. Newer portable glucose meters—analytical improvement compared with previous generation devices? *Clin. Chem.* 45:1821–1825.

52. **Whitley, R. J., P. J. Santrach, and D. L. Phillips.** 2001. Establishing a quality management system for unit-use testing based on NCCLS proposed guideline (EP18-P). *Clin. Chim. Acta* 307:145–149.

53. **Wians, F. H., J. A. Balko, R. M. Hsu, W. Byrd, and W. H. Snyder.** 2000. Intraoperative vs. central laboratory PTH testing during parathyroid surgery. *Lab. Med.* 31:616–621.

54. **Winkelman, J. W., and M. J. Tanasijevic.** 2002. Noninvasive testing in the clinical laboratory. *Clin. Lab. Med.* 22:547–558.

55. **Winkelman, J. W., D. R. Wybenga, and M. J. Tanasijevic.** 1994. The fiscal consequences of central vs. distributed testing of glucose. *Clin. Chem.* 40:1628–1630.

APPENDIX 23.1   Websites with Information Relating to POCT

Critical and Point-of-Care Testing Division of the AACC
(http://www.aacc.org/divisions/cpoct/)
Information about educational programs and other resources.

College of American Pathologists (CAP)
(http://www.cap.org)
Checklists and information about laboratory inspections, articles and instrument surveys in *CAP Today*, and information from the POCT Committee.

Children with Diabetes
(http://www.childrenwithdiabetes.com)
Information about new developments in the field of diabetes including POCT devices.

DiabetesMonitor.com
(http://www.diabetesmonitor.com/meters.htm)
Information about POCT devices and technologies useful for testing diabetics.

U. S. Food and Drug Administration
(http://www.fda.gov/cdrh/oivd)
Website of the Food and Drug Administration, providing a list of approved diagnostic devices and devices classified as waived.

Point of Care
(http://www.poctjournal.com)
Website for the journal *Point of Care*; access to articles requires subscription.

PointofCare.net
(http://www.pointofcare.net)
Website with many links to other sites related to POCT.

24

Principles of Preanalytic and Postanalytic Test Management

Rebecca Katsaras, Adarsh K. Khalsa, Rebecca A. Smith, and Michael A. Saubolle

OBJECTIVES

To familiarize readers with the principles of selection, assessment, and incorporation of diagnostic tests

To review principles of test evaluation and utilization and their effect on patient outcomes

To describe major elements of requisition and test menu formats

To review principles of formatting of reports of test results

To review the needs for record storage

The artist may well be advised to keep his work to himself till it is completed, because no one can readily help him or advise him with it . . . but the scientist is wiser not to withhold a single finding or a single conjecture from publicity.

JOHANN WOLFGANG VON GOETHE

THE PRIMARY FUNCTION of a clinical laboratory is the provision of accurate, clinically significant data for the diagnosis of medical conditions in patients. Once available, the data can be used to provide the individual patient with a management plan to increase the probability of achieving a desirable outcome (29). The production of laboratory data is a culmination of sequential processes including preanalytic, analytic, and postanalytic laboratory activities that begin with a clinician's request for specific studies on an individual patient (36). These sequential processes are also known as "path of workflow" and have been described and defined by the NCCLS guidelines and Clinical Laboratory Improvement Amendments (CLIA) regulations (Table 24.1).

The level of quality of service provided by a laboratory could affect patient care outcomes considerably, either positively or negatively (29). To achieve optimal patient outcomes, it is imperative to evaluate the effect of preanalytic and postanalytic activities on the clinical significance and medical impact of laboratory tests (33).

Processes and procedures implemented within the laboratory should be understood as to their impact on workflow. Their design should have the level of quality needed to minimize errors and resource waste, while maximizing efficacy. Quality standard guidelines and regulatory accreditation requirements have been published and need to be met (19, 23, 24, 36, 51, 52).

To achieve quality processes, dynamic laboratory management requires both pre- and posttest analysis of laboratory studies. It is not adequate to evaluate tests solely from the laboratory-centered perspectives of accuracy,

Table 24.1 Description of processes in the clinical laboratory[a]

Process type[b]	Description or definition
Preanalytic	Steps taken before test actually performed (pre-examination phase). Processes beginning with test request and its format; patient preparation; specimen collection, transportation, and receipt in the laboratory; and preparation for testing.
Analytic	Activities related to the performance of laboratory testing or examination of specimens (examination phase).
Postanalytic	Steps that occur after a laboratory test has been performed (postexamination phase). Processes include data review, report formatting, result interpretation and presentation, permission for release, result transmission, and sample storage.

[a]Compiled from references 19 and 36.

[b]Path of workflow: sequential sum of all preanalytical, analytical, and postanalytical processes, beginning with test order and culminating with laboratory data output.

rapid turnaround time, low cost, and high sensitivity/specificity. The laboratory medical director should have the responsibility for the assessment of the effects of test results on patient outcomes and therapeutic protocols (31). After careful test selection and implementation, the laboratory should evaluate both test utilization and appropriateness of test ordering to best affect cost containment and to achieve the most positive effect on patient outcomes. Because subsequent to laboratory testing, various actions or interventions may occur that are not under laboratory control, it is important for laboratory management to interact with teams of nonlaboratory specialists (such as infectious disease clinicians, hospitalists, infection control epidemiologists, radiologists, pharmacists, clinical case managers, and the nursing staff) to ensure quality care and follow-up for the patient. The reporting format of test results and the accompanying interpretation also play crucial roles in assisting clinicians to best serve their patients.

Preanalytic Activities

The preanalytic phase refers to all steps taken before actual testing is performed on a patient's specimen. It includes the ordering of tests, collection, transportation, handling, storage, and/or referral of specimens, and assessment of all preanalytic activities.

Test Selection and Implementation

Test complexity. The Clinical Laboratory Improvement Amendments were passed by Congress in 1988 (CLIA '88) to establish quality standards for laboratory testing and to ensure the accuracy, reliability, and timeliness of patient test results. Initially, laboratory tests were categorized by CLIA '88 as waived, of moderate complexity, or of high complexity. A "final rule" was published in the *Federal Register* in 2003 recognizing only waived or nonwaived cate-

gories of tests (11). Waived tests are defined as simple laboratory examinations and procedures that are cleared for home use by the U.S. Food and Drug Administration (FDA), have simple methodologies, or pose no reasonable risk of harm to the patient if performed incorrectly (19). Nonwaived tests have more difficult methodologies and require greater amounts of training of the personnel performing them. Thus, the latter also requires more rigorous regulatory compliance. When determining whether to add a specific test to the menu, laboratories must decide into which of these categories the test fits and whether or not the laboratory meets the requirements to perform this level of testing. Further information regarding categorization of tests may be found within the FDA's website (http://www.fda.gov/cdrh/clia/). Laboratories performing nonwaived testing must be certified or licensed under CLIA regulations. They must operate with guidelines in place for proper patient test management and must set specifications for all areas that can affect specimen integrity and positive identification throughout preanalytic, analytic, and postanalytic processes. The laboratory must maintain an adequate number of qualified employees to perform these tests (19).

Types of tests. At the most basic level, laboratory tests are tools to gain information about a patient (14). Tests are commonly ordered for a variety of reasons, including diagnosis, screening for disease, or patient management (Table 24.2) (21). Clinicians' self-described reasons for ordering tests are usually slightly different, in that tests are often ordered to establish a baseline, assess prognosis, reassure patients, and help with treatment decisions. Appropriateness of ordering and effects of testing often go beyond diagnosis or immediate treatment decisions in this setting (13). Thus, understanding testing needs from the clinicians' point of view can help in developing strategies to maximize patient care and enhance cost savings. Testing that may appear unnecessary to the laboratory

Table 24.2 Applications of laboratory tests[a]

Basic screening

Establishing (initial) diagnosis

Differential diagnosis

Estimating prognosis

Evaluation of current medical case management and outcomes

Evaluating disease severity

Detecting disease recurrence

Monitoring course of illness and response to treatment

Selecting drugs and adjusting therapy

Group and panel testing

Regularly scheduled screening tests as part of ongoing care

Testing responding to specific events or certain signs and symptoms (such as sexual assault, drug screening, postmortem)

[a]Adapted from references 14 and 37.

may be based on physical findings known only to the physician (2).

The diagnostic process in patient care is critical in that it leads to prognosis and treatment (21). Unfortunately, in general, there are no perfect diagnostic laboratory tests. A clinician may inappropriately order diagnostic tests because the tests appear to pose minimal risk while providing possible further useful information. This type of overuse may burden the laboratory unnecessarily, may cause the patient avoidable harm, and does not contribute to improved quality of medical care, shorter hospital stays, or reduced mortality (34). An unexpected result may lead to unnecessary additional testing or inappropriate care for a particular patient (21). It has been shown that even for a healthy person, the greater the number of tests ordered, the greater the probability that some of the test results will be outside of the "normal" range. Table 24.3 lists the properties of useful diagnostic tests (28, 37).

Screening tests (such as lipid panels for evaluation of risk for coronary artery disease, prostate-specific antigen for prostate cancer, and carriage of group B *Streptococcus* during the 35th to 37th week of pregnancy as a risk factor for neonatal infection during delivery after premature rupture of membranes) are those that may show previously undetected disease in asymptomatic persons or identify risk factors for a disease (21, 37). Table 24.4 lists various parameters for ideal characteristics for diagnostic screening tests. When these criteria are applied to measure the efficacy of screening tests, it becomes evident that only a few such tests are appropriate and only for a handful of diseases. Persons shown to have an increased risk of disease by a screening test are usually advised to consult a physician for follow-up when appropriate (6).

Input from clinicians and other healthcare providers is vital for optimum selection of tests. Diagnostic and monitoring criteria can be established through collaboration with specialists in each area of clinical practice. From these criteria, essential tests for a particular clinical setting can be chosen. It is also crucial to work with managed care leaders, case managers, contract providers, insurance payors, and government representatives, as certain types of testing may not be covered by insurance or other financial reimbursement.

Needs assessment should also consider the testing environments, of which there are many more options than in the past. Testing may be "in the field," commonly known as

Table 24.3 Properties of useful diagnostic tests[a]

Methodology well described and easily reproducible

Accuracy and precision have been ascertained

Established reference range

Sensitivity and specificity established based on an appropriately wide spectrum of clinical presentations and patient types (including age, where necessary)

[a]Adapted from reference 37.

Table 24.4 Parameters for ideal characteristics for screening tests[a]

Characteristics of population
- Sufficiently high prevalence of disease
- Likely to be compliant with subsequent tests and treatments

Characteristics of disease
- Significant morbidity and mortality
- Effective and acceptable treatment available
- Presymptomatic period detectable
- Improved outcome from early treatment

Characteristics of test
- Good sensitivity and specificity
- Low cost and risk
- Confirmatory test available and practical

[a]Adapted from reference 37.

point-of-care, or may be at a clinician's office, a clinic, a hospital, or a freestanding diagnostic facility (14). Collection of specimens or administration of some tests may require hospital admission, albeit normally as outpatient status.

There is increasing interest, both by consumers and laboratories, in patient-directed orders for testing. Direct access testing (DAT) is initiated by an individual patient, without evaluation or order by a clinician. Results are returned directly to the patient ordering the test rather than to a clinician. Reimbursements for DAT come directly from the patient and not from third-party payors (e.g., Medicare or managed care plans). This type of testing is becoming increasingly popular due to a more health-conscious society that wishes to be more proactive in its health management. Avoiding the cost of the copay or the cost of the entire physician visit is another reason that DAT is becoming popular in the outpatient setting. Self-initiated testing is a natural progression to that offered at health fairs and with home test kits (17).

Laboratories must be aware of some of the issues related to offering DAT. Many states allow the test ordering and result release only to appropriately licensed practitioners. State regulations must be reviewed to ascertain local regulatory constraints because releasing results to unauthorized persons, including the patients themselves, may be a violation.

Many of the tests performed at DAT centers are classified as waived. However, there are tests offered at these facilities that are categorized as more complex, requiring regulatory compliance.

Laboratories considering offering DAT may damage their relationships with their physician clients. Although it appears that corporations are welcoming this type of testing as a business opportunity, physicians may be more concerned about its ramifications and effects. Laboratories will have to find ways to bridge the gap between these differing opinions.

Test sensitivity, specificity, and predictive values. The parameters of sensitivity, specificity, and predictive value of a test in essence describe the clinical value of a test. Numerous detailed descriptions and analyses are available (14, 15, 21, 25). Sensitivity is the percentage of individuals who have the particular disease for which the test is used and for whom positive test results are found. Expressed as a formula, percent sensitivity equals the quotient of the number of persons with the disease who test positive using the test in question divided by the total number of persons tested with disease multiplied by 100. Specificity is the percentage of individuals who do not have the particular disease being tested and for whom negative test results are found (14, 15). Expressed as a formula, percent specificity equals the quotient of the number of persons without disease who test negative by the test in question divided by the total number of persons tested without the disease multiplied by 100.

While sensitivity and specificity do not change with various populations of ill or healthy persons, predictive values can vary considerably depending on age, gender, or geographic location of those tested. The positive predictive value provides the probability that a positive result indicates the presence of disease. Conversely, the negative predictive value provides the probability that a negative result indicates the absence of disease.

Test reimbursement. To remain viable, laboratories need to be reimbursed appropriately for the testing they perform, and test reimbursement by Medicare or other third-party payors must be considered when deciding on a test menu (51). To be reimbursable, the FDA must have approved the test. The test must also have received recognition by the American Medical Association (AMA) by being assigned a Current Procedural Code (CPT-4) by the AMA's CPT committee. When a laboratory performs a test deemed experimental by the AMA or that is not approved by the FDA, the Centers for Medicare and Medicaid Services (CMS), previously known as the Health Care Financing Administration, will not allow reimbursement for that test, and Medicare will not reimburse the laboratory. Managed care providers generally follow this pattern as well.

Thus, laboratory managers must review AMA's official CPT-4 Code Book, which is published and updated yearly, to keep current with the available chargeable tests. Failure to do so may compromise the financial viability of the laboratory due to the performance of tests whose expense is incurred solely by the laboratory. Beyond the initial evaluation, it is imperative to consistently monitor the reimbursement of frequently ordered tests. Laboratories need to reevaluate the reimbursement of individual tests and use this during negotiation for managed care contracts in order to be appropriately compensated and to be able to continue offering the tests.

Available technology. Advancements in science and technology have and will continue to allow laboratories the opportunity to increase and enhance test menus in order to aid the clinician in his endeavor to monitor and provide medical services to patients. Improvement in diagnostic capability and decreasing turnaround times have brought clinical medicine to the verge of "real time" diagnosis, in which early intervention has a real chance to improve outcomes significantly. Molecular-based technology and computerized automation will continue to improve diagnostic capability. Often, clinicians will request diagnostic tests whose overall effect and efficacy on patient care has not been well evaluated and whose reimbursement by third-party payors is in doubt. It is imperative that the laboratory evaluate such innovations and categorize them as to clinical and diagnostic efficacy and financial feasibility. Fiscal and clinical responsibility is paramount when making decisions on implementing newer tests (Table 24.5).

Cost studies. Cost-benefit analysis is imperative for the evaluation of test implementation. Several methods are available to assist with the cost accounting process. The "instrument cost accounting technique" was originally published by Travers in 1989 and is presented elsewhere in detail (51). This method takes into account instrument-related costs, direct materials costs, and labor costs. The process is sufficiently generic to apply to any department in the laboratory. As the cost for each test is determined, total cost for patterns of disease-related groupings can be calculated.

Table 24.5 Factors affecting decision to implement or discontinue a test

Category	Reasons to implement	Reasons to discontinue
CLIA	• Have staff with adequate education and experience • Have system to ensure accurate results	• Staff fails to meet CLIA guidelines
Managed care/Medicare reimbursement	• Assay reimbursed by Medicare and managed care	• Inability to obtain adequate reimbursement from managed care or Medicare
Testing technology	• Ease of use with test kits • More readily obtained • Technology advanced	• Testing becomes obsolete • Manufacturers discontinue test kits/reagents
Cost-effective	• High-volume ordering • Increase in reimbursements from managed care	• Test volumes too low

Procedural analysis can also be implemented using published NCCLS guidelines (35). These guidelines include methods for analysis that can justify or refute addition of new procedures, assist in determining the frequency of test runs, and supply information regarding the performance of staff or instrumentation. The guidelines provide detailed definitions of terms, numerous sample forms, examples of different scenarios, relevant variables, and frequently asked questions. The importance of first having a functional model of the laboratory in place is stressed. The model should include component working departments and laboratory cost centers, as well as availability of ancillary data from finance, payroll, and purchasing departments.

A formula has been described for determining cost-effectiveness of screening tests (47). Each of the factors (prevalence of the disease, cost of the test, and benefit of detecting the disease) is assigned a numerical value, yielding a benefit-cost ratio. To be cost-effective, the ratio should be greater than 1.00.

The consideration of whether to perform a test in-house or to send it to a referral laboratory s influenced by several issues (30). One issue is the comparison of the estimated total cost of performing the test in-house versus the estimated total revenue for that test. The costs must include capital expenditure for equipment, instrument maintenance, reagents, consumables, controls, and personnel expenses. Expected test volume must be considered in the equation. Other issues concern the technical expertise of existing staff, space availability in the laboratory, frequency of test performance, time and complexity of processing the specimen for referral, and the test's clinical acceptance (i.e., is it likely to become commonplace or remain esoteric).

Additional factors in the decision making on in-house performance of testing include consideration of required turnaround time, accreditation and quality of the available reference laboratories, specimen transport issues, reporting format, and method of report delivery (computer, fax, mail, or courier). Because of variances in individual laboratories and the population or community that they serve, there will also be variances in needs for and utilization of tests among laboratories.

As noted above, reimbursement from Medicare, managed care plans, or any third-party payors must also be considered when determining if a test is considered cost-effective or not. As utilization increases for a particular test, a conclusion can be drawn as to the cost-effectiveness of that assay. Although reimbursement is important, there are other ways in which to measure a test's cost-effectiveness. A test's contribution to patient care and appropriate patient outcomes also plays a crucial role in the decision of whether to perform a test. A test that in itself may be a financial loss may contribute significant savings to institutions from either a patient-safety standpoint or in financial savings by other means. As an example, a nonreimbursable, rapid molecular-based test of sputum that is smear-positive for acid-fast bacilli can show the absence of *Mycobacterium tuberculosis*, thus obviating the need to isolate the patient and providing a significant cost savings to the institution. To recognize such financial savings to other areas of the institution, the laboratory must work closely with other clinical departments.

Test implementation: verification and validation. CLIA '88 specifies that a laboratory process must be in place to initially verify the capability of an introduced or revised test methodology and then to periodically validate its performance (12, 19). The topic, including discussion of methods for verification and validation, is well reviewed elsewhere (12). Verification includes evaluation of the performance of a new or modified test being introduced into the laboratory. It focuses on the determination of new performance characteristics or confirmation of commercially determined and published characteristics for a test. Specifically, in verification, test sensitivity, specificity, and perhaps predictive values must be determined or confirmed. Verification results must be available for physician review during the tenure of the test method in the laboratory (12, 42). Validation, on the other hand, as a component of an ongoing laboratory quality assurance program, periodically evaluates and documents the performance of a test over time to ensure its continued provision of expected results established during verification. Guidelines from manufacturers and accreditation agencies may be used to determine validation frequency for a test; CLIA '88 suggests 6-month intervals.

Appropriate Test Utilization

In the patient-oriented, cost-effective laboratory, periodic evaluation of test utilization and appropriateness of test ordering is mandatory. Inappropriate or excessive testing takes scarce laboratory resources that could be used elsewhere (51). In 1990, the Joint Commission on Accreditation of Healthcare Organizations (JCAHO) set the foundation for laboratory responsibility for clinician education in test appropriateness. In its standards (*Accreditation Manual for Hospitals*, standard PA 1.2.7) (24), JCAHO stresses that the medical director of clinical and pathological laboratory services should ensure that an active policy for the monitoring and evaluation of the quality and appropriateness of the services provided is in place (23, 24). Because laboratory tests are a form of clinical intervention, the laboratory medical and administrative management teams have a professional and moral responsibility to clinicians to advocate for the patient (31, 32). Legal and ethical implications also dictate providing the patient information to aid in understanding the risks and benefits of testing (14).

It may appear difficult to determine which tests should be evaluated. There are many examples of tests for which monitoring of testing practices is mandatory to ascertain appropriateness. These examples may include, but are not limited to, repetitive testing on the same specimen sites within short time periods (e.g., 24 h), excessive number of cultures (e.g., more than 2 to 4 blood cultures per episode, daily sputum cultures), cultures of superficial sites (e.g., pressure ulcers), and cultures of inappropriate specimens (nasal swabs for enumeration of etiologies of pneumonia). If available, technical specialists or other senior personnel in each area may encounter situations through studies, day-to-day tracking duties, quality assurance, recently published articles, interdepartmental interactions, meetings, or other problem-solving circumstances that indicate which tests are good candidates for further appraisal. Input from bench technologists concerning clinician-laboratory interactions, usually from telephone calls, may also be a source of potential problems suggesting additional test evaluation.

Some suggest that the Pareto principle, also known as the 80/20 rule, can be applied (35). This rule is commonly employed in many types of industries and states that 80% of an entity's total revenues are produced by 20% of its products. For the laboratory, this means first listing all tests performed by the lab and ranking them according to total annual revenues produced by each test. NCCLS's *Basic Cost Accounting for Clinical Services; Approved Guideline* gives further details of using the principle along with definitions and examples (35).

Laboratory tests may be overutilized, underutilized, or misutilized (39). Overutilization occurs when extraneous tests are ordered; underutilization implies that relevant tests are not ordered. Misutilization occurs when results are ignored or interpreted improperly. Various studies have shown both that increased laboratory testing does not enhance quality of patient care and that there are no serious negative consequences with reduction in testing (48). A potential problem with superfluous testing is that with a larger volume of information to read and comprehend, a clinician may overlook the more important and relevant test values.

Utilization and appropriateness issues are related. While utilization may have more to do with frequency of testing, appropriateness is concerned with use in the right patient in the correct setting for the proper diagnostic, monitoring, or therapeutic reasons. Improving utilization has the ability to reduce laboratory costs, while precluding several less pleasant alternatives such as rationing laboratory tests or eliminating some altogether (55). Several published studies serve to illustrate types of changes possible by reviewing utilization and appropriateness. In 2000, Jacobs et al. questioned whether all trauma victims being admitted to the hospital required, per hospital protocol, a complete battery of 11 laboratory tests (22). To examine alternatives, trauma patients were divided into two categories with established criteria: those with defined severe injuries and those with severe injury unlikely. A team leader or attending physician placed each patient in one of the two groups. Patients with severe injury unlikely received only two laboratory tests, while those with severe injury received five. Evaluation after the 3-month study period showed no patient care problem, no change in quality of patient care, and a cost savings for the organization.

Toubert et al. assessed possible overutilization or inappropriate use of various thyroid tests within their hospital network (50). Thyroid test needs vary, whether for disease screening, diagnosis, or monitoring. In a trial period subsequent to an information campaign, physicians were asked to provide justification and clinical information if tests other than thyroid-stimulating hormone were ordered. Order forms were collected and analyzed for appropriateness by the endocrinology staff. With only the processes of education and requirement of justification, appropriateness of ordering was increased by approximately 30% for most tests.

At times, studies involving multiple institutions may be suitable. In the mid-1990s, Valenstein et al., working with the College of American Pathologists (CAP) and 601 institutions, assessed the use of routine stool microbiology tests in the hospital setting (53). Nearly 60,000 specimens were evaluated, leading to the establishment of guidelines to limit routine bacterial stool cultures to the first 3 days of hospitalization.

In a final example, panels of preoperative laboratory tests appeared to have high usage with low yield and little change in patient management (45). Studies at a variety of facilities led to new guidelines based on patient age and history, thus reducing automatic use of large preoperative panels while not adversely affecting patient outcome.

It has been described in the past to be very difficult, if not impossible, to change physicians' test-ordering patterns (25, 38, 42, 51). Physicians often have prior experience with hospital "quality" programs under various guises and may feel that, in the end, beyond "harassment" and poorly disguised cost-cutting, little occurred to improve patient outcome (8). For these reasons, it becomes imperative to include clinical specialists and service leaders when attempting to alter laboratory utilization patterns.

In spite of the reported past failures to modify physician test ordering, a plethora of articles has been published containing salient points and methods to consider when working with clinicians concerning utilization and appropriateness of testing. One hurdle to overcome is the use of diagnostic testing to purportedly reduce the risk of malpractice liability (10). Analysis has shown that "defensive testing," as it is known, appears rational but is actually costly and harmful to patients. The incremental knowledge gained does not affect the course of treatment but more often leads to misdiagnosis and inappropriate treatment. Physician education offers the simplest solution to this situation.

Consensus between medical staff and laboratorians can help effect positive change. Of primary importance are communications and establishing professional relationships (51). In a first step, it is necessary to examine patterns of clinical thinking, clinical pathways, local and national peer guidelines, preferred practice patterns and, if available, clinician algorithms for decision making (8, 34, 42, 51). This examination can lead to the establishment of customized groupings of laboratory tests for various specialties, which can provide quality results for the lowest cost (e.g., hepatitis serology panel for acute hepatitis and Epstein-Barr virus serology panel for acute mononucleosis). Outdated tests may be eliminated and sequential protocol testing may be developed in line with diagnostic algorithms (38). Validated best-practice information has been shown to be accepted by physicians and to facilitate actual change (18).

Other helpful steps include having recurring meetings with medical staff committees to explain policies, new tests, or changes in protocol; publishing schedules or timetables of particular assays; publishing practice guidelines; integrating the laboratory information system (LIS) into clinician workflow; issuing handbooks (hard-copy or web-based); and education by clinical leaders or respected peers (1, 5, 8, 39, 44). The laboratory physician may also use consultation, interpretive reporting, cumulative laboratory reports, and narrative statements about particular tests (51). One laboratory created a Clinical Laboratory Information Consulting Center, staffed by a medical technologist and a clinical pathologist, that offers availability of a consult by telephone on weekdays and by e-mail or fax on weekends (43). By providing information, interpretation of testing, and, if needed, clinical advice, the center assists in combating unnecessary testing while establishing relationships with the medical staff.

In another idea, Winkens et al. have made individual feedback to family doctors a routine healthcare activity (54). The purpose was to improve the quality of test-ordering behavior. What is unique in their setting is the use of thorough and personal feedback over the course of many years, not just in a temporary study setting. Feedback is provided in a report by respected clinical specialists and looks at both overuse and rationality (in accordance with guidelines or standards). This system requires the enlisting of experts to give feedback and a requisition form that allows for input of basic patient clinical data.

The availability of more sophisticated software programs has been used by some institutions to assist with ordering compliance and appropriate test utilization (18). Essentially, these systems use information technology to enhance clinical decision making, allow compliance to increase reimbursement rates, and speed the processing of orders. As with other solutions described previously, the

software must be designed with cooperation leading to mutual confidence. It must employ legitimate expert information, be monitored by specialists, and provide information in real time when test ordering is taking place. In the organization discussed by Hawkins et al., the computerized order entry system utilizes initial screen views designed to look like the paper order forms they replaced (18). Indicator lists then guide the clinician to lists of most appropriate choices for test ordering for the specific situation at hand. The system is continually evolving as new procedures become available, as professional guidelines are updated, and as the users provide feedback.

House staffing provides a unique environment for influence and training in optimal test ordering. Clinical service leaders, in cooperation with the laboratory, can track frequency and volume of testing by residents and use this as an instructive tool (51). An investigation by Ruangkanchanasetr found that education, peer review, and feedback were most helpful in combination to alter house staff test utilization (40). Part of the education concerned information about the cost of tests, while the feedback showed residents their own results by tracking the numbers of tests per patient. Studnicki et al. also showed a reduction in the number of tests exceeding frequency guidelines by using a feedback system comparing resident test ordering patterns against predetermined guidelines (48). Feedback may also be used for nonresident physicians. Feedback seems to be most constructive when it contains cost-audit information and shows clinicians how their test usage compares to that of their peers (13).

Pharmacists play a role in selecting laboratory tests as well and, when appropriate, should be consulted by the laboratory for input (7). Not only may they order laboratory tests pursuant to consult with a clinician, they also need to interpret and apply test results when making recommendations concerning therapy. Their role as intermediary between laboratory and clinician should be taken advantage of for any applicable evaluations or studies.

Algorithms can be applied to track utilization. Schubart et al. studied the use of algorithm-based decision rules to employ appropriate intervals for repeat testing for some commonly ordered laboratory tests. As an example, for serum potassium testing in their hospital, application of the established algorithm allowed for a 34% reduction in testing for the first 5 days of hospitalization without a reduction in quality of care (41). Even the model laboratory compliance plan can assist in control of redundant testing (26). With the passage of the Health Insurance Portability and Accountability Act of 1996, and later the Medicare Integrity Program, laboratory managers may now have legal liability for inappropriate test utilization. The development of an institution's individual compliance plan is an occasion to incorporate processes for tracking utilization and making appropriate changes. The most successful plans should define the roles of various departments in compliance monitoring and tie the hospital laboratory to the compliance office, usually with the use of the LIS. Commonly, LIS records have the ability to show test usage rates and patterns. Follow-up to potential compliance problems is best effected by meetings with physician and nursing or other staff involved. Through this venue, any noted opportunities for improvement in utilization can be discussed.

Specimen Acquisition, Transport, and Storage

There has been a tendency in today's medical climate to place more emphasis on primary care clinicians seeing more patients and making fewer referrals to the specialists or subspecialists. Often, this emphasis encourages use of more diagnostic tests to ensure quality patient care but decreases the time allocated to evaluation of the patient or to researching diagnostic test ramifications. One of the laboratory's roles and responsibilities is to ensure that adequate information is provided to the clinician-client to make appropriate choices in specimen collection and test ordering.

Written policies and procedures should be in place in the laboratory detailing not only the tests available but also describing for each test the specific patient preparation process, the specimen collection process, and specimen labeling with source (when applicable) and patient name. Additionally, exact criteria should be delineated for specimen storage and preservation and for conditions during transportation and processing. Criteria for specimen acceptability and rejection should be specified and adhered to by the laboratory. For each test offered, the laboratory must be able to provide the appropriate collection materials and instructions together with adequate transport systems and suitable equipment to process and/or store the specimen (Fig. 24.1) (21).

It is the submitting laboratory's responsibility to make sure that the reference laboratory receiving the specimen is appropriately certified (30). When tests are to be referred to another laboratory, all pertinent information should still be provided to the clinician, including the destination of the referred specimen. Written instructions should be available for the client to be able to get additional assistance for unusual circumstances or special specimen handling situations. Standard texts for each laboratory specialty area are excellent sources for specifics along with package inserts for various testing kits and reagents. Special instructions and testing schedules can be obtained from the individual reference laboratories.

For quality improvement, the laboratory must document its policies and procedures for monitoring, assessing, and when necessary, correcting problems identified in specimen submission by clinicians. It must also document attempts to modify clinicians' ordering patterns or behavior when consistent problems in specimen submission occur.

BORDETELLA CULTURE (WHOOPING COUGH) [Includes *B. pertussis* and *B. parapertussis*]

Specimen: Submit 2 nasopharyngeal swabs in Regan Lowe transport media. Specimens should be stored refrigerated until and during transport to the laboratory. Other transport media are not suitable for maintaining the viability of pertussis organisms.

Method: Conventional culture

Setup: Monday through Sunday

Available: Negatives 7 days

CPT: 87081

Reference Ranges: None isolated

Note: Cultures are not useful in adults. Serologies or PCR studies should be considered. All positives are called upon isolation.

Collection: Use a mini-tipped culturette to collect 2 nasopharyngeal swabs. The swab is gently inserted through the nose to the posterior nasopharynx where it is gently rotated. It should remain in this position for several seconds. The withdrawal should be slow to minimize irritation. Place in Regan-Lowe Transport Media. Specimens should be stored refrigerated (2–8° C) until and during transport to the laboratory.

Figure 24.1 An example of information and instructions in a laboratory users' manual for collection and submission of specimens for evaluation of whooping cough.

Test Ordering

Test requests may be received in a variety of manners but must be in either written or electronic form and must originate from an authorized person. Such authorization is prescribed by state law and may vary from state to state. Oral requests for laboratory tests are acceptable if followed within 30 days by written orders (19). The laboratory must document its attempts to obtain written authorization in cases where oral requests are not followed by written ones in a timely fashion.

A thorough requisition enables the laboratorian to provide a higher caliber of service to the physician and patient. Timely, accurate, and relevant results are attained with a comprehensive form. Additionally, proper reimbursement is more likely. The form must be easy for the client to complete and must contain all information necessary for proper result interpretation. Phone calls to verify any missing or unclear data severely consume resources of both the laboratory and physician. Therefore, a considerable amount of time should be spent on requisition format and client education for usage.

The conventional multicopy paper request is most common when sending tests from one facility to another, but with today's connectivity, electronic requests are gaining popularity. Electronic requests are frequently utilized in hospital settings where the LIS is connected with either handheld devices or stationary terminals that the medical staff may make use of to order tests. At times, a physician will hand write the desired tests on a prescription pad (script) rather than use a requisition. This practice should be dissuaded, as multipart requisitions are preferred to scripts for a multitude of reasons.

In any laboratory setting, it is imperative to have a downtime procedure for occasions when the standard operating procedure cannot be followed, such as with electrical or computer outages.

Test requisition. Typically, a written or electronic requisition consists of a demographics section and a test section (Fig. 24.2). The general information needed for the demographic section of a test requisition is depicted in Table 24.6. Requisitions must include the patient's name or other unique identifier, as well as the name and address of the authorized person requesting the test (19). It is also recommended that a contact person and phone number be listed in case critical values are obtained.

All applicable diagnosis code(s) for the date of service should be indicated on the requisition. Diagnosis codes are typically referred to as International Classification of Diseases codes, which are published by the World Health Organization. These codes not only help interpret results but may also be required for reimbursement by third-party payors.

Evaluation of specimen stability depends on the date and time of specimen collection. Some demographics affect reference ranges in certain procedures, such as the patient's sex, date of birth, and fasting state. This information also ensures accurate patient identification for appropriate billing and charting of laboratory tests.

Billing information required would depend on the way the client has the account set up with the laboratory. The laboratory can bill the patient, a third-party payor, the client (the client can then bill the patient or his or her insurance provider), or a combination of payors. Thus,

the Social Security number, patient home address, and patient phone number may not be required if billing the client. Likewise, insurance information may not be necessary.

Laboratories often print the most common tests and their test codes in the test-request section of the requisition for user convenience. Not only specific tests but test panels can be preprinted on the requisition. However, due to compliance issues, it is the responsibility of the laboratory to educate the client that although there is a panel or test preprinted on the form, the option to order any profile or component separately is still available.

The test section should include an area to indicate the specimen site or source. This is especially true when handling anatomic pathology or microbiology specimens. In such situations, it is also imperative to know the type of procedure that was performed and the nature of the disease. For Pap smear testing, CLIA '88 requires that the patient's last menstrual period, age or date of birth, and indication whether the patient had a previous abnormal report, treatment, or biopsy be included.

Other information that should be included on a test requisition includes notation of any medications the patient may be on, symptoms or suspected diagnosis, antibiotic allergies (where pertinent), priority of testing (e.g., stat?), and copy-to instructions for additional reports where needed.

Advance beneficiary notice. The CMS developed a new advance beneficiary notice (ABN) form in 2002. The new ABN is intended to provide a standardized form that results in more effective communication to beneficiaries. For limited coverage laboratory tests that Medicare is expected to deny, an ABN must accompany the test request. Patients have the option to ask for an estimated cost and may decline testing if they choose (which is documented on the ABN). An ABN *does not* take the place of a test requisition.

Local Medicare carriers disseminate specific instructions on when and how to order screening tests. If these specific tests are ordered more than is medically necessary as indicated by CMS guidelines, the beneficiary may be held responsible for payment. However, the same test that is used for screening purposes may also be used as a diagnostic tool if specific symptoms or diseases are present. Medicare will cover this testing when the diagnosis code(s) provided supports the necessity requirements.

Table 24.6 Demographic information needed on test requisition[a]

Authorized person ordering test

Individual using test results (when appropriate)

Laboratory submitting specimen (with contact person for stats)

Patient name or unique identifier

Patient sex and age (or date of birth)

Source of specimen (if appropriate)

Time and date of collection of the specimen (as needed)

Patient's last menstrual period, and indication of whether patient had a previous abnormal report, treatment, or biopsy (for Pap smears only)

Additional information that may be needed in specific tests to ensure timely, accurate testing and reporting (with appropriate interpretation)

[a]From reference 19.

Postanalytic Activities

The postanalytic phase refers to all steps taken after actual testing is performed on a patient's specimen. It includes the reporting of test results, result archiving, and specimen and result storage, as well as assessment of all postanalytic activities (Table 24.7).

PLEASE PRINT CLEARLY ALL INFORMATION MUST BE PROVIDED OR CLIENT WILL BE BILLED. USE BLACK OR BLUE INK ONLY

			DATE COLLECTED
			☐ STAT
PATIENT'S LAST NAME	FIRST	MI	SEX	COLL TIME	Phone #:
			☐ M ☐ F	AM / PM	☐ FAX (verify #)
			DATE OF BIRTH		Fax #:

CLINICAL INFO.	CHART/ OTHER I.D.	FASTING	HRS. PP	URINE VOL. 24 HRS.	TIME OF COLL.
				ML.	HR.

PAT. SS#:	ORDERING PHYSICIAN: (FIRST & LAST NAME)	DIAGNOSIS CODE(S):

BILL: ☐ ACCOUNT COMPLETE YELLOW AREAS   ☐ PATIENT COMPLETE YELLOW & GREY AREAS   ☐ PAID AT PSC (RECEIPT ATTACHED)   ☐ INSURANCE (SEE CURRENT LIST) COMPLETE YELLOW, GREY & GREEN AREAS   FOR MEDICARE USE THE MEDICAL NECESSITY REQUISITION

RESPONSIBLE PARTY/INSURED:	INSURANCE COMPANY/UNDERWRITER/CARRIER:
ADDRESS:	CLAIMS ADDRESS:
CITY / STATE / ZIP CODE:	PT. RELATIONSHIP:	CITY / STATE / ZIP CODE:	EMPLOYER:
HOME PHONE NO.:	WORK PHONE NO.:	INSURANCE PLAN NAME/ADMINISTRATOR:	GROUP/PLAN #:
CARBON COPY TO INCLUDE NAME, ACCT. # AND ADDRESS:	INSURANCE I.D. #:

PLEASE CIRCLE DESIRED TEST(S) - ANY PROFILE COMPONENT MAY BE ORDERED SEPARATELY.

CHEMISTRY PANELS (See Back For Components)							
900320 Basic Metabolic Panel	XS	8015	Folate	SS	3305	Urogram	UT
900323 Comprehensive Metabolic Panel	XS	2021	Glucose, Fasting	SS	3300	Urogram w/Reflex to Microscopic	UT
31033 ChemPanel Basic (CPB)	XS	2329	Glucose, Random	SS	23305	Urogram w/Reflex to Culture	UT, GU
35811 ChemPanel Basic (CPB) + CBC w/Diff/Plt. (CBD)	LT, XS	9230	Hemoglobin A1c	LT	33305	Urogram w/Reflex to Culture (OB)	UT, GU
PANELS/PROFILES (See Back For Components)		9235	Hepatitis B Surface Ab (HBsAb)	SS	43305	Urogram w/Reflex to Microscopic &/or Culture	UT, GU
900616 Cystic Fibrosis DNA Screen w/Reflex	LT	8020	Hepatitis B Surface Ag (HBsAg)	SS	53305	Urogram w/Reflex to Microscopic &/or Culture (OB)	UT, GU
102455 Electrolyte Panel	XS	8587	Hepatitis C Ab	SS	8060	Vitamin B-12	SS
900313 Hepatic Function Panel (Liver)	SS	3682	HIV-1 Ab Screen w/Western Blot Reflex	SS	**MICROBIOLOGY (*=ID & SENSITIVITY IF INDICATED)**		
104750 Hepatitis Panel, Acute	SS	2038	Iron	SS	4704	Culture, Group **A** Strep, Site:	
2040 Iron & TIBC	SS	2120	Lithium	RT	4615	Culture, Group **B** Strep Site:	
1877 Lipid Panel	SS	4034	Occult Blood x3 **Diagnostic**		4703	Culture, Stool* Includes Salm/Shig/Campy	
1424 Liver Profile	SS	13223	Occult Blood x3 **Screen**		704705	Culture, Urine*	
1914 Obstetric Panel w/Reflex	ISS, 2LT	8025	Pregnancy, Qualitative, Serum		700399	Chlamydia, Amplified Probe. Endocerv, M Urethral, Urine Only	
38055 TSH w/Reflex to Free T4	SS	8030	Pregnancy, Quantitative, Serum	SS	900400	GC, Amplified Probe, Endocerv, M Urethral, Urine Only	
INDIVIDUAL TESTS		8501	Prostate Specific Antigen (PSA) **Diagnostic**	SS	900398	GC/Chlamydia, Amplified Probe, Endocerv, M Urethral, Urine Only	
2012 Amylase	SS	10157	Prostate Specific Antigen (PSA) **Screen**	SS	5150	Chlamydia, Direct Probe. Endocerv or M Urethral Only	
2920 ANA Screen w/Reflex to Titer	SS	3500	Prothrombin Time (INR)	BT	5152	GC, Direct Probe, Endocerv or M Urethral Only	
3005 Hemogram (CBC w/o Diff w/Plt.)	LT	3505	PTT (BT stable 24 hours)	FP	5154	GC/Chlamydia, Direct Probe, Endocerv or M Urethral Only	
3000 Complete Blood Count w/Diff/Plt. (CBD)	LT	5376	RPR w/Reflex to Titer	SS	**Routine/Aerobic Culture* (Enter Site & Circle for Culture)**		
8599 CEA	SS	1054	RPR w/Reflex to Titer & FTA Abs	SS			
1014 Creatinine	SS	3105	Sedimentation Rate (Westergren)	LT	Site:		
90045 CRP, High Sensitivity	SS	8040	T3 Uptake	SS	**VIROLOGY - COMPLETE VIROLOGY INFO. SHEET**		
8010 Digoxin	RT	8045	T4 (Thyroxine)	SS	Test Code from back of requisition is required		
9201 Estradiol	SS	8899	T4, Free	SS	Test Code:		
9215 Follicle Stimulating Hormone	SS	8055	Thyroid Stimulating Hormone (TSH)	SS			
		800411	Urinalysis, **Diabetic** (Urogram + Microscopic w/rflx)	2UT	Source:		

Q1553 (4/03)

DRAW FEE ☐   GENERAL REQUISITION LAB COPY

Figure 24.2 Sample of a hard-copy requisition.

Table 24.7 Quality assessment of postanalytic systems should include review or evaluation of the following areas[a]

Effectiveness of corrective actions
Procedures and policies to prevent recurrences
Accuracy and completeness of test results and reports
Disposition of unacceptable specimens
Turnaround times
Referral specimens and their reports
Corrected reports
Procedures for notification of test results, including stats
For analyte-specific reagents, test reports should include information necessary for proper interpretation of results, including disclaimers as needed
Assurance of confidentiality of patient information

[a]From references 11 and 19.

The Report

The laboratory must release results only to authorized persons or the individual responsible for utilizing the test results. The reports can be sent to the authorized persons through a variety of means, including verbal, written, or electronic. Clear processes must be in place to allow timely reporting of preliminary, interim or final reports. Written procedures for reporting of results exceeding normal values (stat or critical values) must be published, clearly understood, and followed by laboratory personnel. Any such reporting must have documentation of when, where, to whom, and what was reported.

Report turnaround time. The clinician should have available to him or her the expected turnaround time for a report to be generated from the time the specimen is collected. It is the laboratory's responsibility not only to make available turnaround time information for all tests but also to periodically monitor this to ascertain that reports are going out in a timely fashion and that there are no problems in the process. Corrective action must be documented if excessive turnaround time is noted. If any delay occurs beyond the expected turnaround time for any test, the laboratory must have a process in place to notify the clinician of the status of the specimen.

Types of reports. The main means used for reporting are standard paper reports, electronic medical records (EMR), and web-based reports. The standard paper report will likely survive for an extended period of time, since backup systems may be required during electronic downtimes. With the EMR, laboratory data are transmitted to the hospital information computer system and are integrated with patient demographic information, providing integrated reports for in-house patients. When available, web-based reports have the advantage of multiple access points, and clinicians can access them from any Internet connection. Web-based and EMR reports must be validated initially and periodically to verify that the information transmitted is being translated accurately and correctly.

Result format. The standard test report must include the name and address of the laboratory at which the test was performed, the test that was performed, the test results (including the unit of measurement, if applicable), any information regarding the condition and disposition of specimens that do not meet the laboratory's criteria for acceptability, and the laboratory's reference or normal range for the test. If the latter is not included on the report, it must be available to the authorized person who ordered the test or to the person responsible for utilizing test results.

It is also the responsibility of the laboratory to make available to clients a list of test methodologies, including any information regarding interpretation of test results. Any changes to this testing information that would affect results or interpretation of results must be communicated to physicians. For tests using "analyte-specific reagents" not FDA-approved for use on patients, disclaimers must be added to reports reflecting such investigational use. The disclaimer statement should read, "This test was developed and its performance characteristics determined by (Laboratory Name). It has not been cleared or approved by the U.S. Food and Drug Administration."

"Value-added" textual comments can be added to reports to help the clinician interpret results or better understand how to use the result appropriately (Table 24.8) (33).

The reports should be easy to read, unambiguous, readily interpretable, and use standard terminologies. Heffner and Adair studied a variety of surgical pathology reports and found that subtle nuances in wording of the diagnosis and comment lines could be significant if misinterpreted (20). They stressed using redundancy (restating what might seem obvious), avoiding certain ambiguous words, and enlarging on details if necessary.

Quality assessment and corrected reports. The laboratory must have a process in place to monitor and evaluate its test results and reports for inconsistencies and inaccuracies. Such evaluation must include a review of patient test reports for completeness of patient information, accuracy of test results, normal ranges, correlation between test results, validation of LIS reports to verify accurate transmission and/or transcription, and review of corrected reports (19). There must be a mechanism for correcting an erroneous report and indicating the new report as one that is corrected, while maintaining both reports in the patient's record.

Storage and Retention

Regulatory constraints require that the laboratory have processes and procedures for the retention and storage of specimens and records. Storage regulations may differ

Table 24.8 Sample list of textual "value-added" comments attached to specific laboratory reports.

- Extended-spectrum β-lactamase-producing isolate. Such isolates may be clinically resistant to therapy with most penicillins, cephalosporins, and aztreonam, despite showing in vitro susceptibility. The activities of aminoglycosides, imipenem, cefoxitin, and cefotetan are often retained. Call Microbiology with any questions.
- Antibodies to cardiolipin have been found in a subgroup of patients with autoimmune disorders as well as in some patients with myocardial infarction and acute and other infections, including syphilis and AIDS.
- Immunoglobulin G (IgG) and IgA cardiolipin antibodies have been associated with thrombocytopenia, arterial and venous thrombosis, and recurrent fetal loss, with the predictive value and specificity increasing with the level of cardiolipin antibodies.
- IgM cardiolipin antibody is predominantly found in association with infections, unless a lupus anticoagulant is also present.
- Methicillin (penicillinase-R-penicillin) resistance in *Staphylococcus* species infers resistance to all other penicillins, β-lactamase inhibitor combinations, cephalosporins, and imipenem.
- Additionally, 10 or more percent of clindamycin-susceptible/erythromycin-resistant strains of methicillin-resistant *Staphylococcus aureus* or *S. epidermidis* may convert to clindamycin resistance while on clindamycin therapy. Please call Microbiology if you have any questions or if clindamycin is a primary consideration for therapy.
- In addition to congenital protein C deficiency, decreased protein C activity can be seen in association with vitamin K deficiency, severe liver disease, nephrotic syndrome, disseminated intravascular coagulation, and other disease states in which consumption is increased. Decreased protein C activity is also seen in patients on warfarin therapy or oral contraceptives.
- A low ratio is indicative of activated protein C resistance due to a factor V gene mutation. This could be confirmed by ordering a factor V Leiden (PCR) assay.

between the various agencies. Individual state laws are typically more stringent than those of the federal government or other agencies. In any case, the laboratory should follow the more stringent regulations.

Specimens. A sample list of how long specimens have to be stored is given in Table 24.9 (36). A procedure should be in place for their retention based on the most stringent regulatory requirements for the individual laboratory.

Records. Typically, test requisitions and reports must be stored in a retrievable fashion for a minimum of 2 years. Some records, especially in areas of immunohematology (5 years), histocompatibility (5 years), histology (10 years), cytology (10 years), bone marrow (10 years), and cytogenetics (25 years), may require longer retention periods (36). In this litigious era, many laboratories are opting to hold records and documents for longer periods of time. Record retention is made easier if electronic copies are used.

Assessment of Test Results on Patient Outcomes

The science of outcomes analysis has been in common use by physician, nursing, and pharmacy staff for many years. However, only recently has it gained importance in the laboratory as regulatory agencies focus on laboratory-associated patient safety and outcome issues (49). In its 1996 *Comprehensive Accreditation Manual for Pathology and Laboratory Services*, JCAHO defined quality to include outcomes: "the degree to which patient care services increase the probability of desired patient outcomes and reduce the probability of undesired outcomes, given the current state of knowledge" (24).

Generally, measurable outcomes are defined in two areas: clinical and financial. Clinical patient outcomes, as a result of medical care, relate to the patient's functional status, health status, and quality of life (6). Measures that are often used for outcomes are familiar to those in the hospital setting: length of stay, mortality, morbidity, infection rate, complication rate, readmission rate, and others. Case management or quality management departments are good sources of quality indicators and measures of performance typically used across institutions and within their statistical analyses. Financial outcomes may concern costs to the patient, a particular department within the healthcare institution, the institution itself, the insurer, or even society at large. One author suggests that all tests currently offered by the laboratory need clinical trials with outcome result studies to show whether they are valid or not (32).

Outcome studies may take a narrower perspective in the laboratory. In simpler terms, the question may be

Table 24.9 Example of specimen retention requirements by regulatory agency

Specimen	Retention period required by:		
	CAP	**CLIA**	**JCAHO**
Body fluids, cerebrospinal fluid, serum	24 h		
Bone marrow smears	10 yr	20 yr	
Fine needle aspirates	10 yr		
Histology slides			10 yr
Negative or unsatisfactory cytology slides	5 yr	5 yr	5 yr
Normal blood films, body fluid slides	7 days		
Paraffin blocks	5 yr	2 yr	2 yr
Positive/questionable cytology slides	5 yr	10 yr	5 yr
Wet and formalin-fixed tissue	2 wk		7 days

posed: When the laboratory reports in a specific way a specific result for a specific patient for a particular test, what is the clinician response and subsequent change (if any) in patient management? Actions taken from the more limited focus will, of course, have an effect on the larger measures described above. It may be said that the only true assessment of the quality of laboratory testing is reflected by the quality of patient outcomes (38). The laboratory must come to be seen as playing an integral role in patient management rather than be viewed as an "ancillary" department. Ultimately, various studies may lead to new roles for the clinical laboratory (6).

As with test evaluation, ideas for outcome studies may arise from technical coordinators, technical specialists, bench technologists, technical directors, or laboratory or department directors. They may be pursuant to articles from the literature, discoveries made during annual budget review, or subsequent to discussion with a clinician or other staff. Many good studies focus on a targeted clinical service, such as pharmacy (49). A multidisciplinary team is usually needed to gather all necessary information and complete the analysis. The team may include as needed, but is not limited to, nursing, pharmacy, case management, laboratory, epidemiology or infection control, clinical specialists, statisticians, information technology, medical records, and the finance and legal departments. Data may be derived from medical records, the LIS, the pharmacy information system billing/charge databases, patient account databases, quality improvement studies, and satisfaction survey systems. Generally, information systems are used as well in radiology, respiratory care, dietary, operating room, and other departments and can assist greatly in studies.

For example, Barenfanger et al. sought to examine the impact of a program used to improve interventions involving antibiotic therapy (4). Comparison was made of the manual, paper-based method of pharmacy review with a system using a computer software program that linked immediately to the pharmacy in cases of alerts for possible intervention. Alerts could show patients with a bacterial isolate and no order for antimicrobial therapy, patients with a bacterial isolate resistant to their current therapy, patients receiving a therapy not tested, or patients with no cultures collected but who were receiving antimicrobial therapy. For the group of patients with alerts generated by the computer software program, the physician received more rapid notification of the information in the intervention. Analysis showed that this group had significant differences in lengths of stay, total costs, variable costs, and radiology costs.

Other institutions have had success with comparable programs (16, 46). Some laboratories may have sophisticated algorithms available to search for, among other situations, suboptimal therapy or use of intravenous antimicrobials when an oral agent might be substituted. These systems can provide savings by keeping antibiotic costs down but, more importantly, have been shown to reduce length of stay, days of intubation, number of subsequent laboratory and radiology tests, and days in intensive care for many patients (3). In almost all instances, multidisciplinary teams oversee interference or outcome evaluation programs.

In a second example, Kollef and Ward worked with the microbiology department in a study involving intensive care unit patients who were mechanically ventilated (27). Ventilator-associated pneumonia (VAP) can be a significant factor in the mortality of critically ill patients. By collecting mini-bronchoalveolar lavage cultures, they hoped to determine the best strategies for administration of antibiotics to improve outcomes of the patients with VAP. From their data, they were able to confirm the findings of earlier investigators and develop recommendations for the empiric treatment of VAP.

The CAP has developed a series of patient outcome templates, an education-based information tool set to assist member pathologists in setting up outcome measurement studies at their institutions (9). Each template set contains several modules: a set of text pages reviewing a particular disease, references, a table of applicable indicators for outcome measures, and a PowerPoint slide presentation with tables, charts, and cost saving models. For example, one template works with the underutilization of lipid analysis in identifying patients at risk for coronary artery disease. Additional tools such as these templates will be emerging as laboratories become more routinely involved in patient outcomes.

Summary

The clinical laboratory has an expanding role in today's healthcare setting. It must, first and foremost, provide accurate, timely, quality-minded, and appropriate analytic testing to help clinicians diagnose and manage medical conditions in patients. It must also recognize its responsibility to provide the overall guidance for appropriate test utilization and result interpretation and to assess the impact of its results on patient outcomes. As such, the laboratory is becoming more of a team player and participant in overall patient management. To fulfill its role adequately, it is imperative for the laboratory to outline, measure, and document the processes needed for all phases of work and to be especially cognizant of the crucial role of preanalytic and postanalytic activities in the provision and application of its accurate, quality-assured, and cost-effective end products.

KEY POINTS

- Preanalytic activities include, but are not limited to, test selection, implementation, appropriate utilization, and ordering, as well as to specimen collection, transport, and storage.

- Postanalytic activities include, but are not limited to, reporting of results, storage and retention of specimens and information, and assessment of effect of test results on patient outcomes.

- Preanalytic and postanalytic activities are crucial to accurate laboratory results and to their appropriate interpretation for patient care.

- The role of the clinical laboratory includes assessment of the effect of its results on patient care and outcomes.

GLOSSARY

Analytic activity Pertaining to actual performance of test procedure on a specimen.

Centers for Medicare and Medicaid Services (CMS) Primary federal body responsible for the oversight of clinical laboratory activity and licensure. Previously called Health Care Financing Administration.

Clinical Laboratory Improvement Act Amendments of 1988 (CLIA '88) Passed by Congress in 1988 to establish quality standards for laboratory testing and to ensure the accuracy, reliability, and timeliness of patient test results. Laboratory tests were categorized as being waived, of moderate complexity, or of high complexity. Laboratories performing tests in the latter two categories had to register and comply with a set of regulatory rules to become certified (licensed). In 2003, a Final Rule was issued in the Federal Register that defined some new regulations and changed the categorization of tests into two categories (waived and nonwaived tests).

Current procedural code (CPT-4) Test codes recognized by the American Medical Association and required for filing claims and billing of Medicare.

Food and Drug Administration (FDA) Federal agency responsible for the oversight of commercial tests and for their approval and licensure for use in clinical health laboratories.

Negative predictive value Probability that a negative result indicates absence of disease.

Pareto principle (80/20 rule) Used in many industries; states that 80% of an entity's total revenues are produced by 20% of its products (35).

Path of workflow Combined sequential activities in the laboratory, beginning with the clinician's ability to order a test and culminating in data being generated and reported for use in patient care.

Positive predictive value Probability that a positive result indicates presence of disease.

Postanalytic activity Pertaining to period after the actual testing of specimen. Includes phases such as reporting of results, storage and retention of specimens and data, and assessment of effect of results on patient outcomes.

Preanalytic activity Pertaining to period prior to actual testing of specimen. Includes phases such as test selection and implementation, appropriate test utilization, and specimen collection, transport, and storage, as well as test ordering.

Procedure A prescribed way to carry out an activity.

Process Systematic course of definitive actions or activities culminating in a desired end product.

Sensitivity Ability of test to detect a condition ([number with condition testing positive/number having the condition who are tested] $\times$ 100 = percent sensitivity).

Specificity Ability of test to define a true condition ([number without condition testing negative/total number without condition who are tested] $\times$ 100 = percent specificity).

REFERENCES

1. **Bailey, M. K., L. Blacklidge, C. M. Day, L. S. Garcia, D. Parks, and T. Street.** 1994. Keep tests in or send them out? *Med. Lab. Obs.* **26:**46–47.

2. **Bailey, M. K., L. Blacklidge, C. M. Day, L. S. Garcia, D. Parks, and T. Street.** 1995. How to curb physicians' excessive testing. *Med. Lab. Obs.* **27:**69.

3. **Barenfanger, J.** 2001. Clinical microbiology laboratories can directly benefit patients. *ASM News* **67:**71–77.

4. **Barenfanger, J., M. A. Short, and A. A. Groesch.** 2001. Improved antimicrobial interventions have benefits. *J. Clin. Microbiol.* **39:**2823–2828.

5. **Baron, E. J.** 1996. Development in laboratory informatics. *Clin. Microbiol. Newsl.* **18:**65–70.

6. **Bissell, M. G.** 2000. Introduction: what's in a laboratory outcome?, p. 3–10. *In* M. G. Bissell (ed.), *Laboratory-Related Measures of Patient Outcomes: an Introduction.* American Association for Clinical Chemistry Press, Washington, D.C.

7. **Cannon, B., and M. Lee.** 1996. Clinical laboratory tests: application to daily practice. *J. Am. Pharm. Assoc.* **NS36:**668–679.

8. **Chassin, M. R.** 1996. Quality of healthcare part 3: improving the quality of care. *N. Engl. J. Med.* **335:**1060–1062.

9. **College of American Pathologists.** 2002. Education: CAP Patient Outcome Templates. [Online.] http://www.cap.org/html/member/secure/education/pot/outcome.cfm. (Accessed 9/24/02.)

10. **DeKay, M. L., and D. A. Asch.** 1998. Is the defensive use of diagnostic tests good for patients, or bad? *Med. Decis. Making* **18:**19–27.

11. **Department of Health and Human Services.** 2003. Medicare, Medicaid and CLIA programs: laboratory requirements relating to quality systems and certain personnel qualifications. *Fed. Regist.* **68:**3639–3371.

12. **Elder, B. L., S. A. Hansen, J. A. Kellogg, F. J. Marsik, and R. J. Zabransky.** 1997. *Cumitech 31, Verification and Validation of Procedures in the Clinical Microbiology Laboratory.* Coordinating ed., B. W. McCurdy. ASM Press, Washington, D.C.

13. **Epstein, A. M., and B. J. McNeil.** 1986. Relationship of beliefs and behavior in test ordering. *Am. J. Med.* **80:**865–870.

14. **Fischbach, F.** 2000. *A Manual of Laboratory and Diagnostic Tests,* 6th ed., p. 1–33. Lippincott Williams & Wilkins, Philadelphia, Pa.

15. **Garcia, L. S., G. W. Procop, G. D. Roberts, and R. B. Thomson.** 1998. Selection of diagnostic tests, p. 60–63. *In* B. A. Forbes, D. F. Sahm, and A. S. Weissfeld (ed.), *Bailey & Scott's Diagnostic Microbiology.* Mosby, Inc., St. Louis, Mo.

16. **Gums, J. G., R. W. Yancey, Jr., C. A. Hamilton, and P. S. Kubilis.** 1999. A randomized, prospective study measuring outcomes after antibiotic therapy intervention by a multidisciplinary consult team. *Pharmacotherapy* **19:**1369–1377.

17. **Halsey, J. F.** 2000. Direct access testing in the clinical laboratory: should laboratories offer testing services directly to the consumer? *Clin. Leadersh. Manag. Rev.* **14:**261–266.

18. **Hawkins, H. H., R. W. Hankins, and E. Johnson.** 1999. A computerized physician order entry system for the promotion of ordering compliance and appropriate test utilization. *J. Healthc. Inf. Manag.* **13:**63–72.

19. **Health Care Financing Administration.** 1992. Medicare, Medicaid, and CLIA programs. Regulations implementing the Clinical Laboratory Improvement Amendments of 1988 (CLIA). *Fed. Regist.* **57:**7002–7186.

20. **Heffner, D. K., and C. F. Adair.** 1999. Clarity on the diagnosis line (the devil is in the details). *Ann. Diagn. Pathol.* **3:**187–191.

21. **Howanitz, J. H., and P. J. Howanitz.** 1991. Principles of laboratory medicine, p. 1–10. *In* J. H. Howanitz and P. J. Howanitz (ed.), *Laboratory Medicine: Test Selection and Interpretation.* Churchill Livingston Inc., New York, N.Y.

22. **Jacobs, I. A., K. Kelly, C. Valenziano, A. H. Chevinsky, J. Pawar, and C. Jones.** 2000. Cost savings associated with changes in routine laboratory tests ordered for victims of trauma. *Am. Surg.* **66:**579–584.

23. **Joint Commission on Accreditation of Healthcare Organizations.** 1990. *Accreditation Manual of Hospitals,* p. 137–138. Joint Commission on Accreditation of Healthcare Organizations, Chicago, Ill.

24. **Joint Commission on Accreditation of Healthcare Organizations.** 1996. *Comprehensive Accreditation Manual for Pathology and Laboratory Services.* Joint Commission on Accreditation of Healthcare Organizations, Oakbrook Terrace, Ill.

25. **Kazmierczak, S. C.** 1999. Statistical techniques for evaluating the diagnostic utility of laboratory tests. *Clin. Chem. Lab. Med.* **37:**1001–1009.

26. **Kilgore, M., L. Hensley, C. Howard, J. Craft, and J. A. Smith.** 1999. Curbing overutilization: the silver lining to HCFA compliance. *Med. Lab. Obs.* **31:**26–28.

27. **Kollef, M. H., and S. Ward.** 1998. The influence of mini-BAL cultures on patient outcomes: implications for the antibiotic management of ventilator-associated pneumonia. *Chest* **113:**412–420.

28. **Labeau, K. M., M. Simon, and S. J. Steindel.** Clinical laboratory test menu changes in the Pacific Northwest: an evaluation of the dynamics of change. *Clin. Leadersh. Manag. Rev.* **15:**16–22.

29. **LaRocco, M.** 1995. Quality and productivity in the microbiology laboratory: continuous quality improvement. *Clin. Microbiol. Newsl.* **17:**129–131.

30. **Lewandrowski, K., and D. MacMillan.** 2003. Selection of a clinical reference laboratory: general principles and some observations from Massachusetts General Hospital. *Clin. Microbiol. Newsl.* **25:**33–37.

31. **Linehan, B. J., M. M. El-Nageh, S. Cordner, and A. Richter.** 2002. Ethics in laboratory medicine, p. 134–142. *In* K. D. McClatchey (ed.), *Clinical Laboratory Medicine,* 2nd ed. Lippincott Williams & Wilkins, Philadelphia, Pa.

32. **Lundberg, G. D.** 1999. How clinicians should use the diagnostic laboratory in a changing medical world. *Clin. Chem. Acta* **280:**3–11.

33. **Marcon, M. J.** 2003. "Value-added" reporting in clinical microbiology: using computer-based textual reports and comments as an aid to communicating appropriate utilization and application of test results. *Clin. Microbiol. Newsl.* **25:**25–31.

34. **Mayer, M.** 1991. Unnecessary laboratory tests in diagnosis and treatment. *Harefuah* **120:**66–69.

35. **NCCLS.** 1998. *Basic Cost Accounting for Clinical Services; Approved Guideline.* NCCLS document GP11-A. NCCLS, Wayne, Pa.

36. **NCCLS.** 2003. *Application of a Quality System Model for Laboratory Services; Approved Guideline,* 2nd ed. NCCLS document GP26-A2. NCCLS, Wayne, Pa.

37. **Nicoll, C. D., and M. Pignone.** 2002. Diagnostic testing and medical decision making, p. 1669–1680. *In* L. M. Tierney, Jr., S. J. McPhee, and M. A. Papadakis (ed.), *2002 Current Medical Diagnosis & Treatment,* 41st ed. Lange Medical Books/McGraw Hill, New York, N.Y.

38. **Plebani, M.** 1999. The changing face of clinical laboratories. *Clin. Chem. Lab. Med.* **37:**711–717.

39. **Rodriguez, F.** 1996. Improve microbiology procedures and utilization while saving money. *Med. Lab. Obs.* **28:**60–64.

40. **Ruangkanchanasetr, S.** 1993. Laboratory investigation utilization in pediatric out-patient department Ramathibodi Hospital. *J. Med. Assoc. Thai.* **76**(Suppl 2)**:**194–208.

41. **Schubart, J. R., C. E. Fowler, G. R. Donowitz, and A. F. Connors, Jr.** 2001. Algorithm-based decision rules to safely reduce laboratory test ordering. *Medinfo* **10:**523–527.

42. **Sewell, D., and J. D. MacLowry.** 1999. Laboratory management, p. 4–22. *In* P. R. Murray, E. J. Baron, M. A. Pfaller, F. C. Tenover, and R. H. Yolken (ed.), *Manual of Clinical Microbiology,* 7th ed. ASM Press, Washington, D.C.

43. **Shimetani, N.** 1998. Consultation on laboratory information—from the perspectives of clinical pathologists and medical technologists. *Rinsho Byori* **46:**987–993.

44. **Silverstein, J. C., and A. S. Rothschild.** 1999. Clinical perspectives on the modern laboratory. *Clin. Lab. Med.* **19:**421–432.

45. **Silverstein, M. D.** 2000. Laboratory tests for case-finding and screening for disease in the ambulatory setting, p. 129–146. *In* M. G. Bissell (ed.), *Laboratory-Related Measures of Patient Outcomes: an Introduction.* American Association for Clinical Chemistry Press, Washington, D.C.

46. **Southwick, K.** 2002. Antibiotic alert—labs, pharmacies take on cost and misuse. *CAP Today* **16:**62–71.

47. **Statland, B. E.** 1994. Cost/benefit of screening. *Med. Lab. Obs.* **26:**11.

48. **Studnicki, J., D. D. Bradham, J. Marshburn, P. R. Foulis, and J. V. Straumfjord.** 1993. A feedback system for reducing excessive laboratory tests. *Arch. Pathol. Lab. Med.* **117:**35–39.

49. **Thomas, J. G.** 2000. Outcomes assessment: empowerment for microbiologists. *Adv. Lab.* **9:**54–60.

50. **Toubert, M. E., S. Chevret, B. Cassinat, M. H. Schlageter, J. P. Beressi, and J. D. Rain.** 2000. From guidelines to hospital practice: reducing inappropriate ordering of thyroid hormone and antibody tests. *Eur. J. Endocrinol.* **142:**605–610.

51. **Travers, E. M.** 2002. Business management of the clinical laboratory, p. 49–77. *In* K. D. McClatchey (ed.), *Clinical Laboratory Medicine,* 2nd ed. Lippincott Williams & Wilkins, Philadelphia, Pa.

52. **Travers, E. M., and K. D. McClatchey.** 2002. Basic laboratory management, p. 3–48. *In* K. D. McClatchey (ed.), *Clinical Laboratory Medicine,* 2nd ed. Lippincott Williams & Wilkins, Philadelphia, Pa.

53. **Valenstein, P., M. Pfaller, and M. Yungbluth.** 1996. The use and abuse of routine stool microbiology: a College of American Pathologists Q-probes study of 601 institutions. *Arch. Pathol. Lab. Med.* **120:**206–211.

54. **Winkens, R. A. G., P. Pop, A. M. A. Bugter-Maessen, R. P. T. M. Grol, A. D. M. Kester, G. H. M. I. Beusmans, J. A. Knottnerus.** 1995. Randomised controlled trial of routine individual feedback to improve rationality and reduce numbers of test requests. *Lancet* **345:**498–502.

55. **Wong, E. T.** 1985. Cost-effective use of laboratory tests: a joint responsibility of clinicians and laboratorians. *Clin. Lab. Med.* **5:**665–672.

25

Selection and Implementation of New Equipment and Procedures

Daniel D. Bankson

OBJECTIVES

To list the factors used to select new laboratory equipment and procedures

To review the need for input on the selection of procedures and instrumentation from multidisciplinary committees

To describe the selection criteria used to evaluate laboratory equipment

To describe the components of the decision process used to select instrumentation

> *GainManagement has three major elements: GainPlanning, GainMaking, and GainSharing. GainPlanning is the work managers do to lead and focus the organization on continuous gains and to organize for a high level of employee involvement. GainMaking is the involvement of all employees in a structured process for making continuous performance improvements. Then, as performance improves, everyone associated with the organization shares in the gains, which is GainSharing.*
>
> BOB AND PAUL DOYLE (5)

CONTINUOUS IMPROVEMENT or the achievement of gains in objective measures is a high priority for clinical, research, and industrial laboratory operations. Managing the gains in a laboratory operation, or "GainManagement" (see epigraph), consists of sequential involvement in "GainPlanning," "GainMaking," and "GainSharing" (5). Laboratory managers can customize these terms by substituting the word "Lab" for the word "Gain." The new compound words, "LabPlanning," "LabMaking," and "LabSharing," refer to all processes in the laboratory, including the selection of new equipment and procedures.

Nontechnical and especially human resource variables influence many of the good technical upgrades that laboratorians seek for their laboratories. In addition to the obvious technology-associated information, managers must ask questions that take them beyond their traditional areas of expertise. During the ongoing LabPlanning stages, laboratory managers will need to consult with specialists or learn new skills on the job or through course work. There are many useful resources, including textbooks with general management information applicable to all businesses (6) or specific management texts for laboratory professionals (19, 22).

Because people are running the equipment and directing the laboratory operation, good overall laboratory management includes setting high standards for hiring the best staff, providing for their ongoing training, and creating a desirable work environment. GainMaking or LabMaking utilizes the most precious laboratory resource, its employees, in a structured program of continuous performance improvement. Equipment procurement and procedural changes are ideal areas in which to include staff. The gains achieved by the laboratory in terms of efficiency and cost savings are a source of workplace pride. In addition, laboratory managers who recognize achievements and contributions through objective rewards and incentives create a superior workplace. GainSharing or LabSharing includes not only the distribution of financial gains with coworkers but also the sharing of information, such as the process of selecting and bringing on-line new equipment and methods. Effective communication and presentation skills, used during the process to obtain equipment and later to promote and educate staff, are important for the laboratory manager or "change agent." The acceptance and placement of the new analyzer are followed by the final evaluation steps and the promotion and marketing of new procedures to customers who order testing.

Like equipment decisions, the selection and implementation of new procedures (assays or methods) are critical to the clinical laboratory. Frequently, however, bringing on-line new procedures is dependent upon the already-installed laboratory equipment. This dependency makes knowing a specific analyzer's assay menu and characteristics very important before the laboratory contracts to use the equipment. Selecting new analyzers and procedures is critical to the laboratory remaining relevant and competitive. The stimulus for obtaining new technology and anticipated improvements derives from the hope of achieving decreased labor needs, decreased costs, faster generation of test results, and increased laboratory revenue. Financial success, for the individual laboratory or larger parent organization, directly relates to these decisions. Key indicators of a good operation, discussed in other chapters, are not limited to positive cash flows, financial ratios (e.g., return on investment), or simply staying within a set budget (4, 8, 18). The best laboratory equipment and procedures in the healthcare setting contribute to earlier disease diagnosis, decreased morbidity, decreased lengths of stay, and decreased mortality.

A laboratory manager must balance his or her time between the critical detailed issues and the big-picture direction of the clinical laboratory. Laboratory managers must take responsibility to remain knowledgeable about new technologies and equipment. Technological advances are numerous and include quick-spin centrifuges, robotic specimen transporters, total laboratory automation, and pneumatic tube systems. Other newly marketed products and procedures attract attention, such as modular equipment, reflexive testing algorithms, specimen integrity checks (lipemia, icterus, hemolysis, clots, etc.), updated safety features, sample buffering areas and integrated refrigerated storage, interfacing with front-end sample processing systems (that may include bar code generation of daughter pour-off tubes), centrifugation, decapping, sample pipetting, and transport to specific locations in multipurpose equipment racks. The "lab-on-a-chip" is moving from concept to reality.

As a laboratory manager learns about these technological advances, his or her goal is to investigate the feasibility of integrating them into the clinical laboratory operation. The first question to ask may be if there is market for the product. This and other questions should be an integral part of deciding whether to select a new technology. If a laboratory is at the leading edge of using a new technology, does it gain a competitive advantage over other local laboratories, or does it risk using a product that may fail in the marketplace?

Just Do It

The phrase "Just do it" not only is an important slogan for Nike but also is applicable to the laboratory and the equipment/technology procurement process (15). In the context of equipment procurement, "Just do it" encourages taking responsibility for the process, planning the steps, proceeding with the timeline, making commitments and decisions despite outside distractions, and behaving honorably toward other participants. The absolute final stage is communication to staff, customers (typically via newsletters, website postings, or e-mail), and clinicians at medical center events.

Creating Multiskilled Decision Makers

Laboratory managers develop skills at selecting the appropriate equipment largely through on-the-job experience. The foundation for managing a clinical laboratory operation, however, starts with training, certification, and credentialing programs. Programs in a number of disciplines related to medical technology, clinical chemistry, microbiology, and laboratory medicine expose trainees to the practicalities of managing a laboratory section or even an entire clinical laboratory. Further evidence of mastery can come from certification. For example, the American Society for Clinical Pathology offers a Diplomate in Laboratory Management certification. The recipe for making the ideal lab manager/equipment decision maker would include the addition of portions of scientist (computer, chemist, pathologist, etc.), architect, negotiator, change agent, accountant (managerial and financial), politician, mentor, and coach. Other important skills and attributes include being humble, realistic, focused on the present deliverables, and customer service oriented (10). The decision maker, even one possessing multiple skills, will have trouble, consciously or unconsciously, eliminating his or her own biases. The formation of committees helps to avoid these individual biases.

Committee-Directed Decision Making

New Equipment

The selection of new laboratory equipment frequently requires an oversight committee or laboratory advisory board or council (LAB) (Table 25.1) to provide the final approval. Depending on the institution, there may be a need for maintaining confidentiality during the procurement process. Figure 25.1 shows an example of a certification document signed by all members of the technical evaluation committee (TEC). Equipment selection may occur through a process of voting on recommendations that come from the TEC (Table 25.1). It is much less common to form committees tasked with making decisions on adopting new analytical methods. For low-cost equipment, say, less than $10,000, the recommendation to obtain the new system usually comes from the specific department head rather than a committee. Organizations are moving to incorporate technology and equipment assessment into the capital budgeting process (7, 21, 23). This is important because the final level of equipment decision making typically involves senior managers, and possibly clinicians, who may not be familiar with the technology under consideration. Figure 25.2 reviews one paradigm for how technology assessment interfaces with capital budgeting. The traditional procedure of purchasing new equipment involves developing a budget, accepting requests, voting on and prioritizing the requests, and purchasing the highest-priority items allowed by the budget. Unless there is an urgent need, equipment procurement commonly occurs on an annual cycle, taking as long as a year from the time of the initial request. The long delay is due to annual budgets and a higher-level LAB review of the TEC recommendations. To try to make better decisions, research on new equipment helps to document the current state of the laboratory and provide justification for acquisitions (Fig. 25.2). Without strong justification, the laboratory will be less competitive against capital equipment requests made by other groups. In contrast, equipment placement via operating leases, financial leases, renting, and reagent rental (using cost-per-test or cost-per-reportable-result programs) may be set up over a few months. In both leasing and purchasing situations, it is useful to compare costs of the former with costs of the latter (20).

Previously Owned Equipment

Because the cost of new equipment is so high, many laboratories consider obtaining used, or previously owned, equipment, either remanufactured, refurbished, reconditioned, or repossessed. These terms describe slightly different products. Remanufacturing is the process of the original equipment manufacturer, or an accredited third party, completely overhauling the equipment and returning it to service as if it were new and perhaps with a warranty. The terms "refurbished" and "reconditioned" refer to cleaned and repaired equipment in acceptable working order. Equipment may be repossessed due to payment problems on the part of the potential owner; such equipment may be relatively new and would be made available through the original vendor as "used" equipment. Another potential problem leading to equipment repossession might be related to leased equipment when reagent purchases continually fail to meet lease contract requirements, and the user returns the equipment to the company. Finally, some used equipment passes on to a customer via a reseller who may add little value and sell without significant guarantees. Those laboratories that are accustomed to obtaining newer technology may never buy previously owned equipment. Whether equipment is new or used, the selection committees continue to play a major part in decision making.

Table 25.1 Possible appointees to clinical laboratory equipment committees

TEC members[a]	LAB members[b]
Clinical pathologist	Chief executive officer
Laboratory manager and/or lab director	Chief financial officer
Contracting/procurement officer	Chief operations officer
Fiscal/financial service representative	Chief medical officer/chief of staff
Biomedical engineer	Clinical pathologist
Laboratory or section technical supervisor(s)	Physician/clinician representative(s)
Day shift medical technologist technical experts	Engineering director
Technical generalists (represent 24-h laboratory operation)	Facilities manager
Laboratory computer manager/medical center programmer	Other administrators (nursing, dietetics, human resources, etc.)

[a]The TEC conducts primary evaluation of equipment and technologies. Members are either voting or advisory depending on committee needs. One member is designated the committee chairperson.

[b]The LAB is the final review committee, which takes the recommendations of the TEC for a final vote on the purchase of equipment or new technologies. One member is designated the committee chairperson.

Memorandum
Date:

From: Chairman, Technical Evaluation Committee (TEC)

Subject: Confidentiality Certificate & Conflict of Interest for TEC members

To: Member, TEC

Thank you for volunteering to be a member of the Technical Evaluation Committee (TEC) for the Laboratory Advisory Board (LAB). We anticipate receiving information from potential contract sources that must remain confidential. As part of this responsibility, you are required to sign the following certificate.

CONFIDENTIALITY CERTIFICATE FOR TEC

In anticipation of my participation in the committee formed to evaluate the proposals submitted in response to information requested from potential cost-per-test (per-reportable) sources, I certify that I will not disclose any information concerning the evaluation (including the number, identity, or content of proposals or the deliberations of the committee) to anyone who is not also authorized access to the information by law or regulation, or pursuant to the order of a court of competent jurisdiction, and then only to the extent that such information is required in connection with such person's official responsibilities. Furthermore, I will report to the contracting officer any communication concerning the procurement or the committee composition and activities directed to me from any source outside the committee. I have signed the "PROCUREMENT INTEGRITY" form which is on file in the human resources office.

CONFLICT OF INTEREST CERTIFICATE

I certify that I am not aware of any matter which might reduce my ability to participate in the TEC proceeding and activities associated with the efforts to consolidate and/or standardize laboratory equipment among the network medical centers in an objective and unbiased manner or which might place me in a position of conflict, real or apparent, between my responsibilities as an evaluator or advisor and other interests.

In making this certification, I have considered all my stocks, bonds, and other financial interests, my employment arrangements (past, present, or under consideration), and, to the extent known by me, all the financial interests and employment arrangements of my spouse, my minor children, and other members of my immediate household.

If, after the date of this certification, any person, firm, or organization with which to my knowledge I (including my spouse, minor children, and other members of my immediate household) have financial arrangements submits a proposal or otherwise becomes involved in the subject project, I will notify the contracting officer, and thereafter, based on advice to do so from the medical center ethics counselor, I will agree to not participate further in any way (e.g., by rendering service, making recommendations, scoring proposals, or otherwise) in the particular subject matter or project.

_____   _____

Signature   Date

Printed name: _____   Facility: _____

Title: _____

Please sign and return these forms to Chair of the Laboratory, TEC, and they will become a part of our official procurement documentation.

Chairperson's fax:
Chairperson's telephone:
Chairperson's e-mail:

Figure 25.1 Memorandum: confidentiality certificate and conflict of interest statement for TEC members.

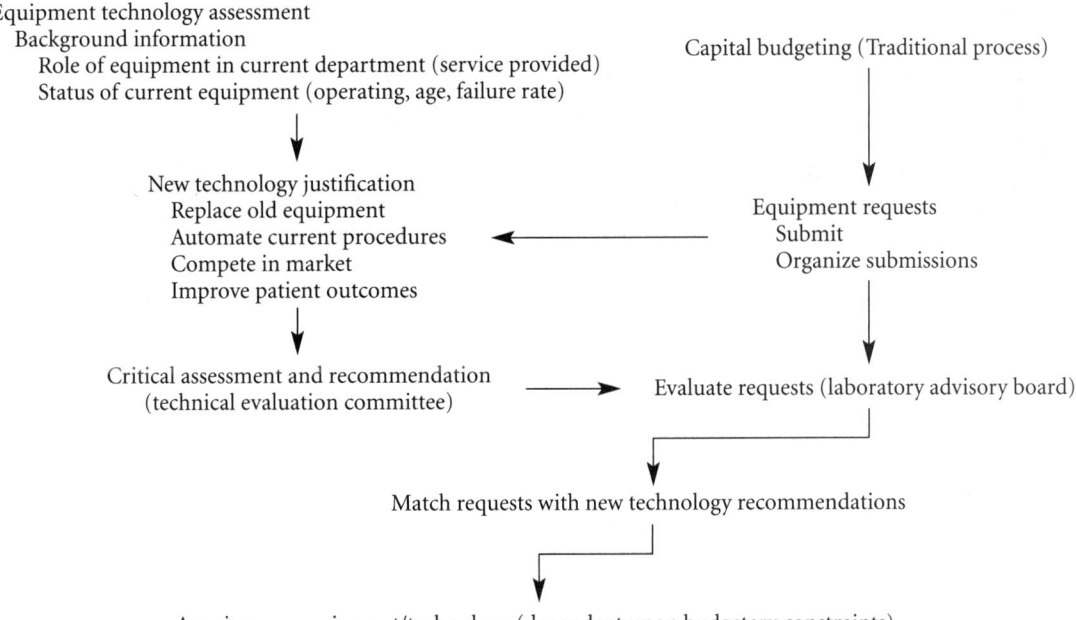

Figure 25.2 Relationship between technology assessment and capital budgeting.

There are extra precautions to take when considering used laboratory equipment (12, 13, 16). Table 25.2 lists cautions such as conducting a vendor background check and looking very carefully at the details of the purchase. The Internet has helped used-equipment resellers market their products nationwide. These businesses no longer need to sell only to their local metropolitan areas. For those laboratories willing to take the risk, some good-value instruments are available from equipment resellers.

Table 25.2 Cautions for buying previously owned equipment as an alternative to new equipment

Conduct a vendor background check.
    Number of years in business
    Number of years in present location
    Educational backgrounds/certifications of employees
    References from current and past clients
    Better Business Bureau membership
    Professional association membership
    License and bonding status

Understand the deal.
    Price of equipment
    Terms of purchase
    Service contract availability
    Warranty period
    Operational status of equipment
        Fully operational but sold "as is"
        Fully operational with preventative maintenance
        Completely rebuilt
        Confirm reliability with last equipment user.

Committee Logistics

Committee dynamics can contribute to a challenging but usually fruitful experience, especially when a multidisciplinary team is involved (Table 25.1). Committees for network or local equipment selection, such as the TEC, may include representatives from contracting/procurement, fiscal/financial services, biomedical engineering, laboratory or section supervisors, day shift bench-level technical experts, technical generalists (perhaps from an off-shift in a 24-h laboratory operation), and computer support/interfacing staff. On a multidisciplinary team, committee members are less likely to know each other. The assigned chairperson has the responsibility of not only focusing the group's efforts but also directing the logistics of determining the appropriate time to meet, deciding on the appropriate frequency of meetings, and reserving a conference room or arranging for a dial-in conference call. The actual scheduling of face-to-face or telephone conference call meetings is difficult. For example, in the summer, committee members may be on vacation or unable to leave a work commitment because staffing in their areas is at a minimum. Travel funds may be unavailable to pay for a central network group meeting or trips off-site to evaluate equipment. For network decisions made for multiple sites and even local decisions, it is advisable to schedule some time for members to become acquainted. Even local committees benefit from some social time. From these initial meetings, a higher level of group trust develops. The hope is that cooperation follows trust. Not many groups, however, want to devote time to team building. This is due to impatience, misunderstanding the importance of team building, and being uncomfortable with the personal stretching that builds relationships. Leadership and team building training can be conducted through contracted consultants or local human resource professionals. In addition, university-based business school programs or community colleges have many appropriate class offerings. As you might expect, there are some situations where decision makers bring their own maverick or quirky personalities to the process. A neutral committee chairperson with enough power to mediate the discussions and detoxify borderline behavior is an important element. In addition, there should be executive-level oversight with the expectation that each member will participate and contribute to the process.

A different organizational structure makes committee formation less relevant in the research laboratory. It is common for a principal investigator to make the decision of whether to purchase equipment. This is because the investigator often has secured his or her own equipment dollars from a governmental agency, a contract, or a private funding source. In contrast, a committee recommendation is more common in a clinical hospital or reference laboratory environment. Individual voting members representing multiple medical centers have the greatest barriers to quick decisions. If the medical centers are the same size and serve the same clientele, then making the decision is an easier task. However, if the medical centers are of different sizes (e.g., from a clinic/doctor office-sized laboratory open Monday to Friday up to a 1000 plus-bed, 24-h, tertiary medical center) or serve different population mixes (e.g., veterans' hospitals compared to children's hospitals), then it is more likely that different equipment or assays are required. Adoption of new procedures does depend on the initial equipment decision. This is because most clinical assays run as proprietary products designed only for use on specific equipment. More good advice is to discount promises of the availability of future assays when making equipment-purchasing decisions.

At some stage in the equipment decision-making process, clinical laboratories may realize that they have become wary of utilizing one equipment vendor for several different product lines. The thought is that distributing purchases or contracts over several vendors avoids possible decreased competitiveness in future pricing. If all things appear equal concerning equipment cost and performance, laboratories will be more likely to stay with their current equipment manufacturer. While this may be an advantage for the equipment seller, contracts through group purchasing organizations can maintain favorable pricing for the laboratory.

Evaluating Vendors and Their Products

During the equipment selection process, much information requires collection and synthesis by decision makers, with input from specialists (1, 2). Examples of questions asked during the decision process include the following:

- What are the initial costs and continuing costs of the new equipment or procedure [*finance*]?

- Do I have room in my laboratory for this new system [*architecture*]?
- Will operators find the equipment easy or difficult to use [*ergonomics, human resources*]?
- Do staff have the background, aptitude, and skill required to operate this equipment [*human resources*]?
- How many operators will be required to run this system [*finance, human resources*]?
- Is the system easy to maintain and reliable, or does it frequently require a backup to perform testing when the primary analyzer is down [*operations*]?
- Are the methods or equipment subject to interferences or anomalies that may result in false-positive or false-negative results [*diagnostic value, malpractice/law*]?
- Do staff enjoy coming to work every day [*human resources*]?

The capabilities of a vendor's instrumentation can be uncovered in a number of ways. The initial stages may include an informal review of up-to-date marketing literature. Information that is more detailed comes from publications like *CAP Today*, published by the College of American Pathologists, which presents yearly analyses of different classes of analyzers appropriate for the clinical laboratory operation. For those more visually oriented, attendance at local and national trade shows enables the laboratory decision maker to see new equipment and methods close up.

A more formal approach is to utilize a set of technically revealing questions sent to vendors as a standardized request for information. As the request for information responses return, a subcommittee must collate the data. Tasks for other committee members include site visits and helping collect additional information from, for example, current user interviews. Figure 25.3 shows an example of a sheet used to gather a variety of evaluative information. Keeping all committee members active and involved requires clearly stated commitments summarized at the conclusion of each committee meeting. Between meetings, the chairperson should distribute minutes by e-mail, along with individual member assignments.

Be sure to poll at least three users of the equipment that you are considering placing in your laboratory. Before making a telephone call or site visit (11), have all your questions outlined and ready to ask. This is important so that you ask each vendor's customers the same questions. Most users are quite open about revealing the advantages and disadvantages of the systems or procedures that they use. Even though the vendor may facilitate your site visit, it is better for you to talk to users alone. This is likely to make for a more candid exchange of information. Keep in mind that each laboratory is unique and made its decision based on the market that was available to them at one point. Setting up evaluation categories and using objective scoring

Manufacturer/Equipment Model	
Evaluation Criteria: (attach pages as needed)	Score
General Questions: • Newness of technology; • Technology licensed or owned; • System footprint; • Lab space available; • Expected lifespan of system; • Large peer group for proficiency testing comparisons	(/5)
Quality of Assays • Between (Within) lot variation (CV); • Interferences; • Carry-over; • Sample stability; • Analytical sensitivity; • High/low linearity; • Reagent stability (manufacturer's expiration date vs. customer experience; Lot to lot variation); • Standardized of assay international std or other manufacturer; • Frequency of reagent reformulations; • Proficiency testing results	(/10)
Assay Menu/Type • Current assays on-line; • Anticipated assay menu; • History of vendor offering new assays as planned; • Need for back up or manual procedures; • Expansion capability; • Methodologies offered; • Control usage and type if supplied; • Open channels or closed system	(/10)
Turnaround Time for STAT/Non-STAT Tests • Chemistry panels; Cardiac assays; Immunochemistry, CBC, Coagulation, Blood gasses, etc.	(/5)
Equipment Operation • Ease of use (tech acceptance); • Complexity of operation; • Walk away capability/labor intensity; • Error alerts (audio/visual); • Ease of trouble shooting; • Maintenance time & frequency (day, week, month, annual); • Ease of adding reagents/supplies/STAT samples; • Safety features (closed tube sampling, reagent exposure); • On board data management; • QC tracking program	(/10)
Equipment Features • On board storage of reagents; • On board refrigeration of reagents if needed; • Bar coded reagents, samples; • Clot detection; • Water system; • External plumbing; • Linking with lab automation systems; • Reagent level detection; • Waste disposal system	(/10)
Variety of Equipment Models Aid in Testing Network Standardization	(/5)
Equipment Down Time • Number of days per year down; • Frequency of down time; • Time to respond to service call; • Uptime guarantee; • Typical problems; • Average time to resolve	(/10)
Computer Interface • Bi-directional, host query; • Ease of maintenance; • Company or third party maintains interface	(/10)

Company Support
1. **Evaluation and Training:** • Off-site/on-site training: • Quality-of-training; • # of staff that can be initially trained;
  • Future training of staff available with/without charge by vendor; • Company helps with evaluation & to what extent;
  • Reagents supplied for initial evaluation & for future assays
2. **Sales Support:** • Ease of obtaining reagents,/supplies; • Visit frequency; • Follow-up on service issues
3. **Customer Support:** • 800 number response/helpfulness; • Hours available
4. **Service Support:** • Skills of service engineers; • Local reps; • # of reps; • ETA of service rep after service call placed;
  • Ability of technical reps to fix problem
	(/10)

Financial • Cost per test; • Cost per reportable; • Cost per year; • Accessory and other supply costs; • Shipping costs covered; • Financial health of company	(/15)
Current Customer Response: • Things you do not like • Would you buy this instrument again?	
Total Score	(/100)

Figure 25.3 Equipment evaluation and rating sheet.

for each category can aid in scoring each vendor's products (Fig. 25.4). In the end, a vote by committee members will lead to the final recommendation by the TEC. This recommendation can go to the final stakeholders, such as the LAB or to decision-making individuals such as the chief executive officer, chief financial officer, or medical center director for final approval.

The scoring from each of the categories results in an objective ranking of the equipment vendors. Some evaluation criteria become critical elements, and a vendor becomes eliminated from future consideration if it fails to meet baseline requirements. Understandably, it is very important requirement that TEC members treat all vendors fairly and equitably.

Continual technology assessment: primary
equipment users/lab managers/directors

↓

Assign multidisciplinary team: team building, commitments,
project management

↓

Document needs of internal/external customers:
constraint analysis

↓

Critical equipment assessment from site visits, peer
interviews, requests for information: Quality of assays, menu,
turnaround time, operational requirements, instrument features,
preventative maintenance, computer interface, company support,
cost and contract issues, backup options, etc.

↓

Request for proposals: specification of contract
options, required deliverables

↓

Selection of system, contract review: specialist study
of details, final clarifications, and negotiations

↓

Formulate final on-line timeline.

↓

Training: key operators

↓

Equipment evaluation: crossover studies, etc.

↓

Training: general users

↓

Communication: staff, providers

Figure 25.4 Instrument selection from technology assessment to active testing.

Figure 25.4 reviews the pathway of instrument selection, including a listing of some of the important evaluation criteria, such as quality of assays, test menu, turnaround time (TAT) for each test, operational requirements, instrument features, preventative maintenance schedules (daily, weekly, monthly, 6 month, yearly), computer interface requirements and capabilities, bar code reading, company support for emergency downtimes, cost and contract issues, and backup options.

Members with specialized training provide focused reviews of their areas of expertise during the evaluation of new equipment. Some participants will be "meeting challenged" and unable to regularly attend. Early in the process, the committee should agree on the desired date for completion of the evaluation. This sets a time horizon for the vendor and for committee members to individually budget their time. In addition, at an early stage, the vendor needs accurate accounting of each laboratory's workload. For example, Fig. 25.5 shows a spreadsheet template for recording annual workload and the cost charged by three different vendors. A vendor with accurate test volume can match up

appropriate instruments with each laboratory. Vendors that sell small, medium, and large analyzers to accommodate different laboratory testing workloads often promote standardized methods and interchangeable reagents. This will allow a laboratory to place a smaller analyzer as a backup if the primary instrument is out of service. It also enables only one set of reference ranges to be in use. The placement of the correct analyzer requires careful interpretation of equipment capacity. Some vendors advertise testing throughput based on the fastest-to-be-completed assay rather than a more realistic variety of sample types that a laboratory may experience during a regular workday. Check any recommendations made by sales staff, as they may use integrated 24-h work period data rather than taking into account hourly or peak testing demand on instrumentation (9). An analyzer undermatched with the workload will frustrate testing staff and elicit complaints from clinicians.

Operational Requirements

There are common logistical questions, such as whether the new assay or instrument is for a 24-h operation or for a specialized purpose on a single shift. Will the assay be available on a STAT basis or scheduled for batch testing at a specific time during the week? How long does it take to turn out a result (TAT)? Are any of the analytes extremely labile upon exposure to extremes of temperature or upon exposure to light or oxygen? Does the analyzer require any specialized power (220 or 110 V) or water (distilled, deionized, type I or II, flow rate)?

Test Characteristics

It is important to gather all the statistics that the manufacturers publish in their product (kit) inserts. You will want to know about test precision (within-run and between-run variability, also called intra-assay variability and interassay variability), linearity/reportable range, reagent stability (before and after opening, and whether the reagent requires reconstitution or is in a ready-to-use format), and analyte stability (at room temperature, refrigerated, and frozen at -20 or $-70°C$) (Fig. 25.6). It is important to collect information such as analytical sensitivity, analytical specificity, reaction type (type of chemical or other measuring scheme), type of detection system (alkaline phosphatase, NAD/NADP linked, radioactive label, biotin/avidin, electrochemical, or chromatographic separation), and other facts so that accurate comparisons can be made between assays and analytical platforms (14).

Equipment Service and Support

Another major selection factor is the availability of local vendor equipment support. Unless the equipment is very easy to service, avoid dealing with third-party contracted service groups, no matter how enticing the potential savings. Third-party service providers may not have received the latest equipment training. Local funding for service

Test Name	Work Load Patient Samples per/ Year	Vendor A Cost per Reportable Result	Vendor A Total Cost/ Year	Vendor B Cost per Reportable Result	Vendor B Total Cost/ Year	Vendor C Cost per Reportable Result	Vendor C Total Cost/ Year
HEMOLYSIS INDEX							
SODIUM							
POTASSIUM							
CHLORIDE							
TOTAL CO2							
GLUCOSE							
UREA NITROGEN							
CREATININE							
TOTAL PROTEIN							
ALBUMIN							
CALCIUM							
PHOSPHATE							
MAGNESIUM							
URIC ACID							
TOTAL BILIRUBIN							
DIRECT BILIRUBIN							
ALK PHOSPHATASE							
AST							
ALT							
CREATINE KINASE							
GGT							
LD							
TOTAL AMYLASE							
CHOLESTEROL							
TRIGLYERIDE							
IRON							
DIRECT HDL							
ALCOHOL							
URINE/CSF TOTAL PROTEIN							
TOTAL IRON BINDING							
ACETAMINOPHEN							
SALICYLATE							
PANCREATIC AMYLASE							
AMMONIA							
LACTATE							
Total Test/Year							
Reagent Total							
Rgt. Cost for Rpts/Cals							
Consumables							
Instrument Cost							
Service contract							
Total Cost/Year							

Figure 25.5 An example of a chemistry laboratory test worksheet for comparison of cost per reportable results and total costs among three different equipment vendors.

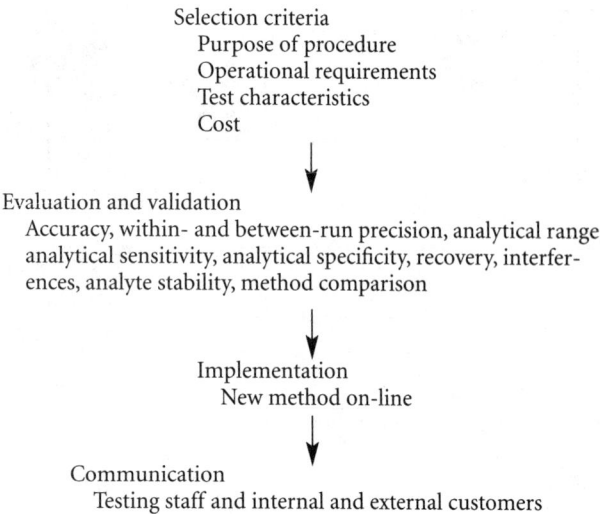

Selection criteria
    Purpose of procedure
    Operational requirements
    Test characteristics
    Cost

Evaluation and validation
    Accuracy, within- and between-run precision, analytical range, analytical sensitivity, analytical specificity, recovery, interferences, analyte stability, method comparison

Implementation
    New method on-line

Communication
    Testing staff and internal and external customers

Figure 25.6 New procedure selection and implementation.

may be out of your hands, and sometimes this encourages the awarding of the service contract to the lowest bidder. Usually you get what you pay for, but in some cases, third-party technicians may be very good, especially when dealing with equipment marketed for a number of years.

Get a guarantee from the vendor that the product will handle the current workload at peak demand and with minimal downtime. Know whether the vendor has an up-time guarantee and whether it will pay for reference laboratory testing if your equipment is down for a significant time. Agree with your vendor about the definition of significant downtime for your laboratory. Map out the number of service technicians in your area and the territory that they have to cover. Get a clear understanding of how long it will usually take to have a service person on-site at your location. It is especially important to know what equipment parts your service technician keeps locally. If the repair requires shipment of parts, know where the parts will be coming from and how long they will take to arrive. Are there other equipment users in your area that would facilitate your helping each other if the needed part or consumable is out of stock, or would the needed part cause you uncomfortable delay in returning to full testing capacity?

Availability in the Community

Relatively few placements of a vendor's equipment in the community can be an indication of its newness or resistance to market penetration because of existing clinical laboratory-vendor contracts. Some laboratories pride themselves on being the first to adopt new technologies or bring on new assays, while other laboratories are more conservative, preferring to wait until the technology is well tested. Very few hospital laboratories are actually developing new assays. Clinical laboratories, for the most part, are buying preformulated diagnostic kits. If a manufacturer's reagents

are usable only by a specific technology, then there needs to be extra effort to justify the placement of the new analyzer.

Cost

There is a rough correlation between the number of workstations and the number of operators and therefore labor costs. The trend for many years has been to decrease the number of workstations in a laboratory to decrease labor costs and counteract the reality of fewer technical staff entering into the laboratory profession. Some manufacturers will promote the feature of greater automation and lower labor costs to justify higher prices for their products. The marketing of a new assay usually results in it commanding premium pricing. The highest prices recently, for example, have been for new molecular biology assays related to genetic, neurological, infectious, and hematological diseases. Many laboratories have brought on-line PCR-based amplification assays or been forced to send out testing to specialized reference laboratories that conduct new assays for which there are few competitors. This occurred in recent years for assays like hepatitis C RNA viral load assays, hepatitis C virus genotyping, and assays for troponin I and T, free prostate-specific antigen, and b-type natriuretic peptides.

Actual test-related costs are broken down in several ways and discussed elsewhere in this book. There can be the cost to purchase the equipment, the yearly cost to lease, or the cost of reagent rental (cost per test or cost per reportable result). Another important cost, sometimes less appreciated, is the cost associated with not proceeding with utilizing the equipment, or lost-opportunity cost. These costs can be either monetary or expressed in terms of morbidity and mortality.

Implementation and Communication

Equipment Placement

The implementation of the new procedure or instrument depends on good site preparation. Typically, in vitro device (IVD) manufacturers ask laboratories to fill out a site questionnaire. Later a company engineer visits the site to make sure that access is possible for transporting the equipment into the laboratory. Factors described earlier in this chapter under "Operational Requirements" are important, along with shielding the instrument from inappropriate electromagnetic sources and smoothing out fluctuations in line voltages. Equipment usually requires proper leveling and the maintenance of set environmental temperatures and humidity.

Following stabilization of the physical setting, the manufacturer's technical representative aids on-site staff in completing the evaluation studies. At the end of the evaluation studies, staff training begins with the help of factory-trained key operators. After the training of a critical mass of medical technologists and medical laboratory technicians, the instrument is nearly ready to go on-line. The final stage of going on-line involves ensuring the completion of bidirectional interfacing between the laboratory information system and the instrument.

Postsale Vendor-Laboratory Relationships

During the selling phase, vendors are extremely visible. After the sale the expectation is that the laboratory and vendor will continue a strong partnership (3). The laboratory wants vendors to provide up-to-date product information. In return, vendors want to continue to present information on their products to the decision makers. Laboratories have to be careful about becoming locked in to one equipment type that makes them less likely to consider other vendors' products. However, working with one vendor across many areas (e.g., chemistry, immunochemistry, hematology, coagulation, microbiology, etc.) may actually improve service for an individual laboratory because the total laboratory account is larger and the service technicians are more likely to be multiplatform trained. Similarly, a laboratory equipment or diagnostic kit vendor may be even more responsive to a laboratory's needs if a group purchasing organization or national laboratory network is involved. One might expect strong positive correlations between better service and the size of the contract or the location of a laboratory in a more densely populated urban setting.

Even with great care, it is not possible for laboratories to predict the continuing availability of presently marketed products. In some situations, vendors pull their products from the market, either by choice or when forced by a regulatory agency, leaving laboratories scrambling to provide a test or service. If a vendor promises labor savings, hold the vendor to it in your contract. Monitor cost per reportable result charge, as accounting errors can affect your profits.

Other Influences on the Decision-Making Process

Creation and Assessment of Provider Interest

An awareness of the value of a new diagnostic test comes from laboratory managers communicating with providers, peers, and vendors. Laboratorians consult with colleagues at other facilities via telephone or e-mail and in person at professional meetings. Further information can come from published literature and advice from colleagues via Internet-based e-mail list servers. The laboratory in a clinical environment can promote new instrumentation and procedures through a number of routes, such as postings on its own laboratory website, medical center newsletters, direct mailings, e-mails to providers, and announcements at local grand rounds or continuing-medical-education events. A more personal way is to pass on information or solicit improvements in services from clinical colleagues as you interact with them during consultations. The distribution of an annual laboratory survey gives providers an opportunity to praise and critique laboratory services and request new procedures or assays. The survey responses returned to the laboratory, either signed or anonymous, enable the gathering of important information on the directions the laboratory should take with the services it offers.

It is becoming more common for diagnostic kit manufacturers, reference laboratories, and instrument companies to market their products directly to clinicians. While it is uncommon to see advertising directed to clinicians concerning large, central laboratory analyzers, it is very common to see marketing materials for point-of-care (POC) devices. A wide variety of devices are sold with an expanding menu of POC tests for cardiac function, human immunodeficiency virus, glucose, blood gases, electrolytes, coagulation, drugs of abuse in urine, lipids, etc. A difficult management situation develops when POC devices are used. Clinicians expect that the central laboratory will maintain the expanding POC program. The reality is that there is generally less appreciation for the scrupulous quality control needed to maintain a POC program (e.g., whole-blood glucose instrument). To encourage the excitement of providers, a marketer of POC products may work directly with a clinical group by suggesting that they use POC products in the emergency room setting for a quicker TAT. In some cases, this may be a very good fit; in others, the TAT from the central laboratory may already be adequate.

Reference laboratories promote new and expensive esoteric tests that only they can perform with the hope that clinician pressure can help develop the market. In a similar way, some researchers outside of the central laboratory evaluate POC-type equipment under a contract with a diagnostic company. The funds for these projects typically come from the IVD manufacturer's marketing group and may influence both the local and national testing markets. These undertakings require the continuing scrutiny over operations remote from the main laboratory in areas such as respiratory care operations, physician office laboratories, community-based outreach clinics, infertility clinics, emergency rooms, operating rooms, urology clinics, etc.

Advertising and literature that are found at IVD vendor-sponsored continuing-medical-education events targeted toward clinical providers may influence clinical providers. Adoption of a new assay occurs when there is a match between clinicians, who are justifiably excited about the potential for diagnostic improvement, and laboratorians, who consider technical and operational advantages. The reverse is to have providers misled by marketing materials or discovering that assays and equipment do not perform adequately. When an instrument does not perform as expected, the laboratory may decide not to bring it online. The ultimate decisions of how the laboratory operates must come from laboratorians focused on being receptive to the needs of their customers.

Medical Value

In the end, outcome research and clinical guidelines determine the medical value of an assay and indirectly the equipment on which the assay runs. Large clinical trials and meta-analysis years after the first use of an assay may or may not give a clear indication of the assay's diagnostic effectiveness. In practical terms, test value comes from evaluation of its sensitivity (not analytical sensitivity), specificity (not analytical specificity), and negative and positive predictive values. Please refer to the previous chapter for a discussion of these indicators or other available discussions (17). The usefulness of a marker changes over time. Early indications that a diagnostic test is useful may later prove incorrect, or better markers become available. For example, the usefulness of quantitating the isoenzymes of lactate dehydrogenase as markers of myocardial infarction has now been supplanted by measures of the creatinine kinase MB subunit and troponin I and troponin T molecules. Different manufacturers have sold similar Food and Drug Administration-released products, used interchangeably by the laboratory community, sometimes against label specifications. For example, Hybritech (now Beckman Coulter) at one time was the only manufacturer that marketed a total prostate-specific antigen assay with a claim for both screening and monitoring of therapy for prostate cancer. Other manufacturers took several more years of clinical studies before they could also make a claim for screening and monitoring, yet many users of the non-Hybritech products in the interim still used the alternate assays for prostate cancer screening. Medical value also may apply only to specified demographic groups based on age, gender, race, etc.

Summary

The selection and implementation of new procedures and instruments are key elements of a well-managed laboratory. Initially, the process must assess the needs of the end users, the availability of the assay in the community, the labor and operational requirements, and the overall cost associated with the implementation of an instrument. The selection process identifies criteria used to evaluate the instruments. After selection of an instrument, analytical evaluation occurs in the laboratory, with each assay validated before integration into the daily testing operation.

KEY POINTS

- End user satisfaction is an important element in the selection of a new instrument or procedure.

- The instrument selection criteria include quality of the assays, TAT, menu selection, manufacturer's support, cost, operational requirements, and computer interface capability.

- Communication with the laboratory and medical staff is essential.

GLOSSARY

GainManagement GainManagement in the laboratory has three major elements: LabPlanning (GainPlanning), LabMaking (GainMaking), and LabSharing (GainSharing).

Group purchasing organization A large group of users banding together to increase their purchasing power and lower procurement costs.

LabMaking The process of involving all employees in a structured process with the goal of making continuous performance improvements (modified from reference 5).

LabPlanning The work managers do to lead and focus the laboratory on continuous gains and to organize for a high level of employee involvement (modified from reference 5).

LabSharing The process of sharing laboratory and organizational gains as overall or specific performance measures improve (modified from reference 5).

Turnaround time (TAT) The time from phlebotomy or receipt of the sample in the laboratory and its accessioning until the time of reporting the result.

REFERENCES

1. Barba, M. V. 2003. Analyzer selection and implementation. *Clin. Lab. Products* **32**(8):34.

2. Cary, E. R., M. Fink, S. L. Stokes, V. L. Simmons, D. A. Kaczor, S. Harmon, L. Quarles, C. Escobar, and D. J. Maier. 2000. Selection and implementation for coagulation instruments/reagents in a multiple hospital/clinic network. *Blood Coagul. Fibrinolysis* **11**(7): 599–608.

3. Cook, J. 1999. Improving vendor, lab manager relationships. *Advance Admin. Lab.* **7**(6):114–118.

4. Crolla, L. J. 2002. Justifying capital expenditures in the laboratory. *MLO Med. Lab. Obs.* **35**:30–31.

5. Doyle, R. J., and P. I. Doyle. 1992. *GainManagement. A Process of Building Teamwork, Productivity, and Profitability Throughout Your Organization.* American Management Association, New York, N.Y.

6. Drucker, P. F. 1985. *Management: Tasks, Responsibilities, Practices.* Harper Collins, New York, N.Y.

7. Fine, A. 2003. Developing an assessment process for new technologies. *Healthc. Financ. Manag.* **57**:84–97.

8. Frantz, D. 1998. Financial tools for clinical chemistry. *Advance Admin. Lab.* **6**(7):16–18.

9. Gonder, J., and L. D. Mell, Jr. 2002. Everything you wanted to know about automated instrument selection but were afraid to ask! *Advance Med. Lab. Prof.* **14**(21):17–20.

10. Hersher, B. 1998. Eye on integration. The glue that holds multidepartmental management together. *Advance Admin. Lab.* **6**(7):23.

11. Johnson, K. C. 1999. Purchasing Strategy: technology travel. Make site visits both smooth and effective. *Diagn. Imaging* **11**:125–126.

12. Johnson, P. 2000. Decisions, decisions, decisions. *Advance Med. Lab. Prof.* **12**(14):14–17.

13. King, D. 2000. Surfing for refurbished equipment. *Advance Med. Lab. Prof.* **12**(22):19–22.

14. Koch, D. D., and T. Peters, Jr. 1999. Selection and evaluation of methods, p. 320–335. *In* C. A. Burtis and E. R. Ashwood (ed.), *Tietz Textbook of Clinical Chemistry*, 3rd ed. W. B. Saunders, Philadelphia, Pa.

15. Lemery, L. D. 2002. "Just do it": moving the box. *Clin. Lab. Manag. Rev.* **16**(3): 204–205.

16. Lindner, J. 1998. Ask the experts. What should a lab expect from a rebuilt equipment supplier? *Advance Admin. Lab.* **6**(7):11.

17. Shultz, E. K. 1999. Selection and interpretation of laboratory procedures, p. 310–319. *In* C. A. Burtis and E. R. Ashwood (ed.), *Tietz Textbook of Clinical Chemistry*, 3rd ed. W. B. Saunders, Philadelphia, Pa.

18. Travers, E. M. 1996. Laboratory manager's financial handbook. The laboratory's importance to the financial stability of a healthcare organization. *Clin. Lab. Manag. Rev.* **10**:56–66.

19. Travers, E. M. (ed.). 1997. *Clinical Laboratory Management.* The Williams and Wilkins Co., Baltimore, Md.

20. Travers, E. M. 1997. *Clinical Laboratory Management*, p. 333–374. The Williams and Wilkins Co., Baltimore, Md.

21. Travers, E. M. 1997. *Clinical Laboratory Management*, p. 717–726. The Williams and Wilkins Co., Baltimore, Md.

22. Varnadoe, L. A. 1996. *Management and Supervision: Operations, Review, and Study Guide.* F. A. Davis Company, Philadelphia, Pa.

23. Watts, D., D. L. Finney, and B. Louie. 1993. Integrating technology assessment into the capital budgeting process. *Healthc. Financ. Manag.* **47**:20–24, 26, 28–29.

APPENDIX 25.1   Websites: Training, Certification, and Credentialing Programs

American Society for Clinical Pathology Diplomate in Laboratory Management certification
http://www.ascp.org/bor/certification/procedures/diplomate.asp

Clinical chemistry
http://www.ascp.org/index.asp; http://www.nrcc6.org/; http://www.aacc.org/abcc/

Laboratory medicine
http://www.abpath.org/homepage.htm

Medical technology
http://www.ascp.org/index.asp; http://www.ascls.org/; http://www.nca-info.org/

Microbiology
http://www.ascp.org/bor/certification/procedures/m.asp; http://www.asmusa.org/acasrc/college.htm

26

Laboratory Safety

David L. Sewell

> **OBJECTIVES**
>
> *To define the essential components of a laboratory safety program*
>
> *To administer the program to meet safety requirements*
>
> *To evaluate the program for regulatory compliance*
>
> *To identify hazardous materials and procedures in the laboratory*

Things that matter most should never be at the mercy of things that matter least.

GOETHE

LABORATORIES, BY THE NATURE OF THE WORK PERFORMED, contain inherent risk to workers that is often difficult to measure and manage because safety is not an intrinsic, absolute, and measurable property (13). Therefore, we must continually assess and manage risk in the laboratory based upon current knowledge and propose and enforce commonsense safety practices to minimize harm or injury to the worker and to prevent laboratory contamination (44). Accidents in the laboratory are often attributable to a person's inability to recognize a hazardous situation, an individual's diminished concern for risk over long periods of time, or excessive risk taking. Thus, an individual's behavior influences the degree of occupational risk present in the workplace (41). Risk takers and individuals who ignore safety precautions not only suffer the consequences from their acts but also pose a risk to their colleagues, families, and friends.

The clinical laboratory environment contains biological, physical, chemical, and radiological hazards that expose workers to risk. Biological hazards (e.g., exposure to blood, body fluids, and other specimens from infected patients who may harbor human immunodeficiency virus (HIV), hepatitis viruses, other newly recognized pathogens such as the severe acute respiratory syndrome [SARS] agent, or agents of bioterrorism) are a major concern for laboratory workers today and have heightened the need for implementation of sound safety practices. Exposure to these pathogens through specimens, aerosols, or droplets may cause an occupationally acquired infection that can be transmitted to other employees, one's family, or the public. Today, the potential use of biological, chemical, and radioactive materials as terrorism agents imposes additional safety and security concerns in the laboratory (7, 20).

Exposure to hazardous chemicals may result in acute and/or chronic disease that may be exacerbated in employees with preexisting medical conditions. Although there is a continuing effort to reduce the number and quantity of laboratory chemicals that are toxic, carcinogenic, caustic, flammable, or radioactive, these compounds cannot be eliminated completely from laboratories.

In addition to biological, radiological, and chemical hazards, fires and electrical accidents may occur, and laboratory instruments and equipment may cause injury to the user. However, the laboratory can be a safe workplace when the risks are recognized and reduced through appropriate training of personnel and implementation of safe work practices, appropriate containment equipment, well-designed facilities, and administrative controls (5, 23, 29, 33, 52).

Safety Management Plan

The key to a safe laboratory environment is the development, implementation, and enforcement of a quality safety management program that considers worker safety as a responsibility of the facility (Table 26.1). The Occupational Safety and Health Administration (OSHA) requires a risk assessment (exposure determination) of each task performed in the laboratory. The safety program begins with a well-written safety manual that defines the program and identifies the individuals responsible for specific tasks (21, 31, 33). Management must commit to the program and provide the necessary resources (e.g., equipment and time) to produce and implement the plan, assign oversight and responsibility for the plan, and communicate the plan and expectations to the employees. The risk associated with each task performed in the laboratory is assessed, and practices are implemented to minimize these risks. These practices include the use of Standard Precautions, personal protective equipment (PPE), engineering and work practice controls, workplace design, vaccination, safe handling and disposal of hazardous waste, and use of safety devices. In addition, the safety plan should include sections on bloodborne pathogens, a medical surveillance program, a chemical hygiene plan, infection control procedures, hazard communications, record keeping, waste disposal, fire safety, and spill cleanup. The federal regulations that directly address general laboratory safety include Hazard Communication Standard 29 CFR 1910.1200 (36), Bloodborne Pathogens Standard 29 CFR 1910.1030 (38), and Occupational Exposure to Hazardous Chemicals in the Laboratory 29 CFR 1910.1450 (37).

To ensure that the laboratory safety policies and procedures are active and enforced, a safety officer and safety committee should be established. All sections of the laboratory should be represented on this committee. These individuals ensure that the safety program's policies, procedures, and training programs are uniform throughout the laboratory and that the laboratory is in compliance with all state and federal safety regulatory requirements. In larger organizations the laboratory safety officer also participates on the other institutional safety-related committees. It is essential that employees review the safety manual, receive annual training based on the hazards and risks present in

Table 26.1 Elements of a safety management plan

Administrative support

Appoint a safety officer and members of the safety committee

Provide for occupational health services

Provide funds and time for surveys, meetings, education, and development of a safety management plan. The plan should address safety and security, exposure control, emergency preparedness, waste, utilities, and equipment management.

Risk assessment

Perform safety audits and risk assessments

Obtain MSDS and other necessary safety information

Develop chemical inventory lists

Identify safety needs and controls

Training

Provide safety training for new employees, annual training for all employees, and training as needed for workers assigned to a new workstation

Plan review and record keeping

Review all audits, surveys, and accident reports to measure the effectiveness of the plan and make changes to reduce the probability of additional occupational exposures

Update the plan when new information is available or new hazards are introduced

Maintain records of all surveys, accidents, and inspections and the resulting corrective actions

the laboratory, and understand the specific safety precautions required for each procedure or workstation.

Laboratory Hazards

The laboratory contains numerous hazards that fall into four general classes: biological, chemical, physical, and radiological. A hazard is any material, condition, or action that may result in physical harm or impairment to employees. The management of these hazards poses a significant challenge due to the complexity of the work and the diversity of the hazards that are present in the laboratory environment. The risk from these hazards is related to exposure levels, duration of exposure, toxicity or pathogenicity of the hazardous material, safety controls present, and other factors such as the general health or age of the laboratory worker. In general, the risk of suffering an adverse event from a laboratory hazard is decreased by minimizing the exposure to the hazard, storing only small quantities of the hazard in the laboratory, and storing hazardous materials in appropriate containers. Whenever possible, a less hazardous material should be substituted for highly toxic or dangerous chemicals.

Biological Hazards

Biological hazards include infectious agents such as bacteria, parasites, fungi, and viruses that may be transmitted through contaminated body secretions, tissue, or other materials. All clinical specimens are potentially infectious, and the isolation and culture of pathogenic microorganisms from these specimens increases the risk to the clinical microbiologist. Bacteria cause the majority of laboratory-acquired infections (LAI), followed by viruses, rickettsia, fungi, and parasites. Today, 96% of all LAIs are caused by bacteria, viruses, and rickettsia (22). The major routes for acquiring an infection in the laboratory are from exposure to a specimen containing a potential pathogen and the procedures used to culture and identify the agent. Agents that are transmitted by aerosols cause most of the serious LAIs and include *Mycobacterium tuberculosis, Bordetella pertussis, Corynebacterium diphtheriae, Neisseria meningitidis, Bacillus anthracis, Brucella* spp., *Francisella tularensis, Burkholderia pseudomallei,* and *Yersinia pestis* (8, 33). The factors that influence the risk of acquiring an infection from blood, body fluids, or other potentially infectious material (OPIM) are related to the quantity of specimen involved in the exposure; the concentration, prevalence, and type of pathogen in the specimen; the number and types of contact experienced by the worker; the susceptibility and behavior of the host; and the routes of exposure (e.g., percutaneous exposure, splashes to mucous membranes, splashes to intact or nonintact skin, oral ingestion, or aerosol inhalation) (2, 22). Aerosols are especially problematic because they are generated by numerous procedures performed in the laboratory such as sonication, homogenization, centrifugation, mixing, pipetting, heating inoculation loops, streaking agar plates, opening lyophilized ampoules, and expelling bubbles from a syringe (33, 42). Because symptoms of infection are often delayed following an exposure, the person generally cannot recall the specific event that caused the infection but only that he/she was working with the agent or was in the laboratory (22). Traditional safety guidelines have emphasized the use of safe work practices, well-designed laboratories, containment equipment, and management controls (5). Today, laboratories also need to prevent unauthorized entry to the laboratory areas and removal of bioterrorism agents (7).

Chemical Hazards

Chemical hazards include all chemicals that may be toxic or irritating and include solids, liquids, and gases such as mercury, acetone, xylene, stains, and formaldehyde. The diversity of chemical hazards found in the clinical laboratory is as great as the biological hazards. The risk and severity of an exposure to a chemical is influenced by the amount of chemical to which one is exposed (dose), the route of exposure (i.e., inhalation, ingestion, absorption through or contact with mucous membranes and intact/nonintact skin), the chemical properties of the compound, the susceptibility of the individual, and the duration of exposure (45).

Because containment procedures are based on the chemical hazard class, laboratory chemicals are labeled and described by their hazard classification, such as irritant, corrosive, flammable (gas, liquid, solid), poison (toxic), or carcinogen. Reactive chemicals must be segregated for storage. Acids are not stored with bases, oxidizers are not stored with reducing agents or organics, and flammables are stored in flammable-safe cabinets. Poisons or toxic compounds can cause acute or chronic symptoms when ingested, inhaled, or absorbed through the skin and can affect the nervous, respiratory, or reproductive systems. Carcinogens may cause malignant neoplasms in humans or animals long after exposure to the compound. Use of highly toxic chemicals or carcinogens should be restricted, and they should be handled only in a designated area by well-trained personnel.

When possible, disposable PPE should be used when handling toxic chemicals. A chemical hygiene plan (required for all laboratories) details the specific safety measures (i.e., engineering and work practice controls, PPE, exposure monitoring, waste management) required for each class of chemicals used in the laboratory.

When exposure monitoring is required, a trained industrial hygienist can measure the chemical level as the work is performed and determine whether the level exceeds the permissible exposure limit (PEL) (3, 23, 32). PELs represent the maximum concentration of a chemical to which an employee may be exposed over an 8-h workday or 40-h workweek (time-weighted average). PELs may also be expressed as a short-term exposure (15-minute period) or a ceiling limit not to be exceeded. These limits are set so that the employees are not exposed to chemical levels that may cause acute or chronic symptoms.

Physical Hazards

Physical hazards abound in the laboratory and include such things as ergonomic issues, fire, electrical hazards, noise levels, equipment, accidents (e.g., slipping, falling, and lifting), UV light exposure, and compressed gases (18). Accidents often occur from overcrowding in the work area, poor lighting, poor maintenance, and lack of attention to detail by the employee. All accidents should be investigated with the intent of identifying the cause of the accident and correcting the problem. For example, back injuries are reduced by training employees on the correct method for lifting heavy objects. Falling is often caused by slippery floors, obstructed vision, or obstacles. Electrical safety relies on the proper grounding of equipment, the availability of adequate electrical outlets, and the prohibition of the use of extension cords. UV lights should be installed according to the manufacturer's instruction to avoid skin or eye injuries. Also, the laboratory should be evaluated for ergonomic problems, excessive noise, and excessive stress on employees. Workers under excessive stress tend to make more mistakes and have more frequent accidents.

Radiation Hazards

The implementation of a radiation safety program monitored by a radiation safety officer can minimize the occupational exposure to ionizing radiation from radioactive material or ionizing radiation-producing equipment (28). The degree of risk from ionizing radiation is related to the type of radiation (i.e., alpha, beta, or gamma) emitted, the quantity of radioactive material present, and the source of exposure (i.e., internal or external). Engineering and work practice controls are essential to minimizing the risk of working with radioactive material. Three factors must be considered: (i) time, (ii) distance, and (iii) shielding. The goal is to minimize the length of exposure, maintain the greatest distance between the radioactive material and the worker, and use an effective shield (i.e., lead, Plexiglas). Work practice controls for radiation, including a dedicated area for working with radioisotopes, are similar to other laboratory hazards and include appropriate PPE (e.g., lead aprons) and monitoring badges (28). Today, most tests that were once performed by radioimmunoassay are now performed by enzyme immunoassay, and so many clinical laboratories no longer handle any radiolabeled compounds.

Standard Precautions

All laboratories should adhere to the concept of Standard Precautions, which states that all patients and all laboratory specimens are potentially infectious and should be handled accordingly (24, 33). This concept arose from the observation that infections are often unrecognized in patients. "Standard Precautions" replaces earlier terms such as "Blood and Body Fluid Precautions," "Universal Precautions," and "Body Substance Precautions" found in OSHA documents (38, 39). The OSHA documents place the emphasis on blood-borne pathogens such as HIV, hepatitis B virus (HBV), and hepatitis C virus (HCV) whereas the concept of Standard Precautions recognizes that all infectious agents and all OPIM, except perspiration, pose risk to the healthcare worker (15, 16).

OSHA identifies a number of practices that should be implemented to protect the worker from exposure to blood-borne pathogens, including an exposure control and risk assessment plan (33). Methods that can be implemented to minimize exposure to infectious agents shield the laboratory worker from infectious material through a set of engineering and work practice controls and the use of PPE. In addition, the OSHA regulations require that employers provide HBV vaccination, postexposure evaluation, and follow-up; communicate the hazards to employees; and maintain appropriate records (2, 6, 33). Employees who decline immunization against HBV are required to sign a HBV vaccine declination form (Appendix 26.1).

Hazard Prevention and Containment

Risk Assessment

The risk associated with handling hazardous material should be assessed, and an exposure control plan should be implemented. Rather than retrospectively analyzing problems, laboratory managers need to proactively assess risk and institute the necessary procedures to reduce the potential risk. For chemical, physical, and radiological hazards, the classification of the hazard is straightforward and usually the risk can be determined. For biohazardous material, the assessment of risk is more difficult, is often qualitative, and is based on the pathogenicity and concentration of the agent, the infectious dose, the route of transmission, the viability of the agent in the environment, and the availability of treatment or prophylaxis (5, 13, 27).

Two lists of risk groups have been published to facilitate the assessment of risk from different microorganisms and to recommend the appropriate safety practices for handling infectious agents (5, 53). The World Health Organization (WHO) lists four groups of biohazardous agents based on the level of risk to the individual and community and the availability of effective treatment and prevention (Table 26.2). The Centers for Disease Control and Prevention/National Institutes of Health (CDC/NIH) guidelines propose four biosafety levels (BSLs) and recommendations for appropriate containment practices for a list of agents known to cause LAIs. Each BSL is based on the increased risk associated with the factors listed earlier (Table 26.3). Each BSL consists of combinations of PPE, engineering and work practice controls, and laboratory design that are appropriate for work with a particular infectious agent (Table 26.4). The BSL numbers (1 to 4) imply increased occupational risk from exposure to an agent and the need for additional containment for work with that agent. A conservative approach should be used when safety information is not available for a microorganism or new laboratory procedure. Generally, routine clinical laboratories operate with BSL 2 practices or BSL 3 practices for some mycobacterial or fungal agents (5). Additional information can be found on websites listed in Appendix 26.2.

A risk assessment and exposure plan for the clinical laboratory should identify the appropriate safety practices for handling infectious material that may contain any of a variety of pathogenic microorganisms (Table 26.5). Risk assessment must take into account the agent, the host, and the work activity in the development of a comprehensive safety plan (13). Management must monitor the plan, document accidents in writing, and make adjustments based on

Table 26.2 WHO's risk groups[a]

Risk group	Characterization
1	Unlikely to cause disease. Not considered infectious.
2	Moderate individual and low community risk. Unlikely to cause serious disease or be transmitted. Effective treatment and prevention available.
3	High individual and community risk. Causes serious infections but not readily transmitted. Effective treatment and prevention usually available.
4	High individual and community risk. Readily transmitted and no effective treatment or prevention available.

[a]From reference 53.

Table 26.3 CDC/NIH guidelines for assigning microorganisms to BSL[a]

BSL	Characterization
1	Well-characterized agents not known to consistently cause disease in healthy adult humans. Minimal potential hazard to laboratory personnel and the environment.
2	Agents of moderate potential hazard to personnel and the environment.
3	Indigenous or exotic agents that cause serious or potentially lethal disease as a result of exposure by the inhalation route.
4	Dangerous and exotic agents that pose a high individual risk of aerosol-transmitted laboratory infections and life-threatening disease.

[a]From reference 5.

accidental exposures to infectious agents and new information. Laboratory accidents should be discussed at the quality assurance or safety committee meeting (preferably quarterly but no less than yearly) and immediately with the staff in the section where the accident occurred. The accident report and corrective action is documented in the minutes of the committee meeting. Common safety mistakes or compliance issues are listed in Appendix 26.3.

Laboratories that use or store Select Agents (Table 26.6) under BSL 2, 3, or 4 practices must address the following security and safety concerns:

- risk and threat assessment
- facility security plans
- physical security
- security of data and electronic technology systems
- security policies for personnel
- access controls to the laboratory
- procedures for agent inventory and accountability
- shipping, transfer and receiving of Select Agents

- emergency response plans; and
- reporting of incidents, unintentional injuries, and security breaches.

The Select Agents plan must be part of the daily operation of the laboratory, and all employees must be knowledgeable of the plan (7). For security of Select Agent areas and public safety, access to the laboratory should be limited and restricted to individuals who have a legitimate purpose for entering the work area. Laboratory entrances should be locked by keypads, keys, or identification card keys. Laboratory employees should continuously monitor entrances that remain open. The laboratory should have a policy that defines who may visit and a procedure for removing unauthorized persons. Visitors and service workers should sign an entry log, be issued an identification badge with an expiration date, wear a laboratory coat, and be accompanied by a laboratory employee. Laboratory supervisors should ensure that all visitors and service workers understand the laboratory's security and safety requirements, safety signage, and areas that are posted off-limits to visitors.

Maintenance workers and cleaning staff must also understand the laboratory's security and safety procedures, sign the entry log, and ideally, perform their tasks when laboratory employees are present. The laboratory supervisor should instruct the maintenance and cleaning staff on the restricted areas of the laboratory (e.g., mycobacteriology laboratory) and precisely define their duties (e.g., do not handle biohazardous material). When work is required in the restricted areas, a laboratory worker should escort or monitor the person.

Handwashing

Handwashing is the most important procedure to reduce the duration of exposure to an infectious agent or chemical, prevent dissemination of an infectious agent, and reduce

Table 26.4 BSLs, practices, and equipment[a]

BSL	Practices	Safety equipment and facilities
1	Standard microbiological practices	None required
2	BSL 1 practices Limit access Display biohazard signs Sharps precautions Staff trained with pathogens Safety manual available	BSC used for specimen processing and work producing aerosols or splashes; PPE (coats, gloves, face shields) as needed; autoclave available
3	BSL 2 practices Controlled access Collect baseline serum for all personnel	BSL 2 equipment/facilities; BSC used for work with all specimens and cultures; PPE (gowns, masks) as needed; negative pressure airflow; self-closing double doors; exhausted air not recirculated
4	BSL 3 practices Clothing change before entering Shower on exit Decontaminate all waste on exit	BSL 3 equipment/facilities; separate building; BSC and full-body, air-supplied positive pressure suit for all procedures; specialized ventilation and decontamination system

[a]From reference 5.

Table 26.5 Risk assessment and exposure control plan for clinical microbiology laboratory[a]

Laboratory section and task	Exposure risk from: Blood and body fluids	Cultured biological agents	PPE[b] Gloves	Lab coats/ gowns	Face/splash shields	Engineering controls[c] BSC	Sharps containers available[d]
General							
Supplies inventory	Low			Coat			
Clerical: computer entry, telephones, records, etc.	Low		P	Coat			
Instrument maintenance:							
Parts contaminated	High	Variable	R	Gown			
Parts not contaminated	Low	Variable	D	Coat			
Surface decontamination	Low	Variable	R	Coat			
Waste disposal	High	Variable	R	Gown	A(D)		Sharps
Bacteriology[e]							
Specimen processing	High	BSL 2	R	Coat		R	Sharps
Subculture blood culture bottles	High	BSL 2	R	Coat	A[f]	A[f]	Needles
Subculture colonies or broth cultures	Low	BSL 2[e]		Coat			Sharps
Prepare, fix, stain, and read slides	Low	BSL 2		Coat			Slides
Identification tests and antimicrobial susceptibility testing	Low	BSL 2		Coat			Sharps
Mycology and Mycobacteriology[e]							
Specimen processing	High	BSL 2/3	R	Gown	R[e]		Sharps
Prepare smears, wet mounts; fix slides	High	BSL 2/3	R	Gown	R		Slides
Read wet mounts from specimens	High	BSL 2	R	Coat			Slides
Read wet mounts from cultures	Low	BSL 2/3	R	Coat			Slides
Examine sealed cultures	Low	BSL 2/3[g]		Coat			
Stain fixed smears, read	Low			Coat			Slides
Handle yeast cultures, smears, and fixed slides	Low	BSL 2		Coat		D	Slides
Handle molds and mycobacteriology cultures	Low	BSL 2/3[h]	R	Gown		R[e]	Sharps
Virology[i]							
Specimen processing	High	BSL 2	R	Coat	R		Sharps
Feed and manipulate uninoculated cells	Low			Coat			Pipettes
Read cells for cytopathic effect	Low	BSL 2		Coat			
Feed and manipulate inoculated cells	High	BSL 2	R		Coat	R	Pipettes
Perform identification tests	High	BSL 2	R		Coat	D	Sharps
Stain fixed slides and read	Low				Coat		Slides
Parasitology							
Concentrate fecal specimens, smears, wet mounts	Low	BSL 2	R		Coat		Pipette, sticks
Read fecal wet mounts	Low	BSL 2	R		Coat		Slides
Prepare blood smears; fix slides	High	BSL 2	R		Coat	A	Slides
Stain and read slides	Low				Coat		Slides
PCR/DNA probes/antigen detection							
Specimen processing	High	BSL 2/3	R	Coat	A[j]	A[j]	Pipettes
Cultured microorganism	Low	BSL 2	D	Coat		R	Sharps
		BSL 3	R	Gown		R[k]	Sharps
Serology							
Manipulate serum	High	BSL 2	R	Gown	A		Pipettes
Arrange tubes; prepare and dispense reagents	Low			Gown			
Mix serum and reagents; read and discard tests	High	BSL 2	R	Gown	A[j]	A[j]	Pipettes

[a]Adapted from reference 19. Abbreviations: R, required; D, discretionary; P, prohibited; A, one of the required alternatives.

[b]Remove PPE when leaving the laboratory. Gowns must have a solid front and be impervious to liquid.

[c]Recapping of needles is prohibited. Carry tubes in racks or use plastic tubes. Plan each task to minimize known hazards. Wash hands before leaving the laboratory.

[d]Sharps include needles, scalpels, pipettes, sticks, syringes, slides, plastic loops, and coverslips.

[e]Requires surveillance and action plan for occasional isolation of BSL 3 organism (e.g., *Brucella* spp., *Francisella* spp., *Mycobacterium* spp., and systemic fungi), especially when plates are held more than 3 days. *M. tuberculosis* requires the use of a safety centrifuge, a BSC, and a HEPA-filtered mask or respirator.

[f]Use a BSC or acrylic splash shield.

[g]Requires a contingency plan for breakage of culture containers.

[h]Mycobacteria other than tuberculosis can be handled at BSL 2; however, use BSL 3 practices because most manipulations precede organism identification.

[i]Special precautions for BSL 4 agents (e.g., hemorrhagic fever virus, smallpox) should be arranged through CDC's emergency number (770-488-7100).

[j]Vortexing or other splatter-generating steps require use of a BSC or safety shield.

[k]Requires BSL 3 practices if there is potential for aerosols.

451

Table 26.6 Select Agent list[a]

Bacteria	Viruses (continued)
Bacillus anthracis	Monkeypox virus
Brucella species	Rift Valley fever virus
Burkholderia mallei and *B. pseudomallei*	South American hemorrhagic fever viruses
Clostridium botulinum	Tick-borne encephalitis complex viruses
Francisella tularensis	Variola major and minor virus (smallpox virus)
Yersinia pestis	Venezuelan equine encephalitis virus
	Viruses causing hantavirus pulmonary syndrome
Rickettsiae	Yellow fever virus
Coxiella burnetii	
Rickettsia prowanzekii and *R. rickettsii*	**Toxins**
	Abrin
Fungi	Botulinum toxins
Coccidioides immitis and *C. posadasii*	*Clostridium perfringens* epsilon toxin
	Conotoxins
Viruses	Diacetoxyscirpenol
Crimean-Congo hemorrhagic fever virus	Ricin
Eastern equine encephalitis virus	Saxitoxin
Ebola virus	Shigatoxin
Equine morbillivirus (Hendre, Nipah)	Staphylococcal enterotoxins
Herpesvirus 1 (herpes B virus)	Tetrodotoxin
Lassa fever virus	T-2 toxin
Marburg virus	

[a]From reference 49.

overall infection rates in a healthcare facility. Hand contamination occurs during manipulation of specimens and contact with work surfaces, telephones, and equipment. Laboratory personnel should wash their hands:

- immediately after removing gloves,
- after obvious contamination,
- after completion of work,
- before leaving the laboratory, and
- before hand contact with nonintact skin, eyes, or mucous membranes.

Handwashing sinks should be located at each entry/exit door, and ideally the faucet should be operated by a knee/foot control. If these controls are not available, the faucet should be turned on and off using a paper towel. Handwashing should be performed using a soap or antiseptic compound, starting at the wrist area and extending down between the fingers and around and under the fingernails. Hands should be rinsed from the wrists downward (51). Recently, CDC recommended that in addition to traditional soap and water handwashing, healthcare personnel can also use alcohol-based gels (Table 26.7) (9).

Barrier Protection
PPE shields the individual from contact with a particular hazard. OSHA standards require that PPE shall be provided, used, and maintained for all hazards found in the workplace, including biological, environmental, chemical, and radioactive compounds, and mechanical irritants capable of causing injury or illness through absorption, in-

halation, or physical contact. Employees must be trained in the appropriate use of PPE for a specific task, the limitations of PPE, and procedures for maintaining, storing, and disposing of PPE.

Gloves. Gloves protect the wearer from exposure to potentially infectious material and other hazardous material and are available in material designed for specific tasks. Gloves must be provided by the employer and should be of the proper size and appropriate material for the task. Gloves are available in wrist, elbow, and shoulder length. Thin latex, vinyl, or nitrile gloves offer protection from exposure to potentially infectious material and should be changed frequently. Because of latex hypersensitivity in some workers, only powder-free latex gloves should be used, or better yet, gloves should be made of nitrile, polyethylene, or other material. The prevalence of latex allergy in healthcare workers ranges from 6 to 16% and usually presents as a type of allergic reaction (e.g., skin rashes; hives; flushing; itching; nasal, eye, or sinus symptoms; asthma; and rarely, anaphylaxis). While removal of latex products from the workplace is the final solution, other exposure control measures include education of new employees on latex allergies, screening high-risk employees for latex allergy symptoms, and frequent cleaning and changing of ventilation filters in latex use areas. When an employee suffers from the more serious Type I hypersensitivity to latex, latex cannot be used in the employee's work area, which should be posted as "latex free."

When working with chemicals, the gloves should be of a material known to resist the particular chemicals. Gener-

Table 26.7 Characteristics of hand-hygiene antiseptic agents[a]

| | Bacteria | | | | | Speed | |
Group	GP	GN	Mycobacteria	Fungi	Viruses	of action	Comments
Alcohols	+++	+++	+++	+++	+++	F	Optimum concentration 60 to 95%; no persistent activity
Chlorhexidine (2% and 4% aqueous)	+++	++	+	+	+++	I	Persistent activity; rare allergic reactions
Iodine compounds	+++	+++	+++	++	+++	I	Causes skin burns; usually too irritating for hands
Iodophors	+++	+++	+	++	++	I	Less irritating than iodine
Phenol derivatives	+++	+	+	+	+	I	Neutralized by nonionic detergents
Triclosan[b]	+++	++	+	−	+++	I	Acceptability on hands varies
Quaternary ammonium compounds	+	++	−	−	+	S	Used only in combination with alcohols; ecological concerns

[a]From reference 9. +++, Excellent; ++, good, but does not include entire bacterial spectrum; +, fair; −, no activity or not sufficient; F, fast; I, intermediate; S, slow; GP, gram positive; GN, gram negative.

[b]phenoxyphenol.

ally the material will be neoprene, nitrile, or a butyl rubber. General purpose utility gloves should be used for housekeeping chores. Insulated gloves are available for handling hot or cold items. Puncture-resistant gloves should be used in the autopsy suite or when handling scalpels or other sharp objects.

Protective clothing. Laboratory workers should wear fully closed long-sleeved coats or gowns that extend below the level of the workbench. When there is a potential for splashing or spraying, the material must be fluid resistant. Fluid-proof clothing (plastic or plastic lined) must be worn when there is the potential for soaking by infectious material. When handling chemicals, clothing must be composed of a material that is resistant to the particular chemical. Laboratory workers should not wear laboratory clothing out of the laboratory. All protective clothing should be changed immediately when contaminated to prevent the potentially infectious material or chemical from contacting the skin. Coats and gowns should not be taken home for cleaning but should be laundered by the institution. When handling highly toxic compounds, complete body suits should be worn.

Face and eye protection. Face and eye protection should be used when splashes or sprays of infectious material or chemicals may occur. Face and eye protection equipment includes goggles, face shields, and splash guards. Face shields provide the best protection for the entire face and neck. Splash guards provide an alternative method for face and eye protection. If only goggles are worn, the user should also wear an appropriate mask to prevent contamination of mucous membranes. Hazardous materials such as corrosives should always be manipulated behind splash guards or while wearing appropriate PPE.

Engineering and Work Practice Controls

Engineering and work practice controls are designed to prevent or minimize exposure to infectious material and injury from sharps. These controls include mechanical pipettes, bench tops impervious to liquids and chemicals, biohazard bags, centrifuge safety cups, eye wash stations, ventilation systems, biological safety cabinets (BSCs) and fume hoods, plasticware, and plastic collection devices (e.g., vacutainers, hematocrit tubes) (10). An OSHA standard requires that safety needle devices or needleless systems be used whenever possible (35, 40). All hazardous chemicals should be stored below eye level and transported in safety carriers. Incompatible chemicals should be stored apart, and flammables should be stored in a safety canister and a flame-resistant cabinet. The maximum quantity of flammable material that can be stored in a cabinet is defined by the manufacturer (23). Flammables requiring refrigeration can only be stored in an explosion-proof refrigerator. Compressed gas cylinders must be moved with the valve safety cover in place and secured to a handcart. When stationary, the cylinder must be secured upright with bottom and top restraints. Open-toed shoes or sandals should not be worn in the laboratory to prevent accidental spillage on bare skin. Movements that bring the hand to the mouth, eyes, or mucous membranes should be discouraged. Therefore, employees should not eat, drink, apply cosmetics or contact lenses, etc., in the laboratory. Visitors should be discouraged or accompanied by an employee.

Respiratory Protection

Respiratory devices are available to prevent inhalation of chemical dust or fumes and infectious aerosols. The type of mask used depends on the specific hazard. For example, a properly fitted N95 mask is employed for protection against aerosolized *M. tuberculosis* (33). A chemical fume mask employs cartridges that are designed to reduce exposure to a particular chemical, but the cartridge must be replaced periodically. A self-contained breathing apparatus offers the greatest degree of protection and is used when toxic levels are high or the danger is unknown (23).

Immunization

The current CDC guidelines on immunization of healthcare workers, including laboratory personnel, provide recommendations for agents of bioterrorism (Table 26.8) and other microorganisms (33). There are no generally available vaccines against *Brucella* spp. or viral hemorrhagic fever agents, and immunization of laboratory workers against the other bioterrorism agents is not recommended at this time. It is also not recommended that clinical labo-

ratory personnel be immunized routinely against *M. tuberculosis*, hepatitis A virus, *N. meningitidis*, rabies virus, or *Salmonella typhi*. However, immunization should be considered when an individual processes a large number of specimens containing one of these agents, performs research on an agent, or in the case of rabies or hepatitis A viruses, works with infected animals.

Warning Signs and Labels

Warning signs and labels are designed to provide a universal policy to alert visitors and employees to potential laboratory hazards and hazardous areas in the laboratory. OSHA-specified signage should be used whenever applicable (31, 36, 37). The color of the sign identifies the level of risk: a) danger (red, white, and black), b) caution (yellow and black), or c) safety instruction (green and white) (31).

Table 26.8 Vaccines[a]

Disease/agent	Immunity by natural exposure	Vaccine type	Vaccine efficacy (aerosol exposure)	Comments
Anthrax	Yes[b]	Human: Cell-free culture filtrate of an avirulent, non-encapsulated derivative of a bovine isolate designated V770 Animal: Spore suspension of an avirulent, nonencapsulated live strain	2-dose efficacy against 200–500 LD_{50}[c] in monkeys	**Required for level A lab[d]:** No **Laboratory-acquired cases:** None reported since the late 1950s, at which time the human vaccine was introduced. **Immunity:** Combined vaccine efficacy against both forms of anthrax (inhalational and cutaneous) = 93%.
Brucellosis	Yes	Human: No human vaccine available in U.S. Animal: In 1996, RB51, a live attenuated strain of *B. abortus* replaced the S19 strain, which was also a live attenuated vaccine	No vaccine	**Required for level A lab:** None available **Laboratory-acquired cases:** It is the most commonly reported bacterial infection acquired in laboratories. One of the largest reported incidents involved 45 cases with 1 death. Protection is based on adherence to BSL 3 precautions. **Immunity:** Studies in humans demonstrate that immunity is acquired after active infection; both cellular and humoral responses are required.
Botulism	No	Pentavalent (ABCDE) toxoid[e]	3-dose efficacy 100% against 25–250 LD_{50} in primates	**Required for level A lab:** No **Laboratory-acquired cases:** There has been 1 report of laboratory-associated botulism. **Immunity:** In food-borne exposures, immunity does not develop even with severe disease, and its repeated occurrence has been reported.
Tularemia	Partial	Live attenuated vaccine	80% protection against 1–10 LD_{50}	**Required for level A lab:** No **Laboratory-acquired cases:** Over the past 50 years, it has been the third most common bacterial infection acquired in laboratories, mostly among research labs. **Immunity:** Multiple episodes of reinfection have been documented among vaccinated laboratory personnel and in unimmunized individuals.

(continued)

Table 26.8 Vaccines (continued)

Disease/agent	Immunity by natural exposure	Vaccine type	Vaccine efficacy (aerosol exposure)	Comments
Plague	Partial	Suspension of killed (formalin-inactivated) *Yersinia pestis*	Has yet to be measured precisely in controlled studies; at least 2 vaccinated persons contracted pneumonic plague following *Y. pestis* exposure	**Required for level A lab:** No **Laboratory-acquired cases:** Few lab-associated cases have been reported; since 1936 only 3 cases of pneumonic plague have been documented. **Immunity:** Indirect evidence, mainly from the military, indicates that the plague vaccine is effective for preventing flea-borne transmission of disease.
Smallpox	Yes	Vaccinia (smallpox) vaccine[f] (grown in the skin of vaccinated bovine calves)	Vaccine protects against large doses in primates	**Required for level A lab:** No **Laboratory-acquired cases:** None **Immunity:** If a smallpox sample is handled at level A, vaccination within 3 days postexposure is considered effective in preventing serious infection and death. Vaccinia immune globulin may also be considered but may compromise postexposure vaccination efficacy.
Viral hemorrhagic fever	?[g]	None available	No vaccine	**Required for level A lab:** No **Laboratory-acquired cases:** Skin/mucous membrane exposure to virus-laden material, i.e., blood, cell cultures, body fluid/secretions, has been responsible for most recognized cases among humans. **Immunity:** To be determined.

[a]From http://www.bt.cdc.gov.

[b]Some degree of immunity is conferred following cutaneous anthrax, i.e., the lethal dose is below that required for an immune response.

[c]LD$_{50}$, Amount of a toxic agent sufficient to kill 50% of a population.

[d]Sentinel (level A) laboratories are located in hospitals and clinics and primarily function at BSL2.

[e]Distributed by the CDC under an investigational new drug protocol and used to protect high-risk laboratorians actively working with *C. botulinum* or the toxins.

[f]Distributed by the CDC.

[g]Immunity to Lassa fever reinfection occurs following infection, but the length of protection is unknown.

Containers of hazardous reagents, radionuclides, chemicals, and waste must be labeled with the chemical name and appropriate hazard label (e.g., flammable, corrosive, carcinogen, irritant).

Biological Safety Cabinets and Chemical Fume Hoods

Chemical fume hoods should be used when there is risk of exposure to hazardous fumes or splashes while preparing or dispensing chemical solutions. Airflow is generally controlled by a movable sash and should be in the range of 80 to 120 feet per minute (23, 37). Objects in the hood should not obstruct the airflow or the workspace. Chemical fume hoods are certified annually.

Biological hazards are best contained within a class IIA or class IIB BSC. BSCs are the most important containment equipment in the microbiology laboratory. Class III cabinets are used with infectious agents requiring BSL 3 or 4 containment. BSCs operate at a negative air pressure, with air passing through a HEPA filter. The vertical airflow serves as a barrier between the cabinet and user. More detailed information on the selection and use of BSCs can be found in Appendix 26.2 and references 4, 5, and 33.

Sterilization and Decontamination

When discussing germicides, sterilants, disinfectants, and decontamination, it is important to understand the differences between the terms (10, 33, 51). A germicide is a substance that kills pathogenic organisms on inanimate surfaces. Disinfectants destroy all microorganisms, but not necessarily their spores, on inanimate surfaces. Sterilants are agents that kill all microbial life, including spores, on inanimate surfaces. Prions (abnormal host proteins) are not covered by these definitions.

Decontamination is a procedure that eliminates or reduces microbial or toxic agents to a safe level with respect to the transmission of infection or other adverse effect. Routine decontamination of the work environment is usually performed with disinfectants (Table 26.9). It is important that the manufacturer's instructions for preparation and use be followed carefully. The selection of a disinfectant depends on the degree of microbial killing required, the effectiveness against an extended spectrum of pathogens, compatibility with the surface or device being decontaminated, toxicity, residue activity, and odor. Disinfectants can be hazardous compounds when not used properly (Table 26.9). No single product is adequate for all decontamination purposes. Appropriate PPE (i.e., gloves, impervious gowns, eye protection, masks) should be worn when cleaning and decontaminating equipment. Alcohol should not be used in a poorly ventilated area or near flames, and corrosive sodium hypochlorite solutions should not be used on metals.

Prions, the causative agents of Creutzfeld-Jacob disease and transmissible spongiform encephalopathies, are resistant to standard disinfection and sterilization procedures (1, 10, 12, 33). The disinfection procedures for high-risk specimens (central nervous system tissue), medium-risk specimens (cerebrospinal fluid, lymph node, spleen, pituitary gland, and tonsil) and low-risk specimens (bone marrow, liver, lung, thymus, and kidney) or equipment contaminated with these specimens differ according to the level of risk (12, 33). Devices or material contaminated with high-risk tissue should be discarded or decontaminated by steam sterilization at 121°C for 1 h or soaked in 1N NaOH for 1 h or in 0.5% sodium hypochlorite (2% free chlorine) for 2 h before cleaning and sterilization by conventional means (33). Conventional heat, chemical, or gas sterilization or high-level disinfection can sterilize devices contaminated by medium- or low-risk specimens. Formaldehyde (3.7 to 4.0%)-fixed brain tissue (<5 mm thick) is soaked in 95 to 100% formic acid for 1 h followed by immersion in fresh 4% formaldehyde for 48 h before preparing histological slides for examination.

Spill Management

Biological

The management of biohazardous spills in the clinical laboratory must account for the specific infectious agent, the volume of infectious material spilled, and the presence of aerosols. Spills involving BSL 3 agents are serious because aerosols can transmit these agents. Occupants should hold their breath, evacuate the area immediately, close the doors, and not reenter the area for 30 to 60 min (14, 33). When breakage occurs in a centrifuge, the equipment must remain closed for at least 30 min before decontamination is undertaken. A tuberculocidal disinfectant should be used for decontamination (10). A low-level disinfectant such as a quaternary ammonium compound should not be used. Additional factors that influence decontamination of the spill site include the type of infectious material (blood, culture medium), the concentration and virulence of the infectious agent, the protein content of the material, and the spill surface (porous or fluid resistant). Initially, spills should be absorbed with paper towels, gauze pads, or commercial absorbents such as granular or silica gel absorbents.

Table 26.9 Activity levels and hazards of selected germicides[a]

Procedure/product	Aqueous concentration	Activity level	Hazards
Sterilization			
Glutaraldehyde	Variable	NA	Dermatitis, toxic
Hydrogen peroxide	6–30%	NA	Irritant
Formaldehyde	6–8%	NA	Irritant, toxic, sensitization
Chlorine dioxide	Variable	NA	Irritant, gas toxic
Peracetic acid	Variable	NA	Irritant
Disinfection			
Glutaraldehyde	Variable	High to intermediate	Dermatitis, toxic
Hydrogen peroxide	3–6%	High to intermediate	Irritant
Formaldehyde	1–8%	High to low	Irritant, toxic, sensitization
Chlorine dioxide	Variable	High	Gas toxic, irritant
Peracetic acid	Variable	High	Irritant
Chlorine compounds	500–5,000 mg/liter free available chlorine	Intermediate	Gas toxic, irritant
Alcohols	70%	Intermediate	Toxic (isopropyl)
Phenolic compounds	0.5–3%	Intermediate to low	Leukoderma, depigmentation
Iodophor compounds	40–50 mg/liter free iodine; up to 10,000 mg/liter available iodine	Intermediate to low	Skin irritation
Quaternary ammonium compounds	0.1–0.2%	Low	Dermatitis, sensitization

[a]From references 17, 33, 51. NA, not available.

Generally, the spill cleanup should be performed by the individual who accidentally spilled the infectious material or by persons specifically trained in the cleanup of biohazardous materials. Appropriate protective equipment must be used in decontaminating spills involving BSL 2 or BSL 3 agents. The PPE includes disposable gloves (heavyweight and puncture resistant), fluid-impermeable shoe covers, coats or gowns with long sleeves, and facial protection. When the spill involves a BSL 3 agent, a respirator or HEPA-filtered mask should be used. In this situation it is usually best to call the spill emergency response team, which is trained to handle this type of spill.

Any broken glass in the spill area should be removed and discarded without contact with the hands. This is accomplished with rigid cardboard, tongs, forceps, hemostats, or a plastic scoop (dustpan). Glass is discarded into a puncture-resistant container, and other contaminated material is discarded into a biohazardous waste container.

After the absorbent material is discarded, the spill site can be cleaned with an aqueous detergent solution to dilute any remaining infectious material and to remove excess protein. You should use a tuberculocidal disinfectant that remains on the site for 20 min. Then absorb any remaining disinfectant with absorbent material, rinse the area with water, and dry.

When spills occur in a BSC, do not turn off the cabinet fan. Minor spills can be absorbed with absorbent paper, and the area can be decontaminated with a disinfectant. When the infectious material has flowed into the grille, all items in the cabinet should be wiped with a disinfectant and removed. The drain valve should be closed and disinfectant should be poured onto the surface and through the grille into the drain pan. You should allow 20 min of contact time with the disinfectant and then absorb the disinfectant with paper towels. Attach a hose to the drain valve and drain into a container with disinfectant. Remove the grille and rinse the drain pan with water. For major spills involving BSL 3 agents, a service consultant should be contacted for decontamination.

All materials necessary for the cleanup of a biohazardous spill should be assembled and stored as a biohazard spill kit (Appendix 26.4). The kit should contain an appropriate disinfectant (e.g., 10% household bleach), absorbent material (e.g., paper towels, gauze pads, and granular material such as BioZorb [Ulster Scientific, Inc., Highland, NY] for large spills), PPE (e.g., puncture-resistant utility gloves, water-impermeable shoe coverings, gown, mask, face shield, or eyewear), and autoclavable dustpan, tongs or forceps, plastic scoop and pusher, and bags. For BSL 3 agents a full face respirator or HEPA-filtered mask should be available. The biohazard spill kit can be stored in a puncture-resistant biohazardous waste container. Examples of spill cleanup procedures may be found in various guidelines

(5, 10, 14, 33) and Appendix 26.5. Following the spill cleanup, a report should be completed and submitted to the safety committee.

Chemical

The laboratory should have adequate spill response equipment readily available as a chemical spill kit (31). In the event of a chemical spill or leak, an initial determination on the need for an evacuation is made based on the immediate danger to life or health or when employees experience severe discomfort. Any or all of the following conditions usually warrant an evacuation:

- injured or ailing personnel
- symptoms of irritation reported by employees
- large volume spill
- flammable or explosive material spilled
- carcinogen spilled
- presence of strong odors

When an evacuation is required, close off the area, notify employees in the immediate vicinity of the spill, and report the situation to the emergency response team. Provide location, nature of the spill, personnel injured or trapped, and the hazard involved. Do not attempt to rescue patients or employees if your life or health may be endangered.

For minor spills (not involving flammables, explosives, or carcinogens), contain the spill, close off the spill area, and contact the emergency response team. An example of a chemical spill cleanup procedure for minor spills is shown in Appendix 26.6. A trained person should clean up the spill using appropriate PPE (gloves, gowns, and shoe covers resistant to the chemical, plus a face shield). Contain the spill with spill pads, pillows, or socks. Clean the spill using approved absorbents and neutralizing agents. Package the waste appropriately for pickup, labeling the container with the substance, date, and amount of material. As with biological spills, the response is dependent on the chemical hazard and volume of the spill. Prepare a spill report and submit it to the safety committee. The Material Safety Data Sheets (MSDS) contain information on the hazard classification, appropriate PPE, symptoms arising from exposure, and instructions for the safe handling, disposal, and cleanup of laboratory chemicals. OSHA requires that MSDS for all laboratory chemicals be readily available to all employees.

Waste Management

The laboratory is a major generator of chemical and biohazardous waste in the healthcare facility. Procedures for the handling of chemical waste are well defined because the hazardous substance is usually identifiable. However, medical or infectious wastes are not well defined and include categories such as contaminated sharps, cultures and stocks of infectious agents, blood and body fluids, and pathological waste (26, 34).

Regulatory Oversight

There are numerous federal, state, and local regulations governing the management of biohazardous waste:

- Federal regulations
  - OSHA's Blood-Borne Pathogen Standard (38): applies to the handling and packaging of regulated waste and the implementation of procedures to protect employees against potential exposure to infectious medical waste
  - Department of Transportation (DOT) (46, 47): sets requirements for transport of hazardous materials and regulated medical waste
- Guidelines and standards
  - CDC/NIH (5): management of infectious waste
  - NCCLS (34): management of waste generated by a clinical laboratory
  - Joint Commission on the Accreditation of Healthcare Organizations: requires a waste management plan for the institution that is in compliance with all federal, state, and local regulations
  - State and local regulations: many state and local jurisdictions have passed regulations governing the handling, treatment, and disposal of biohazardous waste.

Management Program

The laboratory's waste management plan should be part of the overall facility plan and must comply with the numerous federal, state, and local regulations. Most plans address the following elements.

Identification of hazardous waste. Although no generally acceptable definition of medical waste is available, there are categories of waste that are considered potentially infectious, namely human blood, body substances, and blood products; contaminated sharps; cultures and stocks of microbial agents; contaminated laboratory waste; PPE grossly contaminated with blood, body fluids, or microbiological cultures; and pathological waste (5, 11, 33, 34, 38).

Segregation. Knowledgeable personnel segregate waste into designated categories (i.e., chemical, routine trash, radiological, and infectious) at the point of generation to reduce the cost of disposal and to protect employees and others from exposure to hazardous material.

Packaging and labeling. Appropriate containment of hazardous material is the key to minimizing personnel and public exposure. Chemical and radioactive waste is separated and handled differently from other regulated medical waste. Containers for liquids are leakproof. All containers must have secure closures and maintain their integrity throughout the handling and transportation process. Containers must comply with the OSHA requirements for the category and volume of waste and treatment, transportation, labeling, and disposal method. For example, sharps must be placed in impervious, rigid, leakproof, color-coded, puncture-resistant containers with secure lids. Other medical waste may be placed in containers that are leakproof and labeled or color-coded as to hazard and have secure closures.

Storage. All waste should be treated as soon as possible. The waste storage area should be posted as to the hazard, be sited near the treatment area or loading dock for off-site treatment, and maintain a temperature and duration of storage that prevents spoilage. Access should be limited to authorized personnel.

Transport. Waste is transported in labeled and leakproof containers or carts appropriate for the hazard. When shipped to an off-site treatment facility, the containers must meet the specifications established by DOT. Transportation containers or carts should be routinely disinfected.

Treatment and disposal. The treatment and disposal of waste must comply with all federal, state, and local regulations. Most institutions contract with companies licensed to treat and dispose of hazardous waste. A number of waste treatment techniques and disposal methods are available for organizations that produce a small amount of waste (11, 34), but they must meet all regulatory requirements.

Contingency planning. The waste management plan should include a written plan for alternative treatment and disposal in the event of the failure of the normal waste management process. This plan must provide for increased storage or include an agreement with another generator to handle the waste in an emergency.

Training. Employee training must comply with OSHA's requirements and should include exposure risk information, safety policies, procedures for handling waste, required PPE, and the duties and responsibilities of the position. Training occurs annually for all employees, immediately for new employees, and before workers assume new duties or tasks.

Shipment of Infectious Substances

A complex and confusing set of national and international guidelines and regulations governs the shipment of clinical specimens and cultures of microorganisms (25, 46, 48, 53).

Recently, the DOT revised regulations for shipment of hazardous material were finalized (50). These regulations dictate the packaging and labeling of infectious material that is shipped via commercial carriers with the stated goal of protecting employees in the transportation industry and the general public. This protection is based on packages that are unlikely to leak or be damaged during shipment, labels affixed to the package that identify the particular hazard, and trained personnel who are responsible for the shipment of infectious material. These regulations and guidelines are constantly evolving as the various groups and organizations attempt to agree on one set of standards.

Infectious Substances

Classes of Dangerous Goods that are regulated include explosives, gases, flammables (liquids and solids), oxidizing substances, toxic and infectious substances, radioactive material, corrosives, and miscellaneous (includes dry ice). The two classes encountered in the clinical laboratory are Class 6 Toxic and Infectious Substances and Class 9 Miscellaneous Dangerous Goods (dry ice). Infectious substances are materials known or suspected to contain a pathogen with the potential to cause disease upon exposure. A pathogen is a virus or microorganism (including its plasmids or other genetic elements) or proteinaceous particle (prion) that has the potential to cause disease in humans or animals. The shipper must determine:

- when a specimen or material is considered an infectious substance,
- when a specimen or material is considered a diagnostic specimen, and
- when a specimen or material is exempt.

Material that is infectious to humans or animals, diagnostic specimens, biological products, clinical and medical waste, and genetically modified microorganisms are classified in Class 6, Division 6.2, and assigned to UN 2814 or UN 2900 based on their classification in one of four WHO risk groups (Table 26.2). Assignment to a risk group is based on the known medical condition and history of the patient, endemic local conditions, symptoms of the patient, or professional judgment concerning the circumstances of the patient. The four risk groups are defined by the pathogenicity, mode and ease of transmission, degree of risk to individuals and communities, and reversibility of the disease through known and effective preventive agents and treatment (Table 26.2). Specimens containing Risk Group 4 microorganisms or a Select Agent are considered infectious material. Within 7 days after identification of a Select Agent, CDC must be notified and the Select Agent must be destroyed or transferred to a registered entity (http://www.cdc.gov/od/sap/addforms.asp). Specimens that are shipped for diagnostic or investigation purposes and may contain Risk Group 2 or 3 microorganisms are considered diagnostic specimens for packaging

and shipment. Under this interpretation, many specimens that were previously considered infectious for packaging may be considered diagnostic specimens. This category includes material such as blood and blood components; secretions; tissue and tissue fluids; and excreta that are being transported for investigational or diagnostic purposes and do not require a Shippers Declaration for Dangerous Goods. Risk Group 1 includes organisms unlikely to cause human or animal disease and is not subject to regulation.

The shipper is responsible for correctly classifying the material being shipped. When there is uncertainty as to the infectious nature of the material, it is prudent to declare and ship the material as an infectious substance. The following questions may be helpful for classifying diagnostic specimens and biological products (43) and in determining substances that are regulated.

- Is the substance known or suspected to contain a pathogen?
- Is the sample being shipped for diagnostic or investigational purposes?
- Is there a low probability for the occurrence of Risk Group 4 pathogens in the sample?
- Is the sample known not to contain a pathogen?
- Is the substance a licensed biological product?
- Is the substance being shipped for any other reason?

Packaging, Labeling, and Shipping Regulated Material

All packages containing infectious substances must meet the shipping regulations of various organizations or agencies (25, 50, 53). However, the International Air Transport Association (IATA) requirements are usually acceptable under all regulations. They require triple packaging consisting of a primary receptacle that is leakproof, a secondary packaging that is also leakproof, and an outer package that is durable (Appendix 26.7). These containers are commercially available.

There are specific instructions for labeling packages containing infectious substances, diagnostic specimens, and biological products (30). Under IATA requirements, labeling and marking of the outer package must include (Appendix 26.8):

- an "Infectious Substance" label
- an address label with the shipper's and receiver's name, address, and telephone numbers
- the UN shipping name (e.g., infectious substance affecting humans) and the technical or scientific name of the substance
- the UN number (e.g., humans-UN 2814)

The shipping documents must be affixed to the outer package and include the Shipper's Declaration for Dangerous Goods (Appendix 26.9), a packing list, and an airway bill if shipping by air. IATA also requires notice of the type of packaging (e.g., fiberboard) and the statement "Prepared according to IATA." Orientation labels (arrows) must be placed on all packages containing greater than 50 ml of material.

The Federal Aviation Agency and/or Department of Transportation may inspect any shipper or receiver of dangerous goods unannounced at any time. The inspector may review training records, oversee the actual packaging and labeling of a shipment, and/or call the 24-h emergency number listed on the paperwork. The shipper or receiver may be quizzed on the hazards and characteristics of the dangerous goods, the proper decontamination and disposal of the hazardous material (information found on MSDS), and accident mitigation. MSDS for some microorganisms are available at www.hc-sc.gc.ca/pphb-dgspsp/msds-ftss/index.html. It is critical that the training program for the shipment of dangerous goods emphasizes this safety information.

Personnel Training

Safety training and the education of workers about potential hazards and safe work practices are essential to creating a safe work environment (23, 33). All personnel employed in the clinical laboratory must receive adequate safety training applicable to their position in order to perform their assigned tasks in a safe manner. Safety policies should be applied to work practices. This training is mandated by various governmental regulations and accreditation organizations and is required for new employees and students, individuals assigned new tasks, before the introduction of new hazards or procedures to the work environment, and on an annual basis for all personnel.

Training Program

The size and complexity of a safety training program will vary with the needs of the institution but must cover all applicable safety topics and policies. Some topics include:

- chemical information regarding job-specific hazards (e.g., exposure to formaldehyde or carcinogens)
- management of hazardous material and waste
- blood-borne pathogen information (epidemiology, symptoms, transmission)
- Standard Precautions
- selection, use, and limitations of PPE, safety equipment, and other control procedures
- postexposure management, accident reporting, and investigation of incidents
- emergency preparedness, including bioterrorism issues
- availability of all safety regulations

- medical surveillance program
- the employee's responsibility to follow all safety policies and inform supervisors of potential safety hazards

The laboratory safety training program should be developed with input from the infection control practitioner, industrial hygienist, and other knowledgeable individuals; highlight the potential risk from infectious agents and hazardous chemicals; and emphasize the reduced risk when work is performed according to the safety guidelines. The contents of the training program should be updated frequently as new safety information becomes available or regulations change.

Methods

The training format can be lectures, hands-on demonstrations, safety workshops, videos, computer programs, or distance learning. However, no matter which method is used, the trainer must be available to immediately respond to the trainee's questions during the session. The trainer must be competent in the area of laboratory safety and knowledgeable about current safety regulations, work practices, safety equipment, and hazards found in the clinical laboratory.

Documentation

The date of training, a summary of the presentation (or contents of the session), and attendance should be documented and placed in the employee's record. Training records should be maintained for 3 years.

Monitoring and Evaluation

The effectiveness of the training program can be evaluated with a test but realistically must be assessed by observing the daily practices of the employees for compliance with safety policies. When safety practices are not followed, the individual should be counseled and reeducated on the appropriate practice. Repeated disregard for safety guidelines should trigger strict disciplinary action. It is the employer's responsibility to enforce adherence to safe work practices.

The overall effectiveness of the laboratory safety program is assessed through safety audits (Table 26.10), inspections by outside agencies and organizations, review of incident and accident reports (Appendix 26.10), and observations and suggestions from employees. Audits and inspections should highlight concerns and provide recommendations to improve the safety program. Management provides the resources to address and correct any deficiencies, beginning with the most frequent and severe problem. However, in the end, a safe workplace develops from the efforts of all individuals in the organization.

Table 26.10 Laboratory safety checklist

Date: _____   Location: _____

Housekeeping/signage   **Describe deficiency**

_____ Unobstructed aisle/hallway   _____

_____ Bench tops decontaminated   _____

_____ Doors and storage areas labeled   _____

_____ Warning labels on containers   _____

_____ Handwashing sinks available   _____

Chemical safety

_____ Chemicals labeled and stored properly   _____

_____ Chemicals dated at receipt/opening   _____

_____ Containment for wastes and solvents   _____

_____ MSDS available   _____

_____ Chemical inventory lists   _____

Safety practices and equipment

_____ Eyewash stations checked weekly   _____

_____ BSC and fume hoods certified annually   _____

_____ Fire alarms and extinguishers   _____

_____ Chemical/biological spill kits   _____

_____ Sharps containers   _____

_____ Storage of food and drink prohibited   _____

_____ Leakproof specimen containers   _____

_____ Combustibles >18 inches from ceiling   _____

_____ Gas cylinders secured   _____

_____ Emergency procedures posted   _____

_____ Appropriate BSLs practiced   _____

PPE

_____ Disposable gloves used   _____

_____ Appropriate protective clothing   _____

_____ Eye and face protection   _____

_____ Respiratory masks   _____

Personnel training

_____ Chemical hygiene plan   _____

_____ Emergency preparedness   _____

_____ Blood-borne pathogens   _____

_____ Exposure follow-up procedure   _____

_____ Waste disposal   _____

_____ Standard Precautions   _____

Implement corrective action for any deficiencies and notify the safety committee.

Summary

The laboratory contains many biological, chemical, radiological, and physical hazards, including new infectious agents and the possibility for use of biological and chemical agents for acts of terrorism. However, many tools and practices are available to reduce the occupational risk from exposure to these hazards, including safety devices, Standard Precautions, PPE, BSCs and chemical fume hoods, warning signs and labels, safe work practices, and proper disposal of biological and chemical waste. A well-written safety management plan is a blueprint for implementation of safe practices and includes the necessary training to produce a safe work environment.

KEY POINTS

- Laboratory workers are exposed to biological, chemical, physical, and radiological hazards.
- A well-written and enforced safety management plan can minimize occupational risk.
- All laboratory personnel should adhere to the concept of Standard Precautions and use available barrier precautions.

GLOSSARY (33, 44)

Aerosol A system of respirable particles dispersed in a gas, smoke, or fog that can be retained in the lungs.

Airborne transmission The spread of infection by inhalation of droplet nuclei containing an infectious agent.

Blood-borne pathogens Pathogenic microorganisms that are present in human blood and can cause disease in humans.

Carcinogen Substance capable of causing a malignant tumor in humans or animals.

Ceiling limit The airborne concentration of a substance that cannot be exceeded at any time during the workday.

Contaminated Describes the presence or reasonably anticipated presence of blood or other potentially infectious materials on an item or surface.

Corrosive Any substance that causes visible destruction of human tissue at the site of contact. The U.S. Environmental Protection Agency defines corrosivity as a substance that is highly acidic (pH < 2.1) or highly alkaline (pH > 12.4).

Decontamination A procedure that eliminates or reduces microbial or toxic agents to a safe level with respect to the transmission of infection or other adverse effects.

Disinfectant An agent intended to destroy or irreversibly inactivate all microorganisms, but not necessarily their spores, on inanimate surfaces, e.g., work surfaces or medical devices.

Disinfection A procedure that kills pathogenic microorganisms but not necessarily their spores.

Engineering controls Controls (e.g., sharps disposal containers, self-sheathing needles, safer medical devices) that isolate or remove the hazard from the workplace.

Germicide A general term for an agent that kills pathogenic microorganisms on inanimate surfaces.

International Air Transport Association (IATA) A body of the commercial airline industry that governs international aviation. Publishes *Technical Instructions for the Safe Transport of Dangerous Goods by Air* and regulates dangerous goods for member airlines and anyone who tenders dangerous goods to those airlines.

Infectious waste Waste containing or assumed to contain pathogens of sufficient virulence and quantity that exposure to the waste by a susceptible host may result in a communicable disease.

Latex allergy Allergic reaction associated with latex glove use. The two types of allergic reactions are contact dermatitis (type IV delayed hypersensitivity), due to chemicals used in processing latex, and the more serious immunoglobulin E/histamine-mediated allergy (immediate or Type I hypersensitivity), due to latex proteins.

Material Safety Data Sheet (MSDS) Provides detailed information about hazards and protective measures relative to hazardous chemical substances.

Occupational exposure Reasonably anticipated skin, eye, mucous membrane, or parenteral contact with a hazard that may result from the performance of an employee's duties.

Other potentially infectious material (OPIM) Human body fluids including semen; vaginal secretions; urine; cerebrospinal fluid; synovial fluid; pleural fluid; pericardial fluid; peritoneal fluid; amniotic fluid; saliva; body fluids that may be contaminated with blood; unfixed tissue; HIV- or hepatitis virus-containing cell or organ cultures; blood or tissue from an infected animal; reagents; infectious waste; and cultures.

Parenteral Piercing mucous membranes or the skin through events such as needlesticks, human bites, and abrasions.

Permissible exposure limit (PEL) Maximum allowed exposure during a time-weighted average period (e.g., 8-h workday or 40-h workweek).

Personal protective equipment (PPE) Specialized clothing or equipment worn by an employee for protection against a hazard.

Primary container A vessel, including its closure, that contains a specimen.

Prions Infectious, abnormal host proteins that cause transmissible spongiform encephalopathies and are resistant to a number of standard disinfection and sterilization procedures.

Regulated waste Liquid or semiliquid blood or OPIMs; contaminated items that would release blood or OPIMs in a liquid or semiliquid state if compressed; items that are caked with dried blood or OPIMs and are capable of releasing these materials during handling; contaminated sharps; and pathological and microbiological wastes containing blood or OPIMs.

Secondary container A vessel into which the primary container is placed for transport within an institution; will contain a specimen if the primary container breaks or leaks in transit.

Sharps container A container approved for the containment and transport of contaminated sharps.

Short-term exposure limit Maximum exposure to a hazardous substance allowed at one time (normally measured in a single 15-min period).

Standard Precautions Set of precautions applied to all patients; designed to reduce risk of transmission of microorganisms in the healthcare setting.

Sterilant An agent intended to destroy all microorganisms (viruses, vegetative bacteria, fungi, and a large number of highly resistant bacterial endospores) on inanimate surfaces.

Sterilization A procedure that effectively kills all microbial life, including bacterial spores, on inanimate surfaces.

Universal Precautions Set of precautions designed to reduce risk of transmission of HIV, HBV, and other blood-borne pathogens in the healthcare setting.

REFERENCES

1. **Asher, D. M.** 1999. Transmissible spongiform encephalopathies, p. 1145–1157. *In* P. R. Murray, E. J. Baron, M. A. Pfaller, F. C. Tenover, and R. H. Yolken (ed.), *Manual of Clinical Microbiology,* 7th ed. ASM Press, Washington, D.C.

2. **Beltrami, E. M., I. T. Williams, C. N. Shapiro, and M. E. Chamberland.** 2000. Risk and mangagement of blood-borne infections in health care workers. *Clin. Microbiol. Rev.* **13:**385–407.

3. **Centers for Disease Control.** 1987. *Registry of Toxic Effects of Chemical Substances.* U.S. Government Printing Office, Washington, D.C.

4. **Centers for Disease Control and Prevention and National Institutes of Health (CDC/NIH).** 1995. *Primary Containment of Biohazards: Selection, Installation and Use of Biological Safety Cabinets.* J. Y. Richmond and R. W. McKinney (ed.), U.S. Printing Office, Washington, D.C.

5. **Centers for Disease Control and Prevention and National Institutes of Health (CDC/NIH).** 1999. *Biosafety in Microbiological and Biomedical Laboratories,* 4th ed. J. Richmond and R. W. McKinney (ed.), U.S. Government Printing Office, Washington, D.C.

6. **Centers for Disease Control and Prevention.** 2001. Updated U.S. Public Health Service guidelines for the management of occupational exposures to HBV, HCV, and HIV and recommendations for postexposure prophylaxis. *Morb. Mortal. Wkly. Rep.* **50**(RR11):1–42.

7. **Centers for Disease Control and Prevention.** 2002. Laboratory security and emergency response guidance for laboratories working with select agents. *Morb. Mortal. Wkly. Rep.* **51:**1–6.

8. **Centers for Disease Control and Prevention.** 2002. Laboratory-acquired meningococcal disease-United States, 2000. *Morb. Mortal. Wkly. Rep.* **51:**141–142.

9. **Centers for Disease Control and Prevention.** 2002. Guideline for hand hygiene in health-care settings. *Morb. Mortal. Wkly. Rep.* **51**(RR-16):1–47.

10. **Denys, G. A.** 2004. Section 15, Biohazards and safety. *In* H. D. Isenberg (ed.), *Clinical Microbiology Procedures Handbook,* 2nd ed. ASM Press, Washington, D.C.

11. **Denys, G. A., and J. G. Gordon.** 2004. Section 15.7, Management of infectious waste. *In* H. D. Isenberg (ed.), *Clinical Microbiology Procedures Handbook,* 2nd ed. ASM Press, Washington, D.C.

12. **Favero, M. S., and W. W. Bond.** 2001. Chemical disinfection of medical and surgical materials, p. 881–917. *In* S. S. Block (ed.), *Disinfection, Sterilization, and Preservation,* 5th ed. Lippincott Williams and Wilkins, Philadelphia, Pa.

13. **Fleming, D. O.** 2000. Risk assessment of biological hazards, p. 57–64. *In* D. O. Fleming and D. L. Hunt (ed.), *Biological Safety: Principles and Practices,* 3rd ed. ASM Press, Washington, D.C.

14. **Fleming, D. O.** 2000. Prudent biosafety practices, p. 369–381. *In* D. O. Fleming and D. L. Hunt (ed.), *Biological Safety: Principles and Practices,* 3rd ed. ASM Press, Washington, D.C.

15. **Garner, J. S.** 1996. Guideline for isolation precautions in hospitals. Part I: Evolution of isolation practices. *Am. J. Infect. Control* **24:**24–31.

16. **Garner, J. S.** 1996. Guideline for isolation precautions in hospitals. The Hospital Infection Control Practices Advisory Committee. *Infect. Control Hosp. Epidemiol.* **17:**53–80.

17. **Gershon, R., and I. F. Salkin.** 1992. Chemical safety, p. 14.2.1–14.2.5. *In* H. D. Isenberg (ed.), *Clinical Microbiology Procedures Handbook,* vol. 2. American Society for Microbiology, Washington, D.C.

18. **Gershon, R., and T. Stimpfel.** 1992. Physical and ergonomic safety, p. 14.4.1–14.4.3. *In* H. D. Isenberg (ed.), *Clinical Microbiology Procedures Handbook,* vol. 2. American Society for Microbiology, Washington, D.C.

19. **Gilchrist, M. J. R., J. Hindler, and D. O. Fleming.** 1992. Laboratory safety management, p. xxix–xxxvii. *In* H. D. Isenberg (ed.), *Clinical Microbiology Procedures Handbook,* vol. 2. American Society for Microbiology, Washington, D.C.

20. **Gilchrist, M. J. R., W. P. McKinney, J. M. Miller, and A. L. Weissfeld.** 2001. *Cumitech 33, Laboratory Safety, Management, and Diagnosis of Biological Agents Associated with Bioterrorism.* Coordinating ed., J. W. Snyder. ASM Press, Washington, D.C.

21. **Gilpin, R. W.** 2000. Elements of a biosafety program, p. 443–462. *In* D. O. Fleming and D. L. Hunt (ed.), *Biological Safety: Principles and Practices,* 3rd ed. ASM Press, Washington, D.C.

22. **Harding, A. L., and K. B. Byers.** 2000. Epidemiology of laboratory-associated infections, p. 35–54. *In* D. O. Fleming and D. L. Hunt (ed.), *Biological Safety: Principles and Practices,* 3rd ed. ASM Press, Washington, D.C.

23. **Hoeltge, G. A.** 2002. Laboratory safety, p. 78–96. *In* K. D. McClatchey (ed.), *Clinical Laboratory Medicine,* 2nd ed. Lippincott Williams and Wilkins, Philadelphia, Pa.

24. **Hunt, D. L.** 2000. Standard (Universal) precautions for human specimens, p. 355–367. *In* D. O. Fleming and D. L. Hunt (ed.), *Biological Safety: Principles and Practices,* 3rd ed. ASM Press, Washington, D.C.

25. **International Air Transport Association.** 2000. *Dangerous Goods Regulations,* 41st ed. p. 57–88.

26. **Keene, J. H.** 2000. Regulated medical waste handling and disposal, p. 403–409. *In* D. O. Fleming and D. L. Hunt (ed.), *Biological Safety: Principles and Practices,* 3rd ed. ASM Press, Washington, D.C.

27. **Knudsen, R. C.** 1998. Risk assessment for biological agents in the laboratory. *In* J. Y. Richmond (ed.), *Rational Basis for Biocontainment: Proceedings of the Fifth National Symposium on Biosafety.* American Biological Safety Association, Mundelein, Ill.

28. **Mahoney, W., and I. F. Salkin.** 1992. Radiological safety, p. 14.3.1–14.3.3. *In* H. D. Isenberg (ed.), *Clinical Microbiology Proce-

dures Handbook, vol. 2. American Society for Microbiology, Washington, D.C.

29. **McGowan, J. E., Jr.** 1999. Nosocomial infections in diagnostic laboratories, p. 1127–1135. *In* C. G. Mayhall (ed.), *Hospital Epidemiology and Infection Control,* 2nd ed. Lippincott Williams and Wilkins, Philadelphia, Pa.

30. **McKay, J., and D. O. Fleming.** 2000. Packaging and shipping biological materials, p. 411–425. *In* D. O. Fleming and D. L. Hunt (ed.), *Biological Safety: Principles and Practices,* 3rd ed. ASM Press, Washington, D.C.

31. **National Committee for Clinical Laboratory Standards.** 1996. *Clinical Laboratory Safety.* Approved standard GP17-A. National Committee for Clinical Laboratory Standards, Wayne, Pa.

32. **National Institutes of Health.** 1985. *Pocket Guide to Chemical Hazards.* U.S. Government Printing Office, Washington, D.C.

33. **NCCLS.** 2001. *Protection of Laboratory Workers from Occupationally Acquired Infections.* Approved standard M29-A2. NCCLS, Wayne, Pa.

34. **NCCLS.** 2002. *Clinical Laboratory Waste Management.* Approved standard GP5-2A. NCCLS, Wayne, Pa.

35. **NCCLS.** 2002. *Implementing a Needlestick and Sharps Injury Prevention Program in the Clinical Laboratory; a Report.* Standard X3-R. NCCLS, Wayne, Pa.

36. **Occupational Safety and Health Administration.** 1990. *Hazard Communication Standard.* 29 CFR 1910.1200. U.S. Government Printing Office, Washington, D.C.

37. **Occupational Safety and Health Administration.** 1990. *Occupational Exposure to Hazardous Chemicals in the Laboratory.* 29 CFR 1910.1450. U.S. Government Printing Office, Washington, D.C.

38. **Occupational Safety and Health Administration.** 1991. Occupational exposure to bloodborne pathogens: final rule. *Fed. Regist.* **56:**64003–64182.

39. **Occupational Safety and Health Administration.** 2001. Pathogens (29CFR 1910.1030) Directives Numbers: CPL 2-2.69; Effective: November 27, 2001.

40. **Occupational Safety and Health Administration.** 2001. Occupational exposure to bloodborne pathogens; needlestick and sharps injuries; final rule. *Fed. Regist.* **66:**5317–5325.

41. **Phillips, G. B.** 1986. Human factors in microbiological laboratory accidents, p. 43–48. *In* B. M. Miller, D. H. M. Groeschel, J. H.

Richardson, D. Vesley, J. R. Songer, R. D. Housewright, and W. E. Barkley (ed.), *Laboratory Safety: Principles and Practice.* American Society for Microbiology, Washington, D.C.

42. **Sewell, D. L.** 1995. Laboratory-associated infections and biosafety. *Clin. Microbiol. Rev.* **8:**389–405.

43. **Snyder, J. W.** 2002. Packaging and shipping of infectious substances. *Clin. Microbiol. Newsl.* **24:**89–93.

44. **Songer, J. R.** 1995. Laboratory safety management and the assessment of risk, p. 257–277. *In* D. O. Fleming, J. H. Richardson, J. J. Tulis, and D. Vesley (ed.), *Laboratory Safety: Principles and Practices,* 2nd ed. ASM Press, Washington, D.C.

45. **Tweedy, J. T.** 1997. *Healthcare Hazard Control and Safety Management.* Lewis Publishers, Boca Raton, Fla.

46. **U.S. Department of Transportation.** 1991. Performance-orientated packaging standards: revisions and response petitions for reconsideration. *Fed. Regist.* **56:**66124–66287.

47. **U.S. Department of Transportation.** 1996. 49 CFR Parts 171-180. Hazardous Materials Regulations: Public Health Service 42 CFR Part 72. Interstate Transportation of Etiologic Agents. U.S. Government Printing Office, Washington, D.C.

48. **U.S. Department of Transportation.** 1996. 49 CFR 173.134(a)(4): Regulated medical waste. U.S. Government Printing Office, Washington, D.C.

49. **U.S. Department of Health and Human Services.** 2002. Notification of possession of select agents or high consequence livestock pathogens and toxins. *Fed. Regist.* **67:**51058–51064.

50. **U.S. Department of Transportation, Research and Special Programs Administration.** 2002. Hazardous materials: revision to standards for infectious substances and genetically modified organisms; final rule. *Fed. Regist.* **67**(157)**:**53117–53144.

51. **Vesley, D., J. L. Lauer, and R. J. Hawley.** 2000. Decontamination, sterilization, disinfection, and antisepsis, p. 383–402. *In* D. O. Fleming and D. L. Hunt (ed.), *Biological Safety: Principles and Practices,* 3rd ed. ASM Press, Washington, D.C.

52. **Voss, A.** 1999. Prevention and control of laboratory-acquired infections, p. 165–173. *In* P. R. Murray, E. J. Baron, M. A. Pfaller, F. C. Tenover, and R. H. Yolken (ed.). *Manual of Clinical Microbiology,* 7th ed. ASM Press, Washington, D.C.

53. **World Health Organization.** 1993. *Laboratory Biosafety Manual,* 2nd ed. World Health Organization, Geneva, Switzerland.

APPENDIX 26.1   Sample Form for Declination of Hepatitis B Vaccination[a]

HEPATITIS B VACCINE DECLINATION

I understand that due to my occupational exposure to blood, or other potentially infectious materials, I may be at risk of acquiring hepatitis B virus infection. I have been given the opportunity to be vaccinated with hepatitis B vaccine, at no charge to myself. However, I decline hepatitis B vaccination at this time. If I haven't been previously immunized I understand that by declining this vaccine, I continue to be at risk of acquiring hepatitis B, a serious disease. If in the future I continue to have occupational exposure to blood or other potentially infectious materials and I want to be vaccinated with hepatitis B vaccine, I can receive the vaccination series at no charge to me.

Prior vaccination _____   No prior vaccination _____

_____   _____
Print full name   Date of birth

_____
Print Social Security number

_____   _____
Signature of employee   Date

[a]Reference: *Federal Register*, **56**:64182, 1991.

APPENDIX 26.2   Information Resources on the Internet

U.S. GOVERNMENT AGENCIES

Centers for Disease Control and Prevention
(http://www.cdc.gov)
Resources related to public health issues in the United States.

U.S. Department of Transportation
(http://www.dot.gov)
Resources related to the transportation of infectious and diagnostic specimens.

U.S. Environmental Protection Agency
(http://www.epa.gov)
Information on general-purpose disinfectants.

U.S. Food and Drug Administration
(http://www.fda.gov)
Information on chemical germicides formulated as antiseptics, preservatives, sterilants, high-level disinfectants, and agents used on the body.

U.S. Food and Drug Administration
(http://www.fda.gov/cdrh/oivd)
A new website for post-marketing problems. There is a new office for in vitro diagnostic devices, and it gives instructions for making a report and provides an e-mail address for reporting (fdalabtest@cdrh.fda.gov.).

U.S. Department of Health and Human Resources
(http://www.hhs.gov)
Information on policies and regulations, disasters and emergencies, safety, diseases and conditions, aging, resource locators, drugs and food, and other topics.

National Institute for Occupational Safety and Health
(http://www.cdc.gov/niosh)
Training materials and information on chemical agents and emergency preparedness.

Occupational Safety and Health Administration
(http://www.osha.gov)
Training materials, standards, and regulations related to safety in the workplace.

Office of Health and Safety
(http://www.cdc.gov/od/ohs)
Training materials and information on safety, biosafety, and safety survival skills.

U.S Government Printing Office
(http://www.access.gpo.gov/nara/cfr/)
A source for federal regulations.

(continued)

APPENDIX 26.2   Information Resources on the Internet *(continued)*

BIOSAFETY RESOURCES

CDC/NIH: Biosafety in Microbiological and Biomedical Laboratories, 4th ed.
(http://www.cdc.gov/od/ohs/biosfty/bmbl4/bmbl4toc.htm)

CDC/NIH: Primary Containment for Biohazards: Selection, Installation, and Use of Biological Safety Cabinets
(http://www.cdc.gov/od/ohs/biosfty/bsc/bsc.htm)

Medical Surveillance and Biosafety Program References
(http://www.cdc.gov/od/ohs/biosfty/bioref.htm)
References on occupational health and laboratory safety with materials on medical screening and surveillance.

International Healthcare Worker Safety Center at University of Virginia
(http://www.med.virginia.edu/epinet/)
Information on the prevention of occupational transmission of blood-borne pathogens and resources for complying with the federal Needlestick Safety and Prevention Act.

BIOTERRORISM

American Society for Microbiology
(http://www.asmusa.org)
Information related to bioterrorism and protocols for the isolation and identification of Select Agents.

Federal Chemical and Biological Warfare/Bioterrorism Websites
(http://www.usuhs.mil/cbw/fed_links.htm)
Information of interest to healthcare providers and emergency response/safety officials. Lists agencies in the Office of Homeland Security.

Health Alert Network
(http://www.phppo.cdc.gov/han/)
Communications to local and state health departments, distance learning offerings from the CDC, and health alerts.

Bioterrorism Preparedness and Response
(http://www.bt.cdc/gov)
Information on bioterrorism preparedness, training materials, and protocols for handling, identifying, and shipping Select Agents.

Infectious Diseases Society of America
(http://www.idsociety.org)
Clinical information related to bioterrorism and Select Agents.

U.S. Army Medical Research Institute of Infectious Diseases
(http://www.usamriid.army.org)
Reference material on biological and chemical warfare agents.

SHIPPING AND PACKAGING OF INFECTIOUS SUBSTANCES

Centers for Disease Control and Prevention
(http://www.bt.cdc.gov/labissues/packaginginfo.pdf)
Instructions for shipping infectious agents.

International Air Transport Association
(http://www.iata.org)
Information on shipping dangerous goods.

APPENDIX 26.3   Common Safety Compliance Failures

STANDARD PRECAUTIONS, PPE, AND CONTAINMENT EQUIPMENT
Laboratory coats worn open
Staff not wearing gloves at the workbenches
Handling contaminated objects with gloves (e.g., telephones)
Wearing laboratory coats outside the work area
Not using splash guards or appropriate eyewear when required
Improper storage of chemicals in fume hoods and BSCs
Improper storage of flammables, corrosives, and acids
Overfilled sharps containers
Sharps containers not properly secured
Gas tanks not properly secured
Eye wash stations not checked on a periodic basis
Disposal of biohazardous waste in routine trash receptacles
Food stored in refrigerators containing laboratory supplies

LABELING AND SIGNAGE
Improper labeling of chemical waste containers
Primary and secondary containers not labeled as to hazard
Lack of signage for biohazardous areas

FIRE
Storage of combustibles within 18 inches of sprinkler heads
Hallways used for storage
Fire doors blocked open

CHEMICAL HYGIENE PLAN
Chemical inventories not current
Employees' exposure to OSHA-regulated substances (e.g., formaldehyde) not monitored

TRAINING/MONITORING
Staff lacks knowledge of MSDS location
Staff lacks knowledge of fire alarm and extinguisher location
Accident/incident reports are not submitted or reviewed

APPENDIX 26.4   Biohazard Spill Kit Sample

Disinfectant (e.g., 10% household bleach or a tuberculocidal agent)

Absorbent material
Small spills: paper towels, gauze pads, etc.
Large spills: granular material (e.g., BioZorb [Ulster Scientific, Highland, NY])

PPE
Puncture-resistant utility gloves
Water-impermeable shoe coverings
Gown

Eyewear (face shield or goggles)
Mask
Full-face respirator or HEPA-filtered mask for BSL 3 agents

Collection material (autoclavable)
Dustpan
Tongs or forceps
Plastic scoop and "pusher"
Biohazard bag

Puncture-resistant biohazardous waste container

APPENDIX 26.5   Biological Spill Cleanup Procedure (possible aerosol)

Alert personnel in area and evacuate.
Close doors and do not reenter area for 30 to 60 min.
Don PPE appropriate for type of spill.
Wear gown, gloves, facial protection (full-face respirator or HEPA-filtered mask for BSL 3 agents).
Remove and discard broken glass or other objects.
Absorb the spill with absorbent material.
Discard contaminated material in the biohazardous waste container.
Clean the spill site with aqueous detergent.

Decontaminate the area with an appropriate disinfectant:
Pour disinfectant on the spill site or wipe down the site with disinfectant-soaked paper towels or gauze pads.
Absorb the disinfectant or permit it to air dry.
Rinse the spill site with water and allow the site to dry.
Place all disposable, contaminated material in the biohazard bag or container. Treat as infectious waste.
Wash hands.
Prepare a spill/incident report, identify the cause of the spill, and determine remedial action.

APPENDIX 26.6   Minor Chemical Spill Cleanup Procedure[a]

Evacuate personnel in the immediate spill area.
Attend to any contaminated individuals.
Extinguish all sources of ignition.
Contain the spill.
Ventilate the area of the spill.
Close off the spill area (call emergency response team when no trained individuals are available).
Notify safety officials.
Review MSDS for appropriate PPE and specific instructions for cleanup and disposal.
Don appropriate PPE (chemical-resistant gloves, gown, and shoe covers; face shield or goggles; mask).

Dike area of spill to prevent further spread of chemical.
Clean the spill area with appropriate neutralizing agent and absorbent.
Place contaminated material in disposal container.
Scrub area with soap and water.
Package all waste appropriately for pickup. Label containers with substance, amount, and date.
Prepare a spill/incident report, identify cause of spill, and determine remedial action.

[a]Spill does not involve flammables, explosives, carcinogens, or life-threatening chemicals.

APPENDIX 26.7 Shipping Containers

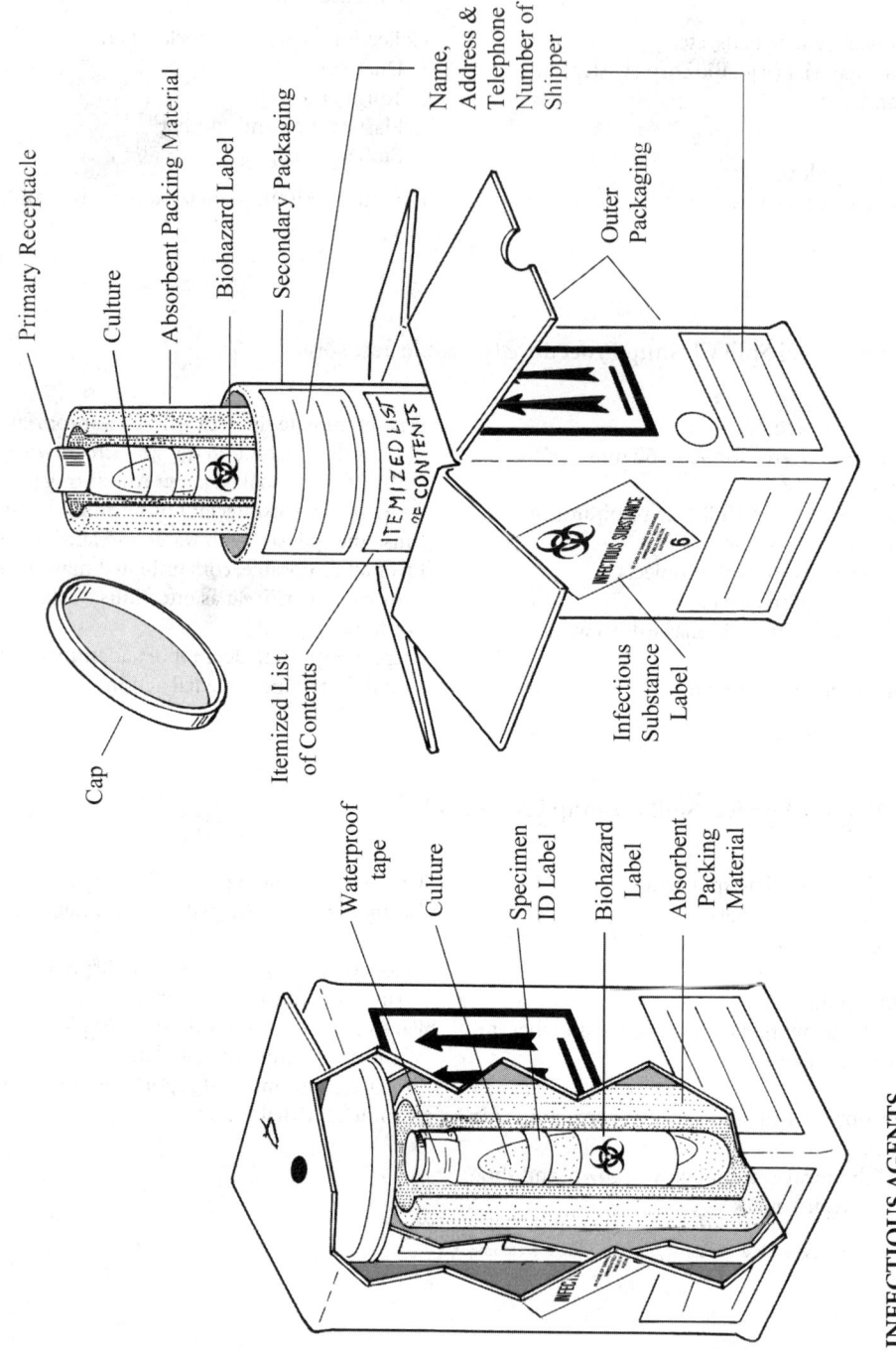

INFECTIOUS AGENTS

(continued)

APPENDIX 26.7   Shipping Containers *(continued)*

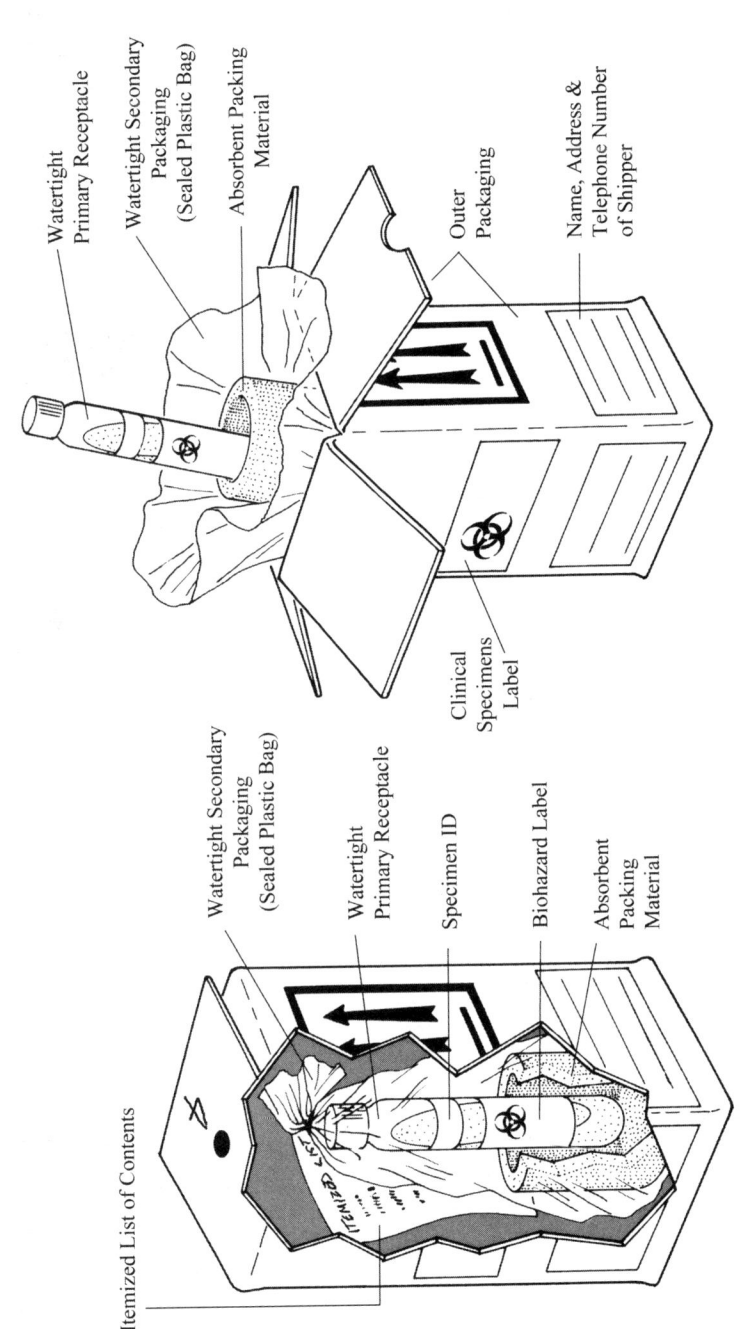

Watertight Primary Receptacle

Watertight Secondary Packaging (Sealed Plastic Bag)

Absorbent Packing Material

Outer Packaging

Name, Address & Telephone Number of Shipper

Clinical Specimens Label

Watertight Secondary Packaging (Sealed Plastic Bag)

Watertight Primary Receptacle

Specimen ID

Biohazard Label

Absorbent Packing Material

Itemized List of Contents

CLINICAL SPECIMENS

APPENDIX 26.8 Shipping Labels[a]

Infectious Substance, Affecting Humans (Human Immunodeficiency Virus [HIV]) UN 2814 ___ mL

Figure A8.1 Marking: proper shipping name, technical name, UN identification number, and quantity.

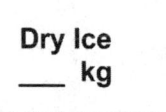

Dry Ice ___ kg

Figure A8.2 Marking: dry ice and weight.

Diagnostic Specimen Packed In Compliance With IATA Packing Instruction 650 UN 3373

Figure A8.3 Marking: diagnostic specimen.

INNER PACKAGES COMPLY WITH PRESCRIBED SPECIFICATIONS

Figure A8.4 Marking: inner packages comply (used only on over-packs).

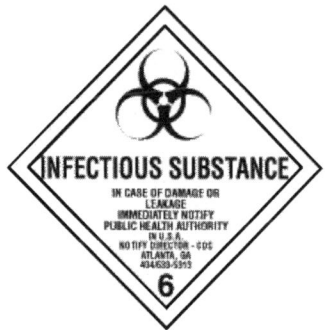

Figure A8.5 Label: infectious substance (class 6).

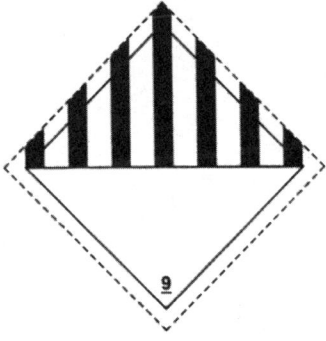

Figure A8.6 Label: miscellaneous dangerous goods (class 9).

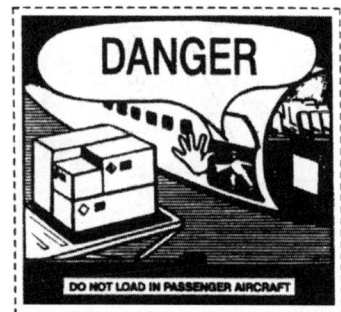

Figure A8.7 Label: cargo aircraft only (figure courtesy of SafTPak®).

Figure A8.8 Label: package orientation.

---

[a]Reprinted with permission of Larry D. Gray.

APPENDIX 26.9   Shipper's Declaration for Dangerous Goods[a]

(Provide at least two copies to the airline.)

SHIPPER'S DECLARATION FOR DANGEROUS GOODS

Shipper	Air Waybill No.
Dr. William Truitt 1234 Blind Lemon Ave. Charlotte, NC 27105	Page **1** of **1** Pages Shipper's Reference Number *(optional)*

| Consignee Acme Laboratory
987 Mt. Vernon Ave.
Cincinnati, OH 45773
Responsible Person: Wm. Truitt (432) 321-4567 | Optional Use
Company Logo, Name, and Address |

Two completed and signed copies of this Declaration must be handed to the operator

WARNING

Failure to comply in all respects with the applicable Dangerous Goods Regulations may be in breach of the applicable law, subject to legal penalties. This Declaration must not, in any circumstances, be completed and/or signed by a consolidator, a forwarder or an IATA cargo agent.

TRANSPORT DETAILS

This shipment is within the limitations prescribed for: *(delete non-applicable)*

PASSENGER AND CARGO AIRCRAFT | ~~CARGO AIRCRAFT ONLY~~

Airport of Departure

Airport of Destination:

Shipment type: *(delete non-applicable)*
NON-RADIOACTIVE | ~~RADIOACTIVE~~

NATURE AND QUANTITY OF DANGEROUS GOODS

Proper Shipping Name	Class or Division	UN or ID No	Subsidiary Risk	Quantity and type of packing	Packing Inst.	Authorization
Infectious substance, affecting humans (hepatitis B virus)	6.2	UN 2814		50 mL Packed in one fiberboard box	602	
Dry ice	9	UN 1845	III	3 kg Overpack used	904	

Additional Handling Information

"Prior arrangements as required by the IATA Dangerous Goods Regulations 1.3.3.1 have been made." Emergency contact: 1-800-123-4567

I hereby declare that the contents of this consignment are fully and accurately described above by proper shipping name and are classified, packed, marked and labelled, and are in all respects in the proper condition for transport by air according to the applicable International and National Government Regulations.

Name/Title of Signatory
William Doe, Supervisor
Place and Date
Charlotte, NC   Feb. 26, 2003
Signature *(see handling notes)*
William Doe

STYLE F83 LABELMASTER, CHICAGO, IL 60646
312/478-0900

[a]Reprinted with permission of Larry D. Gray.

APPENDIX 26.10   **Employee Accident/Incident Report**

Employee information (to be completed by the employee)

Name: _____   Social Security number: _____

Date of birth: _____   Sex: M F   Home phone: _____   Work phone: _____

Address (include city, state, and ZIP code) _____

Job title: _____   Department: _____

Signature: _____   Date signed: _____

Accident/incident information (to be completed by the employee)

Date incident occurred _____   Time: _____   Location: _____

Date incident reported: _____   Reported to: _____

List names of witnesses:

Witness statement:

Description and cause of incident (identify injury and part of body):

Blood/body fluid exposure (identify source patient): _____

Supervisor's report

Name: _____   Work phone: _____

Was employee injured during performance of duty?   Yes _____   No _____ (explain)

Date medical care received: _____

Do medical reports indicate employee is disabled for work?   Yes _____   No _____

Identify corrective actions or safety violations:

Additional comments:

Signature: _____   Date: _____

27

Emergency Management

Patti Medvescek and David L. Sewell

OBJECTIVES

To list emergencies and disasters that could affect the clinical laboratory

To identify the elements of an emergency management plan

To implement the emergency management plan

To evaluate the plan for regulatory compliance

Ignorance more frequently begets confidence than does knowledge.

CHARLES DARWIN

"DISASTER" IS DEFINED in the dictionary as a calamitous event, especially one occurring suddenly and causing great loss of life, damage, or hardship, such as a flood, airplane crash, or business failure, whereas "emergency" is defined as an unexpected situation or sudden occurrence of a serious and urgent nature that demands immediate action (15). In the healthcare arena, external emergencies and disasters generally include meteorological disasters (e.g., tornadoes, hurricanes, hailstorms, snowstorms), landslides, floods, earthquakes, tsunamis, warfare, civil disorder, terrorism, and transportation accidents. Internal emergencies usually include utility failures, hazard spills, fires, bomb threats, and personnel or reagent shortages. A disaster caused by any of these events could ultimately prevent the laboratory from providing test results or services.

Programs or plans that respond to these situations are known as emergency preparedness, emergency management, or disaster plans. In this chapter we will use the term emergency management plan (EMP). Often the EMP developed by the laboratory is part of a larger plan for the entire healthcare organization and may be part of a regional or national EMP.

Emergency planning and preparedness are the keys to preventing interruption or cessation of laboratory services when an emergency or disaster occurs. Understanding the type of external and internal disasters or emergencies fosters appropriate preparation and planning that diminishes or eliminates the disruption of services provided by the laboratory and healthcare facility. The EMP collects in one document the information required by employees to respond appropriately to any emergency. Because disasters or emergencies are unpredictable, an EMP can serve only as a guide. The plan assumes that individuals will use good judgment and adapt the response plan to the unique

473

needs of the situation. A well-written EMP can reduce confusion and panic during an emergency, allow responsible individuals to assess the situation and make information-based decisions, and provide a predictable response for the employees (11).

Emergency Management Plan (EMP)

An organized emergency management program begins with a written comprehensive document that defines the scope and goals of the program and lists the responsible individuals. The College of American Pathologists and the Joint Commission for the Accreditation of Healthcare Organizations require that laboratories and healthcare facilities have an emergency plan in place and be prepared to accommodate and respond to a disaster so that patient care can be provided in an emergency (1, 3). Accreditation guidelines require that the EMP (i) address both internal and external disasters in a general manner such that the facility can respond to multiple scenarios, and (ii) document incidents and training of staff.

The basic EMP should include the following sections.

Purpose or Policy

The purpose or policy states the need for a response plan that deals with the natural or human-caused events that may disrupt normal operations, as well as the responsibility to provide services to patients through effective utilization of limited resources and to assist any injured individuals.

Hazard Analysis

Hazard analysis requires that laboratory personnel prepare a risk assessment for the occurrence of both internal and external disasters or emergencies such as floods, earthquakes, landslides, winter storms, wildfires, volcanoes, windstorms, drought, utility failures, hazard spills, epidemics, reagent shortages, civil disorder, and terrorism. This assessment should attempt to define the direct and indirect impact on the facility and reduce the risk or diminish the damage from an emergency or disaster.

Program Responsibilities

Program responsibilities should define the specific and general responsibilities of each individual in the laboratory.

Incident Management System

The incident management system is used to manage emergency and disaster events through a flexible response regardless of when or where the event occurs. The first employee to discover the problem is in charge of the emergency response until someone higher in the supervision chain arrives. Each employee is expected to provide the leadership necessary to protect life and property and to carry out the responsibilities of the laboratory. He or she will ensure patient, visitor, and employee safety, will report the incident to the proper authorities, and will use proper procedures as outlined in the plan.

Emergency management generally falls into four phases: (i) identification of the emergency (e.g., tornado, transportation accident, electrical failure, etc.), (ii) containment (limit impact of disaster), (iii) response (assist victims and confine the physical damage of the event), and (iv) recovery (restore organization's normal operation). The plan must reflect and include the facility, local, regional, state, and federal requirements for disaster planning. The laboratory EMP should be complete but concise. To be effective, a plan must be well written and easy to execute. Laboratory staff should be familiar with the plan, the location of the plan, and each individual's role in the execution of the plan. Possible disaster scenarios should be covered in the plan based on the probability or frequency of occurrence of an event for a specific laboratory or geographical location or based on the hazardous material and equipment present in the facility. All plans must consider first the safety of employees, patients, visitors, and individuals with special needs and then address alternative sources of utilities and communications, areas for radioactive or chemical isolation and decontamination, and alternative roles and responsibilities of personnel during the emergency.

For example, the plan must address the following questions in emergency planning and recovery.

- Is there sufficient instrumentation to perform testing?

  All instruments (or critical instruments) on emergency power.

- Are there sufficient supplies and reagents to perform testing?

  Supply chain effective, inventories at appropriate levels, alternate sources of materials available.

- Are there sufficient personnel to perform testing?

  Transportation available for weather-related events. Emergency call-back list.

- Is the test menu sufficient to provide requested services?

  Reference laboratory services immediately available for esoteric requests.

- Where will specimens be sent and testing be performed if the laboratory must cease operations?

  Make arrangements for alternative testing sites.

The impact of the emergency or disaster on the staff itself must be considered. Ignoring the emotional response to disasters can create a disaster itself, resulting in staff members who are unable to perform the actions required. At a minimum, employee assistance personnel should be contacted to assist when national or local emergencies or disasters directly affect laboratory staff. Immediate and complete verification of personnel location is important when the staff are involved in the emergency. Open, complete communication with status updates is critical to maintaining laboratory operations throughout the disaster.

To handle a disaster successfully, the laboratory must anticipate and plan for the problems that will arise (Table 27.1). The keys to success include (i) development of flow charts detailing potential events and actions to be taken; (ii) identification of the level of laboratory service required based on the anticipated duration and severity of the emergency or disaster; (iii) projection of the impact of limited service on other hospital services, e.g., emergency room, intensive care units; (iv) establishment of effective lines of communication with laboratory staff and other healthcare providers; (v) identification of alternative sites to provide the necessary laboratory services; (vi) plans for recovery activities, e.g., scheduling and staff changes, alternative test procedures; and (vii) mock drills to test the effectiveness of the plan. Successful planning must involve all of the affected personnel so that they are aware of their individual responsibilities during an emergency as well as activities necessary to maintain essential services to support patient care activities.

The level of service provided by the laboratory dictates the depth and breadth of involvement by the laboratory staff in disaster recovery. A full-service, hospital-affiliated laboratory may be required to play a more comprehensive role in disaster recovery than a satellite facility or rural laboratory. It is important to recognize, however, that national disasters can significantly affect laboratory operations, regardless of the geographic proximity or services offered. Governmental and private agencies that are available to assist in a large community or regional disaster should be listed in the EMP with contact information (Appendix 27.1).

A business failure, such as manufacturer's recall of products, could also prevent the laboratory from providing services. Just-in-time inventory levels absolutely require a dependable delivery system. The receipt of back-up reagents from other sources depends on the availability of transportation and possible reciprocal relationships with local or regional clinical or reference laboratories. Other possible scenarios that may affect the laboratory, and the questions they raise, include:

- A mail or airline strike prevents delivery of reagents or supplies. What is the back-up plan for routine and emergency testing? How quickly can medical staff be notified of a reduction in services based on supply delivery?

- An influx of victims of bioterrorism requires more sophisticated testing than the laboratory has available. Where should the tests be sent? Who should be notified?

- Staffing levels are routinely at or below minimum levels and an earthquake occurs. How and when does the laboratory manager contact additional staff? What testing should be performed until additional staff arrive?

Emergency planning and preparedness allow for more efficient and effective deployment of activities to mitigate the impact of the disaster on laboratory services and staff. The laboratory manager may assign members of the laboratory staff to assist the facility in maintaining patient services. Emergency management requires that all possible events are considered to ensure that appropriate actions are taken to provide laboratory services where needed and to prevent a negative impact on laboratory operations. To do so, emergencies and disasters are categorized as external or internal to the laboratory and by the severity of the event (Table 27.2). External events occur outside of the physical laboratory and can affect the laboratory's delivery of services or require additional services from the laboratory. Internal emergencies occur within the facility or laboratory and significantly influence delivery of services.

Table 27.1 Elements of emergency planning

Element	Action
Identify potential disasters and laboratory's response	Prepare list of authorities to notify
	Identify critical positions and assign individuals
	Identify critical space and supplies
	Prepare security measures
	Develop criteria for evacuation
Define level of service and impact on patient care	Full service (normal operations)
	Limited service (prioritize testing)
	Emergency service (prepare minimal test menu)
Develop communication plan	Identify critical healthcare staff
	Identify critical laboratory staff (call-back)
	Identify critical suppliers
Alternative operations	Identify alternative site of operations
	Identify alternative laboratory for service work
	Prepare alternative scheduling or staffing
Mock drills	Assess performance of emergency plan
	Modify plan to correct deficiencies

Table 27.2 External and internal disasters and impact on the laboratory

Disaster	Impact
External	
Severe weather and natural disasters	Staff availability; relocation of patients and services; utilities and supplies/reagents disrupted
Hazardous material spill or contamination	Staff availability; laboratory services required to treat patients; implement decontamination protocols
Community illness	Staff availability; increase in patient and test volume
Transportation accident	Staff availability; increase in patient volume and specialty requirements (i.e., transfusion services)
National disaster	Supply/reagent availability
National recall of product	Supply/reagent availability
Terrorism	Staff availability; necessary laboratory services for patient care; implement decontamination protocols; increased safety precautions; notification of authorities
Internal	
Utility failure	Services interrupted; relocation or assistance from another laboratory
Hazardous material spill, fire, bomb threat	Personnel affected; testing delayed; special testing may be required; relocation or assistance from another facility
Shortage of personnel	Testing delayed or cancelled; assistance from another laboratory
Shortage of reagents or supplies	Testing delayed or cancelled; assistance from another laboratory
Civil disorder	Staff availability; supplies/reagents and utilities may be disrupted
Computer issues (security breach, downtime, data loss)	Delay or manual test reporting, incomplete database

Each laboratory, regardless of size or affiliation with hospitals or clinics, may be required to participate in emergency or disaster recovery in response to national or regional events that include terrorist acts, acts of war, or accidents threatening public safety.

Elements of an EMP

Emergency Operations Center

The emergency operations center (EOC) represents the situational leadership that is necessary to manage the emergency, protect life and property, carry out the function of the laboratory, and assist in other areas of the facility. Generally, individual employees are empowered to manage the event until relieved by someone higher in authority as defined by the order of succession of management. This concept means that individuals must step up and accept responsibility to perform tasks and supervise areas outside of their normal duties. The EMP (Table 27.3) defines who will automatically return to the facility (e.g., department chairperson, laboratory manager), describes the emergency call list, and defines the level of service that will be provided and how personnel will be deployed. Appendixes 27.2 and 27.3 show examples of an EOC checklist and a status report.

Communications

Communication is the most critical and difficult aspect of managing an emergency. The EMP must define the communication lines and how employees will be notified of the emergency. Communication by telephone, cell phones, runners, two-way radios, and other means provides links to internal and external events, responses to the event, and the recovery operation. Generally, a bell code system or the public address system is used to identify the location of a fire.

The EMP should identify who is notified of internal and external disasters (e.g., on-duty staff, off-duty staff, organizational staff, etc.) and should include a list of emergency phone numbers for external agencies and organizations (e.g., local law enforcement agencies, local and regional emergency management organizations, the Federal Bureau of Investigations (FBI), the state health laboratory, the Centers for Disease Control and Prevention [CDC]) that can assist the facility or that may need to be contacted during the emergency (Appendix 27.1). The plan should identify key personnel, their alternates, and their responsibilities. A part of communications involves assessing the nature of the emergency and the potential impact on patients, employees, and the public and developing a plan to include employee meetings, internal dissemination of information, and public releases. Inquiries from outside sources (e.g., press, employee family members) should be forwarded to the individual responsible for addressing these concerns. Accurate information must be provided to prevent rumors and to inform individuals involved in the event.

Medical Treatment Areas

The laboratory staff must be aware of the areas in the facility that are designated as medical treatment areas in the event that they require treatment or specimens need to be transported to the laboratory.

Table 27.3. Elements of a laboratory EMP

Element	Function
Emergency operation center	Describes leadership hierarchy
	Constructs emergency call-back list
	Defines level of service required
	Deploys laboratory personnel
	Maintains supply level
	Establishes communication services
Communication	Defines communication lines
	Identifies individuals for notification
	Maintains list of emergency numbers
	Disseminates information to employees and authorities
Medical treatment areas	Locates medical treatment areas
	Provides service to the medical treatment areas
Damage assessment	Conducts a damage assessment of laboratory
	Reports assessment to facility's command center
	Determines need to evacuate
Evacuation	Posts evacuation routes
	Identifies evacuation leaders
	Notifies facility's command center
Personnel pool	Assesses availability of personnel
	Assigns personnel to laboratory or where needed
Locator system	Develops system for tracking location of employees, patients, and visitors
	Communicates locations to facility's command center
Security	Assigns individual to provide laboratory security until relieved by security personnel
	Restricts access to laboratory
Training	Addresses personnel responsibility, role in an emergency, communication system, and supply system
	Conducts mock drills
Monitoring and evaluation	Documents deficiencies during drills
	Corrects deficiencies

Damage Assessment

A damage assessment should be performed as soon as possible following a disaster. The assessment can be rapid (5 to 10 min) or more detailed (1 to 2 h) and should determine whether an area can be used safely or must be evacuated. The plan must identify who will assess structural damage, equipment failures, hazard contamination, etc. The assessment should provide uniformity in assessing damage due to structural problems and fire and should address life safety and the status of the environment (e.g., gas, water, electrical power, lighting, etc.). Results are reported to the organization's command center. Appendixes 27.4 through 27.7 contain examples of assessment checklists for a healthcare organization, but the forms can be modified for the laboratory.

Evacuation

Evacuation may be necessary if a fire, hazardous spill, or structural damage occurs. The immediate area should be evacuated, the affected area should be isolated, and the command center should be notified. Evacuation routes must be posted and can be in a vertical or horizontal fashion. Individuals should be identified who are responsible for the safe evacuation of other employees, visitors, patients,

and anyone who requires assistance. Employees should not return until authorized by a designated individual.

Personnel Pool

The incident manager (e.g., laboratory manager) will decide which personnel can be released from their normal responsibilities to assist elsewhere in the laboratory or facility.

Locator System

The EMP must address the problem of communicating the location and status of employees, patients, and visitors to a central location so that the public can locate family and friends quickly (Appendix 27.8). Often victims of a disaster may be spread over an entire metropolitan area or region.

Security

An individual should be assigned responsibility for providing direction to the staff regarding security and crowd control until the security personnel arrive in the affected area. Access to the laboratory is restricted to allow employees and emergency staff to respond to the emergency. The individual with temporary security duty provides information to security personnel and may determine whether to evacuate the laboratory.

Training

The EMP outlines an orientation and education program for facility personnel, including interaction with other emergency organizations in the region. The training addresses (i) specific roles and responsibilities during an emergency, (ii) the information and skills required to perform duties, (iii) the back-up communication system used during disasters, and (iv) the system to ensure that supplies and equipment are delivered where needed. The most important element of training is mock drills that are conducted to test whether the EMP works as anticipated. A challenging aspect of emergency planning and training is the assignment of responsibilities to the various participating community agencies and organizations, especially when there are competing agendas among the groups.

Monitoring and Evaluation

The EMP must address ongoing monitoring of performance regarding staff knowledge and skills, level of staff participation, inspection activities, incident reporting, and interagency cooperation. Corrective measures must be implemented for any deficiencies noted from these activities.

Disasters

Fire

All staff must be familiar with the potential fire hazards within the laboratory and be aware of the procedures necessary to ensure the safety of personnel in the area. These procedures include minimizing working supplies of flammable material, storing flammables in a flammable-safe cabinet, and identifying and controlling ignition sources. Training should emphasize response according to the RACE (rescue, alarm, confine, evacuate/extinguish) approach, sounding the alarm, knowing the preferred and alternative exit route from the work area, which may be dark and smoke-filled, using a fire extinguisher, knowing the fire codes, and closing all fire/smoke barrier doors. When a fire is discovered, the RACE approach is as follows.

Rescue. Immediately notify others on the floor or in the area. Rescue any patients or victims in the fire area and close the door to the room or area involved. Do not reopen door.

Alarm. Activate the alarm by pulling the nearest fire alarm. Next, report the fire to the emergency center and give the location (room number, building, etc.) and the type of fire (type of material burning, how extensive, etc.). Generally, this information is relayed to the responding fire department so they can be properly prepared when they arrive.

Confine. Close all windows and doors on the floor as appropriate. Advise patients and visitors to keep the doors closed until notified otherwise. Keep calm and try to reassure patients. Check to make sure all fire/smoke barrier doors have been closed and are not blocked. Clear corridors.

Evacuate/extinguish. Attempt to extinguish only small fires. Do not attempt to fight large fires. Your best defense is to close the door and evacuate the immediate areas. When using a portable fire extinguisher, PASS guidelines should be followed (11):

- Pull the pin on the extinguisher.
- Aim the nozzle at the base of the fire.
- Squeeze the handle firmly.
- Spray in a sweeping motion.

Hazardous Materials

Hazardous materials are any substances cited as a health and physical hazard by OSHA. Laboratory hazards are usually identifiable and quantifiable, and personnel should be knowledgeable about hazardous materials, be familiar with procedures to follow in an emergency, and be aware of measures to ensure the safety of personnel. Laboratories are required to maintain a chemical inventory list that identifies the type of hazard, the location, and the quantity present. This list should be posted in the laboratory and submitted to the facility's industrial hygienist or the local fire department. The plan should identify and assign responsibility to responders (i.e., safety officer, industrial hygienist) who can shut off utilities to prevent spread of the hazard through the ventilation system and to minimize the potential for fire or explosions. Individuals must be trained to clean up spills and to decontaminate individuals exposed to chemical, radiation, or infectious agents. The telephone number for the regional hazmat team should be posted.

Generally, the industrial hygienist or safety officer can make a prompt evaluation of the hazard severity and based on information available determine what action is necessary. The severity of the hazard is based on room size, type of chemical, and volume of material released. The decision to evacuate and notify the region's hazmat team is based on assessment of imminent danger to life or health as marked by injured or ailing personnel, symptoms of severe irritation, evidence of a large volume spill, gas leaks, fire hazard, presence of carcinogens, or presence of very strong odors beyond the immediate area. When it can be done safely, individuals should be posted at entrances to prevent other people from entering the hazard area. When possible, response personnel will disconnect any heat- or flame-generating equipment. The RACE approach to hazardous materials incidents should be followed.

Rescue. Rescue only when applicable and safe to do so. Provide first aid (eye wash or showers) to victims and control access to the spill area.

Alarm. Activate the emergency response system. Report the spill to the responsible person and provide relevant information such as who, what, when, where, and how much.

Confine. Contain the spill, if possible, but only if trained to do so.

Evacuate. Evacuate when there is immediate danger to life or health.

Radioactive Material

Sources of toxic, ionizing radiation in the laboratory include devices and reagents containing radioactive material. Policies should restrict access of untrained individuals to areas containing radioactive substances. The EMP should describe appropriate responses in the event of a spill, such as preventing spread by covering the spill with absorbent paper, limiting movement of contaminated individuals, shielding the radioactive source if possible, closing and locking the room, or otherwise securing the area. The individual is decontaminated by removing contaminated clothing and flushing contaminated skin with lukewarm water and then washing with mild soap. The affected area should be evacuated when the spill is large. Only trained persons should decontaminate an area, and they must wear protective clothing, gloves, and eye protection. After decontamination, the area must be checked for residual radiation. Each spill incident and decontamination must be documented (Appendix 27.9).

Utility Failure

Utility failures may be long or short in duration, may require an alternative means of providing service, or may require evacuation of the laboratory or facility.

Water. The EMP must address the need for emergency water for both equipment and potable water. The Department of Homeland Security (www.ready.gov) recommends 1 gal of water per person per day and at least a 3-day supply. The potable water should be replaced every 6 months (www.redcross.org). Areas requiring water must be prioritized, and nonessential water consumption must be curtailed.

Electrical. Because loss of electrical power can paralyze a modern clinical laboratory, essential equipment must be attached to lines powered by emergency generators. Battery-powered lighting must be available in the event that the emergency generators fail so that employees can safely exit the premises. Plans must anticipate the loss of ventilation and airflow to chemical and biological safety cabinets (BSCs). Loss of ventilation in the laboratory may cause instruments to overheat and accumulate noxious or toxic fumes. Inoperative chemical hoods and BSCs prevent the performance of procedures requiring their use. BSCs should have a safety mechanism that automatically prevents backflow of air through the filter when the fan shuts off.

Sewer. The EMP should address a failure in the sewer system due to lack of water or inability to discharge effluent. Priority is given to infection control measures (e.g., handwashing), direct patient testing, and meal preparation.

Bomb Threat

All threatening telephone calls should be taken seriously. The employee must remain calm, attempt to keep the caller on the line without increasing his or her antagonism, record details of the call, and notify police immediately (Appendix 27.10). Often, a colleague can notify the security personnel while the first employee talks to the caller. Security personnel will decide whether the facility should be evacuated.

Natural Disasters

Earthquakes, tornadoes, floods, hurricanes, and similar weather-related disasters usually arrive with little warning and can have a major impact on the hospital or clinic and the surrounding community. The EMP should contain definitions of storm warnings used in the local area, provide instructions for employees (e.g., take cover under sturdy furniture or in a doorway during initial earthquake shaking), and establish an early release from work for nonessential employees. When structural damage is suspected, clinical operations should not resume until a qualified inspection of the premises has occurred. The effects of a natural disaster include damage to the facility, interruption of communications, inability of employees to leave or return to the facility, and injured individuals requiring treatment. Initially, a survey of the area should be performed to identify trapped people, structural damage, inoperative equipment or systems, unsafe or unhealthful conditions, and hazardous locations. Damaged containers of chemicals must be removed and infectious material must be bagged and safely discarded. Visitors, patients, and employees within a dangerous area should be evacuated.

Terrorism Threats

Terrorism threats pose a very complex problem for laboratories, facilities, communities, and the nation. Sources of expert information on chemical and biological agents should be readily available (Appendix 27.11). The laboratory EMP must outline procedures for handling terrorism material (e.g., chemical, radiological, or biological) in the laboratory and for managing a large number of walk-in patients and subsequent clinical specimens (Appendix 27.11)

(4, 5, 12, 13, 14). Key elements of an effective terrorism EMP include issues such as prompt recognition of an event; identification of individuals who are first responders (e.g., staff who have received smallpox vaccination), staff and facility security; obtaining assistance from community and federal agencies (e.g., hazmat teams, FBI, local police, CDC, state laboratory); coordination of activities with other external emergency response agencies or organizations; release of public information; and decontamination plans for patients and staff. The administration should address physical security, airflow and ventilation, and maintenance of the facility's structure (7). Security officers must plan for crowd control, directing the flow of casualties and vehicles, and preventing unauthorized entry to decontamination and treatment areas. Plans need to be in place to rotate staff into work areas and to provide food, psychological support, and rest for employees.

CDC's Bioterrorism Preparedness and Response Program addresses a unified public health response to bioterrorism events that includes measures for disease surveillance, laboratory diagnosis of biological agents, communication between various public health authorities, epidemiological investigations, and readiness assessments (www.bt.cdc.gov). The Laboratory Response Network links local, state, federal, military, veterinary, and environmental laboratories and classifies laboratories based on their anticipated role in the event of a biocrime or bioterrorism event and on their capacity to safely handle and identify agents of bioterrorism (2, 6, 9). The original Laboratory Response Network model involved four levels of laboratories (levels A, B, C, and D) but currently contains three classification levels (Sentinel, Reference, and National Laboratories). Sentinel Laboratories (formerly level A) include most clinical and commercial laboratories, whose function is to recognize, rule out, and refer potential agents to the Reference Laboratories (formerly levels B and C). Reference Laboratories are generally local or state public health laboratories, whose function is confirmatory testing and processing of environmental samples. There are presently only two National Laboratories (CDC and U.S. Army Medical Research Institute of Infectious Diseases) that can operate at a biosafety level 4 capability.

Clinical microbiology laboratories must develop protocols for the recognition and identification of the potential agents of bioterrorism and procedures for management of these events. These protocols should be part of the routine bench procedures so that potential agents are not misidentified or improperly handled and can be rapidly referred to a Reference Laboratory for confirmation (8). Protocols developed by authorities are available on various websites (www.bt.cdc.gov, www.asmusa.org) and in publications (10). Sentinel Laboratories should not process specimens for smallpox or viral hemorrhagic fever from high-risk patients. These samples should be sent to CDC after consultation with the state public health division. CDC maintains an emergency number (770/488-7100) that provides instructions for the collection and shipment of specimens. In addition, Sentinel Laboratories should not process environmental samples (e.g., suspicious powder for *Bacillus anthracis* spores) or animal specimens but rather contact the FBI and Reference Laboratory for instructions. Often the latter samples involve a chain of custody procedure.

Civil Disorder

In most situations, the local law enforcement agency is aware of planned demonstrations and arranges for control measures. Unplanned acts of civil disturbance are handled by the facility security personnel in cooperation with the local law enforcement agency. An effective communication system must be in place to keep the employees and public informed.

Summary

Emergency preparedness planning and management must involve the entire healthcare organization, the community, and with the present threat of terrorism, the nation. Effective disaster planning requires anticipation of any type of disaster that prevents the laboratory from providing services. The laboratory manager may be involved in overall disaster recovery, providing laboratory resources as needed for patient care and facility support. Disasters can be external (e.g., weather, failures in transportation services) or internal (e.g., facilities breakdowns, equipment malfunctions, lack of personnel). Consideration should be given to the impact on laboratory personnel, depending on the nature of the disaster. Planning, preparation, and communication will improve the laboratory's response to a disaster if and when it occurs.

KEY POINTS

■ Disasters may stem from a variety of root causes but result in consistent impact on operations—failure to provide services.

■ EMPs should be comprehensive and included in laboratory policy and procedures.

■ Guidelines are available from many resources, based on local, regional, and national regulations.

GLOSSARY

Biohazard An agent of biological origin that has the capacity to produce deleterious effects on humans, e.g., microorganisms, toxins.

Disaster Any incident that interferes with a facility's ability to operate in a normal manner.

Emergency A natural or human-caused event that suddenly or significantly disrupts the environment of care, disrupts care and treatment, or changes or increases demands for the organization's services.

External disaster An event external to the physical laboratory location that may affect operations by limiting available staff or supplies or changing laboratory workload (e.g., influx of patients, uncommon tests required). Examples include major storms, earthquakes, transportation accidents, or acts of terrorism.

Facility A healthcare organization (hospital, clinic, physician's office) that includes an on-site laboratory.

Hazardous material A substance or material that has been determined by the U.S. Department of Transportation to pose an unreasonable risk to health, safety, and property when transported in commerce.

Hazmat team Group of individuals who are trained to respond to and clean up hazardous material spills.

Internal disaster An internal event within the laboratory or facility that affects patient care and facility operation, including power failure, hazardous chemical spill, fire, or lack of personnel.

Laboratory A facility that provides services including specimen collection, testing, and results reporting.

RACE Acronym describing the appropriate approach by first responders to a fire or disastrous situation: rescue, alarm, confine, evacuate/extinguish.

Reference laboratory An on- or off-site laboratory performing tests on behalf of a clinical laboratory or facility, typically including rare or esoteric test menus.

Service levels Test menu, results reporting, and ancillary assistance provided by the laboratory to hospitals, clinics, physicians, and patients.

REFERENCES

1. **College of American Pathologists.** 2002. *Laboratory Accreditation Program, General Laboratory Checklist,* August. College of American Pathologists, Northfield, Ill.

2. **Gilchrist, M. J. R., W. P. Mckinney, J. M. Miller, and A. S. Weissfeld.** 2000. *Cumitech 33, Laboratory Safety, Management, and Diagnosis of Biological Agents Associated with Bioterrorism.* Coordinating ed., J. W. Snyder. ASM Press, Washington, D.C.

3. **Joint Commission for the Accreditation of Healthcare Organizations.** 2000. *Standards for Accreditation, Laboratory Services,* October. Oakbrook Terrace, Ill.

4. **Londorf, D.** 1995. Hospital application of the incident management system. *Prehosp. Disaster Med.* **10:**184–188.

5. **Macintyre, A. G., G. W. Christopher, E. Eitzen, Jr., R. Gum, S. Weir, C. DeAtley, K. Tonat, and J. A. Barbera.** 2000. Weapons of mass destruction events with contaminated casualties: effective planning for healthcare facilities. *JAMA* **283:**242–249.

6. **Miller, J. M.** 2001. Agents of bioterrorism: preparing for bioterrorism at the community health care level. *Infect. Dis. Clin. North Am.* **15:**1127–1156.

7. **National Institute for Occupational Safety and Health.** 2002. *Guidance for Protecting Building Environments from Airborne Chemical, Biologic, or Radiological Attacks.* DHHS publication no. NIOSH2002-139. U.S. Government Printing Office, Washington, D.C.

8. **Shapiro, D. S., and D. R. Schwartz.** 2002. Exposure of laboratory workers to *Francisella tularensis* despite a bioterrorism procedure. *J. Clin. Microbiol.* **40:**2278–2281.

9. **Snyder, J. W.** 2003. Role of the hospital-based microbiology laboratory in preparation for and response to a bioterrorism event. *J. Clin. Microbiol.* **41:**1–4.

10. **Snyder, J. W., and A. S. Weissfeld.** 2003. Laboratory detection of potential agents of bioterrorism, p. 121–128. *In* P. R. Murray, E. J. Baron, J. H. Jorgensen, M. A. Pfaller, and R. H. Yolken (ed.), *Manual of Clinical Microbiology,* 8th ed. ASM Press, Washington, D.C.

11. **Tweedy, J. T.** 1997. Emergency planning and fire safety, p. 121–157. *Healthcare Hazard Control and Safety Management.* CRC Press, Boca Raton, Fla.

12. **U.S. Department of Health and Human Services.** 1996. *Health and Medical Services Support Plan for the Federal Response to Acts of Chemical/Biological (C/B) Terrorism.* U.S. Government Printing Office, Washington, D.C.

13. **U.S. Army Medical Research Institute of Chemical Defense.** 1995. *Medical Management of Chemical Casualties Handbook.* Fort Detrick, Md.

14. **U.S. Army Medical Research Institute of Infectious Diseases.** 1996. *Medical Management of Biological Casualties Handbook.* Fort Detrick, Md.

15. **Webster's American College Dictionary.** 1998. Random House, New York, N.Y.

APPENDIX 27.1   List of Selected Emergency Preparedness Agencies and Organizations

GOVERNMENTAL AGENCIES
Centers for Disease Control and Prevention
Domestic Preparedness Information Line
Federal Bureau of Investigation
Federal Emergency Management Agency
Homeland Security Operations Center
National Centers for Environmental Predictions
National Hurricane Center
National Oceanic and Atmospheric Administration
National Response Center
National Weather Service

U.S. Army Corps of Engineers
U.S. Geological Survey National Earthquake Information Center
U.S. Public Health Service

NONGOVERNMENTAL ORGANIZATIONS
American Red Cross
Church charities
Corporation for National Service (disaster services)
National Emergency Management Association
Salvation Army

APPENDIX 27.2   Emergency Operations Center (EOC) Checklist

_____ Determine status of the emergency and implement emergency management plan as appropriate.

_____ Set up EOC in the designated area. Determine the presence of all key personnel in the EOC and triage areas.

_____ Establish command activity and direct all emergency relief activities.

_____ Identify the departments needed to support the relief activity and ensure that each department knows what is expected of it.

_____ Ensure that the triage area is functioning.

_____ Ensure that appropriate call-back is progressing and all necessary supplies are delivered to the triage area. Utilize personnel pool to ensure that appropriate assistance is maintained.

_____ Request necessary assistance from state or local agencies (i.e., fire, police, ambulance, bomb squad, hazmat team, etc).

_____ Notify other divisions of the emergency and request aid or place staff on standby.

_____ Brief all individuals reporting to the EOC. Dismiss individuals that are not required for the relief effort.

_____ Ensure that all departments (e.g., security, safety) that automatically respond to external and internal emergencies are notified and responding.

_____ Ensure that internal communication is established.

_____ Ensure that recorders are assigned to key response functions to document activities for the incident manager.

APPENDIX 27.3 Operating Status Report Form

Name of hospital: _____   Date/time report given: _____

Contact person: _____   Title/location: _____

Contact method: _____   Contact number: _____

Questions	**Comments**
1. Y N Can you continue to treat incoming patients?	If no, why not?
2. Y N Any patients evacuated to outside the hospital?	If yes, why?
	Total # evacuated
	# unstable or critical patients
3. Y N Any patients or staff injured?	# of injured people. Deaths?
4. Y N Any structural damage?	Partial or total collapse?
5. Y N Any major non-structural problems?	List
6. Y N Power from any source?	
7. Y N Can generator power essential areas?	
8. Y N Can you communicate with the outside world?	
9. Y N Access to all essential areas?	Anyone trapped?
10. Y N Sufficient number of elevators working?	
11. Y N Water lines intact to essential areas?	
12. Y N Natural gas lines intact to essential areas?	
13. Y N Sewage system intact in essential areas?	
14. Y N Adequate staff at the hospital?	What do you need?
15. Y N Adequate supplies and equipment?	What do you need?
16. Y N Any outside assistance needed?	What?
17. Y N Need structural engineer?	

APPENDIX 27.4 Damage Assessment Chart[a]

Damage assessment	Report	Post:
Rapid evaluation by department	Safe	Inspected
	Questionable	Limited entry
	Unsafe	Unsafe
Detailed evaluation by engineering	Safe	Inspected
	Questionable	Limited entry
	Unsafe	Unsafe
Engineering evaluation by consultants	Safe	Inspected
	Unsafe	Unsafe

[a]Adapted from reference 11.

APPENDIX 27.5   Rapid Evaluation Safety Assessment Form[a]

Building/area description:	**Overall Rating:**
Area name: _____	**Inspected**
Room numbers: _____	**Limited entry**
	Unsafe
Primary occupancy:	**Inspector:**
Patient care Office	Name: _____
Laboratory Mechanical	Date: _____
Research Engineering	Time: _____
Other _____	

_____

Instructions: Review area for the conditions listed below. A "yes" answer is grounds for posting an area UNSAFE. If more review is needed, post LIMITED ENTRY.

Condition

1. Collapse, partial collapse, or building off foundation	Yes	No	Review Needed
2. Building or floor leaning	Yes	No	Review Needed
3. Severe cracking of walls, severe damage and distress	Yes	No	Review Needed
4. Ceilings, light fixtures or other non-structural hazards	Yes	No	Review Needed
5. Hazmat spill	Yes	No	Review Needed
6. Other hazard present	Yes	No	Review Needed

Recommendations

No further action required

Detailed evaluation required (circle one)   Structural   Hazmat   Other

Barricades needed in the following areas: _____

Other: _____

Comments:

_____

_____

[a]Adapted from reference 11.

APPENDIX 27.6 Safety Considerations for Fixed Equipment[a]

Item	Principal concern
Boilers	Sliding, broken gas/fuel lines; broken exhaust, steam, and/or relief lines
Refrigerator/freezer	Sliding; loss of function; leaking refrigerant
Emergency generators	Failed isolation mounts; sliding; broken fuel, signal, and/or power lines; broken exhaust lines
Fuel tanks	Sliding or overturning; leaks; broken fuel lines
Fire pumps	Anchorage failure; misalignment between pump and motor; broken piping
On-site water storage	Tank or vessel rupture; pipe break
Communication equipment	Sliding, overturning, or toppling leading to loss of function
Transformers	Sliding; leaking; loss of function
Electrical panels	Sliding or overturning; broken or damaged conduit or electrical bus
Elevators	Counterweights out of guide rails; cables out of sheaves; dislodged equipment
Radiation equipment	Breach of containment
Toxic chemicals	Spills; fumes in ventilation system
Liquid oxygen tanks	Sliding or overturning; leaks; broken lines
Infectious hazards	Overturned incubators; broken culture bottles
Equipment	Sliding or overturning leading to loss of function or damage to adjacent equipment

[a]Adapted from reference 11.

APPENDIX 27.7 Equipment Checklist[a]

General Items	Equipment Damaged		Comments
	No	Yes	
Boilers	——	——	———————————
Refrigerator/freezer	——	——	———————————
Emergency generators	——	——	———————————
Fuel tanks	——	——	———————————
Fire pumps	——	——	———————————
On-site water storage	——	——	———————————
Communications equipment	——	——	———————————
Transformers	——	——	———————————
Electrical panels	——	——	———————————
Elevators	——	——	———————————
Radiation equipment	——	——	———————————
Chemical storage:			
———————————	——	——	———————————
———————————	——	——	———————————
Gas tanks:			
———————————	——	——	———————————
———————————	——	——	———————————
Other equipment:			
———————————	——	——	———————————
———————————	——	——	———————————
Comments:			

———————————————————————————————

———————————————————————————————

———————————————————————————————

———————————————————————————————

———————————————————————————————

[a]Adapted from reference 11.

APPENDIX 27.8   Patient Locator Information Form

Provide the following information by telephone to the Patient Locator System on each new or readmitted disaster victim during the emergency status.

1. Patient name: _____

2. SSN: _____

3. Date of birth: _____

4. Age: _____

5. Patient's sex: Male   Female

6. Patient's condition: Critical   Serious   Fair   Good   Excellent   Deceased   Not Sure

7. Treated by: _____

8. Released from care: Yes   No   Date of release: _____

9. Patient's Address: _____

       City: _____ State: _____ Zip: _____

10. Person to notify: _____

       Relationship: Husband ____   Wife ____   Father ____   Mother ____

                Brother ____   Sister ____   Other ____

       Address: _____

       City: _____ State: _____ Zip: _____

       Phone: Home _____ Work: _____

Name of person filling out form: _____

Information called in: Date: _____ Time: _____

Patient condition update called in:

       Date: _____ Time: _____ Condition: _____

       Date: _____ Time: _____ Condition: _____

APPENDIX 27.9 Radioactive Spill Report

The spill occurred at _____ : _____ (am/pm)   on _____ / _____ / _____ bldg _____ room _____

Instrument used to check for personnel contamination: _____

Meter manufacturer _____ Meter model___ _____

Meter S/N _____ Probe model _____ Probe S/N _____

Personnel present   Personnel contamination results*

_____

_____

_____

*On the back of this sheet, indicate any personnel decontamination or care instituted. Please be detailed.

Survey the spill area to identify hot spots and then begin decontamination. When finished, conduct a post-cleaning contamination wipe test.

Radioisotopes present or suspected in the spill:

_____ mCi of _____ as _____

_____ mCi of _____ as _____

_____ mCi of _____ as _____

Provide a brief description of the accident: _____

_____

_____

_____

_____

Provide a brief description of actions taken to prevent a recurrence: _____

_____

_____

_____

_____

Name: _____

Date: _____

APPENDIX 27.10   Bomb Threat Checklist

Date and time of call: _____

Words of caller:

_____

_____

_____

Questions to ask:

1. When is the bomb going to explode? _____

2. Where is the bomb? _____

3. What does it look like? _____

4. What kind of bomb is it? _____

5. What will cause it to explode? _____

6. Did you place the bomb? _____

7. Why? _____

8. Where are you calling from? _____

9. What is your address? _____

10. What is your name? _____

Caller's voice (circle)

Calm   Disguised   Nasal   Angry   Stutter   Sincere   Lisp   Rapid

Deep   Crying   Squeaky   Excited   Stressed   Accent   Scared

Normal

If the voice was familiar, whom did it sound like? _____

Were there any background noises? _____

Remarks _____

_____

_____

Person receiving call _____

_____

APPENDIX 27.11   Selected Information Resources on the Internet

EMERGENCY PREPAREDNESS WEBSITES

Joint Commission for Accreditation of Healthcare Organizations
(http://www.jcaho.org)
Guidelines on emergency management standards

Occupational Safety and Health Administration
(http://www.osha.gov)
Training materials, standards, and regulations related to safety in the laboratory

U.S. Government Printing Office
(http://www.access.gov/nara/cfr)
Source for federal regulations

Federal Emergency Management Agency
(http://www.fema.gov/areyouready)
Source of materials for emergency preparedness

National Institute for Occupational Safety and Health
(http://www.cdc.gov/niosh)
Resources on chemical agents and emergency preparedness

Office of Health and Safety
(http://www.cdc.gov/od/ohs)
Resource on safety, biosafety, and safety survival

BIOTERRORISM WEBSITES

Department of Homeland Security
(http://www.ready.gov)
Information on preparedness for all terrorism events

American Society for Microbiology
(http://www.asmusa.org)
Training materials, laboratory protocols, and regulations related to bioterrorism preparedness

College of American Pathologists
(http://www.cap.org)
Links to other websites on bioterrorism preparedness

Centers for Disease Control and Prevention
(http://www.bt.cdc.gov)
Training materials, laboratory protocols, regulations, guidelines for laboratory and healthcare facilities preparedness

Infectious Diseases Society of America
(http://www.idsociety.org)
Resources related to bioterrorism preparedness

U.S. Army Medical Research Institute of Infectious Diseases
(http://www.usamriid.army.mil)
Reference material on biological and chemical warfare agents

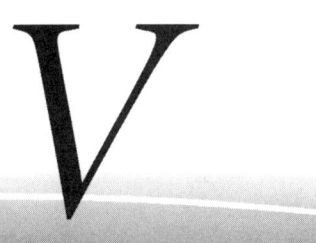

Financial Management

(Section Editor, *Washington C. Winn, Jr.*)

Financial Management: Setting the Stage

Ronald B. Lepoff

OBJECTIVES

To establish the importance of the environment in which the laboratory operates

To review the constraints placed upon management in the hospital and independent laboratory settings

To introduce the fiscal considerations that may be important for laboratory management in these settings

All the world's a stage,
And all the men and women, merely Players;
They have their Exits and their Entrances,
And one man in his time plays many parts. . .

WILLIAM SHAKESPEARE
AS YOU LIKE IT, ACT II, SCENE VII

THERE ARE APPROXIMATELY 175,000 clinical laboratories in the United States. Roughly 98,000 of these laboratories are located in physician offices; of these, 44,000 perform only Clinical Laboratory Improvement Amendments (CLIA)-waived testing (see Glossary) and 31,000 do only provider-performed microscopy. In contrast, there are approximately 6,000 hospitals with associated laboratories in this country. Of the remainder of laboratories, about 3,000 are independent. The demographics of the laboratory industry are summarized in Table 28.1.

The drivers of financial performance are different for these three groups (physician offices, hospitals, and independent laboratories). In this chapter we will concentrate on hospital and independent laboratories. These facilities usually perform moderate- and high-complexity testing and are most likely to have professional laboratory-trained personnel and management. In contrast, testing in most physician office laboratories is limited, of lesser complexity, and performed by individuals whose primary training and responsibilities are not in laboratory medicine.

The most important contributors to financial performance in the laboratory industry are:

- Leadership
  - Operations management
  - Information management

Table 28.1 The demographics of the laboratory industry[a]

Laboratory type	No.
Total clinical laboratories	174,000
Physician office laboratories	97,300
Performing CLIA-waived testing only	44,000
Performing provider-performed microscopy only	31,000
Other physician office laboratories	22,300
Hospitals	6,000
Hospital-associated laboratories	8,500
Independent laboratories	3,000
Others (includes public health, insurance, etc.)	65,200

[a]All numbers approximate.

- Marketing
  - Laboratory specialty niches
  - Service area
  - Competition
- Customer service
  - Couriers
  - Phlebotomy
  - Client services
  - Billing
  - Availability of consultation/expertise

This section of the book deals with the operational management of the laboratory, including strategic planning, human resource management in the operational units, cost analysis, and financial decision making. Before discussing the details, it is worthwhile to consider the broad outlines of the challenges that face laboratory man-

agers and workers in the industry as a whole and in the major segments.

The Hospital Environment

In the hospital institutional environment, the laboratory usually operates as a division under a vice-president or director of operations. Along with other operational divisions such as pharmacy and dietary, the laboratory must compete for resources with direct patient care divisions such as nursing (Fig. 28.1). Because the laboratory is usually not directly represented at the table where administrative and fiscal decisions are made for the institution, and because the work of the clinical laboratory is relatively invisible compared to direct patient care, it is at a relative disadvantage in these negotiations. Consequently, it becomes even more important for laboratory management to be perceived as a team player in the hospital—to be seen as clinically responsive and fiscally responsible. These attributes become increasingly important when large capital expenditures or program expansions are sought.

In these situations the role of the laboratory medical director becomes critically important. To be most effective the director must speak for the medical needs of patients, particularly as they relate to laboratory services, but must also present a credible front to the hospital administration when addressing the business aspects of the laboratory, such as budgeting, billing, and planning.

For certain sections of the laboratory, such as anatomic pathology and the blood bank, the director must be a physician. The directors of all sections—and especially the laboratory director—will be able to function best, no matter what the nature of their degree, if they have a medical or clinical background that gives them credibility with the

Figure 28.1 The organizational chart of a hospital that is organized in a traditional manner. Note that the chief operating officer, who is parallel in reporting responsibility to the VP nursing, is responsible for all ancillary services through a director who is responsible for operations.

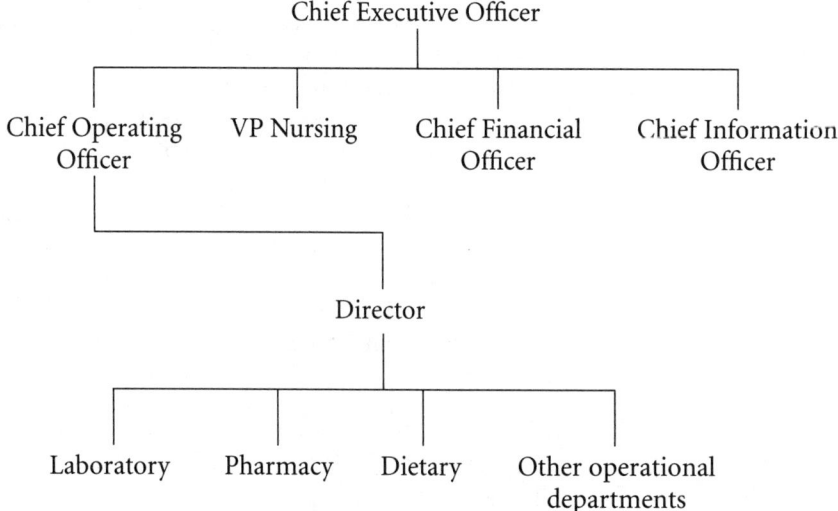

medical staff. Similarly, the relationship with the hospital administration may be enhanced if the laboratory director has a business degree or at least demonstrable training in business matters.

The ideal director, who satisfies fully both sides of the equation, may be difficult to find. In fact, it is not essential that all that talent be manifest in one individual if the director can take advantage of other resources within the laboratory. It is essential, however, that the person at the top have a balanced view of the laboratory world.

Operating in the Inpatient Hospital Setting

The major differences in the cost and operational structures of independent and hospital laboratories lie in the patient populations and the nature of the services provided. The two are dramatically different in their institutional missions, patient populations, hours of operation, percentage of tests requiring rapid turnaround ("stat" testing), communication and reporting requirements, and the need for highly specialized testing. In this section we will explore the environment of the hospital laboratory and how these factors may affect financial performance (Table 28.2).

Hospital laboratories have primary responsibility for an inpatient population of seriously ill people. Care has shifted to the outpatient environment and lengths of hospital stays have dramatically decreased in the United States since the introduction of diagnosis-based reimbursement. As a consequence, the acuity of illness of hospitalized patients has increased. More than ever, hospital laboratories must dedicate significant resources to 24-h-per-day, 7-day-per-week support for critically needed testing, often with a rapid turnaround time, to care for these patients. The simultaneous requirement to support the care of an increasing population of patients who are seeking emergent care further adds to the burden.

In this environment, the primary mission of the institution requires staffing, procedures, and instrumentation that support rapid production of testing results around the clock. The financial consequence of this mission is relatively low productivity for both instruments and personnel; as a consequence, costs are relatively high. Fortunately, the per-unit cost of equipment and reagents for most of the required tests is low. Additionally, economies can be achieved if additional nonemergent testing can be used to fill in excess capacity.

The high acuity setting also leads to its own set of requirements for communication and information technology. The frequent need to transmit highly abnormal results to clinicians who care for critically ill patients often requires staff to leave the work space, both to call in results on the telephone and to answer requests for results. As the laboratory obtains more critically abnormal results, more tests must be repeated or additional procedures must be performed. For example, the percentage of routine blood counts that require a manual differential count in the usual outpatient setting is less than 10%, while in a hospital, especially one seeing a substantial number of patients with cancer, that proportion may reach 30 to 35% or more. Balancing the demanding requirements for testing among sites with critical needs, such as intensive care units and emergency departments, often becomes very difficult to manage. The factors that detract from the efficiency of hospital-based laboratories are summarized in Table 28.3.

Of course, hospital laboratories, depending on their size, do also find it financially feasible to add batch processing for tests that need not have a rapid turnaround time. Cutting-edge technology, such as molecular diagnosis and molecular genetics, does not at present require immediate response. Thus these laboratories tend to have a portion of their staff devoted to relatively low complexity, rapid turnaround testing operating around the clock and a second component of staff devoted to batch production of relatively high complexity testing that requires special expertise, high cost reagents or instrumentation, and longer turnaround times (5). It should be noted that even in the sophisticated arena of molecular testing the pressure is growing to produce speedy results using real-time amplification technology.

The two components of staff needed for these two categories of testing are not interchangeable. Cross-coverage for vacations, illness, or other mandated benefits, such as attendance at conferences, is really impractical because the skill sets (and mind sets) for the two forms of testing are so different. In some hospitals, laboratories support decentralized testing in or near operating rooms, intensive care units, and emergency departments, again increasing cost and lowering productivity of staff. Table 28.4, which is derived from the College of American Pathologists Laboratory Management Index Program, indicates a clear, inverse relationship between the per-test cost of labor and laboratory size; larger laboratories are more productive.

The cost of reagents and supplies is the second largest component of laboratory cost, after personnel. In this case

Table 28.2 Components of diagnostic laboratory testing

Category of testing	Examples
Stat; immediate response required	Blood gases; frozen sections
Intermediate response; same day or shift	Routine chemistry and hematology
"ASAP" response; depending on technology	Microbiology, surgical pathology, molecular testing

Table 28.3 Factors that produce inefficiency in hospital-based laboratories that serve inpatients

Requirement for rapid laboratory response

Necessity for frequent repetition of tests

Need to telephone emergent or critical results to providers

Table 28.4 Laboratory productivity and volume[a]

Expense per billed test	Quartile[b] ($)				All laboratories
	1	2	3	4	
Consumables	2.96	2.65	2.31	2.14	2.74
Labor	6.03	5.51	4.99	4.65	5.02
Direct test	10.22	8.78	8.05	7.34	8.43

[a]Data from Laboratory Index Management Program of the College of American Pathologists (1994).

[b]Quartile values are the means of independent distributions. The sum of mean consumable and labor expense is not necessarily the same as direct expense.

there is a clear relationship between laboratory size, as measured by test volume, and supply cost. Larger laboratories have lower per-test supply costs than do smaller laboratories. Table 28.4 presents the cost-effectiveness ratios for the four quartiles of participating laboratories in the Laboratory Management Index Program of the College of American Pathologists. The relative decrease in the cost of consumables with increase in laboratory size presumably occurs because larger purchasers get better pricing from vendors; the development of group purchasing alliances such as Novation and Premier may well have blunted some of this effect.

Reimbursement of hospitals for inpatient stays is based on one of the following schemes, depending on the payor (Table 28.5):

- Percent of charges
- Per diem reimbursement
- Reimbursement for diagnosis-related groups (DRGs)

The second and third of these schemes are the most common in the United States, where reimbursement based on charges has almost disappeared for inpatients. As discussed earlier, payment schemes affect the financial performance of hospital laboratories in complex ways. For example, the intent of diagnosis-based reimbursement for hospital care is to create incentives for hospitals to minimize unneeded expenditures for all aspects of hospital care (commonly measured as length of stay), including laboratory testing (2). The efficacy of this incentive is illustrated by two changes in health care. Length of hospital stay dropped rapidly, almost precipitously, from around

Table 28.5 Reimbursement mechanisms in the inpatient, outpatient, and independent laboratory settings

Inpatient laboratories	Outpatient and independent laboratories
DRGs	Percent of charges negotiated reimbursement
Per diem reimbursement	
Percent of charges reimbursement	Fee schedule negotiated with payors
	Capitation
	Ambulatory payment classification groups (APCs)

7.5 days before DRGs to approximately 5 days or less now, a change of around 35%. Additionally, de novo systems of less expensive home care, including the ongoing administration of intravenous medications, for example, have proven very popular (1).

Generally, reimbursement for care of hospitalized patients that is not driven by DRGs is done on a per diem basis. For the laboratory, the consequence of both payment schemes is that inpatient revenue is unrelated to the quantity of testing. The institution gains if the cost of stay declines and if the number of laboratory tests done on each inpatient is reduced. Under this scenario, however, physicians are faced with the need to care for increasingly more ill patients quickly. It is estimated that upwards of 80% of the patient data in hospitals comes from the clinical laboratory. The bulk of laboratory testing during a hospital admission occurs in the first few days, when the patient is most acutely ill and when diagnoses are being tested and rejected or established. The financial gain for the laboratory produced by earlier discharge after these initial intensive days may, therefore, be minimal. Pressures to reduce length of stay will tend to compress the same amount of testing into a shorter period, leading to little if any reduction in laboratory cost (6).

Laboratory administrators are often surprised at the amount of indirect cost borne by the laboratory in the hospital setting. The laboratory is one of the few hospital departments that bills for services directly; other charges include those for pharmaceuticals, medical supplies, and "hotel" functions (bed charges). The simplest way to approach these costs is to examine the hospital's annual Medicare cost report, which allocates all indirect costs in a uniform way to departments. Often, direct laboratory cost for labor and supplies may be only half of total cost, with the remainder resulting from these charges for institutional indirect costs (4).

Operating in the Outpatient Hospital Setting

Many hospital laboratories, especially in academic medical centers, serve significant numbers of outpatients. These encounters with the outpatient facility may be associated with prior or future inpatient stays, for example, before or after surgical procedures. Here one might suppose the turnaround time must be less than in the hospital. In fact, the need for high-volume outpatient clinical operations is as varied and complex as is the inpatient facility. In some cases the need for rapid turnaround of test results may be surprising. It results from the increasing shift of sophisticated patient care from the hospital ward or operating room to the outpatient medical clinic, dialysis unit, or surgery. Oncology clinics, for example, often need the results of laboratory testing to decide if a patient may receive chemotherapy that day and at what dose. The complexity and sophistication of testing in this environment actually tends to be higher than in the inpatient setting; complex endocrinology diagnoses, for example, are usually sought in the outpatient setting. In this instance the tests do not usually require rapid turnaround and are best batched.

Hospital reimbursement in the outpatient setting is based on (Table 28.5):

- *Percent of charges*–contractually negotiated by the hospital with payors
- *Fee schedule*–contractually negotiated with payors, or prescribed as by government for Medicare
- *Capitation*–a contractual scheme in which the healthcare system (in some cases including both hospital and physician) undertakes to provide needed care to a defined population at a certain fixed rate per month, regardless of volume of care
- *Ambulatory payment classification groups* (APCs) (3)

The first two methods are straightforward and traditional. Capitation first appeared to any significant degree after the failed Clinton-era attempt at reconstruction of healthcare. Health maintenance organizations and other payors found that their market power enabled them to demand favorable, often capitated contracts from providers in many areas of the country. At one point, capitation of laboratory testing was paid at $0.60 per member per month in some areas. Over the past 6 years, as excess capacity has been wrung out of the healthcare system, providers have regained some of their market power and the pendulum has swung back toward the first two approaches. Medicare now reimburses hospital outpatient services on a modified diagnosis-related scheme (APCs).

In this outpatient arena, hospital laboratories compete with the commercial laboratory sector for business. In recent years the market share of hospital laboratories has increased at the expense of the commercial sector. While serving hospital outpatients has its own set of service demands, as indicated earlier, hospital laboratory outreach programs require, in addition, marketing, courier and phlebotomy services, business services such as billing and accounting, and customer support. Hospital laboratories often have excess technical capacity for testing, resulting from their need for rapid turnaround and their diurnal variation in demand (highest during the day and lowest at night). The unused capacity in the evening may allow the addition of outreach testing at minimal marginal cost. While most hospitals in the United States are still not-for-profit, laboratory operations in the for-profit sector are basically similar to those in the not-for-profit sector.

The Nonhospital Environment

The breadth of testing provided by independent laboratories generally mirrors that of hospital-associated laboratories. The major differences lie in the population served, hours and scope of operation, turnaround time require-ments, and need for ancillary functions, such as business operations. Some of these facilities do a substantial amount of reference (esoteric) testing for hospitals and other laboratories.

Most of the testing done by the independent laboratories is for outpatients of physicians and clinics. Some may provide phlebotomy services at or near the offices and clinics they serve. Most will provide couriers for the transportation of specimens back to the home laboratory. Except for work that requires rapid turnaround, which is unusual in this setting, most specimens are transported during the daylight hours and arrive at the laboratory in the late afternoon or evening, or even later at night, depending on distance. Thus the major testing effort takes place during the night in one large batch, and most results of routine tests are available before the next morning.

This type of workload and scheduling influences the laboratory's staffing and even its instrumentation choices. For example, the setting requires batch instrumentation that can process large numbers of samples relatively expeditiously, but with no need for rapid turnaround of any individual sample. An instrument that operates in a batch mode, then, may be better suited to this setting than one that may be somewhat slower but allows the interposition of "stat" samples at any time.

To the extent that these laboratories do esoteric work, for which a longer turnaround time of up to a week is often acceptable, that work is usually done separately during a day shift. If the marketplace justifies provision of the service, some independent laboratories perform forensic, veterinary, or environmental testing. A number of highly specialized niche laboratories still operate in such areas as cytogenetics, molecular genetics, forensic toxicology, and other areas that the large national laboratories have been reluctant to enter because of cost or need for specialized expertise.

For the most part independent laboratories serve an outpatient population. To be sure, in some, mostly rural, areas an independent laboratory may contract with a hospital to supply laboratory services. The reimbursement schemes for this sector of the industry are the same as those listed above for hospital outpatient work (Table 28.5). Major requirements for these laboratories include, in addition to the aforementioned courier and phlebotomy services, medical consultation, billing, accounting, client relations, marketing, sales, and information services functions. In the hospital setting these functions are usually performed mostly outside the laboratory.

The small independent laboratory has the advantage of flexibility and the ability to move quickly to adapt to the market; it is not burdened with hospital administrative overhead and cumbersome decision-making processes. Of course, management decisions are reflected rapidly in the bottom line, for better or worse. Because diagnosis-related reimbursement is not an issue in this market segment and because the prevalence of capitation is declining, it is in the best interest of the independent laboratory to maximize laboratory utilization and thus revenue.

As the independent laboratory industry has rapidly consolidated, the number of independent laboratories has plummeted; two large public corporations now dominate the industry and consolidation continues apace (7). Operating in the corporate setting involves less local autonomy and more centralized decision making. Local choices of tests offered, instrumentation, reagents, and so forth are likely to be very limited. On the other hand, the corporation will supply a centralized purchasing capability and likely similar data processing functions, releasing the local laboratory from these duties. On the revenue side, while the small independent laboratory must negotiate with providers or with payors who still permit local contracting, the large national corporations negotiate national contracts with payors when possible.

Summary

The objectives of laboratory management must reflect the demands of the laboratory's clients and the clinical and financial environment in which it operates. There are fundamental and striking differences in clinical need and demand, financial constraints and considerations, and laboratory mission and cost structures, which depend on the laboratory's situation. Whether inpatient or outpatient hospital or independent laboratory, each has its own set of functional drivers of which laboratory management must be acutely conscious.

KEY POINTS

- The demands for capable, effective management differ in the hospital inpatient, hospital outpatient, and independent laboratory settings.

- Laboratory management must be able to demonstrate intimate knowledge not only of the clinical needs for laboratory testing in various situations, but also the fiscal constraints of the institution in which it operates, and be able to communicate this understanding to higher administration.

- Reimbursement mechanisms vary according to setting, and laboratory management must have a clear understanding of all of the relevant mechanisms, payor requirements, and limitations.

GLOSSARY

CLIA '88 The Clinical Laboratory Improvement Amendments of 1988 and their implementing regulations, as published since 1992.

CLIA-waived testing A category of laboratory test complexity under CLIA (q. v.) which applies to tests that (i) are cleared by the U.S. Food and Drug Administration for home use; (ii) employ methods that are so simple and accurate as to render the likelihood of erroneous results negligible; or (iii) pose no reasonable risk of harm to the patient if the test is performed incorrectly.

Provider-performed microscopy A category of moderate-complexity tests under CLIA (q. v.) involving a patient care provider using a microscope for testing, such as urine microscopic examinations.

REFERENCES

1. **Centers For Disease Control And Prevention.** 2001. National Hospital Discharge Survey. Centers for Disease Control and Prevention, Atlanta, Ga.

2. **Centers for Medicare and Medicaid Services.** Acute Inpatient Web Page (http://cmshhs.gov/providers/hipps).

3. **Centers for Medicare and Medicaid Services.** Hospital Outpatient Perspective Payment System Web Page (http://cms.hhs.gov/providers/hopps/).

4. **Travers, E. M.** 1997. *Clinical Laboratory Management,* p. 154–155. Williams & Wilkins, Baltimore, Md.

5. **Travers, E. M.** 1997. *Clinical Laboratory Management,* p. 435–480. Williams & Wilkins, Baltimore, Md.

6. **Valenstein, P., A. Praestgaard, and R. Lepoff.** 2001. Six year trends in productivity and utilization of 73 clinical laboratories: a College of American Pathologists Laboratory Management Index Program Study. *Arch. Pathol. Lab. Med.* **125:**1153–1161.

7. **Washington G-2 Reports.** 2003. Laboratory Industry Report, vol. 12, no. 4, April 2003.

29

Strategic Planning

Paul Valenstein

OBJECTIVES

To define strategy and contrast strategic planning with the management of operations

To describe the competitive structure of the laboratory industry

To articulate the elements of competitor analysis

To characterize strategic positions commonly used by clinical laboratories

To explain how strategies are sustained and how they commonly fail

---

The essence of strategy is choosing what not to do.

MICHAEL E. PORTER

Introduction: What Is Strategy?

Strategy is an elusive concept for the typical manager of a clinical laboratory, who is often more comfortable working with operational issues. The word "strategy" evokes images of generals planning vast military campaigns, a process that would appear to have little relevance in the quiet and measured atmosphere of the diagnostic laboratory.

Business strategy complements the management of operations, which comprises the main focus of this book. Operational management consists of optimizing individual business processes. It may involve the efficient use of human resources, supply chain management, financial planning, or quality control. Managing laboratory operations includes the oversight of marketing, client services, specimen processing, billing, safety, and information technology, as well as the testing operations that constitute the heart of the diagnostic clinical laboratory.

In contrast, business strategy is about equipping an organization to withstand competitive market forces. Whereas the operational manager seeks to maximize the effectiveness of each part of a business, the business strategist seeks to arrange the parts into a whole that will succeed in a competitive environment and to toss out any parts that do not fit with a firm's strategy, no matter how well the part seems to function. The business strategist concerns herself with understanding the structure of her industry and her firm's competitors, defining a unique market position for her laboratory, and creating interlocking processes that provide her laboratory with a sustainable competitive advantage

499

in its target market. The business strategist values focus over growth; she is creative but also disciplined and not easily distracted.

Operational effectiveness and sound business strategy both produce competitive advantage. However, neither stands on its own. If all laboratory competitors enjoy excellent operational effectiveness and produce test results that are equally accurate, inexpensive, and timely, none of the competitors will enjoy a healthy financial return. Competition within the market will drive out profitability and lead to commoditization of laboratory services. Conversely, a laboratory may have a well-developed strategy to serve a defined group of customers that is not being well served by others, but at the same time lack the operational wherewithal to execute the strategy and keep its target customers satisfied. It, too, will flounder.

Business strategy includes several elements (Table 29.1). These are (i) understanding of the underlying structure of the industry in which an organization competes, (ii) assessment of a firm's particular strengths, weaknesses, assumptions, and goals, as well as those of its nearest competitors, (iii) identification of a distinctive market position that the firm can occupy more successfully than its rivals, (iv) development of interlocking and reinforcing business activities that drive the organization toward its desired position in the market, and (v) avoiding common traps that upend the best-laid strategy. These five elements will form the basis of this chapter.

Readers may believe that special characteristics of the clinical laboratory industry make it unsuitable for strategic planning. In this view, the concentration of laboratories within not-for-profit hospitals, a regulatory environment that imposes a high degree of uniformity on testing practices, and the strong market power of payors such as Medicare make it impossible for individual laboratories to uniquely position themselves in the market. However, this chapter will show that clinical laboratories have developed a variety of distinctive strategic positions to differentiate themselves from rivals.

Evidence to Recommend Strategic Planning

Randomized Controlled Trials

The process of strategic planning has not been tested in randomized controlled trials. Business leaders are not willing to subject the fates of their companies to experiments

Table 29.1 Elements of strategy

Understanding industry structure
Assessing a firm's and competitors' strengths and weaknesses
Identifying a distinctive market position
Adopting business activities that reinforce a market position
Avoiding common strategy traps

in which their firms are randomized to either using or not using a particular business strategy.

Moreover, strategic planning is not a standardized, well-defined intervention that can be dispensed to corporate leaders in the same manner as a pill or diet. A strategic plan must take account of the unique strengths and vulnerabilities of competitive adversaries and will therefore be different for every business.

As a result, the strongest type of research evidence—the randomized controlled trial—has not been applied to strategic planning. If strategic planning were a medical device, it would not be approved for sale. If it were a drug, it would not be licensed or prescribed.

Case Studies

A number of studies carried out by faculty of business schools have evaluated the role of strategy in business. For example, Porter evaluated the 35-year diversification histories of 33 large U.S. companies, using annual reports, 10K forms, Moody's ratings, and several other sources (7). Porter concluded that a large number of acquisitions were later divested as a result of their poor strategic fit with the acquiring firm. Studies such as Porter's rely on qualitative examination of an individual company or, in this particular example, a series of companies. Many of the case studies have been conducted in considerable depth; it is not unusual for an industry case study to be drawn from hundreds of pages of interview transcripts and financial data. Still, case studies are subject to two types of bias. There are likely to be selection biases in the firms authors choose (or are permitted) to study. Authors may also demonstrate interpretive bias when deciding which attributes of a company led to its market success or failure.

In addition to the case studies published by academicians, consultancies involved in strategic planning have published articles attesting to the importance of strategic planning for organizational success. These publications are subject to the same selection and interpretive biases that beset academic case reports and may additionally be troubled by conflicts of interest when the consultancies derive revenue from helping firms develop strategic plans.

In published case studies and reviews, academicians have identified strategy as a critical component in the success of particular firms (8). For example, Southwest Airlines' strategy of flying only short-haul, point-to-point routes between midsized cities and secondary airports of larger cities has been linked to its ability to attract price-sensitive travelers while maintaining profitability. Jiffy Lube International's strategy of limiting its product line to lubrication services has allowed it to offer faster service and thereby attract time-sensitive customers.

When a particular firm is identified in a case study as having a successful business strategy and the firm later stumbles in the marketplace, readers may conclude that the study author misinterpreted the facts of the case. However, authors argue that the identification of a company with a successful business strategy does not represent an endorsement of the company in all respects or indicate that the company's strategy will be successful for all time. Case studies of strategy represent an analysis at a particular point in time and under specific business circumstances. In this sense, a business author's work is analogous to that of an historian who asserts that a specific historical figure was able to effect political reform at a particular time in history, without also arguing that the subject was a model citizen in all respects or would have been successful in promoting reform under different historical circumstances.

Economic Theory

Classical economic theory provides indirect support for the value of strategy in business. Economic theory suggests that when one firm earns profits that are larger than average, other organizations will emulate the firm's practices until the increased competitive pressure brings the firm's profits down to an average level. The more benchmarking rivals in an industry perform and the more rivals outsource similar activities to third parties, the more alike their operations become (8). Even if operational efficiency improves for the first firm, it will not be able to maintain a relative productivity advantage over its rivals. Therefore, classical economics predicts that the profitability of firms in an industry should tend to equalize over time, as firms' products become commoditized.

The fact that some firms are able to outperform their adversaries consistently suggests that factors other than increased operational effectiveness are at work in the marketplace. Business authors suggest that strategy—the ability of firms to stake out and defend unique market positions—explains the capacity of some firms to earn returns that consistently exceed those of their competitors. A successful business strategy tends to weaken competitive pressure and allows organizations to achieve above-average returns for extended periods of time.

Developing and Maintaining a Business Strategy: The Strategic Planning Process

There is little consensus in the business literature about how strategies are best developed. Bruce Henderson, founder of the Boston Consulting Group, describes the development of strategy as "an iterative process that begins with a recognition of where you are and what you have now. Your most dangerous competitors are those that are most like you. The differences between you and your competitors are the basis of your advantage" (2). Henderson does not require that all of the stakeholders in an organization participate in developing a business strategy or

that it be contained in a written document. He requires only that a business strategy take into account existing differences between a firm and its competitors and purposefully build upon these differences.

Other business authors also downplay the importance of developing a written strategic plan, and some maintain that a formal strategic planning process can lead organizations astray. Campbell and Alexander argue that the planning frameworks managers use to develop strategy often yield disappointing results because business strategy is about insights and not about plans, which tend to be operational in nature (1). Kim and Maugorgne believe that when an inclusive planning process is used to formulate strategy, the competing agendas of an organization's various stakeholders limit development of a clear sense of purpose (3).

Others authors recommend a more formal procedure in which input is solicited from a firm's owners, board of directors, managers, employees, and customers and incorporated into a written document called a strategic plan. Not-for-profit companies tend to be particularly attracted to a formal, inclusive planning procedure. This may be the result of discomfort that many not-for-profit organizations experience in framing their business in competitive terms. Mission-based organizations also lack the direct feedback that for-profit companies obtain from the market, and a formal strategic planning process sometimes substitutes for the validation that for-profit companies receive in the marketplace.

It should come as little surprise that consultancies engaged in selling strategic planning services recommend a more structured approach to strategic planning. The formal strategic planning process consists of several steps (Table 29.2). The process generally begins with a commitment by leadership to identify a strategic direction for the organization. Typically, a planning committee of a half dozen individuals is created to specify important stakeholders and the information that will be collected in the planning process. The second step of the planning process involves development or refinement of a mission statement—what the organization values and seeks to accomplish. The third step involves a situation analysis, in which the strengths and weakness of the organization are articulated, along with external threats and opportunities. This generally takes the form of a competitor analysis, a process to be described later in this chapter. The fourth step of the strategic planning process involves the development of specific objectives and tactics that will further the organization's mission, given the

Table 29.2 The formal strategic planning processes

Formation of strategic planning committee

Development of a mission statement

Situation analysis

Development of tactics to further the organization's mission

Writing of formal strategic plan

realities that surface during the situation analysis. Finally, a subset of the planning committee summarizes the conclusions in a document called a strategic plan, which is given to the board of directors and senior staff to put into practice.

Whether or not a formal process is used to develop a business strategy, all strategies are shaped by the underlying structure of the industry in which a firm competes. We therefore turn our attention to the organization of the laboratory industry.

Structure of the Clinical Laboratory Industry

Competition in any industry is rooted in economics unique to the industry. Competitive pressure is applied not only from existing rivals, but also from potential entrants, substitute products, customers, and suppliers (6). The clinical laboratory industry has its own underlying structure, which is described in the paragraphs that follow and summarized in Table 29.3.

Size of the Testing Market

Excluding over-the-counter testing products, the clinical laboratory market comprises approximately 1% of the healthcare industry, which in turn represents 15% of the United States gross domestic product. The United States diagnostic testing industry had annual revenues in 2001 of

Table 29.3 Structural elements of the clinical laboratory industry

Market size
   Inpatient vs. outpatient
   Routine versus esoteric
Concentration of competitors
   Mergers and acquisitions of hospitals
   Consolidation of commercial laboratories
Barriers to entry
   Regulations, e.g., CLIA
   Customer (physician) loyalty
   Staff-model hospital systems
   Cost to customers of switching
Barriers to exit
   Local resistance to hospital closing
Separation of payor, purchaser, and beneficiary
Economies of scale
   Supplies, reagents, and testing instruments
   Other laboratory functions
Regulatory restrictions
   Markups
   Kickbacks
Powerful buyers and sellers
   Buyers, e.g., Medicare, Blue Cross
   Sellers, e.g., Red Cross
Substitute products
   Potentially, home diagnostics
Economics of inpatient care

approximately $35 billion. Roughly two-thirds of all testing is performed on outpatients, a fraction that has been growing by 1 to 2% per year over the past decade. Overall, clinical test activity has been growing by 4% per year due to changes in clinical practice, the introduction of new tests, and the growth and aging of the U.S. population. Demand for testing increases with age; testing activity per Medicare beneficiary is four to five times higher than testing per commercial insurance beneficiary. Cumulative revenue for the laboratory industry has been growing at a rate of 4% per year. Growth in revenue is the result of a shift in test mix towards more esoteric tests, including gene-based testing, and increases in test volume, offset by reductions in payor fee screens. Trends in laboratory costs are more difficult to measure than revenue trends. In one report that focused on hospital-based laboratories, the variable cost of testing remained constant over a 6-year period in nominal dollars and declined in real (inflation-adjusted) dollars; increases in the cost of wages and reagents were offset by commensurate increases in productivity (12).

Concentration of Competitors

The clinical laboratory industry is highly fragmented geographically; there are many providers but few that operate over large geographic areas. Within any local market there are relatively few competitors. As of this writing most outpatient markets are served by only one or two national commercial laboratories. There are currently four major national reference laboratories offering specialized testing, a figure that reflects the acquisition and exit of several former participants. Mergers or strategic alliances have also reduced competition among hospital laboratories. Although hospital markets are somewhat difficult to define, most communities are served by no more than three local hospitals. The physician office laboratory market is less concentrated than the commercial and hospital-based laboratory markets. Physician office laboratories, however, typically perform testing only on behalf of their owner's patients and as a result do not compete directly with one another.

Barriers to Entry

State and federal regulations constitute a significant barrier to the entry of new competitors to the clinical laboratory field. Certificate of need laws in many states prevent the construction of new hospitals without regulatory approval. In addition, laws in several states limit the acquisition of not-for-profit hospitals by for-profit companies. Laboratories that wish to serve Medicare beneficiaries—approximately 20% of the testing market—must pass regulatory and performance hurdles specified in the Clinical Laboratory Improvement Amendments of 1988 (CLIA) and elsewhere. Most laboratories meet this requirement by participating in the College of American Pathologists (CAP) Laboratory Accreditation Program or the Joint Commission for Accreditation of Healthcare Organizations accreditation program, both of which enjoy deemed status from the Center for Medicare and Medicaid Services of the U.S. federal government. CLIA regulations specify that laboratory directors and workers must meet certain education and experience standards and impose other requirements that limit entry to the laboratory industry.

Little capital is required to enter the laboratory industry; capital is not a significant barrier to entry. Depreciation accounts for less than 7% of the operating costs of most clinical laboratories, even after analytical instruments obtained on a reagent rental basis are capitalized and the cost of information systems are amortized.

Because physicians order the vast majority of laboratory tests, doctors represent an important distribution channel that must be accessed by any new entrant in the laboratory business. Most physicians in private practice who participate in managed care arrangements are accustomed to using several different laboratories for patients enrolled in different health plans. These physicians are fairly easily introduced to new laboratory services. However, physicians employed in staff-model practices or who are affiliated with tightly integrated independent practice associations may not be available to new laboratory entrants and therefore represent a barrier to entry into the testing market.

Switching costs—the cost incurred by a customer switching from one producer to another—may constitute a barrier to entry. In the specialty laboratory market, the effort required to configure and test new laboratory-to-laboratory computer interfaces tends to lock in customers and reduce competitive pressure. Community-based physicians do not currently experience difficulty switching laboratories, but difficulties may increase as laboratories develop sophisticated interfaces with practice management systems and the electronic medical records increasingly common in office practices.

Barriers to exit also influence industry economics. Unprofitable hospitals supported by local communities may not be permitted to close, perpetuating an oversupply of hospital-based laboratories. Specialized staff in unprofitable clinical laboratories who are reluctant to leave their employers or retrain may also produce a surplus of competitors.

Separation of Payor, Purchasing Agent, and Beneficiary

The healthcare industry is characterized by an unusual separation of roles that are typically combined in other businesses. The beneficiaries of services (patients) do not generally pay for services directly; less than 20% of care delivered in the United States is paid directly by patients. Most payments for health services are made by government insurance programs (principally Medicare and Medicaid)

or private insurance companies that are supported by employer contributions. To add to the complexity, neither the payors nor the beneficiaries act as purchasing agents of clinical laboratory services. Physicians order almost all laboratory tests. In fact, in many states it is illegal for patients or insurers to order laboratory tests. The separation of beneficiaries, payors, and purchasing agents creates a number of market distortions that have been widely studied. Teisberg et al. review the implications of this separation of roles on competition and incentives in healthcare (11).

Economies of Scale

There is strong evidence that analytical operations in chemistry, hematology, microbiology, gynecological cytology, and blood banking are subject to substantial economies of scale. In the CAP Laboratory Management Index Program, test volume (standardized billable tests/year) was the single factor most closely correlated with labor productivity (tests/full-time equivalent) and with overall efficiency (cost/test). Most laboratories that participate in the CAP program operate with test volumes that are well below the level at which efficiency tended to flatten out. There are insufficient data to determine whether significant economies of scale operate in other aspects of clinical laboratory operations, such as marketing, courier and transportation services, professional oversight, surgical pathology, and informatics.

Restrictions on Markups and Kickbacks

Federal law prohibits physicians and their employers from marking up Medicare and Medicaid charges billed to their practices. Further, antikickback laws prohibit laboratories from providing referring physicians with goods or services of value in exchange for referral of laboratory tests. These restrictions have been enacted to reinforce the fiduciary duties of physicians to their patients by eliminating financial incentives to order unnecessary tests or to select laboratories based on the physician's potential to profit from the transaction. However, these laws dampen market forces that would otherwise pressure laboratories to lower their prices. Some states, such as New York, New Jersey, Michigan, and Rhode Island, prohibit physicians from marking up laboratory charges when billing nonfederal insurance programs. In states that do not have these restrictions, laboratory charges to physicians for patients enrolled in non-Medicare programs tend to be lower and are then typically marked up by the physician before billing an insurer.

Powerful Sellers and Buyers

Powerful sellers of analytical equipment do not generally trouble the laboratory industry. Large purchasing cooperatives have enabled clinical laboratories to impose competitive pressures on the manufacturers of testing equipment and reagents. There are a number of providers of laboratory information systems that compete on the basis of price, support, stability, and functionality. In a few instances, however, specialized vendors of specific tests have strategically positioned their products with consumers (Cytec's positioning of liquid-based cytopathology tests) or with clinicians (Athena Laboratories positioning of neurological tests) so as to blunt competitive pressure and increase cost to purchasers. Perhaps the most powerful seller to the laboratory industry is currently the American Red Cross, which dominates the blood supply in most American communities. As a result of its market power, coupled with increased requirements for testing, blood and blood products have been the fastest growing expense item for hospital-based laboratories (12). Prices for blood products in markets where American Red Cross facilities compete with community blood centers are significantly lower than in markets in which the American Red Cross is the sole supplier.

The laboratory industry experiences significant pressure from powerful buyers, which the industry refers to as "payors." Medicare, the federal government's largest health insurance program, makes up approximately 20% of the clinical laboratory market by volume. In most communities, Blue Cross/Blue Shield and two or three other insurers dominate the remainder of the market. These buyers profoundly shape the clinical laboratory industry through imposition of (i) fee screens that place upper bounds on effective industry pricing; (ii) claims edits that place limits on the frequency or clinical setting in which services can be ordered and the manner in which tests can be billed; (iii) requirements that laboratories offer broad geographic service before they become eligible for exclusive testing arrangements; and (iv) turnaround time or result reporting requirements.

Substitute Products

The clinical laboratory industry is not currently subject to significant pressure from substitute products. However, over-the-counter testing products, point-of-care instrumentation used by nonlaboratory providers, and disease management programs run by pharmaceutical companies that incorporate laboratory testing have the potential to alter the configuration of the laboratory industry. Currently, most clinical laboratory testing is categorized as high or moderate complexity and thereby subject to extensive regulation under CLIA, which makes it unsuitable for displacement by over-the-counter or physician-office testing.

Unique Economics of Inpatient Care

For most inpatient care, laboratory testing is not a separate reimbursable service. More than 80% of inpatient care is reimbursed on a per diem basis or on the basis of diagnosis-related groupings. As a result, inpatient laboratories are inextricably tethered to the providers of inpatient care, most of which have elected to own and manage their inpatient testing operations. If a hospital-based laboratory does not have an outreach testing program, the laboratories will invariably follow the strategic direction set by its parent institution.

Conclusions

The structural elements of the laboratory industry are girders that impose a general shape on any laboratory business strategy. To develop a strategy for a particular laboratory, the strategist should understand the strengths and weaknesses of her firm's closest competitors.

Competitor Analysis

The objective of a competitor analysis is to predict competitors' behavior, both in the case when the competitors are left to their own devices and in response to moves of rivals. The strategy, position, and capabilities of competitors may limit a firm's opportunities for growth in some areas while simultaneously suggesting other areas in which a firm might expand with little challenge.

Popular back-of-the-envelope competitor analysis relies on a procedure referred to as a "SWOT" analysis, an acronym that describes an assessment of an organization's own strengths and weaknesses and external opportunities and threats. This procedure begins with an inward examination of an organization's capabilities and ends with an outward examination of rivals (Fig. 29.1). Through a SWOT analysis a manager may discover opportunities for market expansion or repositioning or identify areas in which a firm is vulnerable. Appendix 29.2 provides a hypothetical example of the sort of competitive information that the manager of a laboratory might receive about rivals during the normal course of business. Interested readers are encouraged to reorganize this information in the form of a SWOT analysis.

In the academic business literature, competitor analysis is a sophisticated process in which the future goals,

Figure 29.1 SWOT analysis.

assumptions, and capabilities of competitors are analyzed with the aim of predicting a competitor's response profile (9). A fully developed competitor analysis is beyond the means of most clinical laboratories, which are generally too small to conduct extensive systematic research about rivals. The following assessments are included in a formal competitor analysis:

Competitors' Goals

What are the business objectives of major competitors and potential competitors? Is the company most interested in generating returns on investment or sales growth? Is short-run or long-run performance most important? What incentive systems are used for management and sales? Does the competitor have noneconomic values that form part of its culture and that help determine how it will behave? If the competitor is a business unit of a larger company, how important is the unit to the overall company strategy? Most hospital-based laboratories are part of not-for-profit hospital companies that have a distinctive culture. Emphasis is often placed on fulfilling a noneconomic social mission for which laboratory success is tangential. Volume of medical center activity is often expressed in "adjusted discharges"—a unit of activity that reflects the historical importance of inpatient care and the secondary consideration of outpatient and outreach efforts. From these two observations, it can be predicted that most hospital companies will not vigorously defend outpatient laboratory operations that are under attack by competitors.

Competitors' Assumptions

Organizations operate with assumptions about their industry and their place within the industry. One laboratory might believe (correctly or incorrectly) that it enjoys greater physician loyalty than its rivals. Another laboratory might believe (correctly or incorrectly) that the testing industry will rapidly integrate genomic testing to the exclusion of more traditional microbiological assays. These assumptions will govern competitor's behavior. When rivals' assumptions are incorrect, they create business opportunities. A laboratory that overestimates its customer loyalty will be vulnerable to discounts. A laboratory that overestimates the importance of offering broad geographic access to managed care plans may lose business in regional markets in which a smaller rival has partnered with a physician group or a group of hospitals.

Competitors' Capabilities

The strengths and weaknesses of a firm determine its ability to meet its goals. A weak rival is unlikely to represent a competitive threat even if its goals overlap with your own. An assessment of a rival laboratory's strengths and weaknesses includes a study of its testing menu and other services it provides clients, the number and loyalty of physician and institutional customers, marketing capabilities,

operational skills (diagnostic speed and accuracy, specimen logistics, and informatics), patents and proprietary research to which the rival has access, cost structure, financial strength (cash flow and access to capital), and organizational strength (reputation, clarity of purpose, management talent, and special structural characteristics that might make it subject to different regulatory pressures).

Interactions of Competitors

In a market operating with what economists term perfect competition, the actions of one producer do not influence the actions of other producers. If one farmer stops growing corn, the price of corn does not rise. However, in the clinical laboratory industry, which has significant barriers to entry and relatively few direct competitors in a given community, the actions of one party are likely to precipitate reactions from rivals. Competitive situations in which actions precipitate reactions are described by game theory, a branch of mathematics pioneered by John von Neumann, Oskar Morgenstern, and John Nash. The theoretical and economic underpinnings of game theory are complex and beyond the scope of this chapter. However, the wise business strategist will consider likely reactions of rivals before making a change in the marketplace. Every move in business has the potential to shift the competitive equilibrium. Armed with an understanding of a rival's goals, attitudes towards risk, and historic behavior, a strategist may be able to predict her rivals' response to moves her firm might make. For example, if a competitor has recently removed a phlebotomist from one of its client's offices, what will be the competitor's reaction to your placing a phlebotomist in the office to woo the client? Will the competitor retaliate by scrapping a joint venture with your laboratory, or will the competitor's loss of volume from the client be the straw that breaks its back in a local market and cause it to exit?

Conclusions

An understanding of a laboratory's and its competitors' aspirations and capabilities prepares the strategist to identify the distinctive needs or customer groups that her organization can satisfy better than its competitors. Defining these groups and needs is the subject of the next section.

Strategic Positions in the Laboratory Industry

What Are Strategic Positions?

The term "strategic position" refers to an organization's commitment to serve many needs of a specific group of customers or specific needs of many customers. This section will describe generic types of strategic positions common in many industries and will then enumerate particular positions held within the clinical laboratory industry. The list of strategic positions that appears in this section is not exhaustive and should not discourage the development of creative new positions. In a competitive environment, the best strategic positions are often those that are off rivals' radar screens.

Types of Strategic Positions

There is no single taxonomy of strategic positions. Porter has identified several types of strategic positions that successful organizations may develop (8, 9). Implicit in his discussion is the tenet that a single company cannot be all things to all people. Strategy involves choices and tradeoffs.

Variety-based positioning. Companies that offer only a single or narrow scope of service and perform the service exceptionally well or inexpensively demonstrate variety-based positioning. For example, Jiffy Lube International has chosen to offer only automotive lubrication services and does not perform automobile repair or general maintenance. The company has been organized to offer faster service at lower cost than rivals that offer a broader spectrum of services.

Need-based positioning. When groups of customers have different needs, a firm can elect to serve many needs of a defined demographic group. Ikea has been organized to meet the furniture needs of young families who seek style but lack resources. Ikea offers services that appeal to its target demographic, such as in-store childcare and extended hours. Costs are kept low by requiring customers to deliver and assemble their own furniture, a trade-off that the target customer is willing to make.

Access-based positioning. Access-based positions arise when different groups of customers must be accessed in different ways. These differences may be due to geography or differences in size of the customer pool. Carmike Cinemas targets customers in rural communities and small towns and has organized its operations around the constraints and demands of this market.

Cost-based positioning. Competitors with lower production costs may be able to profit at market prices that leave other providers without earnings. As of this writing, Dell Computer Corporation has lower production costs than its competitors and has lowered industry pricing to a level that allows it to profit while other firms are forced to exit the industry.

Product differentiation-based positioning. Some producers, through marketing or other distinctive attributes, are able to convince purchasers that their product is superior to their competitors' and thereby command a price premium. It can be argued that the Mayo Clinic enjoys this position in the market for certain elective clinical procedures. As with most firms that differentiate their product

to obtain a price premium, the Mayo Clinic does not command a large share of the market for hospital services.

Strategic Positions of Clinical Laboratories

Diagnostic laboratories have sought a number of distinguishable market positions to differentiate themselves from rivals and defend their operations from competition (Table 29.4).

Outpatient-centered testing. Several laboratories with national scope have organized themselves primarily to serve the testing needs of physicians operating in offices. These companies compete vigorously for exclusive managed care contracts that allow them to become a "one-stop shop" for the office practitioner who treats patients enrolled in a variety of insurance products. The large size of these companies allows testing costs to remain low and permits profitability despite the low payment levels offered by managed care organizations. An extensive courier system and a sophisticated billing system that can handle the insurance requirements of different payors reinforce these companies' strategic position.

Reference-centered testing. A handful of laboratories provide reference testing that smaller hospital-based or regional laboratories cannot economically perform on their own. Successful competitors in this market manage complex shipping logistics, typically by air, and provide electronic interfaces to referring laboratories' information systems. Professional support is provided to the staff of referring laboratories who are unsure which test to order or how to interpret results. Specialized software allows referring institutions to track the status of orders.

Table 29.4 Sample strategic positions in the laboratory industry

Outpatient-centered testing
    Exclusive contracts with multiple insurers
    Large volume to contain costs
    Blood collection and specimen pickup
Reference-centered testing
    Specialized and esoteric tests
    Specimen logistics
    Professional support for referring laboratories
Hospital-centered testing
    Support for inpatients and intensive care
    Participation in hospital planning committees
Discipline-centered testing
    Niche markets serving a particular subspecialty
    Customized reports for specialists
Community-centered testing
    Outreach by hospital laboratories to physicians on medical staff
Multi-hospital core laboratory
    Centralization of routine testing by laboratories of a multi-hospital system
Co-tenancy
    Shared ownership of esoteric laboratory by a group of hospitals
Purchasing and contracting consortia

Hospital-centered testing. Many laboratories have staked out strategic positions serving a hospital's core patient population—inpatients, ambulatory surgery patients, and emergency department patients. These operations are designed to provide rapid turnaround time appropriate to high-intensity patients. Laboratory representatives serve on hospital patient care committees and are attuned to special coordination and communication needs of this demanding patient population.

Discipline-centered testing. Specialized clinical laboratories have evolved to meet the particular needs of physicians within one medical specialty or the needs of one type of commercial concern. Dermatopathology laboratories, forensic testing laboratories, pharmaceutical trial testing facilities, and urological pathology laboratories provide specialized diagnostic skills required by a subset of laboratory purchasers. These organizations typify variety-based positioning; they may offer unique reporting formats appropriate to their customers, such as provision of reports to urologists that include serial prostate-specific antigen graphs alongside prostate biopsy reports.

Community-centered testing. A number of in-hospital testing operations have expanded into the community outpatient market, serving a defined medical staff that sees patients in both the hospital and outpatient setting. These laboratories maintain tight connections with local physicians and often allow seamless access to old test results as patients move through the healthcare continuum. In one variant of this model, best developed by MDS Diagnostic Services, a for-profit company providing management expertise and capital enters into a joint venture with a not-for-profit hospital to provide community testing services.

Multi-hospital core laboratory. Innovative hospital systems have created core laboratories where routine testing from several hospitals is performed. Outpatient testing from each of the participating hospitals or from a separate combined outreach operation is also processed within the core laboratory. This strategic position drives large volumes of testing into the core laboratory, lowering cost beyond levels that can be achieved in many other configurations. The large test volume permits the economical introduction of robotic equipment to handle repetitive testing and transport tasks. Rapid response laboratories remain in hospitals to serve the urgent testing needs of hospital patients.

Co-tenancy. The author is involved in an operation in which a group of not-for-profit hospitals collectively own esoteric testing services as tenants-in-common. This operation amounts to a shared cost center and provides hospital laboratories with governance control, pricing flexibility,

and a cost structure that cannot be acquired from many reference-centered laboratories (10).

Purchasing and contracting consortia. Purchasing and contracting cooperatives have evolved to provide clinical laboratories with more favorable relations with suppliers and payors. Although not performing testing themselves, purchasing consortia allow testing laboratories to obtain favorable pricing on analytical instruments and supplies. Contracting consortia allow testing laboratories to compete collectively for managed care contracts that require a geographic scope of service that individual members cannot offer on their own. In the author's state of Michigan, Joint Venture Hospital Laboratories has allowed hospital-owned laboratories to acquire exclusive laboratory contracts for the major health maintenance organization (HMO) insurers in the state (10).

Conclusions

The design of business strategy is fundamentally the process of identifying a strategic position for an organization, informed by the underlying structure of the industry and knowledge of an organization's and its competitor's capabilities and proclivities. From the brief preceding discussion, the reader will appreciate that clinical laboratories have developed a wide variety of strategic positions to differentiate themselves in the market.

We now turn our attention to implementing a business strategy. Sadly, managers too often content themselves with design and never move on to implementation. It is during implementation that strategy collides with operations and difficult trade-offs must be made.

Implementing Strategy: Activity Fit

What Is Activity Fit?

Academicians who study businesses with robust strategies emphasize the importance of interlocking and reinforcing business processes that sustain the strategy. The activities of a company with a successful strategy must fit with one another and reinforce the strategy.

For example, Southwest Airlines limits itself to short-haul, point-to-point flights between midsized cities and secondary airports. This activity frees the company from having to coordinate connections between flights or to transfer baggage between planes, which in turn reinforces another Southwest activity—15 min gate turnaround of aircraft. The short gate turnaround time achieved by Southwest reinforces yet another activity—more frequent and more reliable departures. All of these activities— point-to-point flights, rapid gate turnaround, and more frequent departures—allow the airline to maintain a lower cost structure and reinforce its market position as the low cost airline. Low ticket prices lead to higher demand, which increases the airline's load factor (percentage of occupied seats) and supports its ability to offer more frequent departures.

The operational activities of Southwest Airlines reinforce one another and make its business model more resistant to competitive pressure. A competitor that copies only one of Southwest's business activities will not be able to emulate the whole. In Porter's view, "fit locks out competitors by creating a chain that is as strong as its *strongest* link" (8). Milgrom and Roberts have studied successful manufacturers and found that they too use complementary manufacturing and inventory processes to defend their market positions (4, 5).

Activity Fit Involves Tradeoffs

A commitment to reinforcing business activities that sustain competitive advantage requires trade-offs. While the successes of Southwest Airlines have been widely commented upon, we might also consider the many markets that Southwest has skipped over to maintain its strategic position. A traveler who wishes to fly first class will not choose Southwest. There are many cities that Southwest does not serve, and travelers who fly to these cities will select other airlines. Travelers who prefer to use travel agents will use other carriers. Southwest's success in one arena excludes the airline from many other markets. Yet Southwest earns a return its larger rivals envy.

Most hospital-based laboratories focus their activities around a small group of local physicians with whom they maintain close relationships. These laboratories strive to meet the broad testing needs of a narrow group of clients. Activities that fit with this strategy may be found in other departments of a hospital, which may be marketing radiology, cardiology, and other services to the same group of community physicians. The hospital-based laboratory that wishes to maintain its competitive advantage will look to other hospital departments for activities that reinforce its strategic position. For example, community physicians might be offered convenient electronic access to the hospital's entire clinical data repository, which will contain radiology and consultation reports as well as laboratory results. Alternatively, a local laboratory and physician group can bid together for a managed care contract that includes both physician and laboratory services. These activities would fit well with other activities that strengthen a hospital-based laboratory's ties with community physicians.

However, the fit of activities that optimizes a laboratory's value to community physicians may not be suited to other strategic positions. Electronic access to a local hospital's clinical data repository would not serve a laboratory seeking to service a statewide commercial contract, the reference testing market, a geographically dispersed group of dermatologists, or businesses in need of forensic drug testing. From a strategic perspective, the hospital-based laboratory that markets a broad bundle of services to local physicians should pass up the opportunity to market a more narrow set of services over a broad geographic expanse because a different set of interlocking activities will be required.

The reverse is equally applicable. In the author's market, Quest Diagnostics has established a working relationship with the United Auto Workers (UAW). The UAW is a powerful influence with large employers that, in turn, influence the direction of major insurance companies in the state. The effort that Quest Diagnostics has spent developing a relationship with the UAW reinforces Quest's strategy of obtaining exclusive managed care laboratory contracts from large insurers on a statewide basis. However, this activity is not a good fit with a strategy aimed at marketing to community physicians who have no particular relationship with the UAW.

Failure of Strategy

The best-laid strategy may fall short through bad luck or external developments that no strategist could reasonably foresee. Business authors, however, have identified three types of preventable errors that account for the majority of strategic failures.

Straddling

The term "straddling" describes an attempt to hold several strategic positions at once. This failure to focus has also been called "mission creep" and "stuck in the middle."

The business consequences of straddling may be severe. Continental Airlines attempted to emulate some of Southwest's business practices by offering point-to-point service with frequent departures, low pricing, and short gate turnaround. It maintained its position as a full service airline, however, using travel agents to book flights and assign seats, operating with a mixed fleet of aircraft, and allowing interflight baggage checking. The results were severe: late flights and lost baggage generated several thousand complaints per day. Payment of commissions to travel agents prevented the airline from competing on price. Ultimately, the new service was withdrawn.

Other examples of straddling may be found closer to the laboratory industry. Premier, a large purchasing cooperative for hospitals, developed a number of strategic partnerships with suppliers of goods and services. The perception of conflict of interest has resulted in negative publicity for Premier and pushback from its hospital owners, significantly reducing Premier's size and market power (13). Quest Diagnostics has attempted on a number of occasions to manage hospital-based laboratories, but in this author's opinion the difficulty of straddling between operations suited for the commercial market and those required for hospital-based operations has resulted in the abandonment of several joint ventures between Quest and hospitals. The adoption of Internet laboratory portals by many community-based laboratories may represent another case of straddling. Laboratory portals that do not include radiology and other ancillary results represent a better strategic fit for a company that offers only laboratory services.

Although many examples of straddling are readily identified in retrospect after a venture has failed, it should be noted that straddling may not be easy to recognize in its early stages. The concept of leveraging existing competencies and current market position to enlarge a business is an accepted competitive practice. Where leveraging ends and straddling begins can be difficult to determine. This dilemma is familiar to anyone who has attempted to rapidly cross a river by stepping on rocks spaced some distance apart. How far is too far may be clear only in hindsight.

Growth Trap

An overemphasis on growth can cause an organization to lose its focus and competitive advantage. The unfocused pursuit of growth causes managers to add features and services without first considering whether they fit with a firm's existing strategy and set of competencies. Often, new types of customers are pursued when an organization has little distinctive ability to serve the new customers. In the testing industry, the occasional community-centered laboratory has attempted to acquire managed care contracts on its own without partnering with other laboratories or other providers. These facilities have little chance of succeeding in the managed-care market on their own. A few hospital-centered laboratories have added expensive forensic or molecular testing operations without acquiring the distribution channels and client services, billing, and logistics infrastructure that are necessary to support these services. These operations will also fail.

Authors who study strategy advocate more deeply penetrating markets in which a firm already has a distinctive presence, rather than "slugging it out in potentially higher growth areas where a company lacks uniqueness" (8). Henderson points out that "chasing market share is almost as productive as chasing the pot of gold at the end of the rainbow. You can never get there. . . . If you are in business, you already have 100% of your own market" (2).

Hubris

Because strategic initiatives are a deliberate perturbation of the competitive equilibrium and because they require explicit tradeoffs that must permeate an organization, strategy is best championed by confident high-visibility leaders with the ability to persevere amid distractions. Excessive confidence, however, may also undermine disciplined analysis and result in a loss of focus. There is evidence that corporate acquisitions that are preceded by favorable business press about the acquiring company's chief executive officer are less likely to be successful than acquisitions made in a publicity vacuum. Accordingly,

hubris must be added to our short list of reasons that strategies frequently fail.

Summary

Business strategy is about equipping an organization to thrive in a competitive market. In competitive markets, producers tend to emulate one another until their products and services become indistinguishable. This process of commoditization benefits consumers through lower costs and higher quality but minimizes profits for producers.

Strategy represents a deliberate effort to resist commoditization and maintain an organization's competitive advantage by defending a distinctive position in the market. A successful strategy is a creative approach that is shaped by the particular industry in which an organization operates and the particular competitors it faces in the marketplace.

A business strategy complements, but is different from, operational efficiency. Both produce competitive advantage. Many authors believe, however, that strategy is more likely to produce sustained competitive advantage than is operational effectiveness, because rivals can more easily emulate operational improvements than good business strategy.

Business strategy is informed by an understanding of the structure of the industry in which an organization competes. It is further advanced by a competitor analysis in which the capabilities and proclivities of individual competitors are analyzed. An essential element of business strategy is the selection of a strategic position that defines the particular customers or needs that an organization seeks to serve. Finally, a strategy is maintained by the implementation of interlocking activities that drive the company towards its strategic position and which are collectively difficult to emulate.

There is no consensus about how good strategies originate. Some argue for a defined strategic planning process in which a formal, written strategic plan is developed following input from a variety of stakeholders. Others believe that the creative insight of a small group of individuals is more likely to produce a successful strategy. Thus, ideas about how to best undertake strategic planning are varied and debated, even though the importance of a well-articulated strategy is widely recognized.

Strategies commonly fail because organizations lose their focus and attempt to emulate competitors. This may be due to straddling—an attempt to assume several strategic positions concurrently—or due to the unbridled pursuit of growth.

In the clinical laboratory industry, a number of distinctive strategic positions are identifiable. These positions allow focused laboratories to maintain a competitive advantage over rivals in a segment of the testing industry the laboratory claims as its own, while ceding the rest of the market to other competitors.

KEY POINTS

- Business strategy is about equipping an organization to thrive in a competitive market. Strategy is distinct from the pursuit of organizational efficiency. Both produce competitive advantage, but neither stands on its own.

- Strategy requires that an organization pursue a defined strategic position, focusing on meeting many needs of a particular set of customers or particular needs of many customers. In the clinical laboratory industry, laboratory competitors have staked out several distinguishable strategic positions.

- The differences between an organization and its rivals are the source of an organization's competitive advantage and the basis of its strategy. Emulating rivals usually weakens an organization's competitiveness.

- Strategy requires trade-offs. Organizations are not well served by pursuing several strategic positions concurrently or by adopting capabilities that are not central to maintaining the organization's strategic position.

- An effective strategy is maintained by interlocking business capabilities that reinforce an organization's market position and that are collectively difficult to emulate. If rivals copy only one or two of these capabilities, they will still remain at a competitive disadvantage.

GLOSSARY

Activity fit Interlocking and reinforcing business practices that define and defend a strategic position.

Commoditization The process by which a product provided by one firm becomes indistinguishable from products provided by other firms.

Competitive advantage Qualities that allow a firm to outperform its rivals consistently.

Competitor analysis Assessment of the capabilities, goals, assumptions, and strategies of competitors, with the aim of predicting competitor behavior.

Economy of scale The reduction in the cost to produce a unit of product when the level of production increases.

Straddling The attempt to execute several distinct business strategies or to hold several strategic positions at once.

Strategic planning An organized process for developing a business strategy.

Strategic position Serving a particular set of customers or meeting a defined set of needs, usually in a manner that is unique.

Strategy Quest for sustainable competitive advantage by means of analysis of industry structure and competitors, identification of a strategic position, and adoption of business practices that defend that position.

REFERENCES

1. **Campbell, A., and M. Alexander.** 1987. What's wrong with strategy? *Harvard Business Rev.* **Nov.–Dec.**:42–51.

2. **Henderson, B.** 1989. The origin of strategy. *Harvard Business Rev.* **Nov.–Dec.**:139–143.

3. **Kim, W. C., and R. A. Maugorgne.** 2002. Charting your company's future. *Harvard Business Rev.* **June**:76–83.

4. **Milgrom, P., and J. Roberts.** 1991. The economics of modern manufacturing: technology, strategy, and organization. *Am. Econ. Rev.* **80**:511–528.

5. **Milgrom, P., and J. Roberts.** 1995. Complementarities and fit: strategies, structure, and organizational changes in manufacturing. *J. Accounting Econ.* **19**:178–208.

6. **Porter, M. E.** 1979. How competitive forces shape strategy. *Harvard Business Rev.* **March–April**:2–10.

7. **Porter, M.E.** 1987. From competitive advantage to corporate strategy. *Harvard Business Rev.* **March—April**:117–150.

8. **Porter, M. E.** 1996. What is strategy? *Harvard Business Rev.* **Nov.–Dec.**:61–78.

9. **Porter, M. E.** 1998. *Competitive Strategy: Techniques for Analyzing Industry and Competitors.* The Free Press, New York, N.Y.

10. **Smart, J.** 2002. Hospitals in Michigan build unique shared laboratory. *Dark Rep.* **Oct. 28**:1–6.

11. **Teisberg, E. O., M. E. Porter, and G. B. Brown.** 1994. Making competition in health care work. *Harvard Bus. Rev.* **72**(42):131–141.

12. **Valenstein, P., A. Praestgaard, and R. Lepoff.** 2001. Six year trends in expense, productivity, and utilization of seventy-three clinical laboratories. *Arch. Pathol. Lab Med.* **125**:1153–1161.

13. **Walsh, M. W.** 2002. More hospitals change the way they buy drugs and supplies. *The New York Times.* 28 Dec.

APPENDIX 29.1 Websites

Alliance for Nonprofit Management
(http://www.allianceonline.org/faqs.html)
The Alliance is the professional association of organizations devoted to improving the management of nonprofit organizations. Their website provides links to strategic planning resources.

Centers for Medicaid and Medicare Services
(http://www.cms.hhs.gov)
This division of the U.S. Department of Health and Human Services maintains an extensive website that provides information about regulations pertinent to the laboratory industry. These regulations shape the competitive landscape and limit strategic options of competitors.

College of American Pathologists
(http://www.cap.org/)
The College of American Pathologists Laboratory Accreditation Program represents the largest laboratory accreditation program approved under the Clinical Laboratory Improvement Amendments. The CAP program and its standards for accreditation are contained in the CAP web site.

A complete list of accrediting organizations approved under CLIA can be found at http://www.cms.hhs.gov/clia/

Securities and Exchange Commission
(http://www.sec.gov/index.htm)
The web site of the U.S. Securities and Exchange Commission provides access to the EDGAR database of company filings. Quarterly and annual statements of publicly traded laboratory companies discuss company strategy and financial performance.

APPENDIX 29.2 SWOT Analysis

To illustrate SWOT analysis in practice, the current position of a hypothetical but fairly characteristic clinical laboratory will be discussed ("Lab A"), along with its major competitors. This illustration contains the typical snippets and fragments of information that every manager receives about its competitors and its own operations during the normal course of conducting business. As an exercise, the reader is encouraged to extract essential competitive information from the narrative that follows and to list strengths, weaknesses, opportunities, and threats in a 2 × 2 SWOT table of the form illustrated in Figure 29.1.

INTERNAL ASSESSMENT

Lab A processes 700,000 billable tests per year and is located in a not-for-profit hospital in a metropolitan area of 300,000 people. The organization has an active outreach program that accounts for 50% of its total test volume.

Strengths

Lab A employs managers who enjoy personal relations with managers in other hospital departments. The pathologists affiliated with Lab A are members of the local hospital medical staff and market to their colleagues, many (but not all) of whom are the laboratory's outreach customers. A recent hospital-sponsored satisfaction survey demonstrated a moderately high level of satisfaction with laboratory services—86% of physicians and nurses considered Lab A performance to be "highly satisfactory" or "excellent." Lab A staff are well represented on hospital committees and are aware of other department's needs for special testing services (rapid myocardial infarction testing in the emergency department and intensive care units, for example). Lab A transmits test results to a hospital clinical information system that is used to treat inpatients. Many of the laboratory's customers are located in a physician office building constructed by the hospital, in which the laboratory has placed a convenient blood drawing station. The hospital is contemplating the construction of a second office building that may bring in more business. The laboratory contracts with reliable outside couriers to serve members of the medical staff with nearby offices. The analytical equipment in chemistry and hematology is used for both inpatient testing (which is run mostly on the day shift) and outpatient testing (which is run mostly on the afternoon shift), which lowers fixed costs. Patients who lack insurance and financial resources are eligible for the hospital's charitable care program, which absorbs the expenses of laboratory testing.

Weaknesses

Because Lab A does not operate its own courier service, it has difficulty adding courier routes on short notice. Compared to commercial laboratories, the relatively small size of Lab A leads to higher testing costs. During the evenings, when outreach laboratory work arrives, stat testing from the intensive care units sometimes interferes with workflow. Although the laboratory has its own information system, all billing is done through a hospital-operated billing system. This system does not handle front-end advanced beneficiary notice and medical necessity checking and does not offer flexible pricing schedules that would allow the laboratory to match competitors' pricing. The hospital does not participate in TrueCare, the second largest preferred provider organization in the state; when physicians send their TrueCare patients to the laboratory the patients are billed directly, which disturbs many referring physicians. Although the hospital participates in the state's largest HMO, BlueChoice, the HMO has carved out laboratory services to a commercial laboratory that offers statewide coverage. The local chapter of the American Red Cross increased the cost of blood products by 18% 2 months ago, after the laboratory's expense budget was approved. As a result the laboratory will exceed its budget, which means that laboratory

(continued)

management will not be able to fill the open phlebotomy position in the physician office building or purchase a blood irradiator. Because of declining professional reimbursement, the pathology group affiliated with Lab A has decided to operate its own anatomic pathology laboratory for nonhospital patients. Lab A's marketing director was told by four busy pulmonologists in the neighboring community that they will not use Lab A because the hospital that owns Lab A cancelled their contract to provide intensivist services to the intensive care unit. The hospital's chief operating officer has indicated that the hospital's big push for the new fiscal year will be strengthening the hospital's cardiovascular surgery program; he wants the laboratory to open a phlebotomy site in the new ambulatory heart center, even though projected demand for laboratory tests at this site will be low.

EXTERNAL ASSESSMENT

An external assessment begins with the identification of specific rivals that compete with the organization for business. In this particular example, we will limit our external assessment to two hypothetical rivals—a large commercial laboratory that operates in the same community as our hospital laboratory ("OmniLab") and a second hospital laboratory that is part of a seven-hospital system in the process of building a core laboratory ("Lab B").

Opportunities

Word-of-mouth indicates that Lab B is likely to be spending significant effort during the next 2 years planning its core laboratory and installing a robotic system to reduce costs. Lab B has left its outpatient marketing director position open while it recruits a new manager for its laboratory information and robotics system. Lab B has also pulled a phlebotomist from a physician client's office. The physician is now offering to change to any laboratory that provides him with a phlebotomist. Lab B is part of a consortium that is bidding for the BlueChoice laboratory contract in the next calendar year. There may be an opportunity for Lab A to join this consortium. OmniLab recently closed a phlebotomy station in the community, presumably due to slack demand. Wages paid by OmniLab are below those paid by Lab A, and two technologists were recently lured away from the competition's testing center 30 mi away. There are rumors that OmniLab's testing center may be closed, which will mean that OmniLab will have to transport specimens to its next nearest testing site, across the state border.

Threats

Lab B has hired two dermatopathologists and appears to have a stranglehold on dermatology biopsies in the community. Hospital administrators overseeing Lab B wish to partner with a laboratory management company that has significant interest and experience in the outreach business, a prospect that would increase competitive pressure in the local market. Lab B participates in TrueCare and therefore has access to patients who cannot be served by Lab A. OmniLab recently interfaced its computer system with the practice management system used by a group of five family practitioners; office staff no longer have to copy insurance information onto test requisitions and can have advanced beneficiary notices printed automatically at the time of ordering. The practice's office manager is telling other family practitioners in the community about the labor she hopes to save. In addition, OmniLab has started making test results available to physicians and patients over the Internet. A group of gastroenterologists who are important clients of Lab A want to know why Lab A cannot offer the proprietary ultrasensitive quantitative hepatitis C test that OmniLab offers.

30

Human Resources at the Local Level: an Important Component of Financial Management

Washington C. Winn, Jr., and Fred Westenfeld

OBJECTIVES

To establish the importance of managing personnel resources effectively at the individual unit level as well as at the institutional level

To review the constraints on the ability of a manager to lead his crew optimally

To review some important tools for getting the most out of employees

To consider some of the classic problems that may face a unit manager

To provide some specific examples of ways that a manager may get the biggest return from the investment in personnel resources that the institution has made

If my boss calls, be sure to get his name.

-ANONYMOUS ABC EXECUTIVE, QUOTED BY WILLIAM S. RUKEYSER, 1986

THE TWO MOST IMPORTANT *manageable* components of any business enterprise are the costs of personnel and materials. The relative importance of these two factors depends on the business of the organization. A highly automated producer of expensive physical products will have very high materials costs and lower personnel costs. In contrast, for a service industry that produces no physical products, the cost of materials will be minimal, but the highly trained, competent workers who are required to run a successful enterprise will probably come at high cost.

In the laboratory industry, managers are faced with perhaps the worst situation—an information product for which a highly trained workforce must operate expensive equipment and reagents. On the other hand, the fact that both sides of the equation are important means that there are opportunities for savings in two very different managerial areas. In this chapter we will concentrate on personnel costs because they are the ones over which a manager can exert the greatest influence. Although careful negotiation of contracts and searches for alternate suppliers can reduce the expense of materials, these costs are even more heavily driven by volume than are the salaries of workers.

Selected examples of manageable and unmanageable costs are summarized in Table 30.1. It must be recognized that there are aspects of manageable cost components that are beyond a manager's control. Examples of such "acts of God" are sickness, occupational injury, pregnancy, or military conscription of employees. Although these factors cannot be avoided and often cannot be predicted, the consequences can be managed within the budget that has been

Table 30.1 Manageable and unmanageable cost components

Manageable	Unmanageable
Number of employees	Employee fringe benefits
Skill mix of employees	Legal or institutional limitations on permitted duties of employees
Scheduling and cross-training of employees	Injury, illness, pregnancy, and military duty
Competitive bidding and selection of cost-effective materials	Volume requirements for materials
Direct costs of operation	Indirect costs assessed by institutional management

approved. A forward-looking organization will make provisions for such exigencies in the budget process.

Strong leadership is essential at all levels of the organization if costs are to be kept in line with institutional plans and goals (6). The many theories and practical approaches that are useful for good management have been covered in other sections of this book and in a variety of excellent books on management (1, 8, 10, 11). In this chapter we will attempt to address some practical issues that face the manager on the front lines. There is no "correct" way to deal with the problems that come up in daily life, so this discussion will reflect our prejudices and experiences.

A frontline manager must function within the rules established by the organization. The first and most important task, therefore, is to review thoroughly the personnel policies and procedures of your organization. In addition, it is critical to understand the written and unwritten culture both of the organization as a whole and of the smaller unit to which you belong, presumably the laboratory or one of its subunits. Most rules and regulations are open to interpretation. A manager must understand that flexibility in interpretation of the rules is part of the job. Understanding the culture of the organization, however, will help avoid going out on a poorly supported limb, only to find out there is nobody behind to extend a helping hand.

At the start of a new job it is useful to look around and identify those managers who appear to have mastered the system. They will serve as invaluable aids until you gain enough experience to become a resource for other subsequent neophytes.

Even an experienced manager must maintain regular contact with superiors. There should be a sixth sense about the possibility of trouble, depending on the nature of the problem and the nature of the employee(s) involved. Areas that are controversial, such as repetitive stress injuries, and employees who are considered difficult or potentially litigious should elicit early rather than late discussions with superiors. When a recurrent problem is moving towards a final confrontation, it is absolutely essential that both superiors and institutional contacts in human resources be involved. The most valuable manager

is the one who takes the initiative in dealing with problems without burdening superiors unnecessarily, yet keeps upper-level managers in touch with what is going on.

Constraints on Managerial Function

The first potential constraint on a manager is implied in the introduction. If upper-level leaders lack vision, steadfastness, and consistency, it may become extremely difficult or even impossible for subordinates to do their jobs (2, 5). The higher up the organization the problem extends, the greater the odds against correcting the problem quickly. The manager in this situation has only two options: to do the best with the tools available and/or to look for a position in another organization.

The presence or absence of a unionized workforce will dramatically affect the way a manager interacts with workers. Depending on the quality of labor-management relationships, a unionized workforce is not necessarily a constraint on managerial function. The challenges are often substantial with or without a union representative, but the rules may be very different in the two situations, and the manager must constantly keep the specifics of the union contract in mind. We have never worked with a unionized workforce, so we have no personal experience from which to draw. We do suspect, however, that the talented manager will be successful in either situation and that the marginal manager will struggle in each.

Finally, there may be significant constraints placed on a manager by the past history and culture of the unit and perhaps by the capabilities of the employees. In this case, however, the appropriate way to view the situation is as a challenge rather than a constraint. Given support from above, a capable manager should be able to work through any difficulties that may detract from optimal function of the unit (Table 30.2).

The Cardinal Rules for Optimizing Performance

In very simple and straightforward terms, following the biblical golden rule by all concerned is the surest way to motivate employees. A manager must ask whether subordinates are being treated the same way he/she wants to be treated by superiors. Among the employees, it is obviously in everyone's best interest if cooperative activity is the order of the day.

Table 30.2 Constraints on unit managers

Quality of upper-level management
Adequacy of financial and accounting support
Adequacy of human resource support
Quality of work force available
Unionized workforce
Past practices (culture) of the unit

Get It Right at the Outset

A manager will be presented with a group of employees who were selected by previous incumbents. Unless the workforce is totally ossified, however, there will be turnover. When that happens, the new manager has an opportunity to influence the tone of the laboratory unit. Technical competence is obviously an important consideration in a production worker, and a certain base level of ability is essential. From years of experience, however, we are convinced that an indefinable characteristic called "attitude" is even more important. The team player who hits singles consistently and furthers the position of the organization will, in the long run, be far more valuable than the flashy home run hitter who denigrates fellow workers. Often that slugger is, in reality, not so competent as the hyped self-image would make one think. One of the most difficult managerial decisions is to defer hiring the ready applicant if the right candidate is not immediately available. In the long run, however, it pays to wait. The challenge is to convince coworkers of the need to continue the search. If a mistake is made in the initial hiring decision, it is critical to recognize the problem during the evaluation or trial phase that is used by many organizations. A divorce is always easiest when the partners have not been married very long.

Expect Cooperative Behavior and Best Possible Performance

If the expectations are clear, it will be impossible for anyone to plead ignorance (7). Most people respond to high expectations. If nothing else, expecting less is likely to produce less. Expecting the best may not be easy for the manager. It is entirely too easy to make value judgments about individuals and expect only those things that are implicit in the assumption. Moving beyond initial prejudices, however, is an early step to success.

Lead by Example

Employees will adopt the outlook and habits of their manager, just as children emulate their parents. If workers are expected to pitch in and work collaboratively to get the work done, they must see their supervisor doing the same thing. It is important to remember, however, that good habits do not come equally easily to everyone. Some will take more encouragement and coaching than others (3).

Involve All the Members of the Team

Most work groups consist of individuals with differing backgrounds and talents. It will not be possible for everyone to pitch in on every project or in every way. There should be an opportunity, however, for all to contribute their abilities to make the unit function optimally. Even those individuals who find it most difficult to excel should be challenged. If any employee is not given the opportunity to do his best, there is a risk that the individual will feel undervalued or inferior and that colleagues will feel

they have a shirker in their midst. The reluctant or recalcitrant employee will require special attention and a firm, but gentle insistence on participation. On the other side, any employee who feels they are being taken advantage of will require gentle counseling to see that, in fact, everyone is pulling an appropriate load (3).

Perceived Fairness More Important than Rigid Equality

It is impossible to interact with each individual in the same way all the time. Circumstances change and individuals vary in their needs. Judgment is essential when applying rules and regulations to a specific situation. The essence of leadership is making everyone feel valued and a part of the process (13).

Maintain Communication in All Directions

It is extremely important that subordinates feel comfortable talking to each other and to their supervisor. The best way to prevent rumor and innuendo is to avoid secrets by facilitating open discussion. Most importantly, free interchange of ideas and concerns is the best way to quash the development of cliques, the most destructive phenomenon in any group. If a topic cannot be discussed because of institutional strategy or employee confidentiality, it may be possible to indicate that there are constraints, but that full information will be made available at the first opportunity. Managers and supervisors should be seen regularly out in the open, mingling with staff, not tucked away in their offices.

Communication naturally should proceed in multiple directions. It is just as essential that the lines of communication upward be free and clear as that lateral and descending channels be protected.

Keep Your Eyes and Ears Open

The recommendation to keep your eyes and ears open is a companion to the one above. The best way to detect short circuits in the communication network is to observe and listen closely in the course of going about the normal routine of daily business. Body language is as important as speech as clues to incipient problems.

Act Quickly and Decisively

The best way to turn a brewing crisis into one that has boiled over the top of the pot is to ignore it. Action need not be manifested by confrontation. On occasion, judicious temporizing may reduce the heat sufficiently to abort the overflow, but unless the basic problem is addressed a recurrence is guaranteed.

When Problems Surface, Involve Laboratory Manager Immediately

As discussed above, the art of management includes knowing when to involve superiors in a problem. Alerting upper-level management to a potential difficulty does not necessitate their involvement. In fact, the better the interaction, the more likely a manager will be left alone to solve the problem.

Involve Human Resources if Appropriate

If a problem has progressed to a final stage, everyone will be best served if the human resource department knows of the potential for confrontation in advance. Where personnel actions are possible, countermeasures, including legal challenges, are also possible.

A summary of the cardinal rules of personnel management and potential consequences of breaking them is given in Table 30.3.

Classic Situations that May Interfere with Optimal Performance

Some classic personnel situations are described in Table 30.4.

The Underperforming Employee

The first challenge in dealing with an underperformer is to understand why the employee is not reaching potential. If it is a lack of confidence, counseling should be directed at boosting self-esteem. Encouraging involvement in a special project may be a useful tack. If the problem is bore-

Table 30.3 The cardinal rules and possible consequences

Cardinal rule	Potential consequences
Get it right at the hiring stage	An underperforming employee or troublemaker who will consume managerial resources
Expect cooperative behavior	Employees who are not so inclined will not feel constrained to modify behavior
Lead by example	"If gold ruste, what shal iren do"—Geoffrey Chaucer describing the Parson in *The Canterbury Tales*
Team involvement	A solution that is perceived as imposed may be less readily accepted.
Perception of fairness	A decision with unpleasant consequences will be better received if perceived as fair.
Open communication	Without communication, problems will arise and proliferate.
Eyes and ears open	Brewing problems may boil over if not recognized early.
Act quickly and decisively	Matters are likely to deteriorate if not addressed forthrightly.
Involve superiors	Support in a difficult situation will be more difficult if your superior is not prepared.
Involve institutional human resources	A problem that escalates will be more difficult to manage if your support system is not activated early.

Table 30.4 Classic personnel situations

Situation	Necessary action
The underperforming employee	Identify the reason for the failure to reach potential and tailor counseling accordingly.
The overperforming employee	Channel energy in productive ways. Watch for the potential consequences of performance at a level above pay grade.
The underground troublemaker	Attempt to convert the employee to productive behavior. If unsuccessful, attempt to isolate the troublemaker.
The cabal	The single troublemaker magnified. Break up the clique if possible by reassignment or introduction of others into the group.
Weakness at the top	Same approaches as for lower level personnel but with more urgency

dom, once again an additional challenge may be useful. If, on the other hand, the employee has tired of the job or was never truly committed, the direction of counseling may be towards an honest and critical evaluation of career opportunities and challenges. In any event, thorough documentation must be kept throughout the period of evaluation.

The Overperforming Employee

It may seem strange to consider an overperforming employee a problem. In most situations, of course, the response should be to encourage the star to attempt ever greater feats. However, when the employee is capable of work beyond that defined in the job description, or is limited by official rules based on paper qualifications (degrees and/or licensure), a difficult conundrum arises. Should the employee be limited strictly to the tasks defined in the job description? That course may well result in a bored and frustrated employee who will seek a job that is more challenging. The other option is to allow the employee to advance to the limits of intellectual ability rather than bureaucratic guidelines. The result may be an employee who is enriched cerebrally by the expanded experience, but not monetarily due to the salary restrictions of the job description. It is an exceptional individual who does not eventually resent colleagues who do the same tasks, perhaps less well, for significantly higher pay. The decision as to which road should be taken must be guided by the rigidity of institutional or union rules and by frank and open discussion with the employee. Those discussions should not be one-time only, but should continue to assure that resentment does not arise.

The Intrusion of Personal Issues

One of the potential causes of friction in the workplace is carryover from previous experience, either on the job or outside. If a manager senses that personal antipathy may be at the root of a problem, or if that information is volunteered, the response should be the same. The only acceptable behavior in the workplace is collegial or at least tolerant. Past personal experiences must be parked at the door each day. Rarely, the problem is more remote, the result of a perceived similarity of a coworker to someone with whom the employee had had a previous negative interaction. If it is possible to separate the parties physically, lack of interaction may solve the problem. Should separation not be possible, transfer or resignation may be the only alternative for an employee who cannot exert self-control.

The Underground Troublemaker

A very difficult problem is the employee who stirs up trouble surreptitiously—outside of work, on breaks, or in the hallway. Usually the promotion of cliques is the tactic chosen. It is a recalcitrant problem because it is underground and the fomenter will usually deny such activities. The only recourse of the manager is to counsel the disruptive employee and deal with the problems that arise. If the employee cannot be induced to join the team, the only option is an isolation strategy. With patience and care, eventually other employees will see what is going on. It is particularly important not to make the troublemaker a martyr, so the counseling must be done so as not to appear punitive, to the extent possible (12).

The Cabal

A particularly virulent version of the underground troublemaker is the cloned version. A small group of workers, acting in concert, can make life miserable for fellow workers, for superiors, and for those in lower personnel classifications. In addition to the actions recommended for the individual troublemaker, there are a couple of other possibilities for the cabal. If it is possible to separate the group, either spatially or temporally, the problem may be alleviated. An attempt should be made to isolate any obvious leader(s). Alternatively, it may be possible to introduce a new actor into the play, someone who is equal in stature to the members of the cabal but has the proper outlook.

Weakness at the Top

Personnel problems can occur at any level in the organization. The higher up the problem is, the more difficult it is to pinpoint the issue. It may take considerable effort and persistence to determine that the problem is with a supervisor or assistant supervisor, rather than with the lower-level employees. The symptoms may well be manifest at a level below that of the person who is truly responsible. It is often difficult to deal with problems in managers. For a start, it is important to keep an open mind as to where the difficulty lies because the cure is dependent on correct diagnosis of the dysfunction.

Practical Issues in Utilization of Personnel Resources

There are relatively few means available to a manager for optimizing the workforce of a unit. The success of these means will depend to a significant extent on the efficacy of the management approaches described above (Table 30.5) (4).

Skill Mix of Personnel

It is important to examine on a regular basis the skills required for accomplishment of the goals set for the unit. At the least, the question should be raised each time there is a new vacancy. Hiring incompletely trained or educated workers for complex tests is false economy (although the intrinsic intelligence of the individual may be as important or more important than the credentials). Conversely, it is not good stewardship to use overqualified individuals. Some simple testing may be assigned to technicians, who, along with laboratory assistants, can perform other support functions, such as maintenance and accessioning of specimens (9).

Cross-Training and Rotation

Some degree of cross-training (or competence in multiple areas) and rotation through multiple areas is necessary in most laboratories to assure constant coverage with competent workers. The breadth of coverage of an individual worker depends on the depth of experience and knowledge required for the tests. Workers in a small laboratory in a rural hospital may need to perform many simple tests in a variety of scientific disciplines, whereas a technologist working in a large university hospital will probably be responsible for a restricted number of very sophisticated procedures. Even in a large unit, cross-training within the unit is important. The important goal is to strike a balance between what is needed to get the work done, the needs of employees, and the ability for each worker to perform a sufficient number of procedures to maintain proficiency.

Table 30.5 Practical approaches to optimization

Parameter	Approach
Skill mix	To the greatest extent possible consistent with good practice, utilize lesser trained individuals for more routine or menial duties.
Cross-training and rotation	Give employees the stimulation of multiple tasks or areas, being careful not to stretch them too thin.
Scheduling	Make clear what is needed to do the job. To the extent possible, allow employees to work out the details among themselves.
Use of overtime	Within the constraints of the budget, allow overtime if required to get the job done but always look for other options.

Coverage of Vacations, Holidays, and Routine Shifts

In some instances institutional policies or contractual obligations will determine the rules of coverage for vacations, holidays, and routine shifts. Often, however, the procedure is undefined and will vary with each unit. Consistent with the cardinal rules, a manager might adopt the following policy.

1. Define the minimum personnel requirements for each type of work situation, e.g., weekday, weekend, holiday.
2. Define positions so as to provide the most flexible coverage. When a new position opens, give the existing workers a chance to review their schedules. If a worker wants to increase or decrease hours or to change the distribution of work among the daily time periods that must be covered, attempt to balance the request with the needs of the department, but make it clear that all requests may not be possible. Getting the work accomplished well and expeditiously is the first priority.
3. Entrust development of the schedule to the involved workers, preferably with a single individual as coordinator. That individual may be an assistant manager or senior technologist, but should not be the unit manager. It is important that the coordinator have the support of the group as a whole.
4. Solicit requests for vacation time well in advance (as much as 6 months). Make clear that it may not be possible to grant everyone his or her first choice. Try to even out assignment of priority vacation times over a period of years. It may be necessary for the group to make a decision as to whether they will pitch in and work harder during the vacation months to allow everyone to have desired time off. Getting the work done must be the first priority for all concerned.
5. Publish the work schedule far enough ahead for people to make plans (at least 1 month).
6. When holes appear in the schedule, ask for volunteers to fill in. Encourage switching of shifts or use of part-time workers with overtime as a last resort. It should be clear that the possibility of assigning the slot to a nonvolunteer lurks in the background, but avoid resorting to that tactic if at all possible.

Use of Overtime

The objective of every manager should be to get the work done in the most efficient manner with the least expenditure of financial resources necessary. On occasion it may be necessary to use overtime to complete necessary work. When possible, however, an attempt should be made, within the rules of the institution and the government, to use any other methods available, such as compensatory time.

Conversely, there may be occasions when work has been completed expeditiously, leaving free time at the end of the shift. It is useful to have a plan for such occasions. There are usually odds and ends of maintenance, writing of procedures, etc., that could be completed at these times. Another option is to offer the possibility of early departure, leaving the residual time for use on another occasion as regular time.

Summary

Unit managers can make important contributions to the success of an organization by exerting careful control over manageable components. Although economies can be realized in both materials and personnel, the optimization of personnel resources will present the greatest challenge and the greatest opportunity for a manager. To accomplish this goal there is a series of mainly commonsense rules. The savvy manager must recognize some classic personnel challenges, including overperforming and underperforming employees and individuals who work at cross-purposes to the goals of the team. Specific areas where financial economies may be accomplished include careful scheduling, cross-training and/or rotation, and judicious utilization of employees with varying backgrounds and skills.

KEY POINTS

- Provide compassionate, interactive leadership so that employees will understand the goals of the unit as well as the challenges and barriers to achieving those goals.
- Involve all employees in the process so that they feel a part of the solutions that you discover jointly.
- Acknowledge the constraints under which the unit operates and accommodate plans accordingly.
- Recognize at an early stage problems in performance that will interfere with achievement of goals, and take appropriate action.
- Identify the practical issues that will allow employees to use their time most efficiently and get the job done with a minimum of disruption.

GLOSSARY

Cabal A group of people working secretly and underhandedly to overthrow a regime. An acronym for a group of ministers chosen by Charles II of England in 1667: Clifford, Arlington, Buckingham (of *Three Musketeers* fame), Ashley Cooper (later Earl of Shaftesbury), and Lauderdale.

Constraints Factors that limit the flexibility of action.

Cross-training Training of individuals to perform more than one task.

Manageable components A parameter over which a manager has control. Scheduling and use of overtime are manageable. Vacation time and work breaks are defined by government or the institution and are thus not manageable (although the number of employees eligible for these benefits may be).

Rotation Movement of personnel through the tasks for which they have been trained, often on a regular, sequential basis.

Skill mix The variable backgrounds of personnel all of whom will contribute to the operation. The nature of the work will define the required proportion of workers of each background.

REFERENCES

1. **Baron, R. A.** 1986. *Behavior in Organizations. Understanding and Managing the Human Side of Work,* 2nd ed. Allyn and Bacon, Inc., Boston, Mass.

2. **Kanter, R. M.** 1992. Power failure in management circuits, p. 449–461. *In* J. M. Shafritz and J. S. Ott (ed.), *Classics of Organization Theory.* Brooks/Cole Publishing Company, Pacific Grove, Calif.

3. **Kotter, J. P.** 1990. What leaders really do. *Harvard Business Rev.* **May-June:**103–111.

4. **Martin, B. G.** 1985. Cost containment: strategies and responsibilities of the laboratory manager. *Clin. Lab. Med.* **5:**697–707.

5. **Mechanic, D.** 1992. Sources of power of lower participants in complex organizations, p. 424–431. *In* J. M. Shafritz, J. S. Ott, (ed.), *Classics of Organization Theory.* Brooks/Cole Publishing Company, Pacific Grove, Calif.

6. **Rodgers, T. J.** 1990. No excuses management. *Harvard Business Rev.* **July-August:**84–98.

7. **Schaffer, R. H.** 1991. Demand better results–and get them. *Harvard Business Rev.* **March-April:**142–149.

8. **Schuler, R. S., and S. E. Jackson.** 1996. *Human Resource Management. Positioning for the 21st Century,* 6th ed. West Publishing Company, Minneapolis/St. Paul, Minn.

9. **Snyder, J. R.** 1992. Technician or technologist? sorting out overlapping roles in the lab. *Med. Lab. Observ.* **June:**36–41.

10. **Snyder, J. R., and D. A. Senhauser.** 1989. *Administration and Supervision in Laboratory Medicine,* 2nd ed. J.B. Lippincott Company, Philadelphia, Pa.

11. **Szilagyi, A. D., Jr., and M. J. Wallace, Jr.** 1990. *Organizational Behavior and Performance,* 5th ed. Scott, Foresman/Little Brown Higher Education, Glenview, Ill.

12. **Umiker, W. O.** 1991. Turning around the behavior of uncooperative employees. *Med. Lab. Observ.* **October:**59–66.

13. **Umiker, W. O.** 1992. How to qualify as a praise master. *Med. Lab. Observ.* **July:**41–46.

APPENDIX 30.1   Operational Costs for a Hypothetical Hospital Laboratory

	OP LAB	MICRO	IMMUNO	CYTO	HEMA	CHEM	CGEN
Expenses							
1 6000089 NON PRODUCTIVE REG SAL	13575.59	123638	30086.09	91611.04	95316.26	153612.6	24795.79
2							
3 6000090 PRODUCTIVE REG SAL	107872.17	761781.9	257916.1	724866.6	705635.5	1107954	174039.6
4 6000093 STAFF SAL COST RECOVERY							
5 6000104 PRODUCTIVE OT SAL	305.27	3196.43	4581.07	50.89	15265.43	18533.98	1811.64
6 Staff Salaries	121753.03	888616.4	292583.3	816528.5	816217.2	1280101	200647
7 6000101 EMPLOYEE APPRECIATION	127.98	770		525	907.82	200	
8 Other Personnel Expense	127.98	770		525	907.82	200	
9 Salaries	121881.01	889386.4	292583.3	817053.5	817125	1280301	200647
10 6030102 ALLOCATED FRINGE - STAFF	31485.31	229796.2	75662.03	211154.3	211073.8	330889.6	51887.34
11 Allocated Fringe Benefits	31485.31	229796.2	75662.03	211154.3	211073.8	330889.6	51887.34
12							
13 6030165 FRINGE COST RECOVERY							
14 General Fringe Benefits							
15 Payroll Tax & Fringe	31485.31	229796.2	75662.03	211154.3	211073.8	330889.6	51887.34
16 Salaries & Fringe Benefits	153366.32	1119183	368245.3	1028208	1028199	1611191	252534.3
17							
18 6300310 MEDICAL SURGICAL	492.52	1704.07	1232.37	996.34	2516.87	4411.72	848.76
19 6300320 LAB SUPPLIES	9303.09	576924.1	404501.9	315576.3	339253.8	1814630	30315.87
20 6300337 PACKAGING SUPPLIES							
21 6300340 OXYGEN		2549.56				360	173.16
22 6300370 SUTURES							
23 6300380 INSTRUMENTS AND NEEDLES		349.79					72.12
24 Med/Surg Supplies	9795.61	581527.5	405734.3	316572.6	341770.7	1819401	31409.91
25							
26 6320320 PHARMACEUTICALS	20.19	30.59	84.6		376.77		
27 6320330 DRUGS - IV SOLUTIONS							
28 6320331 BLOOD SERVICES							
29 6320336 IV-IRRIGATING SOLUTIONS	17.63	42.44				10.61	
30 Pharmaceuticals	37.82	73.03	84.6		376.77	10.61	
31							
32 6340510 FOOD SUPPLY					14.63		
33 Nutrition Supplies					14.63		
34							
35 6660410 OFFICE SUPPLIES	997.49	1142.28	376.89	618.41	627.79	1395.69	369.18
36 6660420 SUPPLIES OFFICE-PRINTED	289.87	2376.22	52	48	2426.98	−481.24	
37 6660490 SUPPLIES OFFICE-GENERAL	44.58	466.67	60.61	333.28		13.81	
38 6662470 CHINA GLASS AND FLATWARE							
39 Supplies Other	1331.94	3985.17	489.5	999.69	3054.77	928.26	369.18
40							
41 6600710 TELEPHONE							
42 6600770 MAIL & PRODUCTION		534.44	480.24	219.95	257.54	269.75	0.63
43 Utilities		534.44	480.24	219.95	257.54	269.75	0.63
44							
45 6663810 BOOKS/SUBS/DUES NONMD		455.8		9936.7	107.41	517.46	75
46 6663830 TRAVEL/MEET/DUES-GENERAL	272	463.59	1651.97	14991.38	1014.35	2520.33	862.52
47 6664880 FREIGHT CHARGES			51.36	144.96	7.22		
48 6665910 MAINTENANCE-CONTRACT	345		15248.13	11319.61	54183.56	28264.9	17863.27

Spreadsheet detailing operational costs for a hypothetical hospital laboratory. Indirect costs assessed by the institution for support of other departments (housekeeping, cafeteria, security, etc.) are not included. Some items are composed of both manageable and unmanageable components. For instance, fringe benefits and, to a large extent, unproductive time, are determined by the institution as a matter of policy but are also affected by the levels of staffing achieved by the manager (row 14). Supply costs (row 67) are determined by the vol-

APPENDIX 30.1   Operational Costs for a Hypothetical Hospital Laboratory *(continued)*

BB	NIGHTS	HISTO	AUTOPSY	CUSTOMER SERVICE	MANAGEMENT	ADMIN SUPPORT	SPECIMEN ACCESSION
57440.8	33441.37	84119.52	5740.41	73610.14	31795.47	24169.47	124167.95
436089.6	284039.9	663721	65880.1	592448.8	265803.9	177384	1226795.59
		-7689.84					-4035
8408.45	6700.22	18429.32	2927.79	20125.28	463.44	739.98	35618.18
501938.8	324181.5	758580	74548.3	686184.22	298062.81	202293.4	1382546.72
125	50	50		1225		150	2833.78
125	50	50		1225		150	2833.78
502063.8	324231.5	758630	74548.3	687409.22	298062.81	202443.4	1385380.5
129801.4	83833.32	198157.4	19278.17	177447.23	77079.04	52313.08	358570.06
129801.4	83833.32	198157.4	19278.17	177447.23	77079.04	52313.08	358570.06
		−1922.4					
		−1922.4					
129801.4	83833.32	196235	19278.17	177447.23	77079.04	52313.08	358570.06
631865.2	408064.8	954864.9	93826.47	864856.45	375141.85	254756.5	1743950.56
31751.08		47933	9212.7			1312.97	739.14
96331.27	582.23	279392.6	6073.04				2255.07
							1843.6
5228.52							
		140.92					
		3810.34	843.57				
133310.9	582.23	331276.8	16129.31			1312.97	4837.81
32277.11		50.9					16.66
64.4							
3106854							
1612.73		3566.04					
3140808		3616.94					16.66
	833.08				27.55	0.92	5.52
	833.08				27.55	0.92	5.52
17.85		314.21	353.12	2363.73	−243.01	66630.27	4549.26
8673.91		710.72	−21.51	74851.56		64747.81	−1065.11
2.44		2998.34	731.75	2.12	41.75	86.14	1931.47
8694.2		4023.27	1063.36	77217.41	−201.26	131464.2	5415.62
				5043.03	1078.64		249.07
23.29		144.29		4752.77	177.9	17852.26	937.61
23.29		144.29		9795.8	1256.54	17852.26	1186.68
1241.13		428.36		418.16	12455.14		254.03
1705.89		2813.73		6470.12	10022.58		1919.47
7.22				237576.97	56.13	7053.03	−77.25
4495.04		21872.99				23922.44	

ume of testing, which is beyond the control of a unit manager, but are also affected by the acumen that the manager brings to the selection of brands and negotiation of contracts. Note the wide variation by department in the proportion of the total operating costs that are represented by salary and fringe benefits (row 69). Much of this variation is easily understood. The very low percentage (16%) in the blood bank is a reflection of the very high (and ever-increasing) cost of purchased blood components. Some seemingly anomalous values,

APPENDIX 30.1 Operational Costs for a Hypothetical Hospital Laboratory *(continued)*

		OP LAB	MICRO	IMMUNO	CYTO	HEMA	CHEM	CGEN
	Expenses							
49	6665911 UVM MAINT/REPAIR OFFICE							
50	6665920 MAINTENANCE-NONCONTRACT	39	2749	364.6	6143.77	2953.31	8433.39	2472.8
51	6666930 MEDICAL EQUIPMENT							
52	6666940 NON-MEDICAL EQUIPMENT							
53	6666946 RENT - BUILDING							
54	6669603 CAFETERIA		202.9		693.69	296.75		45
55	6669606 CELEBRATION FUNDS		382.43	59.25	248.24	275.28	281	81.25
56	6669611 PROFESSIONAL DEVELOP NON		265	425	13167	2324	3289	490
57	6669612 PROF DEV MD							
58	6669616 SMALL EQUIPMENT	42	561.32		1420.46	1943.28	1997.43	479
59	6669715 INSPECTION & SURVEY							
60	6669890 GENERAL OTHER					43.05		
61	Other Expenses	698	5080.04	17800.31	58065.81	63148.21	45303.51	22368.84
62								
63	Salaries & Fringe Benefits	153366.32	1119183	368245.3	1028208	1028199	1611191	252534.3
64	Total Non-Salary Expense	11867.37	591200.2	424588.9	376503.2	408622.6	1906743	54148.56
65	Total Expense	165233.69	1710383	792834.2	1404711	1436821	3517934	306682.9
66	% Total Expense Represented by Salary	93	65	46	73	72	46	82
67								
68	Staffing FTEs							
69	Productive-Regular FTEs	3.50999	16.93094	5.609384	15.97089	15.55726	25.05952	3.754425
70	Productive-Overtime FTEs	0.006543	0.051802	0.072023	0.001596	0.228296	0.293781	0.025841
71	Non-Productive FTEs	0.418664	2.804622	0.676676	2.107071	2.158297	3.571413	0.545735
72	Total FTEs	3.944092	19.80035	6.438611	18.32687	18.09794	29.07904	4.329848
73								
74	Productivity Labor Hours							
75	Productive-Regular Hours	7300.85	35216.7	11667.63	33219.76	32359.42	52124.31	7809.28
76	Productive-Overtime Hours	13.61	107.75	149.81	3.32	474.86	611.07	53.75
77	Non-Productive Hours	870.83	5833.67	1407.5	4382.75	4489.3	7428.61	1135.14
78	Total Hours	8203.79	41185.12	13392.4	38120.25	37644.08	60484.99	9006.17

such as the relatively low value for administrative support (58%), are artifacts of the assignment of a large maintenance contract to that division. The low percentage in the highly automated chemistry laboratory (46%) is a reflection of the high cost of reagents and instruments and the relatively few technologists required to operate that equipment. Divisions that do little actual testing or use few supplies

APPENDIX 30.1 Operational Costs for a Hypothetical Hospital Laboratory *(continued)*

BB	NIGHTS	HISTO	AUTOPSY	CUSTOMER SERVICE	MANAGEMENT	ADMIN SUPPORT	SPECIMEN ACCESSION
795.5		2672.5		88.31			
		18121					
348					114.1		
					92		
		315		92.02	1744.24	261.85	5.2
123.39		252.06	14	342.27	8072.85		289.28
510	145	3197		2434	4923.45	150	1199
					75		
150		6750.41		4678.2	3520.15	941.99	1010.73
					82889.89		
9376.17	145	56423.05	14	252100.05	123965.53	32329.31	4600.46
631865.2	408064.8	954864.9	93826.47	864856.45	375141.85	254756.5	1743950.56
3292213	727.23	427841	18706.67	347303.64	127137.15	182959.7	1162299.86
3924078	408792.1	1382706	112533.1	1212160.09	502279	437716.2	2906250.42
16	100	69	83	71	75	58	60
9.954823	5.011668	15.96944	1.938246	17.342612	3.863934	5.941154	49.599201
0.130773	0.097893	0.313276	0.06586	0.491793	0.011779	0.015981	0.957457
1.373799	0.696099	2.004755	0.215681	2.211859	0.483779	0.827843	5.076326
11.51179	5.822968	18.38805	2.219786	20.171744	4.436414	6.835458	55.856348
20706.23	10424.37	33216.75	4031.59	36072.98	8037.06	12357.72	103167.33
272.01	203.62	651.62	136.99	1022.94	24.5	33.24	1991.53
2857.53	1447.9	4169.93	448.62	4600.71	1006.27	1721.93	10558.86
23944.76	12111.89	38247.51	4617.2	41957.63	9227.83	14217.89	116182.32

have high personnel costs, e.g., the outpatient laboratory, specimen accession, customer service, and the autopsy service. Similarly, divisions in which the testing is more frequently manual have relatively high personnel costs, e.g., microbiology, cytology, and cytogenetics. The percentage of operation budget represented by personnel costs in the microbiology division is 65%.

APPENDIX 30.2 Budgetary Effects of Use of Overtime in Three Hypothetical Laboratories with Different Mixes of Staff

	FTE	Full Time Workers	Part Time Workers	Full Time Hours	Part Time Hours	Hours Worked	Scheduled Salary Cost ($)	Additional Regular Hours Available	Additional Hours Required	Additional Regular Hours Used	Additional Overtime Hours Used	Additional Regular Salary Cost ($)	Additional Overtime Salary Cost ($)	Total Salary Cost ($)
Lab A Base	20	20	0	1600	0	1600	32000	0	0	0	0	0	0	32000
Lab B Base	20	19	2	1520	80	1600	32000	80	0	0	0	0	0	32000
Lab C Base	20	15	10	1200	400	1600	32000	400	0	0	0	0	0	32000
Lab A Expanded	20	20	0	1600	0	1600	32000	0	120	0	120	0	3600	35600
Lab B Expanded	20	19	2	1520	80	1600	32000	80	120	80	40	1600	1200	34800
Lab C Expanded	20	15	10	1200	400	1600	32000	400	120	120	0	2400	0	34400
Lab A Catastrophic	20	20	0	1600	0	1600	32000	0	400	0	400	0	12000	44000
Lab B Catastrophic	20	19	2	1520	80	1600	32000	80	400	80	320	1600	9600	43200
Lab C Catastrophic	20	15	10	1200	400	1600	32000	400	400	400	0	8000	0	40000

Base Salary = $20/hr.
Overtime Salary = $30/hr.
Pay Period = 80 Hours

Budgetary effects of the need to use overtime in three hypothetical laboratories with differing mixes of full-time and part-time personnel. Lab A is staffed entirely by full-time workers. Lab B has two half-time workers. The full-time equivalents in Lab C are a mix of 75% full-time workers and 25% half-time workers. For normal operation, the salary costs of all three laboratories are the same. When unexpected factors (e.g., additional workload, unexpected illness, pregnancy, disability, etc.) require additional work, the expenses are highest in Lab A and least in Lab C, which has the greatest number of part-time workers available to work at regular pay. When catastrophic conditions prevail, the differences are even more pronounced. This hypothetical example assumes, of course, that some or all of the part-time workers are willing and/or able to work additional hours. Other factors that must be considered when selecting full- and part-time staff include possible detrimental effects of having too many individuals whose expertise is diminished by part-time employment.

31

Costs, Budgeting, and Financial Decision Making

Geoffrey C. Tolzmann and Richard J. Vincent

OBJECTIVES

To learn the types and behaviors of costs, how to measure them, what data are needed to generate a cost analysis, and how to cost a basic laboratory test

To understand the relationships among cost, volume, and profits; calculate contribution margin and break-even point

To apply time value of money concepts to capital acquisition plans using net present value

To understand the three common types of budgets, the budgeting process, and how budgets are used to measure financial performance and to control costs

To be able to analyze the causes of differences in actual financial performance from budgeted amounts and understand how this information is used for management control

To learn about the three primary financial statements: the balance sheet, the income statement, and the cash flow statement

To learn how to calculate key financial ratios that reveal information about an organization's financial health

To understand the basic ways a company raises capital from outside the organization

Accounting is the most useful "information system" for managers, because it organizes and accumulates related information over time and aligns it with initial objectives and requirements, called "budgets." Principles of accounting must be applied to other types of information managers use in order to make "information technology" useful.

PETER F. DRUCKER, AT THE FORBES CEO FORUM
"MANAGEMENT IN THE 21ST CENTURY," JUNE 1997

ALL TOO OFTEN the financial aspects of the laboratory business intimidate managers who have a scientific background. With equal frequency the "bean counters" do not understand the scientific underpinnings of the industry in which they work. The resultant dysfunction at best detracts from the efficient operation of the enterprise and at worst produces devastating results for both the financial and scientific sides of the operation. While it is important to have experts in each field, in the best run businesses, each side understands the principles and therefore the problems of the other. Classically, economics is divided into study of an economy at a global level (macroeconomics) and from a more detailed perspective (microeconomics). It is the microeconomic aspect of a business that will be most relevant to the daily function of departmental, divisional, or unit managers. Every manager must understand and participate in cost accounting and budgeting. In addition, everyone must understand the principles of financial accounting and financial analysis. This chapter will provide an overview of these extensive and complex activities (1–4).

A note on accounting conventions:

- Variances that are "favorable" are depicted unmodified. A favorable variance would be an expense that is less than budgeted or revenue that is greater than budgeted.

- Variances that are "unfavorable" are depicted in parentheses. An unfavorable variance would be an expense that is greater than budgeted or revenue that is less than budgeted.

- Profit is depicted unmodified and in black ink; loss is depicted in parentheses and in red if a colored document is employed.

- "Productive" labor is labor that actually produces a product directly (be it a physical product or an intellectual one).

- "Nonproductive" labor may be necessary for proper functioning of the organization but is not *directly* involved in production of the product. Vacation, conferences, sick time, all management functions, and support activities such as financial analysis and marketing would be examples of nonproductive labor. Note that "nonproductive" is not a pejorative term in accounting lingo. This situation is not to be confused, of course, with the other (sometimes all too frequent) kind of nonproductive labor, which is actually an ineffectual productive labor.

Cost Accounting

Cost accounting is a system of measuring and reporting information about costs. Its purpose is to generate information sufficient for managers to make intelligent decisions. A common challenge of cost accounting systems is balancing the degree of specificity needed with the amount of work required to reach that specificity in light of the decisions to be made. A good system does not require unnecessarily detailed information.

Cost accounting is useful for several purposes:

- Profitability analysis.

- Cost control. Cost accounting helps define the relationship between cost and activity and can help align responsibilities with incurred costs.

- Planning. Cost accounting helps us understand what happens to costs as activity changes.

- Decision making. Cost accounting aids in setting prices, negotiating capitation rates, staffing decisions,

and make versus buy decisions (for example, whether or not to perform a laboratory test in-house or send it to a reference laboratory).

Classification of Costs

Costs can be categorized in many different ways, but the most critical distinction is direct cost versus indirect cost. Direct costs are those costs clearly associated with the item being costed (be it a patient, a service, a department, or an individual assay). In the laboratory, direct costs include testing supplies and reagents, instrument depreciation, maintenance and repairs, and the labor involved in performing testing. Indirect costs are those costs that are not directly associated with the item being costed. The most common types of indirect costs are general laboratory supplies; labor costs associated with supervision, administration, and training; and hospital overhead. The full, or total, cost of an item includes its direct costs and an allocated portion of indirect expenses.

Behavior of Costs

Costs behave in four basic ways depending on their relationship to the relevant range of activity. Variable costs vary in direct proportion to the volume or level of activity, such as reagent cost. Therefore, variable costs are constant per unit of service (UOS), which is the logical measure of work for a given area. Fixed costs, such as rent, are constant regardless of changes in levels of activity. Therefore, fixed costs per UOS change with volume. Semivariable costs have a fixed and a variable cost component. An example is telephone service, for which customers are usually charged a fixed amount per month that may include a specified amount of service above which a per-unit charge is incurred. Step-fixed costs are fixed over a relatively small range of activity and then change to a new fixed level over another relatively small range of activity. Labor costs often exhibit step-fixed behavior, as a certain staffing level supports a range of activity beyond which additional staffing must be added. The behaviors of most costs are fairly intuitive. Figure 31.1 illustrates these behaviors.

Measuring Full Cost

There are four steps to the process of measuring full costs.

1. Identify the responsibility centers into which costs may be appropriately grouped. For a hospital, these areas might be laboratory, radiology, laundry, etc. Within the laboratory, these centers might be chemistry, hematology, microbiology, central receiving, etc. Within chemistry, the centers might be individual analyzers or testing modalities.
2. Trace all revenues and expenses to the responsibility center incurring them.
3. Allocate the costs of supporting responsibility centers to the revenue-producing centers. There are several

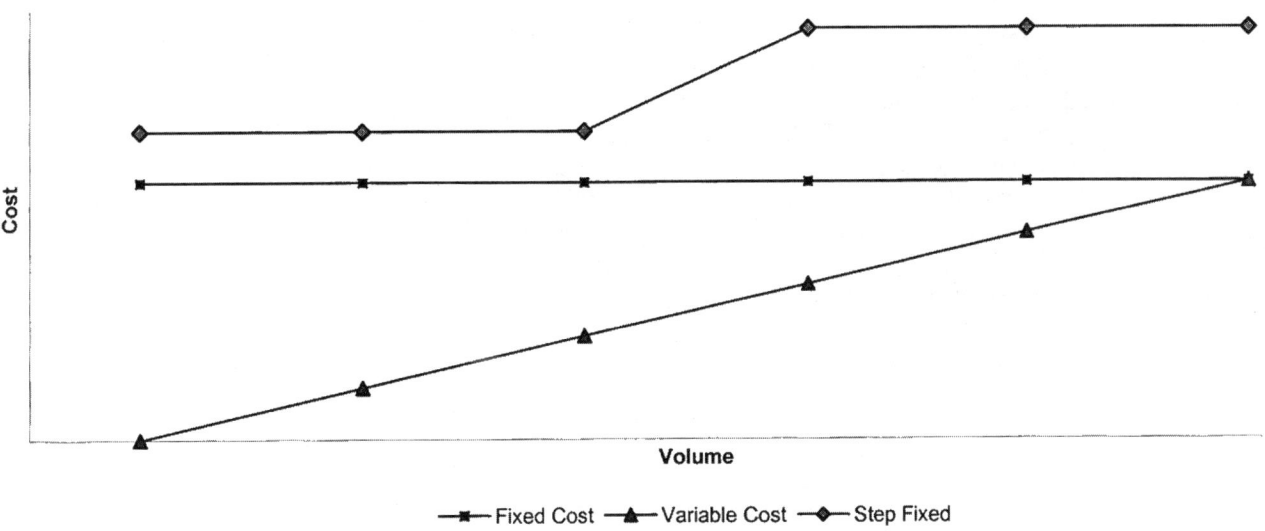

Figure 31.1 Cost behavior.

techniques by which this allocation may be accomplished:

- Direct allocation
- Step-down allocation (which usually entails starting with allocating the costs of centers that provide the most services to all other centers, then allocating the costs of those that provide the next level of service, including those costs that were just allocated in the first round, to all others, etc.)
- Algebraic allocation (used by sophisticated cost accounting systems).

Allocation also requires some sort of basis, such as cause and effect, or facilities provided, or ability to bear the allocated costs. Examples of bases include square footage, utilization, visits, number of personnel, revenues, and payroll expense.

4. Determine the average cost of each procedure or service by dividing the responsibility center's costs by the measure of activity (in the laboratory, the measure is usually the number of procedures or billed tests). The average cost per procedure for the laboratory center might be $10, while the average cost per procedure for the chemistry center might be $5, and the average cost per procedure for a specific analyzer center within chemistry might be $2.

Average versus Marginal Costs

As noted above, the average cost equals the full costs divided by the UOS. Marginal cost equals the change in total cost relative to the change in volume. It is the variable cost plus any additional fixed costs incurred because the volume change exceeds the relevant range. In most instances, there are no additional fixed costs. Marginal costs are also

called incremental costs. Over the long run, average revenues must be greater than or equal to average costs for an organization to survive, but in the short run, decisions should be made based on marginal costs. For example, the incremental cost of adding another sample to a chemistry analyzer that is under capacity is very low. If adding another sample requires the purchase of another analyzer, however, its incremental cost is very high.

Actual Cost versus Standard Cost

Standard costs represent what a given item should cost under normal circumstances. Standard costs are useful for comparison to actual cost experience when analyzing cost variances and for budgeting.

Costing Issues

When performing cost accounting, it is always worthwhile to examine the results and ask: Is it fair? Is it equitable? Is it understandable? Do the benefits justify the effort required to ascertain cost?

A Formula for Developing Laboratory Costs

Direct costs of test (instrument depreciation, maintenance and repair, reagents, calibration, quality controls, direct labor)

+

Indirect costs (general laboratory supplies), indirect labor (such as supervision, training), other indirects (such as research and development expenses)

=

Laboratory section cost

+

General laboratory overhead (specimen collection, report distribution, information systems, management, education, quality assurance, sales, marketing)

=

Laboratory test total cost

Laboratory Costing Examples

Tables 31.1 through 31.6 are examples of the types of information that need to be collected and some of the calculations involved in generating unit costs. Table 31.1 shows the key variables that are needed to generate unit cost, including staff costs that are both variable (tester) and fixed (nontester), plus indirect fixed divisional, overall laboratory, and overall hospital costs.

Table 31.2 is an example of the calculation involved in generating a per-unit cost for a test that is run in a batch with other tests. It is an example of a step-fixed cost.

Should the threshold of 250 tests per run be exceeded, another run would need to be instituted, along with its concomitant expenses. The "step" is the period jump in costs with each new test run, whereas the cost per test progressively decreases within each test run as more samples are added. The most efficient position would be the inclusion of 250 tests in *every* run, the situation in which no further savings could be achieved without increasing the capacity of the run. In Table 31.2, the average number of tests per run was 228, a point that approaches the most economic efficiency possible.

Table 31.1 Key variables for a hematology laboratory with static volume

Position	Type	Average Salary	FTEs	Total Salary Exp	Fringe Expense	Total Salary & Fringe
Lab Specialist	Tester	$ 27,000	1.00	$ 27,000	$ 6,750	$ 33,750
Medical Technologist	Tester	$ 33,500	3.00	$ 100,500	$ 25,125	$ 125,625
Medical Lab Technician	Tester	$ 28,500	1.00	$ 28,500	$ 7,125	$ 35,625
Laboratory Supervisor	Non-Tester	$ 40,500	1.00	$ 40,500	$ 10,125	$ 50,625
Total			6.00	$ 196,500	$ 49,125	$ 245,625

Avg Tester Salary & Fringe Benefit Expense	$ 39,000
Total Non-Tester Salary & Fringe Benefit Expense	$ 50,625

Divisional Indirect Costs	Amount	Cost/Test	
Non-Tester Salary & Fringe	$ 50,625		
Office Supplies	$ 10,000		
Books/Subs/Dues	$ 15,000		
Travel Meeting Dues	$ 15,000		
Total	$ 90,625	$ 0.69	Amount Divided by Total Volume

Lab Indirect Costs	Amount
Management	$ 115,000
Central Receiving	$ 625,000
General Support	$ 100,000
Administrative Support	$ 75,000
Subtotal	$ 915,000

Hospital Indirect Costs (Lab Portion)	Amount
Patient Financial Services	$ 500,000
Human Resources	$ 300,000
Management	$ 100,000
Finance	$ 100,000
Subtotal	$ 1,000,000

Table 31.2 Test run calculation for a hematology laboratory with static volume

Division	Test Description	CPT Code	Total Volume	Test Run Volume	Current Runs/Week	Maximum Tests/Run	Avg Tests per Run	Test Run Minutes	Total Year Salary & Fringe Expense	Total Year Supplies & Reagent Expense	Salary & Fringe Expense per Test	Supplies & Reagents Expense per Test
	Partial Thromboplastin Time	85730	25,973									
	Prothrombin Time	85610	33,318									
HEMATOLOGY	HEMA001 Test Run			59,291	5	250	228	180	$ 14,625		$ 0.25	$0.09

Table 31.3 Cost calulation for a hematology laboratory with static volume

Division	Test Description	CPT Code	Total Volume	Additional Volume	Revised Volume	DIRECT COST — Variable Cost — Test Minutes	Test Salary & Fringe	Test Supplies & Reagents	Step-Fixed Cost — Test Run Sal & Frg	Test Run Supp & Reag	INDIRECT COST — Fixed Cost — Divisional Cost	Lab Cost	Hospital Cost	Variable Cost	Fixed Cost	Total Cost
HEMATOLOGY	Fibrinogen	85384	2,057	-	2,057	5	$ 1.56	$ 1.00	$ -	$ -	$ 0.69	$1.04	$1.14	$ 2.56	$ 2.87	$ 5.43
HEMATOLOGY	Heinz Body Preparation	85441	10	-	10	5	$ 1.56	$ 1.00	$ -	$ -	$ 0.69	$1.04	$1.14	$ 2.56	$ 2.87	$ 5.43
HEMATOLOGY	Hematocrit, Spun	85013	107	-	107	5	$ 1.56	$ 1.00	$ -	$ -	$ 0.69	$1.04	$1.14	$ 2.56	$ 2.87	$ 5.43
HEMATOLOGY	Kleihauer Test	85460	342	-	342	3	$ 0.94	$ 0.50	$ -	$ -	$ 0.69	$1.04	$1.14	$ 1.44	$ 2.87	$ 4.31
HEMATOLOGY	Leukocyte Alkaline Phosphatase	85540	29	-	29	3	$ 0.94	$ 0.50	$ -	$ -	$ 0.69	$1.04	$1.14	$ 1.44	$ 2.87	$ 4.31
HEMATOLOGY	LA Confirm Test	85613	133	-	133	3	$ 0.94	$ 0.50	$ -	$ -	$ 0.69	$1.04	$1.14	$ 1.44	$ 2.87	$ 4.31
HEMATOLOGY	Hemogram	85027	63,600	-	63,600	5	$ 1.56	$ -	$ -	$ -	$ 0.69	$1.04	$1.14	$ 2.06	$ 2.87	$ 4.93
HEMATOLOGY	Partial Thromboplastin Time	85730	25,973	-	25,973	-	$ -	$ 2.00	$ 0.25	$ 0.09	$ 0.69	$1.04	$1.14	$ -	$ 3.21	$ 3.21
HEMATOLOGY	Platelet Aggregation	85576	17	-	17	10	$ 3.13	$ -	$ -	$ -	$ 0.69	$1.04	$1.14	$ 5.13	$ 2.87	$ 7.99
HEMATOLOGY	Prothrombin Time	85610	33,318	-	33,318	-	$ -	$ 2.00	$ 0.25	$ 0.09	$ 0.69	$1.04	$1.14	$ -	$ 3.21	$ 3.21
HEMATOLOGY	Protein C, Functional	85303	181	-	181	10	$ 3.13	$ 2.00	$ -	$ -	$ 0.69	$1.04	$1.14	$ 5.13	$ 2.87	$ 7.99
HEMATOLOGY	Protein S, Functional	85306	175	-	175	10	$ 3.13	$ 2.00	$ -	$ -	$ 0.69	$1.04	$1.14	$ 5.13	$ 2.87	$ 7.99
HEMATOLOGY	Sed. Rate, Westergren	85652	5,527	-	5,527	15	$ 4.69	$ 4.00	$ -	$ -	$ 0.69	$1.04	$1.14	$ 8.69	$ 2.87	$ 11.56
	Total		131,469	-	131,469											

Cost Capture Check

Total Calculated Cost	$ 584,586
Total Actual Cost	$623,500
Cost Capture Percent	93.8%

Table 31.4 Key variables for a hematology laboratory with additional volume

Position	Type	Average Salary	FTEs	Total Salary Exp	Fringe Expense	Total Salary & Fringe
Lab Specialist	Tester	$ 27,000	1.00	$ 27,000	$ 6,750	$ 33,750
Medical Technologist	Tester	$ 33,500	3.00	$ 100,500	$ 25,125	$ 125,625
Medical Lab Technician	Tester	$ 28,500	1.00	$ 28,500	$ 7,125	$ 35,625
Laboratory Supervisor	Non-Tester	$ 40,500	1.00	$ 40,500	$ 10,125	$ 50,625
Total			6.00	$ 196,500	$ 49,125	$ 245,625
Avg Tester Salary & Fringe Benefit Expense						$ 39,000
Total Non-Tester Salary & Fringe Benefit Expense						$ 50,625

Divisional Indirect Costs	Amount	Cost/Test	
Non-Tester Salary & Fringe	$ 50,625		
Office Supplies	$ 10,000		
Books/Subs/Dues	$ 15,000		
Travel Meeting Dues	$ 15,000		
Total	$ 90,625	$ 0.65	Amount Divided by Total Volume

Lab Indirect Costs	Amount
Management	$ 115,000
Central Receiving	$ 625,000
General Support	$ 100,000
Administrative Support	$ 75,000
Subtotal	$ 915,000

Hospital Indirect Costs (Lab Portion)	Amount
Patient Financial Services	$ 500,000
Human Resources	$ 300,000
Management	$ 100,000
Finance	$ 100,000
Subtotal	$ 1,000,000

Table 31.3 combines all the costing information thus far to calculate a unit cost for a given volume. After generating this cost information it is important to validate the model by running a check on the total cost captured by the model. This total is measured by multiplying the unit costs by the volume over a given period of time and comparing that to actual costs for the same time period, which were generated in Table 31.1.

Table 31.4 through 31.6 are the same as the previous examples, except they show the effects of adding an additional 7,500 partial thromboplastin time tests to the mix. Clearly, the additional tests make all the indirect fixed costs less expensive because the same fixed costs are now being divided over a larger number of tests. This relationship is important when generating pricing proposals for new business.

Table 31.5 Test run calculation for a hematology laboratory with additional volume

Division	Test Description	CPT Code	Total Volume	Test Run Volume	Current Runs/Week	Maximum Test Run	Avg Tests per Run	Test Run Minutes	Total Year Salary & Fringe Expense	Total Year Supplies & Reagent Expense	Salary & Fringe Expense per Test	Supplies & Reagents Expense per Test
	Partial Thromboplastin Time	85730	33,473									
	Prothrombin Time	85610	33,318									
HEMATOLOGY	HEMA001 Test Run			66,791	6	250	214	180	$ 17,550	$ 6,240	$ 0.26	$ 0.09

Table 31.6 Cost calculation for a hematology laboratory with additional volume

						DIRECT COST					INDIRECT COST					
						Variable Cost			Step-Fixed Cost		Fixed Cost					
Division	Test Description	CPT Code	Total Volume	Additional Volume	Revised Volume	Test Minutes	Test Salary & Fringe	Test Supplies & Reagents	Test Run Sal & Frg	Test Run Supp & Reag	Divisional Cost	Lab Cost	Hospital Cost	Variable Cost	Fixed Cost	Total Cost
HEMATOLOGY	Fibrinogen	85384	2,057	-	2,057	5	$ 1.56	$ 1.00	$ -	$ -	$ 0.65	$ 0.99	$1.08	$ 2.56	$ 2.72	$ 5.28
HEMATOLOGY	Heinz Body Preparation	85441	10	-	10	5	$ 1.56	$ 1.00	$ -	$ -	$ 0.65	$ 0.99	$1.08	$ 2.56	$ 2.72	$ 5.28
HEMATOLOGY	Hematocrit, Spun	85013	107	-	107	5	$ 1.56	$ 1.00	$ -	$ -	$ 0.65	$ 0.99	$1.08	$ 2.56	$ 2.72	$ 5.28
HEMATOLOGY	Kleihauer Test	85460	342	-	342	3	$ 0.94	$ 0.50	$ -	$ -	$ 0.65	$ 0.99	$1.08	$ 1.44	$ 2.72	$ 4.16
HEMATOLOGY	Leukocyte Alkaline Phosphatase	85540	29	-	29	3	$ 0.94	$ 0.50	$ -	$ -	$ 0.65	$ 0.99	$1.08	$ 1.44	$ 2.72	$ 4.16
HEMATOLOGY	LA Confirm Test	85613	133	-	133	3	$ 0.94	$ 0.50	$ -	$ -	$ 0.65	$ 0.99	$1.08	$ 1.44	$ 2.72	$ 4.16
HEMATOLOGY	Hemogram	85027	63,600	-	63,600	5	$ 1.56	$ 0.50	$ -	$ -	$ 0.65	$ 0.99	$1.08	$ 2.06	$ 2.72	$ 4.78
HEMATOLOGY	Partial Thromboplastin Time	85730	25,973	7,500	33,473	-	$ -	$ -	$ 0.26	$ 0.09	$ 0.65	$ 0.99	$1.08	$ -	$ 3.08	$ 3.08
HEMATOLOGY	Platelet Aggregation	85576	17	-	17	10	$ 3.13	$ 2.00	$ -	$ -	$ 0.65	$ 0.99	$1.08	$ 5.13	$ 2.72	$ 7.85
HEMATOLOGY	Prothrombin Time	85610	33,318	-	33,318	-	$ -	$ -	$ 0.26	$ 0.09	$ 0.65	$ 0.99	$1.08	$ -	$ 3.08	$ 3.08
HEMATOLOGY	Protein C, Functional	85303	181	-	181	10	$ 3.13	$ 2.00	$ -	$ -	$ 0.65	$ 0.99	$1.08	$ 5.13	$ 2.72	$ 7.85
HEMATOLOGY	Protein S, Functional	85306	175	-	175	10	$ 3.13	$ 2.00	$ -	$ -	$ 0.65	$ 0.99	$1.08	$ 5.13	$ 2.72	$ 7.85
HEMATOLOGY	Sed. Rate, Westergren	85652	5,527	-	5,527	15	$ 4.69	$ 4.00	$ -	$ -	$ 0.65	$ 0.99	$1.08	$ 8.69	$ 2.72	$ 11.41
Total			131,469	7,500	138,969											

Cost Capture Check

Total Calculated Cost	$ 589,479
Total Actual Cost	$623,500
Cost Capture Percent	94.5%

Comparing Table 31.5 with Table 31.2 shows the effects of adding additional tests to the cost of a test run. In Table 31.2 we were able to run the batch of tests five times a week and still be under the test run maximum of 250. With the addition of 7,500 tests, one can see in Table 31.5 that the batch now needs to be run six times a week, which adds more cost and increases the per-unit cost of the tests. Thus, the cost for these tests was fixed within a certain volume level (250 tests per batch), but when the volume went over that level, the costs shifted upward, an example of a step-fixed cost.

Break-Even Analysis

Contribution margin is the revenue per UOS less the marginal cost per UOS, and is often written as contribution margin = price − variable costs. As long as the contribution margin is positive, the organization benefits. The margin can go to supporting fixed costs (or to supporting items or activities whose contribution margin is negative), and if fixed costs have been covered, it represents profit.

The break-even point is the volume of activity required for all fixed costs to be covered. Therefore, the break-even point equals the total fixed cost divided by the contribution margin.

$$\text{Volume break-even point} = \frac{\text{Total fixed costs}}{\text{Contribution margin}}$$
$$= \frac{\text{total fixed costs}}{\text{price} - (\text{variable costs})}$$

This equation underscores the relationships among costs, volume, and profits. In the previous section, we discussed cost behavior and displayed the relationships of fixed and variable costs to volume. A given responsibility center incurs both fixed and variable costs, and its total costs are the sum of the two, as illustrated in Fig. 31.2. Adding the revenue line, which increases at a rate equal to the revenue per unit, yields Fig. 31.3.

If the revenue per unit is greater than the variable cost per unit, the revenue line and the total cost line must cross at some point, where revenues = costs, the break-even point. Note that the graph illustrates not only the break-even volume, but also the unit revenue required to reach break-even. Figure 31.4 shows this calculation for a hypothetical hematology division.

Equipment Purchase

When considering expensive equipment purchases, it is critical to know the point at which the volume of procedures performed on the equipment covers its annual depreciation and maintenance costs, compared to the projected demand for the procedures, as illustrated in Fig. 31.5.

Capitation Contract

Under "capitation," healthcare providers are paid a fixed revenue per member per month (PMPM). Revenue varies, therefore, with member enrollment, not with the volume of procedures performed. To understand what the break-even point is in terms of the number of members, a provider must first understand the expected utilization by those members (see Fig. 31.6). The provider, not the health plan, is at risk for variations in utilization. This risk can be ameliorated by negotiating utilization corridors into the contract, whereby the PMPM revenue is adjusted up or down if utilization is over or under budget by a certain amount. If not, the provider can incur significant losses if utilization is over budget.

Capital Acquisition Concepts

Time Value of Money

Before evaluating potential capital acquisitions, it is important to understand the concept of the time value of money. Most people prefer current consumption to future consumption. Similarly, investors expect to be rewarded for their patience by receiving a rate of return on an investment, which could be interest, dividends, or capital

Figure 31.2 Variable, fixed, and total cost.

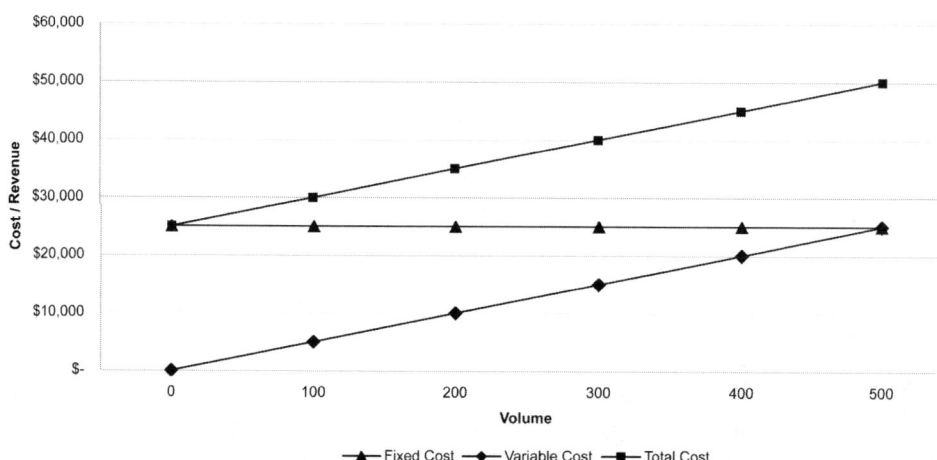

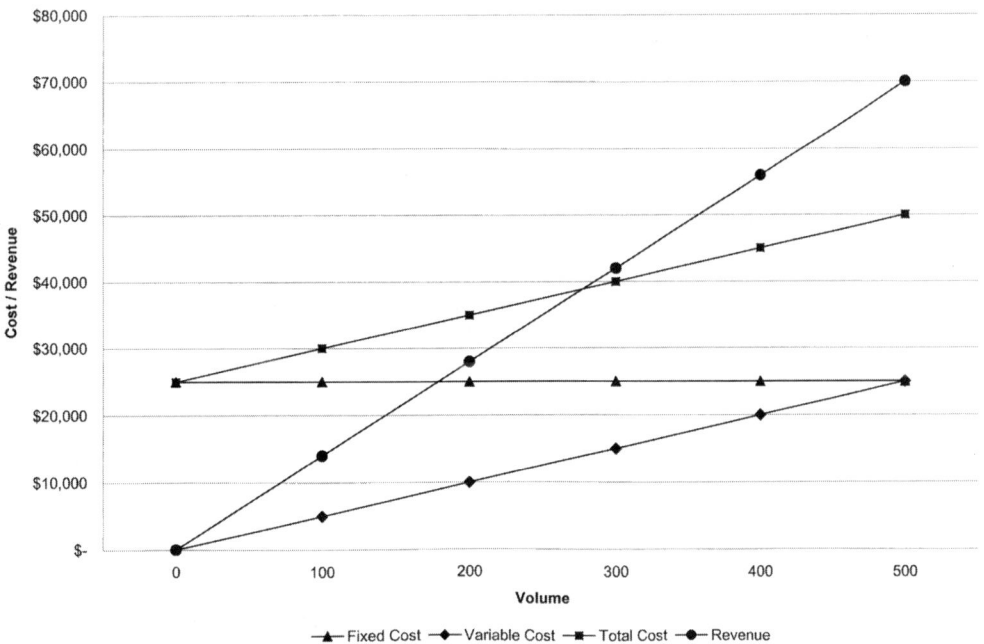

Figure 31.3 Variable, fixed, and total expense and revenue.

gains. Intrinsic in this is the notion that money received in the future is not as valuable as money received today. We can quantify this. The future value (FV) of an investment = its present value (PV) multiplied by (1 + interest rate, k) raised to the number of investment periods, n (usually expressed as years), or

$$FV = PV \times (1 + k)^n$$

The future value in 3 years of $100 invested at 5% interest = $100 \times (1 + 0.05)^3 = 115.76. This formula becomes useful in considering capital acquisitions when we rearrange the terms:

$$PV = \frac{FV}{(1 + k)^n}$$

Here, the rate k is called the discount rate (not the interest rate), and the practice is called discounting (we are discounting the value of money, not to be confused with discounting, or reducing the price of, a test charge). This approach allows us to value different investments in today's dollars in relation to their future values. Which would you rather receive, $115.76 in 3 years or $120.34 in 4 years? At a 5% discount rate, we already know the present value of $115.76 after 3 years is $100.00. For $120.34 after 4 years,

$$PV = \frac{\$120.34}{(1 + 0.05)^4} = \$99.00$$

Therefore, the first choice (3 years) has a higher value.

Investments are evaluated based on their cash flows (CF), where CF = cash revenues − cash expenses. The **net**

present value (NPV) of a project = the sum of the PV of the CF of the project.

$$NPV = \sum_{t=0}^{n} \frac{CFt}{(1 + k)^n}$$

Here, the rate k is referred to as the required rate of return, the cost of capital, or the hurdle rate. If the NPV is >0, the investment is warranted. If NPV < 0, it should not be pursued. If you are comparing two alternatives, pick the one with the higher NPV. A special case is when the NPV = 0. The rate k that induces this is called the internal rate of return (IRR). Instead of calculating the NPV for two competing investments, you can calculate their internal rates of return. Pick the investment with the higher IRR as long as the IRR is greater than your cost of capital (if it is not, then your capital would be better invested elsewhere). For example, a new analyzer costs $100,000 and will allow the laboratory to perform testing it does not perform today, so it will generate $35,000 in net cash flow per year for the next 4 years. If our required rate of return is 10%, is this a worthwhile investment?

Time	Cash flow
0	−$100,000
1	$35,000
2	$35,000
3	$35,000
4	$35,000

$$NPV = \frac{-\$100,000}{(1 + 0.10)^0} + \frac{\$35,000}{(1 + 0.10)^1} + \frac{\$35,000}{(1 + 0.10)^2} +$$
$$\frac{\$35,000}{(1 + 0.10)^3} + \frac{\$35,000}{(1 + 0.10)^4} = \$10,945$$

Figure 31.4 Graphical representation of the break-even point for a hematology division.

Fixed Cost	$	397,700
Variable Cost	$	1.42
Price	$	10.00

Break-even Point = $\dfrac{397,700}{(10.00 - 1.42)}$ = 46,381

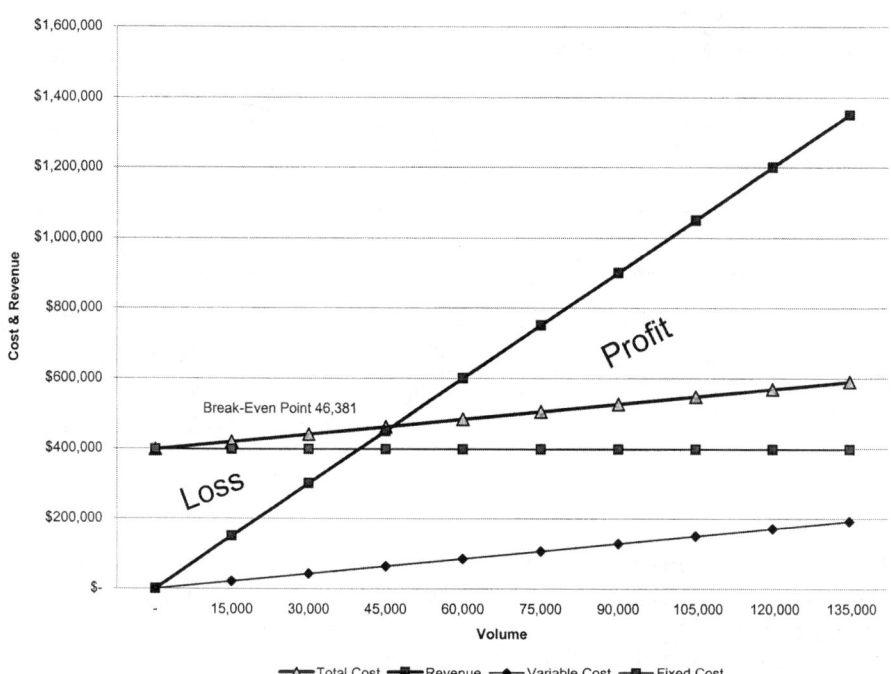

Solving for the internal rate of return (spreadsheet software and most financial calculators automate this):

$$0 = \frac{-\$100,000}{(1 + \text{IRR})^0} + \frac{\$35,000}{(1 + \text{IRR})^1} + \frac{\$35,000}{(1 + \text{IRR})^2} + \frac{\$35,000}{(1 + \text{IRR})^3} + \frac{\$35,000}{(1 + \text{IRR})^4}$$

IRR ≈ 15%. This IRR would then be compared with the other possible returns the company might get with the money if it were invested in other projects.

Many laboratory investments do not create new revenues, but these same techniques can be applied to calculating net present *cost* and then choosing the option with the lowest cost.

Depreciation

Depreciation is associated with capital investments, so it is worth commenting on. Depreciation is the allocation of the cost to acquire an asset that has a useful life of greater than 1 year into each year of the asset's life. It is common to use a "straight line" method in healthcare, whereby the depreciation is evenly allocated across the item's useful life. For example, if a piece of equipment costs $100,000 and has a useful life of 10 years, after which it is worth nothing, an annual depreciation expense of $10,000 per year would be recorded for each of the 10 years. There are other methods of depreciation that are driven by tax laws and usually allow for a more accelerated treatment of this expense.

Investment decisions are based on cash flows, and depreciation is not a cash flow. The relevant cash flow is the purchase event. From an accounting standpoint, the organization is simply exchanging one asset, cash, for another, the asset. Depreciation serves to reduce the value of the asset over time on the organization's financial statements, but it should be *ignored* when evaluating capital acquisitions.

Table 31.7 evaluates a direct purchase versus an installment purchase, where payments are made over time, as an example of a net present cost application. Assume the following: direct purchase price = $200,000; installment purchase = $40,000 per year with a useful life of 7 years; discount rate = 10%. In this example it would be less expensive to purchase the equipment directly versus an installment purchase, $200,000 versus $213,397.

Table 31.8, the evaluation of two different pieces of laboratory equipment that serve the same function, is an example of calculating their NPVs. Equipment #1 costs $200,000 and generates $60,000 of net cash flow per year for the 7-year useful life of the equipment. Equipment #2 costs $300,000 and generates $90,000 per year for the 7-year useful life of the equipment. The cost of the

Cost of Equipment	$	300,000
Annual Depreciation	$	42,857
Maintenance Contract	$	4,286
Variable Cost	$	4.00
Price	$	8.00

Break-even Point $= \dfrac{47,143}{(8.00 - 4.00)} = 11,786$

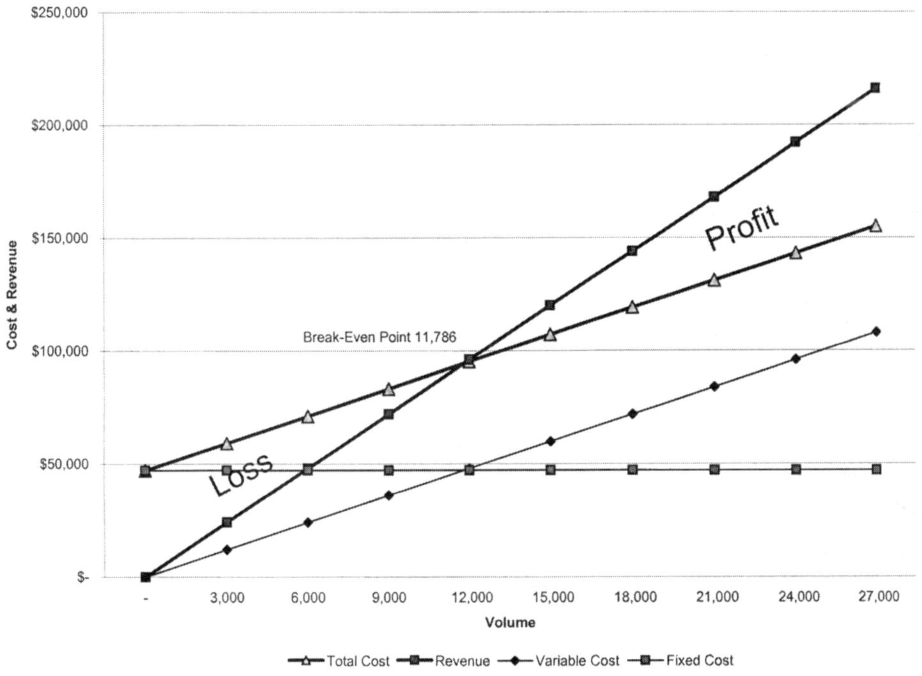

Figure 31.5 Break-even point for equipment purchase.

equipment and depreciation is spread evenly over the 7 years of useful life. Based on these figures, equipment #2 would be chosen over equipment #1 because of its higher NPV, $125,598 versus $83,732.

Budgeting

It is through budgeting that an organization turns its strategic plans into daily operations. A budget expresses planned revenues and expenses, as well as the volumes of services and amounts of resources required to realize them. Through the budget process the organization establishes priorities for its plans, allocates its resources, and controls its costs. It authorizes new programs and services

and sets performance standards for existing ones. A budget thus serves as a tool and a benchmark for monitoring the performance of the organization throughout its fiscal year. In addition it is a mechanism for imposing discipline on the organization.

There are two key concepts that are integral to healthcare budgeting, full-time equivalents (FTEs) and UOSs. An FTE is one or more employees paid for a total of 2,080 h per year (based on 8 h per day $\times$ 5 days per week $\times$ 52 weeks per year); this is the standard labor measure. An employee who is paid for two 8-h days per week represents 0.4 FTE, while an employee who is paid for two 12-h days per week represents 0.6 FTE. Together, they represent 1.0 FTE to the organization. Labor is divided into productive

Table 31.7 NPV of direct purchase versus installment purchase

Project	Year 0	Year 1	Year 2	Year 3	Year 4	Year 5	Year 6	Year 7
Discount Rate	10%							
Direct Purchase	$ 200,000							
Installment Purchase	$ 40,000	$ 40,000	$ 40,000	$ 40,000	$ 40,000	$ 40,000	$ 40,000	$ 40,000
NPV of Installment Purchase	$ 213,397							

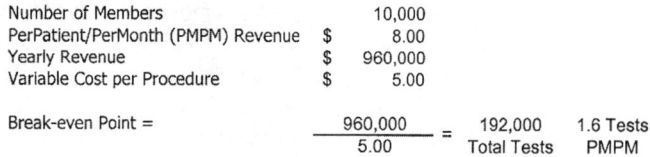

Break-even Point = $\dfrac{960,000}{5.00}$ = $\begin{array}{c}192,000 \\ \text{Total Tests}\end{array}$ $\begin{array}{c}1.6 \text{ Tests} \\ \text{PMPM}\end{array}$

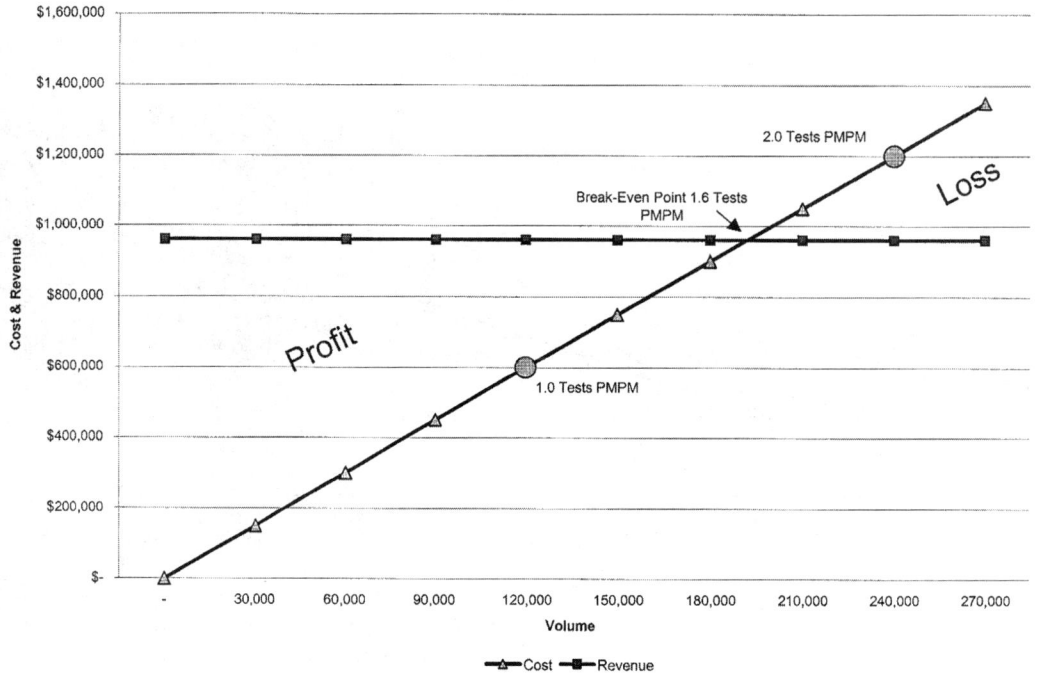

Figure 31.6 Break-even point for a capitated contract.

time, the time spent working on job-related activities, and nonproductive time, which includes vacation, holidays, and sick time. Depending on an organization's fringe benefits policies, it will need 1.1 or more FTEs to realize 1.0 FTE of productive time.

Each area of the organization needs a way of quantifying its productivity. As stated earlier, a UOS is the logical measure of work for a given area. In the laboratory, it is usually either the number of billed tests or the number of procedures performed. For the operating room, it may be the number of surgeries; for a physician office, it may be the number of patient visits. UOSs are useful for measuring and comparing resource consumption, such as total expenses per billed test, or billed tests per FTE, as we saw in the cost accounting section.

Types of Budgets

Three separate budgets are developed during the budgeting process.

The first, and the one with which you are probably most familiar, is the *operating budget*. These are prepared at the level of the cost center, usually by those managers who have direct responsibility for managing the cost center and who can affect its operations. The operating budget can be broken down into three components:

- *statistical budget*, which is the forecast of activity for the unit,
- *revenue budget*, which determines the gross charges that will be generated by the forecasted volume, and
- *expense budget*, which projects the amounts of resources that will be required to produce the forecasted volumes.

The *capital budget* is the second type of budget. Its development can occur simultaneously with the operating budget. It is usually prepared at the organization level and includes new or replacement property, physical plant, and equipment needs of the organization for the coming year. Most organizations have a system in place to collect information on these needs from departments across the organization and then arrange the priorities centrally with respect to acuity of need, organizational goals, and available funding. Capital budgeting is separated from the operating budget because the impact of capital purchases is

Table 31.8 NPV of two different pieces of equipment

Project	Year 0	Year 1	Year 2	Year 3	Year 4	Year 5	Year 6	Year 7
Discount Rate	10%							
Equipment #1								
Cost of Equipment	$ (200,000)							
Incremental Revenue		$ 100,000	$ 100,000	$ 100,000	$ 100,000	$ 100,000	$ 100,000	$ 100,000
Incremental Expense		$ (68,571)	$ (68,571)	$ (68,571)	$ (68,571)	$ (68,571)	$ (68,571)	$ (68,571)
Depreciation		$ 28,571	$ 28,571	$ 28,571	$ 28,571	$ 28,571	$ 28,571	$ 28,571
Net Cash Flow	$ (200,000)	$ 60,000	$ 60,000	$ 60,000	$ 60,000	$ 60,000	$ 60,000	$ 60,000
Net Present Value of Cash Flows	$ 83,732							
Equipment #2								
Cost of Equipment	$ (300,000)							
Incremental Revenue		$ 150,000	$ 150,000	$ 150,000	$ 150,000	$ 150,000	$ 150,000	$ 150,000
Incremental Expense		$ (102,857)	$ (102,857)	$ (102,857)	$ (102,857)	$ (102,857)	$ (102,857)	$ (102,857)
Depreciation		$ 42,857	$ 42,857	$ 42,857	$ 42,857	$ 42,857	$ 42,857	$ 42,857
Net Cash Flow	$ (300,000)	$ 90,000	$ 90,000	$ 90,000	$ 90,000	$ 90,000	$ 90,000	$ 90,000
Net Present Value of Cash Flows	$ 125,598							

predominantly on cash, with only the depreciation expense affecting the operating budget (see the previous section's discussion of depreciation).

With the operating and capital budgets prepared, an organization can develop the third type, the *cash budget*. This is usually prepared by the organization's finance department and predicts the cash flows in and out of the organization and the resultant cash availability. While obscure to most, it is the most critical of the three budgets. In order to remain solvent and thus stay in business, the organization must carefully plan its cash reserves, timing of cash disbursements, and any borrowing and investing activities.

The Budget Process

Creating a budget entails a fairly linear set of sequential steps, some of which occur at the organizational level and some that are done at the departmental or cost center levels.

Step 1. Establish organizational goals and objectives. Although the senior management usually sets these, it is not uncommon for departments to develop their own objectives in support of the broader organizational goals. For instance, a hospital may set a goal to "expand market share in ABC County by 3%." This, in turn, might lead to a goal of establishing a satellite facility in that county. The laboratory might then establish objectives for equipping and running a laboratory or phlebotomy station at that satellite.

Step 2. Review key environmental factors, such as demographics, political and regulatory issues, competition, technology, and the economy. This function is usually performed at the organizational level, although the laboratory may have unique information about its particular niche, such as the marketing activities of a regional reference laboratory with which it is competing for outpatient testing.

Step 3. Determine starting assumptions about inflation, payment levels, admissions, and other key volumes. This function is usually performed at the organizational level.

Step 4. Develop the statistical budget for each UOS in the organization. This budget is completed at the department level using the information garnered in steps 1 to 3. The laboratory manager will need to consider projections of the number of admissions and the length of stay to forecast volumes of inpatient laboratory tests and will have to estimate the activity for various outpatient departments to forecast volumes of outpatient laboratory tests. If the laboratory is freestanding or has nonaffiliated clients, managers must develop forecasting methods for these markets as well.

Step 5. Develop the revenue budget, based on the statistical volumes forecast in step 3 multiplied by the applicable charges per UOS, resulting in the gross revenue budget. In most organizations, consideration of contractual allowances, writeoffs, and bad debt occurs at the organizational level, for purposes of estimating the net revenue budget. These reductions to gross revenue are usually quite significant, often from 20% to as much as 60%.

Step 6. Prepare the expense budget on the basis of the data gathered in steps 1 to 4. Because labor often constitutes roughly 70% of a healthcare organization's budget, the expense budget is frequently broken down separately into a staffing budget and a nonpersonnel expense budget. The staffing budget takes into account the numbers and types of employees, pay rates, and FTEs required in each cost center. Nonpersonnel expenses include the various supplies consumed and services utilized to produce the UOS forecasted.

Step 7. Assuming the capital budget was produced in parallel with the previous steps, there is usually a process of negotiation and revision between department heads and senior managers once all of the departments' budgets are rolled into one organizational budget and the operating income is calculated.

Step 8. Develop the cash budget.

Step 9. Continue negotiations and revisions across the organization.

Step 10. Submit the budget to the organization's board of directors for approval. Most commonly, current year and prior year results form the basis on which the new budget is developed. This process is called incremental budgeting. An alternative used in some organizations is zero-based budgeting. Under this approach, each and every expenditure must be justified as if the service was starting from scratch, as well as why other ways to provide it are not more cost-effective. While this can be time-consuming, it forces a regular reexamination of why things are done they way they are and whether or not they still fit with the organization's mission.

Another refinement to the budget process is the use of flexible budgets. The process that has been described so far results in a fixed budget, one in which an annual budget is developed and approved, after which this agreed-upon budget acts as the yardstick against which monthly performance is monitored. Recall, however, the earlier discussion about cost behavior (fixed, variable, etc.). It is relatively straightforward to divide an organization's expenses into those that vary with changes in UOS and those that do not. Subsequently, the variable portion of the budget may change with volume for purposes of monitoring performance. This approach is known as flexible budgeting.

Budget Examples

Table 31.9 is an example of a staffing worksheet that is prepared to calculate how many FTEs a laboratory division would need for the upcoming fiscal year and the costs associated with those FTEs. In practice, more detailed information is required than just FTEs and hourly rates to generate an accurate staffing budget. A manager also has to break down each employee's hours into the different shifts that he or she works, so that any differential rates can be applied. Examples of typical differential rates would be for weekends, evenings, nights, holidays, overtime, etc. In this example, the manager is requesting 19.36 FTEs, which equates to $853,203 in salary expense and $220,638 in fringe benefit expense (such as payroll taxes, health insurance premiums, etc.). Notice that the salary expense is broken down into productive and nonproductive components. This allocation is commonly done to track nonworked but paid hours versus the actual worked hours.

Table 31.10 is an example of a worksheet that is used to analyze a budget being requested by a manager. In this example, the starting point is a pro forma budget that was calculated by (i) projecting any changes in volume, and (ii) using the revenue and expense per UOS from the previous budget (FY02 ACTUAL) to adjust both revenues and costs.

This calculation allows for a comparison between what one would expect for revenue and expense, given a certain volume level, and what the manager is actually requesting (VARIANCE). The manager will need to present a valid case for deviating from the pro forma budget. Once the differences between the pro forma budget and the requested budget, i.e., the variance, have been resolved with senior management, the last step in the process is to apply inflation factors (INFLATION ADJUSTMENT) to the approved budget (FY03 REQUESTED, if all the variances have been accepted) and generate the final budget for the upcoming fiscal year (FY03 BUDGET).

Variance Analysis

Management reporting is a process of communicating actual versus budget performance throughout the organization to identify necessary corrective actions and help make decisions. Distribution of reports usually follows the organizational structure. Detailed line item reports are analyzed at the cost center level. These reports roll up into more and more summaries as one moves up the chain of command. For example, a chemistry supervisor reviews more detail than does the laboratory manager, who looks at summary reports across the laboratory, while the vice president for ancillary services looks at summary reports for the laboratory, radiology, pharmacy, etc.

Variance analysis is critical to the control function of management. Having established a budget, the extent to which actual experience differs from the budget represents a variance. Controllable variances can be resolved by management action. Vendors may be substituted, contracts may be renegotiated, or alternative methodologies may be pursued. Other variances are not controllable, such as a flu epidemic that drives up demand for services above what was budgeted, but as a result, may require management to make changes to more discretionary expenditures to offset the uncontrollable epidemic factor. Variance analysis commonly focuses on the company's actual results versus budgeted expectations on a line-by-line basis for each cost center. It is important that the line manager who has the understanding of the cost center and the ability to make any necessary changes actually perform this analysis. It is the job of the manager to explain the variances to superiors. Table 31.11 is an example of a typical variance report for a laboratory division.

Cost variances can have several causes. Volume variances result from a change in the volume of services performed, either up or down. A flexible budget, described in the previous section, takes account of these variances. At the top of Table 31.11, you can see that volume is under

Table 31.9 Staffing worksheet

JOB			FY 2002 FTE Budget	FY 2003 FTE Budget	Hourly Rate		Total Pay	
Code	Title	Employee Name						
078J	Charge Technologist	Employee Name	1.02	1.01	$	25.77	$	54,138
078J	Charge Technologist	Employee Name	1.02	1.01	$	25.71	$	54,012
078J	Charge Technologist	Employee Name	-	1.00	$	23.34	$	48,547
078J Total			**2.04**	**3.02**			**$**	**156,696**
078K	Medical Technologist	Employee Name	0.35	0.35	$	20.16	$	14,676
078K	Medical Technologist	Employee Name	0.76	0.76	$	22.28	$	35,220
078K	Medical Technologist	Employee Name	0.82	0.81	$	20.24	$	34,100
078K	Medical Technologist	Employee Name	0.97	0.97	$	22.44	$	45,275
078K	Medical Technologist	Employee Name	1.02	1.02	$	15.72	$	33,352
078K	Medical Technologist	Employee Name	0.53	0.65	$	20.71	$	28,000
078K	Medical Technologist	Employee Name	0.66	0.77	$	22.71	$	36,372
078K	Medical Technologist	Employee Name	0.63	0.75	$	20.23	$	31,559
078K	Medical Technologist	Employee Name	0.87	0.87	$	22.66	$	41,006
078K	Medical Technologist	Employee Name	0.93	0.96	$	16.59	$	33,127
078K	Medical Technologist	Employee Name	0.35	-	$	18.11	$	-
078K	Medical Technologist	Employee Name	0.35	0.35	$	20.10	$	14,633
078K	Medical Technologist	Employee Name	0.53	0.53	$	18.92	$	20,857
078K	Medical Technologist	Employee Name	1.02	1.02	$	18.41	$	39,059
078K	Medical Technologist	Employee Name	0.27	1.01	$	16.50	$	34,663
078K	Medical Technologist	Employee Name	0.27	0.76	$	16.14	$	25,514
078K	Medical Technologist	Employee Name	-	-	$	19.48	$	-
078K Total			**10.33**	**11.58**			**$**	**467,413**
078L	Medical Lab Technician	Employee Name	0.20	0.08	$	18.33	$	3,050
078L	Medical Lab Technician	Employee Name	-	-	$	16.20	$	-
078L Total			**0.20**	**0.08**			**$**	**3,050**
900A	Sr Medical Technologist	Employee Name	0.30	0.27	$	23.51	$	13,203
900A	Sr Medical Technologist	Employee Name	0.78	0.78	$	22.52	$	36,536
900A	Sr Medical Technologist	Employee Name	0.63	0.63	$	23.51	$	30,808
900A	Sr Medical Technologist	Employee Name	-	-	$	20.01	$	-
900A Total			**1.71**	**1.68**			**$**	**80,547**
B474	Lab Assistant II	Employee Name	1.01	1.00	$	14.19	$	29,515
B474	Lab Assistant II	Employee Name	-	-	$	12.18	$	-
B474 Total			**1.01**	**1.00**			**$**	**29,515**
L314	Supervisor Laboratory	Employee Name	1.00	1.00	$	23.36	$	48,589
L314	Supervisor Laboratory	Employee Name	-	-	$	25.94	$	-

Exhibit 15: Example of a Staffing Worksheet for a Hypothetical Laboratory Division

L314 Total			**1.00**	**1.00**			**$**	**48,589**
L437	Chief Technologist - Lab	Employee Name	1.00	1.00	$	32.40	$	67,392
L437	Chief Technologist - Lab	Employee Name	-	-	$	28.63	$	-
L437 Total			**1.00**	**1.00**			**$**	**67,392**
			17.29	**19.36**			**$**	**853,203**

NON PRODUCTIVE REG SAL	$	93,852
PRODUCTIVE REG SAL	$	759,351
PRODUCTIVE OT SAL	$	-
	$	853,203

ALLOCATED FRINGE - STAFF	$	220,638

Table 31.10 Worksheet for constructing a budget

CATEGORY	FY02 PROJECTED	FY02 ACTUAL	VOLUME ADJUSTMENT	FY03 PROFORMA	FY03 REQUESTED	VARIANCE	INFLATION ADJUSMENT	FY03 BUDGET
VOLUME								
Inpatient Volume	155,415	159,897	-	159,897	159,897	-	-	159,897
Outpatient Volume	133,572	130,887	1,000	131,887	131,887	-	-	131,887
Total Volume	288,987	290,784	1,000	291,784	291,784	-	-	291,784
REVENUE								
Inpatient Revenue	3,079,451	3,124,187	-	3,124,187	3,124,187	-	62,484	3,186,671
Outpatient Revenue	2,540,748	2,471,015	19,022	2,490,037	2,490,037	-	49,801	2,539,837
Gross Patient Revenue	5,620,199	5,595,202	19,022	5,614,224	5,614,224	-	112,284	5,726,508
Est Deductions from Revenue	(1,967,070)	(1,958,321)	(6,658)	(1,964,978)	(1,964,978)	-	(39,300)	(2,004,278)
Net Patient Revenue	3,653,130	3,636,881	12,364	3,649,245	3,649,245	-	72,985	3,722,230
EXPENSE								
NON PRODUCTIVE REG SAL	95,979	84,823	332	85,155	93,852	8,697	1,877	95,729
PRODUCTIVE REG SAL	726,993	686,298	2,516	688,813	759,351	70,538	15,187	774,538
PRODUCTIVE OT SAL	10,016	16,011	35	16,046	-	(16,046)	-	-
Salaries	832,988	787,132	2,882	790,014	853,203	63,189	17,064	870,267
ALLOCATED FRINGE - STAFF	215,411	203,584	745	204,329	220,638	16,309	4,413	225,051
Payroll Tax & Fringe	215,411	203,584	745	204,329	220,638	16,309	4,413	225,051
Salaries & Fringe Benefits	1,048,399	990,716	3,628	994,344	1,073,841	79,497	21,477	1,095,318
MEDICAL SURGICAL	2,633	3,594	9	3,603	3,000	(603)	60	3,060
LAB SUPPLIES	256,982	328,640	889	329,529	320,000	(9,529)	6,400	326,400
PHARMACEUTICALS	350	312	1	313	300	(13)	6	306
OFFICE SUPPLIES	2,382	3,054	-	3,054	3,000	(54)	60	3,060
SUPPLIES OFFICE-PRINTED	1,892	-	-	-	-	-	-	-
MAIL & PRODUCTION	67	500	-	500	500	-	10	510
BOOKS/SUBS/DUES NONMD	-	250	-	250	250	-	5	255
TRAVEL/MEET/DUES-GENERAL	3,043	3,349	-	3,349	3,349	-	67	3,416
MAINTENANCE-CONTRACT	34,808	44,000	-	44,000	64,891	20,891	1,298	66,189
MAINTENANCE-NONCONTRACT	2,681	900	-	900	900	-	18	918
CAFETERIA	180	350	-	350	350	-	7	357
CELEBRATION FUNDS	543	345	-	345	345	-	7	352
PROFESSIONAL DEVELOP NON	2,067	1,624	-	1,624	1,624	-	32	1,656
SMALL EQUIPMENT	2,174	2,647	-	2,647	2,647	-	53	2,700
Total Non-Salary Expense	309,802	389,565	900	390,465	401,156	10,692	8,023	409,180
Total Expense	1,358,202	1,380,281	4,527	1,384,808	1,474,997	90,189	29,500	1,504,497
Contribution Margin	2,294,928	2,256,600	7,837	2,264,437	2,174,248	89,586	43,485	2,217,733
STATISTICS								
Contribution Margin Percent	62.8%	62.0%	63.4%	62.1%	59.6%	-2.5%	0.0%	59.6%
Total FTEs	18.30	17.29	0.06	17.35	19.36	2.01	-	19.36
Hours per UOS	0.13	0.12	0.12	0.12	0.14	0.01	-	0.14
Revenue per UOS	12.64	12.51	12.36	12.51	12.51	-	-	12.76
Expense per UOS	4.70	4.75	4.53	4.75	5.06	0.31	-	5.16
Contribution per UOS	7.94	7.76	7.84	7.76	7.45	(0.31)	-	7.60

budget by 1,797, or a little less than 1%. Price variances are due to a change in the price of a supply or service versus what was anticipated in the budget. In Table 31.11, laboratory supplies are budgeted at $1.13/UOS, but the actual is $0.89, a $0.24 favorable price variance. Quantity, or efficiency, variances represent differences in the amount of inputs (labor and/or supplies) used to produce each UOS. The budget in Table 31.11 considers 16,818 tests per FTE (290,784 tests divided by 17.29 FTEs), and the actual is only 15,792/FTE, so more employee hours are required than was budgeted, an unfavorable quantity variance that helps explain the unfavorable salary dollar variance.

Any variance can be broken down into one of three main causes: volume, price, or quantity. If the cause of the variance is understood, a manager can tailor the response rationally and appropriately. Analysis and reporting of variances are ongoing processes and should be conducted monthly in order to respond quickly. As with cost accounting, however, the effort should be justified by the information gained in the process. Normal random fluctuations will cause small variances, so it is useful to establish triggers to indicate when further investigation is warranted. Control charts, as illustrated in Fig. 31.7, are useful tools for this purpose. In this chart the budget monthly test volume serves as the median line. The upper and lower limits represent an (arbitrary) figure that is 5% above and below the budgeted volume.

Variations in labor, which can be further analyzed, are important because labor costs constitute such a large portion of expenses. Both labor costs and hours can be divided into worked and paid categories. The duties of workers who are vacationing, attending conferences, sick,

Month	OCT	NOV	DEC	JAN	FEB	MAR	APR	MAY	JUN	JUL	AUG	SEP	TOTAL
Actual Volume (Number of Tests)	10,600	10,400	10,800	12,000	10,500	10,600	11,000	10,700	11,500	11,800	12,200	11,700	133,800
Monthly Budget Volume	11,000	11,000	11,000	11,000	11,000	11,000	11,000	11,000	11,000	11,000	11,000	11,000	
Monthly Budget Volume + 5%	11,550	11,550	11,550	11,550	11,550	11,550	11,550	11,550	11,550	11,550	11,550	11,550	
Monthly Budget Volume -5%	10,450	10,450	10,450	10,450	10,450	10,450	10,450	10,450	10,450	10,450	10,450	10,450	

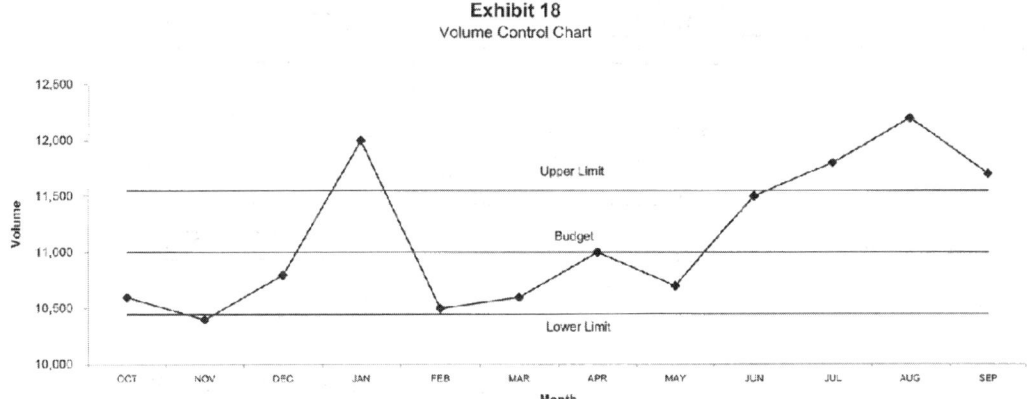

Exhibit 18
Volume Control Chart

Figure 31.7 Example of a volume control chart and associated calculations.

or injured must be assumed by others; the proportion of costs due to a reduction in worked versus paid time may be important for the organization. Worked time can be further subdivided into productive and nonproductive. The variance due to assuming the duties of staff who are attending a conference is considered non-productive worked time. Only if such expenses are adequately identified and characterized can a rational decision be made as to whether they are justified by sufficient benefit to the organization. At the bottom of Table 31.11, one can see that in this example FTEs are over budget by 1.01 or 5.86%.

Laboratory productivity, defined as the UOSs produced divided by the laboratory inputs required to produce them (in either hours or cost), should be benchmarked against regional and national peers to gauge the laboratory efficiency of the organization. At the bottom of Table 31.11, you can see that for this example hours per UOS are over budget by 0.01 or 6.51%. This variance is caused by a combination of volume being slightly under budget and FTEs being over budget.

Accounting Basics and Financial Statements

In the previous section, we discussed internal reporting and variance analysis, which management uses to control expenses and help make decisions. In this section, we turn to external reporting of an organization's finances. The various groups of people interested in the financial health of an organization include stockholders who have invested in the company (or potential stockholders), creditors who

might loan the company money, and government agencies that regulate the company. In healthcare, such agencies include prominently the Medicare and Medicaid programs. Management itself also uses financial statements to help monitor the activities of the firm.

Basic Accounting Concepts

Before discussing the standard financial statements organizations use to describe their financial condition, we must first take a look at some basic accounting concepts. All accounting activity is recorded in what is called the general ledger. From the general ledger, various financial statements can be produced, such as the three primary statements—the balance sheet, the income statement, and the cash flow (CF) statement. All accounts in the general ledger have either a natural credit or natural debit balance. Natural credit balance accounts are revenue accounts (on the income statement), liability accounts (on the balance sheet), and stockholder equity accounts (on the balance sheet). Natural debit balance accounts are expense accounts (on the income statement) and asset accounts (on the balance sheet). All transactions within the general ledger must have both a credit entry and a debit entry so that the general ledger always remains in balance. A fiscal year is the year on which the general ledger is based; this can be different from the calendar year. Healthcare industry fiscal years typically run from October 1 to September 30 because the Medicare program uses that standard.

Figure 31.8 is an example of an accounts receivable transaction. The first entry in the general ledger (#1) reflects a patient bill being sent out to an insurance company for services performed. The $100 would be recorded in the

Table 31.11 Variance report

CATEGORY	FY02 ACTUAL	FY02 BUDGET	VARIANCE	PERCENT VARIANCE
VOLUME				
Inpatient Volume	155,415	159,897	(4,482)	-2.80%
Outpatient Volume	133,572	130,887	2,685	2.05%
Total Volume	288,987	290,784	(1,797)	-0.62%
REVENUE				
Inpatient Revenue	3,079,451	3,124,187	(44,736)	-1.43%
Outpatient Revenue	2,540,748	2,471,015	69,733	2.82%
Gross Patient Revenue	5,620,199	5,595,202	24,997	0.45%
Est Deductions from Revenue	(1,967,070)	(1,958,321)	(8,749)	0.45%
Net Patient Revenue	3,653,130	3,636,881	16,248	0.45%
EXPENSE				
NON PRODUCTIVE REG SAL	95,979	84,823	11,156	13.15%
PRODUCTIVE REG SAL	726,993	686,298	40,695	5.93%
PRODUCTIVE OT SAL	10,016	16,011	(5,995)	-37.44%
Salaries	832,988	787,132	45,856	5.83%
ALLOCATED FRINGE - STAFF	215,411	203,584	11,827	5.81%
Payroll Tax & Fringe	215,411	203,584	11,827	5.81%
Salaries & Fringe Benefits	1,048,399	990,716	57,683	5.82%
MEDICAL SURGICAL	2,633	3,594	(961)	-26.74%
LAB SUPPLIES	256,982	328,640	(71,658)	-21.80%
PHARMACEUTICALS	350	312	38	12.26%
OFFICE SUPPLIES	2,382	3,054	(672)	-21.99%
SUPPLIES OFFICE-PRINTED	1,892	-	1,892	0.00%
MAIL & PRODUCTION	67	500	(433)	-86.64%
BOOKS/SUBS/DUES NONMD	-	250	(250)	-100.00%
TRAVEL/MEET/DUES-GENERAL	3,043	3,349	(306)	-9.14%
MAINTENANCE-CONTRACT	34,808	44,000	(9,192)	-20.89%
MAINTENANCE-NONCONTRACT	2,681	900	1,781	197.91%
CAFETERIA	180	350	(170)	-48.57%
CELEBRATION FUNDS	543	345	198	57.42%
PROFESSIONAL DEVELOP NON	2,067	1,624	443	27.28%
SMALL EQUIPMENT	2,174	2,647	(473)	-17.88%
Total Non-Salary Expense	309,802	389,565	(79,763)	-20.47%
Total Expense	1,358,202	1,380,281	(22,079)	-1.60%
Contribution Margin	2,294,928	2,256,600	38,328	1.70%
STATISTICS				
Contribution Margin Percent	62.8%	62.0%	0.8%	1.25%
Total FTEs	18.30	17.29	1.01	5.86%
Hours per UOS	0.13	0.12	0.01	6.51%
Revenue per UOS	12.64	12.51	0.13	1.07%
Expense per UOS	4.70	4.75	(0.05)	-0.99%
Contribution per UOS	7.94	7.76	0.18	2.33%

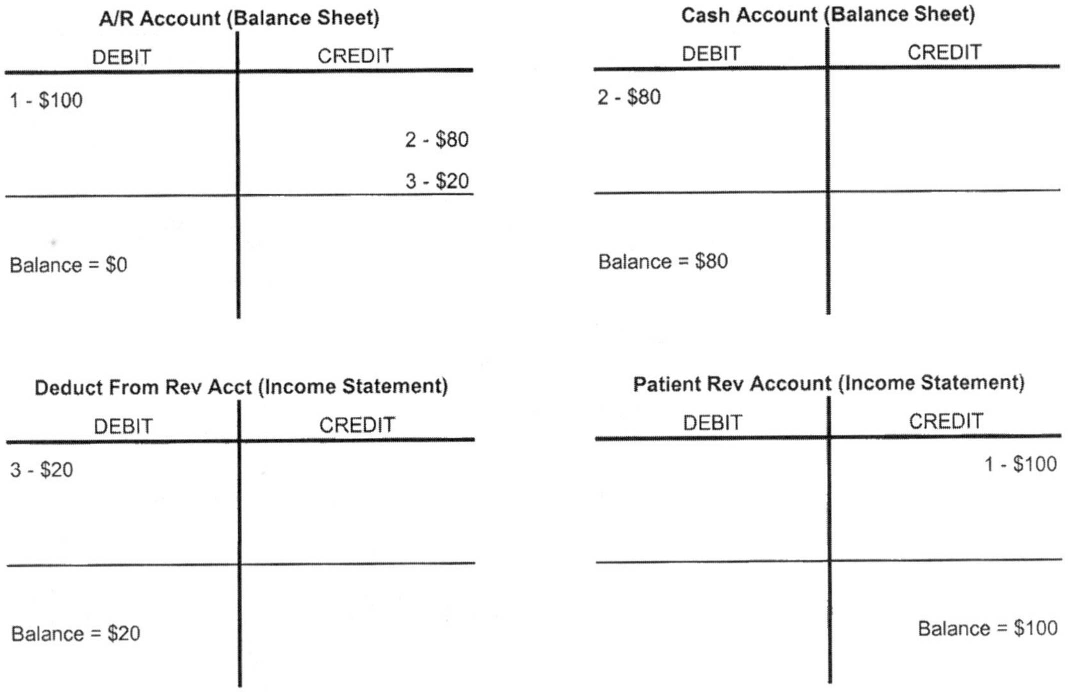

Figure 31.8 Accounts receivable transaction.

accounts receivable account (as a debit), showing that the insurance company owes money, and the same $100 would be recorded as revenue in the patient revenue account (as a credit). The second transaction shows that the insurance company sent $80 on the $100 charge. That means the $80 would be recorded as cash coming in the door in the cash account (a debit) and as an equal reduction in the amount of money that the insurance company owes in the accounts receivable account (a credit). As you can see in the example, that leaves the $20 that the insurance company did not pay, which needs to be recorded as a deduction from revenue in the third transaction (#3) (a debit). This transaction balances out the remaining receivable and reflects the fact that $80 was received instead of the original $100 that was originally recorded when the bill was sent out.

Accounting systems can be based on either an accrual or cash method. The accrual method records revenue and expenses as they occur, whereas the cash method records these items when the cash for them is either paid out or collected. With the accrual method, when a bill for $100 is generated for services performed, the general ledger would record $100 as revenue on the income statement, whereas with the cash method, that same $100 would not be recognized as revenue until the cash for that bill had actually been received. Almost all companies operate under the accrual method.

Generally accepted accounting principles (GAAP) are the set of accounting rules used by businesses in the United States, specifically publicly traded for-profit com-

panies. The GAAP rules were established to give consistency to accounting methods so that one company's financial statements could be compared to another company's. The rules are not cast in stone, and they undergo continuous evaluation and modification when necessary. In the wake of several accounting scandals in the early 2000s, adherence to these standards is being scrutinized increasingly closely.

Not-for-profit companies and agencies that depend primarily on funding from grants use fund accounting. Some companies use a combination of the two methods, using GAAP accounting for operational tracking and fund accounting for tracking their grant activities. The basic premise of fund accounting is that revenues and expenses must always be equal. For instance, a department in a university receives a certain amount of money every year from the university. The allocation is deposited into its fund balance, which the department then uses to support departmental activities. The amount spent, however, cannot exceed the amount in its fund. When the fund is depleted, spending must cease.

Financial Statements

The three primary financial statements are the balance sheet, the income statement, and the CF statement. The balance sheet (Table 31.12) is a snapshot of a firm's financial position at a particular point. It has two sections, assets and equities. Assets are economic resources that are expected to benefit the company's activities. Equities are claims against or interests in the assets. Equities are di-

Table 31.12 Balance sheet for an organization as of September 2000

Assets / Liabilities & Stockholder Equity	Sept 30 1999		Sept 30 2000	
ASSETS				
Current Assets				
Cash	15,000,000		13,200,000	
Short-Term Investments	50,000,000		42,000,000	
Accounts Receivable	140,000,000		145,000,000	
Contractual Allowance Reserve	(60,000,000)		(62,000,000)	
Inventories	5,000,000		5,500,000	
Prepaid Expenses	2,000,000	152,000,000	1,500,000	145,200,000
Fixed Assets				
Equipment	300,000,000		320,000,000	
Furniture & Fixtures	150,000,000		160,000,000	
Leasehold Improvements	200,000,000		205,000,000	
Accumulated Depreciation	(400,000,000)	250,000,000	(419,000,000)	266,000,000
Other Assets		7,000,000		7,500,000
Total Assets		409,000,000		418,700,000
LIABILITIES & STOCKHOLDER EQUITY				
Current Liabilities				
Accounts Payable	8,000,000		7,000,000	
Accrued Expenses	20,000,000		19,000,000	
Short-Term Portion of Notes Payable	5,000,000	33,000,000	4,500,000	30,500,000
Long-Term Liabilities				
Capital Lease Obligations	1,000,000		750,000	
Long-Term Portion of Notes Payable	90,000,000	91,000,000	85,000,000	85,750,000
Stockholder Equity				
Common Stock	185,000,000		185,000,000	
Retained Earnings	100,000,000	285,000,000	117,450,000	302,450,000
Total Liabilities & Stockholder Equity		409,000,000		418,700,000

vided into liabilities and owners' equity. Liabilities are economic obligations of the organization. Owners' equity (usually called stockholders' equity) is the ownership claim against the total assets. The balance sheet shows assets on the left side and liabilities and equity on the right side (although it is often displayed as assets on top and liabilities and equity on the bottom). Balance sheet account balances carry over from year to year, whereas income statement account balances start from zero at the beginning of each new fiscal year.

The income statement in Table 31.13 reports the results of a firm's operations over a period of time by matching its revenues to its expenses, while the CF statement in Table 31.14, also called the statement of changes in financial position, reports the impact of operating, investing, and financing activities over a period of time. Its purpose is to present the results of financial management, as opposed to the operating management reflected in the income statement.

Financial Ratios

Several key indicators, expressed as ratios, can help us understand the financial health of an organization as represented in its statements. There are four categories of financial ratios:

- Liquidity ratios measure the ability of a firm to meet its immediate obligations, i.e., the relationship between a firm's cash and other current assets to its current liabilities.

- Asset management, or activity, ratios measure how effective a firm is at managing its assets.

- Debt management, or leverage, ratios measure both the extent to which the firm is financed with borrowing and its likelihood of defaulting on its debt obligations.

Table 31.13 Income and expense statement for an organization, year-to-date September 2000

Revenue & Expenses	YTD Actual	YTD Budget	YTD Variance	Percent Variance
REVENUES				
Patient Service Revenue				
Inpatient Revenue	250,000,000	260,000,000	(10,000,000)	-3.85%
Outpatient Revenue	120,000,000	105,000,000	15,000,000	14.29%
Physician Revenue	170,000,000	160,000,000	10,000,000	6.25%
Total Patient Service Revenue	540,000,000	525,000,000	15,000,000	2.86%
Deductions From Revenue				
Blue Cross	26,000,000	25,000,000	1,000,000	4.00%
Medicare	58,000,000	57,000,000	1,000,000	1.75%
Medicaid	16,000,000	16,000,000	-	0.00%
Commercial	26,000,000	25,000,000	1,000,000	4.00%
Managed Care	25,000,000	25,000,000	-	0.00%
Contractual Allowance Reserve	9,500,000	9,500,000	-	0.00%
Total Deductions From Revenue	160,500,000	157,500,000	3,000,000	1.90%
Net Patient Service Revenue	379,500,000	367,500,000	12,000,000	3.27%
Other Revenue	10,000,000	9,500,000	500,000	5.26%
Total Revenue	389,500,000	377,000,000	12,500,000	3.32%
EXPENSES				
Salary & Fringe				
Physician Salary	60,000,000	59,500,000	500,000	0.84%
Staff Salary	125,000,000	124,000,000	1,000,000	0.81%
Physician Fringe	18,000,000	17,850,000	150,000	0.84%
Staff Fringe	31,250,000	31,000,000	250,000	0.81%
Total Salary & Fringe	234,250,000	232,350,000	1,900,000	0.82%
Medical Supplies	30,000,000	28,500,000	1,500,000	5.26%
Pharmaceuticals	15,000,000	14,000,000	1,000,000	7.14%
Utilities	8,000,000	7,500,000	500,000	6.67%
Insurance	7,000,000	6,500,000	500,000	7.69%
Purchased Service	14,000,000	14,000,000	-	0.00%
Other Expenses	28,000,000	27,500,000	500,000	1.82%
Depreciation	19,000,000	19,000,000	-	0.00%
Interest Expense	5,000,000	5,500,000	(500,000)	-9.09%
Provision for Bad Debt	16,000,000	15,750,000	250,000	1.59%
Total Expense	376,250,000	370,600,000	5,650,000	1.52%
Income From Operations	13,250,000	6,400,000	6,850,000	107.03%
NONOPERATING GAINS				
NonOperating Gains				
Unrestricted Gifts	400,000	500,000	(100,000)	-20.00%
Investment Income	12,000,000	13,000,000	(1,000,000)	-7.69%
Income from Affiliates	(200,000)	100,000	(300,000)	-300.00%
Unrealized Gain/Loss	(8,000,000)	(5,000,000)	(3,000,000)	60.00%
Total NonOperating Gains	4,200,000	8,600,000	(4,400,000)	-51.16%
Revenue & Gains in Excess of Expenses	17,450,000	15,000,000	2,450,000	16.33%

Table 31.14 Cash flow statement for an organization, September 2000

CASH FLOWS FROM OPERATING ACTIVITIES & GAINS

Revenue & Gains in Excess of Expenses	17,450,000
Depreciation & Amortization	19,000,000
Unrealized Gain/Loss	8,000,000
Decrease (Increase) in Accounts Receivable	(5,000,000)
Decrease (Increase) in Inventories	(500,000)
Increase (Decrease) in Contractual Allowance Reserve	2,000,000
Increase (Decrease) in Accounts Payable	(1,000,000)
Increase (Decrease) in Accrued Expenses	(1,000,000)
Net Cash Flow Provided by Operating Activities & Gains	38,950,000

CASH FLOWS FROM INVESTING ACTIVITIES

Purchase of Fixed Assets	(35,000,000)
Increase (Decrease) in Notes Payable	(5,500,000)
Increase (Decrease) in Capital Lease Obligations	(250,000)
Increase (Decrease) in Common Stock	-
Net Cash Provided by Investing Activities	(40,750,000)
Cash at Beginning of Reporting Period - 09/30/99	15,000,000
Cash at End of Reporting Period - 09/30/00	13,200,000

- Profitability ratios measure the combined effects of liquidity, asset management, and debt management policies on operating results.

Although the financial ratio values themselves, or their trends over time, provide useful information, their greater value is to compare them to industry averages. As an example, the automotive industry, with its well-established firms, will have a very different financial structure than firms in the Internet industry. A negative profitability ratio in the automotive industry would be viewed as a sign of poor financial health, but in the Internet industry it may not be so viewed (or, at least, so it was once thought). Table 31.15 contains the financial ratios for the financial statements shown in Tables 31.12 through 31.14.

Capital Financing

It is not unusual for an organization's capital needs to exceed its available cash generated from operations. Capital investments such as new buildings can rarely be funded solely from operating profits. To fund these investments, the company must turn to other sources for capital.

An organization's ability to access the capital markets, and just how much that capital will cost, depend on the company's credit rating. Rating agencies evaluate creditworthiness based on past and projected financial performance, an assessment of the management, and an evaluation of the external business environment, such as the market position of the organization and the quality of the medical staff.

Table 31.15 Ratio analysis for an organization, September 2000

Financial Ratios	Equation	September 30, 1999	Ratio	September 30, 2000	Ratio	Industry Average Ratio
LIQUIDITY RATIOS						
Current Ratio	Current Assets / Current Liabilities	152,000,000 / 33,000,000 =	4.6	145,200,000 / 30,500,000 =	4.8	4.0
Quick Ratio	Cash + Accts Receivable / Current Liabilities	95,000,000 / 33,000,000 =	2.9	96,200,000 / 30,500,000 =	3.2	3.0
ACTIVITY RATIOS						
Days in A/R	Accts Receivable X 365 / Sales	51,100,000,000 / 370,000,000 =	138	52,925,000,000 / 389,500,000 =	136	140
Days Cash on Hand	Cash + ST Investments / (Expense - Deprec) / 365	65,000,000 / 957,397 =	68	55,200,000 / 978,767 =	56	52
DEBT MANAGEMENT RATIOS						
Debt Ratio	Total Liabilities / Total Assets	124,000,000 / 409,000,000 =	30.32%	116,250,000 / 418,700,000 =	27.76%	35.00%
Times Interest Earned	Net Profit Before Interest / Interest Expense	10,150,000 / 5,000,000 =	2.0	12,450,000 / 5,000,000 =	2.5	1.5
PROFITABILITY RATIOS						
Return on Total Assets	Net Profit / Total Assets	15,150,000 / 409,000,000 =	3.70%	17,450,000 / 418,700,000 =	4.17%	3.50%
Return on Stockholder Equity	Net Profit / Stockholder Equity	15,150,000 / 285,000,000 =	5.32%	17,450,000 / 302,450,000 =	5.77%	7.00%
Return on Permanent Capital	Net Profit / Equity + LT Liabilities	15,150,000 / 376,000,000 =	4.03%	17,450,000 / 388,200,000 =	4.50%	4.00%
Profit Margin	Net Profit / Sales Revenue	15,150,000 / 370,000,000 =	4.09%	17,450,000 / 389,500,000 =	4.48%	6.00%

The primary vehicle for capital financing in healthcare is long-term debt. This debt may be from a bank in the form of a loan or a mortgage, which is a loan collateralized with real estate, or from a line of credit. The latter is more commonly used for short-term capital needs than for long-term needs. Tax-exempt organizations, which include most not-for-profit healthcare organizations, can issue debt in the form of long-term, tax-exempt bonds. The issue can be to the public or be placed privately directly with investors. These bonds pay a lower interest rate than taxable commercial bonds because of their tax advantage and therefore cost the issuing organization less. They must be issued by a state or a political subdivision of a state. The interest rate is a function of the credit rating of the organization and its ability to manage the debt. Two key ratios that rating services look at are the debt to equity ratio and the debt service coverage ratio. In our previous example (from Table 31.12), the debt to equity ratio is $95,000,000/$285,000,000 (the sum of the short-term portion of notes payable and the

long-term portion of notes payable divided by stockholder equity), or 0.33, and

$$\text{Debt service coverage} = \frac{(\text{Net income} + \text{depreciation} + \text{interest expense})}{(\text{Principal payments} + \text{interest expense})}$$

or ($17,450,000 + $19,000,000 + $5,500,000) / ($5,000,000 + $5,500,000) = 4.0

Purchasing bond insurance or having the bonds guaranteed by a financial institution may enhance creditworthiness. While one or both of these tactics may be necessary for companies with lower credit ratings, they come at a cost that must be weighed against the improvement in interest rate they achieve.

A second way to fund capital investment is through equity. A company takes this approach internally every time it uses its excess revenues over expenses to reinvest in the company. External equity financing results from the sale of stock, and therefore, a portion of ownership, in the company. This route is available to for-profit organizations only. Most companies can usually raise more capital through equity than they could through debt, but it generally costs more to do so, and there is the risk of loss of control if significant amounts of stock are sold.

An increasingly common way to fund capital projects in healthcare is through joint ventures, often between a not-for-profit organization and a for-profit company and frequently targeted at a specific market niche (such as esoteric laboratory testing). Another mechanism is through capital leases, whereby the lessee retains ownership of the asset at the end of the lease period (see previous section on capital acquisition).

Summary

In this chapter, we began with cost accounting and discussed the types and behaviors of costs. Direct costs are clearly associated with the item being costed, while all other costs are indirect. Behavior of costs relative to changes in volume can be variable (in direct proportion to volume) or fixed (constant regardless of volume) or some combination thereof. We reviewed how to measure full cost and how it differs from marginal cost, which is the change in total cost relative to a change in volume. An extensive costing example showed what data are needed to generate a cost analysis and how to cost a basic laboratory test.

Understanding the relationships among cost, volume, and profits allowed us to calculate contribution margin—the revenue per UOS less its marginal cost—and break-even point, which is total fixed cost divided by the contribution margin per UOS. These concepts were applied to an equipment purchase and to evaluating a capitation contract. The equipment purchase decision was then augmented by applying time value of money concepts to capital acquisition plans using the NPV and IRR calculations. These techniques allow for acquisitions with different future CF patterns to be compared in today's dollars. We looked at purchasing versus leasing and compared two pieces of equipment using these techniques.

We then turned to budget process and reviewed the three common types of budgets: the operating budget (which consists of a statistical, or volume, budget; a revenue budget; and an expense budget), the capital budget, and the cash budget. We learned the concepts of FTE and UOS, two key building blocks in budget development. We walked through the 10 steps of the budgeting process and illustrations of staffing and budget worksheets. With the budget as the baseline, we looked at management reporting and how to analyze the causes of differences in actual financial performance from budgeted amounts. We broke variances down into one of three causes: volume, price, or quantity variances. Finally, we discussed the importance of understanding which factor is responsible in order to direct the manager's response.

After a brief summary of basic accounting concepts and an example of how double entry accounting works, we learned about the three primary financial statements. The balance sheet is a snapshot of the company's financial condition at a given point in time and is a cumulative statement. The income statement reports the results of the company's operations over a period of time, while the CF statement presents the results of financial, as opposed to operating, management of the company. We used four types of financial ratios to reveal information about an organization's financial health from its financial statements: liquidity ratios, asset management ratios, debt management ratios, and profitability ratios. Ratios are best used in comparison to other companies in the same industry. Finally, we reviewed the basic ways a company raises capital from outside the organization.

KEY POINTS

- Cost accounting is an important tool for controlling expenses and making good resource allocation decisions.
- Marginal costs and the break-even point are relevant when considering taking on additional work.
- Capital investments, such as equipment purchases, require an NPV approach to decision making.
- Budget creation and monitoring should be vested in the managers responsible for implementing the changes that affect the budget.
- Regular variance analysis, especially in regard to labor, is critical to managing within a budget.
- Financial statements and their corollary financial ratios are useful for benchmarking against other organizations in the same industry.
- Successful capital financing can be obtained with strong financial statements that result from carefully crafted and managed budgets that are underpinned by a sound cost accounting system.

GLOSSARY

Accounts receivable Money that is owed to the firm by outsiders.

Accrual accounting System that records revenue and expenses as they occur.

Asset (and asset accounts) Represent the resources owned or used by the firm.

Asset management ratios Measure how effective the firm is at managing its assets.

Average cost Full cost divided by the unit of service.

Bad debt Recorded as an expense for gross charges that are deemed uncollectable from self-payors.

Balance sheet Shows assets on the left side and liabilities or claims against assets on the right side. The balance sheet shows a firm's financial position at a particular point in time.

Break-even point The level of activity at which revenue and total costs are exactly equal.

Capital budget The financial plan for the acquisition of capital assets.

Capital lease A lease in which the firm retains ownership of the asset at the end of the lease period.

Capital markets The markets for long-term debt and corporate stocks.

Capital The cash required to purchase the firm's property, plant, and equipment.

Capitation A reimbursement mechanism in which the service provider receives a fixed payment based on the number of covered lives. The payment does not fluctuate with the level of activity.

Cash accounting Records revenue and expenses when the cash has either been paid out or collected.

Cash budget The cash management plan for how the operational and capital budgets will be supported.

Cash flow (CF) Cash revenues less cash expenses; excludes non-cash expenses such as depreciation.

Cash flow statement Reports the impact on cash flow of a firm's operating, investing, and financing activities over a period of time.

Contractual allowances Discounts on gross charges given to third-party payors who have a negotiated contract with the billing provider.

Contribution margin The excess of revenue over variable costs.

Cost accounting A system of measuring and reporting information about cost.

Credit rating The creditworthiness of a firm based on past and projected financial performance, an assessment of the management, and the external business environment.

Debt management ratios Measure both the extent to which the firm is financed with borrowing and its likelihood of defaulting on its debt obligations.

Depreciation An annual charge of an asset's cost into each year of the asset's useful life, for assets that have a useful life of greater than 1 year.

Direct allocation Allocates costs of each service department directly and only to revenue-producing responsibility centers.

Direct cost A cost that can be traced to, or caused by, a particular service, product, segment, or activity of the department.

Discount rate The rate used to calculate the present value of future cash flows.

Equity Claims against, or interests in, the assets of a company, divided into liabilities and owners' equity.

Equity financing Results from the sale of stock, and therefore, a portion of the ownership in the company.

Expense budget The amount of resources that will be required to produce the forecasted activity.

Fiscal year The year on which the general ledger is based. It can be different from the calendar year. The fiscal year used by a firm is usually based on the norm of the industry to which it belongs.

Fixed budget A budget in which the budgeted amounts do not fluctuate with the volume.

Fixed costs Costs whose total remains constant regardless of changes in level of activity.

Flexible budget A budget in which the variable portion of the budget fluctuates with the level of volume.

Full-time equivalent (FTE) The proportion of an employee's paid hours per year to the standard labor measure, which is typically 2,080 h (5 days $\times$ 8 h $\times$ 52 weeks per year).

Fund accounting A form of accounting in which revenues and expenses must always be equal and expenses are stopped when revenue is exhausted.

Future value (FV) The amount to which a given amount of cash will grow at the end of a given period of time when compounded at a given rate of interest.

General ledger The system that records all accounting activity.

Generally accepted accounting principles (GAAP) The set of accounting rules established to bring consistency to accounting methods so that one firm's financial statements can be compared to another's.

Income statement Reports the financial results of a firm's operations over a period of time.

Incremental budgeting Uses prior year results as a basis for building the current year budget.

Indirect cost A cost that cannot be traced to a particular service, product, segment, or activity.

Interest rate The amount charged by lending institutions for the use of the money borrowed by a firm.

Internal rate of return (IRR) The rate that equates the present value of a project's expected cash inflows to the present value of the project's costs.

Liabilities (and liability accounts) Represent the debts or obligations owed to outsiders.

Liquidity ratios Measure the firm's ability to meet its immediate obligations; thus, the relationship between a firm's current assets and its current liabilities.

Long-term debt The firm's obligations that are due more than a year later.

Management reporting A process of communicating actual versus budgeted performance throughout the organization to identify necessary corrective actions and help make decisions.

Marginal cost The change in total cost relative to the change in volume, i.e., the cost of producing one more unit of service; incremental cost.

Natural credit balance accounts General ledger accounts that have negative balances as established by GAAP rules.

Natural debit balance accounts General ledger accounts that have positive balances as established by GAAP rules.

Net present value (NPV) The present value of future net cash flows, discounted at the cost of capital.

Nonproductive time Paid time for non-job-related activities such as vacation, holidays, and sick time.

Not-for-profits Companies whose primary purpose is something other than generating a profit. Typical not-for-profits are hospitals and charitable organizations. These organizations may make more money than they spend (excess revenue over costs), but there are no shareholders to receive that money, which instead may be donated or reinvested in the business.

Operating budget The financial plan for managers with direct responsibility for managing the operations of a responsibility center(s). The operating budget is made up of a statistical budget, a revenue budget, and an expense budget.

Overhead costs Costs that are from non-revenue-generating departments.

Owners' equity The ownership claim against the total assets of a company (also called stockholders' equity).

Present value (PV) The value today of a future cash flow.

Price variance The difference between the price of a supply or service versus the price that was budgeted.

Productive time Paid time for job-related activities.

Profitability ratios Measure the combined effects of liquidity, asset management, and debt management policies on operating results.

Quantity variance The difference between the amount of inputs (labor and/or supplies) used to produce each unit of service versus the quantity that was budgeted.

Required rate of return Known as the hurdle rate or cost of capital, it represents the minimum return on investment a firm requires on capital expenditures.

Revenue budget The revenue that will be generated by the forecasted activity for a responsibility center.

Semi-variable costs Costs that include both variable and fixed-cost elements.

Standard cost A measure of how much an item should cost, rather than a record of how much it actually did.

Statistical budget The forecast of activity for a responsibility center.

Step-down allocation Distributes the costs of the service departments providing the most services to all departments. All remaining service departments' costs are then allocated in descending order determined by the amount of service they render.

Step-fixed costs Costs that are fixed over a range of activity and are then increased when activity levels go up.

Stockholder equity accounts Represent the difference between a firm's assets and liabilities (claims against assets). The accounts are reported on the balance sheet and have natural credit balances.

Time value of money A concept that recognizes that a dollar of cash today is worth more than a dollar of cash to be received at some time in the future.

Unit of service (UOS) The logical measure of work for a given area. In the laboratory, it is usually either the number of billed tests or procedures performed.

Variable costs Items of cost that vary, in total, directly and proportionately with volume or level of activity changes.

Variance analysis The process of analyzing differences in actual versus budgeted performance to identify necessary corrective actions and help make decisions.

Volume variance The difference between the volume of services performed versus the volume that was budgeted.

Writeoffs Recorded reductions in revenue for gross charges that are deemed uncollectable from third-party payors.

Zero-based budgeting A budgeting methodology in which every expenditure must be justified regardless of the prior year's results.

REFERENCES

1. Finkler, S. A. 1994. *Cost Accounting for Health Care Organizations.* Aspen Publishers, Inc., Gaithersburg, Md.

2. Horngren, C. T. 1984. *Introduction to Management Accounting,* 6th ed. Prentice-Hall, Inc., Englewood Cliffs, N.J.

3. Joy, O. M. 1983. *Introduction to Financial Management,* 3rd ed. Richard D. Irwin, Inc., Homewood, Ill.

4. Richard D. Irwin, Inc., and E. J. Pavlock. 1994. *Financial Management for Medical Groups.* Englewood, Colo.

32

Financial Decision Making: the Endgame of the Planning and Analytical Process

Washington C. Winn, Jr.

OBJECTIVES

To place the financial decision-making process in the context of the laboratory and institution as a whole

To dissect the various stages of effective decision making, concentrating on the financial arena

To discuss some specific issues in the process

every cloud
has its silver
lining but it is
sometimes a little
difficult to get it to
the mint

DON MARQUIS, FROM "CERTAIN MAXIMS OF ARCHY," IN *ARCHY AND MEHITABEL*, 1927

FINANCIAL DECISION MAKING is more than a matter of money. The astute executive or manager will, at a minimum, bring all the issues discussed in this section to bear on the thought processes that lead to a final decision. Skills and techniques that are covered in virtually any aspect of management may be relevant. The reader should refer to "Relevant Economic and Business Concepts" by Ann L. Harris (chapter 3) and "Finance and Decision Making in Outreach" by Michael G. Bissell (chapter 37) when contemplating the universe of approaches to financial decision making.

This chapter will serve as a synthesis of the approaches considered in earlier chapters in the section. The goal is to connect the dots, not to reinvent them.

The Background for Financial Decision Making (Preanalytical Phase)

A sophisticated financial analysis may be technically accurate but completely misleading if all the critical elements of the process are not considered. In laboratory parlance, these factors could be characterized as preanalytical and postanalytical variables (Table 32.1). In the laboratory a technically superb determination of clinically significant antimicrobial resistance in an important human pathogen isolated from blood is rendered meaningless or worse if the specimen was mislabeled and actually came from another patient (preanalytical problem)

Table 32.1 Financial decision making at various stages

Preanalytical phase	Analytical phase	Postanalytical phase
Well-developed vision	Cost analysis	Implementation of decisions—capability of personnel
Realistic strategic plans	"Make vs. buy," "perform vs. send out," etc.	Involvement of multiple areas of the institution
Careful assessment of competitive environment	Budgeting	Monitoring results with benchmarking
Evaluation of the nature of the local institution	Variance analysis	
Communication among upper-level management, financial analysts, and scientific personnel	Communication between financial and scientific personnel	

or if the result never reaches the individual who must make a decision about treatment of the patient (postanalytical problem).

The preanalytical issues are a function of the quality of laboratory leadership. There must be a realistic and fully developed vision (as opposed to a "vision statement") of the goals, competitive position, and strategic aims of the laboratory to have informed financial decision making. There are dramatic differences in challenges and opportunities among organizations that are differently placed within the laboratory industry, as discussed by Lepoff in his introduction to this section (chapter 28). All of the challenges noted by Valenstein in his discussion of strategic planning (chapter 29) pertain to defining the problems that will be addressed during the decision-making process. In other words, the preanalytical phase is a function of the quality of leadership at both the organizational and departmental levels. These issues, addressed in section II of this book, include vision, leadership, and communication of the issues both up and down the organizational structure.

The Financial Decision-Making Process Itself (Analytical Phase)

Once the goals have been established and communicated effectively, it is time for the actual analysis. The extensive discussion of cost concepts by Tolzmann and Vincent (chapter 31) serves as a primer for the major techniques that must be brought to bear on the subject. They have essentially provided a "financial MBA in a capsule," so it is no surprise that putting their examples to work in a particular laboratory will take a lot of work and an equal amount of experience. Once again, effective communication is the key to success. Sophisticated analysis of data must be coupled with an understanding of the scientific issues. A broadly trained individual who has both diagnostic and financial expertise can accomplish the linkage. However, a team of laboratory workers and financial analysts can also accomplish the task equally successfully. Who the individuals are is less important than their intelligence, creativity, and ability to communicate with all the affected parties. The collaboration probably works best if the financial personnel are formally a part of the labora-

tory even if their official home is in the front office. With the right culture and the right people, however, the parties may be based in different areas of the organization.

Implementation of Financial Decision Making (Postanalytical Phase)

Once again, communication is the key to success. If the analyst and effector are the same person, there should be no difficulty understanding what needs to be done. If the parties are several, it is critical that the line managers who will implement the decisions understand the rationale for the processes, comprehend the analysis, understand what needs to be done for implementation, and feel free to express concerns or suggestions for improvement in either the preanalytical or analytical phase.

Multiple sectors of the laboratory will be involved in implementation. Many of those involved will have scientific backgrounds and will typically be line managers and supervisors. Others will be members of the administrative sections of the laboratory or of administration. These individuals may be in marketing, outreach, or compliance divisions, to name just a few. These issues are addressed in this volume, in sections on Managerial Leadership (section II), Personnel Management (section III), and Requirements for Effective Laboratory Management (section IV), as well as in this section (chapter 30).

Finally, there must be established processes for monitoring the success (or lack thereof) of the results. Some of these indicators will be obvious to the financial analysts. Others may be achieved through benchmarking (section IX), by internal or external comparisons.

Some Specific Issues in Financial Decision Making

Cost Accounting and Pricing

The scientific managers who know the requirements for labor and materials better than anyone else must do costing of laboratory tests. Pricing, however, is a more complex process that requires input from scientific managers, marketing personnel, strategic planners, and compliance personnel (to ensure that the other parties do not make inappropriate and potentially risky decisions). Cost has to be considered, but which cost is another matter entirely. Is it direct cost, fully loaded cost, marginal cost, etc.? Ultimately, pricing decisions are as much strategic decisions as they are financial ones, if not more so. Offering tests at marginal cost may be a wise strategic plan, but if everything is on the margin, there will be no margin!

When analyzing performance of costing activities, the issues raised in the discussion of benchmarking (chapter 43) come into play. Analyzing performance at the level of the individual test will be less accurate—and usually, therefore, less instructive—than analyzing costs that have been rolled up to the level of a section, division, or even the laboratory as a whole. Similarly, the concept of analysis by unit of service that is critical to benchmarking is also relevant here.

Break-Even Analysis and Capital Acquisition

The keys to success in break-even analysis and capital acquisition are that the options evaluated by the financial analysts are the correct ones and that all of the appropriate choices have been included. If the house is not built on solid ground, the structural integrity assured by the architect and engineer may not be enough to prevent disaster. It goes without saying that the assumptions (often based on marketing data or perceived need) must also be on target.

Budgeting

Budgets are useful tools if applied appropriately. If the assumptions are realistic and honest, the budget will be a useful tool for measuring performance. If the driving forces behind the budget are strategic or political rather than market-based, disastrous results may ensue. Only in government can one get away with "political budgets," and even that assertion is open to legitimate question.

There is no question that capital budgets are a necessity. Each institution must decide how much money it has to spend on infrastructure, operational tools, and physical structures (bricks and mortar). After that decision has been made, the requests of each manager, rolled up to the departmental level, can be evaluated rationally in light of institutional priorities, strategic priorities, and available resources. It is difficult to conceive of an institution surviving without a capital budget.

Operational budgets, however, are another matter entirely. Some administrators swear by them; others see them as will-o-the-wisps or, worse still, smoke and mirrors. The problem can be encapsulated by looking at an actual budget that differs substantially from the proposed budget, either positively or negatively (budget variance). There are, of course, two possibilities: (i) the managers did not perform as expected (whether better or worse), or (ii) the budget was unrealistic at the outset and the managers performed in the only way available to them. Naturally, no one worries too much about a positive budget variance; in fact, they should, because even a positive variance indicates that there are problems with the ability of the decision makers in the organization to predict the future.

The naysayers maintain that an approach that is superior to an operational budget is continuous monitoring of performance (essentially internal benchmarking, as discussed in chapter 43). Whether the monitoring approach is used or a formal operational budget is adopted, results will be more meaningful if performance is analyzed in terms of an objective unit of service (used prominently in benchmarking methodology). For the monitoring group the goal is to maintain constant pressure on operational performance, always striving for better performance than was achieved in the previous time periods. For the budget group, use of units of service results in a volume-driven operational budget that has the advantages of flexibility and responsiveness.

Capital Financing

The area of capital financing is usually reserved for the corporate office and the boardroom. It will be less relevant at the level of individual departments and divisions. The same principles of consonance with vision and strategic analysis still apply, just on a more ethereal plane. In the lower atmosphere, managers can only pray that there isn't an ozone hole at the top.

Summary

The process of financial decision making is unitarian. All aspects of management must be brought to bear to have any hope of success. Vision, strategic planning, leadership, and motivation are all essential. To paraphrase real estate agents, the critical matter is "communication, communication, communication."

KEY POINTS

- The process of financial decision making can be divided into three stages, analogous to laboratory testing.
- The preanalytical phase is the province of institutional and laboratory management. It requires clear delineation of vision, strategic planning based on that vision, and a realistic assessment of competitive forces in the global and local marketplace.
- The analytical phase consists of the nuts and bolts of financial analysis. It is essential that the analysts understand laboratory medicine and/or communicate effectively with someone who does.
- The postanalytical phase is the implementation stage. It requires the coordination of many different parts of the institution and depends on having well-trained, motivated personnel.
- Success in financial decision making can be achieved if all three phases are mastered, coordination is maintained, and communication is both regular and of high quality.

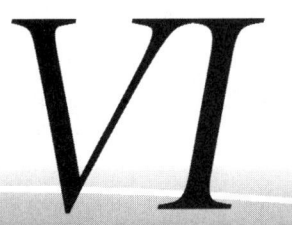

Generation of Revenue

(Section Editors, *Vickie S. Baselski and Alice S. Weissfeld*)

33

Correct Coding of Billable Services in the Clinical Laboratory

Vickie S. Baselski, Alice S. Weissfeld, and Fran Sorrell

OBJECTIVES

To explain the importance of using the standardized coding systems recognized by the payors

To discuss laboratory responsibilities to ensure that correct and complete coding has been done

To describe the importance of the ICD-9-CM coding system and its relationship to proper billing

To discuss the fundamental principles of correct and complete coding

Let the good service of well-deservers be never rewarded with loss. Let their thanks be such as may encourage more strivers for the like.

ELIZABETH I (1533–1603), QUEEN OF ENGLAND (1558–1603)

THE PRIMARY GOAL OF LABORATORY MEDICINE is to provide a variety of laboratory services which facilitate the role of physicians and other direct healthcare providers in the prevention, diagnosis, and treatment of diseases by generating data upon which clinical decisions are made. In fact, it has been estimated that although laboratory medicine accounts for only 5 to 7% or less of total health care costs, the information generated drives 60 to 70% of subsequent resource utilization and is estimated to direct at least 80% of all clinical decision making. In turn, laboratory payments constitute a very low percentage of actual payments to healthcare providers. For example, laboratory services represent only 1.6% of program spending for Medicare Part B outpatient healthcare services. By any standard, this figure demonstrates that laboratory medicine services are a bargain as well as a critical component in the provision of healthcare services. This goal also categorizes the critical parameters that one must specify in accounting for laboratory services: (i) the actual laboratory service (i.e., what test procedures the laboratory performed), (ii) the clinical reason for performing the laboratory service (i.e., why the test procedures were performed), and (iii) the specific laboratory location (i.e., in which laboratory the work was performed). For each of these parameters, the laboratory must use a standard language to communicate with payors and for use in benchmarking comparisons of practices to assess efficiency and effectiveness of services provided.

Procedure Coding: What Test Procedures Have Been Performed?

A number of procedure coding systems have been developed to standardize the documentation of services rendered for financial purposes, although in fact, one particular system is primarily used in the United States and is also in use in many other countries. The predominant procedure coding system is the Current Procedural Terminology system, 4th edition (CPT-4). This system is recognized by the United States federal healthcare payment programs (i.e., Medicare and Medicaid) as the official coding system and has been adopted in entirety as the federal procedure coding system known as the Healthcare Common Procedure Coding System (HCPCS). For procedures or practices not yet defined by a CPT-4 code, HCPCS codes may be established which are used until a CPT-4 code is available. The CPT system is recognized by all other major third-party payors; thus, it is an oft-stated adage that "as goes Medicare, so go others." The CPT system has also recently been named as the Standard Electronic Healthcare Transaction Code Set for procedures under the Health Insurance Portability and Accountability Act of 1996. However, it should be recognized that alternatives do exist, and it was a recommendation of the recent Institute of Medicine report *Medicare Laboratory Payment Policy, Now and in the Future* that "HCFA (Healthcare Financing Administration, now known as the Centers for Medicare and Medicaid Services, CMS) should review alternatives to the current system for coding outpatient clinical laboratory services for claims processing. More accurate, open, and timely coding processes for new technologies as well as tests and services should be sought." Thus, general familiarity with alternatives (e.g., International Classification of Diseases, Version 10, Procedure Coding System [ICD-10-PCS], Logical Observation Identifier Names and Codes [LOINC]) is recommended (3, 10).

The CPT-4 System

Description

The CPT-4 system, a proprietary product of the American Medical Association (AMA), is a listing of five-digit descriptors and numeric or alphanumeric identifiers which are used for documentation of services rendered (Table 33.1). The system was first developed in 1966 and is currently in its fourth edition. The purpose of CPT is to provide a uniform language that accurately describes medical, surgical, and diagnostic services for financial and administrative purposes and to serve as a standard means of identifying and documenting services performed. These codes are multifunctional and serve as the basis for service order documentation and procedure resulting, claim and invoice generation and billing, fee-for-service payment schedules, development of edits that assess the appropri-

Table 33.1 The CPT-4 system

Definition............	The CPT-4 system is a proprietary product of the AMA and is a listing of five-digit descriptors and numeric or alphanumeric identifiers, which are used for documentation of services rendered.
	A "billable service" may be defined as one that is CPT-4 codable.
Purpose..............	The purpose of CPT is to provide a uniform language that accurately describes medical, surgical, and diagnostic services for financial and administrative purposes.
	CPT serves as a standard means of identifying and documenting services performed.
Code uses	Serve as the basis for service order documentation and procedure resulting
	Claim and invoice generation and billing
	Fee-for-service payment schedules
	Development of edits that assess the appropriateness of payment for the service
	Assessing the productivity of laboratories in providing services
	Utilization review and outcomes in specific clinical situations

ateness of payment for the service, assessing the productivity of laboratories in providing services, and utilization review and outcomes assessment in specific clinical situations (4). All aspects of effective financial management of the clinical laboratory begin with correct and complete coding for all services rendered (8). In essence, a "billable service" may be defined as one that is CPT-4 codable.

Types of CPT-4 Codes

All generally accepted laboratory service codes, termed category I codes, are found in a specific pathology and laboratory section which includes both clinical laboratory and anatomic services (Table 33.2). Clinical laboratory services are further divided into discipline-specific subsections (e.g., chemistry, hematology, immunology, transfusion medicine, microbiology). In addition, both technical testing services and professional, physician-provided services may be coded. In general, category I codes represent services that are performed by many healthcare professionals in multiple locations throughout the United States that have received Food and Drug Administration clearance or approval, if required, and that have been shown to have clinical efficacy. Technical category I codes are of several types. Primary codes are those that denote a specific procedure. Add-on codes are those that are performed in addition to a primary code and are indicated by a "+" symbol or by the descriptor language "use in addition to" Organ- or disease-oriented panels represent AMA-approved and Centers for Medicare and Medicaid Services (CMS)-accepted test groupings that are coded as a single

Table 33.2 Types of CPT-4 codes

Category I	All generally accepted laboratory service codes; found in the specific pathology and laboratory section (includes both clinical laboratory and anatomic services)
	Divided into specific subsections (e.g., chemistry, hematology, immunology, transfusion medicine, microbiology)
	Represents services that are performed by many healthcare professionals in multiple locations throughout the United States that have received FDA[a] clearance or approval, if required, and that have been shown to have clinical efficacy
Category II	Developed for performance measurement tools
	Initially released in 2003, with annual updates planned
	Currently, there are no Category II codes which specifically address laboratory practices.
	Use is optional and nonessential for correct coding.
Category III	Were implemented in 2001
	Designed to be a temporary code set for procedures that represent emerging technologies not yet meeting the requirements for assignment of a category I code
	Currently, there are several category III codes that describe laboratory procedures.

[a]FDA, Food and Drug Administration.

billable test and are generally performed conveniently as such on automated instruments. Technical services are generally subject to payment under a defined fee schedule which is updated on a regular basis.

Professional services are identified by specific CPT-4 codes found in the anatomic pathology and cytology subsections, and by two specific codes in a clinical pathology consultation section. In addition, for a few specific clinical laboratory codes requiring clinical interpretation, one may attach a two-digit modifier indicating that the code has both a technical and a professional component that may each be billed by different entities. Coding and billing for professional services are generally subject to payment under a defined fee schedule which is developed through a resource-based relative value system (6, 7, 9).

Category II codes and category III codes are a new component of the CPT system which were developed as a component of the CPT-5 (5th edition) project (Table 33.2). Category II codes were developed for performance measurement tools and were initially released in 2003, with annual updates planned. They are designed to track best practices associated with specific clinical conditions and are thus similar conceptually to Healthplan Employer Data and Information Set (HEDIS) monitors, which are widely used by managed-care plans. However, at this point there are no category II codes which specifically address laboratory practices, although laboratory test use

may be a component of the best practice algorithm associated with a specific category II code. At this time, the use of category II codes is optional and nonessential for correct coding.

Category III codes were implemented in 2001 and are designed to be a temporary code set for procedures that represent emerging technologies not yet meeting the requirements for assignment of a category I code. They are intended to be used to track utilization of these types of procedures and are updated biannually. It is possible that a category III code may eventually satisfy criteria for assignment of a category I code. However, from a correct-coding perspective, if a category III code is available, it must be used. There are currently several category III codes that describe laboratory procedures.

Modifiers

Modifiers are another important component of the CPT system. Modifiers are comprised of two-digit numbers which are attached to a specific code prior to the billing process (Table 33.3) (2). They are "used to indicate that a service or procedure has been altered by some specific circumstance but not changed in its definition or code." In laboratory medicine, there are several modifiers that are critical. The modifier "-26" is used when a certain procedure is a combination of a physician component and a technical component. This modifier for "professional component" is only applicable in selected circumstances, usually involving inpatients, when the professional "interpretative" component is reported separately.

Table 33.3 CPT-4 modifiers

-26	Certain procedures are a combination of a physician component and a technical component; this modifier for "professional component" is applicable only in selected circumstances, usually involving inpatients, when the professional "interpretative" component is reported separately.
-91	Repeat clinical diagnostic test performed on the same patient, on the same type of specimen from the same date of service, to obtain subsequent reportable and clinically useful test values; this modifier may not be used when tests are rerun to confirm initial results (due to testing problems with specimens or equipment) or for any other reason when a normal, one-time reportable result is all that is required.
-59	This modifier (distinct procedural service) identifies distinct and separate multiple services of the same type on the same date of service that "are not normally reported together but are appropriate under the circumstances." This modifier generally refers to different encounters with the same patient or different anatomic sites.
-90	Modifier -90 is used to indicate that a laboratory has referred a procedure it is billing to a reference laboratory. In order to use this code, laboratories must follow a 70-30 rule, which states that no more than 30% of total testing is referred out.

Duplicate services of the same type on the same type of specimen from the same date of service are generally not reimbursed but may be appropriate if modified with "-91" (repeat clinical diagnostic test performed on the same day to obtain subsequent reportable and clinically useful test values). However, this modifier may not be used when tests are rerun to confirm initial results (due to testing problems with specimens or equipment), or for any other reason when a normal, one-time, reportable result is all that is required.

Modifier "-59" (distinct procedural service) identifies distinct and separate multiple services of the same type on the same date of service that "are not normally reported together but are appropriate under the circumstances." This modifier generally refers to different encounters with the same patient or different anatomic sites. Modifier "-59" is also used to report services that may be considered a component of another service but have been carried out in a distinctly unrelated fashion. The modifier is not appropriate if a procedure is repeated due to analytical error or to confirm or verify a result.

Modifier "-90" is used to indicate that a laboratory has referred a procedure it is billing to a reference laboratory. In order to use this code, laboratories must follow a "70-30" rule which states that no more than 30% of total testing is referred out.

Laboratorians must also be familiar with a two-digit alpha character HCPCS modifier set to denote situations for which a CPT modifier does not exist. Modifier "-QW" is used to indicate that a procedure being performed in a Clinical Laboratory Improvement Amendments (CLIA)-waived-status laboratory has received a waiver to be performed as such from the CLIA Committee. Very important are a series of HCPCS modifiers which indicate the status of the acquisition of a "waiver of financial liability" (termed an advance beneficiary notice [ABN]) from the patient. It is of note that in 2002, a laboratory-specific ABN was approved by CMS which cannot be a component of a requisition. An ABN should be obtained whenever it is likely that a service does not meet Medicare payment rules and is therefore likely to be denied.

Use of modifier "-GA" is mandatory and indicates that Medicare is not likely to pay for a service and the patient has signed an ABN. Modifier "-GZ" is optional and indicates that Medicare is not likely to pay for a service but the patient has not signed an ABN. Modifier "-GY" indicates that a service is statutorily excluded from payment and the patient has acknowledged financial responsibility by signing an ABN.

The Process for Change

Since laboratory procedures are constantly evolving, particularly with the emergence of new technology, it is necessary for the CPT-4 system to undergo regular updates (Table 33.4). Updates, which add, delete, and modify existing codes, are issued on an annual basis after an extensive and systematic review process which begins with the submission of a coding change request form by any individual, professional group, or corporation. Each request undergoes a complete review by AMA-appointed specialty committees, general CPT committees (the CPT Advisory Committee and the Health Care Professionals Advisory Committee), and ultimately the CPT Editorial Panel. The time frame to effect a change is usually 15 months or more, with new codes being released in midsummer since 2001, and the completely updated CPT-4 manual released electronically first and then in hard copy in October. Federal payors generally accept new codes beginning in January, with mandatory use by 1 April (1). Other third-party payors generally follow the same timeline, but there may on occasion be disconnects.

HCPCS codes are also published annually but may be developed and issued at any time it is deemed necessary to supplement the CPT system.

Table 33.4 Process and schedules for CPT code revisions

Timing	Action
18 mo prior	Code changes are proposed.
18 to 9 mo prior	Proposals are reviewed by multiple AMA committees
	Healthcare Professionals Advisory Committee
	AMA CPT Advisory Committee and Subcommittees
	AMA CPT Editorial Board
Review schedule	
February prior	Final changes for the next calendar year are approved by CPT editorial board.
Summer prior	Early release of new codes for determination of reimbursement
October prior	Publication of the new edition for the upcoming year
1 January	Medicare implementation of new codes unless instructions specify otherwise
1 April	Date for mandatory use of new codes for federal payment programs
October–1 April	Panic time! Frantic efforts to verify codes, perform new cost analyses, change information systems, etc.

Procedure Coding Guidance

The selection and verification of CPT-4 codes are performed annually, coincident with the release of annual changes by the AMA. Correct coding is clearly the responsibility of the laboratory in which the technical knowledge of the current procedures resides. There is an established hierarchy for choice of codes which places analyte first, followed by method, and then finally the use of a generic "not otherwise specified" code. If no match for analyte and method can be found, then an "unlisted code" (usually ending with "—99") is available. However, as specificity of coding decreases, the probability that a code will not be reimbursed without submission of additional documentation increases. One should also review current HCPCS codes to determine if the procedure in question is located there. One should also ensure that one does not "unbundle codes," that is, select multiple individual codes rather than a comprehensive single code (e.g., when coding for panels). Further, the National Correct Coding Initiative directs that for federal payor programs, "multiple tests to identify the same analyte, marker, or infectious agent should not be reported separately." Keep in mind that the same guiding principles generally apply to other third-party payors.

Procedure Coding Alternatives

The CPT system is obviously firmly entrenched in laboratory management as the primary tool for procedure coding and subsequent billing of laboratory services. However, there are alternatives that may gain wider use at a future date. Foremost among these is a system known as LOINC (10). With input from a consortium of laboratories, information system vendors, hospitals, and academic institutions, the grant-supported Regenstrief Institute developed and maintains LOINC. LOINC is considered a universal laboratory language which is based on the systematic breakdown of the components of a service into more specific units, ultimately creating a highly standardized, typically seven-digit, number, with each possible result from a procedure being mapped to a specific code. The breakdowns take into consideration where performed, the specific analyte type, the method, and the type of result. Unlike CPT, LOINC is publicly available and can be used with no license fee. It is widely used by commercial laboratories to track specific procedures from order to result.

The LOINC system actually formed the basis for the development of the CMS ICD-10-PCS laboratory coding system intended for use as an alternative to CPT (3). This system was developed by 3M under contract to the Health Care Financing Administration (CMS), with substantial input from specialty professional groups. It was finalized and released in 1999 but has remained inactive, as CPT has continued to be used as the "official" procedure code set.

Capitated Services

Beginning in the 1980s, a trend toward paying capitated, or predetermined, amounts for management of a specific disease or in a specific clinical circumstance rapidly emerged (12). This trend began with the development of diagnosis-related groups (DRGs) under Medicare to classify reasons for hospitalization where payment amounts were defined based not on the actual procedures performed but on the final diagnosis, while in other capitated payor plans, hospitalizations were paid for on a per-diem basis. Subsequently, this concept was extended to cover all outpatient healthcare costs, and managed-care plans emerged which paid for all required services under terms like "per member per month" or "per covered life." Finally, Medicare recognized special categories of patients, for whom payments were similarly categorized by the condition or situation of the patient and not by a compilation of individual procedures. Examples may be found in payment for services to patients in skilled nursing facilities (SNF) or being treated in dialysis centers for end-stage renal disease (ESRD). Most recently, Medicare has similarly initiated an outpatient prospective payment system based on defined ambulatory payment classifications (APCs). Needless to say, other third-party payors find inpatient payment by this method to be financially gratifying, and Medicare is seeking to move outpatients into managed-care situations. In other words, the trend is definitely to try to find ways to minimize payment for services.

Under capitated or prospective payment systems, laboratories may find themselves in the situation of representing financial liabilities rather than revenue generators. To balance this perception, it is equally important for laboratories to utilize mechanisms to document all work performed in a given clinical condition. Therefore, correct coding is also a key to success in capitated payment situations. Knowledge of the exact amount of work performed per DRG or APC allows one to justify the allocation of a specific proportion of the total payment to the laboratory. This also allows one to "carve out," or specifically exclude, unique high-cost niche test procedures from the contract. Thus, even in capitated payment situations, laboratorians should seek to code correctly for every laboratory procedure performed.

Diagnosis Coding: Why Is the Service Being Performed?

As previously stated, the purpose of laboratory testing is to facilitate the management of a patient by a physician or other authorized healthcare provider. Thus, to accurately and completely document laboratory testing for both financial and clinical purposes, it is important to also document the reason(s) for performing the test. This, too, requires the use of a standardized and systematic approach if maximum information is to be readily obtained for administrative and financial purposes. The systems currently in use take into account the patient environment (inpatient versus outpatient) as well as the actual diagnosis, signs and symptoms, or other reason for the encounter. It is now both a statutory requirement for Medicare as well as a generally accepted requirement for other third-party payors to provide diagnostic information for claim review prior to payment for services. The information is used to verify that a procedure is clinically necessary for payment purposes and to determine if it is clinically appropriate and useful for patient management in utilization review. It should also be acknowledged that provision of specific diagnostic information with each orderable and billable test is useful in the laboratory to ensure appropriate sample handling.

Inpatient Diagnosis Coding

For inpatient purposes, the DRG system has already been mentioned. Effective in 1983, this system assigns a final diagnosis to each patient admitted to the hospital. Currently more than 500 DRGs have been defined which take into account clinical condition or reason for admission, medical responses, and presence or absence of complications. Each DRG is weighted according to relative costs, inclusive of laboratory costs (although the actual laboratory component is generally quite low), and payment schedules are published annually for a January implementation date. DRGs are now used by many third-party payors to determine payment rates and are the primary basis for developing algorithms for cost-effective management of the condition specified by the DRG. These algorithms are known as "critical pathways," "clinical pathways," or "care paths" and often include delineation of laboratory tests, which should be performed and when (11). Coding of these tests provides the laboratory a means to track utilization as well as costs.

Such tracking has become very important recently, as CMS has begun investigating why certain specific DRGs are consistently increasing both in relative proportion of total admissions and in percentage of total costs in a project dubbed "Project DRG Creep."

One other critical parameter in coding for inpatient procedures pertains to the DRG payment window. At present, any procedure performed by an affiliated laboratory 3 days or less prior to an admission is deemed to be a component of the payment for the admission DRG that should not be billed separately. However, it is still in the laboratory's best interest to continue to code for these procedures to document the actual work performed. Physician professional services are not included in the DRG but are billed separately.

Outpatient Diagnosis Coding

Recently, Medicare has initiated a prospective payment program for outpatient visits similar to the DRG system. As previously discussed, this prospective payment system is based on APCs. However, at this point, laboratory payments are excluded from the APC payments, and tests continue to be billed on a fee-for-service basis. It is likely that at some point in the future, to control costs, the prospective payment may be modified to include laboratory services.

ICD-9-CM

The primary coding system for documentation of the reason for a patient encounter is the International Classification of Diseases, 9th Revision (Clinical Modification) (ICD-9-CM). Whereas the ICD-10 system classifies mortality data in a standardized manner, the ICD-9-CM system classifies morbidity data. The term "clinical" is used to denote its almost universal use to classify morbidity data for medical records, for medical care review, and for basic health and utilization statistics. It is the official CMS system for assigning codes for clinical conditions associated with consequent medical procedures, including laboratory testing. The system is maintained by a consortium of professional clinical medicine groups, professional medical record groups, the National Center for Health Statistics, CMS, and the World Health Organization. Updates are made on a quarterly basis and published for public use. An updated version, ICD-10-CM, was approved in 1998, but implementation has been delayed. The ICD-9-CM is comprised of a tabular numerical list of more than 10,000 codes for diagnoses, signs and symptoms, and clinical conditions or reasons for a physician encounter with a patient as well as an alphabetical list for convenience. It includes both disease conditions and preventative medical reasons for encounters, exposures, and sources of external injury. It also includes a classification system for surgical, diagnostic, and therapeutic procedures.

SNOMED CT

A new clinical coding initiative has recently been completed and released by the College of American Pathologists called SNOMED CT, which is an acronym for a comprehensive and precise "Systematized Nomenclature of Medicine Clinical Terminology." This system was developed in conjunction with the United Kingdom's National Health Service and is expected to gain international acceptance. The system is designed to easily map to other diagnostic terminology systems, but it is unique in its ability to show expected and logical relationships between clinical conditions (5). For example, by the ICD-9-CM a foot ulcer may have diabetes as a contributing diagnosis, but by SNOMED, it is a diabetic foot ulcer. Like the College of American Pathologists' other major coding product, CPT-4, SNOMED will be subject to regular updates and will require a licensing fee for use.

Revenue Codes

The last major issue in correct coding is the assignment of credit for the work performed as well as credit for the revenue generated to the entity performing or billing the services. In most large laboratories, there are multiple departments performing testing, and it is necessary to assign each entity designated as an independent financial center a unique identifier for financial analysis purposes.

Role of CLIA and State Licensing

Under CLIA, each laboratory has a unique license number that validates its status as a billing entity for federal healthcare programs. In fact, most other paying entities also use CLIA licensure as an indicator of the operational validity of the laboratory. Laboratories may only bill for work performed that is compatible with the CLIA service level that they are assigned unless the laboratory is billing reference work properly modified as previously discussed with modifier "-90" and not exceeding 30% of the test volume. Many states also have stringent facility licensing requirements, and in those states, a billing entity must also have the correct state status. CLIA and some states require the license number to appear on claims.

Revenue Codes

Revenue codes comprise a system for categorizing and billing services which is recognized by CMS and most third-party payors. This system is maintained by the National Uniform Billing Committee of the American Hospital Association and is designed to standardize major revenue-producing centers in an institutional setting, particularly hospitals. For each test performed and charge code billed, the institution should determine which revenue code is most appropriate to assign credit. Both charge codes, which map to CPTs, and revenue codes, which map to actual testing location, must appear on claims.

Documentation of Codes

Two types of documents are important in the billing and reimbursement process which allow for the documentation of the procedure, diagnosis, and revenue center appropriate to the testing. First is the requisition, which documents both the order and the diagnosis, and the claim form or invoice, which allows transmission of the bill to a payor. The revenue codes are generally linked to charge codes and appear primarily in financial reports, but they are also required on federal claim forms.

Requisition

Requisitions may be manual (hard copy) or electronic but should be designed to facilitate the capture of all of the required data for accurate processing of an order as well as effective processing of a claim or invoice. Standard elements include demographics for the patient, billing information, ordering provider contact and authenticity information (the unique provider identification number), date of service, and a menu of tests which may be ordered. The

test menu should map to CPT-4 coding information and to diagnostic information justifying payment by a third-party agency, and it should identify those tests requiring an ABN. Any test groupings not strictly defined as a panel by the AMA and any standard reflex protocols should also be clearly delineated. Of course, each orderable test should also have an easily accessible reference defining specimen requirements and clinical utility as well.

Claims

Claims submitted to third-party payors are now commonly electronic in nature, but they may also be done as a manual process. It is also common to engage an independent contractor to perform procedure billings due to the complexity of the process. In any case, claim forms have remarkable similarity in that they all depend on the use of standard coding nomenclature for patient identification, provider identification, laboratory identification, procedures including modifiers, diagnoses, and revenue centers. The forms used by the Medicare program serve as a model for format of claims. The UB-92 is the form required by Medicare for laboratory services submitted through the fiscal intermediary, and the HCFA-1500 is the form required by Medicare Part B for claims submitted to the contractor. Failure to complete all required information on either the requisition or the claim form may result in failure to be reimbursed for otherwise payable services.

Summary

It is of paramount importance for the documentation of services rendered that laboratories employ the standardized coding systems recognized by the payors. While use of each code set is subject to general guidelines provided by the maintaining entity, it is ultimately the responsibility of the laboratory to ensure that correct and complete coding has been done. This pertains particularly to assignment of correct CPT-4 codes for delineation of services and verification that they map to the assigned charge code as well as the determination of circumstances in which appropriate modifiers may be used. Documentation of the ICD-9-CM code provided by the ordering provider is absolutely required for claim processing and may be the responsibility of the laboratory. However, in general, DRGs and APCs are assigned by medical record professionals within institutions, and revenue codes are assigned by appropriate finance personnel within an institution; but it still remains the responsibility of the laboratory to understand the importance of these coding systems to their operations and to verify assignments of codes when appropriate. Without a doubt, all other aspects of billing and reimbursement processes begin with a solid understanding of and application of fundamental principles of correct and complete coding.

KEY POINTS

- It is mandatory that laboratories use standardized coding systems, which are recognized by the payors for documentation of services rendered.

- Although each code set is subject to general guidelines, it is the responsibility of the laboratory to verify that correct and complete coding has been done.

- Documentation of the ICD-9-CM code provided by the ordering provider is required for claim processing and may be the responsibility of the laboratory.

- It is the laboratory's responsibility to understand all aspects of correct and complete coding principles.

GLOSSARY

Advance beneficiary notice A waiver of liability used by the provider to notify Medicare beneficiaries prior to receiving service that it may not be a covered service and that they may have to assume financial responsibility.

Bundling To place codes together in a panel.

Capitation A predetermined, fixed amount paid to providers in return for rendering a specified set of health services. The rate is established per person (per capita) enrolled in the health plan.

Carriers Centers for Medicare and Medicaid Services (CMS) primary third-party contractors who administer Part B payments according to the local medical review policies (LMRP) to physician, ancillary, and commercial laboratory providers.

Carve out To exclude from a capitated contract and bill as fee for service.

Claim The claim form or invoice, which allows transmission of the bill to a payor.

Covered lives Population insured by a managed-care contract.

Current Procedural Terminology, 4th edition (CPT-4) Test codes recognized by the American Medical Association and required for filing claims and billing of Medicare.

Diagnosis code Medical diagnoses are assigned a number code from a book titled International Classification of Diseases, 9th Revision (Clinical Modifications) (ICD-9-CM). The ICD-9-CM code refers to the patient's medical diagnosis.

Diagnosis-related groups (DRGs) Classification system developed at Yale that defines almost 400 major diagnostic categories and places patients into case types based on the ICD-9-CM classifications.

Downcode The use of a lower-reimbursed test, generally coupled with rebundling, to induce unnecessary utilization.

Eligibility/Medicare Part A Federally managed health insurance plan covering Americans over age 65 and Americans under age 65 who have certain disabilities and for most patients with end-stage renal disease (ESRD); established by a 1965 amendment to the Social Security Act. Part A covers hospitalization.

Eligibility/Medicare Part B Federally managed health insurance plan covering Americans over age 65 and Americans under age 65 who have certain disabilities and for most patients with ESRD; established by a 1965 amendment to the Social Security Act. Part B provides supplementary coverage for medical service and supplies, including physician services, outpatient services, and certain home healthcare services, as well as diagnostic laboratory tests and services, X rays, and the purchase and rental of durable medical equipment.

End-stage renal disease (ESRD) The terminology used for Medicare beneficiaries who have permanent kidney dysfunction requiring dialysis treatment.

Fiscal intermediary CMS primary third-party contractors who administer Part A payments according to local medical review policies (LMRP) for hospitals, rehabilitation facilities, and skilled-nursing facilities.

HCFA-1500 The claim form authorized by the Health Care Financing Administration (now CMS) for filing Medicare Part B claims with carriers.

Health Insurance Portability and Accountability Act of 1996 Title I protects health insurance coverage for workers and their families when they change or lose their jobs. Title II requires the Department of Health and Human Services to establish national standards for electronic healthcare transactions and national identifiers for providers, health plans, and employers. It also addresses the security and privacy of health data. Adopting these standards will improve the efficiency and effectiveness of the nation's healthcare system by encouraging the widespread use of electronic data interchange in healthcare.

International Classification of Diseases, Version 10, Procedure Coding System (ICD-10-PCS) Laboratory coding system intended for use as an alternative to CPT.

Logical Observation Identifier Names and Codes (LOINC) LOINC is considered a universal laboratory language which is based on the systematic breakdown of the components of a service into more specific units, ultimately creating a highly standardized, typically seven-digit, number, with each possible result from a procedure being mapped to a specific code. Unlike CPT, LOINC is publicly available and can be used with no license fee. It is widely used by commercial laboratories to track specific procedures from order to result.

Medicaid Program established under Title XIX of the Social Security Act, which provides health insurance to the impoverished; the state and federal governments fund it jointly.

Medical necessity The determination of ICD-9-CM codes for which a CPT code will be reimbursed as reasonable and necessary.

Medicare Federally managed health insurance plan covering Americans over age 65 and Americans under age 65 who have certain disabilities and for most patients with ESRD; established by a 1965 amendment to the Social Security Act.

Modifier Modifiers are composed of two-digit numbers which are attached to a specific code prior to the billing process (see Table 33.3). They are "used to indicate that a service or procedure has been altered by some specific circumstance but not changed in its definition or code."

Neg Reg Negotiated Rulemaking Committee for diagnostic clinical laboratory tests.

Not medically necessary The determination that an ICD-9-CM code does not justify payment for a service.

Prospective payment system (capitated payment) Payment is received prior to the delivery of services. Profit results from care delivered at a total cost below the contract payment; loss results from care delivered at a total cost above the contract payment.

Unbundling To code individual tests rather than using an approved CMS panel.

Upcoding Using a higher-paying code than justified to maximize reimbursement.

REFERENCES

1. **American Medical Association.** 1999. Changing CPT: how it works. *CPT Assist.* **9:**8–9.

2. **American Medical Association.** 2003. *Current Procedural Terminology, CPT 2004,* 4th ed. AMA Press, Chicago, Ill.

3. **Averill, R. F., R. L. Mullin, B. A. Steinbeck, N. I. Goldfield, and T. M. Grant.** 2001. Development of the ICD-10 procedure coding system (ICD-10-PCS). *Top Health Inf. Manag.* **21:**54–88.

4. **Baselski, V., L. Garcia, A. Weissfeld.** 2001. The ABCs of CPT coding in microbiology. *Clin. Microbiol. Newsl.* **23:**37–42.

5. **Brouch, K.** 2003. AHIMA project offers insights into SNOWMED, ICD-9-CM mapping process. *J. AHIMA* **74:**52–55.

6. **Burke, M. D.** 2003. Clinical laboratory consultation: appropriateness to laboratory medicine. *Clin. Chim. Acta* **333:**125–129.

7. **Kratz, A., and M. Laposata.** 2002. Enhanced clinical consulting—moving toward the core competencies of laboratory professionals. *Clin. Chim. Acta* **319:**117–125.

8. **Lorence, D. P., and I. A. Ibrahim.** 2003. Benchmarking variation in coding accuracy across the United States. *J. Health Care Finance* **29:**29–42.

9. **MacMillan, D. H., B. L. Soderberg, and M. Laposata.** 2001. Regulations regarding reflexive testing and narrative interpretations in laboratory medicine. *Am. J. Clin. Pathol.* **116**(Suppl.):S129–S132.

10. **McDonald, C. J., S. M. Huff, J. G. Suico, G. Hill, D. Leavelle, R. Aller, A. Forrey, K. Mercer, G. DeMoor, J. Hook, W. Williams, J. Case, and P. Maloney.** 2003. LOINC, a universal standard for identifying laboratory observations: a year update. *Clin. Chem.* **49:**624–633.

11. **Schubart, J. R., C. E. Fowler, G. R. Donowitz, and A. F. Connors Jr.** 2001. Algorithm-based decision rules to safely reduce laboratory test ordering. *IFIP World Conf. Ser. Med. Inf.* **10:**523–527.

12. **Travers, E. M.** 1997. *Clinical Laboratory Management,* p. 759–760. Williams and Wilkins, Baltimore, Md.

APPENDIX 33.1 Publications, Phone Numbers, Websites, and Guidance Documents

PUBLICATIONS
ICD-9-CM manual (issued every October)
CPT-4 manual (issued every October)
HCPCS manual (issued every January)
Medicare Fee Schedule (issued every November)
National Correct Coding Policy Manual, chapter 10, current version 10 (issued quarterly, National Technical Information Services)
CPT 2003 (updated each year; available November prior to next year's edition)
CPT Companion: Frequently Asked Questions (CAP, 1998)
CPT Changes 2003. An Insider's View (2002, AMA Press, Chicago, Ill.)
CPT Assistant (monthly, CAP)
CPT-4 Professional Edition (St. Anthony's or Medicode; includes relevant citations)
Clinical Laboratory Strategies (newsletter of the American Association of Clinical Chemists Delta Project)
National Intelligence Report (newsletter published by Washington G-2 Reports, Washington, D.C.)
Laboratory Industry Report (newsletter published by Washington G-2 Reports, Washington, D.C.)
Laboratory Compliance Insider (Brownstone Publishers)
The Clinical Laboratory Compliance Alert (Eli Research)
Compliance Hotline (American Health Consultants)

PHONE NUMBERS
Medicode: 1-800-999-4600
AMA: 1-800-621-8335
St. Anthony's: 1-800-621-8353
CMS (formerly Health Care Financing Administration): 1-410-786-3000

WEBSITES
http://www.ama-assn.org/go/cpt: AMA CPT site
http://www.ama-assn.org/ama/pub/category/3117.html: information on the CPT coding helpline
http://www.cms.gov
http://www.cms.gov/medlearn
http://www.cms.gov/medlearn/refabn.asp: ABN
http://www.cms.gov/regulations: CMS and related laws and regulations
http://www.cms.gov/regulations/pfs/2004fc/: Medicare Program, revision to payment policies under the physician fee schedule for calendar year 2004
http://www.cms.hhs.gov
http://www.oig.cms.gov: Compliance Program, Fraud Alerts, Advisory Opinions, Red Book, Work Plan
http://www.labfocus.com: CAP/CLMA Conference on Issues in Medicare Compliance
http://www.medicaretraining.com: Blue Cross Blue Shield Florida training program
http://www.ntis.gov: National Technical Information Service
http://www.cdc.gov/nchswww/data: National Center for Health Statistics
http://www.gao.gov: T-HEHS-00-74, 9 March 2000 (Medicare: HCFA Faces Challenges to Control Improper Payments [HIPAA])
http://www.iom.edu/iom/iomhome/nsf/pages/clinlab+home+page: Institute of Medicine study
http://www.lmrp.net: all contractor LMRPs
http://www.compliance.com: the American Compliance Institute
http://www.columbia.com: the Columbia Compliance Plan
http://www.hcca-info.org: Healthcare Compliance Association
http://www.medpac.gov: Medicare Payment Advisory Commission

FEDERAL REGISTER AND RELEVANT GUIDANCE DOCUMENTS

Category B IDEs
Federal Register. 1995. Medicare program; criteria and procedures for extending coverage to certain devices and related services—HCFA. Final rule with comment period. *Fed. Regist.* **60:**48417–48425.

Analyte-Specific Reagents
Federal Register. 1997. Medical devices; classification/reclassification; restricted devices; analyte specific reagents—FDA. Final rule. *Fed. Regist.* **62:**62243–62260.

Inherent Reasonableness
Federal Register. 1998. Medicare program; application of inherent reasonableness to all Medicare part B services (other than physician services)—HCFA. Interim final rule with comment period. *Fed. Regist.* **63:**687–690.

34

Approaches to Billing Laboratory Services

Vickie S. Baselski, Alice S. Weissfeld, and Fran Sorrell

OBJECTIVES

To illustrate the importance of hiring individuals well versed in all aspects of correct coding, including the rules and regulations

To discuss the importance of having a comprehensive information technology platform and software resources that ensure accuracy and completeness

To explain the need for laboratory personnel to be involved in the billing process and to maintain a close working relationship with members of the billing department

To explain the relationship between complete and accurate billing and the generation of sufficient income to continue to perform expected functions

Alas! How deeply painful is all payment!

GEORGE GORDON NOEL BYRON (1788–1824)

IT IS AN EXTREME UNDERSTATEMENT that the billing of clinical laboratory services is a tedious and complex process. In fact, the billing process can be said to be frequently overwhelming, rarely straightforward, always changing, and never easy. There are a number of variations among providing entities and among paying entities as well as in the actual process of how reimbursement for services is made. The complexity is further increased by the sequential financial relationships between the patient requiring testing, the ordering provider making decisions about which tests to order, the laboratory interpreting the provider's order and verifying the appropriate mechanism to bill for services, and the payor who reimburses an amount generally predetermined per contractual agreement and who may also deny payment based on criteria that are not always readily available or logical. In fact, the laboratory occupies a painful middle position in the entire process, where there is little or no input into the patient-physician process to effect appropriate test ordering and the acquisition of a properly executed requisition and advanced beneficiary notice (ABN) if necessary. However, as the billing entity, the laboratory has total fiscal responsibility and complete financial liability for the procedures the physician may have ordered rightly or wrongly. An understanding of the specific requirements for billing laboratory services and a systematic approach for ensuring that the processes are carried out as specified are key to the financial success of a laboratory (5, 9, 10, 12, 13). Underpayments to providers under their payor agreements are a cause of many thousands of dollars in lost revenue. Providers should devise a plan to make sure that payments made to them are accurate and timely and adhere to other contractual obligations. Specific areas where underpayments are common include underfunding due to late payments, fee schedule changes that are contractually disallowed, miscalculation of performance-based bonuses and errors in risk payment reconciliations, inappropriate denials or inappropriate downcoding of claims, and nonpayments (13). Claim denial management can enhance revenue, particularly in times of declining payment and increasing cost pressures (2). Prospective prevention minimizes denials by defining the scope of service, tracking causes for denials, and improving related processes.

Interactions in the Billing Process

While the entire laboratory test process from test order to test result reporting to payment for services involves several categories of individuals, the actual billing process can be considered in terms of two main categories (Fig. 34.1). The "provider mix" describes those entities that actually perform and/or bill the services, and the "payor mix" describes those entities that have fiscal responsibility for payment for services.

Provider Mix

Since 1992, all laboratory providers must be registered under the Clinical Laboratory Improvement Amendments (CLIA) to provide the type of services they are billing for. CLIA classifies laboratories into four main categories: high-complexity laboratories (capable of providing all services), moderate-complexity laboratories (capable of performing procedures with slightly lower skill requirements and slightly lower patient risk), certificate-of-waiver laboratories (may perform only tests meeting "waived" criteria under CLIA and requiring minimal skill and carrying minimal risk to a patient), and provider-performed microscopy services (applying to only a selected few microscopic procedures when performed by a physician or

other authorized individual). When billing for laboratory services, the laboratory must have the appropriate CLIA status for the service being billed or the service will be subject to denial.

Laboratory services are actually provided in several types of facilities. Hospital-based laboratories perform and bill more tests than the other categories. They provide services for inpatients and often for outpatients in institutionally affiliated clinics, and occasionally for nonaffiliated clinics termed "outreach business." Independent laboratories perform testing for a variety of "clients," including hospitals, physicians, other healthcare providers, patients in areas where direct-access testing is allowed by law, and by contract for nonhealthcare purposes (e.g., employee drug screens). Some independent laboratories perform highly complex procedures not performed in a routine setting and are termed "reference" or esoteric laboratories. Physician office laboratories exist to provide rapid-response-type procedures which may impact immediate clinical decision making. The test mix is generally less complex in a physician office laboratory setting than in the other two settings. The final type of laboratory is the "niche" laboratory, which exists to provide services to specific groups of patients. For example, laboratories may focus on service to end-stage renal disease (ESRD) or skilled-nursing facility (SNF) patients. Each type of laboratory must be prepared to follow the billing processes specified by all of the payors for which it is an approved provider. If the laboratory is not an approved provider, the laboratory services provided will be subject to denial.

Payor Mix

Those entities actually submitting payment fall into several categories. Federal payors include those in the Medicare program for senior and disabled citizens, a program that was initiated in 1965 as a result of the Social Security Act. Medicare pays for services that are "reasonable and necessary for the diagnosis or treatment of illness or

Figure 34.1 Payer-provider interactions in reimbursement. POL, physician office laboratory.

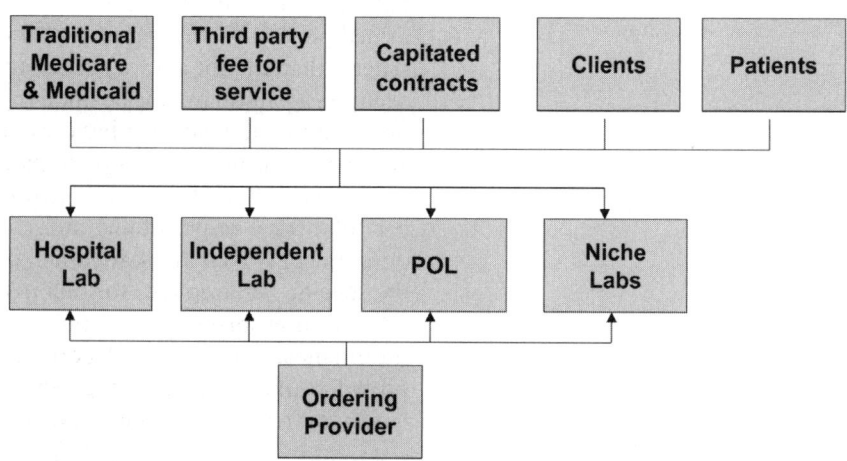

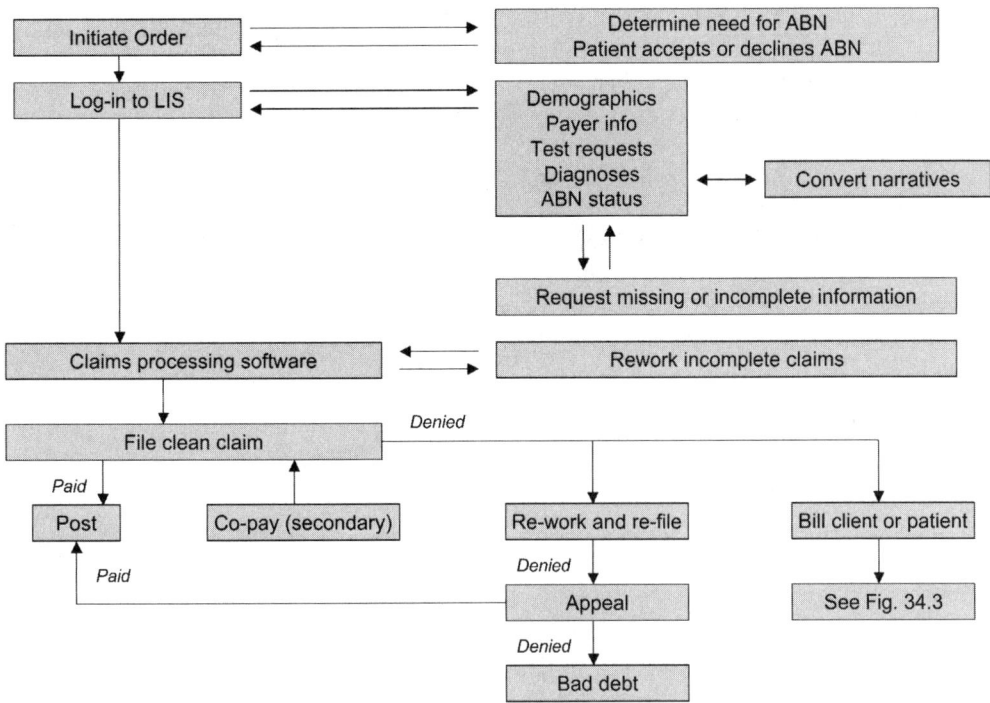

Figure 34.2 Generic billing flowchart: third-party. LIS, laboratory information system.

injury, or to improve the malfunctioning of a malformed body member." Payments are made for either inpatient services, including services provided in an SNF (termed Part A and administered through a contracted fiscal intermediary), or outpatient services (termed Part B and administered through a contracted carrier). In 1972 the Social Security Amendments added coverage to two additional high-risk groups, those disabled and receiving cash benefits from Social Security and individuals suffering ESRD. The Medicaid programs provide federal assistance to states for payment for healthcare for indigent citizens, and the Balanced Budget Act of 1997 created the State Children's Health Insurance Program to assist with healthcare of children.

Figure 34.3 Generic billing flowchart: client or patient. LIS, laboratory information system.

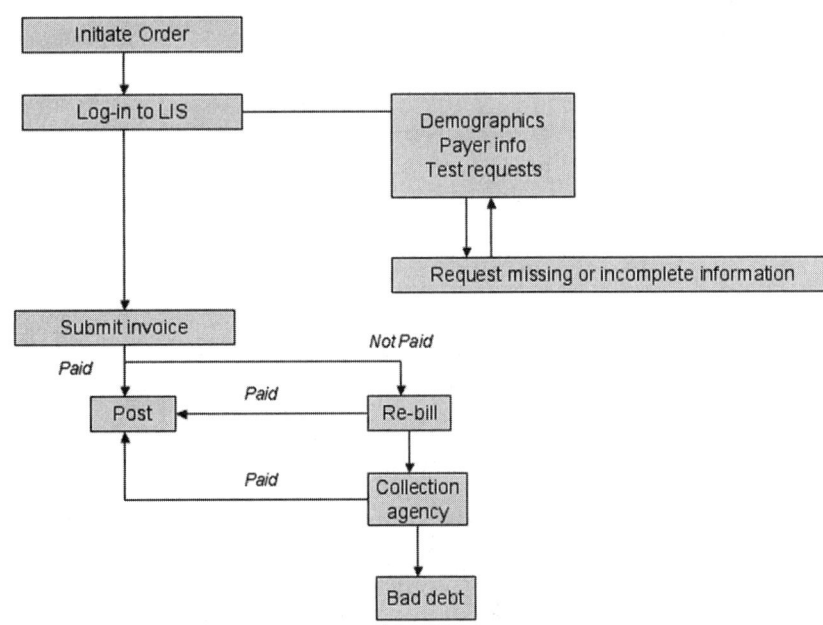

Both Medicare and Medicare are third-party payors; payment for services provided by a healthcare provider to a patient is made by a contracted entity. Many other third-party payors render payment to laboratories as a component of a healthcare benefit plan. These insurance plans require payment of regular premiums so that in the event of a high-cost or catastrophic illness, the third party will cover an agreed-upon percentage or fee for the services provided. There are multiple types of plans, including traditional indemnity, preferred provider organizations, point-of-service plans, and health maintenance organizations. In fact, within the Medicare and Medicaid programs there also exist variations comparable to those seen in the private sector. Adding to the complexity is the frequent presence of a "secondary payor," that is, another healthcare plan that provides coverage on the balance after payment by the primary payor. A generic third-party process is diagrammed in Fig. 34.2.

Laboratories may also receive payments through contract with specific physicians and other healthcare providers who in turn bill third-party payors. These are probably the easiest billing arrangements to execute. A generic client-bill process is diagrammed in Fig. 34.3. Laboratories are also required to bill patients who have no insurance coverage or have received a noncovered service, as well as in any circumstance in which the patient is expected to copay a percentage of the total bill.

Terms of Coverage

Each individual payor sets criteria for payment for services (both which types and under what conditions). Further, each payor is intimately involved in the determination of the actual payment amount. Each payor may interact with each provider through one of two main types of payment: retrospective (or fee for service) and prospective (or capitated).

Types of Services

There are three general categories of laboratory services that are performed based on clinical utility, and payors vary in whether these services will be covered (Table 34.1). The terms "covered services" and "noncovered services" are used to categorize whether a specific type of service will be covered. Diagnostic tests assist in the determination of an etiology for a specific disease or clinical condition. They are almost always covered by third-party payors, although there may be restrictions on which specific tests may be used. In addition, there may be restrictions on when a test may be used based on diagnosis or clinical condition. This type of restriction is generally known as "medical necessity." Monitoring tests are used to follow disease progression or response to therapy or to detect side effects of a therapy. Monitoring tests are generally covered when the therapy is also covered and may also be subject

Table 34.1 Types of laboratory services

Diagnostic tests	These tests are used to identify physiological abnormalities associated with disease.
Monitoring tests	These tests are used to follow disease progression or response to therapy or to detect side effects of therapy.
Screening tests	These tests are performed in the absence of signs, symptoms, complaints, injury, or personal history of a disease to discover potentially treatable or preventable diseases.
Tests requiring prior authorization	In some cases, there may be a requirement for prior authorization from the third-party payor for the test provided.

to restrictions. Screening tests are performed in the absence of signs, symptoms, complaints, injury, or personal history of a disease to discover potentially treatable or preventable diseases. They may or may not be covered by a third-party payor, depending on the particular health plan coverage conditions. A classic example of noncoverage of screening is in the Medicare program, which by historical interpretation of statute allows payment only for "treatment of illness or injury. . ." and not for "screening." For all test types, there may be frequency restrictions which limit the number of times a test may be performed in a given period. In addition, in some cases, there may be a requirement for "prior authorization" for the test service provided. This is, in essence, the obtaining of approval for the service by the third-party payor. If a particular test is deemed noncovered, then the patient generally assumes financial liability for the service if there has been prior notification and acceptance of such.

Payment for Services

There are two general approaches to payment for healthcare services, including laboratory services (Table 34.2). The traditional approach and the one most commonly employed is based on a fee-for-service strategy. This approach is retrospective in that the total amount to be billed is not known until services have been rendered and a cumulative bill is generated. However, the fee schedule used for billing has been prospectively determined and accepted by both

Table 34.2 Payment for services

Fee for service	This approach is retrospective; total amount to be billed is not known until services have been rendered; results in cumulative bill; fee schedule prospectively determined and accepted by provider and payor
Capitation	This approach is prospective; payment amount established on some denominator (per member per month, per DRG[a], or per APC[b]); payment based on average anticipated utilization in the denominator group

[a]DRG, diagnosis-related group.
[b]APC, ambulatory payment classification.

the provider and the payor. Traditional federal payment programs are based on a fee schedule set annually by a specific formula. Other payors generally develop fee schedules after negotiation with providers. Fee schedules may vary considerably based on considerations related to the "cost of doing business" with a particular payor.

The alternative approach is one based on capitation. This approach is prospective in that a payment amount has been established based on some denominator such as "per member per month," per diagnosis-related group or ambulatory payment classification, or per some other patient-related parameter (6). The payment is based on average anticipated utilization by patients in the denominator group. Unusual or very expensive services that are performed outside of the norm are often "carved out" of the agreement and billed separately on a fee-for-service basis. Payment for outpatient services on a capitated basis is not currently common in laboratory medicine. However, in the inpatient population, in SNFs, and in other specialty niches (e.g., ESRD facilities), both Medicare and other payors have moved toward a prospective payment system (14). Thus, the laboratory needs to be familiar with both approaches.

Logistics of the Billing Process

The actual billing process is obviously quite complex considering all of the variations in possible interactions between providers and payors. There are numerous fee schedules, various billing arrangements, multiple payors, multiple forms, multiple coverage conditions, and various rules. Nonetheless, one can outline and compare the general processes involved in billing for laboratory services.

Claim versus Invoice Submission

Claims for payment are generated for submission to third-party payors, while invoices are generated for contractual payment by clients or by patients (Table 34.3). Claims are typically submitted electronically, although the same information may be submitted on a manual claim form. Claims are very complex and require that a great deal of information be accurately and completely provided. This includes date of service, correct codes for services and diagnosis codes, complete patient demographic informa-

tion, complete payor information, and an ABN specific to each service likely to be denied. It is also possible to outsource billing activities to an independent entity that is familiar with the various rules and regulations pertaining to major payors. In contrast, invoices are generally submitted manually and are much less complex, generally including only date of service, patient demographics, and types of services. Thus, billing costs are generally much lower for non-third-party billings.

Invoice Billing

Invoice billing is a relatively simple process (Fig. 34.3). After an order is placed and logged in to a laboratory information system, tests ordered are performed and result reports are generated in the appropriate laboratory department, and a cumulative invoice is generated at some regular interval (e.g., weekly, monthly). The invoice may be based on either a fee-for-service or capitated payment schedule. It may on occasion be necessary to verify information pertaining to an order from the requisition, but the overall process is relatively straightforward. The billed entity either pays or does not pay in the expected time frame. Nonpayment generally results in one or more rebillings and, eventually, action by a collection agency. The amounts due are generally posted upon completion of testing but on occasion may be generated at the time of order. This, however, carries the risk of billing for tests that may not have been completed and requires that a system be in place to issue credits whenever necessary.

Claim Billing

The entire claim process is quite complex, requiring multiple steps conducted over a lengthy period. It also begins with the generation of an order. However, at the time of test order, it is necessary to compare the tests ordered to the diagnoses given to determine if a waiver of financial responsibility (ABN) is required. If it is required, an attempt may be made to contact the ordering provider for additional relevant diagnostic information, but documentation of the attempt must be signed by the patient and maintained on file. Test orders are then logged in to the laboratory information system and samples are routed to the appropriate laboratory for testing and result reporting. During log-in, if any information critical to processing the order for testing or billing is missing, it is again necessary for the laboratory to contact the ordering provider to seek additional documentation. As in invoice situations, a bill for service may be posted at the time of log-in or at the time of result reporting, but if the former is done, there must be a system in place to accurately issue credits when necessary.

Claims are generally processed according to date of service, so multiple services may be submitted on a single claim. However, the ABN, if required, must be both date and test specific. It is also necessary to attach appropriate modifiers to any test code requiring one for payment.

Table 34.3 Billing process: invoice versus claims

Invoice billing	Relatively simple process; can be based on fee-for-service or capitated payment schedule; amounts generally posted upon completion of testing; generated at some regular interval (e.g., weekly, monthly)
Claim billing	Very complex; requires extensive and complete information; careful review prior to payment; payment often denied; need for rechecking all claim information and resubmission for payment

After preparation, each claim is generally subjected to a review using "claims processing software" (11). This kind of review evaluates each claim to determine if all of the information required is complete and accurate, and it also assesses whether a claim is likely to be covered by the particular payor (1, 3, 8). If not, then once again, calls are made to the ordering provider to attempt to obtain appropriate documentation. Once "clean," the claim is actually filed with the payor.

After filing, there are several possible outcomes. In the best case, the claim is paid and the funds are posted to an appropriate account. If denied, the denial documentation may be reevaluated to ensure that everything was in order, and if not, the claim must be corrected and refiled (7). Denial documentation is generally sent to both the laboratory and the patient as an explanation of benefit (EOB) or explanation of medical benefit (EOMB) form. Denials are coded with a generic description outlining the reason(s) for the denial. Careful review of the EOBs can greatly assist in correction of documentation to subsequently obtain payment. If upon review it is determined that payment was appropriate, it is also possible to initiate an appeal for review and reconsideration by the payor.

Alternatively, a new claim or a claim for remaining amounts may be filed with a secondary payor by following the same general pattern. If no payment is forthcoming from any payor, and an ABN or other acceptance of liability is on file, the patient may be billed. It is also necessary to bill the patient in any case in which a copay is part of the process. In cases in which a provider has consistently failed to provide essential information, a laboratory may choose to bill the errant provider. Once a patient or client is billed, the process follows the pathway described for the invoice process. Certainly the billing format and accuracy can play a large role in both client and patient satisfaction and understanding (4).

Summary

With the complexity of the billing process, it is no wonder that in many laboratories, the billing department has undergone rapid expansion in the number of employees. The billing department must employ individuals well versed in all aspects of correct coding and who are knowledgeable about the myriad rules and regulations pertaining to each payor. The billing processes are so complex that it is virtually impossible to develop and submit claims and receive payment without a sound information technology platform and software resources that ensure accuracy and completeness of the process.

However, it is also critical that laboratorians remain involved in the billing process and maintain a close working relationship with members of the billing department. Extensive technical expertise is required to ensure that test procedures are coded correctly, as well as to determine that "best practices" for laboratory medicine are being followed. For clinical laboratories, the key to survival is in complete and accurate billing for all services performed so that timely and comprehensive payment can be made for those services. Regardless of the corporate structure of the laboratory one practices in, the generation of sufficient income to continue to perform expected functions is absolutely essential.

KEY POINTS

- It is mandatory that laboratories hire personnel who are well versed in all aspects of correct coding, including the rules and regulations.

- It is almost impossible to develop and submit claims and receive payment without adequate information technology systems (platforms and software).

- Selected laboratory personnel must be involved in the billing process and work closely with members of the billing department.

- Complete and accurate billing is required in order to generate sufficient income for laboratory operations to continue.

GLOSSARY

Advance beneficiary notice (ABN) A "waiver of financial liability" form used by the provider to notify Medicare beneficiaries prior to receiving a service that it may not be a covered service and that they may have to assume financial responsibility.

APC Ambulatory payment classification.

Capitation A predetermined, fixed amount paid to providers in return for rendering a specified set of health services. The rate is established per person (per capita) enrolled in the health plan.

Claim denial management Can enhance revenue; denials usually arise from process problems leading to inadequate documentation.

Co-pay A fixed dollar amount paid by the subscriber to the provider at the time of services.

Diagnosis-related groups (DRGs) Classification system developed at Yale that defines almost 400 major diagnostic categories and places patients into case types based on the International Classification of Diseases, Ninth Revision (Clinical Modification) code classifications.

End-stage renal disease (ESRD) The terminology used for Medicare beneficiaries who have permanent kidney dysfunction requiring dialysis treatment.

EOB, EOMB Explanation of (medical) benefit form.

Health maintenance organization A prepaid system of healthcare with emphasis on the prevention and early detection of disease and on continuity of care. HMOs generally offer a package of services; however, the choice of physician is frequently limited to those working within the HMO.

Payor mix Describes those entities that have fiscal responsibility for payment of services.

POL Physician office laboratory.

POS Point-of-service insurance plan.

Preferred provider organization A healthcare organization that negotiates set rates of reimbursement with participating healthcare providers for services to insured clients; a type of prospective payment system.

Provider mix Describes those entities that actually perform and/or bill the services.

Regulation Legally binding rules developed to implement a statute.

Secondary payor Another healthcare plan that provides coverage on the balance after payment by the primary payor.

SNF Skilled-nursing facility.

Statute A law passed by the U.S. Congress or a state legislature.

REFERENCES

1. **Adams, D. L., H. Norman, and V. J. Burroughs.** 2002. Addressing medical coding and billing part II: a strategy for achieving compliance. A risk management approach for reducing coding and billing errors. *J. Natl. Med. Assoc.* **94:**430–447.

2. **Alwell, M.** 2003. Stem revenue losses with effective CDM management. *Healthc. Financ. Manag.* **57:**84–88.

3. **Barber, R. L.** 2002. Prompt payment depends on revenue-cycle diligence. *Healthc. Financ. Manag.* **56:**52–59.

4. **Cohen, D., and P. Hoffman.** 2003. When putting patients first fits the bill. *Healthc Financ. Manag.* **57:**90–96.

5. **Eckhart, J., and N. Mathahs.** 2001. Physicians and compliance: developing a system that works. *Clin. Leadersh. Manag. Rev.* **15:**222–229.

6. **Fee, D. N.** 2002. Success with APCs. *Healthc. Financ. Manag.* **56:**68–72.

7. **Hodges, J.** 2002. Effective claims denial management enhances revenue. *Healthc. Financ. Manag.* **56:**40–50.

8. **LaForge, R. W., and J. S. Tureaud.** 2003. Revenue-cycle redesign: honing the details. *Healthc. Financ. Manag.* **57:**64–71.

9. **McNeely, M. D.** 2002. The use of expert systems for improving test use and enhancing the accuracy of diagnosis. *Clin. Lab. Med.* **22:**515–528.

10. **Moss, M. M., and S. M. Schexnayder.** 2001. Coding and billing in the pediatric intensive care unit. *Pediatr. Clin. N. Am.* **48:**783–793.

11. **Segal, M. J., S. Morris, and J. M. Rubin.** 2002. Automated claim and payment verification. *J. Med. Pract. Manag.* **17:**297–301.

12. **Smith-Shoemake, M. A.** 2002. Solving the claims conundrum. *Manag. Care Q.* **10:**13–14.

13. **Welter, T., and P. Stevenson.** 2001. Calculating five types of typical underpayments. *Healthc. Financ. Manag.* **55:**46–50.

14. **Wolf, P.** 2001. Charge-process strategies for outpatient prospective payment. *Healthc. Financ. Manag.* **55:**58–61.

APPENDIX 34.1   Websites

http://www.cms.gov
http://www.cms.gov/medlearn
http://www.cms.gov/medlearn/refabn.asp: ABN
http://www.cms.gov/regulations: Centers for Medicare and Medicaid Services and related laws and regulations

http://www.hhs.gov/medlearn/ncci.asp: Medicare's National Correct Coding Initiative edits
http://www.oig.cms.gov: Compliance Program, Fraud Alerts, Advisory Opinions, Red Book, Work Plan

35

Charges and Fees for Laboratory Services

Vickie S. Baselski, Alice S. Weissfeld, and Fran Sorrell

OBJECTIVES

To discuss the four key concepts related to payment for laboratory services

To explain the relationship between charges and fee schedules and a reasonable profit margin

To describe the uses for profits and how they relate to generating returns on investments

To describe the following terms: market competitive and value-added services

To discuss appropriate ways to avoid the appearance of "kickbacks" and how this relates to compliance

Put money in thy purse.

WILLIAM SHAKESPEARE (1564–1616)

THE ULTIMATE GOAL IN PROVISION OF LABORATORY SERVICES is to make certain that information is delivered to ordering healthcare providers in a timely manner that ensures that quality is maintained, costs are minimized, and clinical relevance is established. At the same time, it is paramount to make sure that the laboratory does not lose money in doing so. This concept applies regardless of the corporate structure. It has been said, "for-profit entities exist to make money, and not-for-profit entities make money to exist, but both need to make money to survive." To make money in the laboratory business, it is critical that one establish charges that at least cover total costs and control expenditures such that low-paying fee schedules do not put the laboratory at risk for significant loss.

Calculating Costs

The responsibility for cost analysis of individual laboratory procedures rests primarily with the laboratorian. Chapters in section V present an in-depth look at the process of cost accounting in the clinical laboratory. However, for purposes of determining a charge structure, it is critical to have a clear understanding of the total costs of a procedure (4, 7). The best parameter to use to make this determination is the "cost per reportable test." In general an "orderable and reportable test" will map to a specific Current Procedural Terminology, 4th edition (CPT-4) code or codes, as well as to the institutional charge code for accounting purposes. The cost per reportable test is a composite of all related costs. These include the obvious costs such as average direct costs (e.g., reagents, equipment), including labor, and indirect costs, including overhead and support services (e.g., housekeeping, couriers, billing, customer service, marketing), but they also include hidden costs such as quality control, calibration, repeats, dilutions, and wastage. The cost per reportable test is considered to be a parameter that allows "apples to apples" comparisons between methods (interassay) and between laboratories (intra-assay).

In addition, the cost per reportable test is a useful tool for setting charges such that the laboratory maintains an appropriate profit margin. The break-even point is the point at which net income equals total costs. Net income takes into account actual payment for services and deducts actual costs as well as "bad debt," that is, the amount that is not reimbursed by any potential payer. Obviously, the goal is to do better than break even. To do so, one must have a clear understanding of both total costs per reportable test as well as expected net income.

Payment Amounts

The amount of payment made for laboratory services may be based on one of three general categories. Actual provider charges may apply to some payors, while payor-defined fee schedules may be the basis for others. In capitated payment agreements, the payment takes the form of a negotiated agreement for a specified level or category of service.

Setting Charges

There are a number of general principles that guide the process of setting a charge. One must consider the actual total costs and the expected reimbursement, so that one can exceed the break-even point. In general, it is never good business to price any service below cost, and in fact, this practice could be viewed as an inducement for ordering providers to submit federally reimbursed testing to a particular laboratory. On the other hand, one cannot charge federal payors "substantially in excess of usual charges." At the same time, one must review the market situation and ensure that charges are comparable to those of competitors unless the service offered has a quantifiable value-added component. It is a common practice in many laboratories to identify tests which are high volume and offer them at a charge below cost (termed a "loss leader"). However, for the same payor, more esoteric, high-cost procedures with lower utilization may be offered with a substantial profit margin to make up the difference. In addition, the billing simplicity of a contractual arrangement in which clients or patients are billed is considered a justification for deep discounts offered in many cases, since billing costs are substantially lower and the percentage of services paid for is significantly higher.

However, the entire area of discounts and multiple fee schedules has come under intense scrutiny recently, and this practice needs to be carefully evaluated for providers doing business with federal payors. Although it is a long-standing interpretation of Medicare law that one cannot charge federal payors "substantially in excess of usual charges," the Office of the Inspector General has issued a proposed rule that defines this concept as 120% greater than a usual charge for the same item or service for any payor. "Usual charge" is defined as either the average or median of charges to all parties for the most recent 1-year period. Thus, determination of charges now has both financial and compliance implications. In addition, a previous Advisory Opinion stated that discounts would be reviewed to determine if they "make business sense standing alone without reference to any other business the provider may receive." In fact, legislation known as the Stark legislation is designed to ensure that laboratories provide services to ordering providers without any evidence of inducement or kickback.

Fee Schedules

Counter to attempts to develop rational charges based on real costs and net income is the concept of payor-established fee schedules. Many payors will arbitrarily establish a fee schedule for defined services, and it is the laboratory's responsibility to determine whether to do business with that particular payor. Fee schedules are generally loosely based on charges; but as previously noted, charges may vary considerably by payor. The quintessential example of payment according to fee schedule is the Medicare Part B payment system.

Medicare Fee Schedule

Medicare currently pays for technical clinical laboratory tests according to a set fee schedule initially established in 1984 and based on 1983 charge data. Fees are assigned based on the CPT-4 or Healthcare Common Procedure Coding System (HCPCS) code established for each procedure (1, 5, 8). The actual Medicare payment is the lowest of (i) the actual charge, (ii) the fee schedule amount set by the contractor, and (iii) the national fee cap, termed the national limitation amount (NLA). For tests established before 1 January 2001, the NLA is currently 74% of the median of local fees, a percentage that has been rapidly reduced from 115% in 1986 to the current level. Local fees are set at 60% of prevailing charges (except for sole community hospitals, which are set at 62%). Thus, Medicare payments can be seen to be substantially lower than actual charges, currently less than 50%. In addition, it can be seen that there may be variation in the actual payment amount based on contractor (6).

Adjustments are made to the NLA on a regular basis. After 2001, as a result of the Balanced Budget Act of 1997, the NLA was set at 100% of the median to allow for improved reimbursement for new CPT-4 codes, ostensibly representing emerging technology. The Centers for Medicare and Medicaid Services (CMS) (formerly the Health Care Financing Administration) adjusts the fee schedule on an annual basis to reflect changes in the consumer price index (CPI). However, from 1998 to 2002, the Balanced Budget Act of 1997 mandated a freeze on the CPI for the NLA, a cost control strategy that was yet again employed in 2004. In addition, on occasion Congress may mandate modifications in fees (increases or decreases) that are viewed as inappropriate or unreasonable. For example, it was recently determined that Pap smear payment amounts were unreasonably low, and the Balanced Budget Reduction Act of 1999 adjusted payments upwards.

It should be noted that while there are occasional decisions that increase payments, the primary trend is to reduce payments. In addition to the increasing percentage reductions in NLA and the CPI freeze already mentioned, CMS has also implemented other strategies to alter payments. One strategy is termed "inherent reasonableness." Under this strategy, CMS may employ "reasonable-charge methodology" to arbitrarily reduce or increase an NLA deemed "grossly excessive or grossly deficient" against market values. In point of fact, reasonable-charge methodology has resulted only in reduced payments. Likewise, the "least costly alternative" approach makes a determination that a new more costly procedure has the same clinical utility as a less costly alternative, and payment is adjusted to that of the older methodology, thus impeding the implementation of new technologies.

For new CPT-4 test codes, fees are assigned based on one of two methods: cross-walking or gap filling. Cross-walking is used when new tests employ a method that is deemed comparable to an existing method or combination of methods, and the fee is simply set according to that of the existing code(s) to which the new code is mapped. Gap filling is used when a new code describes a test using a novel technology for which no comparable code exists. The fee is then set after collection of data by local contractors, who then apply the formulas previously described. Since 2001, the process of assigning fees to new codes has involved open meetings in which laboratorians and professional laboratory groups may present public recommendations on the best method to use.

It is something of a paradox in the Medicare fee schedule process that a laboratory may have to accept a fee lower than its costs but may not set a charge higher than the Medicare fee it accepts. This paradox led the Institute of Medicine to issue 6 of 12 recommendations in its report on Medicare laboratory payment policy pertaining to the fee schedule (Table 35.1). These are (i) that "Medicare payments for outpatient clinical laboratory services should be based on a single, rational, national fee schedule," (ii) that "on an interim basis, relative payments for Medicare outpatient clinical laboratory services should be based on the current NLA," (iii) that "a data driven consensus process" be used to refine the Medicare fee schedule, (iv) that fees be "adjusted for geographic location" and evaluated for other circumstances "likely to affect beneficiary access," (v) that there be processes to "periodically update" the fee schedule, and (vi) that there be an "open, timely, and accessible process" to incorporate new tests into the fee schedule which does not "impede clinical decision making that is essential to providing appropriate care."

Other Fee Schedules

The importance of the Medicare fee schedule is, quite simply, its impact on the fee schedules developed by other third-party payors. Medicare fees are often a starting point for negotiations with other payors, which leads to discounts and special pricing situations already discussed. Alternatively, forced acceptance of lower fees may result in setting higher charges for noncontracted entities (e.g., patients) to attempt to achieve a break-even status. The adage "as goes Medicare, so go other payors" is of particular relevance in the realm of payment for services.

Capitated Contracts

Capitated contracts for laboratory services are somewhat uncommon in outpatient arenas, but they may play a major role in provision of laboratory services in extremely cost-constrained markets. In federal programs, there are a number of examples of capitation for lab services in managed-care Medicaid programs, and capitation will likely emerge in the managed-care Medicare Part C programs. The Medicare ambulatory payment classification and payment system for clinical services may also in the future encompass laboratory testing services (2, 3). In other managed-care environments, like health maintenance organizations, laboratories may also be asked to develop a

Table 35.1 Recommendations related to fee schedules[a]

Recommendation 1	Medicare payments for outpatient clinical laboratory services should be based on a single, rational, national fee schedule.
Recommendation 2	On an interim basis, relative payments for Medicare outpatient clinical laboratory services should be based on the current NLA
Recommendation 3	A data-driven consensus process should be used to refine the Medicare fee schedule.
Recommendation 4	Fees should be adjusted for geographic location and evaluated for other circumstances likely to affect beneficiary access.
Recommendation 5	There should be processes to periodically update the fee schedule.
Recommendation 6	There should be an open, timely, and accessible process to incorporate new tests into the fee schedule.

[a]Institute of Medicine report on laboratory medicare payment policy.

capitated payment scheme. In laboratories, a common payment mechanism is a "per-member-per-month" basis for provision of the most common laboratory services, with a fee schedule generally attached for esoteric services carved out of the capitated contract.

Inpatient service reimbursement may also be considered a type of capitated payment, since hospitals are generally reimbursed a total amount based on either a diagnosis-related group or a per diem. To document input and obtain appropriate credit for services, laboratories should keep complete documentation of all activities.

Certain specific environments represent a hybrid between retrospective and prospective payment systems. End-stage renal disease dialysis facilities are reimbursed a composite amount, which includes some laboratory services, while other additional services may be billed separately. Testing done for patients in skilled-nursing facilities is usually done by contract with an independent laboratory, while the actual stay is reimbursed as a Medicare Part A capitated amount, and other third-party payors generally follow the Medicare model.

Keys to Success in Reimbursement

Regardless of the type of payment situation, there are a few key actions that can help guarantee that a laboratory will be able to attain a reasonable profit or, at the least, avoid any significant losses. Integral to this process is a firm understanding of coding for procedures performed as well as complete knowledge of all billing rules promulgated by a given payor (Table 35.2).

Retrospective Payment

The primary key to success in a retrospective (fee-for-service) payment situation is to obtain payment for all services that a physician orders and that you perform and for which you report the result. Therefore, you should code correctly and completely for all that you do and bill for all that you code for. In any situation in which more than one code applies, or if a procedure is added on by request or as a reflex, the associated codes should be added

Table 35.2 Key concepts related to successful reimbursement

Costs	Know your real/total costs for any given orderable and billable procedure.
Charges and fee schedules	Set charges and accept fee schedules or other payments to guarantee a reasonable profit margin.
Market competition	Set charges to be market competitive and provide services which are equivalent to or better than those of your competitors (value-added services).
Compliance	Avoid any appearance of kickbacks.

to the bill. You should obtain the diagnosis, preferably as an International Classification of Diseases, Ninth Edition, Clinical Modification (ICD-9-CM) code, but translation of a narrative diagnosis into an ICD-9-CM code is generally acceptable. The diagnosis will help to satisfy any documentation requirements that a payor may have to determine whether a service is covered. One should obtain a waiver of liability (an advance beneficiary notice for Medicare Part B) from the patient in any situation in which there is a question as to whether the payor will cover the services. Finally, make every effort to price at a level at least equal to cost per reportable test and preferably at a level that maintains a reasonable profit while remaining competitive in the marketplace.

Prospective Payment

The primary key to success in prospective (capitated) payment is also correct and complete coding. To determine if a proposed payment amount is acceptable, you must know (or project) the utilization rates for services, including rates of use of add-on and reflex tests. You should understand the patient mix according to diagnoses and/or medical subspecialty to help project utilization of specific, especially niche, tests. You must certainly know your costs by CPT-4 code and must project total expenditures based on the terms of the contract. If certain niche tests are extremely high cost, you may wish to carve out those services and amend the agreement with a separate fee schedule for specific services. As for retrospective payment situations, if the proposed terms of the agreement are not financially favorable, you can decline to provide service.

Summary

In considering payment for laboratory services, there are four key concepts to remember. First, know your real costs for any given orderable and billable procedure, and make sure the terms of the payment agreement allow the recovery of costs. Second, set charges and accept fee schedules or other payments to guarantee that a reasonable profit margin has been attained. In order to continue to develop any laboratory business unit, it is essential to generate revenue that can be used to enhance the services offered. Beyond simply paying the bills, profits are essential for additional research and development, for facility improvements, for professional development of employees, and, in the case of a for-profit entity, for generating returns on investments. Third, set charges to be market competitive and provide services which are equivalent to or better than those of your competitors. "Better than" is a relative term but includes developing a strong and knowledgeable customer support team. Finally, avoid any appearance of kickbacks. Under the Office of the Inspector General compliance program for clinical laboratories, it is essential to avoid any appearance of inducement of ordering providers to submit testing from patients under federal payment programs. All of these concepts make for good clinical laboratory practice and also ensure that one is equipped to make good business decisions.

KEY POINTS

- The responsibility for cost analysis of individual laboratory procedures rests primarily with the laboratorian.

- In order to have a clear understanding of the total costs of a procedure, the best parameter to use is the cost per reportable test.

- The determination of charges has both financial and compliance implications; one generally does not charge below cost (may be construed as an inducement for ordering providers) or substantially in excess of usual charges.

- The Medicare fee schedule is quite complex and is adjusted regularly, and payments can be substantially lower than actual charges. A laboratory may have to accept a fee lower than its costs but may not set a charge higher than the Medicare fee it accepts.

- The importance of the Medicare fee schedule is its impact on the fee schedules developed by other third-party payors.

- The laboratory must maintain a thorough understanding of coding for procedures performed, as well as complete knowledge of all billing rules for each payor.

- Payment for laboratory services is based on four key concepts: (i) know your real test costs, (ii) set charges and accept fee schedules that guarantee a reasonable profit margin, (iii) set charges to be market competitive and provide services that are better than those of your competitors, and (iv) avoid any appearance of kickbacks.

GLOSSARY

Actual charge The amount of money a doctor or supplier charges for a certain medical service or supply. This amount is often more than the amount Medicare approves.

Approved amount The fee Medicare sets as reasonable for a covered medical service. This is the amount a doctor or supplier is paid by you and Medicare for a service or supply. It may be less than the actual amount charged by a doctor or supplier. The approved amount is sometimes called the "approved charge."

BBA '97 Balanced Budget Act of 1997.

BBRA '99 Balanced Budget Reduction Act of 1999.

Break-even point Point at which net income equals total costs.

Capitation A predetermined, fixed amount paid to providers in return for rendering a specified set of health services. The rate is established per person (per capita) enrolled in the health plan.

Carriers Centers for Medicare and Medicaid Services (CMS) primary third-party contractors who administer Part B payments according to the local medical review policies (LMRP) to physician, ancillary, and commercial laboratory providers.

Carve out To exclude from a capitated contract and bill as fee for service.

Claim The claim form or invoice, which allows transmission of the bill to a payor.

Covered lives Population insured by a managed-care contract.

Cross-walking The fee is set at the same rate as that for another CPT code (or codes) deemed "equivalent" and to which it is "mapped."

Current Procedural Terminology, 4th edition (CPT-4) Test codes recognized by the American Medical Association and required for filing claims and billing of Medicare.

Diagnosis-related groups (DRGs) Classification system developed at Yale that defines almost 400 major diagnostic categories and places patients into case types based on the International Classification of Diseases, 9th Revision (Clinical Modification), code classifications.

End-stage renal disease (ESRD) The terminology used for Medicare beneficiaries who have permanent kidney dysfunction requiring dialysis treatment.

Gap filling A new code is deemed novel and not adequately described by an existing code. Payments are set by individual contractors based on existing charges, and these payments are then used to subsequently set a national limitation amount (NLA).

HCPCS Healthcare Common Procedure Coding System.

Health maintenance organization (HMO) A prepaid system of healthcare with emphasis on the prevention and early detection of disease and on continuity of care; HMOs generally offer a package of services; however, the choice of physician is frequently limited to those working within the HMO.

Inherent reasonableness CMS may employ "reasonable-charge methodology" to arbitrarily reduce or increase a national limitation amount (NLA) deemed grossly excessive or grossly deficient.

International Classification of Diseases, Version 10, Procedure Coding System (ICD-N-PCS) Laboratory coding system intended for use as an alternative to CPT.

IOM Institute of Medicine.

"Loss leader" High-volume test that is charged below cost.

National limitation amount (NLA) The national fee cap for a particular test.

Reflex test Second related test performed automatically when initial test results are positive (susceptibility test on pathogen).

Stark legislation Designed to ensure that laboratories provide services to ordering providers without any evidence of inducement or kickback.

REFERENCES

1. **Centers for Medicare and Medicaid Services CMS, HHS.** 2002. Medicare program; changes to the hospital outpatient prospective payment system and calendar year 2003 payment rates; and changes to payment suspension for unfilled cost reports. Final rule with comment period. *Fed. Regist.* **67:**66717–67046.

2. **Fee, D. N.** 2002. Success with APCs. *Healthc. Financ. Manag.* **56:**68–72.

3. **Gold, M., and S. Snodgrass.** 2001. Calculating pass-through and outlier payments under APCs. *Healthc. Financ. Manag.* **55:**54–57.

4. **Nigon, D. L.** 2000. *Clinical Laboratory Management,* p. 177–188. McGraw-Hill, New York, N.Y.

5. **Reiser, W. S., and B. O. Brunicardi.** 2002. Assessing the impact of Medicare payment changes. *Healthc. Financ. Manag.* **56:** 68–71.

6. **Roselle, G., M. L. Render, L. B. Nugent, and G. N. Nugent.** 2003. Estimating private sector professional fees for VA providers. *Med. Care* **41**(6 Suppl.)**:**II23–II32.

7. **Travers, E. M.** 1997. *Clinical Laboratory Management.* Williams and Wilkins, Baltimore, Md.

8. **Weiss, R. L., D. Sundwall, and J. M. Matsen.** 2002. Estimating the budgetary impact of setting the Medicare clinical laboratory fee schedule at the national limitation amount. *Am. J. Clin. Pathol.* **117:**691–695.

APPENDIX 35.1 Publications, Phone Numbers, Websites, and Guidance Documents

PUBLICATIONS

Medicare Fee Schedule (issued every November)
Clinical Laboratory Strategies (newsletter of the American Association of Clinical Chemists Delta Project)
National Intelligence Report (newsletter published by Washington G-2 Reports, Washington, D.C.)
Laboratory Industry Report (newsletter published by Washington G-2 Reports, Washington, D.C.)
Laboratory Compliance Insider (Brownstone Publishers)
The Clinical Laboratory Compliance Alert (Eli Research)
Compliance Hotline (American Health Consultants)

PHONE NUMBER

CMS: 410-786-3000

WEBSITES

http://www.cms.gov
http://www.cms.gov/medlearn
http://www.cms.gov/medlearn/refabn.asp: advance beneficiary notice
http://www.cms.gov/regulations: CMS and related laws and regulations
http://www.cms.gov/regulations/pfs/2004fc/: Medicare Program revision to payment policies under the physician fee schedule for calendar year 2004
http://www.cms.hhs.gov/glossary/default.asp?Letter+ALL&Language=English#Content: extensive glossary related to CMS
http://www.cms.hhs.gov
http://www.oig.cms.gov: Compliance Program, Fraud Alerts, Advisory Opinions, Red Book, Work Plan
http://www.cms.hhs.gov/opendoor: monthly and bimonthly forums on Medicare and Medicaid
http://www.labfocus.com: CAP/CLMA Conference on Issues in Medicare Compliance
http://www.medicaretraining.com: Blue Cross Blue Shield Florida training program

http://www.ntis.gov: National Technical Information Service
http://www.cdc.gov/nchswww/data: National Center for Health Statistics
http://www.gao.gov: T-HEHS-00-74, 9 March 2000 (Medicare: HCFA Faces Challenges to Control Improper Payments [HIPAA])
http://www.ion.edu/ion/iomhome/nsf/pages/clinlab+home+page: Institute of Medicine Study
http://www.lmrp.net: all contractor local medical review policies
http://www.compliance.com: The American Compliance Institute
http://www.columbia.com: The Columbia Compliance Plan
http://www.hcca-info.org: Healthcare Compliance Association
http://www.medpac.gov: Medicare Payment Advisory Commission

FEDERAL REGISTER AND RELEVANT GUIDANCE DOCUMENTS

Category B IDE2

Federal Register. 1995. Medicare program: criteria and procedures for extending coverage to certain devices and related services—HCFA. Final rule with comment period. *Fed. Regist.* **60:**48417–48425.

Analyte-Specific Reagents

Federal Register. 1997. Medical devices; classification/reclassification; restricted devices; analyte specific reagents—PDA. Final rule. *Fed. Regist.* **62:**62243–62260.

Inherent Reasonableness

Federal Register. 1998. Medicare program; application of inherent reasonableness to all Medicare Part B services (other than physician services)—HCFA. Interim final rule with comment period. *Fed. Regist.* **63:**687–690.

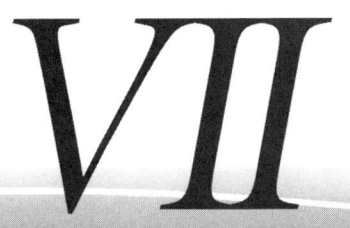

Reimbursement Processes

(Section Editors, *Vickie S. Baselski and Alice S. Weissfeld*)

Rules and Regulations in Reimbursement

Vickie S. Baselski, Alice S. Weissfeld, and Fran Sorrell

OBJECTIVES

To discuss the rules set forth by third-party payors that determine claim payment

To describe the term "medical necessity" and its relationship to reimbursement

To discuss the importance of claim compliance to reimbursement

To describe certain special coverage conditions for which unique billing rules may apply

To discuss national coverage determinations and the relationship between these determinations and local medical review policies

To describe the most common reasons for reimbursement denial and what can be done to correct the problems

---

Call them rules or call them limits, good ones, I believe, have this in common: They serve reasonable purposes; they are practical and within a child's (individual's) capability; they are consistent; and they are an expression of loving concern.

"MISTER" FRED ROGERS (1928–2003)

BEYOND THE BASIC LOGISTICAL ISSUES surrounding the battle for laboratory reimbursement are a number of issues which pertain to the rules of engagement. The logistical aspects include the documentation of what is done through Current Procedural Terminology, 4th edition (CPT-4), and Health Care Common Procedure Coding System (HCPCS) coding, why it is done through International Classification of Diseases, 9th Revision (Clinical Modification) (ICD-9-CM), or alternative diagnosis coding, where it is done through use of revenue and place-of-service codes, and what the actual monetary exchange system and amount of payment are (see section VI). The rules of engagement pertain to the establishment of criteria for the actual execution of payment, also known as conditions for coverage. To evaluate services for appropriateness for coverage and subsequent payment, payors generally employ standard sets of prepay edits, which specify conditions for payment or nonpayment. In addition, payors often conduct postpay audits to evaluate the accuracy of claim payment based on the defined coverage conditions, including prepay edits. While it might be a stretch to compare these rules to the limits imposed upon a child by a parent, they do share some common features. They are basically simple and clearly defined; they are relatively easily applied through an electronic claim review process; and while not an expression of

583

loving concern, they do attempt to place some controls on the rampant spending associated with healthcare, including in laboratory medicine. In addition, one can easily find examples of abuse of the reimbursement system, thus strengthening the need for well-defined limits.

General Criteria

Criteria for coverage of laboratory services historically have as their bases a number of elements. First is the evidence-based-medicine element, which suggests that laboratory services should be covered if shown in the medical literature to be necessary and effective in the management of a particular condition. Second is the medical-ethics element, which suggests that patients should not be denied a procedure proven to be necessary and effective. Third is the medical-judgment element, which places the burden of decision making on the ordering provider, whose training and experience in patient management should serve to justify performance of a procedure. These criteria have been historically adequate to determine coverage. However, as healthcare costs have risen, and rationing of available resources has become a necessity, more rigorous criteria to verify that a service should be covered have emerged in the form of payor rules, which in federal payment programs are based on regulations arising from statutes. These rules are applied through stringent claim review processes in which both procedures and diagnoses are considered in making a payment determination (1, 3, 4, 6).

The primary statute upon which federal programs are based is the Social Security Act of 1967. This provided for healthcare benefits for "the diagnosis or treatment of illness or injury or to improve the functioning of a malformed body part" in the elderly and, subsequently, in disabled individuals. Many regulations have evolved from this phraseology, which serves to limit services to those which have been interpreted by the Centers for Medicare and Medicaid Services (CMS) (formerly Health Care Financing Administration) or its contractors as meeting the intent of the law. Furthermore, many other third-party payors have adopted similar types of payment rules. These rules can be divided into three general categories: those that are basic and review a claim for standard identifying information, those that evaluate the appropriateness of the procedures that are ordered in a given time frame, and, finally, those that assess the "medical necessity" of performing a test in view of the established coverage criteria.

Basic Rules

All claims for laboratory services must meet certain basic requirements for processing. CMS claims are filed using one of two basic forms for laboratory services and are used in entirety or as models for claims submitted to other payors. The CMS-1450 form (formally the UB-92)

is used for institutional (e.g., hospitals, nursing homes) claims for Medicare Part A services. It is designed and maintained by the National Uniform Billing Committee and used by many institutional providers. The CMS-1500 is used by noninstitutional providers (e.g., independent laboratories) to bill Medicare Part B services and some Medicaid services, and it has become a universal claim form for many other third-party payors. The coding requirements for claim transactions have been standardized under the Health Insurance Portability and Accountability Act, which specified all transactions and code sets for electronic transactions.

The major required elements for claim submission and subsequent reimbursement for covered services are as follows (Table 36.1). The patient must be identified using a unique identifier, and all demographic information necessary for subsequent communications, particularly bills for services if indicated, must also be provided. The date of service, which is defined as the date of collection of clinical specimens, must be provided. The ordering provider must be identified using a national provider identifier (previously called the unique provider identifier number), and adequate demographic information must be provided for subsequent communications, including acquisition of additional documentation, test results, and bills for services if indicated (8). The authentication of the laboratory service provider requires a Clinical Laboratory Improvement Amendments number and designation (high complexity, moderate complexity, certificate of waiver, provider-performed microscopy) appropriate to the service being billed. The place of service must be designated, either as a revenue code in the case of an inpatient or using a place-of-service code for outpatient testing. The actual services provided on the specified date must be indicated using the appropriate CPT-4 or HCPCS codes, including units of service and modifiers where appropriate as well as the actual charges for each service. Reimbursement is rarely made at the charge level, but Medicare and other third-party

Table 36.1 Major required elements for claims submission and subsequent reimbursement

Unique patient identifier
Date of service
Bills for services
Ordering provider number (national provider identifier)
Provider CLIA[a] number and designation (high complexity, moderate complexity, certificate of waiver, provider-performed microscopy)
Place of service (either revenue code for inpatient or place-of-service code for outpatient testing)
Actual services provided (CPT-4 or HCPCS codes, including units of service and modifiers where appropriate, and actual charges for each service)
Reason for performing the test (ICD-9-CM diagnosis code for outpatients and DRG or narrative diagnosis for inpatients)

[a]CLIA, Clinical Laboratory Improvement Amendments.

payors use this information for determination of fee schedule payment amounts. Finally, the reason for performing the test must be indicated using an appropriate ICD-9-CM diagnosis code for outpatients and a diagnosis-related group (DRG) or narrative diagnosis for inpatients. Failure to complete all required data fields would result in a denial from a third-party payor (2, 7, 9).

Procedure Code Edits

Basic Edits

The next level of claim review looks at the actual procedures performed as identified by HCPCS or CPT-4 code (Table 36.2). The most basic edit is a determination of whether a service may represent a duplicate service (i.e., same procedure on the same date of service). In the event that a laboratory procedure is performed more than once on a given date of service for a valid medical purpose, an appropriate modifier (-59 or -91) must be amended to the procedure code. Similarly, frequency limits are used to determine how often a particular laboratory procedure may be reimbursed. These types of edits may be problematic for clinical laboratories if a patient has presented to more than one ordering provider or laboratory provider during the time frame for reimbursement. For this reason, it is reasonable to obtain an advance beneficiary notice (ABN) for frequency-limited test procedures.

NCCI

Procedure codes are also reviewed to determine if two or more different codes are appropriately ordered on the same date of service. The Medicare National Correct Coding Initiative (NCCI) provides the most extensive system for this type of claim review process. This program was initiated in 1996 through a contract with a Medicare contractor, AdminaStar Federal. The program was initiated to promote correct coding of healthcare services, including laboratory services, and to control improper payment for incorrect coding. Edits have been developed based on national and local coverage policies, coding guidelines and practice guidelines published by professional societies, and review of provider current coding and billing practice.

The NCCI documents are published on a quarterly basis by the National Technical Information Service and have just recently been made publicly available on the CMS website. The complete document includes a table of contents and 13 narrative chapters, with Chapter X specific to Pathology and Laboratory Services. However, on occasion, there is crossover between chapters in edit pairs, and laboratorians should be aware of all edits pertaining to the laboratory. NCCI is provided to contractors as a set of automated edits which compare all CPT-4 and HCPCS codes submitted on the same date of service. As expected, NCCI serves as a model for claim review by other third-party payors. The edits fall into two major categories termed "comprehensive/component" and "mutually exclusive." The edits also indicate the code pairs in these edit categories for which a modifier (generally -59) may be appropriate to indicate that the tests were in fact appropriate under the circumstances.

Comprehensive/Component Edits

Comprehensive/component edits (also known as column 1/column 2 edits) identify cases in which a specific code has been identified as representing a component of a more comprehensive code documented on the same date of service. The most obvious example is the performance of an American Medical Association-approved panel. In this situation, one would not also code and bill for the individual analytes included in the panel unless a subsequent measurement of a specific analyte was necessary for patient care. In other cases, the descriptor for a procedure may include

Table 36.2 Procedure code edits

Basic edits	Determination of whether a service may represent a duplicate service (review of actual procedures identified by HCPCS or CPT-4 codes)
	Frequency limits (how often a particular laboratory procedure may be reimbursed); it may be necessary to obtain an ABN for frequency-limited test procedures
NCCI	Review to determine if two or more different codes are appropriately ordered on the same date of service. NCCI provides an extensive system for this type of claim review process, administered through AdminaStar Federal (Medicare contractor)
	Documents published on quarterly basis; now available on the CMS website
Comprehensive/component edits	Also known as "column 1/column 2 edits"; these edits identify cases in which a specific code has been identified as representing a component of a more comprehensive code documented on the same date of service (AMA[a]-approved panel—one would not also code and bill for individual analytes included in the panel)
Mutually exclusive codes	Codes for services that are not reasonably performed during the same patient encounter; these codes are considered to provide duplicate information
	Multiple tests to identify the same analyte, marker, or infectious agent should not be reported together.

[a]AMA, American Medical Association.

several related codes. All of the molecular infectious disease codes are considered inclusive of all individual step codes found in the molecular diagnostics section of the CPT-4 codebook. Finally, if after a test was ordered and performed, an additional related procedure was necessary to confirm the result, this would be considered a part of the original ordered test unless a specific confirmatory code is available (e.g., in the case of several serologic tests for infectious agents, including human immunodeficiency virus and *Treponema pallidum*, and for hepatitis B surface antigen). When incompatible comprehensive edit code pairs are billed, the most comprehensive code but not the component codes are generally reimbursed.

Mutually Exclusive Codes

Mutually exclusive codes are those that are not reasonably performed during the same encounter. In essence, these are considered to provide duplicate information. There is a long-standing CMS interpretation of a Medicare statute that has influenced development of mutually exclusive edits. That is that multiple tests to identify the same analyte, marker, or infectious agent should not be reported together. For example, it would not be appropriate to perform an enzyme immunoassay and a nucleic acid detection procedure to detect the same infectious agent from the same specimen on the same date of service, nor would it be appropriate to perform and bill a nonamplified and an amplified nucleic acid test for the same analyte from the same specimen on the same date of service. Again, if additional clinically useful information may be obtained by performing both procedures in a mutually exclusive code set, modifier -59 may be attached. When mutually exclusive codes are billed together inappropriately, in general, the least costly code is reimbursed.

Medical Necessity

The terminology "medical necessity" derives from Section 1862(a)(1)(A) of the Social Security Act of 1965, which stipulates that no Medicare payment will be made for expenses incurred for items or services that are not reasonable and necessary for the diagnosis or treatment of illness or injury or to improve the functioning of a malformed body member. Medicare has consistently interpreted this provision to exclude services that have not been determined to be safe and effective, are experimental, and are not performed in accordance with accepted standards of medical practice as demonstrated through peer-reviewed literature and published professional-society guidelines or practice standards (2). In addition, Section 1862(a)(7) excludes coverage for expenses for routine physical checkups and for testing performed to screen for an illness or an illness precursor in the absence of signs, symptoms, complaints, or personal history of disease or injury except where explicitly allowed by statute (e.g., cervical cytology in women and prostate-specific antigen testing in men).

Medical-necessity edits have been developed which evaluate both the procedures performed and the reason for performing the procedures on a given date of service. These edits may be developed and applied nationally and are known as national coverage determinations (NCDs). Alternatively, where there is not an NCD or where an NCD is silent, local policies may be developed by individual contractors. These are known as local medical review policies (LMRPs). However, a local contractor may not develop an LMRP in conflict with an NCD. Both types of policies define the ICD-9-CM diagnosis codes, which are recognized as providing evidence of medical necessity for coverage of a particular laboratory procedure. As would be expected, private third-party payors have embraced this concept, and while not as extensive as the system used for Medicare reimbursement, medical necessity nevertheless forms the basis for denials of payment in the private sector now too.

NCD

Section 4554(b)(1) of the Balanced Budget Act of 1997 mandated the use of a negotiated rule-making process to develop national coverage and administrative policies for Part B clinical diagnostic laboratory services (Table 36.3). Beginning in 1998 and continuing through 1999, 18 professional groups representing laboratory, physician, and beneficiary interests and the Department of Health and Human Services Medicare Program participated in this process, culminating in the publication of 23 national coverage policies developed through consensus. A Notice of Proposed Rulemaking was published in March 2000, and a final rule was published in November 2001, with an implementation date 1 year hence. These 23 policies are believed to represent 60% of the Part B laboratory outlays and provide consistency in coverage for beneficiaries. Further, a system has been developed to allow for the continuation of the development of new NCDs through a formal process.

The format for an NCD is standardized and is, in fact, very similar to that used for LMRPs. A narrative description of the covered services is given and the associated CPT-4 codes are identified, as well as the ICD-9-CM codes that may be covered, those that are not generally covered, and those that are never covered due to statutory interpretation (e.g., screening tests for diseases or disease precursors). In addition, each NCD has a narrative section that defines indications, coding guidelines, and limitations upon which the coding portions are based. These NCDs have been updated with technical corrections on a regular basis through Program Memoranda issued by CMS. During the claim review process, the procedure codes (CPT-4 or HCPCS) which have been submitted are compared to

Table 36.3 NCDs

Definition	Balanced Budget Act of 1997 mandated the use of a negotiated rule-making process to develop national coverage and administrative policies for Part B clinical diagnostic laboratory services.
Participation	Since 1998, 18 professional groups representing laboratory, physician, and beneficiary interests and the Department of Human Services Medicare Program have participated.
Publications	National coverage policies developed through consensus; 23 policies are believed to represent 60% of the Part B laboratory outlays—provide consistency in coverage for beneficiaries
NCD format	Narrative description of the covered services and associated CPT-4 codes
	Specific ICD-9-CM codes that may be covered, those that are generally not covered, and those that are never covered due to statutory interpretation (e.g., screening tests for diseases or disease precursors)
Content of narrative section	Defines indications, coding guidelines, and limitations
Updates	NCDs have been updated with technical corrections on a regular basis through Program Memoranda issued by CMS.

diagnosis codes (ICD-9-CM) to determine if payment is indicated.

LMRPs

Where a national policy does not exist, or for any aspect of a national policy for which coverage conditions are not specified (e.g., frequency limits), a regional contractor may issue an LMRP. The contents of the LMRPs are very similar to those of NCDs, and each contractor must develop software for claim review, again comparing procedure codes (CPT-4 or HCPCS) to diagnosis codes (ICD-9-CM) to make a payment decision. The Carrier Advisory Committee, or an alternative medical review team in the case of a fiscal intermediary, generally develops LMRPs through a systematic process with review. LMRPs are published in local contractor bulletins for a review-and-comment period (generally 90 days), after which a final policy is developed and implemented. The inequities in coverage promulgated by LMRPs led a recent General Accounting Office report to recommend that new LMRP development be eliminated and existing policies be evaluated to determine if they should be incorporated into national policies or rescinded. At the time of this writing, no action has been taken.

Experimental Testing

Medicare has historically interpreted the "reasonable and necessary" clause to mean that services that were experimental (i.e., for research or investigational use) were not reasonable or necessary and therefore not reimbursed. Further, clearance or approval by the Food and Drug Administration was taken as evidence that a procedure was not experimental. Currently, however, there is much controversy in this area, particularly in the realm of newly emerging molecular technologies. Procedures with a Category B Investigational Device Exemption may be reimbursed at a contractor's discretion, as may routine tests used in support of a new investigational device or procedure in a clinical-trial setting. However, it is still generally accepted that failure to have Food and Drug Administration clearance or

approval if required is justification for denial. In the case of tests using analyte-specific reagents (ASR), the situation is less clear. However, if the ASR is being used in accordance with the ASR rule and all other conditions for medical necessity are met, such assays may be reimbursed at the discretion of a contractor. In the case of other third-party payors, there tends to be more leniency in coverage, as payor-specific independent technology assessment groups make individual coverage decisions.

Administrative Policies

A number of Medicare administrative policies were also negotiated during the rule-making process. These were related to the actual processing of claims and required contractors to accept and evaluate all diagnostic codes submitted before making a medical-necessity determination, allowed a narrative diagnosis to be translated into an ICD-9-CM code if a match could be found, and forbade the use of unpublished frequency edits as a basis for denial of payment. In addition, although the laboratory remains the entity that receives payment and therefore the entity at risk for nonpayment when a claim is denied, the policy did clarify that the ordering providers have a responsibility to submit required medical-necessity documentation. Further, if it is not provided, CMS contractors should notify the ordering provider that additional documentation is required to complete the claim for payment. In the same time frame, a new rule pertaining to the ABN process for clinical laboratories was issued which allowed the use of a laboratory-specific form whenever the ordering provider failed to provide diagnostic information that would support the medical necessity of a test and therefore result in denial of reimbursement. Where appropriate, absent evidence or clear proof of medical necessity, laboratories are encouraged to seek beneficiary signing of an ABN assuming financial liability in the case of denial. Such documents are also common in third-party-payor situations, although the terms of coverage are generally outlined on an annual basis rather than on a date-of-service basis.

Special Coverage Conditions

In a number of clinical circumstances, unique billing rules may apply (Table 36.4). In the Medicare program, special rules apply, particularly in the setting of end-stage renal disease (ESRD) and its management in dialysis centers and in payment for laboratory services in Part A skilled-nursing facilities (SNF). Patients admitted to hospitals with preadmission testing are also subject to a rule called the "DRG payment window." Finally, each individual payor may impose other arbitrary rules that may be discerned only through careful evaluation of denials.

ESRD

ESRD payment rules are rather complex and represent a combination of a capitated system and a fee-for-service system (5). Most clinical laboratory tests are included in a composite rate payment through the fiscal intermediary. In order to bill separately according to the fee schedule, 50% or more of the covered tests must be noncomposite rate tests for a given date of service. In addition, several unique HCPCS modifiers are used to identify a separately billable test.

SNF

The Balanced Budget Act of 1997 altered the manner in which the majority of services are provided to Medicare beneficiaries in a Part A-covered SNF stay. All reimbursement was bundled into a single composite prospective payment. While there are a few exceptions which are separately payable, laboratory services are included in the composite per diem. In a Part B stay in which Part A benefits have been exhausted, certain medical services, including laboratory tests, may be payable according to the previously described rules.

Table 36.4 Special coverage conditions

ESRD	Complex payment rules that represent a combination of a capitated system and a fee-for-service system
SNF	All reimbursement is bundled into a single composite prospective payment; there are a few exceptions, but laboratory services are included in the composite per diem.
Three-day window	Used to prevent transfer of charges from the capitated DRG system to a fee-for-service Part B system
	Specifies that laboratory services performed by a hospital are included in the DRG payment for a related admission
Other private-payor rules	Third-party payors model coverage rules on Medicare; however, each has its own guidelines for reimbursement.

Three-Day Window

Patients admitted to the hospital and eligible for Part A services frequently require preadmission testing. In order to prevent the transfer of charges from the capitated DRG system to a fee-for-service Part B system, Medicare implemented the 3-day payment window, which specifies that laboratory services performed by a hospital or by an entity wholly owned or operated by a hospital are included in the DRG payment for a related admission. In short-term hospital settings, the window is reduced to one calendar day.

Other Private-Payor Rules

While many third-party payors model their coverage rules on Medicare, each has its own guidelines for reimbursement. A large laboratory may interact with several hundred unique payor plans, and the ability to triage claims for compliance with all payment rules absolutely depends on claim processing software. Fortunately, these payors tend to be more liberal in reimbursement for services, yet as healthcare costs rise, such rules restricting payment for services become an attractive means to control costs.

Remittance Advice Review

Beneficiary Documents

The importance of review by the laboratory of the bases for denial or adjustment of claims cannot be overemphasized. For beneficiaries, a specific explanatory statement termed an explanation of benefits or explanation of medical benefits accompanies each denial by any payor. In the Medicare program, a beneficiary receives a Medicare summary notice (previously termed an explanation of Medicare benefits). These documents provide specific and standardized explanatory information which identifies the reason for the denial. This information can be used to attempt to obtain additional documentation from the ordering provider in order to resubmit the claim, initiate an appeal process, or bill an alternative responsible party (i.e., client or patient) if appropriate.

Provider Documents

Laboratories also receive remittance advice reports from Medicare carriers and intermediaries which provide an explanation of the disposition of a claim for specific patients in a given period. These reports list the deficient items that are responsible for preventing expected payment. Under the Health Insurance Portability and Accountability Act of 1996, two sets of standardized codes are now required to convey this information to providers. The claim adjustment "reason codes" communicate why a claim for service was "adjusted" (i.e., paid differently from expected) and are maintained by the American National Standards Institute. The "remark codes" add greater specificity and additional explanatory narrative to the reason codes. CMS is the national maintainer for the standard remark codes.

Auditing Remittance Advice

Careful review of these remittance documents provides a mechanism to identify billing problems that are costly in terms of both labor and lost revenue. Recent publications indicate that the most common reasons for denial include lack of medical-necessity documentation, the fact that the service performed is noncovered (generally used for screening purposes), inadequacy or lack of basic identifying documentation (particularly date of service, ordering provider unique provider identifier number, and patient identification number), and, finally, incorrect coding (both procedure and diagnosis). Study of these reports to identify trends can identify systematic problems often resulting from simple failure to follow the payor rules and can lead to successful interventions to correct the problems and enhance appropriate reimbursement. At least one study has demonstrated significant improvement in reimbursement after implementation of processes to ensure adequate documentation prior to claim submission.

Summary

Thorough knowledge of and understanding of the rules set forth by third-party payors that determine whether a claim submitted for laboratory services will be paid are key to success in the laboratory. Many of the rules emanate from Medicare statutes, with resulting regulations that are designed to ensure that only services that are deemed medically necessary for management of a disease condition are paid for. However, a few statutes deem payment appropriate for certain specific preventative-medicine test procedures (e.g., cervical cytology and prostate-specific antigen testing). Design of a system that attempts to ensure compliance with all of the known rules and regulations from federal and other payors will eliminate costly and time-consuming claim resubmissions. Likewise, the system will ensure timely reimbursement for services that are considered to be covered and allow for alternate billing of the appropriate responsible party in the event of a denial. Indeed, such rules lay a consistent and logical, if not always mutually agreed upon, ground for reimbursement. In addition, since many of these rules are based on statutes, a systematic approach lays a firm foundation for regulatory compliance.

KEY POINTS

- Payor rules are based on regulations arising from statutes; rules are applied through stringent claim review processes.

- Both procedures and diagnoses are considered in making a payment determination.

- Failure to complete all required data fields in a claim for laboratory services will result in a denial from a third-party payor.

- It is important to understand component edits and mutually exclusive codes that can result in claim denials.

- The concept of medical necessity forms the basis for claim denials in both the public (Medicare) and private sectors.

- It is important to understand how your LMRPs are set, where the committee is located, and how to contact the committee members for claim denial clarifications.

- The importance of reviewing all claim denials cannot be overemphasized. A beneficiary receives a Medicare summary notice, which provides specific and standardized explanatory information that identifies the reason for the denial. Follow-up can include obtaining additional documentation, resubmitting the claim, initiating an appeal process, or billing an alternative party.

GLOSSARY

AdminaStar Federal Medicare contractor handling the review of procedure codes to determine if two or more different codes are appropriately ordered on the same date of service. This service was initiated in 1996; these edits are available on the Centers for Medicare and Medicaid Services (CMS) website.

Advance beneficiary notice A waiver of liability used by the provider to notify Medicare beneficiaries prior to receiving services that it may not be a covered service and that they may have to assume financial responsibility.

American National Standards Institute The claim adjustment "reason codes" indicate why a claim for service was "adjusted" (e.g., paid differently from expected) and are maintained by the American National Standards Institute; "remark codes" add greater specificity and additional explanatory narrative to the "reason codes" and are maintained by CMS.

Analyte-specific reagents (ASR) If the ASR is used in accordance with the ASR rule and all other reasons for medical necessity are met, assays may be reimbursed at the discretion of a contractor.

Carrier CMS primary third-party contractors who administer Part B payments according to the local medical review policies (LMRPs) to physician, ancillary, and commercial laboratory providers.

Carrier Advisory Committee LMRPs are generally developed through a systematic approach with review by the Carrier Advisory Committee.

Claim The claim form or invoice, which allows transmission of the bill to a payor.

CMS-1450 (formerly UB-92) Form used for institutional (e.g., hospitals, nursing homes) claims for Medicare Part A services.

CMS-1500 Claim form authorized by the Health Care Financing Administration (now CMS) for filing Medicare Part B claims with carriers.

Current Procedural Terminology, 4th edition (CPT-4) Test codes recognized by the American Medical Association and required for filing of claims and billing of Medicare.

Diagnosis code Medical diagnoses are assigned a number code from a book titled International Classification of Diseases, 9th Revision (Clinical Modifications) (ICD-9-CM). The ICD-9-CM code refers to the patient's medical diagnosis.

Diagnosis-related groups (DRGs) Classification system developed at Yale that defines almost 400 major diagnostic categories and places patients into case types based on the ICD-9-CM code classifications.

End-stage renal disease (ESRD) The terminology used for Medicare beneficiaries who have permanent kidney dysfunction requiring dialysis treatment.

Fiscal intermediary CMS primary third-party contractors who administer Part A payments according to LMRPs for hospitals and rehabilitation and skilled nursing facilities.

Food and Drug Administration clearance Failure to have Food and Drug Administration clearance or approval for a particular test is generally justification for claim denial.

HCFA-1500 Claim form authorized by the Health Care Financing Administration (now CMS) for filing Medicare Part B claims with carriers (*see* CMS-1500).

Health Insurance Portability and Accountability Act of 1996 Title I protects health insurance coverage for workers and their families when they change or lose their jobs. Title II requires the Department of Health and Human Services to establish national standards for electronic healthcare transactions and national identifiers for providers, health plans, and employers. It also addresses the security and privacy of health data. Adopting these standards will improve the efficiency and effectiveness of the nation's healthcare system by encouraging the widespread use of electronic data interchange in healthcare.

International Classification of Diseases, Version 10, Procedure Coding System Laboratory coding system intended for use as an alternative to CPT.

Medicaid Program established under Title XIX of the Social Security Act, which provides health insurance to poor people; the state and federal governments fund it jointly.

Medical necessity The determination of ICD-9-CM codes for which a CPT code will be reimbursed as reasonable and necessary.

Medicare Federally managed health insurance plan covering Americans over age 65 and Americans under age 65 who have certain disabilities and for most patients with ESRD; established by a 1965 amendment to the Social Security Act.

Modifier Modifiers are comprised of two digit numbers, which are attached to a specific code prior to the billing process (see Table 33.3). They are "used to indicate that a service or procedure has been altered by some specific circumstance but not changed in its definition or code."

National Correct Coding Initiative (NCCI) Review of procedure codes to determine if two or more different codes are appropriately ordered on the same date of service. This service was initiated in 1996 through a contract with a Medicare contractor, AdminaStar Federal. These edits are available on the CMS website.

National Technical Information Service Publishes the NCCI procedure code edit documents on a quarterly basis.

NCCI edits Edits fall into two major categories, (i) comprehensive/component and (ii) mutually exclusive. Edits indicate the code pairs in these edit categories for which a modifier (generally -59) may be appropriate.

Neg Reg Negotiated Rulemaking Committee on diagnostic clinical laboratory tests.

Not medically necessary The determination that an ICD-9-CM code does not justify payment.

Program Memoranda National coverage decisions have been updated with technical corrections on a regular basis through Program Memoranda issued by CMS.

Reasonable-charge methodology Based on inherent reasonableness, authority to arbitrarily increase or decrease payment.

Regulation Legally binding rules developed to implement a statute.

Social Security Act of 1967 Provided for healthcare benefits for "the diagnosis of treatment of illness or injury or to improve the functioning of a malformed body part" in the elderly and, subsequently, in disabled individuals.

Statute A law passed by the U.S. Congress or a state legislature.

REFERENCES

1. Alwell, M. 2003. Stem revenue losses with effective CDM management. *Healthc. Financ. Manag.* **57:**84–88.

2. Carter, D. 2002. Optimizing revenue by reducing medical necessity claims denials. *Healthc. Financ. Manag.* **56:**88–94.

3. Cathey, R. 2003. 5 ways to reduce claims denials. *Healthc. Financ. Manag.* **57:**44–48.

4. Murray, M. E., and J. B. Henriques. 2003. Denials of reimbursement for hospital care. *Manag. Care Interface* **16:**22–27.

5. Parker, S., N. Davidson, and R. Gagliano. 2002. Preventing and dealing with ESRD claim denials. *Nephrol. News Issues* **16:**18–21, 25–26.

6. Reed, R. L., II, K. A. David, G. M. Silver, T. J. Esposito, V. Tsitlik, T. O'Hern, and R. L. Gamelli. 2003. Reducing trauma payment denials with computerized collaborative billing. *J. Trauma* **55:**762–770.

7. Reiser, W. S., and B. O. Brunicardi. 2002. Assessing the impact of Medicare payment changes. *Healthc. Financ. Manag.* **56:**68–71.

8. Sutton, J. P., J. Stensland, L. Zhao, and M. Cheng. 2002. Achieving equity in Medicare disproportionate share payments to rural hospitals: an assessment of the financial impact of recent and proposed changes to the disproportionate share hospital payment formula. *J. Rural Health* **18:**494–502.

9. Wallack, S. S., and C. P. Tompkins. 2003. Realigning incentives in fee-for-service Medicare. *Health Aff.* (Millwood) **22:**59–70.

APPENDIX 36.1   Websites

http://www.cms.gov
http://www.cms.gov/medlearn
http://www.cms.gov/medlearn/refabn.asp: ABN
http://www.cms.gov/regulations: CMS and related laws and regulations

http://www.hhs.gov/medlearn/ncci.asp: Medicare's NCCI edits
http://www.oig.cms.gov: Compliance Program, Fraud Alerts, Advisory Opinions, Red Book, Work Plan

APPENDIX 36.2   Medicare's NCCI Edits[a]

PART 1: HELPFUL QUESTIONS AND ANSWERS

How do I obtain a copy of the *CCI Policy and Edits Manual*?

Two ways: (i) through the CMS website at http://www.cms.hhs.gov/physicians/cciedits/default.asp and (ii) purchasing the manual, or sections of the manual, from the National Technical Information Service (NTIS) website at http://www.ntis.gov/products/families/cci (NTIS: 1-800-363-2068).

Are the edits in the *CCI Edits Manual* valid for a whole year?

No, the edits are updated on a quarterly basis. However, the *NCCI Policy Manual* is updated annually in October.

What does the effective date mean for CCI edits?

This date applies to the dates of service on or after a given date.

Do I need to obtain each version update of the CCI in order to manage our coding practices effectively and efficiently?

Yes, there are various numbers of changes in every update.

Do the edits change that much between quarterly updates?

The number of changes depends on the volume of comments received, modifications processed, and edits reviewed.

There are some software coding programs that already contain the CCI edits. Do I still need to purchase the manual from NTIS?

At this time, the official method for providers to receive the CCI edits is through the CMS website or through NTIS. It is up to the hospital and to the physician to be aware of the quarterly updates to the *CCI Edits Manual.*

Is there a list of deletions to each version update available, or do I have to do a comparison between the previous and the current version updates to determine what was actually deleted?

The electronic file that is available on the CMS website has several columns which include the effective dates and deletion dates of the CCI edits. However, the *CCI Manual* (specifically the printed version) available from NTIS does not list the effective and deletion dates of the CCI edits.

How are the CCI edits arranged in the manual?

The edits are arranged by two sets of tables. One table contains the column 1/column 2 correct coding edits (formerly known as comprehensive/component edits), and the other contains the mutually exclusive edits. In both tables, the column 2 codes are not payable with the column 1 codes unless the edit permits the use of a modifier associated with CCI.

If I want to determine what codes/procedures are paired with a certain code, how can I find this out?

NTIS provides the printed versions of column 1/column 2 correct coding edits and mutually exclusive code edits sorted and sequenced in two ways: by column 1 code and by column 2 code. The NTIS electronic version allows you to search for a

code in the database in either position.

What are some of the possible denial messages that may be displayed on the beneficiary's explanation of medical benefits?

"Medicare does not pay for this service because it is part of another service that was performed at the same time."

"Payment is included in another service received on the same day."

Does anyone have input about these edits before they are implemented?

Edit modifications resulting from comments are often referred to medical societies prior to final disposition of the edit. In addition, the American Medical Association receives a listing of all changes at least 1 month prior to the quarterly implementation of a new version of the CCI.

PART 2: TERMS AND DEFINITIONS THAT APPLY TO CCI

What are CCI edits?

CCI edits are pairs of CPT or HCPCS level II codes that are not separately payable except under certain circumstances; the edits are applied to services billed by the same provider for the same beneficiary on the same date of service.

What does it mean when codes are considered mutually exclusive of each other?

Mutually exclusive codes represent procedures or services that could not reasonably be performed at the same session by the same provider for the same beneficiary.

What exactly does "column 1" mean in the coding edits table and in the mutually exclusive edits table?

The column 1 code generally represents the major procedure or service when reported with the column code. When reported with the column 2 code, "column 1" generally represents the code with the greater work relative-value units of the two codes. However, within the mutually exclusive edits table, "column 1" generally represents the procedure of service with the lower work relative-value units and is the payable procedure or service when reported with the column 2 code.

What is the mutually exclusive edit table?

This edit table contains edits consisting of two codes for services which cannot reasonably be performed together based on the code definitions of anatomic considerations. If the two codes of an edit are billed by the same provider for the same beneficiary for the same date of service without an appropriate modifier, the column 1 code is paid.

[a]The information in this appendix is from the website http://www.cms.hhs.gov/. The mailing address for AdminaStar Federal is National Correct Coding Initiative, AdminaStar Federal, Inc., P.O. Box 50469, Indianapolis, IN 46250-0469.

37

Reimbursement Compliance

Vickie S. Baselski, Alice S. Weissfeld, and Fran Sorrell

OBJECTIVES

To describe what constitutes fraud and/or abuse

To discuss specific examples of the most common forms of fraud and abuse found in the public and private sectors

To discuss a prepayment review and its relationship to reimbursement

To describe some of the legal ramifications that might be associated with a postpayment review

To define the seven key elements within a sound compliance program

To list some of the acceptable marketing practices, as well as some that may not be in compliance

To provide several specific examples of potential laboratory fraud and abuse

Money made through dishonest practices will not last long.

CHINESE PROVERB

WITH THE EXTENSIVE ARRAY of statutory, regulatory, and other payor-defined rules that exist with regard to billing for healthcare services, including laboratory medicine, it is no surprise that errors are frequently documented. Errors may occur on the part of either the billing entity or the payor. To minimize and control such errors, including those that are intentional and therefore fraudulent, all entities involved in reimbursement have formal review processes in place. The most extensive review program is that developed by the federal government under "program integrity." In laboratory medicine, program integrity includes elements that ensure both accurate billing by the laboratory and accurate payment by the payor. Similar programs exist for essentially all third-party payors to ensure that appropriate payment is made for covered services but not made in noncovered situations.

Fraud and Abuse

The claim review processes will identify many unintentional errors, particularly those pertaining to inadequate documentation. However, in the last decade, the laboratory medicine industry has been the subject of intense scrutiny for evidence of systematic attempts to receive payment in error. This systematic process of receiving inappropriate payment has been termed "fraud and/or abuse." Abuse may be defined as the receipt of payment for services billed by mistake. This can include a wide range of behaviors including but not limited to billing for a noncovered service, misusing codes on a claim (i.e., not in compliance with coding convention), and inappropriately allocating costs on a cost report (e.g., for diagnosis-related group submission). Fraud is distinguished on the basis of intent and may be defined as the intentional deception or misrepresentation of documentation on a claim to purposely receive reimbursement for services not performed, not necessary, or performed at a higher level or frequency or including more units of service than appropriate. Both fraud and abuse are considered inappropriate and may be subject to criminal and civil penalties as well as payback of amounts determined to be paid in error by both federal payors and private third-party insurers. However, it is important to recognize that innocent errors and mistakes may occur. Only in the setting of actual knowledge of the falsity of a claim, reckless disregard of the truth of the claim, or deliberate ignorance of the correct process will civil or criminal legal action be taken. Truly innocent false or incorrect claims generating overpayment are generally simply subjected to repayment.

Both private insurers and federal payors have defined the most common forms of fraud and abuse. These activities include the following:

- *Providing an incorrect diagnosis or misrepresenting the diagnosis to justify payment.* Providing an incorrect diagnosis or misrepresenting the diagnosis is known as code jamming (i.e., inserting a code that was not provided by the ordering provider but which will justify payment). Another practice is code steering (i.e., providing lists of diagnosis codes that are known to justify payment).
- *Billing for services not performed as ordered.* Performing and billing for tests not ordered is a straightforward incorrect practice, but performing a related test for which the Current Procedural Terminology, 4th edition (CPT-4), code pays at a higher level is also incorrect (termed "upcoding").
- *Routine waiver of deductibles and copayments on non-Medicare patients or offering charges lower than accepted market value.* Any attempt to offer incentives to nonfederal payors to encourage them to also submit federal program testing is termed "inducement" and is a violation of the Stark legislation. The routine offering of waivers for amounts due or the routine billing for a service which pays at a lower level to encourage utilization (termed "downcoding") is similarly inappropriate. Recent Office of the Inspector General (OIG) proposals also indicate the intent to look closely at the common practice of laboratory discounts to determine if the Medicare program payment amounts are excessive relative to the charges to a laboratory's other clients.
- *Soliciting, offering, or receiving a kickback in exchange for receiving business.* The provision of any item of value in exchange for referral of federal business to a

laboratory is also a violation of the Stark legislation. The provision of free testing services to clients (termed "professional courtesy"), free supplies other than those used strictly in the provision of laboratory services, and free data summary reports used for purposes other than evaluation of laboratory utilization (e.g., antibiograms, drug-of-abuse profiles) are unacceptable practices. Also suspect would be clinical trial work done for no charge. Finally, routine leasing of laboratory space, primarily for specimen collection by a laboratory-affiliated phlebotomist, at rates higher than usual is suspect. In fact, one can say that any value-added service has value and should therefore be billed to the client at its fair market value.

- *Unbundling or "exploding" charges by billing for individual codes rather than using a Center for Medicare and Medicaid Services (CMS)-approved comprehensive or panel code or routinely billing mutually exclusive codes.* The National Correct Coding Initiative has been previously discussed (chapter 33) as a system by which all federal claims are subjected to a prepay review process to identify incorrect use of codes as described above. The correct use of "comprehensive" codes rather than "unbundled" individual codes, the routine "bundling" of codes and attaching them to a specific orderable code absent evidence of the medical appropriateness of doing so and with the knowledge and approval of the ordering providers that it is being done, and the routine use of mutually exclusive codes with modifiers to bypass edits absent the same criteria for medical appropriateness and with provider knowledge and approval are all considered suspect.

Authority for Program Integrity

The authority for Medicare program integrity lies in Medicare statutes and resulting regulations which mandate provision of only services that are authorized by law, namely, those described in Section 1828(a)(1)(A), which states that Medicare will pay for services "that are reasonable and necessary for the diagnosis or treatment of illness or injury or to improve the functioning of a malformed body member." Thus, this program does not, in general, cover preventative medicine services. However, there are a few selected preventative services covered at specific frequencies under additional statutes (e.g., Pap smears, prostate-specific antigen testing). Medicaid coverage is generally based on criteria established by states administering the program, and other third-party payors establish their own coverage criteria. Failure to comply with and abide by the rules established by any payor may put a laboratory at risk for legal action.

To enforce compliance in the Medicare program, in 1981, Congress added Section 1128A (the Civil False Claims Act and the Civil Monetary Penalties Law), which authorized the Secretary of Health and Human Services to impose civil monetary penalties (CMPs) for violations of Medicare rules and regulations as well as additional assessments for statutory violations of Medicare law. In addition, the Secretary could specifically exclude an individual or entity determined to be in violation from participation in provision of services to federal program beneficiaries for designated periods. In 1994, the responsibility for enforcing Medicare statutes was realigned between both CMS (the Health Care Financing Administration at that time) and the OIG. The Health Care Financing Administration was given responsibility for program compliance, and the OIG was given responsibility for CMPs involving fraud and abuse. The climate created by increasing recognition of deliberate false claim filing was now such that in the event of suspected fraud, criminal indictments were also a genuine possibility for an offending healthcare provider.

Finally, in 1996, the Health Insurance Portability and Accountability Act (HIPAA) increased maximum CMPs to $10,000 per item or service in noncompliance (increased from $2,000) and increased assessments to three times the amount claimed (increased from two times the amount). HIPAA also established a formal Health Care Fraud and Abuse Control Program to combat such activities in claims filed by both public and private payors. Under this program, Medicare has awarded contracts to specific Program Safeguard Contractors who have formal responsibility for the Medicare Integrity Program. It is noteworthy that HIPAA also paved the way for better enforcement of billing compliance for non-Medicare payors.

In 2000, another comprehensive program integrity activity was initiated by CMS designated the Comprehensive Error Rate Testing Program. In this program, a designated contractor has responsibility for random review of selected claims processed by federal payors to verify that contractor decisions were accurate and based on sound policy compliant with statutes and regulations. The goal is to generate national paid claim error rates, claim processing error rates, provider compliance rates, and benefit-specific error rates. The purpose is to provide benchmark data which can be utilized to identify emerging trends and implement effective corrective action.

It should also be noted that CMS has authority and responsibility under the Clinical Laboratory Improvement Amendments (CLIA) to ensure compliance by registered laboratories with all applicable federal rules and regulations. On a yearly basis, CMS publicly makes available a listing of laboratory providers who have failed to comply with regulations pertaining to billing and reimbursement. The listing includes those laboratory providers to which the following apply:

- They have been convicted under federal or state laws of fraud and abuse.
- They have appeals and hearing pending for the same.

- They have been excluded from participation in federal programs.
- They have had CMPs that have been imposed.

New under HIPAA's Privacy Rule is a proposed system termed the Automated Survey Processing Environment Complaints/Incidents Tracking System, which proposes to track and process complaints and incidents reported against laboratory providers in a federal payor program. The complaints, incidents, allegations, investigations, and dispositions may be logged by any beneficiary or participant in a federal program and are tracked by CLIA number to generate provider-specific data. In sum, there are numerous lines of authority that govern and enforce compliance with billing and reimbursement statutes and regulations. The lines are well established, and specific entities, primarily CMS and the OIG, carry the authority to impose both civil and criminal penalties as appropriate to the situation. New program integrity enforcement and monitoring enhancements are being added on a regular basis, and such programs apply not only to federal payor programs but also to private payors. Such programs, if judged by indictments and payments, may be deemed highly successful. In 2002 alone, the federal government won or settled for more than $1.8 billion, much of which was returned to the Medicare Trust Fund. Federal prosecutors filed 361 criminal indictments, with 480 convictions. The Department of Health and Human Services also excluded 3,448 individuals or entities from participation in federally funded programs. In addition, there have been a few cases of contractor indictment or settlement arising from failure to follow rules pertaining to payment of federal healthcare claims. Compliance should and must obviously be taken seriously if a laboratory is to succeed.

Payor Integrity

While much of the focus has been on laboratory provider error in the claim submission process, contractors or third-party insurers paying claims also have an obligation to develop medical review processes to ensure that appropriate payment has been made. Under Medicare program integrity, the goal is simply to "pay it right." That means "pay the right amount to the right provider for the right service to the right beneficiary." There are two main categories of review processes designed to ensure that this goal is met: those performed prepayment and those performed postpayment.

Prepayment Review

Prepayment review is the preferred approach for a very obvious reason. It eliminates the need to "pay and chase," i.e., attempt to recoup payments made in error. Prepayment review is ordinarily accomplished through a computer-based system of defined edits similar to those used by laboratory providers to submit "clean claims." Prior to payment, claims are assessed for complete documentation, correct coding, and evidence of medical necessity (i.e., meets criteria as a covered service). As already discussed (chapter 33), a variety of edits are currently in place and include those published as frequency limits, National Correct Coding Initiative edits, national coverage determinations (NCDs), and local medical review policies (LMRPs). In a small percentage of cases, claims may actually be manually reviewed to ensure that the edit process is correct, and medical record documentation may be requested from both the ordering provider and the laboratory provider. In addition, any laboratory provider that has been identified as having problems with correct claim submission may be placed on routine prepayment review status.

Postpayment Review

Postpayment review is also an important component of the claim review process. This process focuses on statistical evaluation of subsets of claims (i) to check claims on a random basis to function as a deterrent for fraud and abuse, (ii) to identify aberrant patterns of utilization and billing that may indicate a general emerging or provider-specific problem, and (iii) to determine the extent of a particular kind of problem that has been previously identified. When a review is performed to detect aberrancies or specific problems for a particular laboratory or other healthcare provider, it is termed a focused medical review. In turn, a focused medical review may identify a problem that results in development of a prepayment LMRP.

Postpayment review may be performed on individual claims or on samples of claims. From review of a statistically valid sample, the payor can estimate the extent of overpayment made without necessarily undertaking a complete medical record review. However, the possibility exists that complete evaluation of all individual documentation associated with testing may be performed whenever a postpayment review identifies a significant problem associated with large expenditures.

Laboratory Provider Integrity

While payors have an obligation to pay it right, laboratory providers obviously have an obligation to "do it right" in the first place. The continuing recognition of costly systematic billing errors, including some categorized as fraudulent, led the OIG to issue a Compliance Program Guidance for Clinical Laboratories in August 1998 (1–3, 5, 8, 10, 12, 13). This document, which updated a previous Model Clinical Laboratory Compliance Plan published by the OIG in 1997, is designed primarily to ensure that appropriate reimbursement is made through federal programs, that is, to ensure that payors pay it right. However, it also provides commonsense principles for conducting laboratory business in general by promoting the concept of doing it right. It provides guidance for "doing the right thing" (through compliance with all regulatory and statutory rules and regulations), for "getting paid for doing the right thing" (through correct coding and billing practices), and for "making sure the right thing is done" (through a systematic approach to ensuring that rules and regulations are followed). Its purpose, therefore, is to make certain that laboratories function as business entities providing laboratory services in an ethical and legal manner.

The Seven Essential Elements

The OIG compliance guidance specifies that at a minimum, a sound compliance program should include seven key elements. These are as follows:

- There should be written standards of conduct. These standards should promote the laboratory's commitment to the accurate, ethical, and legal practice of laboratory medicine.
- There should be a chief compliance officer (CCO) charged with procedure and protocol development, education, and monitoring. The CCO should interact with a formal corporate (or institutional) compliance committee (CC) composed of key individuals who are charged with approval of compliance policies and with oversight of all other elements of the compliance program. Both the CCO and the CC should report directly to the chief executive officer.
- There should be an effort to provide standardized education about compliance. Compliance training should be a mandatory component of an employee's initial orientation as well the annual competency assessment process.
- There must be a defined process for receipt and documentation of complaints, including an opportunity for anonymity, if desired, via a hotline.
- There must be a system to respond to allegations of possible fraud or abuse, as well as disciplinary policies which clearly delineate consequences for violations of compliance policies. In fact, it is expected that a zero-tolerance approach to violations will be taken.
- The compliance program must include the use of ongoing monitoring and auditing tools to detect possible compliance problems as soon as possible and to measure the effectiveness of interventions designed to minimize the occurrence of such problems.
- The program must specify the processes for remediation of systemic problems identified and address individuals or other business associates who are sanctioned from participation in federal programs due to a known previous violation.

Specific Areas of Concern

To guarantee that the overall goals of the above elements are met, there are a number of specific areas that the plan identifies as critical to address. Each area should ideally be discussed in a specific compliance policy, with protocols or procedures for implementing the policies developed for each. In addition, each policy area should be specifically monitored using defined audit criteria. Table 37.1 provides a listing of areas commonly requiring compliance policy development. However, these may be divided into five main general areas of concern:

- Coding and billing issues
- Medical necessity issues
- Record retention
- Marketing practices
- Compliance with OIG and CMS compliance issuances

Coding and Billing Issues

Key to any successful compliance program is a clear understanding of the principles of procedure coding as well as the accurate and complete application of those principles. The laboratory should be familiar with the HIPAA standard data sets, particularly those used for billing. These include CPT-4 codes, International Classification of Diseases, 9th Revision (Clinical Modification) (ICD-9-CM), codes, diagnosis-related groups, revenue center and provider type codes, and remittance advice codes.

CPT-4 Coding

The laboratory must have access to a current copy of the American Medical Association (AMA) CPT-4 codebook as well as to current supplementary Healthcare Common Procedure Coding System codes. A comprehensive annual review of procedure coding must be conducted to ensure that additions, deletions, and modifications made by the CPT Editorial Panel and published by the AMA each fall are incorporated by the laboratory into the current recommended coding beginning 1 January but no later than 1 April. This also provides an opportunity to ensure that previous code selections are compatible with coding convention and reimbursement rules. All associated documents such as requisitions, service manuals, charge masters, and fee schedules must also be updated to reflect any changes. It is also recommended that at the time of the annual CPT-4 review, laboratories review and update their cost analyses for use in setting laboratory charges for procedures. In November, CMS generally publishes a Program Memorandum that sets the national limitation amounts (NLA) for Medicare reimbursement of each CPT-4 code, thus allowing revenue projections to be made for budget purposes. In addition, it is necessary to submit actual current charges on Medicare claims so the lowest amount of the actual charge, the NLA, or the contractor fee schedule amount may be

Table 37.1 Summary of areas requiring compliance policies[a]

ABN	Home health service client arrangements
Ambiguous test orders	ICD-9 codes, obtaining and using
Anonymity and nonretribution	Indigent care
Billing for calculations	Medical-necessity guidelines
Claim submission, postsubmission review of EOMBs	Monitoring utilization of laboratory services by clients
Claim submission, presubmission review	Nonemployment of sanctioned individuals
CLIA regulations	Notices to physicians
Client contracts	Nursing home client arrangements
Client supplies, provision of and monitoring	OSHA regulations
Confidentiality of medical information	Placement of equipment or products in client offices
Contracts with third-party billing companies	Professional courtesy
Cost reporting, laboratory component	Record retention
Courier service	Reflex testing
CPT coding	Release of test results by phone, fax, and or other nonroutine methods
Custom panels and physician acknowledgment	Removal of hazardous waste for clients as inducement
Data summaries as a free service	Rental or lease of space from healthcare providers
Diagnosis information, translation to ICD-9 codes	Reporting compliance issues and open-door policy
Discounts and special prices	Requisition design
Education and training for customers as inducement	Sales and marketing
Employees, phlebotomists in client offices	Sales proposals
ESRD arrangement	Standing orders
Excused charges and adjustments	Test not ordered and/or not performed
Fraud Alerts, review and compliance	Test ordering by authorized individual
Gifts, contributions, and entertainment	Test orders, requisitions, and electronic order review
Health fairs as inducement	Verbal and add-on test orders

[a]EOMBs, explanations of medical benefits; OSHA, Occupational Safety and Health Administration.

paid. Of course, it is absolutely essential that all payors be informed of any coding or charging changes.

Modifiers

The laboratory has the responsibility for the appropriate use of modifiers. In general, these are added at the time of billing. However, it is up to the laboratory to review coverage rules and edits to determine when use of a modifier is indicated. The most common modifiers used are those which designate advance beneficiary notice (ABN) status (GA, GY, and GZ), those that designate replicate use of a code (-59 and -91), and one that indicates CLIA waived status (QW).

ICD-9-CM Coding

ICD-9-CM codes are updated on a quarterly basis. While the ordering provider rather than the laboratory provider selects diagnostic codes used for a test order, it is still necessary that the laboratory maintain updated data files for claim review. In addition, laboratories do have the authority to translate a narrative code provided on a requisition into an ICD-9-CM code if an exact match is available. Under HIPAA, a narrative diagnosis is absolutely required on all claims submitted, and laboratories must make a serious attempt to obtain this information if not provided.

The Requisition

The requisition, whether electronic or manual, represents the major tool used by ordering providers to select tests for use in patient management. Thus, it should be designed to be user-friendly and include all data elements required for billing. All orderable tests must be clearly defined and represent only AMA- and CMS-approved codes representing procedures, individual tests, or panels. If a special situation exists (as described below), this too should be indicated on the requisition. However, the actual CPT-4 code does not need to be on the requisition if readily accessible elsewhere (e.g., in the service manual). In the event of receipt of an ambiguous order, the laboratory is required to take action to clarify the order. An ambiguous order is one that does not match the test description or conditions in the laboratory. In these cases, a laboratory should not attempt to guess the ordering provider's intent. Rather, it is necessary to make contact with the physician to determine the exact procedure desired.

Special Ordering Situations

There are several situations in which an orderable procedure may be represented by more than one code, and these must be clearly indicated on a requisition as such (Table 37.2). First is a reflex procedure. A reflex test is defined as a second related, codable test, which is performed automatically when initial tests are positive or abnormal. It does not include duplicate testing performed per protocol or repeat testing performed to confirm or verify a result (9).

Second is a composite procedure. This terminology is most commonly used to describe the battery of tests that are included under end-stage renal disease (ESRD) payment, but the term can also be used to describe the routine use of two or more unique codes simultaneously to meet accreditory guidelines or in accordance with an accepted standard of practice (e.g., microbiology: test 1, microbial stain; test 2, microbial culture). Under compliance guidance, these two types of multiple code situations typically meet medical-necessity requirements. However, what is actually done and its associated codes must be clearly communicated to the ordering provider, generally through the requisition and service manual, and there should be documentation of such notification. In addition, each ordering provider must have the clear choice to not have the testing performed in that manner, rather to order only specific codes if desired.

The third multiple-code situation is the custom panel. This is a grouping of several independent codes made available as a single orderable procedure, usually as an ordering convenience, and generally specifically requested by a physician to meet his or her own style of practice. These kinds of test order groupings must meet the same medical-necessity determination requirements as the individual

Table 37.2 Examples of reflex test procedures[a]

Laboratory category	Primary test	Reflex test
Immunology	RPR or VDRL, positive	Specific treponemal serology and RPR titer
Microbiology	Primary culture, positive	Identification and susceptibility
Molecular diagnostics	Pap smear with ASCUS	HPV DNA
Toxicology	Qualitative drug screen, positive	Drug confirmation, each procedure
Urinalysis	Nonculture bacteriuria screen *or* biochemical urinalysis, positive	Urine culture
Chemistry (7)	Quantitative RT-PCR for HCV	If quantitative test result is below limit of detection, qualitative RT-PCR for HCV is performed.
Hematology (14)	Reticulocyte count, erythrocyte morphology, bilirubin, haptoglobin (help diagnose hemolytic anemias)	If acute intravascular hemolysis is suspected, plasma and urinary hemoglobins and a DAT may be ordered.

[a]HPV, human papillomavirus; RT-PCR, reverse transcriptase PCR; HCV, hepatitis C virus; DAT, direct anti-human globulin test.

components and require that a physician formally acknowledge in writing his or her understanding of such.

Lastly, one should address the issue of "standing orders." This practice is most common for chronically ill individuals with extended courses of treatment, as in a skilled-nursing facility or ESRD setting. Although not prohibited, the practice is discouraged. The reason is that the tests included in the order must meet medical-necessity requirements for the date of service, and that information may not be known in advance. At a minimum, laboratories should ensure that standing orders have a fixed term, defined in writing, and that such arrangements are renewed at expiration. The term of expiration should be no more than 1 year and preferably a shorter interval.

Medical Necessity Issues

"Medical necessity" as defined by CMS is an assessment by CMS or another payor of whether the ordering provider's reason for ordering a test represents a condition which meets criteria for coverage and reimbursement at the appropriate level. The term does not indicate whether a particular test is medically appropriate or believed to be necessary for management of an individual patient by a physician. From the CPT-4 and ICD-9-CM codes, the laboratory should be able to make a determination of whether a claim will be paid for by a third-party payor based on its knowledge of the particular billing rules of the payor. The complexity of the rules, and the numbers of payors that any given laboratory may do business with, is such that electronic rule-based claim review is essential to accomplish this task. If it is determined that payment is unlikely, then the laboratory should obtain a waiver of financial liability from the patient (e.g., the Medicare ABN) (4). In the setting of specimen collection by the ordering provider, the ordering provider should make this determination and obtain the waiver. It is acceptable for laboratories to make copies of LMRPs, NCDs, and National Correct Coding Initiative edits, including in the form of a software application, available to ordering providers to facilitate this process. It is recommended that laboratories clearly indicate on requisitions tests that are likely to be noncovered or have limited coverage (i.e., LMRPs and NCDs).

Indeed, it is the responsibility of the laboratory to ensure that physicians are aware of all Medicare and other payor rules for coverage. For Medicare, it is also necessary that an annual notice be sent to physicians describing laboratory practices with respect to coding and billing and reaffirming the concept of medical necessity in making a payment determination.

Record Retention

Adequate record retention is an extremely important component of a compliance program. All records should be maintained as required by applicable federal statutes and regulations for use if needed in the investigation of potential fraud or abuse. It should be noted that there might also be additional requirements based on voluntary accreditation standards and state laws and regulations. Federal statutory retention times include the following:

- *42 CFR 482.24(b)(1).* Condition of participation for hospitals in federal programs specifies 5 years.
- *42 CFR 488.5(a).* Discussion of accreditation standards deemed to meet Medicare conditions of participation indicates variable times of at least 5 years.
- *42 CFR 493.1105.* CLIA of 1988 (CLIA '88) specifies 2 years for test requisitions.
- *42 CFR493.1107.* CLIA '88 specifies 2 years for testing records.
- *42 CFR 493.1107 and 1109.* CLIA '88 specifies that transfusion medicine records should be held for a minimum of 5 years.
- *42 CFR 493.1257(g).* CLIA '88 specifies that cytology slides should be held for 5 years.
- *42 CFR 1003.132.* The False Claims Act specifies that claims related to civil actions may be initiated up to 6 years after the date of claim presentation.

While most laboratorians are aware of the CLIA requirements, few understand the need to maintain records that document test orders and test performance for a longer period in the event that civil or criminal legal action is taken.

Marketing Practices

All marketing efforts in a laboratory setting should adhere to strict principles of offering clear, correct, nondeceptive, and fully informative guidance and pricing regarding testing services. It is quite simply good laboratory medicine practice to ensure that all parties understand both the testing and billing processes.

Pricing and Inducements

No free supplies, equipment, or services of any kind should be offered that are not an essential component of performing and reporting laboratory tests. No other services or items should be provided which may be construed as an inducement for the submission of federally reimbursed work. Rather, any special services should be billed to a client at a fair market value rate. Similarly, prices charged to physicians and other payors should represent fair market value and be based on careful and consistent cost accounting practices for each test procedure. For Medicare in particular, you cannot establish a charge to be substantially in excess of any charge offered to another payor. "Substantially in excess" has been redefined in a recent proposal as 120% of the average charge to all payors for each test. Although you will likely not be reimbursed at your charge rate, the data are used in the determination of the NLA. In fact, Medicare laboratory reimbursement is made at the lower amount of the charge, the NLA, or the local fee schedule. Discounts below costs, particularly if offered to match competitor pricing, may be viewed as an inducement. In addition, failure to attempt to bill patients for services that were denied on the basis of medical necessity may also be viewed as an inducement. Any form of inducement is a violation of the Stark Amendments and therefore represents a federal offense.

Ordering Provider and Patient Communication

To ensure that all parties understand the testing and billing processes, it is critical that a laboratory establish clear and consistent lines of communication. For ordering providers, coding information should be readily accessible through a service manual or other test-listing document. The laboratory must send an annual notice to each client detailing the ordering and billing processes and must clearly document any special ordering or billing situations. The laboratory may provide any relevant limited-coverage or noncoverage test information to assist in determining the need for an ABN. Open lines of communication regarding billing must be maintained during regular business hours. Finally, the name of the individual who serves as the CLIA clinical consultant for a specific laboratory should be readily available. For patients, open lines of communication must similarly be available. It may be helpful to have written patient information readily available that describes unfamiliar terms such as medical necessity and ABN. As in all endeavors, a thorough, consistent, and honest approach is the best one to take.

Fraud Alerts and Advisory Opinions

A number of guidance documents are issued on a regular basis by both CMS and the OIG. Each laboratory CCO and CC should be aware of the issuance of any such documents. Obviously, laboratories should remain abreast of any new coverage decisions and edits which are issued by any payor. Other documents that should be reviewed include relevant Program Memoranda and Transmittals from CMS, specific Fraud Alerts from the OIG, and Advisory Opinions issued by the OIG which are specific to a given provider situation but which may set important precedents. Also important are annual reports from the OIG called the Red Book, which describe proposals designed to reduce reimbursement for services which have been assessed to be at risk for overpayment, and, issued later in the year, the OIG Work Plan, which actually defines the areas targeted for intervention. Careful review of these documents will prepare a laboratory to effectively manage a situation with emerging compliance ramifications.

Auditing and Monitoring

To demonstrate that a compliance program is effective, it is essential to have in place a series of monitors and audits (6, 11). Monitors simply measure a parameter that can be used to assess some aspect of compliance. The most common monitor is test utilization. The OIG recommends that annual review of the top 30 test codes ordered be performed to determine if any significant pattern changes (i.e., greater than 10%) are noted. Further investigation should be performed to ascertain the reasons for the change. In most cases, the change can easily be explained by test volume growth, new-procedure implementation, or correct-coding adjustments. However, if not explainable, additional review of the reasons for testing may be indicated.

Audits are a more comprehensive and systematic review of a specific compliance policy to determine that the policy is in fact being followed. For each compliance policy in place (Table 37.1), there should be some measurable parameter that assesses its effectiveness. The most common audit is one that simply reviews a statistically significant sampling of claims to determine the tests that were ordered, that they were actually performed and the results were reported, and that the tests were billed correctly. This audit technique encompasses the entire process. Other audits may be applicable to a specific policy. For example, one might review the accuracy of translation of narrative diagnoses to ICD-9-CM codes, the frequency and appropriateness of obtaining ABNs, and whether a high percentage of supplies for sample collection are being returned with samples and requested services. The overall effectiveness of the training program might be assessed by examination of employees after training, and the effectiveness of the overall program might be determined by an employee survey. Careful and complete audits are a time-consuming task and are often outsourced to external parties. This is an acceptable practice, although review of findings and plans for improvement remain the responsibility of the CCO and the CC.

Response to the Possibility of Fraud or Abuse

Every laboratory must have plans in place to evaluate complaints received that indicate the possibility of fraud or abuse. If a complaint is determined to actually indicate receipt of unwarranted reimbursement, the OIG Compliance Program clearly specifies the actions that must be taken. If the overpayment represents a true mistake, caused by misunderstanding or misapplication of rules, the laboratory should take prompt action to correct the problem and to make voluntary repayment as outlined in the OIG Compliance Program. If a specific employee is found to be responsible, standard disciplinary actions should be taken. If, however, there is evidence of intent to defraud a payor, the potential violation should be reported to the Department of Justice. All subsequent actions will then be directed as part of a legal investigation process, with outcomes including both settlements and indictments. For individuals, laboratories should maintain a zero-tolerance policy toward deliberate disregard for compliance policies. In the event of an indictment, both facilities and individuals will be listed on the OIG sanction list and prohibited from doing further business with or for the federal government. Other nonfederal payors may similarly file suits, and they may also exclude an entity from participation when evidence of a systematic error representing fraud or abuse is found.

Laboratories must also be prepared to deal with a legal process emanating from an external complaint reported by a "whistle-blower" directly to the Department of Justice. There should be a well-defined plan of action in which employees are advised as to the correct course, particularly with regard to notification of superiors. Certainly, cooperation is expected and any type of obstruction is to be avoided. However, laboratories should take steps to legally protect their interests. For example, categories of documents protected by client-attorney privileges should be clearly marked as such and maintained separately, and legal counsel should be sought as soon as possible after recognition of fraud or abuse, or the allegation thereof.

Laboratory Examples of Fraud and Abuse

Sadly, there are many examples of deliberate attempts by a low number of healthcare providers to obtain improper and illegal reimbursement for services. While some have resulted in indictments, many more are settled out of court when it is recognized that there may be actions that could be construed as evidence of impropriety. Some of the more dramatic and visible laboratory compliance cases have involved the following practices:

- Billing for tests not performed, e.g., billing for identifications and susceptibilities on "no growth" urine samples
- Routinely performing additional tests that were not part of the original order, e.g., adding a chemistry test to an approved panel
- Improper billing for panels, e.g., when not all components of a chemistry panel were performed
- Routinely performing reflex testing that was not subject to a defined review process, e.g., performing microscopic analysis on a urine sample with abnormal urinalysis
- Routinely reporting results for and billing tests when quality control was out of range and therefore in violation of CLIA
- Routinely performing procedures, including laboratory testing, in specific DRGs to artificially inflate the

payment, e.g., in the setting of pneumonia, organism not specified

Unfortunately, these isolated episodes of improper billing influence the overall view that many who hold political office share: that is, that (i) laboratories cannot be trusted and must be subjected to close scrutiny and (ii) overpayment is rampant and therefore payment reductions are justified. To combat these negative opinions, it is paramount that laboratorians adopt the attitude that a successful compliance program that guarantees that laboratories "get paid right" is essential to survival.

Summary

Compliance has assumed a new meaning in the last decade as laboratories have been accused of and found guilty of fraud and abuse. The actual concept of adherence to rules and regulations is not new, however. Laboratories must comply with the rules and regulations promulgated by many government entities. What is new is the concept that laboratorians must also comply with rules and regulations pertaining to reimbursement. A sound knowledge of coding and billing practices is an absolute key to success. The OIG Compliance Program Guidance for Clinical Laboratories published in 1998 provides the basis for development of policies and procedures that ensure that laboratories are paid appropriately for what they do. In essence, the document provides the basis for application of commonsense principles for receiving requests for laboratory services, performing those services, and getting paid for those services.

KEY POINTS

- Compliance has taken on a new meaning during the last few years as laboratories have been accused of and found guilty of fraud and abuse.
- Laboratories and laboratorians must comply with rules and regulations related to reimbursement.
- It is mandatory that laboratory personnel maintain a thorough understanding of coding and billing practices.
- All laboratories should have in place a comprehensive compliance program, with its key provisions and requirements in effect at all times.
- It is critical and appropriate that laboratories be paid for the services they provide within the framework of the compliance regulations.

GLOSSARY

Advance beneficiary notice A waiver of liability used by the provider to notify Medicare beneficiaries prior to receiving services that it may not be a covered service and that they may have to assume financial responsibility.

Automated Complaints/Incidents Tracking System Tracks and processes complaints and incidents reported against laboratory providers in a federal payor program.

Bundling To place codes together in a panel.

Civil False Claims Act and the Civil Monetary Penalties Law Authorizes the Secretary of Health and Human Services to impose civil monetary penalties (CMPs) for violations of Medicare rules and regulations, as well as additional assessments for statutory violations of Medicare law.

Code jamming Inserting a code that was not provided by the ordering provider but which will justify payment.

Code steering Providing lists of diagnostic codes that are known to justify payment.

Compliance Program Guidance for Clinical Laboratories (1998) Updated Model Clinical Laboratory Compliance Plan (1997); designed to ensure that appropriate reimbursement is made through federal programs, to ensure that payors "pay it right"; provides guidance for doing the right thing (through compliance with all regulatory and statutory rules).

Comprehensive Error Rate Testing (CERT) Program A designated CERT contractor has responsibility for random review of selected claims processed by federal payors to verify that contractor decisions were accurate and based on sound policy compliant with statutes and regulations; the purpose is to generate national paid claim error rates (benchmark data).

Current Procedural Terminology, 4th edition (CPT-4) Test codes recognized by the American Medical Association and required for filing of claims and billing of Medicare.

Custom panel Grouping of several independent codes made available as a single, orderable procedure, usually as an ordering convenience.

Diagnosis related group (DRG) Classification system developed at Yale that defines almost 400 major diagnostic categories and places patients into case types based on the International Classification of Diseases, 9th Revision (Clinical Modification) (ICD-9-CM), code classifications.

Downcode The use of a lower-reimbursed test, generally coupled with rebundling, to induce unnecessary utilization.

End-stage renal disease (ESRD) The terminology used for Medicare beneficiaries who have permanent kidney dysfunction requiring dialysis treatment.

Fraud and abuse The receipt of payment for services billed by mistake.

Health Insurance Portability and Accountability Act of 1996 (HIPAA) Title I protects health insurance coverage for workers and their families when they change or lose their jobs. Title II requires the Department of Health and Human Services to establish national standards for electronic healthcare transactions and national identifiers for providers, health plans, and employers. It also addresses the security and privacy of health data. Adopting these standards will improve the efficiency and effectiveness of the nation's healthcare system by encouraging the widespread use of electronic data interchange in healthcare.

Inducement Offering incentives to nonfederal payors to encourage them to also submit federal program testing; violation of the Stark legislation.

Kickback The provision of any item of value in exchange for referral of federal business to a laboratory.

Medical necessity The determination of ICD-9-CM codes for which a CPT code will be reimbursed as reasonable and necessary.

Modifier Modifiers are composed of two-digit numbers which are attached to a specific code prior to the billing process. They are "used to indicate that a service or procedure has been altered by some specific circumstance but not changed in its definition or code."

National Correct Coding Initiative (NCCI) Review of procedure codes to determine if two or more different codes are appropriately ordered on the same date of service. This service was initiated in 1996 through a contract with a Medicare contractor, AdminaStar Federal. These edits are available on the Centers for Medicare and Medicaid Services (CMS) website.

Pay it right Pay the right amount to the right provider for the right service to the right beneficiary.

Reflex test Second related, codable test, which is performed automatically when initial tests are positive or abnormal.

Standards of conduct Standards should promote commitment to the accurate, ethical, and legal practice of laboratory medicine.

"Substantially in excess" Defined as 120% of the average charge to all payors for each test.

Unbundling To code individual tests rather than using an approved CMS panel.

Upcoding Performing a related test for which the CPT-4 code pays at a higher level; using a higher-paying code to maximize reimbursement.

REFERENCES

1. Beatty, M. F. 1999. A survey measuring the degree of model compliance plan for clinical laboratories implementation in small/rural hospital laboratories. *Clin. Lab. Manag. Rev.* **13:**81–86.

2. Belton, P. R., and S. E. Roughton. 1999. The ideal compliance world: integrating physicians into the compliance program. *QRC Advis.* **16:**4–10.

3. Campen, R. B., and D. DiLoreto. 2000. Here to stay: health care compliance. An overview. *Med. Group. Manag. J.* **47:**30–33.

4. Carter, D. 2003. Obtaining advance beneficiary notices for Medicare physician providers. *J. Med. Pract. Manag.* **19:**10–18.

5. Eckhart, J., and N. Mathahs. 2001. Physicians and compliance: developing a system that works. *Clin. Leadersh. Manag. Rev.* **15:**222–229.

6. Keoppel, P. 2001. Performing laboratory compliance audits. *Clin. Leadersh. Manag. Rev.* **15:**368–375.

7. **Kukuczka, S., and L. E. Grosso.** 2002. Effective management of hepatitis C molecular testing improves test use without compromising patient management. *Arch. Pathol. Lab. Med.* **126:**100–102.

8. **Lovitky, J. A., and J. Ahern.** 2002. Using the OIG model compliance programs to fight fraud. *Healthc. Financ. Manag.* **56:**64–68.

9. **MacMillan, D. H., B. L. Soderberg, and M. Laposata.** 2001. Regulations regarding reflexive testing and narrative interpretations in laboratory medicine. *Am. J. Clin. Pathol.* **116**(Suppl.)**:**S129–S132.

10. **Matusicky, C. F.** 1998. Fraud and abuse. Building an effective corporate compliance program. *Healthc. Financ. Manag.* **52:**77–80.

11. **Mesaros, F., Jr.** 2000. The remittance advice, auditing for compliance. *Clin. Leadersh. Manag. Rev.* **14:**69–71.

12. **Saner, R. J.** 1999. Third-party biller compliance guidance emphasizes risk awareness. *Healthc. Financ. Manag.* **53:**43–45.

13. **Saum, T. B., and J. Byassee.** 2000. Effective health care corporate compliance. *Physician Exec.* **26:**56–59.

14. **Schwabbauer, M.** 1999. The anemias, p. 391–402. *In* B. G. Davis, D. Mass, and M. L. Bishop (ed.), *Principles of Clinical Laboratory Utilization and Consultation.* W. B. Saunders Company, Philadelphia, Pa.

APPENDIX 37.1 Websites

http://www.cms.gov/medlearn/refabn.asp: ABN
http://www.cms.gov/regulations: CMS and related laws and regulations
http://www.oig.cms.gov: Compliance Program, Fraud Alerts, Advisory Opinions, Red Book, Work Plan
http://www.labfocus.com: CAP/CLMA Conference on Issues in Medicare Compliance

http://www.compliance.com: the American Compliance Institute
http://www.columbia.com: the Columbia Compliance Plan
http://www.hcca-info.org: Healthcare Compliance Association

38

Determination of Profitability

Vickie S. Baselski, Alice S. Weissfeld, and Fran Sorrell

OBJECTIVES

To describe those items that are included in the true costs of a laboratory procedure

To discuss possible reasons why cost analyses rarely account for all expenditures

To list the three primary tools used in the laboratory to assess profitability

To describe several of the key indicators used to evaluate an institution's performance (benchmarking)

To discuss the term "outcome assessment"

To discuss the concept of human profitability and its relationship to quality patient care

---

If you don't do it excellently, don't do it at all. Because if it's not excellent, it won't be profitable or fun, and if you're not in business for fun or profit, what the hell are you doing there?

ROBERT TOWNSEND (FROM *FURTHER UP THE ORGANIZATION*),
1988, HARPERCOLLINS, NEW YORK, N.Y.

IN ANY BUSINESS, including laboratory medicine, the ultimate goal is to be profitable. From financial profits come funds for enhancements in facilities, equipment, and personnel. From profits also come the means to continue to exist as either a for-profit or nonprofit entity. A laboratory must certainly be profitable as a business unit, and there are well-defined financial monitoring tools to demonstrate this. However, profits in medicine are measured by more than simply dollars made or lost and dollars spent or saved. A profitable laboratory is also one that contributes positively to patient care. In the current healthcare climate, the term "outcome assessment" has been used to describe the success or failure of a disease management strategy with regard to both financial and medical measures (7). Profitability of an institution arises at least in part from effective and efficient patient care, including laboratory medicine. Therefore, in laboratory management today, one must be able to discuss both the individual profitability of a laboratory unit and the contribution of the laboratory to the profitability of patient care. Finally, it must be appreciated that at least in part, one can also measure the satisfaction of making a positive contribution to patient care as a measure of human profitability.

Inaccuracies in Cost Accounting

Integral to any determination of profitability is a clear understanding of the true costs of a procedure. Cost accounting is dealt with in chapter 35 in detail, but a few key concepts justify review here. First is that a complete cost analysis should consider all identifiable costs for a service. One must consider many factors, including all of the following:

- Direct material costs, including all consumables, quality control, repeats, and wastage
- Direct labor costs, including benefit costs
- Equipment and other capital costs, either leasing or depreciation based on purchase as well as maintenance and repair costs
- Laboratory-specific indirect costs, generally based on an allocation method and including licensure and accreditation maintenance (e.g., inspections, documents, proficiency testing) and training or continuing-education costs
- Facility indirect costs, also based on allocation of a percentage of costs due to utilities, rent or purchase notes, housekeeping and infectious-waste disposal, and information technology and communication systems
- Administrative indirect costs, again allocated and including courier services, marketing, customer service, and financial processes (e.g., billing, collections, payments)

Careful consideration of all of these factors in a systematic manner will allow a laboratory to make reasonable decisions regarding price structure for testing services. However, costs analyses in any business, including in a laboratory, are rarely able to account for anywhere near 100% of expenditures. There are frequently many unpredictable variables, particularly in areas in which the laboratory has little or no control. For example, supplies provided for collection and submission of samples are rarely accounted for 100% on return, and rates of recollections due to preanalytical issues, repeats due to analytical issues, and wastage due to insufficient product in a kit lot to complete an additional run all contribute to inaccuracies in projecting total technical expenses. In addition, allocated costs are similarly subject to changes associated with unanticipated events.

In a like manner, attempts to account for anticipated revenue are also subject to inherent inaccuracies. Inability to obtain critical documentation, misunderstanding or misapplication of payor rules or issuances of new rules, failure to obtain patient waivers of financial liability, and failure to collect billed amounts due all contribute to reduction in anticipated revenues.

In order to determine true costs and revenues, and to subsequently assess profitability as well as efficiency, it is necessary to measure resources actually expended, including through amortization, and compare that measurement to amounts actually collected. Simply stated, revenues less expenses equals profit and revenues divided by expenses equals profitability.

Laboratory Profitability

Analyses to assess laboratory profitability are usually performed on a regular basis, not less than quarterly and typically monthly. To accomplish this there are three primary tools used in the laboratory setting: the balance sheet, the income statement, and the cash flow statement (5, 6).

Balance Sheets

The balance sheet provides an indicator of an organization's overall financial well-being. It compares an organization's total assets to its total liabilities. In the laboratory, assets include not only cash holdings and accounts receivable but also facilities and all possessions used to create services (e.g., equipment and supplies). Liabilities include all money owed and, in the case of a for-profit institution, shareholder equity amounts. Simply stated, a balance sheet should at least balance. However, in order to be profitable, total assets should exceed total liabilities. From a laboratory management perspective, while a positive balance sheet is critical to success and may certainly be reassuring to employees and shareholders, it provides little information which may be used to improve operational efficiency in an individual laboratory setting.

Income Statements

An income statement is used to demonstrate profitability over a given period. These statements are also known as "profit and loss" statements because they compare the net profit for a specified period to the total expenses of doing business during the same period. Calculating total gross income and subtracting total expenses determine net profits or losses. The net profit may also be expressed as a percentage of gross income and may be referred to as the profit margin. The net profit should not be considered an absolute value, however. This figure is generally determined prior to consideration of taxes and interest amounts due and is referred to as earnings before taxes and interest. Clearly, an accurate determination of profit requires considerations of these expenses as well.

Income statements also frequently include figures reflecting budgeted and expected revenue and expense amounts. Thus, they allow a laboratory to assess whether there are significant variances from the amounts expected in both categories. In general, variances of more than 3 to 5% require evaluation to determine if other downstream adjustments may be necessary. For example, loss or gain of a major client may necessitate renegotiation of standing reagent orders for delivery of a more appropriate quantity of supplies.

As with the balance sheet, the income statement often reflects the overall financial situation of a laboratory and therefore is most useful to upper management for determining profitability for the entire laboratory. However, this statement may be configured to reflect the income and expenses of a specific department as well. In this configuration, individual department heads may find the document useful to assess whether expenses and income are as expected and to assess whether an individual department is profitable.

Cash Flow Statements

Cash flow statements demonstrate exactly what the name implies. They provide a summary of the amounts paid out and to whom (accounts payable) and the amounts received in payment for services or other items and activities (accounts receivable). Again, simply stated, accounts receivable should exceed accounts payable.

Key Indicators

In addition to these institutional summary reports, most laboratories employ the use of key indicators to assess not only profitability but also overall operational efficiency. Such indicators are often financial or other ratios (i.e., a numerator/a denominator) that may be used to evaluate an institution's performance over time or in comparison to that of like institutions. This practice is known as benchmarking and can provide very useful information for operational improvement leading to financial benefit (8). Key indicators most often look at both sides of doing business: income and expenses.

Key Income Indicators

Key income indicators are used to determine whether a laboratory is financially successful. They measure both success in an institutional sense and success from an investment perspective. In a business sense, monitors generally compare assets to liabilities, or revenue to expenses. Clearly the expectation is that in each case the ratio should exceed 1. In addition, it is customary to track volume indicators that translate into income. Most laboratories track daily numbers of billable tests and look for significant deviations that may have a financial impact. For independent laboratories, new sales or lost business can also be used to monitor potential for future financial success or failure.

From an investment perspective, for-profit laboratories must also demonstrate earning potential for investors. This is usually done by comparing price per share to earnings per share. Here as well, data on volumes may be used to demonstrate earning potential.

Key Expense Indicators

While income monitors should show favorable performance in order for a laboratory to be considered profitable, monitors that assess efficiency or effectiveness over time are more useful to individual laboratory managers seeking to ensure that their departments contribute to overall prof-

itability. While it is useful to monitor indirect and fixed expenses for deviation and for comparability to those of similar institutions, of most importance to laboratorians are those monitors that assess an aspect that can be adjusted or controlled. Both labor and material expenses are considered useful for development of such monitors.

Monitors for labor efficiency generally focus on productivity. It has become customary to use billable tests (i.e., Current Procedural Terminology, 4th edition, codable tests) produced per full-time equivalent for this purpose, although the monitor may also be inverted and expressed as time paid or time worked per billable test. There is a wide variation in expectations for productivity based on the department being evaluated. Obviously, an automated-testing department will show higher output than a laboratory employing more manual processes. For this reason, productivity assessments are most useful when used for benchmarking either temporally to assess performance of a single institution over time or when comparing laboratories that have been determined to be comparable in both scope and processes for services provided.

Another commonly used labor effectiveness monitor is percentage of overtime used. In a properly staffed laboratory, overtime usage should be minimal (<3%). Excessive overtime payments, generally paid at an elevated hourly rate, reduce profitability.

Expense monitors generally focus on actual costs per billable test. These monitors may be constructed to be comprehensive and include all direct costs (materials and labor) as well as an allocated indirect cost. However, material costs as a stand-alone item should also be evaluated. A monitor of material cost per billable test is, as for labor cost per billable test, most useful for temporal evaluations or in comparison to that of a like laboratory.

This kind of analysis is distinct from an actual cost analysis for a specific billable test in that it measures the actual and not simply the expected cost. A wide variation between calculated cost and actual cost per billable test is cause for concern regarding possible inefficiencies.

One monitor for material use efficiency is actual versus potential utilization rates for specific high-cost items. With all kit products, it is common for wastage to occur when small amounts of product remain that are insufficient for a complete run including controls and patient samples. Utilization rates of substantially less than 100% may indicate a need to redesign work flow processes to improve efficiency.

Institutional Profitability

It is clear that each individual laboratory must be able to operate efficiently within a defined budget and that each laboratory manager must continue to seek ways to operate more effectively to decrease overall costs in an era of ever-continuing decreases in available revenues. However, laboratory medicine is unique in that the product, which has defined costs and specific individual value, may also have a positive financial impact in a manner not directly financially benefiting the laboratory. In other words, the results of a specific test may be used to improve the clinical outcome for a patient such that the total costs of providing care for that patient are decreased. Thus, the beneficiary of the savings is the payor and not the laboratory providing essential information. Therefore, laboratory managers and payors must not be shortsighted in making a decision to perform and pay for a particular test based simply on the laboratory economics of the situation. The term "outcome assessment" has been used to describe the process of determining whether a particular measure will have a positive clinical and presumably financial impact on patient care.

In laboratory medicine, there are several well-designed studies that demonstrate healthcare system savings emanating from the performance of a particular laboratory procedure. For example, implementation of rapid antimicrobial susceptibility testing via an automated system has been shown to decrease length of stay, use of additional services and drugs, and overall hospital charges compared to an overnight system (2). In a nursing home setting, implementation of rapid influenza virus antigen testing has been shown to decrease the numbers of secondary cases through prompt implementation of appropriate prophylaxis, thereby reducing total costs of caring for ill residents (1, 3). In an outpatient setting, testing for *Chlamydia trachomatis* using a rapid method, while less sensitive than an overnight method, was shown to reduce the occurrence of costly secondary salpingitis cases and allowed immediate treatment in a patient population at risk for such due to failure to present for follow-up care (4). In fact, acceptance of routine testing for *Chlamydia* in at-risk patient populations in order to prevent costly sequelae has achieved status as a Healthcare Employer Data Information Set monitor for effectiveness of healthcare under various payor plans.

In the future, decisions regarding whether to implement costly new technologies in a laboratory will have to take into consideration the financial impact on healthcare in a more comprehensive sense as well as the immediate financial impact on a given laboratory.

Human Profitability

Through all discussions of profitability, one must not lose sight of the reason for the existence of laboratory medicine as an accepted discipline. The role of the laboratory is to provide data used for effective management of patients. In doing so, laboratory professionals feel a sense of pride and accomplishment in assisting in patient care that cannot easily be measured in financial terms. However, a life saved or salvaged from a serious illness does have a lifetime earning value, which can be calculated, and additional value in terms of human existence that cannot be calculated. Our hope is that the human profit margin will take precedence over strictly financial terms in the provision of quality laboratory medicine services. Further, it is fervently hoped that some degree of rationale and logic will be applied in the realm of reimbursement for laboratory services, including in setting appropriate compensation for laboratory scientists performing the work, such that the ultimate financial and human benefit may be reaped.

Summary

Absolute profitability or lack thereof in laboratory medicine may be easily measured within an individual laboratory or laboratory department. To do so, one may use a number of standard accounting tools to compare real expenses to real revenues. However, profitability in laboratory medicine may also extend beyond the boundaries of the laboratory by allowing clinical decisions to be made that have an overall positive impact on a patient's clinical outcome, which may also be measured in financial terms. In addition, a positive clinical outcome may result in many nonquantifiable benefits to patients, their families, and their healthcare providers. Therefore, while laboratory professionals must necessarily make sound financial decisions, which allow their facilities to operate with a reasonable profit margin, administrators and other purchasers of laboratory services must remain cognizant of the overall importance of laboratory medicine to profitability in provision of healthcare services.

KEY POINTS

- A complete cost analysis must include all identifiable costs for a service.

- Although cost analyses rarely account for all expenditures, it is important to understand what some of these unpredictable variables may be.

- Analyses to assess laboratory profitability usually include balance sheets, income statements, and cash flow statements.

- Key income and expense indicators are required to assess not only profitability but also overall operational efficiency.

- Future decisions regarding implementation of expensive technologies will have to take into consideration the financial impact on healthcare in a more comprehensive sense.

GLOSSARY

Analytical time   Time for the labor required to analyze the specimen or specimens and to perform all routine procedures up to reporting of results. This time includes any required calculations and checking but does not include test repeats.

Balance sheet   Shows assets on the left side and liabilities and claims against assets on the right side. The balance sheet shows a firm's financial position at a particular point in time.

Billable test (Current Procedural Terminology, 4th edition, codable tests) Tests performed and charged to a patient, physician, or third-party payor account that generates revenues. The billable test is the focal point in laboratory cost accounting for laboratories that generate revenue.

Cash flow Case revenues less cash expenses; it therefore excludes noncash expenses such as depreciation.

Cash flow statement Reports the impact on cash flow of a firm's operating, investing, and financing activities over a period of time.

Cost accounting A system of measuring and reporting information about costs.

Direct cost A cost that can be traced to, or caused by, a particular service, product, segment, or activity of the department. Examples are labor and consumables.

Fixed costs Costs that remain constant in total regardless of changes in the level of activity. Fixed costs are only fixed in relation to the given time period and are only fixed within a relevant range of activity.

Full-time equivalent The proportion of an employee's paid hours per year to the standard laboratory measure, which is typically 2,080 h (5 days × 8 h × 52 weeks per year).

Healthcare Employer Data Information Set Monitors for effectiveness of healthcare under various payor plans.

Income statement Reports the financial results of a firm's operations over a period of time.

Indirect cost All expenses that cannot be directly assigned to a billable test but contribute to the production of a test and the provision of an adequate work environment. Examples are lease or rental contracts, maintenance contracts, maintenance for physical plant, utilities, etc.

Not-for-profits Companies the primary purpose of which is something other than generating a profit. Typical not-for-profits are hospitals and charitable organizations.

Outcome assessment The process of determining whether a particular measure will have a positive clinical, and presumably financial, impact on patient care.

Overtime Time worked before or after regularly scheduled working hours or pay for such time worked.

Postanalytical time Time for labor required to report results, as well as the sorting, filing, and telephoning related to final reports.

Preanalytical time Time for specimen collection, work list and label preparation, start-up, sample-cup, and daily quality controls and standards.

Profitability ratios Ratios that measure the combined effects of liquidity, asset management, and debt management policies on operating results.

Revenue budget The revenue that will be generated by the forecasted activity for a responsibility center.

Unit of service The logical measure of work for a given area. In the laboratory, it is usually the number of billed tests or procedures performed.

Variable costs Cost items that vary, in total, directly and proportionately with volume or level of activity changes.

REFERENCES

1. **Church, D. L., H. D. Davies, C. Mitton, H. Semeniuk, M. Logue, C. Maxwell, and C. Donaldson.** 2002. Clinical and economic evaluation of rapid influenza A virus testing in nursing homes in Calgary, Canada. *Clin. Infect. Dis.* **34:**790–795.

2. **Doern, G. V., R. Vautour, M. Gaudet, and B. Levy.** 1994. Clinical impact of rapid in vitro susceptibility testing and bacterial identification. *J. Clin. Microbiol.* **32:**1757–1762.

3. **Drinka, P. J., P. Krause, L. Nest, S. Gravenstein, B. Goodman, and P. Shult.** 2002. Delays in the application of outbreak control prophylaxis for influenza A in a nursing home. *Infect. Control Hosp. Epidemiol.* **23:**600–603.

4. **Gift, T. L., M. S. Pate, E. W. Hook III, and W. J. Kassler.** 1999. The rapid test paradox: when fewer cases detected lead to more cases treated: a decision analysis of tests for *Chlamydia trachomatis. Sex. Transm. Dis.* **26:**232–240.

5. **NCCLS.** 1998. *Basic Cost Accounting for Clinical Services.* Approved guideline GP11-A. NCCLS, Wayne, Pa.

6. **Travers, E. M.** 1997. *Clinical Laboratory Management,* p. 259–283. Williams and Wilkins, Baltimore, Md.

7. **Wilkinson, D. S.** 2000. Technology assessment: measuring the outcomes of laboratory practice. *Clin. Leadersh. Manag. Rev.* **14:**267–271.

8. **Wilkinson, D. S., and D. D. Reynolds.** 2003. Using benchmarking to manage your laboratory. *Clin. Leadersh. Manag. Rev.* **17:**5–8.

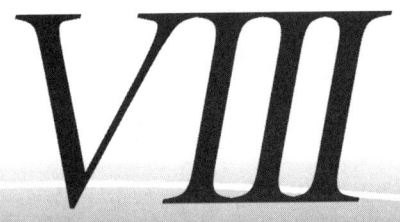

Outside Marketing and Expansion

(Section Editor, *Dale A. Schwab*)

39

Outreach Considerations and Overall Goals

Charlene H. Harris

OBJECTIVES

To determine initial interest and make a position assessment

To perform in-depth market and operational assessment

To develop a business plan

To implement the outreach plans

To assess program progress

To evaluate program growth

To provide examples of letters, forms, graphs, questionnaires, etc., that support guidance

Our mission: to boldly go where no man has gone before.

JAMES T. KIRK, CAPTAIN, STARSHIP *ENTERPRISE*

A LABORATORY OUTREACH PROGRAM can broaden the scope of services for any hospital laboratory and meet the outpatient needs of the community if it is well researched prior to implementation. Hospital-based laboratory outreach can describe everything from patients coming to the hospital out-patient services to have laboratory work done to a stand-alone reference laboratory with draw sites and courier services. Referrals can come from people ranging from the hospital medical staff to providers with patients who will never use the sponsoring hospital's services. The structure of each outreach program is as unique as the set of customer needs that it satisfies. The key to success is in-depth planning and administrative support. In this chapter, we'll provide you with practical, step-by-step guidance on setting up your outreach program, including

- Initial interest and position assessment
- In-depth market and operational assessment
- Business plan construction
- Implementation plan
- Program assessment
- Program growth

Considering an Outreach Program

The implementation of outreach programs can present many opportunities:

- Restructuring and strengthening the role of the hospital laboratory in the community

- Redefining the relationship with various reference laboratories
- Increasing market share
- Marketing the laboratory's specialty or niche testing
- Establishing potential mergers and affiliations with other outreach programs
- Providing true STAT testing for outpatients
- Instituting systems to evaluate new revenue opportunities
- Managing quality across a continuum of care

Administrative Interest

No outreach program can be successful without the complete support of your facility's administration, including the associated pathologist. This support must include not only operational funding but also strategy, understanding, and backing. Prior to approaching administration with the idea of an outreach program, you need to perform an industry analysis, a situational analysis, and a SWOT (strengths, weaknesses, opportunities, and threats) analysis.

Industry analysis. An industry analysis recognizes unique factors within the industry, outside the direct control of the healthcare institution, that affect the survival of the program.

Barriers to entry. Each industry has its own set of entry requirements that must be met by any organization or program desiring to function within that industry. This is also true for an established organization, such as your healthcare institution, which introduces new services into the industry in your market area.

The medical laboratory industry is highly regulated by the United States government. These regulations address such operational areas as personnel requirements, quality control and improvement activities, proficiency testing, methodology validation, etc. The Center for Medicare and Medicaid Services (CMS), the federal agency that administers the Medicare program, and the Food and Drug Administration (FDA), which has oversight of medical devices and licensure of blood banks and blood donor services as well as all laboratories involved in interstate commerce, are the two main federal regulatory agencies. Many states also have statutes covering laboratory operations and personnel.

In addition to regulations dealing with certification or accreditation, several other federal initiatives further affect the laboratory industry and must be considered. Job safety regulations are applied by the Office of Safety and Health Administration (OSHA), including recent directives dealing with needle safety and transport of hazardous materials. The Equal Employment Opportunity Commission (EEOC) oversees employee recruitment and relations. The landmark Stark legislation, prohibiting certain types of physician self-referrals, and *Medicare Fraud and Abuse Alerts*, released by the Office of the Inspector General (OIG) and defining illegal inducements to clients by medical laboratories, have further structured how laboratories do business. Recent Medicare requirements related to Advanced Beneficiary Notices (ABNs), determined by Local Medical Review Policies (LMRPs) and National Coverage Decisions (NCDs), and Medicare Secondary Payor (MSP) questionnaires have had an effect on consumers as well as medical laboratories.

Nongovernmental regulations are also present within the laboratory industry. Outreach programs are subject to inspection by the Joint Commission on the Accreditation of Healthcare Organizations (JCAHO) as part of an overall hospital accreditation program. Many laboratories undergo voluntary inspections by the College of American Pathologists (CAP) to meet accreditation requirements through "deemed status." This means that one accrediting agency recognizes another accrediting agency's certification in lieu of its own certification, i.e., CAP has deemed status for JCAHO.

The advent of managed-healthcare plans has added another barrier that many outreach programs must overcome. Many plans that are national or regional in scope have contracted with a single laboratory testing entity to perform all the testing for their insured individuals. The large, national laboratories are in a good position to provide services over a large geographical area. In effect, this capability prevents many local or regional outreach programs from even bidding on a contract due to their geographical limitations. The direct impact of these laboratory changes is summarized in Table 39.1.

The managed-care picture, however, is not totally dark. Successful outreach programs have discovered several segments of opportunity:

- Test utilization
- Linkages with other hospitals
- Providing superior service
- Relationships with community providers: physicians, home health, hospice, nursing home
- Matching laboratory services to changing patient needs

Table 39.1 Direct impact of laboratory changes in the current healthcare environment

From	To
Revenue center	Cost center
Test-based payment	Capitated payment
Limited utilization controls	Strong utilization controls
High quality	Commodity pricing
Centralized testing	Point-of-care and satellite testing
Internal laboratory	Core laboratory
Semiautomated processing	Fully automated processing
Reputation facilitates referrals	Value-added facilitates referrals

Opportunities for cost management or reductions are readily available through alterations to the staff mix, levels in the organizational structure, and relationships within the organization. Cost analysis becomes a necessity. Supply and equipment costs may be examined. Make-versus-buy decisions are made. Process improvement and work redesign are examined.

The capital requirements in the medical laboratory industry are high. To offer a new service or open a new site, the most recent technology must be available to gain a competitive edge. This technology refers not only to laboratory testing equipment but also to the implementation of highly sophisticated information systems including local area network (LAN) and Internet-based systems.

Another factor deals with the availability of qualified personnel. For years, there has been a shortage of qualified laboratory personnel, and that shortage has now grown to include a shortage of training programs. As with other professions, such as teaching, the number of new technicians and technologists entering the personnel pool is less than the number of individuals approaching retirement. Not only is it difficult to recruit personnel, but once they are hired, their learning curve for each laboratory takes weeks, sometimes months. There is very little transfer of process knowledge from facility to facility.

Determinants of supplier power. Medical suppliers are very powerful within the medical laboratory industry. A few vendors dominate the supplier distribution. This power is readily demonstrated by the inability to solve the continuing problems with reliable shipments and repair service from vendors.

The advent of purchasing networks, such as the Voluntary Hospitals of America (VHA), plus the added emphasis of cost-effectiveness, have contributed to the increased number of laboratories that have aggressively negotiated more-favorable purchasing agreements. These same factors are active in the increased use of multiple vendors by individual laboratories. The luxury of dealing with one vendor is outweighed by the need for the best pricing available, although convenience is regained with the awarding of aggregate bids to a single distributor.

Usually the suppliers of the most recent technologies are not obliged to contend with substitutes for their products because very few, if any, substitutes exist. Therefore, switching costs are high. To counteract this high substitution cost, many laboratories are negotiating "packaged deals up front" with the vendors for stable or no-cost maintenance contracts and/or training and continuing education on the equipment at no cost.

Determinants of substitution threat. Medical laboratories have seen their activity base within the industry erode. In the past, medical laboratories were the only places where consumers/patients could have laboratory testing done. These laboratories were either in the physician office, in the core hospital laboratory, or associated with a reference laboratory. Micro technology (which utilizes very small sample sizes and more compact testing equipment) and patient education have allowed laboratory testing to move to alternate substitution sites. The introduction of home testing for pregnancy often allows a woman to know she is pregnant before her physician knows. Most diabetics now do their own glucose testing in the privacy of their own home. Laboratory testing at the patient's bedside rather than in a designated place called "the laboratory" is available, and utilization is growing at a geometric rate. Many physician office laboratories or outreach satellite labs are now performing analyses that formerly were done only by hospital laboratories.

These alternate sites provide care at a low price, thereby competing with most medical laboratory charges for the same services. They also provide a convenience factor for the client that is not always present with a stationary core hospital laboratory. In many cases, the insurance industry's emphasis on cost reduction through a reduction in both patient hospitalization days and outpatient care also encourages use of these substitutes.

Determinants of buyer power. The medical laboratory industry shares a unique characteristic with the rest of the healthcare industry: the ultimate consumer, the patient, is usually not the final purchaser or payor. Payor or buyer may refer to one of many groups, including patients, individual physicians or physician group practices, employers, federal and state governments through Medicare and Medicaid, insurance companies, and business coalitions. Thus, discussion of buyer power is complex, especially when one considers the use of forward integration within the industry by some buyers such as physician-owned joint ventures with insurance companies and independent practice associations with their own laboratories.

The components of buyer power are varied. Buyers are powerful if they purchase large volumes of products or services relative to the total provider's volume. The majority of laboratory testing is ordered by physicians, who act as the gatekeepers to the laboratory industry, although there is a growing national trend toward self-ordering of tests by patients. The major buyers/payors have begun directing the flow through the gatekeepers with direct provider contracting—the use of preferred-provider organizations (PPOs), managed-care programs that can include capitation or "at-risk" arrangements or possibly competitive bidding as considered by Medicare. Because most outreach programs are not well differentiated from other outreach programs, it is relatively easy for any payor to switch to another provider.

Price sensitivity. The medical laboratory industry, in relation to the entire healthcare industry, has a history of moderate to high price sensitivity. However, in relation to other U.S. service industries, it has had a sluggish response to price sensitivity. This situation is changing.

Until recently, price has not been a major concern for patients, either because they had insurance coverage or because the costs of laboratory testing had been small in proportion to the entire picture. As individual healthcare consumers have become responsible for larger portions of the bill payment, their concern about price has increased. Corporate and government consumers are increasingly concerned about the rising costs of laboratory testing in relation to their total budgets. Consumer demand for lower prices is increasing. Managed-care contracts demand lower prices. Insurance companies have progressed from encouraging their enrollees to use outpatient healthcare services, rather than inpatient, to price-shopping among the laboratory providers. Because of the cutbacks in physician reimbursement, physician practices are searching for lower laboratory prices. Although some individuals have raised quality of care as a concern, the overwhelming tide of concern is associated with price.

Rivalry determinants. When the growth of new providers within an industry is rapid, the level of competition is also high. Many hospital laboratories have entered into the outreach industry segment. The character of the industry itself is changing in response to the aging of the population, the diagnosis of newly discovered maladies, and the development of the field of molecular pathology.

Although brand identity or product differentiation is just now emerging on the national level, low switching costs, little competitor diversity, and local concentration of outreach providers have increased the rivalry between laboratories. Buyers tend to select outreach programs according to

- Low pricing
- Good customer service, which includes timely consultation services by respected pathologists
- Rapid test turnaround time
- The availability of electronic data entry, including interfacing with office electronic medical records
- Accurate billing practices
- The range of testing provided

Just as hospitals are beginning to negotiate regional and sometimes national relationships, outreach programs are forming loose organizational networks aimed at securing regional managed-care contracts for physician office laboratory work. The sharpest competitive edge that hospital-based laboratory networks enjoy is the potential to offer physicians a comprehensive, integrated clinical database containing inpatient, outpatient, and physician office laboratory data. However, competing hospitals seeking to form laboratory networks also face the task of overcoming long-standing rivalries and antagonisms to unify behind a composite strategy. Despite these challenges, many networks are slowly but surely making inroads into the regional outreach market. For an individual laboratory to survive the current industry changes, it must be responsive both to the fluctuation of its local environment and to industry-wide restructuring.

Situational analysis. Answering the question "Does an outreach program fit with who we are?" is the purpose of a situational analysis. It describes the major features of the local environment influencing the program's operation. It also describes where the organization is and where it might go.

Background. This summarizes the organizational factors affecting the potential success of the proposed program. It includes a brief history of the organization or institution with an emphasis on founding purpose, mission, values, and community need. A description of the events leading to the laboratory's decision to look into establishing an outreach program is desirable.

Current activity and normal forecast. The background information is followed by a summary of key performance indicators for the past few years and a forecast of future volume under normal conditions. This assumes no major changes in the marketing environment or strategies. The forecast may be done first without considering the proposed outreach volume and then with that projected volume. The comparison of the two forecasts provides important information needed to decide if the costs outweigh the benefits of establishing an outreach program. It gives your administration a picture of what to expect. The basis of the forecast could be statistical curve fitting, conducting focus groups of potential clients, or other accepted marketing procedures. The forecast needs to be revised if there are changes in environmental conditions or strategies. At times, depending on the location of the market you're in and its volatility, trying to do a "normal" forecast is like trying to build a castle with dry oatmeal.

Market description. Another picture is painted for Administration with the market description. A primary purpose is to clarify the market in which the outreach program will be operating. Some of the elements that may be included are

- A map of the proposed service area
- A list of the targeted clients or customers
- A demographic profile of the service area
- A discussion of other competitors within the market including current activity, services, and location
- Results from a satisfaction survey of the area's providers and patients

Product review. We have worked our way down from a broad view of the local environment (background), through a prediction of what future performance could be, to a picture of what the potential market looks like. Now we need to examine the product itself: the laboratory. Discussion may include

- The current services of the department, both inpatient and outpatient
- How those services fit into the portfolio of the institution
- The value that both providers and patients place on the service
- The life-cycle position, both within the community and within the organization
- A breakdown of potential product lines such as physician office services, nursing home collection, or service center establishment.

SWOT analysis. Both external (outside the organization) and internal (inside the organization) factors that will influence the successful implementation of an outreach program need to be considered. This is the SWOT analysis, and it answers the question "Can we do this?"

External factors can be categorized as opportunities or threats. An opportunity is a positive element of the market in which an organization is likely to enjoy superior competitive advantage. A proposed outreach service center location convenient to a large number of prospective patients would be an opportunity. A threat is a challenge posed by an unfavorable trend or competitor which would lead, in the absence of purposeful marketing action, to the stagnation, decline, or end of a program or product. An example would be the establishment of a regional reference laboratory within your market area by a competitor.

Internal factors are addressed through examination of strengths and weaknesses inside the organization. Strengths need to be supported and maximized, while weaknesses need to be corrected. A weakness could be the inability to determine test costs, thereby inhibiting the establishment of a pricing methodology. A strength is exemplified by the presence of state-of-the-art technology within the testing laboratory. Special consideration needs to be given to factors dealing with specimen transport, information systems including reporting functionalities and remote order entry, marketing and sales availability, and customer service capabilities.

Although opportunities, threats, strengths, and weaknesses describe different factors, the presentation of these factors may have common elements. All are written to suggest some actions that might be needed. The person preparing the analysis may be asked to rate each for its potential impact and to determine which deserve the most planning attention. All have implications for strategy formulation.

Exploring the Market

Having a picture of your market that is accurate and as complete as possible prior to making the decision to start an outreach program is a must. This will serve as a foundation for all subsequent actions.

Determination of the service or market area is needed. This may be accomplished by looking at the area from a functional and geographic viewpoint. Within the hospital organization itself, especially if a healthcare system is involved, a determination of what services the core laboratory will provide (and where) as compared to what services Outreach will provide (and where) must be determined. Some questions to be answered are

- Who will do the reporting and how?
- Where and by whom will testing services be provided?
- Who will provide customer services support?
- How, where, and by whom will the specimens be processed?

Geographically, the outreach program's service area may be different from that of the hospital or healthcare system. A primary service area (specimen transport within 2 hours of collection) may be structured around local providers such as physicians and home health agencies. A secondary service area (specimen transport within 2 to 24 hours) is best developed after the initial market share involving the primary service area is gained.

Market segments need to be identified. There are a number of resources that can provide demographic information concerning market segments such as

- Physician practices
- Home healthcare agencies that can also assist in determining a possible need for a home draw program
- Hospice programs
- Long-term-care facilities
- Dialysis centers
- Mental health facilities
- Occupational health programs
- Other hospitals
- Veterinary practices

Your hospital marketing department may already have this information. If not, a list of demographic resources appears in Appendix 39.1.

Assessing the market segments may be done by several methods. Since medical staff physician referrals is the most easily accessible segment and offers the most potential return on investment for the beginning outreach program, we will use this segment as an example; however, similar strategies may be utilized with each market segment. Initial focus needs to be on the specialties that usually provide most of the test referrals: Family Practice,

Internal Medicine, and Obstetrics/Gynecology. In some markets, Pediatrics may be added to this list.

Information concerning the community need for outreach laboratory services may be gathered by interviews with 10 to 15 carefully selected physicians and a mail-in survey to all medical staff. Generally, the return on mail-in surveys is about 10% to 15%, but the responses can be improved by active promotion by pathologists and hospital/medical staff committees through individual discussions, a newsletter to local offices explaining the purpose of the survey, and announcements in hospital or medical society newsletters. Focus groups made up of physician office staff members who regularly interface with a laboratory are also useful. In addition, it is also valuable to identify physicians who, based on their specialties and/or their ability to influence other physicians within the medical community, may serve as champions for the outreach program.

The survey questionnaires or interview and focus group guides need to solicit responses about issues related to laboratory testing which are important to the physicians and office staff. Sample forms are provided in Appendixes 39.2 to 39.4.

Another useful tool in exploring the market is an image analysis. An organization's image is a function of its deeds (services) and its communication (public relations). It is the organization's image, not necessarily its reality, to which people respond. This has strategic implications for the development of any new program. Services can be designed to be more responsive to the consumer when thought has been given to the structure of the image desired for the new program. Consequently, the level of customer satisfaction can be expected to be higher because of the great congruence between expectations and actual service features.

Many methods have been proposed for measuring images. The last section of the sample questionnaire in Appendix 39.4 is designed to provide information to measure image. Each characteristic listed is an image element.

The last step prior to presenting your findings to administration is to develop a plan for planning. It establishes a planning framework by determining the specific planning steps to be followed, identifying the internal and external constituencies which need to be involved, and specifying the roles of the individuals on the planning team. It also establishes the planning time schedule. The plan for planning is summarized below:

- *Planning objectives:* These are statements that describe the goals or objectives of the planning exercise or why a plan is being made. Examples include "develop functional and useful strategic, business, and implementation planning documents" or "gather support for the development of a laboratory outreach program."

- *Planning environment:* These factors, both positive and negative, will influence the planning process. Examples include "the amount of time available for the planning

process" or "the management style prevalent within the organization."

- *Planning approach:* This describes how the planning will take place, who will do it, and which stakeholders are involved. The planning might be done through a collaborative approach by a planning task force or team involving such stakeholders as Registration, Billing Services, Information Systems, and Laboratory as the process progresses.

- *Course of action:* A brief description of the events leading up to the determination that there was a need to investigate the development of an outreach program is valuable in providing background in the plan for planning reader. Individuals involved in developing the planning documents need to be identified, along with their areas of responsibility. Future activities including the structure of the planning documents need to be outlined.

- *Planning schedule:* A plan of action needs to be roughed out. It should include the broad planning steps and a Gantt chart outlining expected timelines and responsibilities for the planning process only. Remember, this is a plan to plan—not a strategic plan or an implementation plan.

It is now time to return to your administration with the information you have gathered to solicit support for further planning, including a strategic plan, business plan, sales plan, and implementation plan. Without administrative support, both financially and strategically, any outreach program is doomed to fail.

Strategic Plan

Strategic planning entails making intelligent choices in determining future programs and goals. Although it is a continuous process of taking a long view of the planning horizon, it can also involve an immediate response to a sudden shift in circumstances. It can be considered a blueprint for dealing with changing circumstances. Planning is important for no other reason than it forces us to think about how we are going to remain or become a viable entity under different sets of assumptions and circumstances—whether they are related to the government, community, or market.

Strategic planning poses such questions as

- What is the purpose of this program?

- What is its mission?

- What major category of clients or patients will it serve next year? In fifteen years?

- What will be the program's major geographic area next year? In the future?

- What are the upcoming trends in delivery of outreach and hospital services?

- What major services should we pursue?

- At what point would changes in funding or demography affect these plans?
- What alternative services would have to be introduced to deal with the new situation?
- What effect would these alternatives have on the original purposes of the program?
- Will a new mission statement have to be defined?

Once a commitment to strategic planning has been made, a strategic-planning team needs to be formed. The team needs to be large enough to represent all outreach stakeholders but small enough for an exchange of ideas. Seven to 10 members is ideal. A common denominator should be their problem-solving ability and their knowledge of the market from their own unique perspective. Suggested stakeholders include representatives from Hospital Administration and Finance, Patient Access or Registration, Billing and Collection Services, Physician Services, Information Systems, Marketing and Public Relations, affiliated hospital services such as Home Health and Hospice, and, of course, the laboratory, including Pathology. After completing the strategic plan, this group could easily become the outreach advisory group discussed later in the business plan of this chapter.

The process of strategic planning is best accomplished over a relatively short period to ensure continuity of purpose and participants as well as maintain the momentum that the process generates in its early phases. Consensus is essential to the implementation of a strategic plan. It cannot be achieved if one or two people dominate the planning process. The plan that evolves from the process should provide a framework for orderly decision making. It should make it possible for problems and services to be examined with a sense of perspective.

An effective strategic plan needs to include the following sections:

1. *Mission statement.* A program's mission statement is its fundamental purpose or reason for existence. The mission statement should not be so vague as to provide no direction, nor so restrictive as to inhibit the strategic-planning process, nor so broad as to substitute for the final planning document. The future should be discussed as well as the present. The outreach program mission statement must be compatible with the institution's mission statement. The process should be part fact-finding, part brainstorming, and part evaluation of the present situation.

2. *Goal development.* Based upon the information from the industry, situational, and SWOT analyses, strategic goals need to be developed. Goals reflect the results that the outreach program seeks to achieve and are the means for achieving the mission. Goals translate the mission into concrete terms. To be effective, the goals established need to be prioritized and stated in quantitative terms so progress may be measured.

3. *Strategy formulation.* A strategy is a broad course of action designed to achieve a program's goals and objectives. Strategy formulation is a decision-making activity for choosing between alternative courses of action. Strategies may include focusing on target markets, such as physician offices or long-term care, or deciding what the outreach program's portfolio will include regarding product, price, place, and promotion. A truly effective strategic plan should facilitate the day-to-day decision-making process so that decisions are not agonized over but seem inevitable. In addition to defined strategies, a broad timeline needs to be developed to provide a background for expectations.

4. *Control procedures.* Missions, goals, and strategies are not written in stone—or they shouldn't be. Even the most carefully designed plans require periodic review and revision if results deviate from objectives. The establishment of control procedures ensures that strategic planning is a continuous process. The plan should include a mechanism for evaluating new and ongoing services so that criteria for success are defined before the services are initiated. The plan should include a process for scanning the environment to make sure that the program's strategies and even its mission are still desirable and feasible given changing circumstances.

Business Plan

Although we have come a long way from just thinking about starting an outreach program, we still have unanswered questions that must be addressed before we are ready to implement the program. Based on the information previously gathered, a plan is developed defining organizational structure and relationships, compliance issues, fee schedule policies, and a cost-benefit analysis.

How will the outreach program be structured and organized? The types of organizational structures are as numerous as the number of outreach programs. Each is unique to the needs of the particular program and market, but it is vital that all responsibilities be clearly described and assigned, keeping in mind that the program must be able to respond rapidly to changes in the marketplace, whether they are opportunities or threats. Many hospitals choose to establish the outreach program as a separate business entity with its own provider ID and tax ID to facilitate this responsiveness to the market.

The administrative structure of the outreach plan is, like the organizational relationship, structured to meet the unique needs of the market.

1. An advisory group, composed of the same stakeholders involved in the strategic plan plus the outreach director, is often beneficial. In addition to providing feedback about the performance of the outreach program and related activities within the service area from their unique perspectives, these individuals may assist with coordinating services with other hospital

departments, monitoring quality assurance and customer/client satisfaction, and providing ideas for future program development based on client needs. Having support and buy-in from these key stakeholders and utilizing them as champions for outreach is valuable to ensuring broad support for the program from the entire facility.

2. The outreach program is driven primarily by the external customer base, not the internal operations of the hospital or laboratory. It is vital that the outreach director not only be capable of operationally managing the program but also be able to communicate clearly the needs of the clients to administration. In addition, the director must have prior experience in marketing and sales to be able to successfully balance the needs of the clients with the needs of the outreach operations. A sample job description is included in Appendix 39.5.

3. Depending on the size and scope of the planned outreach program, additional administrative or managerial personnel may be needed. Usually a client services or operations coordinator is needed to supervise the day-to-day activities of the patient service center(s) and personnel, including functions such as order entry and registration, telephone or call center operations, and interaction with the testing laboratory, usually the hospital laboratory. A logistics coordinator may be needed if the number of couriers warrants a supervisor unique to the specimen pickup function. If the service area is large enough to require more than one person to provide adequate client sales and account management, a sales representative may be needed to assist the director. It is often advisable to consider hiring a financial assistant to oversee billing and collections, both client and patient, if that function is done by the outreach program rather than the hospital billing office. Sample job descriptions may be found in Appendixes 39.6 to 39.9.

4. The front-line staff will have the most contact with patients and clients. It is through them that the constituents of the market see the outreach program, and they are the major determinants of what image is formed. Again, depending on the services offered by the outreach program, phlebotomists, couriers, and customer service associates may be needed. Hospital registration, if necessary, may be performed by either the registration department or Outreach, and the function may be combined with the phlebotomy process. Sample job descriptions are found in Appendixes 39.10 and 39.11.

An operational assessment of the facility's and laboratory's abilities to provide the types and level of services defined by the prior market and client needs analyses is absolutely necessary to determine the cost and operational impact that the outreach program will have. Service requirements may include

- Efficient and extremely reliable courier service for both routine and STAT testing
- Effective methods and appropriate equipment to register patients, order tests, and process specimens
- Reporting capabilities and turnaround times that meet most customer needs
- Knowledgeable, personable, and customer-focused client service representatives for problem-solving activities
- An adequate telephone system to handle the volume of different types of calls, from courier dispatch to information about location or hours of operation
- Information systems that support efficient patient registration and test ordering, remote order entry, interface with client electronic medical records, flexibility of reporting types and format (electronic and hard copy), call center management including telephone call workflow and customer service software, and timely program evaluation based on volume, process, and financial indicators including utilization data
- Requisition forms, preferably customized by client or specialty, that address not only testing designation but also test status (STAT or routine), compliance needs, billing assignment/information, and special requirements.
- Regular and consistent client contact done in person
- Sales literature explaining the outreach program's services, technical updates, and periodic newsletters
- A complete and up-to-date directory of services that includes not only phlebotomy instructions but also specimen-handling requirements
- Customer- and client-focused educational programs
- Market-driven, competitive fee schedules which may include multilevel client fees based on discounting levels due to client volume (Please note that a methodology of establishing charges based on test cost *must* be in place to meet the most basic of OIG compliance requirements.)
- Flexible billing options including the typical third-party requirements, monthly client billing, managed-care billing for capitated contracts, and individual patient billing

Each outreach program is uniquely structured to meet the needs of its targeted market. Not only does this apply to administrative and organizational structure, it also applies to physical arrangement and processes. If there is a need for patients to have their blood drawn at a site convenient to them rather than solely at the hospital, service centers need to be developed. If there is a need for patients to have their blood drawn within a physician's practice, a phlebotomist needs to be placed at that service site, given the presence of adequate volume to justify the associated costs. The physical layout for specimen processing and testing also needs to be examined from the outreach viewpoint rather than solely from a hospital inpatient perspective.

A clear, explainable process for the establishment and periodic review of the outreach fee schedule and associated Current Procedural Terminology (CPT) codes must be developed. Without the presence of a competitive fee schedule and correct coding, your outreach program has little chance for success. The charges developed should be based on marginal, per-test costs, leveraging off the already present capacity of the hospital laboratory. Usually, this means that only the supply and reagent costs of performing the test are used as the foundation of the fee schedule. The testing personnel costs do not need to be included for most outreach programs, especially in their initial development, because they would be part of the hospital laboratory budget whether or not the outreach program was in existence. The direct costs, such as salaries, gasoline, postage, and space rental, and indirect costs, such as education, marketing, and equipment service agreements, of operating the outreach program need to be added to the test cost. Other indirect facility costs, such as the cost of billing a test, may also be added. Markups to the base cost for both patient and client charges need to be developed, but be cautious of using anything lower than a 10% markup. Client pricing is based on various volume categories, which can be as sophisticated as a per-test determination (i.e., volume discounts calculated by number of individual tests) to a total client volume (i.e., volume discounts calculated by total number of tests). It is imperative that these client volume categories be strictly adhered to so that no hint of inducement is present. Based on the volume figures from the normal forecast done previously, a projection of both the costs and billed revenue needs to be done to assure the profitability of the program.

Processes related to compliance issues must be addressed. CLIA (Clinical Laboratory Improvement Amendments) certification is required. Certification by CAP, JCAHO, or your state may also be necessary. A documented, usable compliance plan must be constructed. Service agreements that outline what outreach services are provided to which clients and have been approved by your facility's legal department need to be drafted for later signature as clients are developed. A mechanism to obtain descriptive diagnosis or *ICD-9* (*International Classification of Diseases, Ninth Revision*) codes prior to registration and billing needs to be formulated. Medicare patients must have ABNs and MSPs documented prior to testing. The advent of NCDs in addition to LMRPs will make Medicare patient registration and billing even more complex.

Customer service processes need to be developed. Usually, customer service issues relate to client education, client problem solving, quality assurance monitors, quality improvements, and problem reporting.

Marketing and sales functions also need to be examined and assigned. Broadly, marketing functions include

- Developing, conducting, and evaluating market research
- Identifying market changes and developing strategies to address them
- Developing and implementing professional-standard sales literature
- Promoting the outreach program within the service area

Many hospital laboratories will find marketing and sales to be a new function that may necessitate additional staff, especially for sales, which requires one-on-one contact with the clients, sometimes at very short notice—a requirement not easily addressed by most laboratory managers due to their already full schedules. Sales personnel are usually compensated with a competitive base rate of pay plus clearly defined incentives for accomplishing defined sales objectives. In addition, the question of mileage reimbursement versus a car provided by the institution needs to be decided.

Sales Plan

Development of a sales plan is also valuable. The sales plan not only needs to outline sales expectations such as targeted markets and/or clients, test volume, number of patient contacts/registrations, and billed revenue for the coming year, but it also needs to discuss the sales approach adopted by the outreach program. The concept that salespeople have about their role influences their attitude about themselves and the client, the behavior demonstrated in the approach to the client, and whether or not the client believes that the salespeople and/or the program they represent are there to serve that client. If salespeople believe that their role is simply to make the sale, they will focus on their own needs rather than the client's needs. On the other hand, if the sales force personnel see themselves as resources and problem solvers, they will focus on the client and will seek ways to meet the client's needs.

There are four basic steps in the sales approach to developing a client.

1. *Relating.* The first step is to build a solid relationship. The salesperson must address the client's initial lack of trust and act to reduce the feeling of anxiety or discomfort that we all have about other people when we first meet them. One way to accomplish this is to communicate why we are meeting, how the meeting will proceed, and how we both will benefit from this meeting.
2. *Discovery.* During the discovery phase, the salesperson needs to uncover all the factors that would affect the client's decision to utilize the outreach services. The outcome should summarize the gap between what the

client has and what the client wants. The process is similar to peeling an onion. It is accomplished one layer at a time until the core is uncovered.

3. *Advocating.* The purpose of the advocating phase is to assist a client in understanding how the outreach services will aid them in meeting their business needs. The sales force will also develop a stronger, more lasting relationship with the client because they are able to demonstrate appreciation and understanding of the client's problems and needs.

4. *Supporting.* From the first three steps, the salesperson gains the information and develops the client relationship to meet the client's expectations after the sale. Supporting the client is built upon four principles: support the buying decision, manage the implementation, deal with dissatisfaction, and enhance the relationship.

The role of service has never been more important than now. Outreach programs can no longer rely solely on price or test menu to differentiate themselves from their competitors. Most competing programs offer comparable test menus at similar prices and can quickly copy any innovations. Today, the emphasis is on service, and service is the key business strategy for gaining and keeping the competitive advantage. In addition, more and more clients are not only demanding higher levels of service but are also placing more and more emphasis on value added as the basis for deciding where to look for services and what to retain. In short, this growing emphasis on service means that organizations will rely even more heavily on the quality of their service, the success of their service providers, and the effectiveness of their sales force.

Prior to making a sales call, a list of prospects and information about the prospects must be developed. Several questions can be used to facilitate this part of the process:

- Who are your prospects?
- Where do you get names of prospects?
- How do you qualify prospects?
- How do we know their potential?
- How does the salesperson get the information to qualify the prospects?
- What is the ideal prospect?
- How long does it take to turn a prospect into a client?
- Who are the top five prospects?
- What will it take to sell them?

Once the prospects are identified, the "Probability Pipeline" scale for rating prospects is used in true territory management. The theory behind the Probability Pipeline is that the salesperson needs to have enough prospects evenly distributed through the Pipeline to flow through to consistently completed sales. Prospects may be graded as seen in Table 39.2.

Table 39.2 "Probability Pipeline" scale for rating prospects

Prospect status	Score
All prospects—any possible client	0.00
Initial contact—left literature, gathered information, set appointment	0.25
Secondary contact—met with prospect, prospect interested	0.50
Client setup—ready to send business	0.75
Specimen received from client	1.00

Each prospective client is unique in not only the services they desire but also the rate at which the account may be developed. Some prospects will become clients during the first meeting, while other prospects will require numerous meetings before they reach client status; however, some overall guidelines may be used in developing the "typical" visit scenarios (see Appendix 39.12).

Promotional literature is a necessity. It can range from basic (business cards and handbook) to sophisticated. A list of promotional literature which may be considered for the salesperson is in Appendix 39.13.

Client profiles need to be built on each prospect by the salesperson and updated upon each contact. The profile will be the complete story about each prospect/client, from initial contact to current or most recent sales interaction. The minimum information that should be contained in the client profile can be seen in Table 39.3.

One of the tenets of being a successful salesperson is the development of strong relationships with existing clients. Communication and personal service are the keys. To facilitate the use of these keys, a schedule for client visits by the salesperson can be developed based upon the volume generated by each client and the preference of the client as to visit frequency. The visits may be as often as once a week or as infrequently as once a quarter.

Communication about sales activity is vital to the coordination of an integrated outreach program. It is the re-

Table 39.3 Minimum information that should be contained in the client profile

- Provider/physician name
- Mailing address
- Voice phone number
- Specialty
- Hospital affiliations
- Original service agreement date
- Method of reporting results
- Organization name
- Pickup/delivery address
- Fax number
- Contact person and position
- Beginning service date
- Last service agreement renewal date
- Check-off of equipment issued

sponsibility of the salesperson to keep Outreach management and personnel informed of prospect development and client relations. In addition, it is the salesperson who will play a major role in coordinating the outreach program's sales efforts with other areas of the hospital or health system that are also involved in sales. A monthly report of sales activity may facilitate the communication. The report should also include prospects rated according to the Probability Pipeline, visit summaries for current clients, and any issues of importance.

Now it is time to put together a budget based upon the people, processes, equipment, facilities, and fee schedule. Most hospitals already have a budget template that may be used. Usually, additional expense categories that may not be routinely addressed by the facility need to be developed, including

- Marketing/sales/public relations
- Rent
- Gasoline
- Utilities (electricity, natural gas, water)
- Postage
- Printing
- Billing service
- Courier service

In concert with the budget, a cost-benefit analysis must be done to look at the expected profitability of the program, including the test volume and revenue (sales), both billed and collected, that are needed for the program to break even.

Commitment from All Relevant Parties

Feasibility Report

Final commitment for the outreach program from the facility's administration must be solicited before implementation can occur. A feasibility report or business plan, based on the data previously acquired, provides valuable information for the administration to use in making the "go or no-go" decision. The report is a summary of

- The market assessment
- The service assessment
- The cost-benefit analysis
- Operational options
- Recommendations

Philosophical Understanding

Commitment from administration must not only provide financial and human resource support; it must also provide a philosophical understanding of the plans and goals of the outreach program—both short term and long term. Administration must also have a clear understanding of the nature of the volatile outpatient outreach industry and

how it differs from the traditional inpatient hospital industry.

Service and Financial Support

The commitment should include service support for issues related to information services, marketing, sales, and billing and collections. Once this commitment is firmly in place, you are ready to plan the implementation of the outreach program.

Implementing the Outreach Program

After all the time and effort spent on researching the possibility, probability, and need for your outreach program, planning the implementation of the program seems fast and effortless in comparison. It's the juggling of the different areas of implementation and bringing them to fruition in a coordinated manner by the required deadline that is challenging: people, processes, facilities, equipment, and supplies. No one part of the implementation plan is more important than any other. Each is integral to a successful startup. Use of some sort of project management software is strongly suggested due to the complexity of the coordination needed.

People

In his book *Good to Great*, Jim Collins asserts that it's not just the people, but the right people, who are important to the success of a company. He compares the company to a bus. If the right people are on the bus and in the right seats, then no matter where the bus goes, that group of people can adapt to the challenges facing the bus. Job descriptions are the seat designs. The more defined and complete they are, the more likely you are to find the right person to fill the seat. Recruitment must follow job description development, not precede it. The training program needs to adequately prepare the people for the seats they will be taking, and it is an investment in the future operational efficiency of the outreach program. Too many programs find out the hard way that although skimping on training puts personnel in their seats faster, it also leads to increased error rates, patient and client dissatisfaction, and employee dissatisfaction. Competency testing, mandated by several accrediting organizations, is the documented story of training success.

Processes

The processes that the outreach program will use need to be consciously thought out, documented, and communicated, not only to the outreach people hired but also to interfacing departments such as the laboratory staff, Information Systems, and Billing—possibly through a series of presentations outlining the program development. Workflow, including physical layout and process steps, needs to be developed and documented. The use of flow charts can point out redundant steps and bottleneck points. Policies and procedures must be written and shared with all involved staff. Planning and implementation of a process improvement program, including quality control, quality indicators, quality improvement, and compliance audits, is necessary in addition to processes related to patient and client services.

Facilities

Depending on the goals and size of the outreach program, some attention will need to be paid to the facilities in which the people and processes will be functioning. Many organizations have personnel within their engineering or facilities management departments who may be helpful. Example questions to be considered include

- Will service centers or draw sites be necessary? If so, where will they be located? What size and space arrangement is necessary?
- Will any construction or renovation be necessary if existing structures are to be used?
- What requirements are there related to utilities, patient access, patient parking, and courier parking?
- What look and feel does the program want to project to its clients and their patients? To the community as a whole?
- What resources are available to announce new service center openings?

Equipment

The equipment required, like the facilities required, will be unique to each outreach program. You must decide what is best for your program when evaluating equipment for information services, technical areas (such as phlebotomy chairs or telephone systems), testing (waived or more-complex testing), and specimen transport (contracted courier services or your own). The materials management department may be able to assist in those selections, and many organizations have already-existing contracts with multiple vendors. Remember that installation and training, as well as repair, need to be considered in your equipment selections.

Supplies

Now that you've hired the people, outlined the processes, designed the facilities, and selected the equipment, it's time to address the subject of supplies. Most outreach programs not only stock supplies for their own use, but they also provide supplies at no charge for clients to use in collecting specimens which will later be sent to the outreach program. The OIG of CMS has issued a fraud abuse alert specifically on this subject. Supplies may be provided free of charge to clients only if those supplies are used exclusively for the collection of specimens sent to the outreach program providing those supplies. Supplies such as tourniquets or syringes that may be used for procedures

other than venipuncture may not be provided free because they are not exclusive to venipunctures. By what method will the clients order their supplies? How and when will the supplies be delivered? How will you monitor client supply usage versus tests ordered?

Outreach Indicators

Once the outreach program is up and running, it is time to monitor its performance by developing outreach indicators. To date, there is very little in the literature concerning outreach benchmarking, so it is difficult for one program to assess how it compares to other programs. However, month-to-month progress can be tracked in terms of service, finance, efficiency, and sales (Table 39.4)

Growing the Outreach Program

Congratulations! Your data gathering and planning have paid off. The outreach program is set up and is a success! Now what happens? The market, competition, and operational processes must continually be monitored to uncover changes and make improvements.

Market Assessment

Ideally, market assessments (Appendix 39.4) should be done on a yearly basis, although in some markets, biannually is sufficient. Anyone who has contact with the customers—sales personnel, couriers, service representatives—needs to provide continuous feedback about the concerns of patients and providers (Appendix 39.14). The key to the prolonged success and growth of an outreach

Table 39.4 Outreach indicators

Service
- Customer satisfaction surveys
- Clinical errors
- Missed specimen pickup
- Days in accounts receivable
- Telephone call center summary

Finance
- Cost/revenue per patient contact
- Test volume
- Test cost-to-charge ratio
- Net collections
- Tests per requisition

Efficiency
- Patient wait times
- Test-to-report turnaround time
- Staff hours per patient contact
- Ratio of patients to specimens

Sales
- Pipeline report
- Current client visit summary
- Client billing report

program is responding quickly to market changes and the needs of the customers.

Client Needs

If the expectation is to have a successful outreach program, then development and implementation cannot be haphazard or casual. It is not something that a laboratory does in its "spare time." It is a business and must be operated as such. It must be customer-focused. Services and processes must be structured from the customer's point of view rather than from a traditional, inpatient laboratory viewpoint. Once this is accomplished, the successful laboratory outreach program is an asset not only for the parent facility but also for the community it serves.

- Each laboratory outreach program is unique, depending upon the particular needs of its customers, the market environment, and the resources available. The structure and processes of the outreach program must be designed to meet those needs for sustained success.

- Meeting customer needs is not rocket science. It is primarily listening to customers, whether patients or providers, and addressing their concerns—sometimes successfully, sometimes not—but always demonstrating your desire to provide them with solutions.

- The successful outreach program contains a strong yet flexible infrastructure constructed to meet the ever-changing market needs through efficient processes, placement of the right people in the right jobs, and strong commitment to the program from hospital administration.

- Outreach is a business and, as such, needs to be operated as a business, with strong fiscal policies, effective operational procedures, accurate market research, and enlightened strategic management.

Summary

We have seen how a laboratory outreach program can broaden and enhance the scope of services for a hospital laboratory and meet the outpatient needs of the community. However, development of such a program must be thoroughly researched prior to implementation. Important aspects of planning include an initial interest and position assessment, an in-depth market and operational assessment, construction of a detailed business plan, timely implementation, an ongoing program assessment, and an ongoing commitment to the program's growth and improvement.

Commitment from all relevant parties must be ongoing, including both service and financial support. Implementation requires comprehensive understanding and cooperation on the part of all involved, with a solid commitment to growth potential; component parts will include people, processes, facilities, equipment, supplies, and financial support.

KEY POINTS

- Several issues must be considered prior to obtaining administrative commitment for the implementation of an outreach program. These include determination of administrative interest, a thorough exploration of the market potential, and development of potential strategic, business, and sales plans.

- Once a detailed feasibility report has been reviewed and discussed by all relevant parties, then there should be some confirmation of philosophical understanding and service and financial support required from all parties, particularly the administration.

- Detailed plans related to people, processes, facilities, equipment, and supplies must be developed and reviewed by all relevant personnel and then implemented using a detailed timeline.

- Indicators for ongoing assessment of the program's progress must be reviewed on a continuous basis, with anticipated growth being a critical component of the overall plan.

GLOSSARY

Advanced Beneficiary Notice (ABN) Advises Medicare beneficiaries, before items or services are actually furnished, when Medicare is likely to deny payment for them.

Business plan A financial and operational analysis of the feasibility of the implementation of a program.

Center for Medicare and Medicaid Services (CMS) A federal agency within the U.S. Department of Health and Human Services that runs the Medicare program, Medicaid program, and State Children's Health Insurance Program (SCHIP).

Clinical Laboratory Improvement Amendments (CLIA) CMS regulates all laboratory testing (except research) performed on humans in the United States through the Clinical Laboratory Improvement Amendments (CLIA). In total, CLIA covers approximately 175,000 laboratory entities. The Division of Laboratory Services, within the Survey and Certification Group, under the Center for Medicaid and State Operations has the responsibility for implementing the CLIA program. The objective of the CLIA program is to ensure quality laboratory testing. Although all clinical laboratories must be properly certified to receive Medicare or Medicaid payments, CLIA has no direct Medicare or Medicaid program responsibilities.

College of American Pathologists (CAP) The principal organization of board-certified pathologists, CAP serves and represents the interests of patients, pathologists, and the public by fostering excellence in the practice of pathology and laboratory medicine.

Cost-benefit analysis A projection of the resources needed to implement a program and the benefits derived from such a program.

Equal Employment Opportunity Commission (EEOC) The EEOC was established by Title VII of the Civil Rights Act of 1964 and began operating on July 2, 1965. The EEOC enforces the following federal statutes:

- Title VII of the Civil Rights Act of 1964, as amended, prohibiting employment discrimination on the basis of race, color, religion, sex, or national origin

- The Age Discrimination in Employment Act (ADEA) of 1967, as amended, prohibiting employment discrimination against individuals 40 years of age and older

- The Equal Pay Act (EPA) of 1963, prohibiting discrimination on the basis of gender in compensation for substantially similar work under similar conditions

- Title I and Title V of the Americans with Disabilities Act (ADA) of 1990, prohibiting employment discrimination on the basis of disability in the private sector and state and local governments

- Section 501 and 505 of the Rehabilitation Act of 1973, as amended, prohibiting employment discrimination against federal employees with disabilities

- The Civil Rights Act of 1991, providing monetary damages in cases of intentional discrimination and clarifying provisions regarding disparate impact actions

Food and Drug Administration (FDA) The FDA Modernization Act of 1997 (PL 105-115) affirmed the FDA's public health protection role and defined the agency's mission:

- To promote the public health by promptly and efficiently reviewing clinical research and taking appropriate action on the marketing of regulated products in a timely manner

- With respect to such products, to protect the public health by ensuring that foods are safe, wholesome, sanitary, and properly labeled; human and veterinary drugs are safe and effective; there is reasonable assurance of the safety and effectiveness of devices intended for human use; cosmetics are safe and properly labeled; and public health and safety are protected from electronic product radiation

- To participate through appropriate processes with representatives of other countries to reduce the burden of regulation, harmonize regulatory requirements, and achieve appropriate reciprocal arrangements

- As determined to be appropriate by the Secretary, to carry out paragraphs above in consultation with experts in science, medicine, and public health and in cooperation with consumers, users, manufacturers, importers, packers, distributors, and retailers of regulated products

International Classification of Diseases, Ninth Revision (Clinical Modifications) (ICD-9-CM) Based on the official version of the World Health Organization's ICD-9, which classifies morbidity and mortality information for statistical purposes, for the indexing of hospital records by disease and operations, and for data storage and retrieval.

Image analysis An evaluation of the customer's beliefs, ideas, and impressions of an organization.

Industry analysis An evaluation of an industry that recognizes unique factors within the industry that have an impact on the survival of an organization. It includes barriers to entry, determinants of supplier power, determinants of substitution threat, determinants of buyer power, price sensitivity, and rivalry determinants.

Joint Commission on the Accreditation of Healthcare Organizations (JCAHO) The Joint Commission evaluates and accredits nearly 17,000 healthcare organizations and programs in the United States. An independent, not-for-profit organization, JCAHO is the nation's predominant standards-setting and accrediting body in healthcare. JCAHO's evaluation and accreditation services are provided for the following types of organizations:

- General, psychiatric, children's, and rehabilitation hospitals

- Critical-access hospitals

- Healthcare networks, including managed-care plans, preferred-provider organizations, integrated delivery networks, and managed behavioral healthcare organizations

- Home-care organizations, including those that provide home health services, personal care and support services, home infusion and other pharmacy services, durable medical equipment services, and hospice services

- Nursing homes and other long-term-care facilities, including subacute-care programs, dementia special-care programs, and long-term-care pharmacies

- Assisted-living facilities that provide or coordinate personal services, 24-hour supervision and assistance (scheduled and unscheduled), activities, and health-related services

- Behavioral healthcare organizations, including those that provide mental health and addiction services, and services to persons with developmental disabilities of various ages, in various organized service settings

- Ambulatory-care providers, for example, outpatient surgery facilities, rehabilitation centers, infusion centers, and group practices, as well as office-based surgery

- Clinical laboratories, including independent or freestanding laboratories, blood transfusion and donor centers, and public health laboratories

Local Medical Review Policies (LMRP) Local policies outline how contractors will review claims to ensure that they meet Medicare coverage requirements. The CMS requires that LMRPs be consistent with national guidance (although they can be more detailed or specific), developed with scientific evidence and clinical practice, and developed through certain specified federal guidelines. Contractor medical directors develop these policies.

Marketing Determining the customer's needs and wants.

Market segment A portion of the market where consumers share a group of common characteristics.

Medicare Secondary Payor (MSP) A Medicare provider, whether a physician, nonphysician practitioner, laboratory, or other supplier (durable medical equipment supplier, etc.), is required to indicate if there is other insurance that may be primary to Medicare when submitting a Medicare claim for payment. The purpose of this questionnaire is to determine whether Medicare or the other insurance has primary responsibility for meeting the beneficiary's healthcare costs. The goal of these MSP information-gathering activities is to identify MSP situations rapidly, thus ensuring correct primary and secondary payments by the responsible parties.

National Coverage Decision (NCD) An NCD sets forth whether Medicare will cover, or not cover, specific services, procedures, or technologies on a national basis. Medicare contractors are required to follow NCDs. If an NCD does not specifically exclude an indication or circumstance, or if the item or service is not mentioned at all in an NCD or in a Medicare manual, it is up to the Medicare contractor to make the coverage decision (see Local Medical Review Policy).

Office of Safety and Health Administration (OSHA) The mission of OSHA is to save lives, prevent injuries, and protect the health of America's workers. OSHA and its state partners have approximately 2,100 inspectors, plus complaint discrimination investigators, engineers, physicians, educators, standards writers, and other technical and support personnel spread over more than 200 offices throughout the country. This staff establishes protective standards, enforces those standards, and reaches out to employers and employees through technical assistance and consultation programs.

Office of the Inspector General (OIG) The mission of the OIG, as mandated by Public Law 95-452 (as amended), is to protect the integrity of Department of Health and Human Services programs, as well as the health and welfare of the beneficiaries of those programs. The OIG has a responsibility to report to both the Secretary and the Congress program and management problems and recommendations to correct them. The OIG's duties are carried out through a nationwide network of audits, investigations, inspections, and other mission-related functions performed by OIG components.

Operational assessment An evaluation of the organization's ability to provide the types and levels of services defined by prior market needs.

Situational analysis Description of the major features in a local environment that affect an organization; includes a background,

current activity, normal forecast, market description, and product review.

Stark legislation The Stark legislation prohibits a physician from referring his or her patients to entities with which the physician or his or her family members have a financial relationship, such as an ownership interest or compensation arrangement. The initial Stark legislation, known as Stark I, was enacted in 1989 and applies only to clinical laboratory services. In 1993, Congress enacted the Stark II legislation, which extends the prohibition to referrals made by a physician to an entity for the furnishing of "certain designated health care services" if the physician or his or her family member has a financial relationship with that entity.

Strategic plan Documentation of a process that develops the organization's future goals and programs within the context of a changing industrial and market environment. The plan includes a mission statement, goal development, strategy formulation, and control procedures.

SWOT analysis An evaluation of internal (strengths, weaknesses) and external (opportunities, threats) factors that may influence the successful implementation of a program.

Target market The market segment(s) chosen by the organization to focus on.

REFERENCES

1. *Be Our Guest.* 2001. Disney Editions, New York, N.Y.

2. Collins, J. 2001. *Good to Great: Why Some Companies Make the Leap and Others Don't.* HarperCollins Publishers Inc., New York, N.Y.

3. Harris, C. 1988. An Image Analysis of Hospitals in the Austin, Texas, Area Market. Master's thesis. Southwest Texas State University, San Marcos, Tex.

4. Kotler, P. (ed.) 1987. *Strategic Marketing for Nonprofit Organizations,* 3rd ed. Prentice-Hall, Inc., Englewood Cliffs, N.J.

5. Magrath, A. J. 1992. *The 6 Imperatives of Marketing.* American Management Association, New York, N.Y.

6. Nigon, D. L. 1997. *Within Your Reach: a Manual for Developing a Laboratory Outreach Program.* Clinical Laboratory Management Association, Inc., Wayne, Pa.

7. Romig, D. A. 2001. *Side by Side Leadership.* Bard Press, Austin, Tex.

8. Rubin, B. (ed.). 1991. *The Department of Pathology Outreach Program Proposal.* The University of Iowa Department of Pathology, Iowa City.

APPENDIX 39.1 Resource List for Obtaining Provider Demographics

Directory of Board Certified Medical Specialists
American Board of Medical Specialists
Available at most public libraries or http://www.abms.org/

Guide to Hospitals
American Hospital Association
Available from the American Hospital Association
(312-422-3000 or http://aharc.library.net/)

Physician Socioeconomic Statistics
Available from the American Medical Association
(312-464-5000 or http://www.ama-assn.org/ama/pub/
article/3375-5361.html)

Physician Select
Available from the American Medical Association
(312-464-5000 or http://www.ama-assn.org/aps/amahg.htm)

State and County QuickFacts
Available from the U.S. Census Bureau (301-763-4636 or
http://quickfacts.census.gov/qfd/index.html)

APPENDIX 39.2 Model Letter for Interview

Dear Dr. _____ :

_____ Medical Center is assessing how well we meet the needs of the medical staff for medical laboratory services. As part of this research, we would like to get the opinion of physicians and their staff concerning the provision of inpatient, outpatient, and office-based testing services and how we can improve those services.

We value your opinion as a user about how these services can be provided. Would it be possible to set up a brief interview of no more than 30 minutes with you to discuss laboratory issues? This interview, of course, can be conducted at any time and place that is convenient for you.

I will be contacting you by phone within the next few days to set up an appointment. We appreciate your setting aside time for this brief interview. I look forward to talking with you.

Sincerely,

APPENDIX 39.3 Model Cover Letter for Market Survey

Dear _____ :

We are very interested in what you think about outreach laboratory services for health-care providers in the _____ *(geographic location)* medical community. Every two years we survey current and potential clients, so we can tailor our services to meet your specific needs. Your assistance in completing the enclosed brief questionnaire will be a great help.

In appreciation for returning the completed survey, we will send you a coupon for _____ *(pizza, cookies, donuts, etc.)* per physician. For those respondents outside the _____ *(city)* metropolitan area, we will be glad to bring the _____ *(pizza, cookies, donuts, etc.)* to you. Please return your completed questionnaire by _____ *(due date about two weeks from mailing)*. You may fax it to _____ *(fax number)* or mail the survey by using the fold-over option.

Thank you for your assistance!

APPENDIX 39.4   Model Questionnaire for Interview, Focus Group, or Market Survey

Practice Name _____   Specialty _____

Number of Physicians _____ Location _____

How many laboratory tests are ordered in your practice during a typical month? _____

Estimated percentage of total testing performed as in-house laboratory testing? _____

Primary reference laboratory:

Name _____

Location _____

Principal reason used _____

If _____ (*your outreach program*) is not your main reference lab, have you used it for any testing?   Yes ____   No ____

Would you be willing to consider a proposal to use _____ as your primary reference lab?   Yes ____   No ____

What would _____ need to do to be considered? _____

Please rate, on a scale of 1 to 5, the importance of the lab services listed below.

   5 = critically important, 4 = very important, 3 = moderately important, 2 = somewhat important, 1 = not important

Also, please rate the quality of your current laboratory and of _____ (if you have used our service).

   5 = outstanding, 4 = good, 3 = satisfactory, 2 = poor, 1 = extremely poor

Services	Importance	Quality of current reference laboratory	Quality of _____
Overall satisfaction	1 2 3 4 5	1 2 3 4 5	1 2 3 4 5
Price	1 2 3 4 5	1 2 3 4 5	1 2 3 4 5
Courier	1 2 3 4 5	1 2 3 4 5	1 2 3 4 5
Specimen-collection site	1 2 3 4 5	1 2 3 4 5	1 2 3 4 5
Telephone communication	1 2 3 4 5	1 2 3 4 5	1 2 3 4 5
Quality of testing	1 2 3 4 5	1 2 3 4 5	1 2 3 4 5
Availability of Path/tech consult	1 2 3 4 5	1 2 3 4 5	1 2 3 4 5
Request forms	1 2 3 4 5	1 2 3 4 5	1 2 3 4 5
Test ordering manual	1 2 3 4 5	1 2 3 4 5	1 2 3 4 5
Reports	1 2 3 4 5	1 2 3 4 5	1 2 3 4 5
Billing accuracy	1 2 3 4 5	1 2 3 4 5	1 2 3 4 5
Participates in Ins/Mng care	1 2 3 4 5	1 2 3 4 5	1 2 3 4 5
Computer interface	1 2 3 4 5	1 2 3 4 5	1 2 3 4 5

APPENDIX 39.5 Sample Job Description—Administrative Director

- **Reports to:** Vice President, Clinical Services
- **Jobs reporting to this position:** Direct reports include Operations Coordinator, Logistics Coordinator, Financial Coordinator, and Sales Associate. Indirect reports include the Pathologist and Hospital Lab Director. Works very closely with Main Lab, Business Office, Registration, and Medical Records. Responsible for approximately _____ full-time employees and an annual budget of approximately _____ dollars in revenues.

JOB SUMMARY

Responsible for the overall operations, marketing, and sales activities of lab outreach services. Ensures that personnel adhere to all regulatory standards and guidelines. Works to ensure that the identified needs of the medical staff, patient, family, coworkers, and other customers are addressed in a timely and efficient manner within the medical center. Acts as a liaison between clients and the Hospital Lab. Accountable for forecasting, developing, and meeting strategic marketing plans and sales goals.

JOB QUALIFICATIONS

- **Education:** B.S. degree in Medical Technology or a related field. Additional degree/education or prior experience in marketing, sales, or a related field is desirable.
- **Licensure:** Required as Medical Technologist.
- **Experience:** Five years' experience in all phases of the clinical laboratory. Two years' experience in management. Successful track record in marketing and sales.
- **Skills:** Works well with people, organizes and plans well, good management skills. Strong interpersonal communication skills, written and oral. Problem-solving skills and good judgment skills. Demonstrates ability to organize, orient, train, and develop staff. Demonstrates the ability to plan and improve the processes and functions of Lab Outreach. Able to interact effectively with physicians, patients, family, vendors, hospital staff, and other customers. Must be able to deal fairly and consistently with personnel under his or her supervision. Communicates effectively with administration, medical staff, department directors, subordinates, hospital staff, and other providers. Deals with patients in a caring, professional manner and ensures the same approach by his or her staff. Additional skills in salesmanship and customer service.

ESSENTIAL PHYSICAL AND MENTAL FUNCTIONS AND ENVIRONMENTAL CONDITIONS

- Frequently exposed to moving objects and loud noise. Occasionally exposed to dust and radiation. Rarely exposed to blood, body tissue/fluids, hazardous materials, chemicals, high elevations, slippery surfaces, special clothing and safety equipment, vibration, wetness, potential electrical hazards, and potential burns.
- Able to see objects closely, as in reading, frequently. Able to see objects far away occasionally. Able to discriminate color occasionally. Able to perceive depth frequently. Able to hear normal sounds with some background noise, as in answering a telephone, frequently. Able to distinguish sounds, as in voice patterns, continuously. Able to give and receive verbal communications continuously. Able to read and write written communications continuously.
- Able to lift objects weighing 10 pounds or less occasionally, 35 pounds or less rarely. The highest point of any lift, the shoulder; the lowest point of any lift, the floor. Able to carry objects weighing less than 10 pounds occasionally.
- Able to sit 45 minutes consecutively, 5 hours per shift. Able to stand in place 10 minutes consecutively, per hour per shift. Able to remain on feet 10 minutes consecutively, 2 hours per shift.
- Able to perform motor skills frequently such as grasping, finger manipulation, feeling perception. Occasionally climbing stairs, reaching out, fast response. Rarely bending, twisting, turning, kneeling, squatting, reaching in, wrist turning/torquing, pinching. Able to perform tasks that require hand-eye coordination continuously, arm-hand coordination and upper body coordination frequently, lower body coordination occasionally.

(continued)

- Needs to attend to task/function for 45 minutes at a time or less frequently, 60 minutes at a time or less occasionally, 60 minutes at a time or more rarely. Able to concentrate on fine detail with constant interruptions occasionally. Able to concentrate on moderate detail with constant interruptions frequently. Able to understand and relate to the theories behind several related concepts continuously. Able to remember multiple tasks/assignments given to self and others over long periods of time continuously.

JOB DUTIES

The following description of job responsibilities and performance expectations is intended to reflect the major responsibilities and duties of the job, but is not intended to describe minor duties or other responsibilities that may be assigned from time to time. Requirements are representative of minimum levels of knowledge, skills, and/or abilities. To perform this job successfully, the incumbent will possess the abilities or aptitudes to perform each duty proficiently. All requirements are subject to possible modification to reasonably accommodate individuals with disabilities.

Responsibility

Maintain a staffing level that is consistent with quality patient care.

Standards

- Provide for the recruitment of prospective employees following the guidelines of the Department of Human Resources.
- Ensure that quality staff is hired according to licensure regulations and the Human Resources policies.
- Ensure that coaching, counseling, and disciplinary action are performed according to the Human Resources policies.
- Monitor staff scheduling to ensure proper coverage of the work area.
- Provide pertinent and complete orientation for new employees.
- Coordinate the preparation and/or update of criteria-based performance evaluations annually.
- Ensure the annual performance evaluation of personnel according to the established time frame.
- Delegate authority and work assignments, taking into consideration priority of work and skills of the employees.
- Monitor the system maintenance of timekeeping mechanism to ensure correct payroll.

Responsibility

Direct, supervise, and administer the outreach program to maintain high-quality technical work and good working conditions.

Standards

- Maintain compatible working relationships with personnel of other departments, as demonstrated by the cooperation between departments in providing patient services.
- Participate in department and medical center committees and task forces relative to areas of practice or interest.
- Develop and meet goals and objectives that support department and medical center goals.
- Demonstrate ability to use all channels of communication to address inter- and intra-departmental concerns, solve problems, and address conflicts.
- Inform the Vice President of any unusual concerns, situations, or conditions relative to staff, patients, families, or physicians.
- Assess new products and equipment to promote and ensure quality patient care and meet medical center cost-effectiveness goals.

(continued)

- Demonstrate effective time management by completing commitments within negotiated time frames.
- Coordinate and collaborate with the Safety Committee and Infection Control Committee to ensure a safe workplace.
- Participate in 80% of the department head meetings.
- Conduct a departmental meeting monthly as indicated by meeting minutes.
- Communicate changes in philosophy, goals, procedures, plans, and activities of the department and of the medical center to the staff in a timely manner, as demonstrated by the department implementing changes.

Responsibility

Plan and implement marketing and sales activities for Outreach.

Standards

- Conduct market research and analyze data gathered to serve as basis for annual strategic marketing and sales plans.
- Develop annual marketing and sales plans in accordance with medical center strategic initiatives.
- Act as a resource on legislative, regulatory, reimbursement, and competitive issues for all medical center laboratory services and Outreach client providers.
- Develop promotional activities and printed materials including brochures, fee schedules, and directory of services.
- Develop pricing strategy based on cost per test in accordance with medical center guidelines to maximize collections and assure competitive position in the market.
- Act as a sales representative for outreach activities to client providers, visiting providers on a regular basis as dictated by testing volume.

Responsibility

Responsible for the annual management plan and budget, which includes a 5-year capital equipment and system management plan.

Standards

- Actively participate in the medical center retreat and preparatory meetings for the annual plan.
- Establish goals and objectives for the department that are compatible with and enhance those of the medical center.
- Demonstrate effective time management by completing the annual plan within the allotted time frame.
- Review and take action when necessary on the monthly budget reports.
- Inform the Vice President of staffing needs or changes.
- Review workload recording to monitor staffing needs or trends.

Responsibility

Responsible for quality assurance activities for the department.

Standards

- Prepare an annual report of the quality assurance activities for the Quality Assurance Committee.
- Ensure that variance reports and client problem reports involving the department are researched, including documentation of root cause and improvement actions.
- Formulate plans for improvement of outreach services that will enhance quality patient care.

(continued)

APPENDIX 39.5   Sample Job Description—Administrative Director *(continued)*

- Keep abreast with CAP and state inspection requirements.
- Ensure the maintenance of files of CAP and state inspection materials, communicating with these agencies as necessary.

Responsibility
Responsible for inventory control of supplies for the department and clients.

Standards
- Ensure that an adequate amount of acceptable supplies are on hand for collection of specimens.
- Oversee the monitoring of inventory so that no excessive outdating or overstocking occurs.
- Minimize the need for emergency supply orders.
- Direct cost-comparison analysis to ensure cost-effective purchasing.
- Request bids for supplies on like products to ensure cost-effective purchasing.

Responsibility
Demonstrate commitment to professional growth and competence.

Standards
- Attend at least 60% of the monthly laboratory in-service education classes.
- Review current literature in field, as demonstrated by contributing this knowledge in the workplace.
- Attend at least two area workshops annually in field of need or interest.
- Attend 75% of the management development seminars offered by the medical center.
- Establish and meet annual individual goals that are developed to assist the department and medical center in achieving their established goals or projects.
- Collaborate with supervisor to suggest and/or contribute to the monthly laboratory in-service programs.

APPENDIX 39.6 Sample Job Description—Operations/Client Services Coordinator

- **Reports to:** Laboratory Outreach Director
- **Jobs reporting to this position:** Patient Service Specialists, Technical Support Specialists

JOB SUMMARY

Provides supervision for all applicable outreach staff, which involves assigning workload, scheduling, staffing, training, resolution of problems, etc. Liaison to providers, Hospital Laboratory, and patients. Oversees overall daily functions of patient service centers and sites.

JOB QUALIFICATIONS

- **Education:** B.S. degree in Medical Technology or an equivalent combination of an associate's degree and experience.
- **Licensure:** Required as Medical Technologist.
- **Experience:** Five years of clinical laboratory experience to include rotation through the technical areas. Supervisory experience and a demonstrated performance in sales and outreach program support a plus.
- **Skills:** Highly motivated, good organizational skills, proactive in problem solving and processing of information. Must work well with people and possess excellent communication skills. Ability to deal with internal and external customers in a courteous, professional manner at all times. Must have computer experience.

ESSENTIAL PHYSICAL AND MENTAL FUNCTIONS AND ENVIRONMENTAL CONDITIONS

- Continuously exposed to blood, body tissue/fluids, hazardous materials, and chemicals, requiring special clothing and safety equipment. Occasionally exposed to loud noise. Rarely exposed to radiation, potential electrical hazards, and potential burns.
- Able to see objects closely, as in reading; to see objects far away; and to discriminate color and perceive depth continuously. Able to hear normal sounds with some background noise, as in answering a telephone, continuously. Able to hear job-specific sounds and to give and receive verbal communications continuously. Able to read and write written communications continuously.
- Able to lift objects weighing 10 pounds or less continuously, 35 pounds or less rarely. The highest point of any lift, overhead; the lowest point of any lift, the floor. Able to carry objects 10 pounds or less frequently, 50 pounds or less rarely. Able to push and pull objects using minimum effort occasionally.
- Able to sit 2 hours consecutively, 6 hours per shift. Able to stand in place 10 minutes consecutively, 30 minutes per shift. Able to remain on feet 1 hour consecutively. Able to sustain awkward position 5 minutes consecutively.
- Able to perform motor skills continuously such as bending, twisting, turning, reaching out, reaching up, wrist turning/torquing, grasping, pinching, finger manipulation, feeling perception. Frequently fast response. Occasionally kneeling, squatting. Able to perform tasks that require arm-hand, hand-eye, and upper and lower body coordination continuously.
- Needs to attend to task/function for 45 minutes at a time or less frequently, 60 minutes at a time or less occasionally, 60 minutes or more at a time rarely. Able to concentrate on fine detail with some interruptions continually. Able to understand and relate to the concepts behind specific ideas continuously. Able to understand and relate to the theories behind several related concepts frequently. Able to remember multiple tasks/assignments given to self and others over long periods of time continuously.

JOB DUTIES

The following description of job responsibilities and performance expectations is intended to reflect the major responsibilities and duties of the job, but is not intended to describe minor duties or responsibilities that may be assigned from time to time. Requirements are representative of minimum levels of knowledge, skills, and/or abilities. To perform this job successfully,

(continued)

APPENDIX 39.6   Sample Job Description—Operations/Client Services Coordinator *(continued)*

the incumbent will possess the abilities or aptitudes to perform each duty proficiently. All requirements are subject to possible modification to reasonably accommodate individuals with disabilities.

Responsibility
Supervise the staff to ensure the quality of work and workflow is maintained.

Standards
- Assign staff workload, taking into consideration the priority of work, training, and skill of the employee.
- Assess the number and level of personnel necessary to provide quality services; adjust staffing and assignments as workload and workflow dictate.
- Constantly monitor the job performance of each employee and evaluate annually.
- Complete all employee annual performance appraisals in the required time frame.
- Initiate counseling and/or disciplinary action according to medical center policy.
- Recruit, interview, and hire employees according to the guidelines and policies of the medical center and department.
- Keep staff informed of events and changes that affect their jobs. Conduct regular staff meetings.
- Effectively serve as a consultant and role model for Outreach personnel.
- Inspire confidence from others by performing and communicating in a highly professional manner at all times.
- Ensure that all staff members have a clear definition of their work responsibilities and management's expectations for performance.
- Always provide recognition for good work performance; give positive feedback both verbally and in writing to staff members when their performance and/or special efforts are deserving.
- Regularly encourage staff participation and communication in decision making. Demonstrate the ability to be creative and maintain an environment conducive to optimal efficiency where employees are encouraged, reinforced, and supported for their desire to contribute fully.

Responsibility
Manage the workflow of the department to ensure the completion of work assignments.

Standards
- Ensure that policies and procedures manuals are current and are reviewed regularly by all staff members; review and revise policies and procedures manuals on an annual basis or as necessary.
- Assess new products and equipment that may benefit the quality of care of the patient.
- Demonstrate professional communication skills and grammar. Maintain calm and professional manner.
- Demonstrate ability to adapt to increasing or changing department workload and duties.
- Effectively coordinate and oversee the ordering of supplies. Regularly monitor the use of supplies and identify potential savings through the appropriate use or substitution of products.
- Demonstrate knowledge and ability as "resource" contact for Outreach. Provide accurate and complete testing and lab information. Find answers for customers in a reasonable amount of time.
- Promptly investigate complaints concerning outreach services and take appropriate actions.
- Maintain awareness of "potential" accounts; promptly communicate with Sales Associates, Director, and Hospital Laboratory staff.

(continued)

Responsibility
Perform specific responsibilities assigned to the Coordinator.

Standards
- Demonstrate effectiveness in maintaining a well-organized operation to ensure efficiency and accuracy of the work and information flow; monitor procedures and implement corrective actions as required.
- Ensure that equipment is maintained and that staff is familiar with the operation and maintenance of the equipment.
- As part of the management team, participate in maintaining a current, complete directory of services on an annual basis or as needed.
- Provide a general orientation of new employees. Oversee rotation and review performance in each section. New employees are assigned a mentor and provided with a verbal and written overview of Outreach and Hospital Laboratory operations.
- Be responsible for the coordination of orientation and training of all students.
- Assist the department Director in administering a program of continuous quality improvement—accept assignments to monitor, measure, and report on Outreach processes for continuous quality improvement.
- Assist the Director in coordinating laboratory efforts in preparation for announced inspections from regulatory agencies. When assigned, provide a plan for ensuring compliance, inform Director and Pathologists of problem areas or concerns.
- Evaluate contract cleaning services routinely and provide comments on performance.
- Maintain an adequate inventory of supplies.
- Ensure balance of petty cash box.
- Administer and monitor continuing education program for employees.
- Maintain payroll and time and attendance.
- Assist the Director in the preparation and monitoring of the budget.
- Proactively monitor the computer system for problems that may culminate in downtime.
- Provide input that develops procedures and policies for downtime procedures and make recommendations during downtime for course of action.
- Perform a Laboratory Information System troubleshooting consistent with the extent of training or recognize need for and request assistance when necessary.
- Provide support for personal computers.

Responsibility
Manage and regulate all departmental safety activities.

Standards
- Serve as departmental Safety and Chemical Hygiene Officer.
- Lead the departmental Safety Committee.
- Coach employees to ensure and maintain compliance of the department with all regulatory requirements for safety, note problems and concerns with compliance regarding safety issues. Inform the Director, make recommendations, and offer solutions.
- Administer departmental safety orientation to new employees and/or students. Employees and students are tested on knowledge. Inform Director of any problems or concerns.

(continued)

APPENDIX 39.6   Sample Job Description—Operations/Client Services Coordinator *(continued)*

Responsibility
When designated, perform the duties of the Director in his or her absence.

Standards
- Accept the additional responsibility of acting department Director; demonstrate good judgment and decision-making skills when confronted with problems, inquiries, or concerns— act as department Director when designated. Address problems and concerns and answer inquiries. Report to the department Director upon return.
- Attend meetings when requested by the department Director. Effectively listen and take detailed notes. Inform the department Director of the content and outcome.
- Accept special assignments as requested by the department Director. Keep the Director informed of progress and concerns. Usually complete assignments by the deadline. Provide a report on the project.

Responsibility
Demonstrate commitment to professional growth and competence.

Standards
- Attend the required number of continuing education meetings per year and keep records.
- Equitably schedule supervised employees for continuing education.
- Review code and safety manuals annually.
- Attend the departmental management team meetings.
- Establish and meet annual individual goals.
- Remain informed and up-to-date in all technical aspects of the department through literature, workshops, seminars, courses, and conferences with other laboratory professionals.

APPENDIX 39.7 Sample Job Description—Logistics/Courier Coordinator

- **Reports to:** Laboratory Outreach Director
- **Jobs reporting to this position:**—Couriers (directly), Patient Service Specialists (indirectly)

JOB SUMMARY

Supervises and directs logistics and reverse-logistics activities and personnel related to the procurement, receipt, shipment, and disposition of materials in a variety of areas such as inventory management, warehousing, supply and delivery-chain management, material control, transportation activities, and technical documentation in a highly demanding and time-sensitive work environment. Coordinates safe, reliable transport of specimens and scheduling and provision of venipuncture services to nursing homes and homebound patients throughout the service area. Establishes and maintains customer relations as it concerns service levels to ensure the ability to resolve day-to-day operating issues with customers. Work is performed independently under the general guidance and direction of the department Director.

JOB QUALIFICATIONS

- **Education:** Bachelor's degree in logistics, transportation or supply-chain management, or related field or an equivalent combination of an associate's degree and experience.
- **Licensure:** Valid state driver's license.
- **Experience:** Two years of experience in performing related work.
- **Skills:** Highly motivated, good organizational skills, proactive in problem solving and processing of information within a multitasking environment. Must work well with people and possess excellent communication and customer service skills, demonstrating an ability to deal with internal and external customers in a courteous, professional manner at all times. Knows and applies a broad knowledge of principles, practices, and procedures of inventory control and material management in providing logistics support services. Must have clear understanding of or demonstrated success in route planning and be able to use analysis skills to develop and manage transportation projects in anticipation of the organization's needs. Experience may be necessary for those aspects of transportation efforts that relate to the handling of hazardous materials for domestic shipments. Must have computer experience with Microsoft Word, Excel, and Access.

ESSENTIAL PHYSICAL AND MENTAL FUNCTIONS AND ENVIRONMENTAL CONDITIONS

- Occasionally exposed to loud noise. Rarely exposed to radiation, potential electrical hazards, and potential burns.
- Able to see objects closely, as in reading; to see objects far away; and to discriminate color and perceive depth continuously. Able to hear normal sounds with some background noise, as in answering a telephone, continuously. Able to hear job-specific sounds and to give and receive verbal communications continuously. Able to read and write written communications continuously.
- Able to lift objects weighing 10 pounds or less continuously, 35 pounds or less rarely. The highest point of any lift, overhead; the lowest point of any lift, the floor. Able to carry objects 10 pounds or less frequently, 50 pounds or less rarely. Able to push and pull objects using minimum effort occasionally.
- Able to sit 2 hours consecutively, 6 hours per shift. Able to stand in place 10 minutes consecutively, 30 minutes per shift. Able to remain on feet 1 hour consecutively. Able to sustain awkward position 5 minutes consecutively.
- Able to perform motor skills continuously such as bending, twisting, turning, reaching out, reaching up, wrist turning/torquing, grasping, pinching, finger manipulation, feeling perception. Frequently fast response. Occasionally kneeling, squatting. Able to perform tasks that require arm-hand, hand-eye, and upper and lower body coordination continuously.

(continued)

APPENDIX 39.7 Sample Job Description—Logistics/Courier Coordinator *(continued)*

- Needs to attend to task/function for 45 minutes at a time or less frequently, 60 minutes at a time or less occasionally, 60 minutes or more at a time rarely. Able to concentrate on fine detail with some interruptions continually. Able to understand and relate to the concepts behind specific ideas continuously. Able to understand and relate to the theories behind several related concepts frequently. Able to remember multiple tasks/assignments given to self and others over long periods of time continuously.

JOB DUTIES

The following description of job responsibilities and performance expectations is intended to reflect the major responsibilities and duties of the job, but is not intended to describe minor duties or responsibilities that may be assigned from time to time. Requirements are representative of minimum levels of knowledge, skills, and/or abilities. To perform this job successfully, the incumbent will possess the abilities or aptitudes to perform each duty proficiently. All requirements are subject to possible modification to reasonably accommodate individuals with disabilities.

Responsibility

Direct personnel to achieve prescribed business objectives while contributing to the promotion of personal employee career goals.

Standards

- Coordinate and schedule Couriers for specimen pickup and supply and report delivery, and coordinate and schedule Patient Service Specialists for nursing home and/or home draw programs to include contingency plans supporting the consistent and timely provision of services.
- Meet with Couriers and Patient Service Specialists to discuss base transportation issues, monitor performance, and review current practice versus potential improvements.
- Monitor and follow up on logs of Couriers and Patient Service Specialists daily to ensure compliance with operational standard.
- Monitor compliance with pickup, delivery, and sample-collection requirements to provide event history to client if needed.
- Assure personnel comply with both internal and external issues relating to company policy and procedures.
- Develop, coordinate, and provide training for Couriers and Patient Service Specialists for Courier duties, resulting in capable, well-rounded employees.
- Develop and maintain a productive staff of Couriers by hiring, training, and professional development; matching the skill and background of Couriers to the work required; applying sound communication and motivational techniques to supervise and counsel staff and implementing in timely fashion the performance evaluation system for recommending promotions, wage increases, and terminations.

Responsibility

Provide flawless execution of transportation services to clients.

Standards

- Hold monthly review meetings or contacts with customers and provide summary to Director by the fifth working day of the month.
- Interface daily with Operations to resolve any problems associated with scheduling and dispatching.
- Notify customers of status and delivery changes.
- Improve outbound and inbound customer service while minimizing transportation expense.
- Effectively communicate with associates, customers, and personnel in person or via computer or phone to accomplish necessary objectives.

(continued)

APPENDIX 39.7 Sample Job Description—Logistics/Courier Coordinator *(continued)*

Responsibility
Provide input to Director related to areas of responsibility on day-to-day operations, process improvement, and budget.

Standards
- General responsibilities include total cost reduction, total supply-chain process improvement, OSHA and Department of Transportation hazardous materials compliance, and ISO and FDA compliance.
- Develop and operate an effective transportation information reporting system; ensure the accurate and timely preparation, processing, distribution, and retention of all necessary reports and records regarding transportation operations; and develop additional and/or enhanced reports to support customers' changing needs.
- Direct development of transportation studies for analyzing trends and make recommendations to improve the flow of information, costs, and delivery-cycle times.
- Evaluate customer service efficiency and design new processes to reduce nonconformances such as supply returns, missed specimen pickups, and customer complaints.
- Responsible for forecasting workload volume, determining client distribution alignments, determining the number of Couriers and routes needed, identifying the timing and location of new routes, and analyzing the impacts of changing distribution strategies.
- Recommend programs to the Director that improve the transportation function, including reduction of cost and delivery/pickup time.

Responsibility
Responsible for inventory control system and supply ordering and delivery system.

Standards
- Provide leadership for the effective use of the inventory control system for all inventory movement, supply, and distribution.
- Develop system to monitor and reconcile, by client, test volume and supply usage to meet requirements issued by the CMS Office of the Inspector General (OIG).
- Direct all warehousing activities, including receiving, stocking, order picking, replenishment, intradepartmental shipping, cycle count, manpower planning, budget development, capital equipment management, and customer service level goals.
- Direct and supervise the scheduling of supply shipments to ensure the most economical utilization of Couriers based on service parameters.
- Develop service contingencies to support the entire supply chain.
- Monitor and develop financial controls related to scheduling personnel, pickup of specimens, and filling and delivering supply orders.

Responsibility
Demonstrate commitment to professional growth and competence.

Standards
- Attend the required number of continuing education meetings per year (one regional), and record attendance—no more than two instances of failing to record continuing education or missing no more than two of the required continuing education meetings.
- Review code and safety manuals annually.
- Attend the departmental management team meetings—no more than two instances of missing the meetings or failure to communicate with the Director or failure to follow up and obtain distributed information.
- Establish and meet annual individual goals.
- Remain informed and up-to-date in all technical aspects of the department and Core Labs as needed to provide a basis for sales promotions through literature, workshops, seminars, courses, and conferences with other laboratory professionals.

APPENDIX 39.8   Sample Job Description—Billing/Financial Coordinator

- **Reports to:**   Laboratory Outreach Director
- **Jobs reporting to this position:**   With expansion-information system and/or financial techs

JOB SUMMARY

Responsible for compliance and reimbursement auditing, information gathering and analysis, and revenue structure for third-party and client reimbursement. Duties include development and implementation of coding, billing, and reimbursement audits based on federal, state, and regulatory guidelines; review, analysis, and updating of fee schedules to insure reimbursement commensurate with cost and revenue goals of outreach; and analysis of accuracy and integrity of information between Laboratory and Hospital Information Systems, to include coordination of development of Hospital and Laboratory Information Systems to meet Outreach's operational and information needs. Job requires considerable knowledge of general accounting practices, healthcare coding, regulatory guidelines, and information systems. Work is performed independently under the general guidance and direction of the department Director.

JOB QUALIFICATIONS

- **Education:**   Bachelor's degree in business administration, accounting, or related field.
- **Licensure:**   Registered Health Information Administrator, Certified Coding Specialist, or Certified Professional Coder preferred; Certified Patient Accounts Representative required within two years.
- **Experience:**   Three to five years of experience in performing related work, to include revenue management, information systems, and regulatory compliance guidance. Job requires considerable knowledge of general accounting practices, healthcare coding, regulatory guidelines, and information systems.
- **Skills:**   Highly motivated, good organizational skills, proactive in problem solving and processing of information. Must work well with people and possess excellent communication skills. Ability to deal with internal and external customers in a courteous, professional manner at all times. Must have computer experience with Microsoft Word, Excel, and Access.

ESSENTIAL PHYSICAL AND MENTAL FUNCTIONS AND ENVIRONMENTAL CONDITIONS

- Occasionally exposed to loud noise. Rarely exposed to radiation, potential electrical hazards, and potential burns.
- Able to see objects closely, as in reading; to see objects far away; and to discriminate color and perceive depth continuously. Able to hear normal sounds with some background noise, as in answering a telephone, continuously. Able to hear job-specific sounds and to give and receive verbal communications continuously. Able to read and write written communications continuously.
- Able to lift objects weighing 10 pounds or less continuously, 35 pounds or less rarely. The highest point of any lift, overhead; the lowest point of any lift, the floor. Able to carry objects 10 pounds or less frequently, 50 pounds or less rarely. Able to push and pull objects using minimum effort occasionally.
- Able to sit 2 hours consecutively, 6 hours per shift. Able to stand in place 10 minutes consecutively, 30 minutes per shift. Able to remain on feet 1 hour consecutively. Able to sustain awkward position 5 minutes consecutively.
- Able to perform motor skills continuously such as bending, twisting, turning, reaching out, reaching up, wrist turning/torquing, grasping, pinching, finger manipulation, feeling perception. Frequently fast response. Occasionally kneeling, squatting. Able to perform tasks that require arm-hand, hand-eye, and upper and lower body coordination continuously.
- Needs to attend to task/function for 45 minutes at a time or less frequently, 60 minutes at a time or less occasionally, 60 minutes or more at a time rarely. Able to concentrate on fine detail with some interruptions continually. Able to understand and relate to the concepts behind specific ideas continuously. Able to understand and relate to the theories behind

(continued)

APPENDIX 39.8 Sample Job Description—Billing/Financial Coordinator *(continued)*

several related concepts frequently. Able to remember multiple tasks/assignments given to self and others over long periods of time continuously.

JOB DUTIES

The following description of job responsibilities and performance expectations is intended to reflect the major responsibilities and duties of the job, but is not intended to describe minor duties or responsibilities that may be assigned from time to time. Requirements are representative of minimum levels of knowledge, skills, and/or abilities. To perform this job successfully, the incumbent will possess the abilities or aptitudes to perform each duty proficiently. All requirements are subject to possible modification to reasonably accommodate individuals with disabilities.

Responsibility

Coordinate financial and reimbursement monitoring, auditing, and reporting.

Standards

- Review and process requests for clinical and financial records and information accurately and promptly.
- Working with Outreach management and facility directors, analyze record requests and complete corrective-action plans based on internal and external audit results. Monitor action plans and provide summaries as needed.
- Perform random audits on a statistically significant number of accounts for compliance, from physician order through third-party reimbursement documents. Prepare and present audit analyses to department and facility directors as requested.
- Working with Outreach management and ancillary department management, prepare and revise corrective-action plans. Review all plans annually and report as requested.
- Prepare, analyze, and provide information to internal auditors as requested.
- Coordinate specialized financial audits as needed within specified time frames.

Responsibility

Coordinate financial compliance auditing to insure Outreach's adherence to federal, state, and regulatory guidelines.

Standards

- Working with Outreach management, train personnel on compliance needs for outreach functions.
- Audit and analyze daily, monthly, and annual reporting, including billing to third-party payors, to determine and document compliance with federal, state, and regulatory guidelines.
- Develop policies and procedures as well as corrective-action plans as necessary.
- Perform and report on topic audits as required by Director and Corporate Compliance. Act as Outreach's representative in absence of Director for financial or compliance issues.
- Educate outreach clients regarding regulatory issues and monitor adherence to said regulations. Prepare and present corrective-action plans as necessary.

Responsibility

Responsible for information management, including all Outreach databases, Hospital Information Systems patient clinical and financial data, and Laboratory Information Systems system coordination, including patient and customer satisfaction, medical necessity, clinical documentation and compliance, service, and other performance.

(continued)

APPENDIX 39.8   Sample Job Description—Billing/Financial Coordinator *(continued)*

Standards
- Oversee existing database maintenance to insure data integrity and compliance with pertinent regulatory guidelines.
- Develop new databases as needed.
- Develop database training policies and procedures for new users.
- Prepare and provide data analysis and reports for Outreach databases as requested. Coordinate, review, and develop reports from Hospital and Laboratory Information Systems to meet informational needs of Outreach and facility directors.

Responsibility
Maintain revenue structures for third-party payment, including government programs, commercial insurers, and client payors.

Standards
- In collaboration with the Director, determine and document pricing schema for all payors and services.
- Maintain and update fee schedule and related databases and spreadsheets.
- Prepare and provide notification to customers and clients of changes in pricing at least 30 days prior to effective date.

Responsibility
Coordinate the billing and reimbursement cycle for all payors.

Standards
- Prepare and distribute client statements by the 15th of each month.
- Research and analyze client accounts as requested by clients within 48 hours. Correct revenue assessed as necessary.
- Submit client billing summary to Director by 10th working day of each month.
- Review and reconcile client problem accounts daily. Respond to clients and patients concerning billing and reimbursement concerns within 24 hours.
- Review and correct account referrals and reporting exceptions on a daily basis.
- Work with Outreach management to educate clients concerning appropriate billing practices and industry guidelines.

Responsibility
Demonstrate commitment to professional growth and competence.

Standards
- Establish and meet annual individual goals.
- Review code and safety manuals annually. Attend mandatory medical center in-services.
- Maintain confidentiality of information and ensure disposal of confidential records and documents according to established practices.
- Demonstrate effective time management by completing commitments within negotiated time frames.
- Attend the departmental management team meetings.
- Attend the required number of continuing education meetings to maintain professional licensure requirements.

APPENDIX 39.9 Sample Job Description—Sales Associate

- **Reports to:** Laboratory Outreach Director
- **Jobs reporting to this position:** Future Sales Representatives

JOB SUMMARY

Assists in the marketing and sales activities of Regional Lab Outreach. This person is the primary liaison between Outreach and customers and is responsible for maintaining superior client relationships.

JOB QUALIFICATIONS

- **Education:** B.S. degree in Medical Technology or an equivalent combination of an associate's degree and experience.

- **Licensure:** Required as Medical Technologist.

- **Experience:** Two years of clinical laboratory experience to include rotation through the technical areas. Supervisory experience and a demonstrated performance in sales and outreach program support a plus.

- **Skills:** Highly motivated, good organizational skills, proactive in problem solving and processing of information. Must work well with people and possess excellent communication skills. Ability to deal with internal and external customers in a courteous, professional manner at all times. Must have computer experience.

ESSENTIAL PHYSICAL AND MENTAL FUNCTIONS AND ENVIRONMENTAL CONDITIONS

- Continuously exposed to blood, body tissue/fluids, hazardous materials, and chemicals, requiring special clothing and safety equipment. Occasionally exposed to loud noise. Rarely exposed to radiation, potential electrical hazards, and potential burns.

- Able to see objects closely, as in reading; to see objects far away; and to discriminate color and perceive depth continuously. Able to hear normal sounds with some background noise, as in answering a telephone, continuously. Able to hear job-specific sounds and to give and receive verbal communications continuously. Able to read and write written communications continuously.

- Able to lift objects weighing 10 pounds or less continuously, 35 pounds or less rarely. The highest point of any lift, overhead; the lowest point of any lift, the floor. Able to carry objects 10 pounds or less frequently, 50 pounds or less rarely. Able to push and pull objects using minimum effort occasionally.

- Able to sit 2 hours consecutively, 6 hours per shift. Able to stand in place 10 minutes consecutively, 30 minutes per shift. Able to remain on feet 1 hour consecutively. Able to sustain awkward position 5 minutes consecutively.

- Able to perform motor skills continuously such as bending, twisting, turning, reaching out, reaching up, wrist turning/torquing, grasping, pinching, finger manipulation, feeling perception. Frequently fast response. Occasionally kneeling, squatting. Able to perform tasks that require arm-hand, hand-eye, and upper and lower body coordination continuously.

- Needs to attend to task/function for 45 minutes at a time or less frequently, 60 minutes at a time or less occasionally, 60 minutes or more at a time rarely. Able to concentrate on fine detail with some interruptions continually. Able to understand and relate to the concepts behind specific ideas continuously. Able to understand and relate to the theories behind several related concepts frequently. Able to remember multiple tasks/assignments given to self and others over long periods of time continuously.

JOB DUTIES

The following description of job responsibilities and performance expectations is intended to reflect the major responsibilities and duties of the job, but is not intended to describe minor duties or responsibilities that may be assigned from time to time. Requirements are representative of minimum levels of knowledge, skills, and/or abilities. To perform this job successfully,

(continued)

APPENDIX 39.9   Sample Job Description—Sales Associate *(continued)*

the incumbent will possess the abilities or aptitudes to perform each duty proficiently. All requirements are subject to possible modification to reasonably accommodate individuals with disabilities.

Responsibility
Assist Director in managing all marketing functions to achieve the objectives for sales, growth, profits, and visibility while ensuring a consistent marketing message and positioning on a regional basis consistent with the corporate direction.

Standards
- Develop and implement appropriate strategies by
  - Selecting, segmenting, and targeting markets.
  - Promoting services to those markets.
  - Providing enhancements for program development.
- Determine a pricing approach and set prices for services.
  - Maintain and update fee schedule database.
  - Develop and update pricing policy.
  - Provide adequate notification to customers of changes in pricing.
- Set goals in terms of market share and growth.
- Develop plans in relation to advertising, sales promotion, public relations, and sales management by working with Corporate Development to
  - Ensure the proper amount and type of coverage to raise awareness, win reviews, and ensure consistent corporate and product branding and image.
  - Create the media schedule, negotiate the rates, and prepare and execute the deliverables.
  - Follow up and measure the advertising campaign using print and electronic methods.
  - Ensure a consistent look and feel among collateral materials such as sell sheets, product slicks, folders, trade show graphics, and all other program imaging.
- Undertake marketing audits to monitor outreach performance and to ensure that services are demand-driven.
  - Create research methodologies.
  - Design data collection tools.
  - Analyze data collected, prepare reports, and present findings.
- Prepare annual marketing plan.
  - Identify and analyze the organization's strengths and weaknesses and the marketing environment's opportunities and threats.
  - Develop and review (annually) client contracts.
  - Prepare sales collateral, brochures, data sheets, and new-client packets.

Responsibility
Assist Director in coordinating sales activity of Regional Lab Outreach.

Standards
- Develop specific sales plans and strategies to meet laboratory goals.
  - Find new ways to bring in business and prospects.
  - Develop lead-generation strategies including cold calling, direct-mail campaigns, trade shows, and list acquisition.
  - Identify top 20 prospective clients.

(continued)

- Arrange a program of visits to all major potential clients by contacting people and making appointments.
  - Maintain established clients.
  - Provide best follow-up possible consistent with need and arranged schedule.
  - Qualify leads and contacts.
- Determine the best methods of promoting services.
  - Develop and update knowledge of competitors' services.
  - Maintain competitor profiles.
  - Speak with other medical center sales and marketing personnel.
- Assess customers' needs and explain services to them, which may involve providing technical descriptions as well as describing the purposes for which they may be used.
- Quote and negotiate prices within established guidelines, prepare contracts for signature by clients, and maintain client database.
  - Updates must be completed within two working days of client acquisition.
  - Database data must be clean and accessible for direct mailings and client-list preparation.
  - Ensure consistent, accurate data coding.
- Report to Director on sales and acquisition of new clients by the 10th working day of each month.
  - Generate a report of tests ordered by account in table and graphic format within 10 working days of the beginning of the month.
  - Generate a report of sales activity and new-account acquisition within two working days of the beginning of the month.
  - Generate a report summarizing client visits, concerns, and problem resolution within 10 working days of the beginning of the month.
- Coordinate development and production of promotional and informational material.
  - Prepare and carry out formal presentations and/or proposals of services customized to fit individual client needs by using overheads, slides, videos, and other training aids.
  - Represent program at promotional markets such as trade association meetings.
  - Organize services displays.

Responsibility
Perform specific responsibilities assigned.

Standards
- Promptly investigate complaints concerning Outreach services and take appropriate actions.
- Ensure that customers are familiar with the operation and maintenance of the equipment received from Outreach.
- As part of the administrative team, participate in maintaining a current, complete directory of services on an annual basis or as needed.
- Be responsible for the coordination of orientation and training of all customers who are provided with a verbal and written overview of laboratory operations, policies, and procedures.
- Monitor customer orders to see that they are filled promptly and accurately. Maintain timely communication with Logistics Coordinator to ensure no more than one documented instance of supplies not being delivered or failure to communicate problems to the Director or Logistics Coordinator.
- Assist the Director in the preparation and monitoring of the budget.

(continued)

- Monitor budget to determine if the department is operating within allocated funds.
- Provide input that develops procedures and policies for downtime procedures as they relate to customer sites, make recommendations during downtime for course of action. Allow no instances of downtime procedures not being current or failure to communicate an appropriate course of action or failure to update customers on status of repair/rebuild.
- Provide support for customers' personal computers—allow no more than one instance of not responding to a request for assistance on a computer or not notifying Information Systems of the need for assistance.

Responsibility
Demonstrate commitment to professional growth and competence.

Standards
- Attend the required number of continuing education meetings per year, and record attendance—no more than two instances of failing to record continuing education or missing no more than two of the required continuing education meetings.
- Review code and safety manuals annually.
- Attend the departmental management team meetings.
- Establish and meet annual individual goals.
- Remain informed and up-to-date in all technical aspects of the department and Hospital Laboratory as needed to provide a basis for sales promotions through literature, workshops, seminars, courses, and conferences with other laboratory professionals.

APPENDIX 39.10 Sample Job Description—Courier

- **Reports to:** Logistics Coordinator
- **Jobs reporting to this position:** None

JOB SUMMARY

Picks up and/or delivers specimens and supplies for the Laboratory and represents medical center laboratory in a positive, professional manner as contact to the customers. Uses courier logs and appropriate compliance with safety standards. Helps with specimen processing by labeling and packing specimens/requisitions for transport to the Core Lab. Uses Laboratory Information Systems (LIS) in processing and tracking down specimens.

JOB QUALIFICATIONS

- **Education:** High school diploma or equivalent.
- **Licensure:** Valid state driver's license.
- **Experience:** Good driving record, dealing with public.
- **Skills:** Good people skills, customer service skills, and organizational skills. Neat, orderly and conservative appearance.

ESSENTIAL PHYSICAL AND MENTAL FUNCTIONS AND ENVIRONMENTAL CONDITIONS

- Continuously exposed to blood, body tissue/fluids, hazardous materials, and chemicals, requiring special clothing and safety equipment. Occasionally exposed to loud noise. Rarely exposed to radiation, potential electrical hazards, and potential burns.

- Able to see objects closely, as in reading, frequently. Able to discriminate color and perceive depth continuously. Able to hear normal sounds with some background noise, as in answering a telephone, continuously. Able to hear job-specific sounds and to give and receive verbal communications continuously. Able to read and write written communications continuously.

- Able to lift objects weighing 10 pounds or less continuously, 20 pounds or less rarely. The highest point of any lift, overhead; the lowest point of any lift, the floor. Able to carry objects 10 pounds or less continuously, 50 pounds or less rarely. Able to push and pull objects using minimum effort occasionally.

- Able to sit 45 minutes consecutively. Able to stand in place 5 minutes consecutively.

- Able to remain on feet 1 hour consecutively. Able to sustain awkward position 5 minutes consecutively. Able to perform motor skills continuously such as bending, twisting, turning, reaching out, reaching up, wrist turning/torquing, grasping, pinching, finger manipulation, feeling perception. Frequently fast response. Occasionally kneeling, squatting. Able to perform tasks that require arm-hand, hand-eye, and upper and lower body coordination continuously.

- Needs to attend to task/function 10 minutes at a time or less continuously, 20 minutes at a time or less occasionally, 45 minutes at a time or less occasionally, 60 minutes at a time or less rarely. Able to concentrate on fine detail with some interruptions continuously. Able to understand and relate to the concepts behind specific ideas continuously. Able to understand and relate to the theories behind several related concepts frequently. Able to remember multiple tasks/assignments given to self and others over long periods of time continuously.

JOB DUTIES

The following description of job responsibilities and performance expectations is intended to reflect the major responsibilities and duties of the job, but is not intended to describe minor duties or other responsibilities that may be assigned from time to time. Requirements are representative of minimum levels of knowledge, skills, and/or abilities. To perform this job successfully, the incumbent will possess the abilities or aptitudes to perform each duty proficiently. All requirements are subject to possible modification to reasonably accommodate individuals with disabilities.

(continued)

APPENDIX 39.10   Sample Job Description—Courier *(continued)*

Responsibility

Complete courier pickup and delivery.

Standards

- Complete pickup and delivery of specimens, reports, and/or supplies according to accepted procedure, including timeliness and problem resolution resulting from specimen mislabeling or transport delay. Maintain patient confidentiality when delivering reports to clients. Deliver reports according to defined time schedule.
- Notify supervisor of any concerns or conflicts in completing courier duties according to schedule as documented by supervisor.
- Immediately respond to and complete STAT services in a timely manner.
- Modify and adjust courier runs in accordance with priority and direction received from the supervisor as evidenced by correct follow-through.
- Identify and communicate to the supervisor any questions pertaining to run instructions prior to start of run.
- Represent Outreach in a positive, courteous, professional manner regarding "appearance," "attitude," and "communication skills."

Responsibility

Assist with processing, inventory, maintenance, and courier logs.

Standards

- Assist in inventorying and restocking of supplies. Date all supplies when stocking shelves. Rotate stock, keeping most recently received supplies behind older supplies. Notify Logistics Coordinator when supplies reach critically low limits.
- Deliver requests for supplies within 24 hours. Notify clients when supplies are back-ordered.
- Accurately maintain and record all patient names, specimens, times, and special instructions in courier log.
- Receive specimens into LIS, matching patient name with form, complete information, and computer labels.
- Correctly generate order labels from LIS, matching patient name on the forms, complete information, and patient name on the tube(s).
- Correctly label specimens according to the Outreach secondary labeling of specimen policy, matching patient name and information on the patient order label(s) and the patient specimen tube(s).
- Perform duties of appropriate specimen preparation for transport.
- Deliver specimen and labels to appropriate laboratory department, communicating, as necessary, any appropriate information.
- Consistently and in a timely manner, perform maintenance procedures on the client centrifuges, including timer check, tachometer check, and evaluation of centrifuge physical condition.
- Communicate routinely with Biomedical Engineering regarding centrifuge maintenance and record keeping.

Responsibility

Obey outreach and other laws and regulations when operating the courier vehicle.

Standards

- Obey all traffic laws and regulations, as evidenced by lack of citations.
- Allow no one other than an appropriately assigned Outreach employee to operate vehicle.

(continued)

APPENDIX 39.10   Sample Job Description—Courier (*continued*)

- Check tires, water, oil levels, and gas prior to each shift and before operating vehicle, as observed by supervisor.
  - Fill with gas if tank is less than half full.
  - Fill with oil if more than 1 quart low.
  - Keep tires properly inflated.
  - Keep vehicle clean and wash vehicle when needed to maintain professional appearance.
- To ensure security and confidentiality, keep vehicle doors locked when not in vehicle.

Responsibility
Actively contribute to the efficient operation of Laboratory Outreach.

Standards
- Page Couriers in an accurate and timely manner according to accepted procedures. Consistently and accurately document required information on the courier call log.
- Promote the image of Laboratory Outreach by adhering to the medical center policy and departmental guidelines and dress code.
- Participate in computer downtime recovery team, being available when assigned and assisting with specimen labeling and dissemination of work.
- Accept, in a positive manner, delegation of new responsibilities and changes in responsibilities.
- Clarify directions or communications that are unclear.
- Maintain patient privacy at all times according to established procedures.
- Maintain confidentiality of departmental information according to established procedures.

Responsibility
Demonstrate commitment to departmental growth and competence.

Standards
- Willingly perform other duties as assigned according to procedure.
- Attend laboratory in-service education classes when scheduled.
- Attend departmental meetings and/or read and sign corresponding minutes.
- Remain current in field, as demonstrated by proactively contributing this knowledge in the workplace, generally sharing ideas, information, and knowledge of the field.
- Contribute to improving the department's operations.
- Establish and meet annual individual goals that are developed to assist the department in achieving its established goals or projects.
- Review code, safety and infection control manuals annually, as evidenced by knowledge and signature in each manual's log sheet.
- Participate in the JCAHO-required safety procedure review/update annually, as indicated by in-service record.
- Participate in continuous improvement in the department.

APPENDIX 39.11   Sample Job Description—Phlebotomist/Patient Service Representative

- **Reports to:** Operations Coordinator
- **Jobs reporting to this position: None**

JOB SUMMARY

As needed, performs a range of duties that include, but are not limited to, testing patient samples, training new employees or current staff on new procedures, registering patients and specimens, and collecting specimens. Represents Outreach in a positive, professional manner as contact to the customers. Will also assist with insurance verification and management and with the coordination of department operations. Provides patient care for patients of all ages. Uses Hospital and Laboratory Information Systems as needed.

JOB QUALIFICATIONS

- **Education:** Associate's degree in related medical field or high school diploma or equivalent with related applicable experience.
- **Licensure:** Valid state driver's license. Certified Phlebotomist or Certified Patient Accounts Representative-certified preferred.
- **Experience:** Good driving record. Successful completion of medical terminology course or experience in clinical setting preferred.
- **Skills:** Excellent communication skills, both verbal and written; general office skills with computer experience in Microsoft Word, Excel, and Access.

ESSENTIAL PHYSICAL AND MENTAL FUNCTIONAL AND ENVIRONMENTAL CONDITIONS

- Continuously exposed to blood, body tissue/fluids, hazardous materials, and chemicals, requiring special clothing and safety equipment. Occasionally exposed to loud noise. Rarely exposed to radiation, potential electrical hazards, and potential burns.

- Able to see objects closely, as in reading; to see objects far away; and to discriminate color and perceive depth continuously. Able to hear normal sounds with some background noise, as in answering a telephone, continuously. Able to hear job-specific sounds and to give and receive verbal communications continuously. Able to read and write written communications continuously.

- Able to lift objects weighing 10 pounds or less continuously, 35 pounds or less rarely. The highest point of any lift, overhead; the lowest point of any lift, the floor. Able to carry objects 10 pounds or less frequently, 50 pounds or less rarely. Able to push and pull objects using minimum effort occasionally.

- Able to sit 2 hours consecutively, 6 hours per shift. Able to stand in place 10 minutes consecutively, 30 minutes per shift. Able to remain on feet 1 hour consecutively. Able to sustain awkward position 5 minutes consecutively.

- Able to perform motor skills continuously such as bending, twisting, turning, reaching out, reaching up, wrist turning/torquing, grasping, pinching, finger manipulation, feeling perception. Frequently fast response. Occasionally kneeling, squatting. Able to perform tasks that require arm-hand, hand-eye, and upper and lower body coordination continuously.

- Needs to attend to task/function for 45 minutes at a time or less frequently, 60 minutes at a time or less occasionally, 60 minutes or more at a time rarely. Able to concentrate on fine detail with some interruptions continually. Able to understand and relate to the concepts behind specific ideas continuously. Able to understand and relate to the theories behind several related concepts frequently. Able to remember multiple tasks/assignments given to self and others over long periods of time continuously.

JOB DUTIES

The following description of job responsibilities and performance expectations is intended to reflect the major responsibilities and duties of the job, but is not intended to describe minor duties or responsibilities that may be assigned from time to time. Requirements are representative of minimum levels of knowledge, skills, and/or abilities. To perform this job successfully,

(continued)

the incumbent will posses the abilities or aptitudes to perform each duty proficiently. All requirements are subject to possible modification to reasonably accommodate individuals with disabilities.

Responsibility

Provide technical support and front-desk services courteously and in an efficient manner.

Standards

- Answer phone using appropriate phone etiquette with no more than three rings.
- Monitor incoming and outgoing faxes, including confirmation of the receipt of test orders by Outreach within one hour of receiving orders.
- Able to operate copier according to procedure.
- Acknowledge on-site patients in a timely manner according to customer service standards.
- Notify patients of expected wait times upon check-in and every 10 minutes during peak times when longer than 15-minute wait times occur or if a special situation occurs, e.g., patient fainting.
- Communicate with waiting patients on reason for taking STAT patient out of order.
- Dispatch Courier within five minutes of notification and follow up according to procedure.
- Process patient payments according to procedure.
- Ensure that correct forms are completed by patient prior to registration, including the proper signatures on consent form and copy of insurance card and proper identification.
- Notify all back-office areas of arriving patients to ensure that wait times are kept at a minimum, including possible temporary reassignment of job duties.
- Verify status of patient or specimen requirements including STAT, fasting status, legal name, etc.
- Perform accurate clinical quality assurance as required according to procedure and with minimal backlog.
- Call patients and providers concerning re-collects according to procedure.
- Release results to appropriate personnel according to procedure.
- Problem-solve with clients, including issues involving supplies, reports, courier service, and billing.
- Advocate for patients and clients in billing issues with Patient Billing Services, insurance company, etc., including problem solving, issue resolution, and request to resubmit bill if necessary.

Responsibility

Exhibit customer-focused behavior and provide excellent customer service.

Standards

- Follow the safety plan, recognizing that safety always comes first, and proactively take steps to maintain a safe environment.
- Follow guidelines for customer service.
- Meet quality service standards.
- Continuously set the proper environment for customers so that their outreach experience is as positive as possible.
- Follow dress code.
- Meet attendance (tardiness and absences) expectations.

(continued)

APPENDIX 39.11   Sample Job Description—Phlebotomist/Patient Service Representative *(continued)*

Responsibility
Provide clinical testing (testing waived).

Standards
- Perform accurate testing, including quality control and troubleshooting (if necessary), according to established procedure and in a timely manner.
- Report test results according to established procedure and turnaround-time guidelines.
- Alert provider(s) of panic and/or critical values according to established procedure.
- Demonstrate knowledge of principles or concepts related to testing performed.

Responsibility
Collect specimens appropriately and as needed.

Standards
- Label specimens legibly, correctly, and immediately after collection.
- Identify patients correctly according to standards.
- Collect blood specimens using proper technique and in a timely manner by finger stick, heel stick, or venipuncture according to standards, including special collection and/or handling requirements and test priority.
- Label specimens legibly, correctly, and in a timely manner.
- Collect specimens correctly (clinical accuracy).
- Collect other specimens according to procedure, including monitoring and starting glucose tolerances, random urinalysis, 24-hour urine assays, throat swabs, nasal saline washes, semen specimens, stool specimens, sputum specimens, and nasal swabs.
- Instruct patients effectively and correctly in the collection of 24-hour urine, stool, semen, sputum, and clean-catch urine specimens.
- Meet standard for minimum number of re-collects within a 12-month period.
- Maintain patient confidentiality at all times.
- Reassure patients by explaining procedures.

Responsibility
Process specimens appropriately and as needed.

Standards
- Reconcile requisition and testing requirements with specimen received both at front desk and in processing area.
- Order test correctly.
- Be able to cancel test or generate add-ons according to policy and procedure.
- Register patients and specimens correctly (registration accuracy).
- Process specimens in a timely manner, including readiness for transport.
- Process patients in a timely manner, including registration and collection.
- Demonstrate knowledge of billing process steps.
- Make corrections and insurance changes as needed.

Responsibility
Demonstrate knowledge of and participation in outreach process improvement.

Standards
- Actively participate in at least one process improvement group, either at the departmental or institutional level.
- Willingly adjust to change as needed.

(continued)

- Demonstrate ability to be part of the solution rather than part of the problem.
- Demonstrate problem-solving abilities.
- Demonstrate knowledge of and adherence to quality control procedures related to testing.
- Utilize client problem reports, variance reports, and other quality improvement documents as needed and according to established procedure.
- Review distributed professional journal articles to improve job knowledge.

Responsibility
Participate in training of other staff.

Standards
- Model appropriate behavior for new employees, providing advice and counseling.
- Participate in training new employees or existing staff in new procedures, using accepted methodologies and techniques.
- Review and sign off on all manuals on a yearly basis.
- Evaluate trainees at end of module and recommend further training if needed to training coordinator.
- Evaluate other staff during annual competency assessments and recommend further training if needed to Operations Coordinator.
- Attend at least _____ hours of continuing education outside of Outreach.
- Attend seminars as requested, to include a written summary of information and presentation to staff.
- Attend departmental meetings as assigned.

Responsibility
Perform routine maintenance and assist with supplies as required.

Standards
- Perform and document required preventative maintenance on equipment and facilities as assigned.
- Order supplies as needed by clients and when inventory reaches reorder level.
- Receive supplies as needed according to procedure.
- Stock supplies in storage areas as needed according to procedure.
- Stock supplies in work area as needed according to procedure.

APPENDIX 39.12   Guidelines for Client Visits

1. *First contact.* Set up appointment by phone or in person.
2. *Second contact.* In person, determine client needs and leave initial literature. Follow up within two working days with thank-you note.
3. *Third contact.* By phone or preferably in writing, confirm information found during the discovery phase. Set up an appointment to outline how the outreach program can help the client with their issues.
4. *Fourth contact.* In person, present customized services and fee schedule.
5. *Fifth contact.* Within five working days and in writing, send thank-you for opportunity to make presentation. Also notify client of intent to contact client representative about their decision.
6. *Sixth contact.* By phone within five working days, discover client issues—if any. Ask for the business and set up meeting to discuss implementation plans.
7. *Seventh contact.* In person within five working days, develop implementation plan with client.
8. *Eighth contact.* Provide on-site assistance with implementation in person.
9. *Ninth contact.* Within five working days and in person, follow up on implementation and solicit client satisfaction.
10. *Tenth and subsequent contacts.* Schedule periodic visits based upon size of account, client preference, and problem-solving needs to develop strong relationship with client.

APPENDIX 39.13   List of Promotional Literature

Three-fold brochure for patients
Brief history of outreach program
List of participating insurance plans
Sample fee schedule
Services handbook
Business cards
Electronic presentation template
Literature folder

Fact sheet for clients
List of current clients
Sample client service agreement
Sample client bill
Rolodex punchout page
Sample requisition
Proposal cover
Giveaways like pens, notepads, etc.

APPENDIX 39.14   Model Patient Satisfaction Survey

Please take a moment to tell us about your visit to our Patient Service Center. Your comments are important to us and will help us look at ways to make your future visits more comfortable.

We thank you.

Name: _____
(optional)

How did you hear about _____ Outreach?

☐ Relative   ☐ Friend   ☐ Physician

☐ Newspaper/magazine   ☐ Other

Was our staff caring, courteous, and responsive to your needs?

☐ Yes   ☐ No

Would you use _____ Outreach in the future?

☐ Yes   ☐ No

Did you consider your wait time reasonable?

☐ Yes   ☐ No

Can we do anything to improve our services?

☐ Yes   ☐ No

Comments and/ or suggestions:

_____

_____

_____

_____

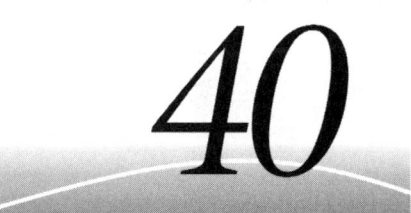

Outreach Implementation Requirements: a Case Study

Frederick L. Kiechle and Joseph E. Skrisson

OBJECTIVES

To describe the planning process to implement an outreach program

To identify potential barriers to acceptance of the implementation plan for an outreach program

To discuss the impact of a successful outreach program on various laboratory sections

To discuss the advantages of computer-assisted routing for couriers

To describe methods for monitoring the financial success of an outreach program

To discuss the advantages of initiating a joint venture with affiliating hospital-based outreach laboratories to obtain contracts with managed-care organizations

The headlines never say good morning any more.
Every day the forecast reads: A chance of showers.
The Tigers keep losing the ballgames.
And Dick Tracy is reported missing.
His smashed wrist-radio recovered
From a burned-out crater of the moon.
The market has plunged again;
Clad dimes and quarters have replaced the real ones.

But you ring the doorbell with a Sunday sunrise
Rolled up casually in one pocket
And a handful of silver coins
With rare mint-marks in the other.

NAOMI LONG MADGETT, "GOOD NEWS" (29)

LABORATORY MEDICINE has been increasingly commercialized since 1950 in three phases (46). Since 1985, the primary focus has been on the business aspects of laboratory medicine. The method of healthcare reimbursement has resulted in decreased revenue for the healthcare provider. Laboratories have responded to this gradual conversion of fee-for-service to managed-care contracts with a fixed fee per member per month by restructuring laboratory operations with a focus on both cost containment and revenue enhancement (22, 26). A variety of methods to improve hospital laboratory efficiency have developed during the continuous evolution to the next iteration of healthcare delivery and reimbursement. Methods have been designed to reduce cost per procedure, which include increased test volume through hospital laboratory mergers, consolidation, or integration (13, 19, 26, 45, 47, 54) and/or development of an outreach program that markets laboratory services to physician offices, nursing homes, and other hospitals (2, 8, 9, 26, 35, 36, 38, 44). Other methods have been designed to reduce the operating costs and increase the efficiency in the laboratory, including the introduction of robotics and/or automation (16, 21, 26, 41, 43), point-of-care testing (23, 24, 25, 26, 30, 40), and a different mix of skill levels in the workforce (10, 15, 24, 26, 28).

Increasing laboratory test volume through the introduction of an outreach program has been described in a variety of settings: a national reference laboratory (36), smaller hospitals (2, 35), larger hospitals (8, 26, 36, 38, 44), and hospitals in Malaysia (38). The success of each of these outreach programs depends on many factors, one of which is the ability of the outreach laboratory to obtain provider status with local and regional insurance carriers and managed-care organizations (8, 44). The following case study describes the implementation of a hospital-based clinical laboratory outreach program, Beaumont Reference Laboratory (BRL), in Royal Oak, Michigan, and its affiliation with a regional hospital laboratory network to secure provider status with major local and regional insurance carriers.

Outreach Plan Approval Process

Barriers to the Plan's Approval

An entrepreneur, or "a person within a corporation who takes direct responsibility for turning an idea into a profitable finished product through assertive risk-taking and innovation" (39), is required to initiate the change process needed to facilitate the implementation of an outreach plan. The entrepreneur must convert the illusion of revenue consisting of clad coinage created by delusional, magical thinking to a coherent outreach program generating genuine profits. Numerous potential barriers may be encountered during this change process, including myths, active inertia, lack of incentive, insufficient support from Financial Analysis and other groups, slow approval process, conflicting visions, and others (22, 26). At times, the task of strategic alliance building (32) required to achieve the goal will seem overwhelming. Capitalize on serendipitous circumstances and use variable-term opportunism (32). For example, the mental visualization of the plan has no effect until the vision is verbalized. An entrepreneur will use every opportunity to introduce the new plan during any conversation or meeting where the problem the new plan will resolve is discussed. Continuous, relentless use of this strategy subtly convinces many individuals that the new plan has been approved, and they will then express dismay that there are apparent delays in their area of responsibility in its implementation. Gandhi said, "Satisfaction lies in the effort, not in the attainment.

Full effort is full victory" (11). Carl von Clausewitz, the 19th-century Prussian general, wrote, "In the dynamics of execution, under the ever-changing conditions of the surroundings (whether terrain and weather in war, or the economy and consumer attitudes in business), the contestants must increasingly evaluate the potential advantages to be gained from shifting their perceptions between any number of polar opposites" (53). Remember to retain the flexibility, fluidity, and dynamic resilience required to "weigh the situation, then move" (50).

Active inertia and myths are two indolent, disruptive barriers to outreach program implementation. Myths represent inaccurate information perceived as truth by major administrative decision-makers. "Fiction, like all operas: a lie, but a lie is sort of a myth, and a myth is sort of a truth" (14). Myths are plentiful and reflect the need for administrators to codify apparent truths, thus eliminating the need for their further evaluation or validation. There are myths related to customers (51), laboratory management (33), and tribal knowledge (22, 26). Does it mean, "There is no such thing as 'truth.' There's only language. There's no such thing as a 'fact.' There is no truth or falsehood, just dominant processes by which reality is socially constructed" (48). However, language is the primary method of communication, and work-arounds may be required. For example, myths within an organization are difficult to dispel by local storytellers. Three efforts to initiate an outreach program at our institution failed because the data were generated and presented by the Department of Clinical Pathology. Myths surrounded the legality of the project, the ability to bill, and the financial analysis. To reverse this indocility, we spent money and hired a consultant who had a global view of many other hospitals, each of which had successfully initiated an outreach program. Field trips for numerous decision-makers were organized to sites with successful outreach programs as a preemptive strike to dislodge the myths. After this drill, the consultant's presentation confirmed the findings of the field trips, thus building administrative enthusiasm for the project. In this situation, the myths were removed from their pedestal by convincing data contradicting their authenticity.

A manifestation of active inertia, which is the insensate repetition of the same behavior pattern without regard to the magnitude of the paradigm shift (49), can effectively destroy all of the efforts outlined above. In this environment, "Do anything, but do something" is the mantra and values become dogma. The combination of active inertia (49) and myths can send the most reasonable plan to a committee for eternity. The decision-makers on that committee have descended to "the lowest level of awareness" in a stepwise manner, as defined by Albert Einstein: "'I know.' Then, 'I don't know,' 'I know I don't know,' 'I don't know that I don't know'" (7). Having achieved the lowest level of awareness through the promulgation of myths and active inertia, the committee members will leave these meetings feeling as if "we, none of us, ever mean anything" (6). Remember that tough financial times make tough decisions easier. A failure to achieve the margin (profit) goal will initiate the change process faster in a hospital administration than any other consequence (26).

Consultants to the Rescue

This is a case study, and certainly there are successful outreach efforts that have been initiated without the aid of consultants. However, with the past history of three failed attempts over 5 years to obtain administrative approval, it was suggested that we needed to try a different approach. In April 1991, we retained the services of a consulting firm to investigate the feasibility of starting an outreach program either as a joint venture with a commercial laboratory or as a stand-alone hospital laboratory outreach program (8). The market was evaluated by first reviewing the subspecialty mix for the more than 1,000 physicians on the hospital staff. Physicians in subspecialties with high laboratory utilization, like Internal Medicine, Obstetrics/Gynecology, Family Practice, and others (Table 40.1), were sent a survey asking if they would be interested in doing business with BRL if it were organized. More than 90% of the physicians responded in the affirmative. Current managed-care contracts were reviewed. The potential for attracting work from local nursing homes and other hospitals was explored. Discussions with several commercial laboratories about potential joint-venture relationships were uniformly unsuccessful. Their primary message was, "We want to run your laboratory." Of course, we began to wonder what our role would be in this takeover strategy. Frankly, we preferred to run our own laboratory.

The positive results of the feasibility study led to a second engagement that produced a market survey and a three-year pro forma financial projection. The pro forma reflected conservative volume increases over the 3-year period in each of the market sectors including physician offices, nursing homes, and other hospitals. Reimbursement was based on payor mix averages for tests frequently ordered in each sector. This plan was approved by Hospital Administration with support from the chairmen of the

Table 40.1 2002 BRL outreach laboratory utilization analyzed by specialty

Specialty	No. of physicians	Total procedures
Family Practice	464	631,086
Pediatrics	219	123,244
Internal Medicine	831	1,347,426
Cardiology	126	82,068
Endocrinology	96	68,880
Gastroenterology	60	60,860
Nursing homes	575	395,742
OB/GYN	309	250,520
Urology	126	16,668

Department of Clinical Pathology and the Department of Anatomic Pathology. The two pathology departments operate independently of each other at William Beaumont Hospital. BRL was defined as a for-profit unrelated business enterprise within a nonprofit hospital. Registered outpatients were excluded from BRL pricing. BRL clients were limited to those who drew their patients' blood or who had adequate volume to justify having BRL provide a phlebotomist in their office.

Bureaucratic Simplification Equals Success

In general, administration in a hospital is focused on inpatient and registered outpatient issues. A large number of middle or upper managers are assigned the task of providing signature approval for procedures, pricing, capital equipment, personnel, and other details. These individuals are usually so far removed from issues related to the request that a lack of urgency will guarantee delays. For example, the delay in approval of open employee positions caused by requests for additional documentation may represent a covert effort by a manager to cook the books and save on total overall personnel dollars for the quarter. Once this objective is attained, approval for filling the open position is very rapid. A successful outreach program must be run more like a business. Approvals must be streamlined from the usual ten managers to three or fewer managers who are very familiar with the operation. The competition for outreach clients is more volatile than the competition for inpatients. The volatile environment requires a method for rapid assessment of options and rapid initiation of a solution.

An outreach program will require continuous, intense support from Financial Analysis, Information Services, Marketing, and Managed-Care Services. Adequate staffing will be required to address the complaints of outreach clients and meet the needs of the program's growth. Hospital Administration provides staff for the cyclic changes anticipated for inpatients and registered outpatients. For example, during the financial cycle, the preparation of the annual budget and end-of-the-year financial reports may completely preoccupy all of the staffing resources for at least 3 months. During this period, the financial analysis department is paralyzed and unable to perform routine evaluations for capital equipment or new personnel. The consequence of this paralysis is that outreach business development grinds to a halt while requests for approval sit on someone's desk. A potential solution is to establish a financial staff that responds only to the needs of the outreach program. These staff members must be sequestered and protected from being removed from their tasks during the crisis of hospital financial analysis. A similar strategy may be required to assure that there are adequate personnel available to handle outreach-related computer issues, such as autofax, outreach billing using a stand-alone system, nursing home setup, new-client setup, requisition scanning, client services, critical values, and others. In short, for the implementation and future success of an outreach program, the departments that support the new program and the laboratory, such as Personnel, Information Services, Financial Analysis, and Marketing, must be attentive, efficient, streamlined, and responsive.

The complexity of establishing an outreach program predicts that a small-scale demonstration project will fail. Abandon any idea of experimenting with outreach. All elements of the outreach initiative, including sales force, couriers, client services, registration, accessioning, result delivery, and patient or client billing, must be in place before its first day of operation is announced. A failed pilot project or small-scale experiment will tarnish the program's reputation, a perception that may take years of hard work to reverse. The goal is to dazzle each customer from the beginning and nurture loyalty through a continuous high level of performance.

Requirements for Outreach Implementation

Figure 40.1 represents the current organizational diagram for BRL. This section will review the development of the sales and marketing department, as well as courier services.

Sales and Marketing Program

Step 1. Design a competitive salary and commission package for sales staff. Base salary should be aligned with the degree of experience the individual brings to the job. For example, the ideal candidate would have had previous experience in a clinical laboratory and in laboratory sales and training (preferably from a national laboratory). The commission program should be competitive when compared to the marketplace in order to attract the top candidates. In addition, the commission structure should be aggressive to promote new-sales efforts and also provide a reward for maintaining existing business. Ideally, the top sales representatives would derive 66% of their yearly earnings from commissions and the remaining 33% from their base salary. Remember, the hardest sell is going to be the hospital administrators, when you tell them that a top laboratory sales representative could make six figures or more a year. If the majority of these earnings come from commissions, then it will be easier to get administrative approval for a competitive sales compensation program.

New-sales and overall business growth targets are set annually at budget time. BRL sales representatives are given their team's annual new-sales target along with their individual minimal sales quota. BRL's commission program rewards sales representatives for new-business sales, existing-business growth (upgrades), and overall maintenance and growth of their territory (bonus). For new-business growth, BRL has an aggressive commission program based on a rolling 3-month average of new-business sales. This program is structured to encourage

sales representatives to bring in new business quickly and steadily, since the higher their 3-month rolling average, the greater the commission that is paid. The new-sales commission program also penalizes the sales representative for lost business. Monthly lost-business numbers are subtracted from monthly new-sales numbers before establishing the 3-month rolling average. BRL has experienced great success with this program and it has been a great motivator for the sales staff.

Sales representatives also get paid an upgrade commission on existing-business growth. These business upgrades are treated separately and paid based on a less aggressive commission structure than new-business sales. Sales representatives are also rewarded quarterly with a bonus based on their overall territory growth and meeting their business sales quota. This sales compensation program has worked well for BRL, as it has kept our sales staff highly motivated in bringing in new business and maintaining (retaining) and growing existing business, as highlighted in our past years' business growth numbers (Table 40.2).

Step 2. Nurture the experience level of staff. Our experience at BRL has demonstrated that there is no substitute for sales training and field experience. National laboratories excel in this area, and most hospital-affiliated outreach programs fall short. Significant time, dollars, and resources are required to train the sales staff in basic sales techniques, compliance training, and end-sell strategies.

Step 3. Develop a new sales and maintenance program. Know your market and make sure your market knows you. To maximize market penetration, first identify prospective clients in the target market, prioritize the most profitable prospects, and then assign those prospects to sales staff members for office calls and/or sales presentations. Prospects lists (physicians, nursing homes, hospitals,

Table 40.2 Beaumont Reference Laboratory's annual client numbers and clinical pathology procedures

Year	Client number	BRL total clinical pathology procedures	BRL procedures as a percentage of hospital's total clinical pathology procedures[a]
1994	170	307,403	14.5%
1995	300	570,014	22.8%
1996	543	598,689	21.6%
1997	677	805,463	28.1%
1998	761	1,484,874	38.0%
1999	841	1,897,526	41.0%
2000	998	2,081,245	44.8%
2001	1,085	2,258,252	41.1%
2002	1,175	2,292,672	46.2%

[a]Total clinical pathology procedures include inpatients, hospital-registered outpatients, and BRL clients.

and other healthcare facilities) can normally be acquired or purchased from your state medical societies, insurance providers (network listings), and third-party research firms. We have found that buying a prospect list from a marketing research firm is worth the investment since the list can be customized to your specifications. For example, request a list of only practicing physicians in a certain county and only their office addresses. Often a state medical society lists all members, both practicing and retired, and their home and office addresses.

Once the target list of prospects/customers is established, your sales staff can focus on contacting these prospects. Sales presentations must be customized for the respective business lines: physician offices and long-term-care/nursing homes. Sales presentations for physician offices should always stress that you are providing information services, highlighting such value-added services as office web-based order entry and result-reporting software. Sales staff should customize their presentations based on the physician specialty and be prepared to discuss the physician's patient mix (disease states), most commonly ordered tests, and emerging new tests that can be of benefit to patient diagnosis and treatment. Up-selling existing and emerging tests helps improve diagnostic efficiency as well as operating margins. Up-selling refers to the practice of informing clients of new or improved laboratory tests that may have superior sensitivity and specificity than the routine screening assays. These new or improved assays may be applicable to patients with a well-defined subset of a certain disease or for patients who have failed the usual therapeutic strategies.

Long-term-care/nursing homes and assisted-living (LTC) facilities create another business opportunity for outreach programs. Most laboratories have shied away from LTC, unable to meet the special needs of skilled nursing homes. For those outreach programs that can customize their services to provide routine and STAT phlebotomy, same-day test results, standby orders, and Medicare Part A billing, then LTC provides a business opportunity with minimal competition. Outreach programs interested in servicing LTC facilities may want to consider partnering with a firm that brokers nursing-home services (i.e., radiology, podiatry, dentistry, psychiatry, occupational therapy, physical therapy, etc.) and contract to have one of these firms market their lab services to the LTC market.

Courier Services: Basics and Logistics

An outreach program's courier service is the front line in terms of customer service and relations (see Fig. 40.1). Couriers act as your ambassadors of good will and your intelligence service in regards to customer satisfaction. At BRL, we train the courier staff to put the customer first, and this emphasis gets results, as demonstrated by their high score on BRL's customer-satisfaction surveys. The following are the key characteristics of a high-performance courier network that consistently meets the expectations and requirements of its customers (external and internal):

- Courier routing/scheduling is performed dynamically to optimize the use of resources (staffing, vehicles, etc.).
- Couriers maintain the integrity of specimens, materials, and supplies transported and handled (keeping frozen specimens frozen and room-temperature specimens at room temperature, performing special handling as required, and ensuring supplies are transported and stored according to manufacturer specifications.
- Couriers maintain confidentiality of patient reports.
- Couriers are responsible and reliable transport agents (vehicles are routinely serviced and checked; couriers complete a driver safety course).
- Couriers are trained to handle, transport, and clean up hazardous materials.
- The courier department assists in monitoring/auditing supplies delivered and utilized by clients.

The courier department serves as the program's representatives to customers, in both the delivery of services and the monitoring of your customers' overall satisfaction.

What is required when putting together an efficient courier network? The first task is to create a routing network that meets customer needs while maximizing the efficient use of resources (drivers, automobiles, etc.). Routing optimization, however, usually occurs in an environment of multiple conflicting priorities. For example, service requirements, especially turnaround times, vary with client type. Delivery of client specimens to the laboratory should be coordinated with the laboratory production schedule to maximize the efficient use of laboratory staff. Courier routing is a dynamic process with many variables, including day and time of service, courier availability, weather conditions, and cyclic traffic congestion. A system needs to be designed to monitor specimen location and to verify specimen pickup. Designing courier travel manually results in routes located in geographically defined sectors without regard to optimization. Courier route optimization can be achieved using commercial software.

In February 1995, BRL introduced routing-optimization (logistics) software. BRL selected a routing package called RouteSmart™ (Boune Distinct Ltd., Columbia, Md.) to assist the courier department with route creation. Operational issues or constraints that management had to consider in route formulation included service-time window, staggered start times, average service duration per client of 2 minutes, drop-box service duration of 1.5 minutes, special deliveries, draw-station sweeps, last pickups (30 minutes after close), maximum route duration (7 hours with breaks), all routes being in by 6:00 p.m., and other special client requirements. By July 1995, BRL was testing the RouteSmart™ routes, and the program was

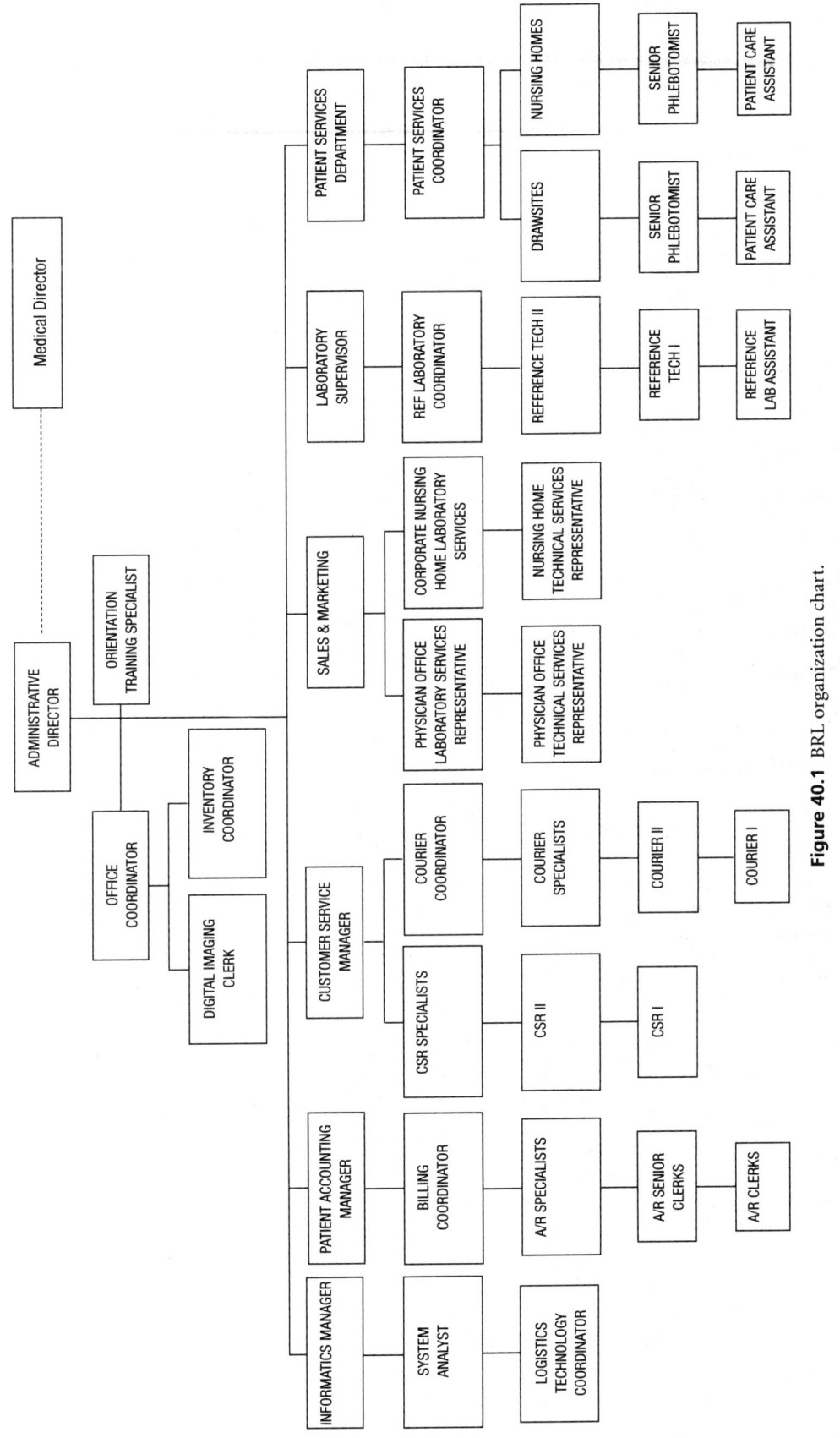

Figure 40.1 BRL organization chart.

Table 40.3 Courier routing-optimization results: the BRL experience

Attribute of courier program	Before May 1995	After May 1996	Change
No. of routes	9	6	−33.3%
No. of accounts	408	471	+15.4%
Full-time employees	16	14	−12.4%

fully implemented by August 1, 1995. Results achieved included a 25% reduction in labor, excess capital resources of 23% (fleet car returned), and more-productive use of staff drivers. In short, BRL realized a savings of $82,094 (see Table 40.3) with a return on its investment in a short 7.5 months (26, 27).

In 1997, BRL moved to a new generation of routing software called RIMMS (Resources In Motion Management System), offered by the Lightstone Group (Mineola, N.Y.). RIMMS is a customizable, Windows-based open-architecture system that supports real-time dynamic routing, or routing "on the fly." In other words, the courier department can reroute in minutes to adjust to staffing shortages, weather, traffic, special events, and/or vehicle breakdowns. RIMMS has made it more convenient to handle client will-calls and STATs and assign them to the appropriate route/driver.

This software permits rerouting for extreme cold-weather conditions (temperature range, 0 to 15°F). Courier management was concerned about specimen integrity when specimens would be left in drop boxes located outside for extended times in this extremely cold weather. To address this issue, courier routes were redefined or reoptimized to pick up all clients' work within 2 hours of closing (or placement in drop boxes). The RIMMS software accomplished this task in real time within minutes and without an increase in resources (Table 40.4). Surprisingly, the cold-weather afternoon-evening (p.m.) route optimization actually saved labor hours.

Other applications for route-optimization software include home-care service, hospital materials management department, and nursing-home phlebotomy service (scheduling and routing). William Beaumont Hospital has had success utilizing RIMMS for home-care services and materials management transportation. BRL's future plans call for utilization of logistics software in optimizing the scheduling, routing, and dispatching of phlebotomists in the long-term-care division (a network of more than 70 nursing and assisted-living homes).

In December 2001, BRL implemented handheld personal computers for its courier staff. These handheld PCs utilize courier-management software for specimen logging (tracking), routing, and supply ordering (inventory) (Fig. 40.2). The software is called Frontline and is offered by Gajema (Charlotte, N.C.). The Frontline product includes integrated call-management, client-services, and courier modules. BRL evaluated and implemented the Frontline call-management module in the fall of 2002. With the Frontline modules, BRL was able to automate and go paperless for incoming and outgoing calls handled by its client services department, including client supply orders, courier will-calls, STATs, add-on tests, and client problem logging. With an interface to Frontline, RIMMS can pass the courier routes to the handhelds and place dynamic or "on the fly" routing right at the courier's fingertips. With the handhelds, the couriers are now able to log or document electronically their entire stop, indicating whether it's a pickup or delivery of specimens, reports, and/or supplies, scan their arrival time and patients, and enter or log the number of specimens and tube types. All this information is downloaded to the courier-management module server when the couriers dock their handhelds back at the lab. In addition, with products such as RIMMS and Frontline, BRL was able to achieve true cross-department integration and communication (Fig. 40.2). The wealth of information captured and retrievable from these software products will have a positive impact in the areas of customer satisfaction, process improvement, compliance, and accountability. The new handhelds required an additional 22 seconds per requisition to enter data and interact with the device. To minimize the impact of this time loss, BRL management reoptimized all the p.m. routes with RIMMS (Table 40.5). It was determined that the new routes were more efficient in spite of the additional time required by couriers to interact with the handhelds. These findings indicate that BRL's courier operations need to reoptimize their routes more frequently.

Beaumont Reference Laboratory: 1993 to 2002

Annual Growth and Its Implications

In the summer of 1993, BRL opened for business in a construction trailer behind the hospital. BRL provides both clinical pathology and anatomic pathology (cytology and biopsy microscopic evaluation) services. For the first 3 to

Table 40.4 Route-optimization results: rerouting for cold weather

Optimization condition	Miles	Labor (min)	Drive time (min)	Vehicles	Routes	Requisitions
Baseline	1,176	65:49	37:26	17	17	1,308
Cold	1,206	55:58	38:10	17	17	1,308
Gain	−30	9:51	−0:44	0	0	0

Figure 40.2 Courier management, client services, and client interaction with software for courier routing, specimen counts, STAT pickups, client supplies inventory, specimen tracking, and client service problem logs.

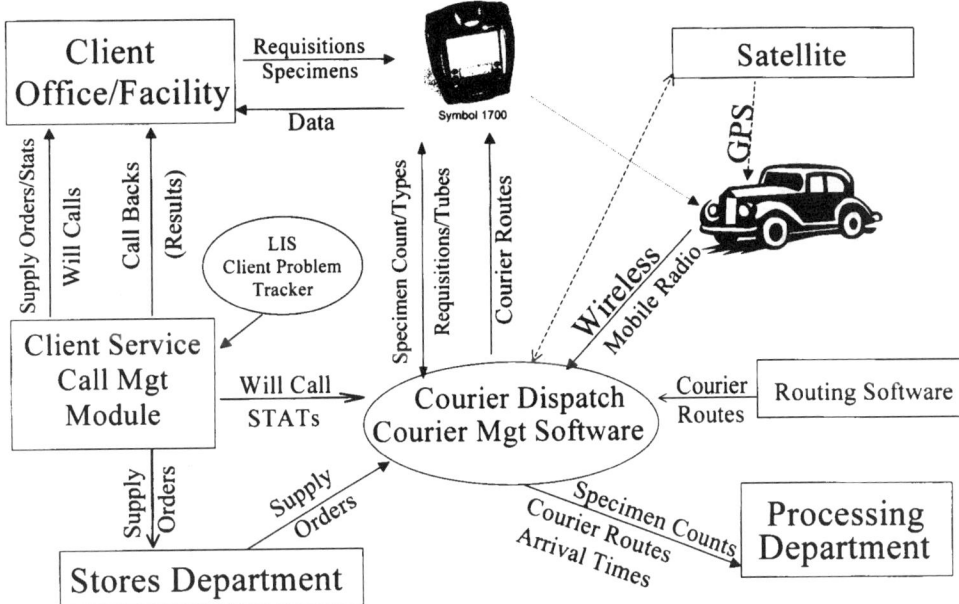

4 years, the majority of clients were physicians on the staff at William Beaumont Hospital. These physicians had computers in their offices connected to the Hospital Information System. As a result of becoming a BRL client, each physician, through the Hospital Information System, had electronic access to results for inpatients, registered outpatients, and patients seen in his or her office all in one location. This convenience factor was a major selling point for many of the early clients. There was no need for an additional computer for laboratory results for their office visit data.

Table 40.2 illustrates BRL's growth in clinical pathology from 1994 to 2002. Currently, BRL volume represents 46.2% of the total clinical pathology test volume. Physician offices represent 81% of total clients and 89.5% of all test requests, while nursing homes represent 19% of all clients and 10.5% of all tests requested. BRL clients generate 82% of the volume in the cytology laboratory.

Table 40.6 demonstrates that there has been a dramatic shift from cervical cytology in Anatomic Pathology evaluated by the conventional Papanicolaou method to the liquid-based method, which provides a specimen compatible for oncogenic human papillomavirus (HPV) detection (52, 53, 56). Approximately 15 of the more than 100 types

of HPV are associated with cervical cancer, especially types 16, 18, 31, and 45 (17, 55). The detection of HPV DNA is reliable and highly sensitive for precancerous lesions of the cervix compared to the insensitivity and subjectivity of the conventional cytology method (41, 44). This relatively rapid shift in physician ordering practice illustrates the need for flexibility in planning for future outreach growth.

BRL's growth has had an impact on the test menu in each laboratory section. For example, the total number of billable procedures has increased each year from 1993 to 2002 in the Molecular Pathology Laboratory under the medical direction of Domnita Crisan (Fig. 40.3). Table 40.7 outlines the specific assays and test volumes for 2002. In late 1992, a royalty agreement was signed with Roche for the clinical use of PCR (polymerase chain reaction). In 2002, the assay for *Chlamydia trachomatis* and *Neisseria gonorrhoeae* in urine was moved from ligase chain reaction to PCR (5, 37). More than 95% of the requests for these two assays are by BRL clients. In late 2001, HPV DNA detection by hybrid capture was introduced, and 2,477 identifications of HPV types with a low and high risk for cervical cancer were completed in 2002. There has been a steady increase in molecular-based tests, from 0.04% (84 assays) of total laboratory test volume in January 1994

Table 40.5 Route-optimization results: reoptimization of Monday p.m. routes

Optimizaton condition	Miles	Labor (min)	Drive time (min)	Route segments	Vehicles/ drivers	Requisitions expected
Baseline	1,233	69:23	40:22	17	17	1,323
Reoptimized	1,014	50:24	33:19	17	13	1,323
Gain	219	18:59	7:03	0	4	0
% Gain	18%	27%	17%	—	24%	—

Table 40.6 Annual volume of tests of cervical cytology at BRL[a]

Year	Conventional Papanicolaou test	Liquid-based cytology	Annual total
2000	54,524	14,359	68,883
2001	39,375	33,795	73,170
2002	17,009	63,973	80,982

[a]Data collected by Jennifer Shimoura.

to 0.57% (28,531 assays) in 2002. This laboratory section has been profitable since 1997. To fulfill the prediction that molecular testing would encompass 5% of total laboratory test volume in the early 21st century (20), a total of 21,000 molecular pathology procedures per month would need to be performed.

Projecting Future Volume

The numbers of BRL clients and test volume have increased each year since 1994 (Table 40.2). Each year a target figure for annual growth is established that is between 8% and 15% of the volume from the previous year. We have utilized several methods to monitor this growth and project its impact on the individual laboratory sections. The number of requisitions received from each of the two major client types (physician offices and nursing homes) is tracked each day. A summary of the month of January 2002 is illustrated in Fig. 40.4. During the Monday-to-Friday cycle, the greatest total volume of requisitions is received on Monday, usually with a nadir in requisitions from physician offices on Wednesday, when many offices are closed in the afternoon. These data provide a global baseline for monitoring fluctuations in volume.

We also monitor the volume generated by nine different practice categories and calculate annually the number of requisitions per physician, the number of procedures ordered per physician, and the number of procedures per requisition (Table 40.8). In 2002, the number of requisitions per year per physician fluctuated from 94 for Urology to 282 for OB/GYN, while the number of procedures per requisi-

Table 40.7 Tests performed in 2002 in the Molecular Pathology Laboratory at William Beaumont Hospital

Test[a]	No. of tests
PCR, RT-PCR	
Chlamydia trachomatis	10,374
Neisseria gonorrhoeae	10,101
HCV qualitative	523
HCV quantitative	1,190
HIV quantitative (standard, ultrasensitive)	968
HBV quantitative	171
CMV	165
ACE polymorphism	212
Angiotensinogen mutation	34
Angiotensin receptor type 1 mutation	36
CYP2C9 genotyping (for Coumadin hyperresponsiveness)	30
Hereditary hemochromatosis mutations	414
Glycoprotein Pl A1/A2 mutation	35
TMA	
Mycobacterium tuberculosis	181
Invader technology	
Factor V Leiden mutation	1,218
Prothrombin mutation	713
MTHFR mutations	448
Apo E genotype	122
Hybrid capture	
HPV low-risk group	1,237
HPV high-risk group	1,240
Hybridization/PCR	
HCV genotyping	376
DNA sequencing	
HIV genotyping for drug resistance	Starting in 2003

[a]RT-PCR, reverse transcriptase PCR; HCV, hepatitis C virus; HIV, human immunodeficiency virus; HBV, hepatitis B virus; CMV, cytomegalovirus; ACE, angiotensin-converting enzyme; TMA, transcription-mediated amplification; MTHFR, methylene tetrahydrofolate reductase; HPV, human papillomavirus.

tion varied from 1.4 for Urology to 10.3 for Internal Medicine. This information is useful when targeting specific physician categories for growth by the sales team. The laboratory sections will require further analysis of the data before they can project their capital equipment and personnel

Figure 40.3 Annual volume of tests, including total tests and five different methods, performed from 1992 to 2002 in the Molecular Pathology Laboratory at William Beaumont Hospital.

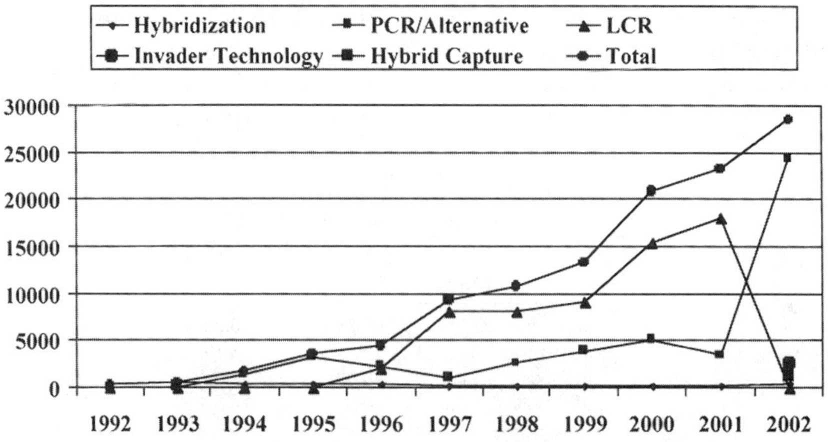

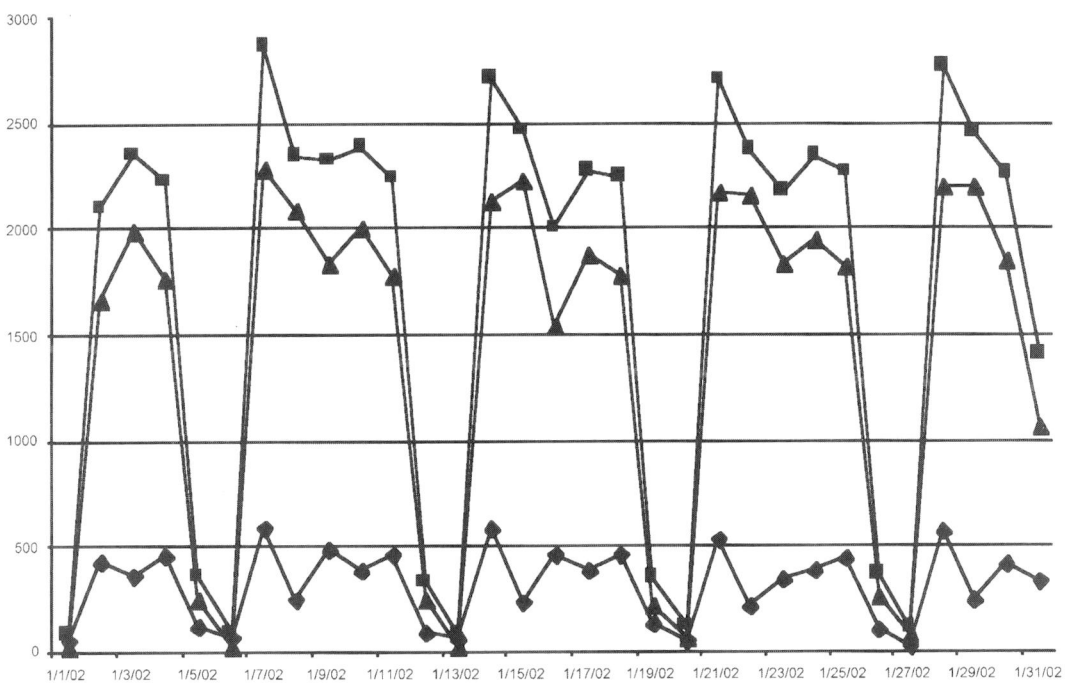

Figure 40.4 The daily requisitions for tests at BRL received by physician offices (▲) and nursing homes (◆), and totals (■), in January 2002.

needs to support the projected additional test volume. Table 40.9 illustrates the distribution within eight different laboratory sections of the tests requested by the nine different practice categories. Given the new client's subspecialty and the number of physicians in the group, these data can be used to estimate the number of procedures each of the eight laboratory sections should analyze over a period of time. The clinical chemistry section receives the greatest volume of test requests from six of the practice categories but fewer than 40% of the total procedures from OB/GYN and Urology. Microbiology procedures are ordered most frequently by Urology. Table 40.10 enumerates the average monthly number of specific tests ordered per physician in each of the nine practice categories in the five most frequently used laboratory sections. Managers of the five laboratory sections,

armed with the expanded data compiled in this manner, can easily begin to project capital equipment and personnel needs based on projected new client volume. In OB/GYN, HPV DNA analysis is requested four times less frequently then the presence of *Chlamydia* or *Neisseria* DNA in Molecular Pathology (Table 40.10).

Send-Out Tests

Send-out tests represent procedures that are not performed in any of the laboratory sections and must be sent to an accredited laboratory. We review the volume of these procedures every 6 months. Cost analysis and the feasibility of bringing assays with increasing volumes into the main laboratory are also evaluated. One of the benefits of an outreach program is the expansion and enhancement

Table 40.8 Summary of tests performed by BRL in 2002 according to specialty

Specialty	No. of physicians	Total requisitions	Total procedures	Requisition/ physician	Procedures/ requisition	Procedures/ physician
Family Practice	464	66,970	631,086	144	9.4	1,360
Pediatrics	219	21,172	123,244	97	5.8	563
Internal Medicine	831	130,460	1,347,426	157	10.3	1,621
Cardiology	126	19,766	82,068	157	4.2	651
Endocrinology	96	11,540	68,880	120	6	717
Gastroenterology	60	6,566	60,860	109	9.3	1,014
Nursing homes	575	108,536	395,742	189	3.6	688
OB/GYN	309	87,004	250,520	282	2.9	810
Urology	126	11,886	16,668	94	1.4	132

Table 40.9 Breakdown of tests performed by BRL in 2002 according to specialty

Specialty (no. of physicians)	Lab area[a]	% Total procedures	Billable procedures	Procedure/ requisition
Family Practice (464)	CHE	86.20	544,822	8.10
	HEM	5.20	35,562	0.53
	IMM	3.50	22,058	0.33
	MIC	2.70	17,096	0.25
	MOL	0.40	2,418	0.04
	FLO	0.10	754	0.01
	BLB	0.10	802	0.01
	CYT	1.20	7,574	0.11
Gastroenterology (60)	CHE	82.00	50,482	7.70
	HEM	8.30	5,092	0.78
	IMM	6.40	3,934	0.60
	MIC	0.50	306	0.05
	MOL	1.70	1,046	0.16
	FLO	–	0	–
	BLB	–	0	–
	CYT	–	0	–
Pediatrics (219)	CHE	72.10	88,800	4.20
	HEM	5.60	6,916	0.33
	IMM	2.60	3,148	0.15
	MIC	18.60	22,902	1.08
	MOL	0.20	232	0.01
	FLO	–	4	–
	BLB	0.03	34	–
	CYT	0.50	644	0.03
Nursing homes (575)	CHE	84.80	335,650	3.10
	HEM	9.20	36,346	0.33
	IMM	0.40	1,756	0.02
	MIC	5.50	21,902	0.20
	MOL	0.01	24	–
	FLO	0.01	56	–
	BLB	–	8	–
	CYT	–	0	–
Internal Medicine (831)	CHE	90.20	1,222,434	9.40
	HEM	4.40	58,878	0.45
	IMM	2.50	34,478	0.26
	MIC	1.40	19,200	0.15
	MOL	0.30	3,916	0.03
	FLO	0.20	1,992	0.02
	BLB	0.03	418	–
	CYT	0.60	8,110	0.06
OB/GYN (309)	CHE	34.50	90,534	1.00
	HEM	6.60	17,286	0.20
	IMM	11.20	29,244	0.34
	MIC	10.40	27,180	0.31
	MOL	4.60	12,162	0.14
	FLO	0.01	20	–
	BLB	6.80	17,776	0.20
	CYT	21.50	56,318	0.65
Cardiology (126)	CHE	94.80	77,926	3.90
	HEM	2.60	2,154	0.11
	IMM	2.20	1,816	0.09
	MIC	0.20	124	0.01
	MOL	0.04	34	–
	FLO	–	0	–
	BLB	0.01	12	–
	CYT	–	2	–
Urology (126)	CHE	38.20	7,320	0.62
	HEM	1.60	306	0.03
	IMM	0.70	128	0.01
	MIC	33.40	6,414	0.54
	MOL	0.60	116	0.01
	FLO	–	0	–
	BLB	–	0	–
	CYT	12.40	2,384	0.20
Endocrinology (96)	CHE	88.60	61,606	5.30
	HEM	1.70	1,202	0.10
	IMM	5.10	3,550	0.31
	MIC	1.00	724	0.06
	MOL	0.10	68	0.01
	FLO	–	0	–
	BLB	1.00	682	0.06
	CYT	1.50	1,048	0.09

[a]CHE, Chemistry; HEM, Hematology/Coagulation; IMM, Immunology; MIC, Microbiology; MOL, Molecular Pathology; FLO, Flow Cytometry; BLB, Blood Bank; CYT, Cytology.

Table 40.10 2002 Frequently ordered tests performed by BRL in 2002 listed in rank order according to specialty

Average no. of specific tests/physician/month[a]

Family Practice (113)

Chemistry		Hematology/coagulation		Immunology		Microbiology		Molecular pathology	
AST	34.00	CBC	39.00	ANA	2.30	Urine Cul	6.50	C. trachomatis	0.89
K	32.00	ESR	2.70	RA	1.60	Prel aerobic Cul ID	3.70	N. gonorrhoeae	0.85
ALT	32.00	Retic	0.41	HBsAg	1.20	Antibiotic Sens	1.20	HPV	0.29
BUN	32.00	PTT	0.19	Anti-HCV	1.10	Smear	1.10	HIV RNA Quant	0.15
Na	32.00	PT	0.19	Anti-HBcIGM	0.92	Def aerobic Cul ID	1.00		

Pediatrics (47)

Chemistry		Hematology/coagulation		Immunology		Microbiology		Molecular pathology	
T Bili	12.00	CBC	13.00	ANA	0.55	β-Hemolytic strep	8.40	C. trachomatis	0.24
AST	12.00	ESR	1.50	EBV VCA IgG	0.46	Prel aerobic Cul ID	7.50	N. gonorrhoeae	0.23
ALT	12.00	Smear (Eos/PMN)	0.84	EBV VCA IgM	0.45	Urine Cul	6.00		
Glu	11.00	Send-out	0.18	Helicobacter pylori	0.43	Infl A DFA	4.80		
CR	10.00	Retic	0.11	Anti-HCV	0.43	Infl B DFA	4.70		

Internal Medicine (135)

Chemistry		Hematology/coagulation		Immunology		Microbiology		Molecular pathology	
T Bili	40.00	CBC	30.00	ANA	2.20	Urine Cul	4.70	C. trachomatis	0.38
AST	39.00	ESR	5.90	Homocyst	1.30	Prel aerobic Cul ID	2.30	N. gonorrhoeae	0.37
K	39.00	Retic	0.58	HBsAg	1.30	Antibiotic Sens	0.94		
Na	38.00	P Bld Smear	0.10	Anti-HCV	1.20	Def aerobic Cul ID	0.65		
CR	38.00	Send out	0.06	RA	1.10	Smear	0.60		

Cardiology (54)

Chemistry		Hematology/coagulation		Immunology		Microbiology		Molecular pathology	
AST	25.00	CBC	8.00	Homocyst	5.40	Urine Cul	0.19	Factor V	0.02
CHOL	24.00	ESR	0.36	HS CRP	0.76	Blood Cul	0.17	ACE	0.02
ALT	24.00			ANA	0.11				
TRIG	24.00								
HDL	24.00								
CPK	20.00								

Endocrinology (60)

Chemistry		Hematology/coagulation		Immunology		Microbiology		Molecular pathology	
GLU	18.00	CBC	5.70	VDRL	2.50	Urine Cul	3.10	HPV	0.15
E2	17.00	ESR	0.25	HBsAb	2.40	Antibiotic Sens	0.26	C. trachomatis	0.09
T Bili	16.00	PTT	0.13	HIV Ab	2.30			N. gonorrhoeae	0.09
ALT	15.00	PT	0.13	Anti-HIV	2.20				
AST	15.00			Rubella IgG	2.00				

Gastroenterology (84)

Chemistry		Hematology/coagulation		Immunology		Microbiology		Molecular pathology	
T Bili	48.00	CBC	36.00	Reticulin Ab	3.40	Urine Cul	0.77	HCV viral load	0.62
ALT	32.00	ESR	5.00	Endomysial Ab	3.40	Clostridium difficile toxin	0.30	HH	0.32
Alb	31.00	Retic	0.67	Gliadin Ab	3.40	Ova/parasites	0.28	Hep C	0.27
AST	31.00	Send-out	0.13	Antiparietal Ab	3.00	Stool pathogens	0.27		
Alk Phos	31.00			HBsAg	2.20	Stool culture	0.27		

Nursing homes (57)

Chemistry		Hematology/coagulation		Immunology		Microbiology		Molecular pathology	
K	34.00	CBC	34.00	HS CRP	0.16	Urine Cul	6.10		
Na	33.00	Hct	33.00	VDRL	0.13	Antibiotic Sens	3.60		
CO2	33.00	Hgb	1.10	Prot Elect	0.11	Def aerobic Cul ID	1.70		
CR	33.00	ESR	1.10	HBsAg	0.11	Clostridium difficile toxin	1.50		
BUN	30.00	Retic	0.62	Anti-HIV	0.10	Urine ID	1.50		

OB/GYN (68)

Chemistry		Hematology/coagulation		Immunology		Microbiology		Molecular pathology	
Glu	10.00	CBC	16.00	VDRL	5.10	Urine Cul	9.60	C. trachomatis	4.90
TSH	9.50	Sickle cell	0.11	Rubella IgG	5.00	Prel aerobic Cul ID	4.90	N. gonorrhoeae	4.90
U/A	6.70	ESR	0.10	HBsAb	4.70	Smear	3.20	HPV	1.20
β-HCG	6.30	PTT	0.06	HIV AB	3.10	Strep B cul	3.00	Factor V	0.03
CHOL	4.00			E3	1.70	Def aerobic Cul ID	1.40		

Urology (11)

Chemistry		Hematology/coagulation		Immunology		Microbiology		Molecular pathology	
PSA	15.00	PT	0.06	Alpha FP	0.07	Urine Cul	18.00	C. trachomatis	0.24
U/A	1.30	Semen	0.73	HSV-2 IgG	0.06	Antibiotic Sens	3.70	N. gonorrhoeae	0.22
Testosterone	1.20	CBC	0.33	HSV-1 IgG	0.06	Def aerobic Cul ID	1.50		
CR	0.94	Hgb	0.07	HIV Ab	0.06	Urine ID	1.40		
BUN	0.88	Hct	0.07	ANA	0.03	Prel aerobic Cul ID	0.15		

[a]E2, estradiol; U/A, urinalysis; ESR, erythrocyte sedimentation analysis; Ab, antibody; Ag, antigen; E3, estriol; Prel, preliminary; Def, definitive; HS, high sensitivity; HH, hemochromatosis gene mutation; ID, identification; Cul, culture.

Table 40.11 Send-out test volumes at William Beaumont Hospital

Year	BRL (% of total)	Non-BRL[a]	Annual total
1998	16,316 (40%)	24,641	40,957
1999	16,924 (34%)	32,777	49,701
2000	16,211 (32%)	34,660	50,871
2001	21,585 (38%)	34,781	56,366
2002	30,719 (46%)	35,837	66,556

[a]Non-BRL represents inpatient, emergency center, and registered outpatient send-out procedures.

of the test menu (26). In our state, send-out laboratory charges cannot be marked up and frequently patients' third-party reimbursement fails to cover the charge or the cost. In general, the reduction of send-out test volume is an excellent project for laboratory cost containment (4). Table 40.11 illustrates the volume of send-out tests for BRL and non-BRL patients from 1998 to 2002. Although BRL's contribution to the total number of send-out tests has fluctuated from 32% in 2000 to a high of 46% in 2002, the total number has steadily increased each year. In 2001, BRL send-out test charges were $996,000. In 2000, we initiated a review of low-reimbursement, high-cost send-out requests from both BRL and non-BRL, as described by Carter and Bennett (4). A resident in Clinical Pathology contacts the admitting physician for inpatients or ordering physician for registered outpatients or outreach customers and explains the cost, clinical value, and alternative tests. Most tests are canceled because the admitting or ordering physician was not aware that a resident or consultant had ordered it. Table 40.12 demonstrates that although the total number of tests called on per year was a fraction of the total number requested (listed in Table 40.11), almost half of the requestors called in 2002 canceled the request, saving approximately $70,000. This program will expand in the future, and BRL will also develop methods for outpatients to pay for these tests with a credit card, check, or cash before they are sent out.

Monitoring Financial Outcome

It is imperative that the financial well-being of an outreach program be monitored frequently. Table 40.13 outlines a few examples of items to monitor, including test volume, supply costs, personnel costs, and revenue cycle (1, 26). We have excluded capital equipment and reagents related to laboratory testing since our clinical laboratory represents

Table 40.12 Review of send-out tests by telephone at William Beaumont Hospital

Year	Canceled (% of total)	Approved	Annual total
2000	77 (27%)	208	285
2001	62 (46%)	73	135
2002	70 (49%)	74	144

Table 40.13 Potential areas to monitor to track financial outcome in an outreach program

Topic area	Specific monitor
Test volume	Requisition count
	Lost-business report
	New-business prospects
Supply costs	Client supply utilization
Personnel costs	Overtime report
	Open positions
	Diversification
Revenue cycle	Financial reports
	Rejection reports
	Accounts-receivable report
	Capitation contracts report
	Ratio of uncollected charges to payment received

a hybrid operation consisting of 50% outreach and 50% non-outreach testing. These supply and capital-equipment costs are charged back to BRL based on annual volumes. Requisition counts from global sites (physician offices, nursing homes, other hospitals) (Fig. 40.4) or more-specific designations can be used to monitor unexpected fluctuations. Potential new clients targeted by Goldmine (42) or other methods, as well as careful review of causes for lost business, should be tracked. Client issues directly related to lost business, if monitored, may lead to quality-improvement projects to prevent repetition. Supplies required for specimen collection are provided to clients and should be returned to BRL. Monitoring the supplies provided to and returned from a client will determine if any of these resources are being diverted for the client's office laboratory use or being sent to another testing site. Personnel costs can be evaluated by reviewing overtime expenses in each of the major job categories, like billing, courier services, client services, phlebotomy, and processing. In general, the greater the number of open positions in these categories, the greater the savings in salary dollars and the more inefficient the operation becomes. Personnel should be hired with adequate training to perform the assigned tasks. Diversification of personnel based on the complexity level of tasks they perform would facilitate the introduction of tiers (layers) within a single job class or reassigning duties from a higher job class to a lower job class (26). The basic principle is that personnel should be assigned a job level, perform only duties defined for that job level, and rarely be required to perform tasks assigned to individuals at lower job levels. This mandate assures that the greatest efficiency for performing high-complexity tasks is achieved.

The revenue cycle is the sequence of events that the provider must monitor to maximize the amount and timeliness of payment from payors. A few examples of areas to monitor are given in Table 40.13 (1, 26). If payment is denied for Part A or Part B reimbursement, a re-

Table 40.14 Annual revenue at BRL

Year	Procedures[a]	Gross revenue	Net revenue
1994	307,043	$7,499,834	$4,539,275
1995	571,014	$15,085,483	$6,174,779
1996	598,689	$20,112,825	$8,115,697
1997	805,463	$26,509,990	$10,934,010
1998	1,484,874	$35,018,448	$13,990,098
1999	1,977,514	$45,387,965	$18,455,008
2000	2,401,202	$66,985,910	$31,401,994
2001	2,731,837	$77,224,829	$32,705,163
2002	2,796,113	$93,499,882	$38,999,895

[a]Total procedures performed by BRL in Anatomic and Clinical Pathology.

Table 40.15 Payor mix for three years at BRL

Payor	Percent of revenue		
	1996	2000	2002
Blue Cross/Blue Shield	30.4	19	28
Medicare	17.3	33	28
Medicaid	1.5	1	1
Selectcare	27.8	8	–
Health Alliance Plan	–	–	7
Patient pay	4.0	5	4
Blue Care Network	–	4	10
Other[a]	19.0	30	22

[a]Comprises capitated and fee-for-service contracts.

jection report from the billing/receivable system will provide data on the reason for denial of payment. Recurrent rejection episodes for the same reason may require direct inquiry of the third-party carrier to resolve the problem.

Table 40.14 reports the gross and net revenue achieved by BRL from 1994 to 2002. Improvements in the efficiency of the current revenue cycle process will improve the level of reimbursement noted in the past. Reimbursement will fluctuate based on contractual arrangements with capitated and noncapitated payors. Table 40.15 lists the payor mix for BRL in 1996, 2000, and 2002. In general, there has been a decrease in Blue Cross and Selectcare and an increase in Medicare and a variety of other providers. The payor mix may be determined for each of the nine physician categories listed in Tables 40.8 through 40.10. Using this information, the average reimbursement for the most commonly ordered tests can be calculated for each of the nine physician groups.

Most financial reports calculate labor per procedure and supply costs per procedure, which have decreased for BRL from $0.86 and $1.72, respectively, in 1997 to $0.58 and $1.59 in 2000 (26). Table 40.16 reviews 6 years of financial data for both clinical and anatomic pathology services provided by BRL. In general, over that time period, the number of requisitions and procedures and the net revenue per procedure increased each year. Therefore,

the goals of lowering unit costs and increasing revenue have been achieved (26).

Joint Venture Hospital Laboratory

History of JVHL

To achieve success, BRL must market and sell its laboratory services. This objective can only be met if BRL obtains provider status with the major insurance carriers and managed-care organizations. Since many of these contracts require one major regional laboratory provider, BRL, as a solo outreach program with a limited coverage area, would be ruled out. To resolve this dilemma, BRL joined a regional laboratory network of other hospital-based laboratory outreach programs, Joint Venture Hospital Laboratory (JVHL), to meet the wide geographic coverage required by third-party payors (26, 44).

Regional laboratory networks are a recent phenomenon and have experienced a dynamic evolution in both development and longevity (3, 12, 31, 34, 47). The purpose of such a laboratory network may be to share testing or to obtain managed-care contracts, but rarely both (26). The participating laboratories are independently owned and operated. A central network administrator coordinates negotiations for managed-care contracts or distribution of laboratory procedures to be shared. In summary, regional laboratory networks provide specific geographic coverage

Table 40.16 Annual statistics relating to procedures performed by BRL

Year	Procedures[a]	Requisitions	Procedures/ requisition	Net revenue/ procedure
1997	1,226,906	279,466	4.39	$8.44
1998	1,600,643	339,028	4.72	$8.36
1999	2,020,721	410,748	4.92	$9.63
2000	2,401,202	535,330	4.49	$13.03
2001	2,731,837	608,066	4.49	$12.10
2002	2,796,113	637,066	4.39	$13.95

[a]Total procedures performed by BRL in Anatomic and Clinical Pathology.

Table 40.17 Comparison of procedures and revenue for BRL and JVHL business

Year	Procedures		Gross revenue		
	BRL	**JVHL**	**Total BRL**[a]	**JVHL and Related**[b]	**JVHL only**[c]
1994	NA[d]	NA			
1995	NA	405,000			
1996	88,000	412,000			
1997	78,000	414,000	$26,265,000	$16,553,000	$1,754,000
1998	113,000	602,000	$35,098,000	$28,945,000	$2,157,000
1999	171,000	987,000	$45,119,000	$38,313,000	$1,873,000
2000	268,000	2,527,000	$66,986,000	$60,636,000	$9,174,000

[a]Refers to all BRL business and all payors (Medicare, Blue Cross, JVHL, etc.)
[b]Refers to the total revenue for clients with JVHL activity and includes JVHL-only gross revenue column.
[c]Refers to JVHL capitated contracts (payments) only and excludes pull-through business.
[d]NA, not applicable.

without consolidation, downsizing, or restructuring among the member laboratories.

JVHL was founded in 1992 by four southeast Michigan hospital-affiliated laboratories (St. John Hospital, Providence Hospital, William Beaumont Hospital, and Oakwood Hospital) in response to the increasing competition by the national commercial laboratories (MetPath, SKBL, and National Health Labs, at that time) for outpatient and physician office (outreach) client testing services. The organization acquired its first contract, 80,000 capitated lives, in 1994, permitting member laboratories to develop their competency in this market environment. In 1996, the managed-care organization renewed its contract and increased the total covered lives to 340,000. By December 2000, JVHL had 15 managed-care contracts representing 2.2 million covered lives (20). In December 2002, JVHL consisted of 123 hospital-affiliated laboratories throughout Michigan with 12,000 physician clients served by 350 patient service centers and a combined fleet of more than 100 courier vehicles (18).

Benefits of BRL's Affiliation with JVHL

What impact has JVHL membership had on the growth of BRL? To answer this question, we need to first compare the overall business growth of BRL, including both procedures and revenue from all payors, to that of BRL's JVHL work and related business (so-called pull-through volume). Table 40.17 indicates that for the years 1997 through 2000, JVHL and related work ranged from 63% to over 90% of BRL's total business. The total revenue for all BRL business compared with the total revenue gained through JVHL (JVHL only) highlights the contribution of JVHL and JVHL pull-through test volume to BRL's overall business growth. It is important to note that in 2000, BRL's procedures numbered 268,000, which represented approximately 10.6% of the total JVHL procedures for that year (Table 40.17). For BRL, JVHL has been a major positive factor in its successful business growth. Other member laboratories will have to evaluate their own situations to determine what financial benefit JVHL membership has achieved.

In conclusion, laboratory networks appear to provide an advantage in increasing pull-through in laboratory volume due to the network's extensive coverage of basic managed-care organizations, thereby providing one-stop shopping for laboratory services.

Summary

This case study has shown how one hospital laboratory outreach program (BRL) has built success through affiliation with a laboratory network, in this case JVHL. The key factor to success in this network affiliation is the ability of the laboratory network to win provider status for its members with the major managed-care organizations. The implementation of the outreach program has led to many benefits, including using spare capacity and thus achieving economies of scale, generating a new revenue stream, lowering unit costs, enhancing the test menu, and creating a new avenue for customer (physician) bonding. The implementation of the outreach program required careful planning. Its success is dependent on efficient support from Financial Analysis, Information Services, Hospital Administration, and the Departments of Clinical and Anatomic Pathology. Improvements in operating efficiency have been implemented: computer-assisted courier routing, on-line test directory, client interaction tracking and report system, and software to identify prospective new clients (26, 27). Remember, the goal is to dazzle all the clients most of the time with excellent service.

KEY POINTS

■ An outreach program will expand the laboratory's core business—providing laboratory services.

■ A champion or entrepreneur is required to facilitate implementation of a new outreach program.

- Hospital Administration is aligned with inpatient issues.
- The aid of a consultant may be of value in developing the outreach program.
- Simplify the bureaucracy surrounding the approval process for new equipment and personnel for outreach program needs.
- Sales and marketing staff require training to design sales strategies specific for client categories.
- Computer-assisted courier routing is more efficient than manual routing.
- Outreach volume growth will increase the test menu in each laboratory section.
- Develop a system to project future volume from prospective new clients to aid in planning for personnel and laboratory equipment.
- Reduce the number of low-reimbursement, high-cost send-out test requests.
- Monitor the outreach program's financial outcome at least monthly, including test volume, supply costs, personnel costs, and revenue-cycle issues.
- Affiliation with a joint venture with other hospital-based outreach laboratories will increase success in obtaining contracts with managed-care organizations.

GLOSSARY

Active inertia Insensate repetition of the same behavior pattern without regard to the magnitude of the paradigm shift.

Clad A coin consisting of an outer layer of one metal bonded to a core of a different metal.

Entrepreneur A person within a corporation who takes direct responsibility for turning an idea into a profitable finished product through assertive risk taking and innovation.

Fee-for-service Provider of services is paid according to the service performed, after the service is delivered.

Managed-care organizations A means of providing healthcare services within a network of healthcare providers.

Medicaid Federal and state matching entitlement program established under Title XVIII of the Social Security Act intended to provide medical assistance to eligible needy individuals.

Medicare Federal health insurance for the aged established under Title XIX of the Social Security Act.

Myth Inaccurate information perceived as truth by major administrative decision makers.

Organization chart Defines the formal lines of reporting and communication.

Outreach program Marketing laboratory services to physician offices, nursing homes, and other hospitals.

Payor mix The preparation of revenue realized from different types of payors.

Revenue Actual or expected cash inflow due to the outreach program's major business.

Revenue cycle Sequence of events that the provider must monitor to maximize the amount and timeliness of payment from payors.

Send-out test Procedure not performed in any of the hospital's clinical laboratories which, therefore, must be sent to another laboratory to be assayed.

Up-selling The practice of informing clients of a new or improved laboratory test that may have improved sensitivity and specificity over the routine screening assay. These new or improved assays may be applicable to patients with a well-defined subset of a certain disease or for patients who have failed the usual therapeutic strategies.

REFERENCES

1. Baker, J. J., and R. W. Baker. 2000. *Health Care Finance. Basic Tools for Nonfinancial Managers.* Aspen Publishers, Gaithersburg, Md.

2. Beatty, M. F. 2001. Marketing the rural hospital-based laboratory: building a customer-centered outreach program. *Clin. Leadership Manage. Rev.* **15**(1):11–15.

3. Boudreau, D. A., W. D. Scheer, J. S. Majonos, F. W. Brazda, and J. P. Strong. 2003. Integration of a statewide public hospital laboratory system. *Clin. Leadership Manage. Rev.* **17**(1):9–15.

4. Carter, E., and B. D. Bennett. 2002. Reference test review by pathology house staff: a cost-containment strategy for the clinical laboratory. *Clin. Leadership Manage. Rev.* **16**(1):3–6.

5. Castriciano, S., K. Luinstra, D. Jang, J. Patel, J. Mahony, J. Kapala, and M. Chernesky. 2002. Accuracy of results obtained by performing a second ligase chain reaction assay and PCR analysis on urine samples with positive or near-cutoff results in the LCX test for *Chlamydia trachomatis. J. Clin. Microbiol.* **40**:2632–2634.

6. Coward, N. 1965. *Hay Fever*, p. 155. *In Three Plays: Blithe Spirit, Hay Fever, Private Lives.* Vintage International, New York, N.Y.

7. Einstein, A. 2000. Attributed to Einstein, p. 321. *In* A. Calaprice (ed.), *The Expanded Quotable Einstein.* Princeton University Press, Princeton, N.J.

8. Fantus, J. E. 1999. Business strategies for hospital outreach programs. *Clin. Lab. Manage. Rev.* **13**(4):188–196.

9. Forsman, R. W. 2001. Joint venture *versus* outreach: a financial analysis of case studies. *Clin. Leadership Manage. Rev.* **15**(4):217–221.

10. Galvis, C. O., S. S. Raab, F. D'Amico, and D. M. Grzybicki. 2001. Pathologists' assistants practice. A measurement of performance. *Am. J. Clin. Pathol.* **116**:816–822.

11. Gehrels, T. 2000. Brains, courage and integrity. Gandhi and Sakharov set us an inspiring example for the twenty-first century. *Nature* **404**:335.

12. Gilbertson, J., P. Mango, S. McLinden, M. J. Becich, and D. Triulzi. 1997. The Pittsburgh Reference Laboratory Alliance: a model for laboratory medicine in the 21st century. *Am. J. Clin. Pathol.* **107**:387–394.

13. Gordini, A., V. Nardi, and F. di Stanislao. 2002. Is there a future for clinical laboratories? Experience in the Marche Region, Italy. *Clin. Chim. Acta* **319**:107–110.

14. **Handler, D.** 2002. Part one, p. 4. *In Watch Your Mouth.* Harper Collins Publishers, New York, N.Y.

15. **Harmening, D. M., B. M. Castleberry, and M. E. Lunz.** 1995. Defining the role of medical technologists and medical laboratory technicians. *Lab. Med.* **26:**175–177.

16. **Hawker, C. D., S. B. Garr, L. T. Hamilton, J. R. Penrose, E. R. Ashwood, and R. L. Weiss.** 2002. Automated transport and sorting system in a large reference laboratory: part I. Evaluation of needs and alternatives and development of a plan. *Clin. Chem.* **48:**1751–1760.

17. **Herrero, R., A. Hildesheim, C. Bratti, M. E. Sherman, M. Hutchenson, J. Morales, I. Balmaceda, M. Greenberg, M. Alfaro, R. D. Burk, S. Wachalder, M. Plummer, and M. Schiffman.** 2000. Population-based study of human papillomavirus infection and cervical neoplasia in rural Costa Rica. *J. Natl. Cancer Inst.* **92:**464–474.

18. **Joint Venture Hospital Laboratories.** http://www.jvhl.org/about.asp, accessed January 15, 2003.

19. **Kastor, J. A.** 2001. *Mergers of Teaching Hospitals in Boston, New York, and Northern California.* University of Michigan Press, Ann Arbor, Mich.

20. **Kiechle, F. L.** 1993. Residency in pathology: the William Beaumont Hospital perspective. *Am. J. Clin. Pathol.* **100**(Suppl. 1): S29–S30.

21. **Kiechle, F. L.** 1999. The William Beaumont Hospital experience with total laboratory automation. *Arab J. Lab. Med.* **25:**163–170.

22. **Kiechle, F. L.** 2001. Hospital laboratory survival in a cost control environment. *J. Clin. Ligand Assay* **24:**235–238.

23. **Kiechle, F. L.** 2002. Point-of-care testing for body fluids, p. 267–283. *In* G. J. Kost (ed.), *Principles and Practice of Point-of-Care Testing.* Lippincott, Williams and Wilkins, Philadelphia, Pa.

24. **Kiechle, F. L., and I. Gauss.** 2001. Provider-performed microscopy. *Clin. Lab. Med.* **21:**275–387.

25. **Kiechle, F. L., and R. I. Main.** 2000. Blood glucose: measurement in the point-of-care setting. *Lab. Med.* **31:**276–282.

26. **Kiechle, F. L., and R. I. Main.** 2002. *The Hitchhiker's Guide to Improving Efficiency in the Clinical Laboratory,* p. 1–128. AACC Press, Washington, D.C.

27. **Kiechle, F. L., and J. Skrisson.** 1997. Computer-assisted courier routing for hospital-based reference laboratories. *Ann. Clin. Lab. Sci.* **27:**313.

28. **Lark, S.** 1997. Patient-focused care. Is it working? Is it here to stay? *Lab. Med.* **28:**644–651.

29. **Madgett, N. L.** 2001. Good news, p. 229. *In* M. J. Boyd and M. L. Liebler (ed.), *Abandon Automobile: Detroit City Poetry 2001.* Wayne State University Press, Detroit, Mich.

30. **Main, R. I., and F. L. Kiechle.** 2000. Point-of-care testing: administration within a health system. *Lab. Med.* **31:**453–460.

31. **Marchwinski, J., S. S. Sullivan, J. B. Castillo, and R. Johnson.** 1996. The Rochester consortium. *Clin. Lab. Manage. Rev.* **10**(5): 486–497.

32. **Meyerson, D. E.** 2001. Radical change, the quiet way. *Harvard Bus. Rev.* **79**(9):92–100.

33. **Michel, R.** 1999. The ten myths of lab management that led clin lab industry astray. *Dark Report* **6**(11):9–13.

34. **More, J. D., S. K. Sengupta, and P. N. Manley.** 2000. Promoting, building and sustaining a regional laboratory network in a changing environment. *Clin. Leadership Manage. Rev.* **14**(5):205–210.

35. **Nigon, D. L.** 1993. Economics of outreach testing in the hospital laboratory: part II. *Clin. Lab. Manage. Rev.* **7**(5):414–418.

36. **O'Sullivan, M. B., and C. L. Bakken.** 1988. A medical center-based tertiary reference laboratory. *Arch. Pathol. Lab. Med.* **112:**953–956.

37. **Palladino, S., J. W. Pearman, I. D. Kay, D. W. Smith, G. B. Harnett, M. Woods, L. Marshall, and J. McCloskey.** 1999. Diagnosis of *Chlamydia trachomatis* and *Neisseria gonorrhoeae* genitourinary infections in males by the Amplicor PCR assay in urine. *Diagn. Microbiol. Infect. Dis.* **33:**141–146.

38. **Riley, P. A.** 1996. Commercialization of health services: implications for the laboratories. *Malaysian J. Pathol.* **18:**21–25.

39. **Sahlman, W. A.** 1997. How to write a great business plan. *Harvard Bus. Rev.* **75**(4):98–108.

40. **Santrach, P.** 2001. Point of care coagulation testing: a targeted approach. *J. Clin. Ligand Assay* **24:**248–252.

41. **Sasake, M., T. Kageoka, K. Ogura, H. Kataoka, T. Ueta, and S. Sugihara.** 1998. Total laboratory automation in Japan. Past, present and the future. *Clin. Chim. Acta* **278:**217–227.

42. **Scott, J.** 2000. Sales forecasting, p. 107–116. *Goldmine for Dummies.* IDG Books Worldwide, Foster City, Calif.

43. **Seaberg, R. S., R. O. Stallone, and B. E. Statland.** 2000. The role of total laboratory automation in a consolidated laboratory network. *Clin. Chem.* **46:**751–756.

44. **Skrisson, J. F., J. Shaw, and F. L. Kiechle.** 2001. Hospital laboratory outreach program builds success through affiliation with a laboratory network. *J. Clin. Ligand Assay* **24:**253–256.

45. **Sodeman, T.** 2001. Elements in merging laboratory operations. *J. Clin. Ligand Assay* **24:**239–244.

46. **Statland, B. E.** 1995. The commercialization of lab services . . . or, make no mistake about it, lab testing is big business. *Med. Lab. Observer* **27**(10):33–37.

47. **Steiner, J. W., J. M. Root, and R. L. Michel.** 1995. *The Transformation of Hospital Laboratories—Why Regionalization, Consolidation and Reengineering Will Lead Laboratories into the 21st Century,* p. 1–33. Hospital Technology Series (AHA 012040), American Hospital Association, Chicago, Ill.

48. **Sterling, B.** 2000. *Zeitgeist,* p. 151. Bantam Books, New York, N.Y.

49. **Sull, D. N.** 1999. Why good companies go bad. *Harvard Bus. Rev.* **77**(4):42–52.

50. **Tzu, S.** 1963. *The Art of War,* p. 102. S. B. Griffin (translator), Oxford University Press, Oxford, United Kingdom.

51. **Ulrich, D., J. Zenger, and N. Smallwood.** 1999. Customer results: building firm equity, p. 107–137. *In Results-Based Leadership.* Harvard Business School Press, Boston, Mass.

52. **Valente, P. T., and H. D. Schantz.** 2001. Cytology automation: an overview. *Lab. Med.* **32:**686–690.

53. **von Ghyczy, T., B. von Oetinger, and C. Bassford (ed.).** 2001. *Clausewitz on Strategy,* p. 1–39. John Wiley & Sons, Inc., New York, N.Y.

54. Wiedbrauk, D. L., and J. Holden. 1998. Laboratory consolidation. Minimizing the angst and aggravation. *Med. Lab. Observer* **30**(7):66–73.

55. Wright, T. C. Jr., J. T. Cox, L. S. Massad, L. B. Twiggs, and E. J. Wilkinson for the 2001 ASCP Sponsored Consensus Conference. 2002. 2001 consensus guidelines for the management of women with cervical cytological abnormalities. *JAMA* **287:**2120–2129.

56. Wright, T. C., Jr., L. Denny, L. Kuhn, A. Pollack, and A. Lorincz. 2000. HPV DNA testing of self-collected vaginal samples compared with cytologic screening to detect cervical cancer. *JAMA* **283:**81–86.

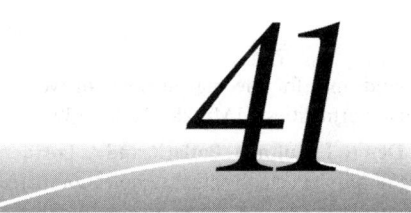

Finance and Decision Making in Outreach

Michael G. Bissell

OBJECTIVES

To provide background on some basic financial concepts related to operational and strategic decision making in laboratory outreach and the logic behind them

To provide formulas and worked examples of calculations in the appendixes

I been rich and I been poor. Rich is better.

SOPHIE TUCKER

Introduction

The Clinical Laboratory as a Business

As a business, the clinical laboratory is unique and complex, sharing the economic characteristics of both a service business and a manufacturing industry (1–6). It is a service industry that is nonetheless responsible for a product: clinical information. The production of laboratory data requires a heavy investment in assets such as scientific instruments and advanced facilities. This heavy endowment of assets is more typical of manufacturing firms. The laboratory's service is characterized by an extremely short service turnaround time compared to many other service industries. Clinical laboratory operations (particularly those that are "24 × 7") require a more constant and demanding management of human and financial resources than does the average service business.

It is often overlooked that laboratory work can have a seasonal component, as, for example, when setting up assays for influenza. When found to be present, seasonality should be an important planning factor, especially in efforts to deploy the usually limited human and financial resources.

Constant technological innovation characterizes the clinical laboratory to a greater extent than in many other service industries. The frequent changes and improvements in techniques and methods of producing laboratory results create much uncertainty in the acquisition of equipment and material, which may have a relatively fast rate of obsolescence.

Some have compared the clinical laboratory business to a bakery or a photo-finishing firm, in that both product and rapid turnaround time are basic components of the service.

The Phases of the Growth Curve

A product, technology, firm, or industry is said to evolve through phases of development during which aspects of its economics may change. The initial or startup phase is a time when the new venture is usually not profitable, and its rate of growth is sluggish at first. This is the phase in which many laboratory or product failures occur. Financial planning for this phase is inherently difficult and challenging because of the number of uncertainties involved.

The growth phase is the phase of fastest expansion and the greatest operational challenge, when a laboratory venture breaks even or a product begins to pay off. The chance of its long-term survival is considered much improved if it has successfully weathered this phase. Financial planning during this phase is exciting because of the unusual growth rate, though some residual uncertainty remains.

During the mature phase, typically operational pains are no longer as great and the rate of growth has slowed. When a laboratory or product reaches this stage, its prospects for survival in the market are favorable. Financial planning becomes routine and continuous.

The declining phase is the phase of negative growth, which presents a special challenge. At the least, it should be anticipated so that it will trigger a search for a new product or technology. The clinical laboratory industry as a whole has often been portrayed as being in the mature phase presently, though foreseeable changes in technology may modify this assessment one way or the other.

Given all of the clinical laboratory's special characteristics as a business, and given the fundamental dynamics of change in the contemporary U.S. healthcare industry, the ongoing challenge is to provide lower prices and easy access to services while reducing per capita cost and maintaining high standards of quality. As more decisions about the cost and volume of health services to be delivered move from the physician and hospital to the purchasers of care, both hospital and physician office clients have focused energy on accounting for and managing costs. The economic mission of the hospital laboratory has shifted from revenue generation per se to managing the cost side of the equation. Hospital laboratories have increasingly replaced labor with technology; creatively dealt with productivity issues; and merged, consolidated, regionalized, and formed joint ventures to achieve economies of scale.

Decision Making in Laboratory Outreach Management

Outreach potentially represents an alternative approach to ensure the survival of the hospital clinical laboratory in the midst of unparalleled industry change. The transition to outreach, however, represents a true change of culture, in that price competition, external service demands, and the quest for market share vie with and may supplant certain of the internal preoccupations of traditional hospital-focused laboratory management. More of the decision making has a distinctly financial character, and a deeper understanding of a variety of cost concepts and cost behavior is the ultimate basis for it.

Types of Costs

Fixed, Variable, and Mixed Costs

Variable costs change in more or less direct proportion to test volume. Examples of variable costs include technologist wages and benefits, reagents, glassware, disposable supplies, and forms. Fixed costs remain unchanged for a given period of time, despite fluctuations in test volume. Examples of fixed costs include supervisory and custodial wages and benefits, required regardless of volume, as well as depreciation of building, space, and equipment. It is appropriate to regard some costs as mixed costs, since costs are often difficult to classify definitively as either fixed or variable. Clerical staff can be reduced upon a decrease in clinical activity, but a certain number of such positions are required regardless of volume. Fixed costs hold constant only over a relevant range of activity. If volume increases or decreases dramatically, as under catastrophic conditions, all fixed costs become variable to some extent.

Direct and Indirect Costs

Direct costs are all costs that can be specifically linked to a test. Examples of direct costs include technical, supervisory, and clerical wages; overtime; on-call payments; and chemicals and supplies related to the test. Service costs are direct costs that are incurred as tests are performed. They represent variable costs plus those fixed costs that are most directly traceable to the testing. The service cost concept is useful in budgeting and analyzing cash flow.

Indirect costs (or overhead) are all costs not directly traceable to the test but included in total laboratory expense. Examples of indirect costs include depreciation, building and equipment maintenance, insurance, utilities, housekeeping, and purchasing and billing services, as well as sales, marketing, and development costs. Many indirect costs are period costs, i.e., costs that represent fixed outlays for the whole laboratory or the whole hospital per unit time. For outreach operations that are integral with hospital laboratories, the details of the allocation formulas by which hospital administration assigns indirect costs from the general hospital operation to the outreach laboratory operation can be the deciding factor in understanding the true profitability of lab outreach. These allocation rules must be explicit, well-justified, and mutually agreed upon at the outset for laboratory outreach to have any hope of success.

Unit Costs

Unit costs are the costs per unit of production or unit of service provided, accountable as fixed and variable costs per unit. Variable cost per unit generally remains the same regardless of volume. As volume increases, total variable cost increases by the same percentage, yet on a per-unit basis variable cost remains unchanged. Fixed cost per unit is generally reduced as the total fixed cost is spread over more tests. Total fixed costs remain the same regardless of volume increases, whereas on a per-unit basis they decline. Economy of scale means that the higher the volume of tests, the lower the overall unit cost.

It is important to be able to differentiate the varieties of unit costs that occur in clinical laboratory operations. Cost per test (or cost per result) is typically the total of the direct (both fixed and variable) costs, as well as allocations of certain of the "more direct" indirect costs associated with the production of a single individual analyte test result: reagents, disposable supplies, equipment, and labor. Cost per reportable result includes the same costs not only for the individual analyte test result itself but also for all the quality control, calibrator, waste, and repeat results necessary to be able to report that result. Cost per billable result accounts for the costs of all the reportable results that are included in a unit of service, such as a test panel or battery, that is made up of multiple individual analyte results but billed as a group, i.e., counts a 12-test panel as 1 result unit, not 12. Cost per relative value unit (RVU) applies to certain results, like surgical pathology reports, that have a labor component involving significant professional time spent on cognitive interpretative tasks. For such results, various systems of RVUs have been devised and implemented by professional organizations to account for these activities in order to bill for them. The laboratory costs associated with these billables can be accounted as cost per RVU.

Additional Cost Concepts for Decision Making

Costs can be accounted in a variety of ways, and the particular cost concepts used in a given situation may differ depending on the nature of the decision to be made, i.e., planning and budgeting, reporting, or monitoring and feedback. Each cost concept thus has a task-specific usefulness.

Out-of-pocket costs represent cash outlays made at or close to the time of a given activity. Timing of cash flows in capital transactions may have out-of-pocket costs as important considerations in decision making. In contrast to out-of-pocket costs, book costs reflect allocations of past outlays to the current period and have more limited usefulness in budgeting and capital decision making.

Historical costs are actual cash payments accounted for and recorded at the time of outlay. They are used extensively in external reporting and represent what are also called sunk costs, since they are not changeable by any management decision and have importance mainly in forecasting trends. Future costs, both fixed and variable, direct and indirect, on the other hand, have the potential to be changed by current decisions and thus represent the most appropriate focus for planning efforts, like budget and capital-acquisition decisions.

Differential or incremental costs represent the change in future fixed and/or variable costs resulting from specific courses of action. A special case is the unit incremental or marginal cost, which is the cost of adding one additional unit of production. Total costs represent the sum of these incremental costs plus those costs that do not change due to the course of action being considered.

Opportunity costs represent benefit that may be missed as a result of rejecting a more profitable alternative use of resources (materials, labor, facilities, or capital) when making a decision. They represent lost revenue, not expenditure, and they are variable costs whose amounts depend on the alternatives under consideration. Imputed costs are all costs (including opportunity costs) that do not involve outlay of cash. An example might be depreciation of capital equipment. For capital-expenditure decisions and in other situations in which investment alternatives are being considered, opportunity or imputed costs become useful concepts. They are not explicitly listed in accounting records, but must be derived.

Controllable costs are fixed or variable costs that can be influenced by a specific individual's decision making. Noncontrollable costs are outside the scope of a specific individual's control. The concepts of controllable and noncontrollable costs are useful in evaluating individuals' performance in terms of fiscal accountability. Thus the statement that an executive has "P and L" (profit and loss) responsibility for any portion of the operation implies that all of its costs are controllable, either directly or indirectly, by that individual.

Characteristics of Laboratory Costs

Fixed costs constitute a large proportion of overall cost in a typical clinical laboratory. This fact has implications for certain key decisions, such as those involving analyses of cost, volume, and margin interrelationships. It also means that in a typical hospital laboratory, the range of alternatives may be limited by the fact that a change in volume does not necessarily result in a directly corresponding change in costs. The existence of this phenomenon may, on the other hand, create opportunity for outreach in terms of the potential for utilizing the de facto marginal excess production capacity these necessary fixed costs may represent when viewed from the outreach perspective. An example might be expanding volume on off shifts in a three-shift operation to "fill the factory" 24 hours per day.

It is essential that an outreach laboratory account explicitly for all of its direct and indirect costs of production. Ideally, each test on its menu should be microcosted to account for each and every category of expense involved in the production of each unit of service at the test volume at which the laboratory is operating. Microcosting can be either bottom-up (built up from known unit-cost inputs;

also known as job order costing) or top-down (unit costs estimated from aggregate expenses divided by units of service; also known as process costing). These methods are reviewed in detail in reference 5. Either way, the availability or nonavailability of cost data by areas or tests may restrict the analysis of cost behavior.

In certain cases, initial estimates may have to be made based on experience and partial studies and then revised as additional cost data are accumulated. Although this situation is not ideal, it enables a laboratory to use fixed- and variable-cost analyses for financial management, most particularly, as a basis for pricing decisions in the creation of the laboratory's fee schedule.

Levels of Decision Making in Outreach Operations

Menu: To Test or Not To Test

Ideally, of course, a hospital clinical laboratory's decision about whether or not to offer a given test on its test menu should be driven by objective evidence of clinical need, by perceived patient benefit, and, ultimately, by measures of patient outcome associated with the test's use. In this context, it is largely a medical-technical decision that depends upon a consideration of the test's potential "contribution to mission" for the institution, and is the responsibility of the laboratory director. Within the hospital, typically the laboratory director is also responsible for participating in the management of utilization of laboratory testing, especially important under managed-care arrangements and increasingly necessary for federal compliance. If offering a given test will result in increased levels of inappropriate utilization (e.g., if its published diagnostic performance is such that a great many false positives or false negatives leading to unnecessary workups are associated with its use), then the laboratory director may face the challenge of educating the medical staff to this by opposing the test's inclusion in the laboratory's menu.

In outreach, while most of these underlying ethical and regulatory considerations are the same, the economic aspects of this decision making can be somewhat different. It will be useful to compare and contrast the situations obtaining in each setting with respect to the important questions associated with test-menu decisions.

First, is the test reimbursed? The decision about including a test in the laboratory's menu will have this as a fundamental consideration, whether the test is offered for hospital inpatients, outpatients, or outreach clients (nonpatients). But whether and how any given test is paid for, and the circumstances under which it may make sense to include an under- or unreimbursed test in the menu, will definitely differ. The subject of clinical laboratory reimbursement is an extremely complex one, requiring knowledge of the detailed history of federal and state healthcare reimbursement programs, third-party payors, and managed care.

In dealing with this issue, first of all, it is essential to know the difference between reimbursements and charges. In the context of outpatient fee-for-service within the hospital, the charge for a given test is the amount associated with it in the institution's charge description master (CDM). It represents the amount the hospital theoretically bills all fee-for-service payors for the test. It is important to realize that this is a purely nominal figure, however, and the "revenue stream" that results from such fee-for-service billings, called gross revenue or gross billed revenue, does not actually exist as such in today's world, except in certain increasingly unusual circumstances. Note, however, that gross revenue is typically the only laboratory revenue data available to laboratory management on in-hospital work.

What the hospital actually gets paid is either directly determined by federal or state government policy (in the case of Medicare/Medicaid) or strongly influenced by it (in the case of other third-party payors). The test's rate of reimbursement by these payors is driven by its billing code, e.g., the Current Procedural Terminology (CPT) code assigned by the American Medical Association and updated annually. To know whether or not a given test is reimbursed, therefore, the first question to be answered is: Does it have a CPT code assigned at this time? If the answer is no, financing the test through the usual channels will be difficult. New tests and locally developed (or "home-brew") tests that are truly novel analytes (as opposed to merely novel methods for accepted analytes) are often assigned to a category of "research use only" or "not for in vitro diagnostic use" until they have been approved for diagnostic use by the U.S. Food and Drug Administration under its 510(k) or pre-market approval processes. Medicare/Medicaid does not reimburse this test category until specific CPT codes are assigned. Attempting to bill under a general "miscellaneous"-type billing code is virtually guaranteed to be unsuccessful.

In contrast to this, the outreach laboratory, in fee-for-service situations, will bill not based on a CDM but rather from a fee schedule. The price at which the test is sold to a client will usually represent a value that is negotiated to include a discount off of the fee schedule list price. These negotiations may often include loss leaders, i.e., tests sold to the client at or below cost in order to meet an overall service need or provide "one-stop shopping." Note, however, that predatory pricing, involving discount of the full fee schedule below the lab's cost, usually done for the purpose of excluding competition, is unethical and may be illegal as well. Clearly, such pricing cannot be sustained over the long run, and it is only the larger laboratories, i.e., the "deeper pockets," that can hold out long enough to drive smaller competitors out of specific markets. In general, the outreach laboratory will be billing other providers (hospitals or physician offices) on an account-bill or client-bill arrangement, or billing patients directly on a patient-bill arrangement, but not billing state or federal agencies directly. Under these circumstances, questions of CPT coding and/or Food and Drug Administration approval need not drive decision making to the same degree, as long as Clinical Laboratory Improvement Amendments (CLIA) and any other applicable regulatory quality requirements are met. In fact, clinical considerations may drive utilization of tests that are under- or unreimbursed within the hospital, so that it may have to buy them from a reference lab or outreach program under an account-bill arrangement.

The amount that either the hospital or the outreach program actually gets paid for a given test (called the net revenue or net collected revenue) is equal to the billed amount minus allowances and bad debt. Allowances include cost-based reimbursements, reductions in payments based on discounted charges, and charity care. Bad debt is other unpaid and uncollected billings. The reimbursement rate depends upon the type of financing in place for the patient on whom the test was ordered (known in the aggregate as the provider's payor mix).

If the service is being provided under a managed-care arrangement, then there is no billing at all for the test— its cost is simply reimbursed as part of the managed-care organization's per capita payments to the hospital or laboratory for its members' care (e.g., a prenegotiated per member per month, or PMPM, rate). Any positive margin earned by the hospital or laboratory under these circumstances is strictly a function of the degree to which it can minimize both unit cost and utilization of testing. Negotiating managed-care contracts is a very specialized subject and is beyond the scope of this chapter.

As previously mentioned, pricing of outreach testing must ultimately be based on the unit cost plus a markup representing profit margin. It must also, of course, reflect what the market will bear, i.e., it must be competitive with the pricing of the other lab providers, including national reference laboratories, operating in the area. Because this is so, it can be crucial that the costing of the test reflect a true sense of the marginal or incremental net cost of its production, given the hospital's sunk costs and excess capacity. These concepts are illustrated in some of the material below.

Operation: To Make or Buy the Test

Given a decision to offer a test as part of the laboratory's menu, the next decision is whether to set up the new test in-house or to send it out to a reference lab. In addition to the logistical considerations of test turnaround time and availability, an essential financial consideration in this decision is the concept of the laboratory's net contribution margin (for in-hospital work) or net profit (for true outreach) for a given test. This is defined as the total net revenue generated by the test minus the total unit cost (both direct and laboratory-related indirect) for which the laboratory is responsible. A sample problem adapted from one presented in reference 5 should make this clear, while also showing how some of the different cost-related concepts above are used in a typical make-or-buy decision:

Suppose a laboratory offers a test on its menu and charges $10.00 per billable result for it. Suppose further that a calculated, fully loaded total cost per billable for this test is $13.00, which includes all test-specific direct costs at $5.00, all laboratory-specific indirect costs at $4.25, and all hospital-wide allocated indirect costs at $3.75. Calculating the test's profit or contribution then gives $10.00 – $13.00 = – $3.00, a loss on each test performed. If the laboratory performs 1,000 of these tests annually, the extended loss becomes $3,000 per year. If the test, offered at $10.00 per billable, were purchased by the laboratory as a send-out from a commercial laboratory at $8.00 per billable instead of being produced in-house, the loss would apparently turn to a profit (handling fee) of $2.00 per billable. Is this what should be done?

The reasoning here needs to be scrutinized by concentrating on exactly which costs of performing this test are relevant in this decision-making process. The test-specific direct costs of $5.00 per billable include $3.52 direct labor, $0.48 direct reagents and disposables, and $1.00 other direct costs. These are out-of-pocket cost savings that will be realized by no longer performing the test on site. The labor cost may be considered fixed in this case, because the technologists are likely to remain on staff. For purposes of this example, assume labor to be a truly variable cost savings. The appropriate analysis, then, would be as shown in Table 41.1. The $8.00 purchase price, if the test is sent out, results in a net increase in out-of-pocket cost of $3.00 per billable above the savings in direct costs of $5.00. Since the indirect costs incurred by the laboratory remain in effect, regardless of this decision, arguably they should not be considered relevant. Therefore, if the test is continued in-house its net profit is greater. If the labor component is treated as a fixed cost (the technologist would remain on staff), then labor, like the indirect costs, would no longer be relevant and the argument for continuing to do this test

Table 41.1 Factors in the decision to make or buy a test

Factor	Make (continue in-house testing)	Buy (from reference lab)
Charge	$10.00	$10.00
Direct costs	$5.00	$8.00
Indirect costs	Not relevant	Not relevant
Contribution	$5.00	$2.00

in-house would become even stronger. The methodology underlying this discussion is called break-even analysis. If the revenue and cost associated with a procedure like this one (or an instrument or a methodology) are both plotted on a graph of test volume (x) versus dollars (y), they will cross at a point representing a net contribution of zero, i.e., the point at which revenue equals cost, called the crossover or break-even point.

Assume for the moment that a hypothetical laboratory is currently operating at the break-even point determined by the calculations above. What about next year? What happens if volume, cost, and/or revenue increases or decreases? The method most often used for exploration of such what-if scenarios is sensitivity analysis. This technique uses data provided from the break-even analysis and provides potential insight into the effects of changes in costs, revenues, volumes, and/or net income. Basically, the calculations are repeated with substitution of the hypothetical change in one variable at a time. For example, consider whether the above decision would be different with any of the following changes in the conditions. Suppose there were a 20% increase in test volume; or a price increase that produces a 20% increase in revenue, assuming no bad debts or allowances; or a 20% reduction in variable labor expense for the same test volume. Virtually any future situation may be simulated with the use of current data. Although sensitivity analysis has the virtue of relative simplicity, it should be applied with some caution. It assumes that all costs are either variable or fixed (i.e., no mixed costs), that variable costs are a linear function of (directly proportional to) volume, and that a relevant range exists for all levels of activity. Though these simplifications make the analysis possible, they may influence interpretation of analytical results, such that an appropriate "taking it with a grain of salt" is always in order.

Note that federal tax and regulatory considerations, the so-called shell laboratory provisions, dictate an effective upper limit for the portion of a laboratory's volume that can be sent out to another laboratory. *Basically, a laboratory that is sending out more than 30% of its work to be performed elsewhere is regarded as not actually being in the laboratory business under federal fraud and abuse regulations.*

Capital: Whether or Not To Acquire New Equipment

Given a decision to "make," i.e., produce test results in-house, the next decisions involve the use or acquisition of any capital equipment that may be involved. This aspect of planning, capital budgeting, may be interdependent in the outreach laboratory with both operational budgeting and strategic planning. It may include allocations for major investments in buildings as well as equipment. In accounting terms, a capital item is commonly defined as a fixed asset that is expected to provide service (i.e., have a useful life) of more than 1 year. Within this broad definition, some important distinctions among concepts should be kept in mind.

Repair and maintenance of capital items, for example, should be differentiated from capital improvements. Maintenance and repair provides ongoing upkeep of the investment and is most appropriately treated as an operating expense. Since capital improvements are just that, that is, they make the items better than when purchased, they are most appropriately treated as capital expenses. Replacing an entire fixed asset should be regarded as a capital expenditure, whereas replacing a component part is best treated as an operating expense.

Leasing arrangements differ in whether they define a given expense as a capital or an operating line item. Relatively inexpensive new items with useful lives of greater than 1 year are often initially classified as capital, but their replacements are treated as operating expenses from then on (e.g., certain furniture items and items costing $500 or less).

The budgeting period is very important for capital budgeting. In outreach work, review of capital needs should occur at least annually. Long-term planning, while always desirable, may often not be possible in today's dynamic marketplace. The longer the time horizon used, the more likely are the predictions involved to be inaccurate, so this process must always be approached flexibly.

Capital budgets typically contain separate categories for minor and major items. Minor capital consists of relatively low-cost items, perhaps under $2,500, requiring less in the way of analysis. This may just be an outline of the costs, along with an indication of whether the item is a replacement, new item, renovation, improvement, or regulatory requirement, along with a brief budgetary justification. These items may just be prioritized numerically or classified into the following categories: (i) needed to continue present service, (ii) needed to support recent volume growth, (iii) providing opportunity for cost savings or profit at the existing volume, (iv) providing opportunity for improvement in quality or service levels, and (v) providing opportunity to implement new programs or initiatives.

Major capital items, e.g., items over $2,500 (or a similar figure), may be split up into annual purchase requests over a longer (3- to 5-year) period and generally require more in the way of analysis. Supporting documentation needs to be more detailed and specific, often involving statements or descriptions of (i) general purpose, (ii) importance, (iii) projected client demand and utilization, (iv) availability of alternatives, (v) estimated useful life, (vi) estimated total acquisition cost, (vii) estimated associated yearly cash outflows, and (viii) estimated yearly cash inflows or savings.

It may be difficult to make these last two projections, but such data on expected cash flows are crucial to the analytic techniques used in evaluating capital alternatives. In performing these projections, consider only incremental amounts. Be concerned only with marginal or additional cash outflows and inflows that will occur as the direct result of the new project above and beyond the current baseline.

Count only *cash* inflows and outflows, bearing in mind that accounting statements of revenue and expense that are maintained on other than a cash basis are likely to yield inaccurate estimates of the actual cash either generated or spent.

In the clinical laboratory business, capital items are vital to financial capability and future viability. An attempt must therefore be made to assure a reasonable return on the investment represented by each capital item. Return-on-investment (ROI) calculations (discussed in some detail in Appendix 41.1) need to start with an estimation of this return percentage, referred to as the required rate of return (or discount rate). In the example adapted from reference 4 and given in the appendix, a 10% rate is used. The actual required rate of return on a given project may be based on any of a number of factors that may include (i) the cost of borrowing new funds (i.e., the interest rate at which the laboratory can borrow money); (ii) the return realized on investments of laboratory profits in short-term liquid investment instruments such as money markets, government securities, or certificates of deposit; (iii) in a for-profit environment, the return on investment expected by stockholders; and/or (iv) a "fudge factor" accounting for possible misestimates in the calculation or the relative riskiness of the project.

Financing Capital: To Lease or Buy Equipment

Given a decision to acquire a new piece of equipment, the next decisions revolve around determining the least costly financing alternative. The lease-or-buy decision is an application of present-value analysis, as described in Appendix 41.2. Following generally accepted accounting principles (GAAP), there are two types of leases, known as cancelable and noncancelable leases. In the first of these, if the laboratory can cancel the lease and cease making payments whenever it chooses without penalty, the lease is called an operating lease and treated as an operating expense. If, for the term of the lease, it cannot be canceled and there is an option to purchase the equipment, then the lease is called a capital lease, is viewed as a form of capital borrowing for a purchase, and is accounted for as a capital acquisition within the capital budget.

Financing alternatives typically are three: (i) to purchase the item from the laboratory's internal funds, (ii) to borrow external funds for its purchase, or (iii) to lease the equipment. The costs associated with each of these approaches can be analyzed side by side using the present-value methodology as described in Appendix 41.2.

Summary

Outreach can represent an alternative path in the development of a hospital laboratory, but it is one in which price competition becomes a basic reality and market share becomes a critical measure of success. The outreach labora-

tory must compete on quality and service, and these are critical success factors that must be invested in. It may also, if it is large enough, have the opportunity to compete on technological innovation, but in reality this applies to relatively few hospital-based startup ventures. Mainly, it will have to compete on price, which means that, of necessity, it must produce as much or more with the same or fewer material and human resource inputs per unit of service than does the competition. It also means that the cost of new sales, in terms of the cost of marketing, sales activity, distribution, client service, and quality enhancements and/or technology improvements, must be managed as actively as are the costs of daily production. In all of this, familiarity with the basic types and interrelationships of costs becomes key.

KEY POINTS

- An understanding of the nature and analysis of cost behavior has fundamental significance for decision making in outreach laboratory management.

- A large proportion of the typical hospital laboratory's costs are fixed, and this can create opportunity for outreach when properly viewed as such.

- Key decisions that are financially driven include pricing and menu decisions, make-or-buy decisions, and decisions about the financing and acquisition of equipment.

GLOSSARY

Accounts payable Obligations or liabilities of a buyer that usually arise from normal operations of a business. They are neither backed up by a negotiable instrument nor considered overdue. Contract obligations owed by individuals or the business on an open account.

Accounts receivable Balances due from debtors on current accounts.

Allowances Amounts to be subtracted from gross billings (along with bad debt) in the calculation of net revenue, including contractual and cost-based reimbursements, reductions in payments based on discounted charges, and charity care.

Assets All money, property, or valuables that are owned by an individual or organization. Assets may be used in whole or in part to pay off liabilities (debts).

Average rate of return (ARR) The average dollar return on a project divided by the average dollar investment it represents, usually calculated on an annual basis.

Bad debt Billings that are unpaid and uncollected and/or uncollectible.

Billing Presenting a statement of charges to another healthcare provider, such as a hospital or physician office (account bill or client bill), or to a patient (patient bill).

Billing code Standardized designation for medical procedures (like laboratory tests) that are billable under federal government reimbursement rules, e.g., the Current Procedural Terminology (CPT) code assigned by the American Medical Association and updated annually.

Book costs Outstanding liabilities counted against the assets of a business as shown on its account books, and reflecting allocations of past outlays to the current period.

Bottom-up microcosting Estimating the unit cost of a laboratory test by summing the estimated unit costs of each of the input components (materials, labor, etc.) for a single performance of that test (also called job order costing).

Break-even or crossover point The point in the lifespan of a business or project at which the revenue it generates equals its cost, and thus represents a net contribution margin or profit of zero.

Capital item A fixed asset that is expected to provide service (i.e., have a useful life) of more than 1 year.

Capital lease A lease that cannot be canceled during its term and that typically includes an option to purchase. It is accounted as a form of capital borrowing for a purchase and is accounted for as a capital acquisition within the capital budget.

Cash flow The patterns of receipts and expenditures of a company (or other entity) resulting in the availability or nonavailability of cash.

Charge In the context of outpatient fee-for-service within the hospital, the charge for a given test is the amount associated with it in the institution's charge description master (CDM), representing the amount the hospital theoretically bills all fee-for-service payors for the test.

Controllable costs Fixed or variable costs that can be influenced by a specific individual's decision making.

Cost per billable result Unit cost of production of all the reportable results that are included in a unit of service, such as a test panel or battery that is made up of multiple individual analyte results but billed as a group.

Cost per reportable result Unit cost of production for all the items necessary to report a test result, including the individual analyte test result itself and all the quality control, calibrator, waste, and repeat results that are necessary to be able to report it.

Cost per test (or cost per result) Unit cost of production of a single individual analyte test result, representing both fixed and variable direct costs as well as allocations of certain indirect costs most closely associated with production: reagents, disposable supplies, equipment, and labor.

Depreciation Estimated allowance made in accounting for the decrease in value of a fixed asset through wear, deterioration, or obsolescence during its useful life; may be calculated by different standard methods.

Differential or incremental costs The change in future fixed and/or variable costs projected to result from changes in production methods, costs of inputs, or other events or specific courses of action.

Direct costs All costs that are incurred directly as a result of producing test results, e.g., technical, supervisory, and clerical

wages; overtime; on-call payments; and chemicals and supplies specifically expended to perform the test.

Economy of scale Positive relationship between increased volume and decreased unit cost of production.

Fee schedule Listing of the prices charged for tests by an outreach laboratory in fee-for-service situations, i.e., in billing individuals who are nonpatients of the laboratory or its parent institution or in billing clients representing nonpatients.

Fixed assets The items of physical property (equipment, buildings, and/or land) owned by a business or other entity; also known as tangible or nonliquid assets.

Fixed costs Laboratory costs that remain unchanged for a given period of time, despite fluctuations in test volume, e.g., supervisory and custodial wages and benefits required regardless of volume, building maintenance and utilities, and depreciation.

"Fraud and abuse" provisions Portions of the Medicare and Medicaid regulations pertaining to definitions of prohibited laboratory business practices, such as physician self-referral and other forms of inducement and conflict of interest.

Future costs Anticipatable costs that potentially can be affected by current budget and capital-acquisition decisions and thus represent the most appropriate focus of planning.

Generally accepted accounting principles (GAAP) A widely recognized set of standard accounting procedures and definitions.

Gross revenue or gross billed revenue The amount of gross income that would theoretically result if a hospital or laboratory could bill and collect all its charges from all its payors.

Historical costs Costs incurred by a business in the form of payments that are accounted for and recorded at the time of actual cash outlay (also known as sunk costs).

Imputed costs Costs incurred by a business in any form that does not involve actual outlay of cash, such as opportunity costs, depreciation, etc., which are not explicitly listed in accounting records but must be derived by calculation.

Indirect costs (or overhead) All general laboratory costs not easily or directly traceable to the production of individual test results but included in total laboratory operating expense, e.g., depreciation; building and equipment maintenance; insurance; utilities; housekeeping; and costs associated with purchasing and billing services, sales, marketing, and development.

Inflation Effective relative increase in the amount of money in circulation, resulting in a fall in its value and a rise in prices over time.

Job order costing *See* Bottom-up microcosting.

Lease A written agreement or contract by which one party (the lessor) gives to another (the lessee) the use and possession of property for a specified time (the term) and for fixed payments.

List price The price of a test listed in a laboratory's fee schedule and representing the nominal price charged to its fee-for-service clients (nonpatients and clients representing nonpatients). The actual price is typically negotiated to include a discount off of the fee schedule list price.

Loss leader A test sold to a client at a price discounted below cost in order to meet an overall service need or provide "one-stop shopping." Note that it is not legal to loss lead entire accounts, but only individual tests within an account. *See also* Predatory pricing, *and* "fraud and abuse" provisions.

Marginal cost The incremental cost of adding one additional unit of test production.

Microcosting Calculating the unit costs of test production to account for each and every category of expense involved at the laboratory's current test volume: performed in either a bottom-up or top-down fashion.

Mixed costs Costs that are somewhat, though not totally, dependent on volume, i.e., are difficult to classify definitively as either fixed or variable, e.g., clerical staff.

Net contribution margin For all hospital inpatient and outpatient testing, the total net test revenue generated by the laboratory, minus the total cost of test production (both direct and laboratory-related indirect) for which the laboratory is responsible, constitutes its contribution to the hospital's bottom line.

Net present value (NPV) The present value of all the cash flows created by a project minus the dollar amount of the initial investment in it (also known as the time value of money associated with the investment).

Net profit For all true outreach nonpatient testing, the total net revenue generated by the laboratory, minus the total cost of test production (direct and indirect) for which the laboratory is responsible, constitutes the laboratory's profit.

Net revenue or net collected revenue The amount either the hospital or the outreach program actually gets paid for a given test is equal to the billed amount minus allowances and bad debt.

Noncontrollable costs Costs outside the scope of a specific individual's control.

Operating lease A lease that can be canceled during its term and that typically does not include an option to purchase. It is accounted as a form of operating expense.

Opportunity costs Imputed costs representing missed opportunity, i.e., the potential financial gain that is missed when a more profitable use of resources (materials, labor, facilities, or capital) is rejected or abandoned in favor of a less profitable one. They are lost revenue, not expenditures, and they represent variable costs whose amounts depend on the alternatives under consideration. (They are related to the concepts of time value of money or net present value, i.e., best use of funds among competing investments.)

Out-of-pocket costs Costs involving immediate expenditures, i.e., incurred as cash outlays occurring at or near the time of purchase; potentially important in capital budgeting.

Patients Individuals receiving care (and laboratory testing) after being registered and seen in clinic (hospital outpatients), after being registered and admitted to the hospital (hospital inpatients), or as clients of the laboratory's outreach business with no other connection to the hospital per se (hospital nonpatients).

Payback period The period of time that a capital investment takes to be completely recovered from its resulting cash flows.

Payor mix The distribution of the different forms of healthcare financing in place among the population served by a healthcare provider, e.g., Medicare, Medicaid, private pay, managed care, uninsured, etc.

Per member per month (PMPM) rate For services provided under a managed-care arrangement, the managed-care organization's per capita payments to the hospital for its members' care. Under such arrangements, laboratory tests are most typically bundled, i.e., there is no separate billing for tests, which are regarded as being reimbursed as part of the overall capitated payment.

Period costs Costs that represent fixed outlays for the whole lab or the whole hospital per unit time.

Predatory pricing Discount of the full fee schedule to a client below the laboratory's cost, and done for the purpose of excluding competition, is unethical and illegal.

Present value (PV) or time value of money The dollar amount which, if it were invested now at a given rate of return, would accumulate to a given specified value at a specified time in the future.

"P and L" (profit and loss) responsibility Individual financial accountability for a business or portion of a business implies that all of its costs are controllable, either directly or indirectly, by that individual.

Process costing A method of microcosting in which unit costs are estimated from aggregate expenses divided by units of service. *See also* Top-down microcosting.

Relative value unit (RVU) Workload units accounted under any of several weighting systems devised and implemented by professional organizations to account for a labor component involving significant professional time spent on cognitive interpretative tasks in the production of certain test results, like surgical pathology reports, in order to equitably bill for them. The laboratory costs associated with these billables can be accounted as cost per RVU.

Return on investment (ROI) Calculation (involving a variety of different methods) of a specified payback amount (also known as the required rate of return, or discount rate) on a given investment.

Sensitivity analysis A method for testing premises used in decision making, i.e., determining the sensitivity of conclusions derived from calculation to the ranges of numerical values chosen as inputs with substitution of the change in one variable at a time to determine their effects (also known as what-if calculations or best- and worst-case scenarios).

Service costs Costs that are incurred as tests are performed, representing variable costs plus those fixed costs that are most directly traceable to the testing, and related to the concept of cash flow.

"Shell lab" provisions Portion of federal fraud and abuse regulations dictating an effective upper limit for the portion of a laboratory's volume (30%) that can be sent out to another laboratory.

Straight-line depreciation Standard accounting method of calculating depreciation of fixed assets that involves equal weighting of time periods.

Sum of the years' digits (SYD) method Standard accounting method of calculating depreciation of fixed assets that involves unequal weighting of time periods.

Sunk costs *See* Historical costs.

Top-down microcosting. *See* Process costing.

Unit costs Costs per unit of production or unit of service provided (test, reportable result, billable result, or RVU), accountable as total of fixed plus variable costs per unit.

Variable costs. Direct or indirect costs that vary in direct proportion to test volume, e.g., technologist wages and benefits, reagents, glassware, disposable supplies, and forms.

REFERENCES

1. Bennington, J. L., G. E. Westlake, and G. E. Louvau. 1974. *Financial Management of the Clinical Laboratory.* University Park Press, Baltimore, Md.

2. Beebe, M, J. A. Dalton, C. Duffy, D. Evans, R. L. Glenn, D. Hayden, G. M. Kotowicz, E. Lumakovska, M. L. Mindeman, K. E. O'Hara, M. R. O'Heron, D. Reyes, D. Rozell, L. Stancik, A. Walker, A. A. Watkins, J. Zacharias. 2002. *Physicians Current Procedural Terminology, CPT 2003.* American Medical Association Press, Chicago, Ill.

3. Shuffstall, R. M., and B. Hemmaplardh. 1979. *The Hospital Laboratory; Modern Concepts of Management, Operations, and Finance.* The C.V. Mosby Co., St. Louis, Mo.

4. Snyder, J. R., and D. A. Senhauser. 1989. *Administration and Supervision in Laboratory Medicine,* 2nd ed. J.B. Lippincott, Philadelphia, Pa.

5. Travers, E. M., D. C. Delahunty, L. L. Hunter, K. D. McClatchey, J. M. Rudar. 1998. Basic cost accounting for clinical services. Approved guideline GP11-A. National Committee for Clinical Laboratory Standards, Wayne, Pa.

6. Ullmann, J. E. 1976. *Theory and Problems of Quantitative Methods in Management. Schaum's Outline Series.* McGraw-Hill, New York, N.Y.

APPENDIX 41.1   ROI Calculation Methods

The calculation of the monetary benefit realized as a result of a given capital expenditure is called a return-on-investment or ROI calculation. When this amount is prespecified, it is known as the required rate of return or discount rate for the investment. Major methods for ROI calculations and typical laboratory examples follow.

PAYBACK METHOD

The number of years that a capital investment takes to be fully recovered from cash flow is called the payback period. The simplest method for calculating the return on an investment is the payback method. When payback periods (number of years necessary for incremental cash inflows to equal the capital acquisition cost) for different candidate items are ranked from shortest to longest, the shortest is the best, and the differences between the shortest payback period and the others represent (at least a portion of) the opportunity cost of each investment.

As an example, consider an immunoanalyzer with a purchase price of $100,000 and an estimated useful life of 5 years. Suppose the estimated yearly incremental cash inflow generated by the machine is:

> Year 1 = $55,000
> Year 2 = $55,000
> Year 3 = $58,000
> Year 4 = $60,000
> Year 5 = $45,000
> Total = $273,000

Estimated yearly cash outflows related to the machine are estimated to be:

> Year 1 = $15,000
> Year 2 = $15,000
> Year 3 = $20,000
> Year 4 = $30,000
> Year 5 = $35,000
> Total = $115,000

Calculated net cash flow for each year is then:

> Year 1 = $40,000 (= $55,000 − 15,000)
> Year 2 = $40,000 (= $55,000 − 15,000)
> Year 3 = $38,000 (= $58,000 − 20,000)
> Year 4 = $30,000 (= $60,000 − 30,000)
> Year 5 = $10,000 (= $45,000 − 35,000)
> Total = $158,000

Payback of the original $100,000 occurs between years 2 and 3:

$$\$100,000 = \$40,000 + \$40,000 + [\$20,000].$$

The payback time is

> Year 1 + Year 2 + Year 3 ($20,000/$38,000) = 2.53 years

This method is most useful when comparing projects with similar useful lives and provides a crude measure of risk in the opportunity-cost estimation. It fails, however, to take into account the effects of depreciation or inflation and, more generally, the time value of money, i.e., the best use of funds, and it does not take into account the impact of any cash flows beyond the payback period.

DEPRECIATION

The rate of depreciation is an additional datum often used in the analysis of capital alternatives. Depreciation recognizes the fact that fixed assets have a finite useful life and accounts for this by charging a fraction of the cost of the capital item as an expense in each accounting period of its use. Useful lives of capital items are difficult to establish precisely, so the rate of depreciation (fraction expensed each year) is usually estimated. Different standard methods for performing this estimation (e.g., for tax purposes) are in use.

Straight-line depreciation is a simple, and therefore very commonly used, method for calculating the expensing of capital items. In the straight-line method, the total cost of the item is simply divided by its estimated useful life in years to give the amount to be expensed as depreciation in each period. For example, in our sample problem, (item's price)/(item's useful life) = $100,000/5 years = $20,000 per year listed as depreciation.

The sum of the years' digits (SYD) method of depreciation is a weighted calculation that assigns a large amount of depreciation in the first year, which then declines uniformly to a small amount for the last year. Under this formula, annual rates are derived as follows.

1. Add the ordinal numbers of the years, i.e.,

$$= 1 + 2 + 3 + \ldots + [n' \, (n' - 1)]/2 = S_n$$

2. Write the numbers of the years in reverse order, i.e.,

$$n', n' - 1, n' - 2, \ldots , 3, 2, 1$$

3. The annual fractional rates of depreciation (d) are

$$n'/S_n, (n' - 1)/S_n, (n' - 2)/S_n, \ldots , 3/S_n, 2/S_n, 1/S_n$$

In our example, S_n would be $1 + 2 + 3 + 4 + 5 = 15$, and the yearly fractional depreciation rates would be 5/15 (= 1/3), 4/15, 3/15 (= 1/5), 2/15, 1/15. The actual dollar amounts of annual depreciation would then be:

> Year 1: $100,000(1/3) = $33,333
> Year 2: $100,000(4/15) = $26,667
> Year 3: $100,000(1/5) = $20,000
> Year 4: $100,000(2/15) = $13,333
> Year 5: $100,000(1/15) = $6,667

AVERAGE RATE OF RETURN

The calculation of the average yearly return on a project divided by the average yearly investment it represents is called the average rate of return (ARR) for that investment. When these ARRs are ranked from highest to lowest positive values, the highest ARR is the best. In our example, the average annual investment return = (sum of net cash flows)/(useful life) = $158,000/5 years = $31,600/year. The average annual investment is calculated as follows:

The initial value of the investment = $100,000, and its useful life is 5 years, so the annual straight-line depreciation = $20,000/year. The yearly value of the investment then is:

> Year 1 = $100,000
> Year 2 = $80,000
> Year 3 = $60,000

(continued)

APPENDIX 41.1   ROI Calculation Methods *(continued)*

Year 4 = $40,000
Year 5 = $20,000
Year 6 = $0

The sum of these values for years 1 through 6 total $300,000, and the average annual investment = $300,000/6 years = $50,000/year. The ARR then equals (average annual investment return)/(average annual investment) = $31,600/$50,000 = 63%. This method accounts for all the cash flows, but it does not recognize the time value of money.

TIME VALUE OF MONEY (PRESENT VALUE)

The present value of all the cash flows created by a project minus the amount of the initial investment is called the net present value (NPV) of that investment, or the time value of money involved with it. Present value (PV) represents the dollar amount, which, if it were invested now at a given rate of return (r), would accumulate to a given specified value a specified number of years (n) in the future. The formula for present value assumes that there are unequal annual rates of cash flow (CF) in years 1 to n:

$$PV = [(CF_1)/(1 + r)^1] + [(CF_2)/(1 + r)2] +$$
$$[(CF_3)/(1 + r)^3] + \ldots + [(CF_n)/(1 + r)^n]$$

When NPVs of different projects are ranked from highest to lowest positive values, the highest NPV is the best. In our example, if the required rate of return r = 10% and the term n = 5

years, the PV would equal the sum of the annual net cash flows according to the above formula:

$$PV = [\$40,000/(1.10)] + [\$40,000/(1.10)^2] +$$
$$[\$38,000/(1.10)^3] + [\$30,000/(1.10)^4] + [\$10,000/(1.10)^5] =$$
$$\$44,000 + \$48,400 + \$50,578 +$$
$$\$43,923 + \$16,105 = \$203,006$$

NPV = PV – initial investment =
$$\$203,006 - \$100,000 = \$103,006$$

This method accounts explicitly for the time value of money and evaluates projects at a common required rate of return, but does not take into account differences in the size of different investments or allow easy comparison of projects with different useful lives. These considerations must be kept in mind in the final analysis.

Inflation, of course, corrects for changes in the value of money itself over time. The effect of inflation can be calculated as follows: If prices increase at a rate of i per year, and if an item costs P0 now, then n years from now it will cost $A_n = P_0 e^{in}$, using a general exponential formula for continuous compounding of interest. In our example, if the rate of inflation is 2% per year, the cost of our $100,000 immunoanalyzer in 5 years will be:

$$A_5 = (\$100,000)e^{[(.02)(5)]} = (\$100,000)e^{(.10)} =$$
$$(\$100,000)(1.1052) = \$110,520$$

APPENDIX 41.2 Financing Alternatives

Methodology based on calculation of the present value is relevant for making choices among alternative sources of funding for capital acquisition.

PURCHASE

In the case of purchase from hospital funds, the present value equals the initial investment. Returning to the example of the immunoanalyzer in Appendix 41.1, purchase with hospital funds involves a cash outflow of $100,000.

For purchase with borrowed funds, the present value equals the annual loan payments plus interest, discounted at the required rate of return for the term of the loan. In the example, for a loan with a term $n = 5$ years, a required rate of return $r = 10\%$, and an annual loan payment CF at 12% interest = $27,168, the PV of loan payments, discounted at 10%, is calculated by using the formula for PV with even cash flows:

$$PV = CF \{[1 - (1 + r)^{-n}]/r\} = \$27,168$$
$$\{[1 - (1.10)^{-5}]/0.10\} = \$27,168(3.7908) = \$102,988$$

LEASE

A 5-year lease with a required rate of return $r = 10\%$ and an annual lease payment CF of $24,000 has a PV of lease payments, discounted at 10%, calculated as follows using the formula for PV with even cash flows:

$$PV = CF \{[1 - (1 + r)^{-n}]/r\} = \$24,000$$
$$\{[1 - (1.10)^{-5}]/0.10\} = \$24,000(3.7908) = \$90,797$$

Here the alternative with the *lowest* present value is the best method, in this case the lease. If this is to be a noncancelable lease and there is no potential opportunity to sell the equipment at the end of the lease term, no further analysis is required. If, on the other hand, the equipment can be sold at the end of the lease (i.e., it has what is known as a salvage market), further analysis is relevant. If the PV for the lease is subtracted from the PV for the purchase, the result will be positive and represent the PV of the amount required to be obtained from the future resale.

This should then be compared with the best estimate of the future market for this resale. If it looks as if the equipment can be sold for more than the required future resale price, then purchase is favored; if not, then leasing is. The lease-or-loan decision can be approached in the same way.

In the example,

PV of resale = PV of purchase – PV of lease =
$$\$100,000 - 90,797 = \$9,203$$

Required future value of resale to provide for PV of resale is

$$PV(1 + r)^n = \$9,203(1.10)^5 = \$9,203(1.61051) = \$14,821$$

which is what the future resale will have to fetch at the end of 5 years. For the choice between lease or loan,

PV of resale = PV of loan – PV of lease =
$$\$102,988 - 90,797 = \$12,191$$

The required proceeds of the resale will then be

$$PV(1 + r)^n = \$12,191(1.10)^5 = \$12,191(1.61051) = \$19,633$$

Thus, if the resale nets $9,202 or less, leasing is favored; at $9,203, there's no difference between leasing and borrowing; in the range $9,204 to $19,622, borrowing is favored; at $19,633, there's no difference between leasing and purchasing; and at $19,634 or greater, purchasing is favored.

Outreach: Obstacles to Hospital Outreach and Enhancing Customer Satisfaction

Beth H. Deaton

OBJECTIVES

To understand the items that must be in place to compete in the outreach market and why some will conflict with hospital practices and policies

To understand how to capitalize on the strengths of the hospital or health system

To understand the obstacles that must be overcome as part of a hospital or health system

To understand all of the pieces that make up customer service

To know when to say yes and when to say no to customers

To be able to plan the customer service aspects of the outreach program

You need to show some insensitivity to the organization's history in order to show the proper respect for its future. Be willing to break with the past.

PRICE PRITCHETT

WINDING THROUGH A COMPLEX HOSPITAL SYSTEM to set up a service that in many respects flies in the face of conventional hospital thinking is a daunting and complex task. Hospitals have many policies in place that work well for them, but hospital laboratory outreach programs compete with large national reference laboratories for their place in the market and need to be able to act and respond in a similar way. This means changing hospital policies or having exceptions made for parts of the outreach business. The level of customer service the laboratory decides to provide will in many cases decide the level of success the outreach program will achieve. What many fail to realize is that this is a decision that is made by the policies put in place and management's actions. The ability of the organization and the staff members to communicate quickly and accurately with its customers and the ability to then respond to issues can be deciding factors in the success of the program.

Making Organizational Changes

A hospital outreach program needs to operate differently than a hospital laboratory department. The laboratory needs to evaluate the test menu, where testing is performed, the turnaround time that is available, as well as its management,

685

equipment, and staffing. In an outreach program, where cost is of primary concern, volume is the name of the game. Because approximately a third of the cost of producing a laboratory test is fixed, the volume of testing that is produced will be paramount to reducing cost on a per-test level. Fixed costs are costs that do not vary with volume. Examples would be depreciation, administration and management, some full-time equivalents (FTEs) (those necessary for coverage), professional fees (Part A coverage), license fees, controls, and standards. To begin to build volume and expand the test menu, look at other entities within the organization. Other hospitals and nursing homes can provide much-needed volume. However, other facilities will not be eager to give up this volume. They will only be willing to participate if they achieve a financial advantage.

Centralize Work

Review the volume of send-out testing by test. By consolidating to one location, the laboratory may have enough volume to bring some testing in-house. Then review the more esoteric testing being performed at other facilities in your organization. If there is more than one hospital, clinic, physician office laboratory, or home health agency in the health system, review the testing that is performed in those settings. Centralize as much of the testing as possible to the central laboratory. Special Chemistry is usually a good place to start. This may need to be done in steps, depending on the politics of the organization and its philosophy about change. Review the testing offered at each site and agree on a standard list of tests that will be performed at each site. In return, the central laboratory will have to agree to and meet stringent service standards. By consolidating the test volume, the laboratory will be able to lower test expenses for everyone by reducing fixed costs on a per-test basis, reducing FTEs, and standardizing.

Place Laboratory Management on Off Shifts

Another area that will need to be reviewed is management. Place appropriate laboratory management personnel on off shifts, because that is where the workload will be the heaviest. Management structure needs to be addressed very early in the analysis of outreach. While the laboratory is reviewing the testing from other system facilities, it may be a good time to entertain complete laboratory integration. If the laboratory is not ready to go that far, it will need to assess its internal management. More laboratory testing will be performed on the second and third shifts than ever before, so management resources need to be in place on those shifts. Technicians who are in charge, but still working the bench, will not suffice. Someone who has leadership qualities and is authorized to make decisions throughout the entire laboratory should be on each shift, at least Monday through Friday. The reporting relationships can be structured in a number of ways. For example, each shift manager can be responsible for the Human Relations duties (hiring, firing, and employment reviews) on the shift he or she is on, as well as be responsible for a specific clinical area (Chemistry, Hematology, Microbiology, etc.). The shift manager can report to a supervisor who has Human Relations responsibilities, while assigning the clinical responsibility to a shift leader or different manager. Another option would be to have all of the staff report to managers who rotate management responsibilities to all shifts.

Give Outreach Its Due

Make Outreach High-Profile

Make sure the outreach laboratory's place in hospital management is high-profile. Outreach programs complicate laboratory operations and increase the level of complexity of every area within the laboratory. For this reason the laboratory needs to ensure it has an appropriate place in the organizational structure of the system or the hospital. The person in charge of the laboratory needs to have the ability to access every major department and to have resources allocated to the laboratory that are important to ensure the business can grow and operate efficiently. The person in charge of the laboratory should be at least a director and should attend the workgroup meetings with hospital leadership. If successful (usually based on revenue), there will be a point where the laboratory should be able to break away from hospital management and operate as an entity on its own. Laboratory management must be at an appropriate level in the organization to communicate what outreach testing encompasses and must be able to enlist the help of senior management when needed.

Manage Outreach as a Business, Not a Department

The laboratory outreach program must be viewed and operated as a business, not as a department (cost center) of the hospital. Laboratories in hospitals are typically treated as cost centers. Depending on how an organization displays department financial statements, revenue is sometimes not even on the statements seen by the department, only expenses. This gives rise to the attitude, and subsequent management, of the laboratory as a cost center. When the outreach business begins to operate, the financial statements need to reflect the revenue procured by the program, the reimbursements, and the expenses. If this cannot be done on the current hospital monthly financial statements produced by Finance, it is imperative that these data be made available for review in order to manage the laboratory.

Information Technology Changes

Hospital Systems versus Separate Systems

Should hospital systems be used to operate the outreach program or would it be better to use different systems? A system that allows separation of the billing and financial operation of the outreach program from the rest of the hospital is optimal. For several reasons, it is best if the laboratory can manage both patient and client billing and receivables separately from hospital-based patients. Hospital systems require a great deal of patient demographic information that is not necessary or cost-efficient to collect for reference laboratory patients. Because other reference laboratories do not require the expanded information, if the laboratory is forced to collect such information, it will be at a disadvantage in the marketplace.

The average revenue per bill is significantly lower for the laboratory than for other hospital services. Hospital patient accounting departments focus on the high-dollar accounts. Often, reference laboratory accounts are below the level for even a cursory review, leaving the laboratory struggling to obtain reimbursement from payors and patients. If these things can be addressed with the current hospital system, then you would be wise to use it. Otherwise, look to the laboratory system or an outsource vendor.

Client billing is an area where the hospital patient accounting department will have little or no experience. The laboratory's ability to accurately bill, adjust, and manage these accounts will be a direct reflection of its ability to compete in the outreach world. Even if the laboratory is unable to convince Finance to relinquish management of the patient accounts, Finance may be happy to have the laboratory manage the client accounts. This is an area that needs monthly management, and the ability to access the laboratory system to review charges and testing performed is advantageous.

Nonstaff Physicians

Nonstaff physicians may present a problem when working with the hospital system. The physician database in the HIS (hospital information system) is built with very few, if any, nonstaff physicians. There is an overriding principal that says that if the medical staff office does not approve the physician, he or she will not be entered into the system. Outreach will require that the laboratory be able to accept, process, and bill for specimens received from nonstaff physicians. The physicians must be put into the database so they can appear on the bill and patient results can be correctly routed. The laboratory must be diligent in updating the database, as physicians will continually enter, leave, and move within the geographic area.

Data Interface

As the program grows, others are going to want the data that can be mined from the system for a variety of purposes. Health Plans will want the data sliced and diced for utilization and for the employer reporting that it is required to deliver. Physician offices will want to interface with the system or an intermediate product so that they do not need to rekey results. Pharmacy will want to review the microbiology susceptibility profile of organisms to review how infections are reacting to drugs. Others will want the data, blind and in other formats, to use for research. The system used will determine, to a large extent, the laboratory's ability to provide data to other systems. After HIPAA (Health Insurance Portability and Accountability Act) considerations are reviewed, the next question is what value the laboratory and outreach programs gain from an interface. It will be the responsibility of the laboratory staff to ensure that the data are crossing the interfaces and displaying properly. Each time a change is made to either system, the laboratory will need to keep the interfaces in mind and ensure that data continue to flow properly.

Patient Registration and Accounting Concerns

The demographic data required for most insurance companies for an outpatient bill include: patient name, date of birth, address, Social Security number, ordering physician, diagnosis, insurance company, insurance address, group number, and member or subscriber identifier. This list is significantly shorter than the list of requirements for an inpatient admission or hospital-based service. This seemingly simple issue can make or break specimen processing. The laboratory must be able to collect only what is absolutely required for outreach billing. The list of information for client billing is even more abbreviated, and a separate process will need to be developed to bill these accounts.

The issue of multiple fee schedules can be problematic because some hospitals believe that multiple fee schedules are a compliance issue. Careful review of the Model Laboratory Compliance Program will reveal this is not true. As long as the laboratory is charging each segment of the business above cost, the compliance standards have been met. After convincing the hospital compliance staff that it is indeed okay to have multiple fee schedules, the laboratory will need to be able to manage the fee schedules. The system chosen for billing must have the capability to have multiple fee schedules, to set up contracts for individual clients, and to apply percentage discounts. It is important to develop and enforce a strict set of fee policies from the beginning. As part of the compliance program, all fees should be reviewed each year against the policies that have been set and in relation to the cost of testing.

The form used for billing will determine, for some insurance companies, how the laboratory is reimbursed. Hospitals bill using a UB92 form, because this is the form required for hospitals. Freestanding laboratories and other Part B providers bill on an HCFA/CMS-1500. Some insurance plans will require that the laboratory bill on a HCFA form and therefore be treated as an outpatient or reference laboratory and not as part of the hospital. These differences are important because they may affect the amount patients are required to pay. Patients' insurance benefits are often different if they visit a hospital versus a reference laboratory. Even if the laboratory testing was picked up from the physician office, the insurance company will have no way to make the distinction between the outreach laboratory and the hospital outpatient. The patient will therefore be charged the hospital copay or coinsurance, which is usually higher than if the testing was sent to a reference laboratory (see Appendixes 42.1 and 42.2).

Populating the Patient Record

Requirements by the hospital to populate the patient record with results may prove burdensome. In most hospital systems, client billing is out of the norm. The patients billed to physician offices are not seen as patients within the system, but only the client account is seen as a patient. Therefore, it is difficult to update the patient record/history that already exists on the system. The laboratory could decide not to populate the patient history with reference laboratory information. This is not the best solution, because one of the advantages sold to customers is the continuum of care. Outreach results in the patient's hospital history offer an advantage that sets an outreach program apart from the stand-alone laboratories. There are numerous information technology solutions that can be applied, but they take planning, capital, and forward thinking.

Physician Office Connectivity

Physician Office Connectivity is a system that allows physicians to register and order their patients' laboratory testing from their offices. The information the office inputs will flow to the laboratory system. Depending on the vendor used, clients can register patients, review results on-line, screen for medical necessity, usually graph results over time, and have on-line lookup to the laboratory test guide, as well as many other functions. The patient registration portion is the piece that will be difficult for the hospital. Allowing nonemployees to create or add to patient records is not normal for most hospitals. This connectivity is critical, however, to procure the large, lucrative clients that are sending testing to the bigger laboratories because those laboratories have computer systems in many offices that allow this functionality. To compete with the reference laboratories for these practices, the laboratory will need to support this technology. It will also help the outreach program obtain better registration information, reduce medical necessity denials, properly identify testing desired, and deliver results. Overall, there should probably be an upside in terms of FTE reductions.

Meeting the Needs

Capital

In most hospital systems capital funding is difficult to obtain, because competition for the limited funds is fierce and because the outreach program may not be a priority for the hospital. It is also sometimes difficult to purchase the things that are vital to outreach programs, such as cars and printers. Finance and Hospital Administration need to be continuously educated about the outreach business and why these items are necessary for program success. Leasing cars and printers is an option, depending on how the organization views these types of agreements. The advantage to leasing is that the leasing company will usually service the equipment for a flat fee. The service is usually worth the price.

FTEs

Anytime the hospital is experiencing a budget crunch, one of the first things to occur is a freeze on FTEs. Even when no freeze is in effect, approval of FTEs can be an arduous process. This is difficult for a growing business. The laboratory must have contingency plans for replacement of key FTEs, like couriers, should open positions occur. Maintaining a few part-time employees is a great option if you can keep these positions filled. A temporary employment service can help with staffing, but keep in mind the lead time required for training. Temp services can help in other areas. If you plan correctly and have portions of jobs that can be easily delegated and require little training, these responsibilities can be given to a temp. The best, but most expensive, option for courier coverage is to have contracts with one or more local courier services. Form relationships with these vendors and share route information in advance of requiring their help.

Hospital versus Outreach Contracting

Defining Insurance Plans

Define the important insurance plans in your area. If the hospital or system owns physician practices, use their information to determine the major insurance companies in the area. If not, the hospital should be able to supply its payor mix. Medicare, Medicaid, and most point-of-service plans accept any provider. If the insurance company allows it, apply for a provider number separate from that of the hospital. If the laboratory is viewed by the insurance company as a laboratory and not just part of the hospital, it is sometimes easier to get a lower copay for patients, but the reimbursement is also reduced. Review the other insurance companies and identify the most important payors.

Ability To Contract on Your Own

Obtain permission to contract on your own within certain parameters. The hospital contracting department can be a tremendous help, but to the extent possible, have someone who knows the outreach business do the contracting. At a minimum, attend the meetings during contract negotiations. This has several benefits. You are the expert about the laboratory outreach business, and you may be able to save a contract that the hospital thinks cannot be administered. The laboratory may also decide, again because you know the business, that the administrative burdens of the contract are too costly for the reimbursement offered. Also, if the laboratory is in control of the negotiations, you should be able to control the timeline to coincide with the volume you want or need for the laboratory.

Acceptance of Payors

The laboratory does not have to accept all payors, but will need to participate with most providers to secure the business of clients. Plan to be shocked as you review the various terms and pricing structures set out by some of the insurance companies. This is another area that the hospital will have difficulty understanding. The idea that the laboratory can accept reimbursement that is significantly below the fee schedule will be difficult to sell. Know and understand the laboratory costs and the reimbursement that can be accepted. Do not accept low capitation rates or fee schedules that do not cover at least the variable cost in the hope that the laboratory will make up the difference on the "pull-through" business. First, this can be a compliance problem, because Medicare may see this as an inducement. Second, there is no way to be assured the pull-through business will materialize. Always request utilization data. For large populations, data should be required.

Failure To Understand Financial Implications and Requirements

Unrelated Business Income Tax

Unrelated business income tax (UBIT) is an income tax that must be filed annually. Make sure that the corporate finance office understands the outreach business and will file this return for the outreach program. The income tax rate is 40% of the unrelated net income. Depending on the practices using outreach services, not all of the income will be taxable. The laboratory may be able to exclude some of the clients because they are corporately "related" to the outreach program. Work closely with the finance tax department to clearly understand the income that can be excluded from the calculation. Keep the work papers and reports used to produce this information. Large changes in not-for-profit companies usually trigger an audit.

Other Taxes

Other taxes that the laboratory may be subject to include sales tax, business license tax, and personal property tax. Depending on the tax status of the parent company and the laws in your locality or state, some or all of these taxes may apply to the outreach business. The hospital may not have detailed information about some of these taxes, because it may not be required to pay them. But the outreach business may be required to pay some or all of these taxes. Investigate which taxes will need to be paid and, if necessary, build these taxes into the expenses for the outreach program.

Understanding the Hospital's Point of View

There are generally some underlying reasons for, or a charter for, an outreach business. The hospital has expectations that must continue to be met, even as the laboratory progresses from a cost center to a product line.

Lower Cost per Test

Securing the laboratory testing of a hospital or hospital system is usually one of the main objectives of an outreach program. A hospital's cost per test is generally high because of fixed costs and underutilized resources. By adding volume to a facility, the cost per test decreases, assuming minimal incremental resources are added. Employees and equipment are not fully utilized on off shifts. The balancing act for outreach is to add testing to fill this void. This will work for a while, during the time the outreach program begins to build its business. As Outreach grows and outgrows the unused capacity, be careful to add testing and resources that make sense. Cost per test should at worst remain static after an initial drop, but even as resources must be added, cost per test should continue to decrease. This will be imperative for long-term success.

Make Money

The hospital will, at worst, expect the laboratory outreach business to break even on direct expenses and make a contribution to hospital and system expenses. It is important to be able to produce financial documents, get them in the hands of the right people, and have a break-even financial position. UBIT will be a factor, but there may be other unrelated business lines that are losing money. The hospital may be able to apply the outreach income against those losses to avoid paying UBIT.

Translating Hospital and Laboratory Compliance for an Outreach Operation

All hospital laboratories should have a written compliance plan in place. A current active compliance plan will help keep the laboratory on track during outreach implementation; however, the plan will need to be modified, and some policies not previously applicable will need to be added.

Physician Communication

The depth and breadth of physician communication will probably need to be improved. This communication must include information related to compliance policies. Medical necessity and advanced beneficiary notices will need to be explained. Billing practices will need to be covered in detail. Specifically, physicians need to know what is included in various panels and when more than one Current Procedural Terminology (CPT) code is billed for a group test. A clinical pathologist contact must be listed, with information on how that person can be reached. Take this opportunity to explain other compliance policies, like supply orders, standing orders, reflex testing, and requisitions (Appendix 42.3).

Medicare Secondary Payor Questionnaires

Medicare secondary payor (MSP) questionnaires are completed in the current hospital setting when patients first present to the hospital. There has been a recent change in legislation that no longer requires hospital outreach programs to complete the MSP questionnaire. There is still the burden of determining if Medicare is the primary payor, but the questionnaire is not mandatory (Appendix 42.4).

Physician Acknowledgments

Physician acknowledgments must be completed if the laboratory is going to allow physicians to order non-CPT-approved panels. For instance, if the laboratory allows a physician group to create a panel that includes all of the components of the basic metabolic panel plus serum glutamic oxalacetic transaminase (SGOT), the group must sign a physician acknowledgment. The acknowledgment must include the CPT codes that will be billed, the charges, and the expected Medicare reimbursement. There is also specific language required. It states (i) that the physician understands that the only laboratory tests that should be ordered are those that he or she believes are medically necessary for the care of the patient; (ii) that he or she is aware that using a customized profile may result in the ordering of tests for which Medicare or other federally funded healthcare programs may deny payment; (iii) that as the ordering physician, he or she will order individual tests or a less inclusive profile when not all of the tests included in the customized profile are medically necessary for an individual patient; and (iv) that as the ordering physician, he or she understands that the Office of the Inspector General (OIG) takes the position that a physician who orders medically unnecessary tests may be subject to civil penalties. These notices must be completed annually (6) (Appendix 42.5).

Advance Beneficiary Notices

Train, train, train, and train some more. This is the only way to have hope that the laboratory will receive advance beneficiary notices (ABNs) as necessary. It is the laboratory's responsibility to properly train the physician offices, when appropriate, to collect and properly complete an ABN. The new instructions for ABNs are more clear and concise than ever before. Even if the laboratory industry does not agree with everything in the new policy, it has opened up some areas for recourse not previously available. Remember, if the physician does not provide the laboratory with a correct diagnosis code or an ABN, and the laboratory does not get paid, the physician is unaffected. However, there is a provision in the instructions that will allow the laboratory to collect an ABN after the specimen has been received but before the test is performed. The patient can be called for authorization to perform the test and then a follow-up ABN can be sent by mail (1). This presents obvious processing problems, but does leave an avenue to pursue for this particular problem.

Beware of physician practices that collect too many ABNs. The ABN should only be collected *when appropriate* (i.e., when there is a valid reason to believe the test will not be paid for by Medicare). Also, remember that the new instructions require a copy of the form be given to the patient. If the laboratory does not prepare the forms in duplicate, the patient will probably not get a copy at the physician office. Remember, it is the laboratory's reimbursement at stake and therefore the laboratory's responsibility to train the physician office to collect this information when necessary.

Requisition Design

The requisition design should be carefully planned and evaluated. If a requisition is already in place, a comprehensive review should be completed before using it for outreach purposes. Ensure that billing for panels is properly represented and that all components of a panel, as well as the panel, can be ordered. Make sure the form flows easily for data-processing purposes. Carefully select the tests that will appear on the requisition. Too many or too few tests can be problematic. Leave space for write-ins, but place instructions on the requisition that detail the required information for write-in tests. There is required language from the Model Laboratory Compliance Program about ordering of tests that must be on the requisition (6). Supply proper space for all of the billing information. Use this opportunity to denote when an ABN might be necessary and when there will be a separate bill from the professional group. And last, make sure the laboratory's phone number is on the form. Provision for storage of requisitions must also be considered; these requisitions/orders will need to be retained for a minimum of 5 years. The requisitions must be accessible for audits, but not necessarily stored on-site, and electronic storage is acceptable.

Pricing

Special pricing should be carefully considered on a case-by-case basis. There should be an overriding policy that dictates pricing and discount guidelines (6). Pricing for any client-bill portion of an account must be determined separately from pricing of other testing that will be received. A client bill is for the testing that is billed directly back to the physician/client rather than to an insurance company. Do not cost-shift between payors (client, Medicare, and other insurance) to win an account. Cost shifting is when the laboratory uses profits from one portion of the account, Medicare for instance, to offset shortfalls in profitability from another portion, for instance the client-bill portion. Each part of the testing received must be profitable.

Add-On Tests

There must be a policy that covers how add-on tests will be processed. An add-on test is a test that is requested on a specimen after the initial requisition is received. When an add-on is called in, it must be followed by a written order and, if needed, the laboratory must be able to produce that order, just as if it were a requisition. An internal process to determine specimen availability and quantity also needs to be considered. This is probably an instance when the technical section should be involved. Even if specimen processing is responsible for locating the specimen, the technical section should assess specimen viability and adequacy before responding to the client. Requiring the order to be faxed before processing the additional test request alleviates the issue of matching the phone order with the written order before billing. Otherwise, a review of the phone orders every 30 days is advised.

National Coverage Policies

The new policies for medical necessity became effective November 25, 2002. A negotiated rule-making process that included members from the laboratory industry, physicians, and officials from Centers for Medicare and Medicaid Services (CMS) developed these policies. Local carriers and financial intermediaries are allowed to add to the policies or add new policies but may not delete parts of the existing policy. It has been about two years since the policies were promulgated, so we can reasonably expect that changes will be requested soon after their implementation.

Sanctioned Physicians

A policy for identification and resolution of specimens received from sanctioned physicians will need to be put in place. Sanctioned physicians are doctors who have been restricted from submitting claims and ordering services for Medicare patients. Most laboratory and hospital compliance programs bar the hospital and laboratory from doing business with sanctioned physicians for any testing. Hospital Admissions uses the medical staff office to research doctors and determine their status and grant privileges, if appropriate. In the outreach business, specimens will be presented to the laboratory from physicians who are not on the medical staff. The laboratory will need to be able to identify physicians who have been sanctioned to know whether or not to process the test. If the test is not going to be processed, the specimen should be made available for pickup.

Contracts

A standard client contract will need to be developed and approved by the legal department. The contract should be signed by all clients, but it will be a requirement for clients who have a client bill. Try to keep the contract short (three pages or less) and include only key points. In the agreement, set the terms of the agreement, including payment terms, compliance guidelines, services offered, fees, requirements concerning retention of records, where to send contract changes, and governing law. The legal department will also have a number of items it will want to include.

Audits and Reviews

Each of the areas discussed here will need to be reviewed annually, and some areas will require an audit. Add-ons, sanctioned physicians, physician acknowledgments, and requisitions should be reviewed or audited annually. Billing (including ABNs and medical necessity forms) should be audited more often. For the items that require an audit there should be a specified format followed and the documentation should be maintained for a minimum of 2 years.

Participation and Cooperation

An outreach program is a large undertaking and will require changes in every area of the laboratory, including Transfusion Services, Anatomic Pathology, Professional Services, Immunology, and Cytology. Each area will need to review its operations, make decisions, and perhaps create new policies to prepare for the new business.

If successful, the second and third laboratory shifts will change from a slower pace to the busiest time of the day. Successful outreach business is based on the ability of the second- and third-shift employees to complete the bulk of the outreach testing on these shifts. Equipment, staffing, and facility design will need to be examined to ensure that a larger volume of testing can be produced in the time frame required. A review of on-site testing will also be necessary. With the additional testing that will be procured, tests that were previously sent out will be able to be, and should be, performed in-house. The decreased turnaround time for these tests will benefit not only the outreach program but the hospital patients as well.

Transfusion services. Although Outreach will not get involved in transfusion of patients, blood typing and screening and ABO and Rh tests will be ordered. Transfusion Services needs to decide how these specimens will be handled in relation to patient history. Because it is widely believed that patient identification is not as carefully monitored in the physician office setting, outreach testing is sometimes excluded from the patient history lookup in Transfusion. If that decision is made, then outreach specimens for transfusion testing must be ordered and processed differently than for hospital patients. The policies for this area need to be developed and communicated before Transfusion Services receives outreach specimens.

Anatomic pathology. Many of the items discussed for the clinical laboratory also apply to Anatomic Pathology. The same shift of workload, in terms of time of day, will occur in Anatomic Pathology. Additionally, Anatomic Pathology may want to evaluate whether it wants a different numbering sequence for the cases received from Outreach. This is an area where the continuum of care is very valuable for clinicians and should be marketed.

Professional services. Reimbursement for professional pathology services needs to be discussed and decided upon prior to beginning sales for Outreach. This is especially true for any client-bill testing. Normally, the professional component for testing is included with the clinical portion for client billing. This means that the laboratory must have a method to capture and pay the professional group for those services. The fee schedule for the professional group must also be completed beforehand so that the fees for the clients can be set to include this cost. If the professional group has a company that does its billing, it may be able to bill the outreach program for the testing. The laboratory may also want to agree with the pathologists about how much the patients will be charged and how the demographic and insurance information for patient billing will be transferred to the pathologist.

Immunology. This department is often separate from the "regular" laboratory, and the department may or may not be willing to accept specimens from the outreach program. Determine if this is a service that can be offered and what hours it will operate. Usually, Immunology's requirements for specimen transportation are very strict, so transportation will need to be arranged outside of that for the clinical laboratory. Immunology may be interested in using the processes the outreach program sets up for delivery of results and client billing.

Cytology (gynecologic and nongynecologic). Pap smears will be an important part of the outreach business. Determine the acceptable turnaround time for the market. If beginning the outreach program as a new program, this is one area where resources may need to be invested. Hospitals do not traditionally perform many Pap smears, so cytology may lack the ability to easily add volume. The laboratory will need to address the issue of liquid-based versus traditional Pap smears. It is my opinion that if the laboratory can afford it and the physician community agrees, you should market only the newest and best technology, the liquid-based Pap. If the hospital offers nongynecologic cytology, this service could be marketed as a niche. Few laboratories have this capability and the professional expertise that is needed, so this is an excellent service to develop as a niche and "get your foot in the door" with many

clients. This testing is expensive, so do not underprice it, but offer short turnaround time and superior professional expertise and the outreach program will have a great place to begin to make its mark.

Enhancing Customer Satisfaction: Communication

It has been said that you need to communicate seven times in seven ways . . . and it still will not be enough. Keep this in mind when implementing a new program or making changes to existing programs and policies for staff and clients. It will help remind those communicating that once, twice, or even three times is probably not enough. There are some things that can be done to help with this endeavor.

Create a consistent format and brand for all communication. This includes the name of the outreach program, the letterhead, the logo, and the format of the newsletter, guidebook, and any other printed material used for the lab program. Use either the hospital logo or one that is created for the laboratory program. If the hospital has good name recognition and a good reputation in the community, the laboratory program should use that advantage. Use a consistent name for the program: ABC Reference Lab, or ABC Lab Services, or Labs "R" Us. It is important that the same name be used consistently. This consistency will help to begin to create an image and recognition for the outreach program.

Newsletter

A newsletter can be a great communication and marketing tool if done correctly. If the laboratory is going to publish a newsletter, it should be published on a regular schedule in a consistent format and should deal with issues that are important to the laboratory and the clients. Do not let the client newsletter double as the employee newsletter. It is acceptable to profile the laboratory director and some of the other managers, but do not list birthdays, weddings, births, etc. The newsletter should be professional in its writing and presentation. Do put the logo and name prominently on the newsletter. Do tell about new procedures performed in the laboratory. It is acceptable to put technical information in the newsletter. Include policy changes that will affect the clients. Do use it as a marketing tool, by telling everyone about proficiency testing excellence, courier on-time information, phone answer times, and turnaround time statistics. However, remember that although the newsletter is delivered faithfully, it will only be read by about 30% of the clients.

Couriers

Couriers can be important assets in communicating with clients, and they can be used to carry short, uncomplicated messages. Generally, they only have a few moments in the office, so the communication must be short and straightforward. To entice the couriers to disseminate information, reward them for results. For instance, we have rewarded our couriers for improvement in the packaging of their clients' specimens. In this case the message was "Fold the requisition and put it in the bag so we can see the patient information at the top of the form." The prize for the courier whose clients had the highest-percentage standardization was a gift certificate to a nice restaurant. The improvement for the laboratory was our ability to sort the specimens before they were unpackaged. Couriers can be great communicators and ambassadors for the laboratory. They are in the clients' places of business every day. They represent the laboratory, so choose them carefully, use them wisely, and praise them for the job they do.

Marketing and Sales Team

The marketing and sales team should be used to communicate more in-depth issues and to reinforce information contained in the newsletter. These employees should be excellent communicators. They need to be comfortable speaking with people of all ages, education levels, and nationalities. There should be a standard communication checklist completed with each client setup. The marketing staff is limited, so they will not be able to visit all of the clients each time a communication is necessary. Also, since this may be the same staff that is responsible for sales, do not consume all of their time communicating to current clients about operations. Use this staff for operational communication only when it is very important.

Laboratory Guidebook

The laboratory guidebook should be complete and concise. Use the guidebook to provide comprehensive information about the laboratory and its operations, policies (including forms), testing, specimen preparation, result reporting, billing, staff, and licensure. The guidebook should serve as the client's primary source of information about the laboratory. If successful in its layout and content, the guidebook should reduce calls to the laboratory. Use the logo and name branding discussed earlier on the cover and throughout the guide.

Take this opportunity to list all of the management staff, the pathologists, and any other specially trained personnel on staff. Give their names, degrees, certification, and phone numbers. Provide information on important policies. Information about the policy on laboratory compliance, medical necessity, inclement weather, how to complete a requisition, patient confidentiality, specimen retention, and ordering supplies should all be available in the guidebook. Give step-by-step instructions for collection and preparation of *all* specimens, not just urine and blood. Publish the list of tests that must be transported frozen and the tests that can be ordered STAT.

The most important portion of the guidebook is the test listing. Make sure that this section is user friendly. Use the names of tests that are typically used across the laboratory industry, not the computer nomenclature used in the laboratory. List the sample size and tube requirement, the CPT code(s), how often the test is performed, the expected turnaround time, the reference range, and any special instructions for collection and preservation. Unfortunately, the minute the directory is published, it will already be out of date. If the guidebook can be posted on a website, updates can be made often. For the printed guidebook, it is very important to send out updates as changes occur and to revise the guidebook every 18 months to two years. If this resource becomes very outdated, the program begins to lose credibility as a reference laboratory in the community.

Website

A website can be a very useful tool. In its most advanced form it can be used to replace the guidebook for many offices and can include interactive communication with the laboratory that the client might require, with the exception of the actual pickup of the specimens. If the local medical community is very computer literate and the laboratory is willing to invest the time and money, the website can enable clients to place supply orders, look up information on tests, register patients, order tests, look up results, print results, request a courier pickup, or change the time of a pickup. The possibilities are endless. Web design should be carefully thought out and again identified with the prominent name and logo. There are many software products available that have the functionality described.

Focus Group

Focus groups can be organized to help the laboratory with marketing and change. A focus group should consist of 10 to 15 clients. The clients selected should be important to the outreach program but not necessarily the largest clients. A particular client may be chosen because he or she represents a specialty that is important or uses a portion of the laboratory that is marketed as a niche market. Include people who are not afraid to be critical. Recognize that they are giving their time for the laboratory program. Make them feel important for being "chosen," but do not forget that they are "donating" their time; do not waste it. The meetings should be about an hour, and the agenda should be comprehensive but clear. This should be not an information session but a fact-gathering session. The clients should do most of the talking, so make sure someone who is comfortable with that format is available to lead the meeting. Use this group to review new print pieces that are in development, the guidebook format and new programs and to let them learn about new testing prior to official publications. Solicit their ideas for improved ways to deliver appropriate information.

Customer Satisfaction Assessment

Surveys

Conduct a survey of the clients annually. There are many topics on which to solicit input from clients. Couriers, turnaround time, test menu, client services, billing, technical staff, professional services, pricing, marketing, print routines, and fax services are a few areas that may be considered. Carefully select the questions for the first survey. Changing the survey questions makes comparison between surveys difficult and not necessarily valid. The survey should be no longer than 40 questions and should include room for client comments. Be prepared for a low response rate. A 30% response rate is considered very successful. Designing ways to improve the response rate is tricky because most respondents also want to remain anonymous. Be prepared to change once the survey is complete and the data are tabulated. Completing a survey is only worthwhile if the laboratory heeds the results and uses them to improve the outreach program.

Quality assurance monitors should be developed for the outreach program. Use the same kinds of measures in the outreach operations that are used in laboratory operations. Know what is expected of the program and measure against that baseline. Establish thresholds for call abandon rate, on-time courier pickup, call wait time, registration accuracy, missed pickups, and lost specimens. Track numbers on a daily basis. The numbers of tests performed by section per day, the number of requisitions processed, and the number of daily courier pickups will help identify staffing requirements and find weaknesses. Outreach volume is not the same every day, not even Monday through Friday. Know the peak-volume times and days and plan resources accordingly.

Problem Reporting and Resolution

Have a defined process for problem reporting and resolution. There are a number of policies that should be written and tested before the first phone call is answered. All calls should be logged. If a system is not available for this purpose, use paper logs. What happens when a client calls for a result, because of a printer problem or missed pickup, or with a specimen collection question? Why did they need to call? What is the laboratory's response? Who handles the call? What about patient confidentiality? How do you track the calls? By patient? By client? By call type? Having someone answer the phone and provide the result quickly and courteously is only the first step. Problem reporting and resolution should be a defined cycle. Responses to the typical questions should be quick, efficient, and automatic.

The use of remote printers and faxes is an effective, efficient means to communicate results. A policy needs to be in place to troubleshoot this equipment over the phone. The policy should detail what to do if the initial troubleshooting does not work and should determine if the marketing representative, the phone company, or the equipment vendor should be called.

Calls for results will be the most frequently received calls. These calls can occur for a variety of reasons, including that the test result is not ready, the result was never communicated to the office, or the office lost the result after it was received. Because patient confidentiality is an issue, the policy should first detail how to identify the person calling and should ensure that the individual is "eligible" to receive patient results. This can be determined by having the caller identify his or her client number, doctor number, or even complete street address. The policy should also state what to do if the caller cannot provide this information. After identity is established, the policy should contain information about how to correctly identify the patient in the laboratory system and how to explain the acceptable methods for communicating the results. Providing long lists of test results and reference ranges verbally is not always the best approach; this is also a problem for microbiology susceptibility results. After the caller is identified, the patient is identified, and the results are appropriately communicated, the laboratory should attempt to determine why the results were not available to the clinician in the office when needed.

Write a policy to describe the process if the wrong test is ordered. When the client calls, determine the patient and test in question. Check to see what test was performed or if a test was missed. In either case, the original requisition will need to be pulled. If specimen processing ordered the incorrect test, the correct test should be ordered. If the physician ordered the incorrect test, a new order will be needed from the physician. For missed tests, the new test should be ordered immediately and performed STAT if possible. In any of these situations, determine specimen adequacy and viability before indicating that the new test will be performed, and include a step to credit incorrectly ordered tests. Employee education may also be required.

There should be a policy for informational requests. These include questions about turnaround time, specimen collection and preservation, location of the laboratory and collection sites, and services available. When the client service representative provides this information, the call should be logged and information provided to the client regarding where the requested information could be found. The policy should outline when, if the client service representative is unable to answer the call, it is appropriate to send the call to the technical section or other resource and how the call will be handled from that point. The best practice is for the client service representative to use three-way calling or conference call capability to have the client and technical section on the line together so he or she can hear the answer and also take care of any follow-up that may be necessary. This provides the advantage of including technical expertise without just passing the call to the technical section, in case there is further follow-up needed. If the client needs a guidebook or some other information that is available, the marketing representative should follow up with the client.

A missed pickup is a difficult service recovery call for the client services staff. The policy for this call will be largely determined by the process in place for making pickup assignments and the client's status for pickups (daily pickup vs. call-in). The specimen(s) should be picked up as quickly as possible, even if specimen viability is not an issue, because the client will view further delay as further lack of customer service. These calls should be logged and tracked for trends that may reveal problems with the predetermined routes or other courier issues.

It is difficult to write a policy for lost specimens, especially ones that cannot be replaced, because service recovery is extremely difficult. If the specimen can be recollected, the laboratory should offer to call the patient and perform the phlebotomy at the patient's home or office if necessary, at no charge. The tests should be performed STAT and results communicated by phone and fax. The good news, if there is any, about specimens that cannot be replaced is that they generally stay viable for an extended period. Search high and low, in all of the courier cars, all of the coolers, the client's lockbox (and their next-door neighbors'), the refrigerators in the laboratory and at the client's office, all of the technical sections, and anywhere else imaginable. If the specimens cannot be replaced, report to the quality assurance department and do whatever service recovery is appropriate for the client and the patient. Also keep in mind this may be the ammunition needed to obtain a specimen-tracking system. Obviously, this kind of situation needs to be logged and studied carefully to determine where the process failed and how this can be prevented in the future.

For problems not covered with a specific policy, there should be a policy that covers how to document an issue and generally what department will handle certain issues. The policy should generally explain the problem-resolution flow and philosophy for handling calls. For atypical or serious problems, there should also be a problem-resolution cycle that includes notification of management as early in the process as possible.

All calls should be logged and the data should be reviewed and trended for system or procedural problems that may need to be addressed. Client services should be able to handle more than 95% of the calls that are placed to the laboratory. If not, the employees and policies in place should be revisited, and these calls should be monitored routinely.

Couriers: the First Line

Couriers are the face of the outreach business to the clients. Clients see their couriers on a daily basis, and couriers are the only people they see except when they have a serious problem or during marketing personnel's quarterly visits. Couriers should be neatly groomed, be in uniform, have two-way radios or cell phones, and be in vehicles identified with the organization's logo (even if they only pick up from lockboxes).

Give the couriers the respect and resources they need, because the clients will look to them for help when problems occur. Make them accountable for their route by designing route sheets that have all the information on it that they need. Provide the couriers with the ability to access the laboratory if they have a question or problem. Remember, the entire cycle starts with the courier. The on-time delivery of results for the specimens they are collecting begins with the courier pickup. If the courier is late or a pickup is missed, it sets in motion a chain of events that may culminate with late results or no results until the second day. Clients expect to have the majority of reports by the next morning when they open. The ability to deliver this level of service depends on all steps in the process being performed quickly and accurately. A delay in any step may not be correctable later in the process.

Give couriers the ability to please their customers—make sure they carry in their car some blank requisitions, some supply request forms, a box of paper, and some SST and lavender tubes. It is a level of service that most laboratories do not provide.

Client Services

Client Services should be open when the physician office staff begins to arrive in the morning. If the laboratory has nursing-home clients, Client Services should be available when the physicians make rounds in those facilities. This is usually before their office hours and occurs around 7:00 a.m. The client services area can be staffed with some "on-the-job-trained" staff but should also be staffed with medical laboratory technicians (MLTs) or Medical Technologists (MTs). At least one MT or MLT should be in Client Services almost constantly and always during peak call hours. The more technical the staff in Client Services, the better the overall service will be. The technical staff has the advantage of understanding all aspects of the testing, including specimen collection and acceptability and testing protocols.

Offer clients flexibility in reporting. They should be able to choose how they want the reports delivered. Delivery can be by printer (if a report's size warrants a printer), by fax, by mail, or by courier. The laboratory should also have the ability to send results at multiple times each day. Decide how to comply with requests for multiple copies of reports. Will you fax it, print it, or call it in to one, two, or three different locations? What are the processing ramifications of providing this kind of service? Does the laboratory system support this kind of request? Results that are to be delivered by the courier need to be ready before the couriers leave each day. Reports are sorted by practice and courier, assembled into the appropriate envelopes, and ready to be delivered. The time schedule needs to be determined so that adequate staff is on hand to ensure that the reports are printed and prepared for delivery before the couriers leave. The couriers cannot wait for results.

Access to Draw Sites and Patient Service Centers

Draw sites and patient service centers will be vital to laboratory outreach success. Decide the overall strategy for access to the laboratory by examining options for each of these areas.

Hospital-owned facilities are a great start for patients to access outreach services. Facility locations are generally known, well marked, and easy to find. However, sometimes that is where the advantage ends. A hospital is not always easily accessible in terms of parking and navigating the inside of the building. Do not eliminate the use of the hospital as a draw site, but, depending on its layout and accessibility, you may not count on it as a primary source for collections.

Large competitor laboratories often have many patient service centers set up and may allow you to contract with them to perform collections for your patients. This gives you geographically broad, ready-made, pay-as-you-go access for patients. However, remember that this is the competition and clients may ask, "If I am sending my patient to Laboratory X to be drawn, why shouldn't I let them do the testing?" Keeping this potential problem in mind, try to open sites specific for your laboratory outreach operation and phase out this type of competitor agreement.

When opening draw sites and patient service centers, remember that location, location, location is critical. Select a location that is highly visible, has easy access, and is in an area where the medical community practices. Staff it with friendly, customer service-oriented staff, and ensure adequate staff support as the volume grows. Keep it clean and well organized. Signage should be large and hours of operation should be listed on the door. Here are a few hints from lessons we have learned recently.

1. Begin communication about the draw site after a firm opening date has been established.
2. Execute a formal marketing campaign to announce and entice practices to use the location. The campaign should be four to eight weeks long. Include flyers, client visits with candy ("We want to be your lifesaver"), invitations to an open house, and perhaps a cholesterol screening. The communication about the new draw site needs to be reinforced continuously, but you must provide various communications for the

marketing representative to take to the clients. Sending the same flyer or using the same verbal message will not keep the clients interested.
3. Use the new site to draw new business. It is the only way the site will pay for itself. Diverting existing business into the site is nice but will not result in overall growth.
4. Continue to visit practices and encourage them to use the site. Expect that the volume will be very slow at first, but, with continued communication, it should grow.
5. Since laboratory staff are available to collect demographic and insurance information, it is not necessary that the client complete all of this information on the form. However, it is recommended that the client use something other than a prescription pad. See Appendix 42.6. A test requisition gives the client the ability to check the tests needed, and there is a map to the draw site on the back for the patient.
6. Employers may let the laboratory put information about the draw site in their employee newsletter.
7. Put an announcement in the section of the newspaper that announces new physicians.
8. Update insurance provider directories with the new site and put an announcement in the member newsletter.

An idea that has been used to improve awareness of such a site was to involve area schools by displaying student artwork. Students were asked to submit artwork to be displayed at the site. Families and friends were able to visit the site to view the artwork, and information was sent home with the children about the display and the site.

If a physician office will allow the laboratory to provide a draw site from the office, there can be potential advantages for both the laboratory and the physicians. The physicians will gain the addition of a phlebotomist to the staff, when they normally might not have been large enough to obtain one from the laboratory. This will be an additional service they can offer their patients. The laboratory will gain the additional draw site and may not have to pay for the waiting area and some of the draw space. The site needs to be carefully considered, and doctors may resist sending their patients to another practice to be drawn. A written agreement should be developed for the protection of both parties.

Building and Retaining Your Client Base

Leverage the Continuum of Care

If the physician community has loyalty to the hospital or hospital system, start the campaign for the outreach business with the medical staff. Find the practices that primarily admit to the facility. Leverage the continuum of care for their patients. The same laboratory can produce results for their patients regardless of the patients' status: inpatients, same-day surgery, or referred specimens from the physician's laboratory. This way there will never be a problem with reference ranges or varying technology when comparing patients' results from one setting to another.

Keep Asking Why

Continually review and understand why decisions are made. The answers that have been standard over the years may no longer apply. Constantly ask customers about their needs for service, supplies, couriers, client services, and turnaround time. This does not have to be done with a formal survey; client service representatives, couriers, and marketing representatives are great sources of information. Make sure the laboratory is meeting the client's needs and make the client feel involved in the process.

Follow Up When Clients Leave

When customers notify the laboratory that they are leaving or when you determine that an account has been lost, follow up as soon as possible to find out why. Even if the account is not salvageable immediately, taking the time to follow up may help you win accounts back in the future. Follow up again about 3 months after the client leaves and then at least annually. Many "new accounts" will be old accounts that have returned. Also remember to review and discuss the information clients shared about why they left and determine if any other accounts are in jeopardy for the same reason.

Professional Marketing and Sales Personnel

Some laboratories use their current technical staff for sales and marketing. If you are able to find laboratory professionals who possess the skills for selling, they should be transitioned into the sales and marketing role. They will require sales training that may not be readily available. Laboratory professionals are trained to be very detail-oriented and very analytical. They like following procedures, and being creative is not encouraged. Not all laboratory professionals fit this cookie-cutter image, but many do, and these are not the same set of skills and traits needed for a sales employee. Hiring sales professionals with proven sales records brings this ready-made expertise to the outreach program. While the laboratory is not an easy area to learn, laboratory professionals with many years of training should be able to help train the sales staff. Don't underestimate the time required to train a new sales representative. Each person should spend at least a month in the laboratory, followed by quarterly training sessions. The time spent in the laboratory will help sales personnel understand laboratory operations so they can communicate effectively when speaking with a client. It also helps them build personal relationships with the technical staff producing the product they sell.

Training should also take place on how to conduct negotiations and set boundaries for what is acceptable. Some of the training is dictated by the laboratory's compliance program, but there need to be additional guidelines set by the sales manager. The sales representative needs to understand that it is acceptable to walk away from a contract, even a large one, if it does not serve the business objectives of the laboratory. These guidelines need to include profitability and service requirements. Negotiations with any given client "should not hinge solely on the negotiator's individual skill level" (2).

Commission Plans

Each commission plan must start with a baseline against which results can be measured. Establishing the baseline, and then being able to continuously and accurately measure against it, is the greatest challenge of any commission plan. It is a good idea to break the commission into several parts. For example, pay a different percentage rate on new sales than on growth of existing territory. Decide how to treat commission for related entities, if, for example, the hospital also owns or has ownership relationships with physician practices or nursing homes. If the laboratory has managed-care contracts, decide if testing received as part of these contracts will be allowed as part of the commission payment. It may be appropriate to pay a "new account" commission for upgrade of an account. An upgrade occurs when the marketing representative is able to obtain a new line of business from an existing account. This could be an account that is currently only sending testing related to a managed-care contract and later adds more payors. Reports needed to calculate commissions must be ready early in the month. The revenue used to pay commissions should be after contractuals, so be prepared to calculate that information. Also, be able to calculate contractuals when the fee schedules change, and change historical data so that the marketing and sales representatives are unaffected either positively or negatively.

Reports

Sales representatives should be encouraged to stay on the road. Assignment of a personal desk in the laboratory may not be a good idea. Office time should be kept to a minimum. This presents certain challenges for staff management. Over time you will be able to tell if the representative is producing sales. However, you need to keep communication open so you can monitor progress, give feedback, track problems or problem patterns, and ensure that the facilities that management defines as important are visited. Weekly and monthly (see Appendixes 42.7 and 4.28) reports are useful to convey information in a consistent format and to track progress. These reports should be in a standard format and should be completed and turned in at appointed times. The weekly report should include information about each visit made with client decision-makers the previous week. Dropping off information to a client office or seeing the receptionist does not count. There should be a minimum number of visits required each week and an accounting of time that is not spent in the field. The monthly report recaps the month's sales efforts. All active prospects should be listed and their status provided. This also serves as the document used to identify accounts that are eligible for commission. Each account in the territory should have a territory card (see Appendix 42.9). The cards should be kept up to date and should be reviewed by the manager a few times a year. The information on the card will vary but should include basic demographic information, contact information, the names of all of the physicians in the group, the hours, and all of the visits made to the account.

Prepackaged Information

Print pieces are a great source of prepackaged information for the sales and marketing team, and a number of pieces should be developed detailing information about the laboratory. Pieces might cover new product offerings, special programs, a niche expertise, and the professional group, if they provide a competitive advantage. Each piece should stand alone, but identify each with the corporate name and logo, as discussed previously.

Technical Expertise Accessibility

Identify how and when to access technical staff. The technical staff is a tremendous resource for client services, marketing, and clients. Use them wisely. This is the same staff the outreach program relies on daily to produce the high-quality, quick results the clients count on. Identify situations when it makes the most sense to involve the technical staff and contact the right person in the technical section for assistance. For Client Services, contacting the technical section should be done according to a policy. There should be other steps to follow before calling the technical section for help. Once it is decided that a technical section needs to be involved, it should be called by Client Services and conferenced in with the client. That way the section can answer the client's question, and the client service representative can record the answer and complete any necessary follow-up. Marketing personnel should build rapport with the technical staff during their training and in subsequent training so they will be able to contact them directly for quick answers to questions.

If it is necessary to take someone from the technical staff to meet with a client, the visit should be well planned. The exact source of questions and problems should be researched before a meeting is scheduled. The marketing representative should complete the follow-up whenever possible so the technical staff member can return to the bench. Use this option only for large clients and when the material warrants this level of attention. For instance, we have a large drug-screen account that has a definite cycle. The company begins to hire a large number of employees each fall. A meeting is scheduled with the client and we know that the doctor who is in charge of the employee health program for the company will be on hand. This is the time to bring a technical staff member from toxicology. He or she will be able to discuss changes that have occurred with the testing and discuss any plans for future changes.

Use the in-area (hometown) availability to your advantage, but do not overburden staff. Being able to provide this level of service to clients is going to be difficult for the competition to match. The large commercial laboratories that have STAT labs in the area do not have this expertise to offer. The technical staff is a powerful weapon when used correctly. Be careful not to let them become overwhelmed with phone calls and client commitments that could have an adverse affect on test turnaround time. For the most part, the technical staff will welcome the opportunity to answer questions and visit with clients occasionally and will be able to help win and keep business.

Accounts That Require Special Care

Each of these account types can be very lucrative but also has specific demands that must be met. Before making a decision to enter any of these market segments, review the demands and ensure the laboratory can meet them and still generate a profit.

Nursing Homes

Nursing homes come in all sizes and are attractive because of the opportunity to collect many specimens in one location and to control the entire account. Marketing representatives like nursing homes and rehabilitation facilities because they produce large commissions. To compete in the nursing-home business, the laboratory must be able to commit a phlebotomist to the facility each day Monday through Friday (for most facilities) and be available on weekends and after hours to collect specimens for emergent situations. Results must be turned around the same afternoon they are collected. The laboratory must have a commitment from the nursing-home staff to provide medical necessity information or pay for the charges that do not meet medical necessity, because collecting an ABN is usually not an option. If the nursing home has Part A patients, a process must be in place to establish the patient's status at the time the specimen is collected and also to check it before a bill is sent. Part A patients are patients for whom Medicare reimburses the nursing home on a case rate that includes all of their ancillary services (laboratory, radiology, rehabilitation). The laboratory will need to bill the facility, not Medicare or other insurance providers, for the testing for these patients. A patient's status can change retroactively. A commitment must exist from the nursing home to collect MSP information and either make and communicate primary payor information or forward the MSP information to the laboratory. This is a demanding business that has some compliance risks, but we have found that it is profitable for mid-sized to large nursing homes.

Drug Accounts

Drug accounts for pre-employment screening also have unique demands. Drug-screen accounts usually require chain-of-custody forms to be completed and can be demanding concerning locations for specimen collection. The more sophisticated employee health programs will want specific testing in place for drugs. Ensure that Marketing and the client understand the difference in testing and pricing between a drug screen and a quantitative drug test.

Home Health Agencies

Home health agencies want easy access to a large number of facilities, quick turnaround time, and delivery of reports to numerous places. Requests to call and send reports to the agency, as well as to a number of doctors, are not unusual. The advantage to this segment of business is that it usually comes to the laboratory. Most home health agencies will deliver the testing to the laboratory. This may be enough of a benefit to offset the requirements of the additional reporting.

Define Service Area and Services

One of the easy mistakes to make is to change the service offered or the service area without enough consideration. Marketing will get excited about the amount of "easy business" that can be retained if you change the business. Adding another courier route, expanding a courier route, offering three-times-a-day pickup, or doing home draws may be all that is needed. After the initial assessment of the service area, do not expand without a marketing and financial analysis. Decisions should be made about the services offered and the territory to be covered based on financial information and resource availability. Stepping outside of the original plan usually means that something else will be done to a lesser extent or that more resources will be needed. Do not presume that extension of services can be accomplished without sacrifice. If the laboratory has an opportunity and the flexibility to change plans, that is great. But make sure careful analysis has been performed prior to such a decision. Flexibility and adaptability are admirable qualities and ones that young businesses tend to be better able to attain than established businesses. Yoke that strength but understand the consequences before a change is made.

Range of Services

What other services will you offer? Once word of the new business lines spreads, departments throughout the hospital system will be anxious to use the service, but not always for the purpose intended. System courier, home draws,

arterial blood gases, and pulse oximetry are some of the services we have provided over the years. We determined that they were not our core business, as they were expensive or administratively burdensome, and since we did not feel we serviced them well, we discontinued these services. Other laboratories have been willing to invest the resources to make this a niche for themselves in their system.

Courier for the system. We have been asked to deliver everything from X rays to office supplies to furniture. If the laboratory decides to take on the responsibility of transporting items other than laboratory supplies and testing, ensure that there is a tracking system in place. X rays cannot be replaced, nor can medical records. Transporting other items while transporting specimens can provide a good business case for a specimen-tracking system, which will be an added benefit to the clients. If the laboratory can adequately provide this service without sacrificing the timeliness of pickup and delivery of specimens, it could be a win for everyone. Remember, though, that if couriers do not have the ability to do their laboratory job well, the laboratory is behind schedule from the time the specimen arrives, and making up that time is not easy.

Pulse oximetry. The laboratory sometimes will take on the responsibility of pulse oximetry, since the same people performing this function also collect arterial blood gases. Pulse oximetry testing is needed to certify patients for oxygen. However, Medicare is currently not reimbursing for this testing when billed by itself. Also, the task is administratively burdensome. The patients often need the equipment delivered and picked up from their homes. Then there is the issue of ensuring the results are reported as needed. This service can be an added benefit for existing clients, but the number of people who will use the service does not usually provide sufficient benefits to distinguish the program in the market.

Arterial blood gases. Some hospital laboratories include this function because it is related to phlebotomy. Someone will need to be available in the hospital at all times for this service. The skills that are required are different from those of phlebotomy. More in-depth training is required to collect arterial blood gases, so the function is generally limited to a subset of the phlebotomy staff. Nursing homes will want this service and will view it as an added benefit of dealing with the outreach program. Most reference laboratories do not provide this service. This draw is usually not scheduled, unlike the daily draws performed for nursing homes, and as discussed, the entire phlebotomy staff will probably not be trained to do this testing, thus making the service difficult to deliver. The respiratory vendor that the nursing home contracts with will also offer this service, and it may be advisable to direct inquiries for this service to them.

Home draws. Doctors far and wide and home health agencies will be very pleased with the laboratory for this service. If the laboratory can rigidly control the service area and hours of operation, meet medical necessity standards, and only provide the service for offices that have signed contracts for their complete business, it may be worthwhile. Profitability is difficult with this business because of the time and distance involved in collecting the specimens and the limited number of tests that will be drawn at each stop. Often, the only billable tests will be a protime, a draw fee, and the travel fee. Remember that unless the patient meets the criteria for being homebound, a travel fee may not be billed. The criteria for being homebound must be confirmed by the physician. A short questionnaire may be helpful.

1. For what reasons do you leave home?

   If the patient leaves the home two or three times a week to eat, go to church, go to work, or go to the doctor, the patient is not considered homebound.

2. Do you drive a car?

   If the patient is able to drive a car, the patient is not considered homebound.

3. When you have a doctor's appointment, how do you get there?

   If the patient is able to have a family member transport him or her to his or her doctor's appointments, proceed to question 4.

4. Is it possible to have a family member transport you to a draw facility?

   If the patient has the ability to have a family member transport him or her to a draw facility, he or she is not considered homebound.

There is also a safety factor to consider for the phlebotomist. Consider the neighborhoods they will be asked to visit and the fact that they are in homes of strangers. Do not ask that they collect funds, even if the patient is a self-pay.

In-office phlebotomy. This is a service that will win accounts quickly. Be careful not to run afoul of the compliance issues and ensure that the physician office is large enough so that the account remains profitable. This service should only be offered to accounts with three or more providers in the office each day and only to certain specialties. Family Practice, Internal Medicine, Oncology/Hematology, Infectious Disease, and large OB/GYN groups are all excellent opportunities for placement of a phlebotomist. Surgical groups are not a good option because although they generate a large volume of work, the blood-bank criteria are hard to meet even if the patient is being admitted to your facility. If the patient is not being admitted to your facility, then you cannot draw most of the testing. Even very large Pediatrics, Psychiatry, Dermatology, and Orthopedic Medicine groups generally do not generate enough volume

to make placement of a phlebotomist profitable. Gastroenterology, Urology/Nephrology, and other specialties may work out, depending on the size of the practice and the types of services they offer. When profitability is calculated, remember to consider not only the time for the phlebotomist who is assigned to the office but also the cost of coverage when that person is sick or on vacation. Also consider what happens to that employee if the office closes for a day on which the employee would normally work.

The Importance of Standardization

Some companies build their reputation on their ability to personalize service and are sometimes able to charge a premium rate for the additional service. To some extent, the laboratory needs to be prepared to personalize service and should determine in advance what personalization could be offered. But, because reimbursement is largely fixed based on a fee schedule or a capitated rate for an insurance company, recouping additional expenses will be difficult.

Product offering. Decisions need to be made about the testing that will be performed and the schedule that will be offered. What testing will be offered STAT? STAT fees can be charged but will not be reimbursed by many insurance companies. In Virginia, the STAT fee cannot even appear on the bill for Medicaid patients. Decide on fees for services and discount schedules. Decide what the discounts will be based on, keeping in mind the compliance restrictions.

Process. Testing referred to the laboratory should be handled in a consistent format for ease and accuracy of processing. However, the laboratory will have many requests to alter the process to accommodate clients. Will clients be required to only use the requisition form the laboratory provides? There may be compliance concerns if they do not, because the laboratory will be required to determine from the client's form what testing needs to be completed. Can clients affix stickers with patient information on the requisition instead of completing the form? This usually allows for better, more legible information, but all of the billing information must be submitted and the client's label may not have all of the information required. If clients want to change how their reports look or if they want specific identifying information on the report, can this be accomplished, and if so, how? The laboratory will need to be prepared to allow the client to submit its own identifying information, and the laboratory will need to determine how that information will appear on the report form. How often will reports for clients print? For clients with faxes or printers, there should be multiple print options available. Can they control when their reports print (if they have a printer or autofax) or choose only to receive final reports? Will you deliver reports to more than one doctor; if so, how is this communicated and accomplished? Will you allow the client to direct where testing is performed? This is a case where pathologist involvement will be advantageous.

What happens when you do not receive all of the information you need to process the specimen for testing or bill the patient? A process will need to be developed to collect information not received on the original request. Two kinds of issues will need to be addressed. First, a policy will need to be established for situations when information needed to run the test (test name, patient name, and patient identifier) is not received. Second, a policy will need to be developed for when proper billing information, including ABNs, is not received. If the test information is not received, the laboratory will need to determine if any testing will be done. For instance, if a lavender tube is received, should a complete blood count be performed? If this is done, billing must be held until an order is received. If an ABN is needed, and not received, and the test is performed, the laboratory will bear the risk of not being paid. Some laboratories will send a comment about the problem on the report and will call the physician office for the missing information.

For every step of the process, the laboratory will receive requests to alter the process. To the extent that the laboratory can customize its service without compromising overall service or quality, the program will be better able to compete. Ensure that the laboratory can consistently deliver the service promised and administer the agreed-upon exceptions.

Courier routes. Practices across the service area will close at approximately the same time and want their specimens picked up as they leave the office. Knowing that is not possible, the laboratory needs to design the routes so that the majority of the specimens are picked up as quickly as possible and returned to the laboratory for processing to begin. Couriers will need to be equipped to handle a number of requests and issues. If a client is not ready when the courier arrives, the courier must decide whether to wait for the specimens, try to come back, or call another courier to pick up the specimens. If a client that usually leaves many specimens in a lockbox does not leave the lockbox out, an attempt should be made to contact the practice by phone. If that is unsuccessful, the courier should have preprinted notes to leave on the door. The laboratory will also need to decide how to handle calls for STAT transports or requests for multiple pickups in the same day. Depending on the size of the account, multiple pickups may be a good idea for both the client and the laboratory, so processing of the specimens can begin sooner. Requests for STAT pickups should be monitored and addressed if problematic.

Summary

Successful establishment of an outreach program can have numerous benefits for the hospital laboratory, the hospital system, the physicians, and the community. Leverage the intellectual and capital assets of the hospital while working internally to offset any challenges that being part of a hospital present. The decisions made regarding how to maintain and service customers while still being able to expand the business are important and will affect the program's overall success. Choose the service offerings and service standards carefully and always be able to deliver what is promised. Saying yes is not always best.

KEY POINTS

- Deciding how to implement an outreach program within the current hospital environment requires decisions at many levels of the organization. Contracting, information technology, finance, and compliance are key areas that require attention. Understanding each of these areas is critical to success.

- Being part of a hospital system offers advantages to the physician base and to the patients. Leverage those advantages to make a winning and profitable business.

- Consider all of the points and options for customer service. Customer service is not only a department or something people do in their spare time. It must be a united, consistent strategy employed to win and keep customers.

GLOSSARY

Advance Beneficiary Notice (ABN) Notice that must be provided to patients for testing that is not medically necessary so that the lab may bill the patient should Medicare deny payment.

Add-on Test that is added on by a physician after the initial lab order is received.

Client bill Bill sent to the client for payment of lab services as opposed to billing the patient or the patient's insurance.

Commission plan A written plan for calculation and distribution of commission payment to marketing staff and other individuals.

Continuum of care A patient's continuum of care would include the hospital, physician office, skilled nursing facility, outpatient surgery, primary care, specialty care, and any other health service a patient may need.

Fixed costs Costs that remain constant in spite of changes in output (3).

Full-time equivalent (FTE) An employee who works full-time hours.

Guidebook A book that provides comprehensive information about the laboratory and its operations, policies (including forms), testing, specimen preparation, result reporting, billing, staff, and licensure.

Health Insurance Portability and Accountability Act of 1996 (HIPAA) A law to improve the flow of information between insurance companies and providers and protect the privacy of patient information (5).

Medical necessity Services that are "covered, reasonable and necessary for the beneficiary, given his or her clinical condition" (6).

Medicare secondary payor (MSP) Information that is collected from the patient to determine when Medicare is not the primary payor.

Model Laboratory Compliance Program A statement of expectations published by CMS (Centers for Medicare and Medicaid Services) for laboratories to use as a model for behavior.

Nonstaff physicians Physicians who are not part of the hospital medical staff.

Physician office connectivity System that allows clients access to the laboratory information, usually via the Web. The system should also provide the client the ability to register patients, order tests, and print results.

Pull-through The testing that is sent to a laboratory because the client already has to use the laboratory for other testing. Usually associated with a laboratory that has a health maintenance organization (HMO) contract. Clients that have a large volume of testing for that HMO may send the laboratory testing for other patients whose insurance does not require a specific laboratory.

Sanctioned physicians Physicians who have been barred from billing Medicare, Medicaid, or other government payors, usually for compliance/billing issues. Other providers and persons can also be barred from the government programs.

UB92/HCFA-1500 Standard billing forms: UB92 is the billing form used by hospitals; HCFA-1500 is the billing form used by physicians and other ancillary nonhospital providers.

Unrelated business income tax (UBIT) An income tax that must be filed and paid annually for net income that is not related to the hospital. Laboratory testing and revenue generated from physician office, clinics, and employers that do not have a corporate relationship with the laboratory or parent company would be considered unrelated. The income tax rate is 40% of the unrelated net income.

REFERENCES

1. Department of Health and Human Services. July 31, 2002. Program Memorandum Intermediaries/Carriers Transmittal AB-02-114.

2. Ertel, D. 1999. Turning negotiation into a corporate capability. Reprint number 99304. *Harvard Bus. Rev.* May–June.

3. Kieso, D. E, and J. J. Weygandt. 1983. *Intermediate Accounting*, 4th ed., p. 347. John Wiley & Sons, Inc., New York, N.Y.

4. National Intelligence Report. March 10, 2003. "Bill Reintroduced for Fee-Setting Process for New Lab Tests."

5. Payne, S. 2003. "A Privacy Law". *https://wavenet.sentara.com/HIPAA/Forms/SEEP.ppt*

6. Taulbee, P. August 1998. The HHS office of Inspector General's Compliance Program Guidance for Clinical Laboratories.

7. United Governmental Service, LLC. March 5, 2003. Changes to the Laboratory National Coverage Determination (NCD) Edit Software for April 1, 2003. Program Memorandum AB-03-030 Change Request 2578.

APPENDIX 42.1 UB92 Insurance Claim Form

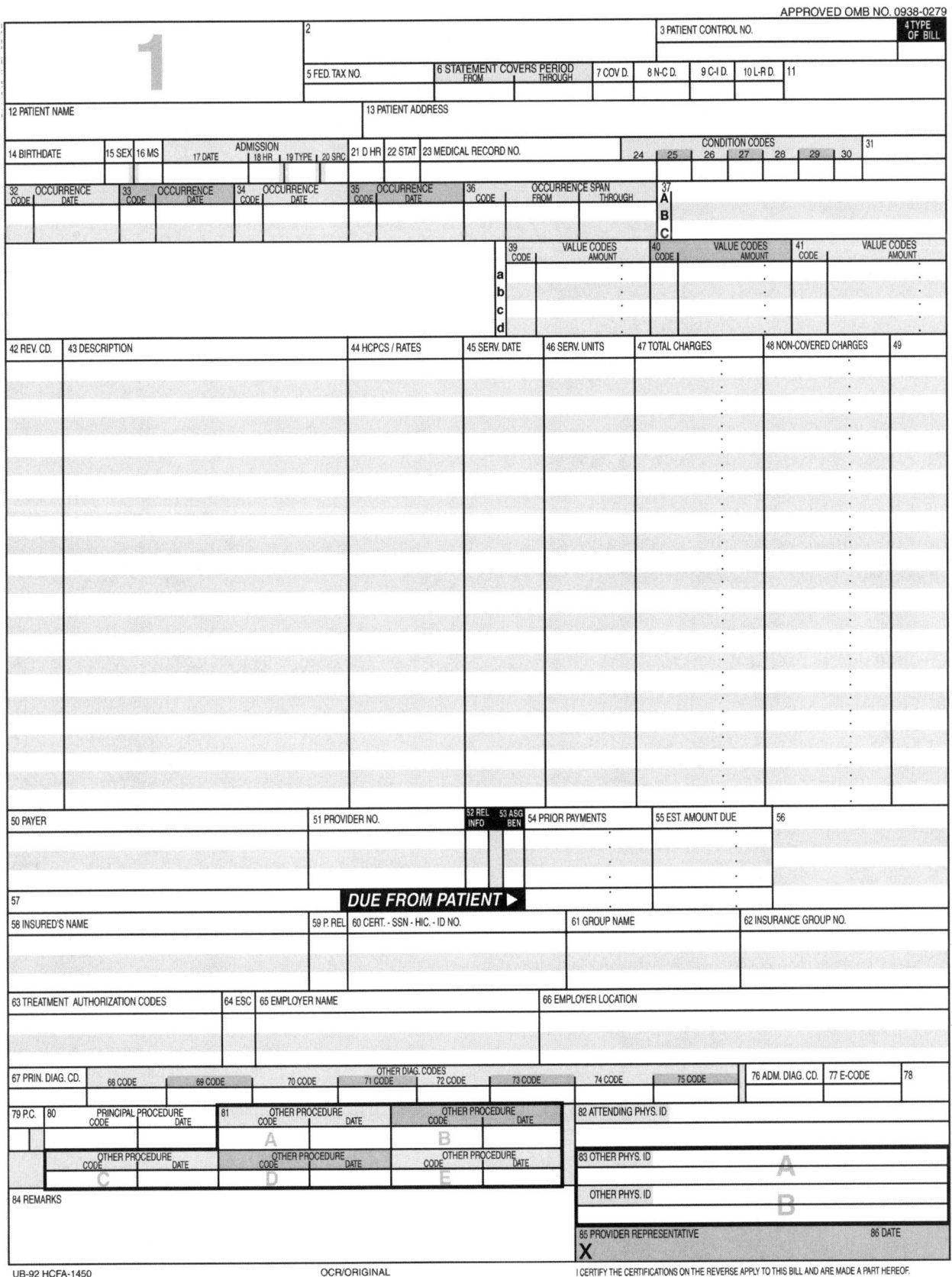

(continued)

APPENDIX 42.1 UB92 Insurance Claim Form *(continued)*

UNIFORM BILL: **NOTICE: ANYONE WHO MISREPRESENTS OR FALSIFIES ESSENTIAL INFORMATION REQUESTED BY THIS FORM MAY UPON CONVICTION BE SUBJECT TO FINE AND IMPRISONMENT UNDER FEDERAL AND/OR STATE LAW.**

Certifications relevant to the Bill and Information Shown on the Face Hereof: Signatures on the face hereof incorporate the following certifications or verifications where pertinent to this Bill:

1. If third party benefits are indicated as being assigned or in participation status, on the face thereof, appropriate assignments by the insured/beneficiary and signature of patient or parent or legal guardian covering authorization to release information are on file. Determinations as to the release of medical and financial information should be guided by the particular terms of the release forms that were executed by the patient or the patient's legal representative. The hospital agrees to save harmless, indemnify and defend any insurer who makes payment in reliance upon this certification, from and against any claim to the insurance proceeds when in fact no valid assignment of benefits to the hospital was made.

2. If patient occupied a private room or required private nursing for medical necessity, any required certifications are on file.

3. Physician's certifications and re-certifications, if required by contract or Federal regulations, are on file.

4. For Christian Science Sanitoriums, verifications and if necessary re-verifications of the patient's need for sanitorium services are on file.

5. Signature of patient or his/her representative on certifications, authorization to release information, and payment request, as required be Federal law and regulations (42 USC 1935f, 42 CFR 424.36, 10 USC 1071 thru 1086, 32 CFR 199) and, any other applicable contract regulations, is on file.

6. This claim, to the best of my knowledge, is correct and complete and is in conformance with the Civil Rights Act of 1964 as amended. Records adequately disclosing services will be maintained and necessary information will be furnished to such governmental agencies as required by applicable law.

7. For Medicare purposes:

    If the patient has indicated that other health insurance or a state medical assistance agency will pay part of his/her medical expenses and he/she wants information about his/her claim released to them upon their request, necessary authorization is on file. The patient's signature on the provider's request to bill Medicare authorizes any holder of medical and non-medical information, including employment status, and whether the person has employer group health insurance, liability, no-fault, workers' compensation, or other insurance which is responsible to pay for the services for which this Medicare claim is made.

8. For Medicaid purposes:

    This is to certify that the foregoing information is true, accurate, and complete.
    I understand that payment and satisfaction of this claim will be from Federal and State funds, and that any false claims, statements, or documents, or concealment of a material fact, may be prosecuted under applicable Federal or State Laws.

9. For CHAMPUS purposes:

    This is to certify that:

    a) the information submitted as part of this claim is true, accurate and complete, and, the services shown on this form were medically indicated and necessary for the health of the patient;

    (b) the patient has represented that by a reported residential address outside a military treatment center catchment area he or she does not live within a catchment area of a U.S. military or U.S. Public Health Service medical facility, or if the patient resides within a catchment area of such a facility, a copy of a Non-Availability Statement (DD Form 1251) is on file, or the physician has certified to a medical emergency in any assistance where a copy of a Non-Availability Statement is not on file;

    (c) the patient or the patient's parent or guardian has responded directly to the provider's request to identify all health insurance coverages, and that all such coverages are identified on the face the claim except those that are exclusively supplemental payments to CHAMPUS-determined benefits;

    (d) the amount billed to CHAMPUS has been billed after all such coverages have been billed and paid, excluding Medicaid, and the amount billed to CHAMPUS is that remaining claimed against CHAMPUS benefits;

    (e) the beneficiary's cost share has not been waived by consent or failure to exercise generally accepted billing and collection efforts; and,

    (f) any hospital-based physician under contract, the cost of whose services are allocated in the charges included in this bill, is not an employee or member of the Uniformed Services. For purposes of this certification, an employee of the Uniformed Services is an employee, appointed in civil service (refer to 5 USC 2105), including part-time or intermittent but excluding contract surgeons or other personnel employed by the Uniformed Services through personal service contracts. Similarly, member of the Uniformed Services does not apply to reserve members of the Uniformed Services not on active duty.

    (g) based on the Consolidated Omnibus Budget Reconciliation Act of 1986, all providers participating in Medicare must also participate in CHAMPUS for inpatient hospital services provided pursuant to admissions to hospitals occurring on or after January 1, 1987.

    (h) if CHAMPUS benefits are to be paid in a participating status, I agree to submit this claim to the appropriate CHAMPUS claims processor as a participating provider. I agree to accept the CHAMPUS-determined reasonable charge as the total charge for the medical services or supplies listed on the claim form. I will accept the CHAMPUS-determined reasonable charge even if it is less than the billed amount, and also agree to accept the amount paid by CHAMPUS, combined with the cost-share amount and deductible amount, if any, paid by or on behalf of the patient as full payment for the listed medical services or supplies. I will make no attempt to collect from the patient (or his or her parent or guardian) amounts over the CHAMPUS-determined reasonable charge. CHAMPUS will make any benefits payable directly to me, if I submit this claim as a participating provider.

ESTIMATED CONTRACT BENEFITS

APPENDIX 42.2   HCFA-1500 Insurance Claim Form

APPROVED OMB-0938-0008

PLEASE DO NOT STAPLE IN THIS AREA

CARRIER

HEALTH INSURANCE CLAIM FORM

PICA   PICA

1. MEDICARE MEDICAID CHAMPUS CHAMPVA GROUP HEALTH PLAN FECA BLK LUNG OTHER	1a. INSURED'S I.D. NUMBER (FOR PROGRAM IN ITEM 1)
(Medicare #) (Medicaid #) (Sponsor's SSN) (VA File #) (SSN or ID) (SSN) (ID)	

2. PATIENT'S NAME (Last Name, First Name, Middle Initial)	3. PATIENT'S BIRTH DATE MM DD YY SEX M F	4. INSURED'S NAME (Last Name, First Name, Middle Initial)

5. PATIENT'S ADDRESS (No., Street)	6. PATIENT RELATIONSHIP TO INSURED Self Spouse Child Other	7. INSURED'S ADDRESS (No., Street)

CITY STATE	8. PATIENT STATUS Single Married Other	CITY STATE

ZIP CODE TELEPHONE (Include Area Code) ( )	Employed Full-Time Student Part-Time Student	ZIP CODE TELEPHONE (INCLUDE AREA CODE) ( )

9. OTHER INSURED'S NAME (Last Name, First Name, Middle Initial)	10. IS PATIENT'S CONDITION RELATED TO:	11. INSURED'S POLICY GROUP OR FECA NUMBER
a. OTHER INSURED'S POLICY OR GROUP NUMBER	a. EMPLOYMENT? (CURRENT OR PREVIOUS) YES NO	a. INSURED'S DATE OF BIRTH MM DD YY SEX M F
b. OTHER INSURED'S DATE OF BIRTH MM DD YY SEX M F	b. AUTO ACCIDENT? PLACE (State) YES NO	b. EMPLOYER'S NAME OR SCHOOL NAME
c. EMPLOYER'S NAME OR SCHOOL NAME	c. OTHER ACCIDENT? YES NO	c. INSURANCE PLAN NAME OR PROGRAM NAME
d. INSURANCE PLAN NAME OR PROGRAM NAME	10d. RESERVED FOR LOCAL USE	d. IS THERE ANOTHER HEALTH BENEFIT PLAN? YES NO If yes, return to and complete item 9 a-d.

READ BACK OF FORM BEFORE COMPLETING & SIGNING THIS FORM.

12. PATIENT'S OR AUTHORIZED PERSON'S SIGNATURE I authorize the release of any medical or other information necessary to process this claim. I also request payment of government benefits either to myself or to the party who accepts assignment below.

SIGNED _____   DATE _____

13. INSURED'S OR AUTHORIZED PERSON'S SIGNATURE I authorize payment of medical benefits to the undersigned physician or supplier for services described below.

SIGNED _____

PATIENT AND INSURED INFORMATION

14. DATE OF CURRENT: MM DD YY ILLNESS (First symptom) OR INJURY (Accident) OR PREGNANCY(LMP)	15. IF PATIENT HAS HAD SAME OR SIMILAR ILLNESS. GIVE FIRST DATE MM DD YY	16. DATES PATIENT UNABLE TO WORK IN CURRENT OCCUPATION MM DD YY MM DD YY FROM TO
17. NAME OF REFERRING PHYSICIAN OR OTHER SOURCE	17a. I.D. NUMBER OF REFERRING PHYSICIAN	18. HOSPITALIZATION DATES RELATED TO CURRENT SERVICES MM DD YY MM DD YY FROM TO

19. RESERVED FOR LOCAL USE	20. OUTSIDE LAB? $ CHARGES YES NO

21. DIAGNOSIS OR NATURE OF ILLNESS OR INJURY. (RELATE ITEMS 1,2,3 OR 4 TO ITEM 24E BY LINE)

1. |___.___| 3. |___.___|

2. |___.___| 4. |___.___|

22. MEDICAID RESUBMISSION CODE   ORIGINAL REF. NO.
23. PRIOR AUTHORIZATION NUMBER

24. A DATE(S) OF SERVICE From To MM DD YY MM DD YY	B Place of Service	C Type of Service	D PROCEDURES, SERVICES, OR SUPPLIES (Explain Unusual Circumstances) CPT/HCPCS MODIFIER	E DIAGNOSIS CODE	F $ CHARGES	G DAYS OR UNITS	H EPSDT Family Plan	I EMG	J COB	K RESERVED FOR LOCAL USE
1										
2										
3										
4										
5										
6										

PHYSICIAN OR SUPPLIER INFORMATION

25. FEDERAL TAX I.D. NUMBER SSN EIN	26. PATIENT'S ACCOUNT NO.	27. ACCEPT ASSIGNMENT? (For govt. claims, see back) YES NO	28. TOTAL CHARGE $	29. AMOUNT PAID $	30. BALANCE DUE $

31. SIGNATURE OF PHYSICIAN OR SUPPLIER INCLUDING DEGREES OR CREDENTIALS (I certify that the statements on the reverse apply to this bill and are made a part thereof.) SIGNED _____ DATE _____	32. NAME AND ADDRESS OF FACILITY WHERE SERVICES WERE RENDERED (If other than home or office)	33. PHYSICIAN'S, SUPPLIER'S BILLING NAME, ADDRESS, ZIP CODE & PHONE # PIN# GRP#

(APPROVED BY AMA COUNCIL ON MEDICAL SERVICE 8/88)   *PLEASE PRINT OR TYPE*   FORM HCFA-1500 (12-90), FORM RRB-1500, FORM OWCP-1500

(continued)

APPENDIX 42.2 HCFA-1500 Insurance Claim Form *(continued)*

BECAUSE THIS FORM IS USED BY VARIOUS GOVERNMENT AND PRIVATE HEALTH PROGRAMS, SEE SEPARATE INSTRUCTIONS ISSUED BY APPLICABLE PROGRAMS.

NOTICE: Any person who knowingly files a statement of claim containing any misrepresentation or any false, incomplete or misleading information may be guilty of a criminal act punishable under law and may be subject to civil penalties.

REFERS TO GOVERNMENT PROGRAMS ONLY

MEDICARE AND CHAMPUS PAYMENTS: A patient's signature requests that payment be made and authorizes release of any information necessary to process the claim and certifies that the information provided in Blocks 1 through 12 is true, accurate and complete. In the case of a Medicare claim, the patient's signature authorizes any entity to release to Medicare medical and nonmedical information, including employment status, and whether the person has employer group health insurance, liability, no-fault, worker's compensation or other insurance which is responsible to pay for the services for which the Medicare claim is made. See 42 CFR 411.24(a). If item 9 is completed, the patient's signature authorizes release of the information to the health plan or agency shown. In Medicare assigned or CHAMPUS participation cases, the physician agrees to accept the charge determination of the Medicare carrier or CHAMPUS fiscal intermediary as the full charge, and the patient is responsible only for the deductible, coinsurance and noncovered services. Coinsurance and the deductible are based upon the charge determination of the Medicare carrier or CHAMPUS fiscal intermediary if this is less than the charge submitted. CHAMPUS is not a health insurance program but makes payment for health benefits provided through certain affiliations with the Uniformed Services. Information on the patient's sponsor should be provided in those items captioned in "Insured"; i.e., items 1a, 4, 6, 7, 9, and 11.

BLACK LUNG AND FECA CLAIMS

The provider agrees to accept the amount paid by the Government as payment in full. See Black Lung and FECA instructions regarding required procedure and diagnosis coding systems.

SIGNATURE OF PHYSICIAN OR SUPPLIER (MEDICARE, CHAMPUS, FECA AND BLACK LUNG)

I certify that the services shown on this form were medically indicated and necessary for the health of the patient and were personally furnished by me or were furnished incident to my professional service by my employee under my immediate personal supervision, except as otherwise expressly permitted by Medicare or CHAMPUS regulations.

For services to be considered as "incident" to a physician's professional service, 1) they must be rendered under the physician's immediate personal supervision by his/her employee, 2) they must be an integral, although incidental part of a covered physician's service, 3) they must be of kinds commonly furnished in physician's offices, and 4) the services of nonphysicians must be included on the physician's bills.

For CHAMPUS claims, I further certify that I (or any employee) who rendered services am not an active duty member of the Uniformed Services or a civilian employee of the United States Government or a contract employee of the United States Government, either civilian or military (refer to 5 USC 5536). For Black-Lung claims, I further certify that the services performed were for a Black Lung-related disorder.

No Part B Medicare benefits may be paid unless this form is received as required by existing law and regulations (42 CFR 424.32).

NOTICE: Any one who misrepresents or falsifies essential information to receive payment from Federal funds requested by this form may upon conviction be subject to fine and imprisonment under applicable Federal laws.

NOTICE TO PATIENT ABOUT THE COLLECTION AND USE OF MEDICARE, CHAMPUS, FECA, AND BLACK LUNG INFORMATION
(PRIVACY ACT STATEMENT)

We are authorized by HCFA, CHAMPUS and OWCP to ask you for information needed in the administration of the Medicare, CHAMPUS, FECA, and Black Lung programs. Authority to collect information is in section 205(a), 1862, 1872 and 1874 of the Social Security Act as amended, 42 CFR 411.24(a) and 424.5(a) (6), and 44 USC 3101;41 CFR 101 et seq and 10 USC 1079 and 1086; 5 USC 8101 et seq; and 30 USC 901 et seq; 38 USC 613; E.O. 9397.

The information we obtain to complete claims under these programs is used to identify you and to determine your eligibility. It is also used to decide if the services and supplies you received are covered by these programs and to insure that proper payment is made.

The information may also be given to other providers of services, carriers, intermediaries, medical review boards, health plans, and other organizations or Federal agencies, for the effective administration of Federal provisions that require other third parties payers to pay primary to Federal program, and as otherwise necessary to administer these programs. For example, it may be necessary to disclose information about the benefits you have used to a hospital or doctor. Additional disclosures are made through routine uses for information contained in systems of records.

FOR MEDICARE CLAIMS: See the notice modifying system No. 09-70-0501, titled, 'Carrier Medicare Claims Record,' published in the <u>Federal Register</u>, Vol. 55 No. 177, page 37549, Wed. Sept. 12, 1990, or as updated and republished.

FOR OWCP CLAIMS: Department of Labor, Privacy Act of 1974, "Republication of Notice of Systems of Records," <u>Federal Register</u> Vol. 55 No. 40, Wed Feb. 28, 1990, See ESA-5, ESA-6, ESA-12, ESA-13, ESA-30, or as updated and republished.

FOR CHAMPUS CLAIMS: <u>PRINCIPLE PURPOSE(S):</u> To evaluate eligibility for medical care provided by civilian sources and to issue payment upon establishment of eligibility and determination that the services/supplies received are authorized by law.

<u>ROUTINE USE(S):</u> Information from claims and related documents may be given to the Dept. of Veterans Affairs, the Dept. of Health and Human Services and/or the Dept. of Transportation consistent with their statutory administrative responsibilities under CHAMPUS/CHAMPVA; to the Dept. of Justice for representation of the Secretary of Defense in civil actions; to the Internal Revenue Service, private collection agencies, and consumer reporting agencies in connection with recoupment claims; and to Congressional Offices in response to inquiries made at the request of the person to whom a record pertains. Appropriate disclosures may be made to other federal, state, local, foreign government agencies, private business entities, and individual providers of care, on matters relating to entitlement, claims adjudication, fraud, program abuse, utilization review, quality assurance, peer review, program integrity, third-party liability, coordination of benefits, and civil and criminal litigation related to the operation of CHAMPUS.

<u>DISCLOSURES:</u> Voluntary; however, failure to provide information will result in delay in payment or may result in denial of claim. With the one exception discussed below, there are no penalties under these programs for refusing to supply information. However, failure to furnish information regarding the medical services rendered or the amount charged would prevent payment of claims under these programs. Failure to furnish any other information, such as name or claim number, would delay payment of the claim. Failure to provide medical information under FECA could be deemed an obstruction.

It is mandatory that you tell us if you know that another party is responsible for paying for your treatment. Section 1128B of the Social Security Act and 31 USC 3801-3812 provide penalties for withholding this information.

You should be aware that P.L. 100-503, the "Computer Matching and Privacy Protection Act of 1988", permits the government to verify information by way of computer matches.

MEDICAID PAYMENTS (PROVIDER CERTIFICATION)

I hereby agree to keep such records as are necessary to disclose fully the extent of services provided to individuals under the State's Title XIX plan and to furnish information regarding any payments claimed for providing such services as the State Agency or Dept. of Health and Humans Services may request.

I further agree to accept, as payment in full, the amount paid by the Medicaid program for those claims submitted for payment under that program, with the exception of authorized deductible, coinsurance, co-payment or similar cost-sharing charge.

SIGNATURE OF PHYSICIAN (OR SUPPLIER): I certify that the services listed above were medically indicated and necessary to the health of this patient and were personally furnished by me or my employee under my personal direction.

NOTICE: This is to certify that the foregoing information is true, accurate and complete. I understand that payment and satisfaction of this claim will be from Federal and State funds, and that any false claims, statements, or documents, or concealment of a material fact, may be prosecuted under applicable Federal or State laws.

Public reporting burden for this collection of information is estimated to average 15 minutes per response, including time for reviewing instructions, searching existing date sources, gathering and maintaining data needed, and completing and reviewing the collection of information. Send comments regarding this burden estimate or any other aspect of this collection of information, including suggestions for reducing the burden, to HCFA, Office of Financial Management, P.O. Box 26684, Baltimore, MD 21207; and to the Office of Management and Budget, Paperwork Reduction Project (OMB-0938-0008), Washington, D.C. 20503.

APPENDIX 42.3 Sample Physician Letter

Sentara Reference Laboratory

June 1, 2002

Dear Physician:

The Office of the Inspector General (OIG) of the United States Department of Health and Human Services has issued a Model Compliance Plan for Clinical Laboratories in 1997 that provides guidelines for various aspects of a clinical laboratory's business. The plan states that laboratories should provide healthcare professionals annual written communication addressing various policies that affect ordering, performing and billing clinical laboratory tests.

Advance Beneficiary Notices (ABN): an Advanced Beneficiary Notice (ABN) should be completed if any of the laboratory services ordered for a Medicare patient is not accompanied by a diagnosis code eligible for coverage by Medicare. Medicare will only pay for services that it determines to be "reasonable and necessary."

Before the laboratory service is performed, the beneficiary should be notified in writing of the likelihood that Medicare will deny payment for the specific service. After reviewing the ABN, the beneficiary has the choice to sign the ABN agreeing to receive the service and to pay for it, or not to receive the service. The ABN must clearly identify the specific test, the date of service, state that payment for the test will likely be denied, and give the reason(s) that payment is likely to be denied. *Requesting an ABN from all Medicare beneficiaries or requesting beneficiaries sign a blank ABN are considered unacceptable practices.*

Sentara Reference Laboratory is committed to comply with the guidelines issued by the OIG-HHS and completing an ABN only when appropriate. A sample of the ABN used by Sentara Reference Laboratory is included as Attachment 1. Additional information or training on the ABN and Medicare coverage can be obtained by contacting your Marketing Representative or Sentara Reference Laboratory Client Services at (757) 668-3621.

Medical Necessity: claims submitted for laboratory services will only be paid by Medicare if the service is covered, reasonable, and necessary for the beneficiary, given his or her clinical condition. Medicare may deny payment for a service you, as a physician, believe is appropriate, but which does not meet the Medicare coverage criteria (such as for screening).

ICD-9-CM diagnosis codes must be provided for each laboratory service ordered. Sentara Reference Laboratory publishes a guide of Medicare Approved Diagnosis Codes for certain tests to help ensure this information is provided correctly and to obtain an ABN when appropriate.
If necessary, Sentara will contact the ordering physician to obtain diagnosis information. To request a copy of this guide of Medicare Approved Diagnosis Codes prepared by Sentara Reference Laboratory contact your Marketing Representative or Sentara Reference Laboratory Client Services at (757) 668-3621.

Revised Requisitions: Sentara Reference Laboratory has revised the standard test requisition to make patient registration, test ordering, and billing quicker and to reduce errors. Specimen labels and the requisition bar code have been relocated to the upper right hand corner of the form. Placing one of these ID labels on each patient specimen will help prevent misidentification and processing errors.

To assist with registration and billing, patient information is now listed horizontally across the top of the form, shaded in pink. Check boxes have been added for client, insurance and Part A Medicare billing. There is also a check box to indicate Medicare Secondary Payer (MSP) information is on file with the physician's office. MSP information should be collected for all Medicare patients. For more information regarding MSP information, please contact Beth Deaton at 668-3376.

(continued)

New to the form is a complete listing of microbiology tests. CPT Codes have also been updated. The Alpha Fetoprotein history has been removed from the back page, and a separate history sheet is required for all AFP maternal #10082 and AFP Triple Screen #10081 tests. A copy of the new requisition is included as Attachment 2. To request a supply of new requisitions or AFP history sheets, or to request additional information or training on these forms, contact your Marketing Representative or Sentara Reference Laboratory Client Services at (757) 668-3621.

Patient Information: complete and accurate patient information is critical for identifying, processing and billing laboratory services. When information is incomplete or incorrect, the laboratory will enter a request for information on the result, or in some cases the test cannot be processed. This not only delays results, but also requires Sentara Reference Laboratory to call physician offices and sometimes patients to gather the missing or incorrect information. If the requested information is not received for completed services, charges may be billed to the ordering physician's practice.

Standing Orders: all standing orders for outpatient testing will be valid for six months. All standing orders older than six months will be verified with the physician that has provided the orders to the lab. Verification will be completed in writing, dated and signed by the test ordering professional and retained at all appropriate locations. Standing orders may be verified through a new written order presented at the collection site or a notice of expiration may be sent to the ordering physician for renewal or cancellation of orders.

Supply Requests: in accordance with OIG-HHS guidelines, Sentara Reference Laboratory provides specimen collection supplies for Sentara lab testing only. To monitor supply distribution, the laboratory audits monthly supply orders and test utilization rates. Please be sure to order Sentara supplies each month based on the amount of Sentara testing you expect to process.

Clinical Consultant: clinical consultant services are available by contacting Stephanie Spingarn, M.D., Director of Clinical Services at (757) 668-3096. All surgical pathology testing will incur separate professional charges. Other clinical tests and pap smears, based on results, may also incur separate professional charges. Professional charges appear on a separate bill from testing. A list of clinical tests that have a separate professional charge is included below.

Clinical Test	CPT Code	Clinical Test	CPT Code
Blood Platelet Aggregation	85576	Hemoglobin Electrophoresis	83020
Crystal Examination	89060	IFE	86334
Darkfield Exam	87164	Protein Electrophoresis	84165
Fibrinolysis or Coag Screen	85390	Smear, Parasites	87207

Test and Medicare Reimbursement Listing: test panels, reflex testing and profiles offered at Sentara Reference Laboratory are listed below with corresponding CPT codes and expected Medicare reimbursements.

Chemistry Panel	Tests	CPT	2002 Medicare Reimbursement
Electrolyte Panel	Na, K, CO$_2$, Cl	80051	$9.69
Basic Metabolic Panel (BMP)	BUN, CO$_2$, Cl, Creatinine Glucose, Na, K, Calcium	80048	$11.70
Creatine Kinase - MB	Total CK CK-MB	82550 82553	$9.01 $15.95
Comprehensive Metabolic Panel (CMP)	Albumin, Alk. Phos., ALT(SGPT), AST(SGOT), BUN, Calcium, CO$_2$, Cl, Creat, Glu, K, Na, Total Bili, Total Protein, Glob	80053	$14.61

(continued)

APPENDIX 42.3   Sample Physician Letter *(continued)*

Chemistry Panel	Tests	CPT	2002 Medicare Reimbursement
Folic Acid, Serum/ Vitamin B_{12}	Folate Vitamin B_{12}	82746 82607	$20.32 $20.83
Hepatic Function Panel	ALT(SGPT), Alk. Phos., AST(SGOT), Total Bilirubin, Direct Bilirubin, Albumin, Total Protein	80076	$11.29
Hepatitis Panel Acute	HAV Ab IgM, HBc Ab IgM, HbsAg, Hep C Ab	80074	$65.82
Hepatitis Panel Chronic	HBs Ag HBs Ab HBc Ab Hep C Ab	87340 86706 86704 86803	$14.27 $10.71 $16.66 $19.73
Immunoglobulins	IgG, IgA, IgM	82784 × 3	$12.85 × 3 = $38.55
Iron Saturation	Iron IBC	83540 83550	$8.95 $12.08
Lipid Panel, Initial	Cholesterol HDL	82465 83718	$6.02 $11.31
Lipid Panel, Complete	Cholesterol, HDL, Triglycerides. If triglyceride is > 400 mg/dl a direct LDL (83721) will be performed and billed separately.	80061 83721 (if indicated)	$18.51 $13.18
Renal Function Panel	Albumin, Ca, CO_2, Cl, Creat, Gluc, Phos, K, Na, BUN	80069	$12.00

Ordered Test CPT Code	2002 Medicare Reimbursement	Reflex Test CPT Code	2002 Medicare Reimbursement
Allergy Inhalant Panel (six separate mixes) 86003 × 6	$7.22 each mix	Additional tests performed depending on positive mix. Allergy Animal - 86003 × 2 Allergy Dust - 86003 Allergy Grass - 86003 × 3 Allergy Mold - 86003 × 4 Allergy Tree - 86003 × 10 Allergy Weed - 86003 × 8	$7.22 × 2 = $14.44 $7.22 $7.22 × 3 = $21.66 $7.22 × 4 = $28.88 $7.22 × 10 = $72.20 $7.22 × 8 = $57.76
ANA Screen - 86038	$16.70	ANA Titer - 86039	$15.43
Anti-neutrophil Cytoplasmic AB - 86255	$16.66	If P-ANCA + = MPO antibody 83516 If C-ANCA + = PR-3 antibody 83516	$15.95 $15.95

(continued)

APPENDIX 42.3 Sample Physician Letter *(continued)*

Ordered Test CPT Code	2002 Medicare Reimbursement	Reflex Test CPT Code	2002 Medicare Reimbursement
Breast Tumor Surgical Pathology Mastectomy, partial/simple 88307 Or Mastectomy, with lymph node 88309	$67.80 $80.70	HER-2/neu 88342, If 2+ positive upon pathologist interpretation then, FISH 88365 88271 88274 ER/PR 86342 X 2	$34.86 $102.96 $29.60 $48.10 $69.72
Cryptococcal Antigen (serum or fluid) 87449	$16.58	Cryptococcal Antigen Titer (serum or Fluid) 86406	$14.70
Culture - AFB 87116 and 87206	$14.45 + $7.42 = $21.87	M. tuberculosis by PCR - 87556	$45.45
Culture - Blood - 87040 Culture - Urine - 87086 Culture - other - 87070, includes respiratory, wound and or abscess Culture - Stool - 87045 and 87046	$14.27 $11.16 $11.90 $4.83 + $1.21 = $6.04	Sensitivity (may be more than one per culture) 87186 Organism ID(may be more than one per culture) 87077	$11.94 $11.16
Culture - Fungus - 87102	$11.61	Fungus identification (may be more than one per culture) 87106	$14.27
Culture - Throat - Strep Only - 87081	$9.16	Organism ID (may be more than one per culture) 87077	$11.16
Direct Antiglobulin - 86880	$7.42	Monospecific Testing - 86880 X 2	$ 7.42 X 2
HIV Ab by EIA - 86701	$12.28	HIV Western Blot - 86689	$26.75
Lyme Abs 86618	$23.54	Lyme Western Blot - IgG & IgM 86617 X 2	$21.40 X 2
Pap Smear, Liquid Based 88142	$28.00	If ASCUS, then HPV titer 87621	$45.45
RPR - 86592	$5.62	RPR Titer - 86593 FTA Ab - 86781	$6.09 $18.30
Streptozyme - 86063	$7.98	ASO Ab - 86060	$9.66
Thyroid Cascade - TSH - 84443	$23.21	T4 Free - 84439 T3 Total - 84480	$12.46 $19.60
Thyroid Replacement TSH - 84443	$23.21	T4 Free - 84439	$12.46
Lipid Complete - 80061	$18.51	If Triglycerides >400, then Direct LDL - 83721	$13.18
Urinalysis - automated 81003, microscopic if indicated	$3.10	If microscopic indicated then 81003 credited and Urinalysis, automated with microscopy - 81001 is billed	$4.37

(continued)

Transfusion Services Test	CPT Codes *some transfusion tests not on Medicare Fee Schedule	2002 Medicare Reimbursement
Immune D Screen	86900, 86901*, 85461	$4.12, *, $9.17
Cord Blood Screen	86900, 86901*, 86880	$4.12, *, $7.42
Crossmatch	86900, 86901*, 86850*, 86920* or 86922*	$4.12, *
Additional Crossmatch	86900, 86901*, 86920* or 86922*	$4.12, *
Indirect Antiglobulin 86850*	if indicated then 86870*, 86905, 86880 × 3, 86970*, 86886	*, $5.28, $7.42 × 3, *, $7.15
Direct Antiglobulin	86880 x 3, 86860* - if indicated	$7.42 × 3, *
Transfusion Reaction	86078*, 81003, 83010* if indicated	*, $3.10, *
Type and Screen	86900, 86901*, 86850*	$4.12, *, $9.17

Frequently Ordered Tests with Multiple Billable CPT Codes	CPT Codes	2002 Medicare Reimbursement
Bacterial Latex Antigens	87147 × 5	$7.15 × 5 = $35.75
Bartonella Antibodies (Cat Scratch)	86611 × 4	$14.06 × 4 = $56.24
Bilirubin, Indirect	82248, 82247	$6.94 + $6.94 = $13.88
Body Fluid Profile	89051, 84315, 84155	$7.61 + $3.46 + $5.06 = $16.13
CD4 W/ CBC/DIFF	88180, 85025	$14.96 + $10.74 = $25.70
CD4/CD8	86360 × 2, 85025	$64.93 × 2 + $10.74 = $140.60
CSF Profile	89051, 82947, 84155	$7.61 + $5.42 + $5.06 = $18.09
Culture, Tissue	87070, 87176	$11.90 + $8.13 = $20.03
DIC Screen	85610, 85730, 85384, 85378	$5.43 + $8.30 + $11.74 + $9.86 = $35.33
DNA Ploidy with Surgical Pathology	88358, 88309 × 2	$16.71 + $80.70 × 2 = $178.11
ENA Antibodies	86235 × 2	$24.78 × 2 eq $49.56
Glucose Tolerance Testing	82950 × 2	$6.56 × 2 = $13.12
Hematocrit and Hemoglobin	85014, 85018	$3.27 + $3.27 = $6.54
IgG Subclass	82787 × 4 , 82784	$11.09 × 4 + $12.85 = $57.21
Immune Complex	86332 × 2	$67.36
Iron Profile	83540, 83550	$8.95 + $12.08 = $21.03
Lead Screen	84202 × 2, 83655	$19.83 × 2 + $16.72 = $56.38
Motor and Sensory Neuropathy	83520 × 7, 86334, 86256, 83883	$17.89 × 7 + $30.87 + $16.66 + $18.79 = $191.55
Ova and Parasites	87177, 87210, 88312	$12.30, $5.90, *
Parvovirus Panel	86747 × 2	$20.77 × 2 = $41.54
Platelet Aggregation	85576 × 5	$29.69 × 5 = $148.45
Sjogren's Antibodies	86235 × 2	$24.78 × 2 = $49.56
Synovial Profile	89051, 82947, 83872, 89060	$7.61 + $5.42 + $8.10 + $9.88 = $31.01
Thyroid Antibodies Profile	86376, 86800	$20.11 + $21.98 = $42.09
I-STAT EG 6+ - Na, K, pH, PCO2, PO2,Hct	84295, 84132, 82803, 85014	$6.65 + $6.35 + $26.74 + 3.27 = $43.01
I-STAT 6+ - Na, K, Cl, BUN, Glu, Hct	84295, 84132, 82435, 84520, 82947, 85014	$6.65 + $6.35 + 6.35 + $5.45 + $5.42 + $3.27 = $33.49
I-STAT EC 4+ - Na, K, Glu, Hct	84295, 84132, 82947, 85014	$6.65 + 6.35 + 5.42 + 3.27 = $21.69
I-STAT G 3+ - pH, PCO_2, PO_2	82803	$26.74
I-STAT E3+ - Na, K, Hct	84295, 84132, 85014	$6.65 + $6.35 + 3.27 = $16.27
I-STAT G - Glucose	82947	$5.42

Note: Any culture with a gram stain will have a separate charge. All wound and abscess cultures will have a gram stain performed to provide rapid clinical information. Gram Stain 87205, $5.90 Medicare Reimbursement. Medicare Reimbursement is based on outpatient fee schedule published by the Medicare Intermediary.

If you have any questions or would like more information about the topics covered in this communication, please contact your Marketing Representative or Sentara Reference Laboratory Client Services at (757) 668-3621.

Beth H. Deaton
Compliance Officer
Sentara Reference Laboratory

APPENDIX 42.4 Medicare Secondary Payor Questionnaire

BENEFICIARY INFORMATION:

Medicare Beneficiary: _____ Patient Account #: _____ HIC:

Dates of Services: From _____ through _____ DCN:

Name of person who supplies the information: _____ Relationship to Patient:

Provider Rep Name: _____ Provider #: _____ Date:

WORKERS COMPENSATION: <u>**Check Yes or No**</u>

1. Per the patient, should this illness/injury be covered by a workers comp claim?   ☐ Yes ☐ No
    If yes, this should be an MSP or conditional claim, not Medicare primary.
    What is the claim number?
    What is the original date of injury?
    What is the name of the workers comp plan?
    What is the address?
    City? _____ State? _____ Zip?

FEDERAL BLACK LUNG:

2. Is the patient covered by the Federal Black Lung Program?   ☐ Yes ☐ No
    If yes, are you able to determine at this time if the claim will be covered by the Department
    of Labor per the acceptable diagnosis list?   ☐ Yes ☐ No
    If yes, this should be an MSP or conditional claim, not Medicare primary.

DEPARTMENT OF VETERAN AFFAIRS:

3. Is the patient entitled to benefits through the Department of Veteran Affairs, due to having
    a service related injury?   ☐ Yes ☐ No
    If yes, does the patient want the VA to be contacted for authorization of these services?   ☐ Yes ☐ No

PUBLIC HEALTH SERVICE:

4. Are the services covered by a Public Health Service (PHS), other than Medicare or Medicaid?   ☐ Yes ☐ No
    If yes, what is the name of the PHS?
    What is the address?
    City? _____ State? _____ Zip?
    What was the time span of the study by the PHS?

ACCIDENT:

5. Are these services the result of an accident?   ☐ Yes ☐ No
    If yes, what type of accident was this (for example; Auto, Slip & Fall (please list location
    of accident), Malpractice, Product Liability, Homeowners)?
    Is Non-Liability insurance available (for example: Premises Medical, Auto Medical
    Coverage, No-Fault, Homeowners Premises)?   ☐ Yes ☐ No
    If yes, what is the name of the Insurance Company?
    What is the address?

    City? _____ State? _____ Zip?
    Does the patient feel someone else is responsible for the accident/injury?   ☐ Yes ☐ No
    If yes, what is the name of the patient's attorney or the responsible party's insurance
    company?
    What is the address?
    City? _____ State? _____ Zip?
    What is the name of the responsible insured party?

(continued)

APPENDIX 42.4   Medicare Secondary Payor Questionnaire *(continued)*

EMPLOYER GROUP HEALTH PLAN:

6.   Is the patient covered by any Employer Group Health Plan (EGHP), including Federal
Employee Health Benefits or any retirement policy?   ☐ Yes   ☐ No
If no, this questionnaire is complete. If yes, continue.

WORKING AGED:

7.   Is the patient 65 years or older?   ☐ Yes   ☐ No
If yes, is the patient and/or spouse currently employed by an employer of 20 or more
employees?   ☐ Yes   ☐ No
If yes, is the patient covered by that Employer Group Health Plan (EGHP)?   ☐ Yes   ☐ No
What is the address?
City? _____ State? _____ Zip? _____
If the beneficiary is no longer employed, give a retirement date if possible:
If the spouse is no longer employed, give a retirement date if possible:

DISABILITY:

8.   Is the patient under the age of 65?
If yes, is the patient entitled to Medicare due to a disability other than end stage renal disease?   ☐ Yes   ☐ No
If yes, is the patient or family member currently employed by an employer of 100 or more
employees?   ☐ Yes   ☐ No
If yes, is the patient covered by that Large Group Health Plan (LGHP)?   ☐ Yes   ☐ No
If yes, what is the name of the LGHP?   ☐ Yes   ☐ No
What is the address?   ☐ Yes   ☐ No
City? _____ State? _____ Zip? _____

END STAGE RENAL DISEASE (ESRD):

9.   Is the patient under 65 years old and entitled to Medicare due to end stage renal disease?
If yes, is the patient covered by any Employer Group Health Plan through a current or
former employer of any size?   ☐ Yes   ☐ No
If yes, is the patient within the 30 month coordination of benefits period?   ☐ Yes   ☐ No
What is the month/year of the first regular dialysis?   ☐ Yes   ☐ No
What is the name of the EGHP that covers the patient?
What is the address?

City? _____ State? _____ Zip? _____
What is insured's name?
What is the policy#? _____ Employer?

DUAL ENTITLEMENT:

10.   Has the patient been identified as either MSP working aged in Question 7 or MSP
Disability in Question 8?   ☐ Yes   ☐ No
If yes, does the patient meet the entitlement criteria for ESRD?   ☐ Yes   ☐ No
If yes, is the patient within the 30 month coordination of benefits period?   ☐ Yes   ☐ No
If yes, the above identified EGHP/LGHP remains the primary payor for the 30 month
coordination of benefits period.
What is the month/year of the first regular dialysis?

Patient's signature: _____ Date:

Witness: _____ Date:

APPENDIX 42.5   Sentara Laboratory Services Physician Acknowledgment Form

---

June 7, 2001

Medical Center
Hampton, Virginia Beach and Chesapeake

Dear Medical Center

Sentara's goal is to provide our physicians with the exact testing required in the delivery of appropriate care for their patients. Within acceptable standards Sentara Lab Services will create any test combination or profile(s) that you desire to meet the medical needs of your patients. You have requested the creation of a custom profile that includes the tests listed below:

TEST NAME	CPT /HCPCS CODE	CHARGE	MEDICARE REIMB
CBC W Diff	85025	$ 43.00	$ 10.74
Comprehensive Met Pan	80053	$ 92.00	$ 14.61
Lipid Complete	80061	$ 44.00	$ 18.51
Thyroxin	84436	$ 61.00	$ 9.50

ACKNOWLEDGMENT:
1. As the ordering physician, you are aware and understand that laboratory tests should only be ordered that you believe are medically necessary for the care of your patient.
2. As the ordering physician, you are aware that using a customized profile may result in the ordering of tests for which Medicare or other federally funded health care programs may deny payment.
3. As the ordering physician, you will order individual tests or a less inclusive profile when not all of the tests included in the customized profile are medically necessary for an individual patient.
4. As the ordering physician, you understand that the OIG takes the position that a physician who orders medically unnecessary tests may be subject to civil penalties.
5. As the ordering physician, you may consult with our Medical Director, Dr. Richard Moriarty at 668-3221 to ensure that appropriate tests are ordered.

Please sign and date to acknowledge the receipt of the above listed information. Thank you for your cooperation in this matter. If you have any questions concerning this form please contact Beth Deaton at 668-3376 or your Marketing Representative. In the event this form is not complete and returned to Lab Services within 15 days the panels listed above will no longer be orderable.

_____ M.D.   Date: _____

APPENDIX 42.6   Sample Test Requisition Form (Front and Back)

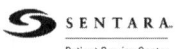

SENTARA
Patient Service Center

Churchland Psychiatric
3300 Academy Avenue • Portsmouth, VA 23701
Tel: (757) 483-6404 • Fax : (757) 483-0737
Client Code: 5040

Patient's Name: _____   Date: _____

PANELS	ICD CODE	PROCEDURES	ICD CODE
☐ Electrolytes	_____	☐ Hep B DNA PCR Quantitative	_____
☐ BMP Basic	_____	☐ HbsAg	_____
☐ CMP Comp	_____	☐ HbsAb	_____
☐ LFT Hep Func	_____	☐ HcAb	_____
☐ Prenatal	_____	☐ HCV RNA	_____
☐ Renal Function Panel	_____	☐ Iron	_____
PROCEDURES	**ICD CODE**	☐ Iron Binding	_____
☐ AFP Tumor	_____	☐ Lipid Initial	_____
☐ Amylase	_____	☐ Lipid Complete Fasting	_____
☐ ANA SCR	_____		
☐ CBC with Diff	_____	☐ PT	_____
☐ CBC w/o Diff	_____	☐ PTT	_____
☐ Ferritin	_____	☐ Sed Rate	_____
☐ H. Pylori Ab, IgG	_____	☐ SGPT (ALT)	_____
☐ Hep A Ab, IgG & IgM	_____	☐ Triglycerides	_____
☐ HBcAb, IgG & IgM	_____	☐ TSH	_____

OTHER: _____

_____

_____

Patients/Physicians: This lab slip only for use at:
Sentara Reference Laboratory Patient Service Center
12695 McManus Boulevard, Suite 7B • Newport News, Virginia 23606
Telephone: 757.890-4783   Fax: 757.890-4778

Aetna, BC/BS, Champus, Trigon, Sentara HMO and PPO, Medicare, Medicaid

---

SENTARA
Patient Service Center

Churchland Psychiatric
3300 Academy Avenue • Portsmouth, VA 23701
Tel: (757) 483-6404 • Fax : (757) 483-0737
Client Code: 5040

Patient's Name: _____   Date: _____

PANELS	ICD CODE	PROCEDURES	ICD CODE
☐ Electrolytes	_____	☐ Hep B DNA PCR Quantitative	_____
☐ BMP Basic	_____	☐ HbsAg	_____
☐ CMP Comp	_____	☐ HbsAb	_____
☐ LFT Hep Func	_____	☐ HcAb	_____
☐ Prenatal	_____	☐ HCV RNA	_____
☐ Renal Function Panel	_____	☐ Iron	_____
PROCEDURES	**ICD CODE**	☐ Iron Binding	_____
☐ AFP Tumor	_____	☐ Lipid Initial	_____
☐ Amylase	_____	☐ Lipid Complete Fasting	_____
☐ ANA SCR	_____		
☐ CBC with Diff	_____	☐ PT	_____
☐ CBC w/o Diff	_____	☐ PTT	_____
☐ Ferritin	_____	☐ Sed Rate	_____
☐ H. Pylori Ab, IgG	_____	☐ SGPT (ALT)	_____
☐ Hep A Ab, IgG & IgM	_____	☐ Triglycerides	_____
☐ HBcAb, IgG & IgM	_____	☐ TSH	_____

OTHER: _____

_____

_____

Patients/Physicians: This lab slip only for use at:
Sentara Reference Laboratory Patient Service Center
12695 McManus Boulevard, Suite 7B • Newport News, Virginia 23606
Telephone: 757.890-4783   Fax: 757.890-4778

Aetna, BC/BS, Champus, Trigon, Sentara HMO and PPO, Medicare, Medicaid

---

SENTARA
Patient Service Center

Behavioral Medical Institute
606 Denbigh Boulevard, Suite 100 • Newport News, VA 23608
Tel: (757) 872-8303 • Fax : (757) 872-6857
Client Code: 5042

Patient's Name: _____   Date: _____

PANELS	ICD CODE	PROCEDURES	ICD CODE
☐ Electrolytes	_____	☐ Hep B DNA PCR Quantitative	_____
☐ BMP Basic	_____	☐ HbsAg	_____
☐ CMP Comp	_____	☐ HbsAb	_____
☐ LFT Hep Func	_____	☐ HcAb	_____
☐ Prenatal	_____	☐ HCV RNA	_____
☐ Renal Function Panel	_____	☐ Iron	_____
PROCEDURES	**ICD CODE**	☐ Iron Binding	_____
☐ AFP Tumor	_____	☐ Lipid Initial	_____
☐ Amylase	_____	☐ Lipid Complete Fasting	_____
☐ ANA SCR	_____		
☐ CBC with Diff	_____	☐ PT	_____
☐ CBC w/o Diff	_____	☐ PTT	_____
☐ Ferritin	_____	☐ Sed Rate	_____
☐ H. Pylori Ab, IgG	_____	☐ SGPT (ALT)	_____
☐ Hep A Ab, IgG & IgM	_____	☐ Triglycerides	_____
☐ HBcAb, IgG & IgM	_____	☐ TSH	_____

OTHER: _____

_____

_____

Patients/Physicians: This lab slip only for use at:
Sentara Reference Laboratory Patient Service Center
12695 McManus Boulevard, Suite 7B • Newport News, Virginia 23606
Telephone: 757.890-4783   Fax: 757.890-4778

Aetna, BC/BS, Champus, Trigon, Sentara HMO and PPO, Medicare, Medicaid

---

SENTARA
Patient Service Center

Behavioral Medical Institute
606 Denbigh Boulevard, Suite 100 • Newport News, VA 23608
Tel: (757) 872-8303 • Fax : (757) 872-6857
Client Code: 5042

Patient's Name: _____   Date: _____

PANELS	ICD CODE	PROCEDURES	ICD CODE
☐ Electrolytes	_____	☐ Hep B DNA PCR Quantitative	_____
☐ BMP Basic	_____	☐ HbsAg	_____
☐ CMP Comp	_____	☐ HbsAb	_____
☐ LFT Hep Func	_____	☐ HcAb	_____
☐ Prenatal	_____	☐ HCV RNA	_____
☐ Renal Function Panel	_____	☐ Iron	_____
PROCEDURES	**ICD CODE**	☐ Iron Binding	_____
☐ AFP Tumor	_____	☐ Lipid Initial	_____
☐ Amylase	_____	☐ Lipid Complete Fasting	_____
☐ ANA SCR	_____		
☐ CBC with Diff	_____	☐ PT	_____
☐ CBC w/o Diff	_____	☐ PTT	_____
☐ Ferritin	_____	☐ Sed Rate	_____
☐ H. Pylori Ab, IgG	_____	☐ SGPT (ALT)	_____
☐ Hep A Ab, IgG & IgM	_____	☐ Triglycerides	_____
☐ HBcAb, IgG & IgM	_____	☐ TSH	_____

OTHER: _____

_____

_____

Patients/Physicians: This lab slip only for use at:
Sentara Reference Laboratory Patient Service Center
12695 McManus Boulevard, Suite 7B • Newport News, Virginia 23606
Telephone: 757.890-4783   Fax: 757.890-4778

Aetna, BC/BS, Champus, Trigon, Sentara HMO and PPO, Medicare, Medicaid

APPENDIX 42.6   Sample Test Requisition Form (Front and Back) *(continued)*

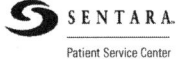

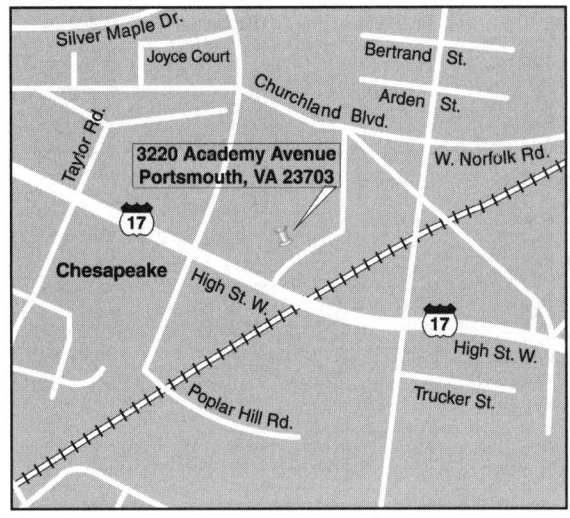

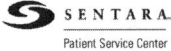

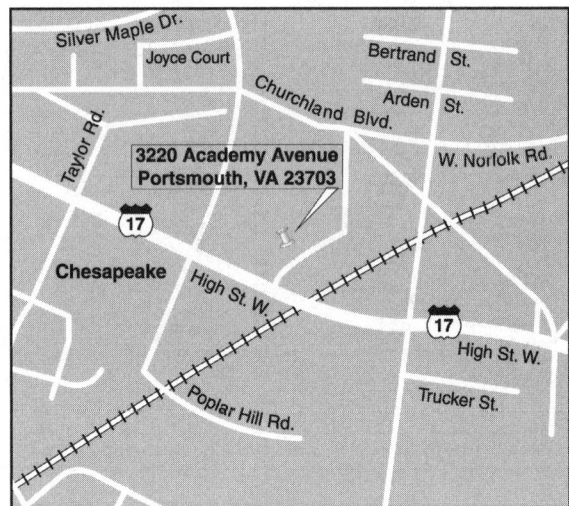

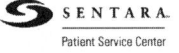

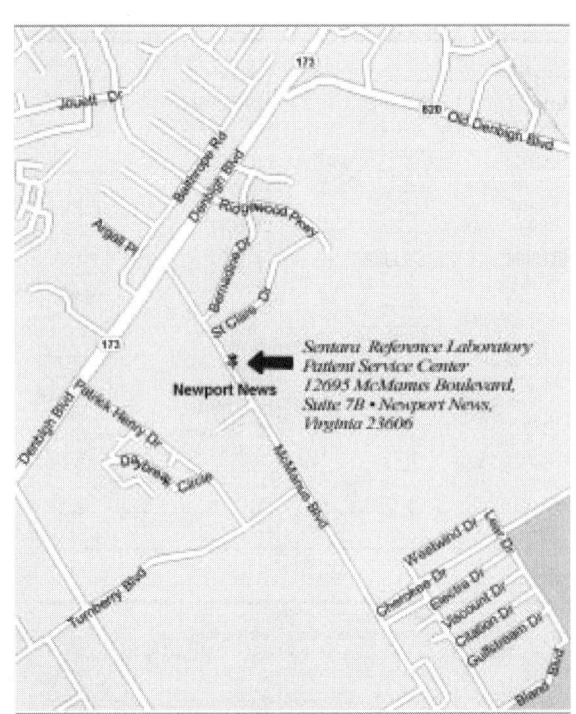

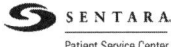

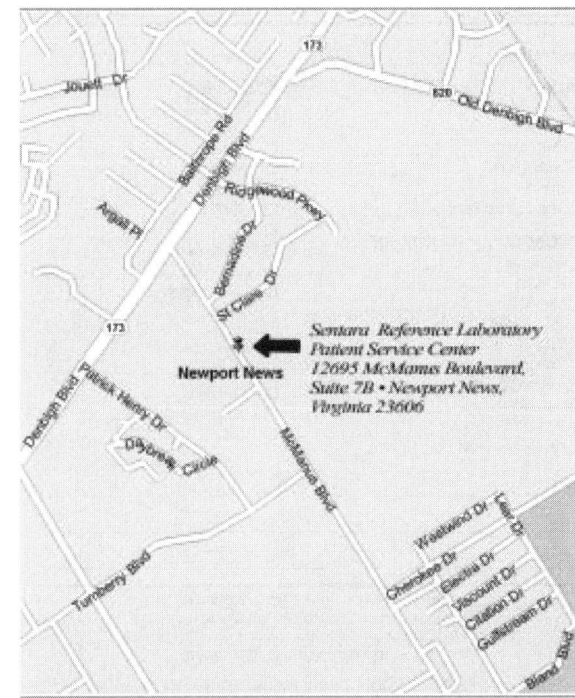

APPENDIX 42.7   Weekly Sales Call Report

Market Rep _____   Page _____ of _____

Week Ending _____

- Fax report by Monday 8:00 a.m. each week to Beth Deaton, Sales Manager.
- Record face-to-face sales and service calls with decision-makers and influencers <u>only</u>. DO NOT record other calls such as telephone inquiries, receptionist contact only, etc.
- Comment required if problem or complaint is encountered. Advise action taken and follow up planned.
- Complete all sections of report. Use as many pages as necessary

Call	Date	Client Prospect	Client #	Name of Decision-Maker seen Face-to-Face	Call Type			Results					
					IV	RV	SC	NQ	SP	NP	SS	COM	Date

Call #	Comments

Date(s) and Time(s) Not Spent in Field/Reasons

KEY

IV = Initial visit   NQ = Not yet qualified   COM = Competitor
RV = Repeat visit   SP = Solid prospect (60-day close)   Date = Follow-up date
SV = Service Call   NP = Not a prospect

APPENDIX 42.8   Monthly Prospect Report

Market Rep _____   Page _____ of _____

Week Ending _____

- The following are fully qualified prospects.
- The decision-makers, decision-influencers, and decision-making processes are clearly identified.
- A "yes" answer has been obtained for each of the qualifying criteria:

Last Month's Prospects (<u>all</u> must be listed):

Name	Clt#	EMV	Current Lab	Close Date	U/N	Next step or reason for deletion

Total _____

New Qualified Prospects, this Month:

Name	City	EMV	Current Lab	Close Date	U/N	Next step or reason for deletion

Total _____

Suspects, this Month:

Name	City	EMV	Current Lab	Close Date	U/N	Next step or reason for deletion

Total _____

Comments: _____

_____

APPENDIX 42.9 Sample Territory Sales Record (Front and Back)

TERRITORY RECORD   Marketing Rep: _____

MARKET TYPE	Client No:	Printer:	☐ Yes ☐ No
☐ Physician	Start Date:	Centrifuge:	☐ Yes ☐ No
☐ Hospital/Clinic	Client Bill: ☐ Yes ☐ No	Lock box:	☐ Yes ☐ No
☐ Medical/Physician Group		In-house draws:	☐ Yes ☐ No
☐ Drug Screen			
Specialty:	Affiliation:	General Location:	

ACCOUNT INFORMATION/BUSINESS CARD

	OFFICE HOURS	
Name:	M –	TH –
	T –	F –
	W –	S –
Street:	Contact:	
City:	Zip:	Title:
		Other Location(s):
Phone No:	Fax:	Volume:
Other Information:		

KEY PERSONNEL

	BEST CALLING HOURS
Physician(s):	
	PAYOR MIX/MANAGED CARE DATA:
Office Manager:	
Nurse:	
Billing Contact:	Other Information:
Other:	

CALL RECORD FOR: _____

DATE	CONTACT	COMMENTS	MATERIALS

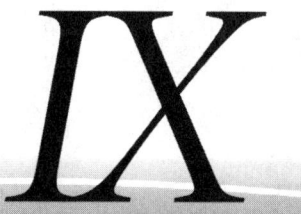

Defining and Measuring Standards for Success

(Section Editor, *Washington C. Winn, Jr.*)

43

Laboratory Benchmarking

Lionelle D. Wells and Washington C. Winn, Jr.

OBJECTIVES

To discuss the reasons for undertaking benchmarking

To review the types of benchmarking activities and where to find benchmarks

To discuss the general approach to the most common type of benchmarking—financial benchmarking for productivity and cost

To discuss the specific approaches to internal and external benchmarking

To discuss the interpretation of internal and external benchmarking data

---

. . . though truth and falsehood bee
Neare twins, yet truth a little elder is;
Be busie to seeke her, beleeve mee this,
Hee's not of none, nor worst, that seekes the best.
To adore, or scorne an image or protest,
May all be bad; doubt wisely; in strange way
To stand inquiring right, is not to stray;
To sleepe, or runne wrong is. On a huge hill,
Cragged, and steep, Truth stands, and hee that will
Reach her, about must, and about must goe;
And what the hills suddenness resists, winne so . . .

JOHN DONNE, SATYRE III

WHAT IS BENCHMARKING? What benchmarks do you use to evaluate your financial performance, human resources activities, customer satisfaction, marketing success, or overall performance? Will you wait for this to pass like other management fads? Will you embrace benchmarking as you previously embraced Total Quality Management (TQM) or will embrace Six Sigma? (5).

Benchmarking is something that should be done continuously on both a personal and professional basis. Benchmarking (with a capital "B") is merely a more systematic and planned approach to our personal "benchmarking." Just as Six Sigma provides a common language and systematic approach to go beyond the 95% or 99% success rate, Benchmarking allows you to compete more effectively, obtain and retain resources for your department, enhance the reputation of your department, and improve the satisfaction of your employees.

Benchmarking is necessary if your laboratory is licensed or accredited by an accrediting organization such as the Centers for Medicare and Medicaid Services

(CMS), the College of American Pathologists (CAP), the Joint Commission for the Accreditation of Healthcare Organizations (JCAHO), the state department of health, or others. (Other organizations that are concerned with quality improvement and implementing standards of performance include the American Association of Blood Banks [AABB], the American Association for Clinical Chemistry [AACC], the American College of Medical Genetics [ACMG], the American Society for Microbiology [ASM], the American Society for Reproductive Medicine [ASRM], the Clinical Laboratory Management Association [CLMA], the Centers for Disease Control and Prevention [CDC], and COLA [formerly the Commission on Office Laboratory Accreditation].) For licensure or accreditation, a laboratory must meet or exceed a series of performance standards. CMS was charged by Congress in the Clinical Laboratory Improvement Act (CLIA) of 1967 and its amendments in 1988 with the task of regulating all laboratories in the United States that perform diagnostic tests on specimens from human patients. All other organizations must be "deemed" by CMS to substantially meet or exceed the standards adopted by CMS. This deemed status is time-limited, and the continuing performance of the accrediting agencies is monitored and evaluated by CMS. A laboratory that is accredited by an organization other than CMS is responsible for ensuring that the deemed status of the certifying agency is current.

The standards range from attracting and retaining qualified personnel to recording and documenting the laboratory's performance in all phases of testing (quality assurance), to compliance with all relevant national, federal, state, local, and industry rules and regulations. Most rules or regulations that pertain to laboratory licensure and accreditation are based on generally accepted principles of good laboratory practice. While regulations may only incorporate the basic or minimal standards for good practice, most voluntary accrediting agencies include far more stringent performance standards, reflecting principles that move an accredited laboratory's performance closer to that of the highest performing laboratories (quality improvement [QI]).

Why Benchmark?

Unfortunately, throughout the world, the cost of available healthcare generally exceeds available resources by a significant margin. As a result, laboratories, much as other healthcare organizations, have limited resources and must maximize their returns on the investment of scarce resources. The returns sought include at a minimum a combination of improved health for the population served, perceptions that they provide high quality of care, and effective and efficient use of allocated resources. If the laboratory is in a market-based system, such as the United States, financial returns are of paramount importance to the survival of the laboratory. Laboratory licensure and accreditation are typically effective in producing high quality care and perceptions of quality. They are not, however, typically focused on effective and efficient use of resources.

Performing well at a price is much more difficult than performing well when price is no object. It requires continuous evaluation and reevaluation of performance. Ensuring the best possible achievement requires a standard against which performance can be evaluated; that standard is a benchmark. Benchmarking is a fundamental process necessary for any laboratory and indeed any healthcare organization with limited resources to survive and thrive.

For best efficiency, each process in the laboratory must perform close to the best balance between what is envisioned and what is possible. What is envisioned are the mission, vision, and goals of the laboratory personnel— why they are there, whom they want to serve, what they hope to accomplish, and how they plan to reach their goals. What is possible reflects the constraints imposed by the customers, equipment, facility, physical space, staff, funding, and organizational culture that the laboratory has acquired over time. Many of these constraints could be changed, but analyzing the effect of changing the constraints is much more than benchmarking. Benchmarking typically involves measuring a process and improving that process. Benchmarking is primarily focused on doing the best that you can with whatever you have today.

The Payoff from Benchmarking

Picking benchmarks and attempting to understand what they mean in terms of your own performance may lead to an analysis of "what if" scenarios (or what could be called *strategic benchmarking*). During the planning for a benchmark activity, you may realize that changes in the mix of customers, laboratory staff, or location of the laboratory would allow performance to reach even higher levels. Thus, benchmarking may eventually include an analysis of strategic changes as well as an analysis of process changes, which may, in turn, alter the mission, vision, and goals of a laboratory. Ultimately, this process represents good business. Benchmarking is but one of many tools that a laboratory or healthcare entity employs to improve performance, focus on customers, survive, and thrive in an environment with limited resources.

The Basic Steps

Begin your benchmarking process by ordering the priorities of your needs for improvement. It is also important to understand what can and cannot be accomplished through benchmarking. Allocate sufficient time to determine the scope of the project. Make sure that the purpose of the project is clear to everyone participating on the benchmarking team. Ensure the support of leadership and the process owner(s). Include a commitment from leadership and process owner(s) to provide time and resources to improve the process and correct any disconnects discovered. Document your findings. Communicate with team members and other stakeholders. Recalibrate or replace benchmarks if necessary. In short, implement good management techniques just as you would for any organizational change—pick your team members well, ensure buy-in of relevant groups, and keep up the team spirit throughout the project.

Once the benchmarking project has started, you must be prepared to communicate findings on an ongoing basis, so as not to surprise the process owner(s). Ensure that data collection and other standards are maintained throughout the measurement period and that there are sufficient resources so that parts of the planned analysis and measurement do not get delayed due to the unavailability of key personnel. Be prepared to expand your analysis and plans for change beyond the scope of the original activity as new or additional relevant findings or needs are uncovered.

Finally, carefully plan and implement changes and ensure adequate piloting of planned changes. Make sure there is adequate training of process owner(s) and staff in new planned processes. Observe and record, document your findings, and plan for additional change(s).

Sometimes during a benchmarking activity, additional items will come up for review that impinge on a process and that may be more relevant to the final solution than was originally expected. Organizational knowledge about processes is usually accurate but may be incomplete. Supervisors and managers can explain in detail the reasons why a process cannot be changed or improved. Often, however, that knowledge does not fully take into consideration some of the less frequent variations that can occur in a process. Changing the way you manage these less frequent, but often very disruptive, variations in a process may result in a substantial but unexpected improvement in the process, although supervisors and managers "knew" that this process could not be improved. The documentation of the project from start to finish is an important tool to finding and using this additional knowledge to improve what cannot be improved and change what cannot be changed.

Where Do We Find Information About Benchmarks?

Business organizations outside of healthcare typically use benchmarking to evaluate performance in the areas of employee development, customer satisfaction, human resources, marketing, and process improvement. If you search the Internet for benchmarks using these terms, you will find between 200,000 and 1,000,000 hits for benchmarks in each of these areas. Notably, only about 75 to 100 hits were found at Yahoo.com. Google.com, Altavista.com, Excite.com, and Lycos.com reported the largest number of valid hits for benchmarks. Thus, to find information about benchmarks, it pays to be expansive rather than limited in

scope. Searching for information in related industries may also yield new insights into processes and introduce further improvements in performance.

Quality Benchmarks

Most laboratories prefer benchmarks that are specifically tailored to the services that a laboratory provides. In the area of quality performance, the CAP's Q-Probes and Q-Tracks programs are excellent benchmarking projects (4, 8). They allow laboratories to share competitive and best practices data in a blind study focusing on areas that typically could be improved in most laboratories. The Q-Probes and Q-Tracks are intended to help laboratories meet the QI standards in accreditation surveys. The Q-Probes are short-term studies that generate a single report without trended data. They tend to be detailed, contain extensive analysis, and require relatively long turnaround times because of the complexity. The Q-Tracks are long-term, focused monitors with tabular and graphic reports; data are submitted quarterly. Analysis is less extensive than in Q-Probes, turnaround time is shorter, and trended data are supplied. Both programs extend beyond the laboratory environment to focus on key processes and areas of concern, including such issues as accuracy of labeling of blood specimens, reducing telephone calls to a surgical pathology department through the incorporation of standardized reporting formats, measures of satisfaction with laboratory services, and effectiveness of services. Many of these studies are published in the *Archives of Pathology* and are also available on the CAP website (http://www.cap.org). If the concerns of highest priority for the laboratory are in these areas, these programs are a good place to start the search for information about benchmarks. They will serve the laboratory well when benchmarking preanalytic and postanalytic activities. These approaches to benchmarking issues of quality have been applied in Great Britain as well as in the United States (2).

Financial Benchmarks

One of the most difficult areas to benchmark is financial performance. However, difficult does not mean impossible; with some thought and creativity, you can find a number of measures that can be used effectively to track the financial performance of a laboratory. The two general categories that are of interest to the directors of laboratories and hospitals are cost data and productivity data. That is, how much does it cost to operate the laboratory and how efficient is the operation?

General Approach to Financial Benchmarking

The Problem of Comparability

One important issue that comes up when looking for financial benchmarks is the lack of comparability of any organization's accounting system with another organization's accounting system. For example, one organization may not allocate a line item for overhead (e.g., for the executive office staff); instead, it loads all these costs, including utilities, into a charge per square foot for laboratory space (approximately $92 per square foot). This approach makes line-by-line budget comparisons with other organizations that analyze costs in a more traditional manner very difficult because the charge per square foot cannot be broken out into the components for utilities, overhead, etc.

In another organization, costs for overhead are taken out and paid before a budget is allocated for the laboratory service. As a result, the laboratory administrators in this organization did not have access to the fully loaded cost of their laboratory services. This type of budgeting process seems to be more prevalent in governmental than in for-profit entities; thus, when seeking comparisons, it is essential to identify organizations that function in a similar manner so that the likelihood of making valid comparisons and consequently drawing valid conclusions is maximized.

This problem is the old issue of comparing apples and oranges or even crab apples and gigantic Red Delicious fruit. Several approaches to the problem will be discussed in the section on implementation.

The Problem of Cost Accounting

Most laboratory professionals will agree that determining the cost of an individual laboratory test is very difficult. For tests performed in one of the relatively automated sections of the laboratory, such as chemistry or hematology, the true cost of a laboratory test will vary substantially with the shift, the day of the week, and the instrument on which it is performed. Most laboratories have multiple instruments or systems that may be used for performing some tests; for example, a test for blood glucose may be performed by point of care instrumentation or with a multichannel analyzer. If the laboratory is responsible for the cost of both systems, what is the true cost of the glucose test? If an attempt is made to analyze performance at the level of methodology as well as analyte, the system becomes very complex. For batched tests, the cost of a test will vary with the size of the batch because the expense exhibits a stepwise, rather than a linear, progression with increasing volume.

For relatively manual sections of the laboratory, such as microbiology and blood bank, the problems are difficult but no more tractable. All microbiology specimens are not created equal. A specimen that yields no bacterial growth will generate costs in labor and materials that are very different from a specimen with several potential pathogens. Similarly, all blood typing and cross-matches do not have identical complexity. Once again, the system becomes very complex if an attempt is made to account for each of the variables.

Workload Recording

The classic attempt to measure laboratory cost and productivity was the workload recording method developed by the CAP. It followed classic industrial methods for assessing productivity, concentrating on productivity of labor. Each laboratory operation was assessed by detailed time-motion studies. The labor required for an individual test was the sum of the labor required for each component of the test. The sum of labor inputs for all tests of that type could then be calculated, after which the labor input for the division could be derived, etc. Eventually, a value for the laboratory as a whole could be determined. The results of the time-motion studies were published and were widely used in the laboratory industry. Theoretically, comparable data would be generated if every laboratory used the same standard. A committee that was broadly representative of the industry was charged with maintaining the program.

After many years of swimming against the stream, the workload recording system was eventually abandoned in favor of a unit-of-service (UOS) approach, as described below. The workload recording approach foundered on the multiple shoals of complexity, variability, and most importantly, the inability to keep pace with the constant changes in methodology. The method made people feel good about measuring all the variables, but it was ultimately nonviable. As it has receded into the mists of distant memory, there has been a tendency to yearn for the "good old days" when we measured everything. Hidden in the mists are all the problems that led to the demise of the workload approach.

The resilience of workload recorders was well demonstrated when a national consultant promised to save an institution millions of dollars by improving efficiency. The method that the consultants employed was workload recording under another name, but unfortunately, the reprogramming did not make the approach work any better. The first attempt at measuring the "efficiency" of the histology laboratory, for instance, resulted in a productivity of greater than 1,000%. There was, of course, a simple explanation for the aberration. The consultants did not realize that the time allotted for performing a single hematoxylin-eosin stain did not translate into a valid number when a whole rack of slides was stained! Eventually, a number for productivity was negotiated between the consultant and the manager of the histology laboratory, but the number was based on guesswork rather than science. Not surprisingly, a new hospital administration finally admitted that the consultants had not only failed to realize the savings that they had promised, they did not even realize enough savings to pay the enormous fee that they had taken home. The more things change, the more they stay the same!

The Search for Simplicity

According to the law of parsimony (Occam's razor), the simplest solution is preferred and should be sought first. Everyone is painfully aware of the complexity of the problems faced in the laboratory; a complex solution, therefore, is intuitively appealing. Settling for a parsimonious solution makes us feel unfulfilled and unappreciated! But, in truth, these good intentions lead to you-know-where. You must look for proxies that can be used on either a global or indirect basis to monitor the financial perform-ance of a laboratory. Programs can determine these costs in various ways; some include benchmark data. Current labo-ratory information systems often include activity-based costing or attempts at workload recording. Various consult-ing firms, including many large accounting firms, also claim to have benchmark data and expertise in this type of analy-sis of the financial performance of a laboratory, as described above. The consultants, although often very expensive, are readily available if needed by any laboratory. But a sophisti-cated laboratory worker should beware of the facile solution to an incredibly difficult problem. For instance, the labora-tory information systems still do not take account of such issues as batch size, work shift, or technical level of the oper-ator. Nor can they keep up with changes in negotiated price of labor and materials without a large amount of time and effort to keep the data current (assuming the presence of an adequate computer system in the first place). It is feasi-ble, although time-consuming and expensive, to develop a snapshot of laboratory cost and efficiency at the test level at a single time point. It is entirely another matter to track performance over time, a process that provides most of the managerial value.

What then are some of the alternatives to detailed and specific financial benchmarks? One alternative is to move to a higher level, so that many of the distortions that occur in pricing individual tests average out across a section, di-vision, or laboratory. One technique that many managers have used successfully in the past is:

1. Determine in some reproducible fashion the total number of laboratory tests done (with or without tests referred to a reference laboratory),
2. Determine the total budget of the relevant laboratory unit, and
3. Finally, use these numbers to calculate an average cost per test.

This approach might be termed "benchmarking by UOS." It is an example of the ratio method described in the next section. Not surprisingly, the greater the number of tests counted, the greater the statistical robustness of the analysis. Thus, cost and productivity at the level of the laboratory will be more accurate and reproducible than divisional data, which will, in turn, be more robust than test-specific data.

Selection of Indicators for Benchmarking

As in epidemiology and financial analysis, ratios are much more useful than raw numbers. Knowing the denominator does not assure that the numbers will be meaningful, but the numerator alone will be useful only rarely. The two general types of instructive ratios may be characterized as cost ratios and productivity ratios. In both cases the most valid denominator is a UOS. The most generally accepted unit is the billed test, because most financial systems cap-ture the data and *Current Procedural Terminology*, 4th ed.

(CPT-4; published by the American Medical Association and updated yearly), allows a relatively standardized char-acterization of laboratory tests among all laboratories, whether for-profit or not-for-profit, whether commercial, hospital-based, or physician office laboratories (1). Labo-ratories may differ in the services for which they actually bill clients; some systems, therefore, use the term "billable test" to describe any procedure for which there is a CPT code and for which a client could have been billed.

Although quality control procedures, repeat tests, and research procedures do not have CPT-4 codes and cannot be billed to insurers, a laboratory could, at its discretion, include these procedures in the denominator of their benchmarking tool if systems are available to integrate the numbers with the officially billed tests. Alternatively, the assumption may be made that the numbers of such tests will be consistent over time and may be excluded from analysis. Commercially available systems for external benchmarking will define the criteria for tests that may be counted in the system.

Examples of variables that are frequently analyzed are summarized in Table 43.1. Commonly used ratios are de-tailed in Table 43.2.

The use of the ratio method to evaluate cost per test, as summarized above, can be applied to the components of the cost. The two major components are labor cost and materials cost. Depending on the scientific discipline and nature of the clientele served by the laboratory, the divi-sion of costs between these two categories can vary greatly. Similarly, the productivity of laboratory labor can be evalu-ated based on worked hours (a component of "produc-tive" labor costs) and paid hours (a component of "non-productive" labor costs and a direct measure of the total labor costs in the laboratory). "Productive" and "nonpro-ductive" are technical terms used to differentiate those ac-tivities that produce test results directly, as opposed to other activities (which may also be very important or even essential).

Problems Associated with Benchmarking by UOS

There are many obvious flaws in a measure such as overall cost per test. One problem is that it is much easier to ac-complish a reduction in cost per test in an environment where there is a substantial increase in the number of tests ordered each year than it is to achieve the goal in an envi-ronment where volume of testing is stable or decreasing. The volume relationship of costs has been well demon-strated and is discussed by Lepoff in chapter 28.

A second drawback is that by giving up nuclear detail in order to get a valid picture of the whole organism, man-agers at the front line may feel shortchanged as they try to address detailed challenges of everyday life. Scientists and physicians should be used to these kinds of tradeoffs. In the microbiology laboratory, for example, we recognize that in standardizing the conditions of antimicrobial sus-ceptibility tests to get reproducibility from day to day and

Table 43.1 Variables that are frequently assessed in benchmarking programs

Variables	Comments
Billable tests - total, on-site, off-site, referred	The most frequently used denominator for cost and productivity. May also be used as numerator when analyzing work by patient population. Separation by testing site allows analysis of costs associated with work done locally or referred.
Billable tests - total, inpatient, outpatient, "non-patient"	Commonly denominator, but may be numerator (see above). Allows analysis of various patient populations. "Non-patients" represent work from outside hospitals or other clients. To be truly useful, it must be feasible to dissect the costs actually incurred for each category (often difficult or impossible).
Inpatient days, inpatient discharges	Denominator for evaluation of workload by patient type. A hospital with a large population of chronically ill patients may have an aberrantly small value when days are the denominator, but discharges will provide a better comparison.
Outpatient visits vs. non-patient encounters	The most problematic distinction because of the variation in how institutions categorize their outpatients vs. physician office patients.
Total FTEs and total hours	Often used as denominator in productivity ratios. Measures "productive" and "nonproductive" labor.
Testing FTEs and testing hours	Measures productive labor only. In comparison programs, each laboratory must count productive labor identically for this variable to be useful.
Worked versus paid hours	Comparing ratios may shed light on the fringe benefits (vacation, sick time, conference time, etc.) granted by a laboratory to employees.
Total and testing labor expense	Defines the cost of productive and total labor. When analyzed with FTE/h, the effects of differing skill mixes, wage rates, and fringe benefits may be evident.
Consumable expense	Costs of supplies and reagents.
Maintenance expense	Reflects the cost of maintenance contracts.
Depreciation expense	The cost of equipment depreciation; may not be broken out by the institution to the level of department or division.
Manageable expense	Those expenses that should be under the control of laboratory managers; usually the sum of labor, consumables, depreciation, and maintenance expenses.
Blood expense	The cost of purchased blood products; increasingly separated from other consumables because of the increasingly high cost. This expense may not be easily managed.

laboratory to laboratory, we are giving up the ability to reproduce the nonstandardized conditions that occur in each individual patient. We have adjusted to that necessary scientific compromise; we must learn to adjust to the similar financial compromise.

UOS Benchmarking in a Competitive Environment

If you use a measure such as overall cost per test in a competitive environment, other laboratories would likely experience similar increases or decreases in their work, un-

less there is a difference in the marketing, service, or customer base of your laboratory leading to significant differences in growth of testing. Again, since overall cost per test is an easily derived number, you should be able to determine if anomalies such as this are influencing your performance against the benchmark. If there are significantly different inter-institution changes in the underlying costs and number of tests used to calculate overall cost per test, you may have to find a new benchmark or perhaps spend time and resources addressing the issues that are causing

Table 43.2 Commonly used ratios in benchmarking

Financial ratios	Productivity ratios	Miscellaneous ratios
Testing (total)[a] expense/FTE (h)	Billable tests/total FTE (h)	Testing FTE/total FTE
Consumable expense/total (on-site) billable tests	Billable tests/testing FTE (h)	Worked hours/paid hours
Total expense/inpatient day (inpatient discharge, outpatient visit)	Billable tests/inpatient day (inpatient discharge, outpatient visit)	
Referred billable test expense/referred billable test		On-site billable tests/total billable tests
Blood expense/total (on-site) expense		Inpatient (outpatient, non-patient) billable tests/total billable tests
Maintenance expense/total (on-site) expense		
Depreciation expense/total (on-site) expense		

[a]Items in parentheses are other, similar parameters.

you to fall behind your goals. For example, if your laboratory is losing market share, you may need to improve the marketing of your laboratory services to meet your goals for overall cost per test.

Implementing Financial Benchmarking

There are several possible approaches to financial benchmarking. They are not mutually exclusive, and each has its pros and cons, which are summarized in Table 43.3.

Internal Benchmarking

The simplest and most straightforward approach to benchmarking is to use your own laboratory as the standard and measure performance over time. What you gain by this maneuver is reproducibility because management has control over the assumptions and can ensure consistency over time. In addition, departments, divisions, and laboratories within the organization that are difficult or impossible to compare against each other can legitimately be compared against themselves. It is not valid to expect the same productivity or expense in a cytogenetics laboratory as is required in an automated chemistry laboratory, but it is valid to ask each of those laboratories to make ongoing improvements in both productivity and cost on a continuing basis.

Internal benchmarking is, in fact, no more than continuous monitoring of performance. An example of such continuing analysis is displayed in Appendix 43.1. A great deal of useful information can be derived from close examination of sequential numerical data. Added value can be obtained if the data can be displayed visually as control charts (Fig. 43.1, 43.2, and 43.3). The control chart is familiar to most members of the laboratory team as a means of tracking quality control of laboratory tests. It is also a commonly used tool by epidemiologists and by managers in general.

By limiting the analysis to a single organization, management loses the value of comparing performance with peers in the industry, some of whom might even be competitors. Although it is not possible to evade this deficiency completely, it is possible to provide surrogates that approach the kind of comparisons found in external benchmarking.

- In truth, the most important external effect of benchmarking is to convince the ultimate institutional authority, whether it is the CEO or a subordinate, that the laboratory is functioning efficiently. If there is a mutually agreeable definition of good performance between laboratory and institutional managers, formal external comparisons become less important.

Table 43.3 Approaches to financial benchmarking

Type	Method	Pros	Cons
Internal	Workload recording	Measures actual work performed.	In practice, difficult or impossible to validate and maintain.
Internal	UOS monitoring	Variables are known and can be controlled; temporal comparisons legitimate; should be done even if external benchmarking performed.	Continuous improvement in financial and productivity indicators can be documented, but performance relative to peers cannot be assessed.
External	Commercial program (laboratory-based)	Standardized reporting form; flexibility in assessing performance relative to peers; program constructed and data analyzed by peers in the laboratory industry.	Required data may be difficult and/or time-consuming to obtain. Peer groups may not be valid and/or peers may not submit their data according to instructions, potentially producing misleading interpretations. Results may be viewed skeptically by institutional administration.
External	Commercial program (hospital-based)	See above; however, program constructed by individuals who may not understand laboratory structure and performance; design may be relatively unsophisticated from a laboratory perspective.	Results may be more useful to institutional managers, who can see them in the context of total institution benchmarking. Results may be more easily accepted by institutional managers.
"External"[a]	Comparison of UOS with selected peers in voluntary group	Control over construction of peer group; contacts for discussing anomalies easily available.	Number of peers may not produce statistically valid comparisons.
"External"[a]	Comparison against "arbitrary" standard	If the standard comes from the institutional leadership, it will be the operative goal from a practical point of view.	Standard may be flawed; it should be validated (carefully and with political sensitivity).
"External"[a]	Comparison with published industry norms	Provides useful comparison data with published recommendations on publicly traded companies.	Ensure that the laboratories are truly comparable or that recommendations come from evaluating comparable laboratories.

[a]These activities involve external comparisons, but they are performed at the local level. They are discussed in the text under internal benchmarking.

Figure 43.1 Control chart for internal benchmarking. The parameter depicted is billable tests, followed over time. Upper and lower control limits are statistical parameters that can be set at any desired value (e.g., ± 1, 2, or 3 standard deviations around the mean). The data are plotted by quarter over a period of 3 years. Note that the laboratory has achieved a steady increase in billable tests beginning in the first quarter of 1995. The trend is going in the desired direction, but it is important to understand the reason(s) for the change. Compare with Fig. 43.2 and 43.3. Data adapted from a report provided to a participant in the LMIP of the CAP.

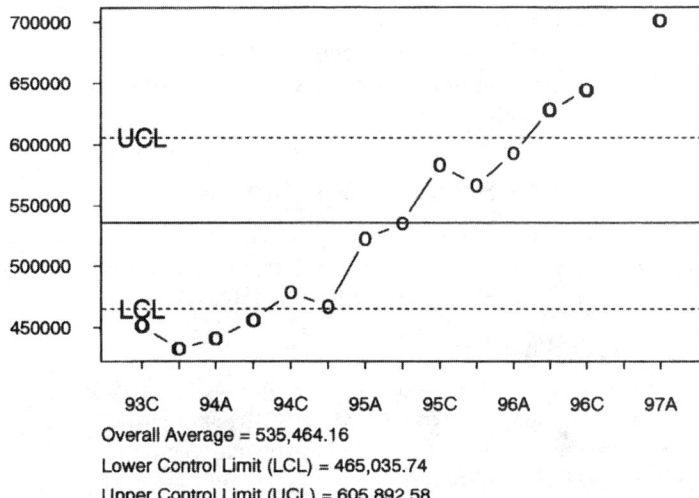

Overall Average = 535,464.16
Lower Control Limit (LCL) = 465,035.74
Upper Control Limit (UCL) = 605,892.58

- Sometimes it is possible to develop voluntary agreements with other institutions to share productivity and cost data (3). Although this approach does not have the statistical rigor of comparison with a large number of institutions, you do have complete control over the comparison group. Appendix 43.2 provides an example of a hypothetical agreement among hospitals.

- Most healthcare institutions and all publicly traded companies are required by law to file financial reports with governmental regulators. The degree of detail and the depth of analysis available in the public records of most hospitals are probably insufficient to provide productivity data that are adequate for the purposes of comparison. The filings of publicly traded laboratories, however, will have much more relevant detail. An example of such an analysis is detailed in Table 43.4.

Several notes on these approaches to comparisons are in order.

1. If a laboratory director takes (or is forced to take) the road of agreed standards with institutional managers, the same issues of comparability that plague external benchmarking will apply. An example may be found in the following brief play, entitled "The Tragical Comedy of the Laboratory Director and the Chief Executive Officer."

Act I [*Office of the Chief Executive Officer (CEO)*]

CEO (a former consultant with a prominent national consultancy): In my extensive experience, a valid laboratory benchmark for productivity is 0.2 h per billed test.

Laboratory Director: That may be difficult to achieve. We are in an academic institution with responsibilities for training residents and medical technologists. In addition, we have active programs that service transplant programs and cancer patients, all of whom are immunosuppressed and very ill, requiring extensive laboratory support.

CEO: That is all very well and good, but my benchmark comes from one of the most prestigious academic institutions in the country, one that far exceeds ours in the amount and sophistication of research and transplant service.

Laboratory Director: May I ask which institution that is, please?

Figure 43.2 Control chart for internal benchmarking. The parameter depicted in this chart is paid hours, followed over time. Note that a dramatic increase in paid hours was recorded in the first quarter of 1995, after which the number of employees stabilized. Such a large increase in personnel might appear undesirable, but it must be understood in the context of other changes in the operations of the laboratory. Compare with Fig. 43.1 and 43.3. Data adapted from a report provided to a participant in the LMIP of the CAP.

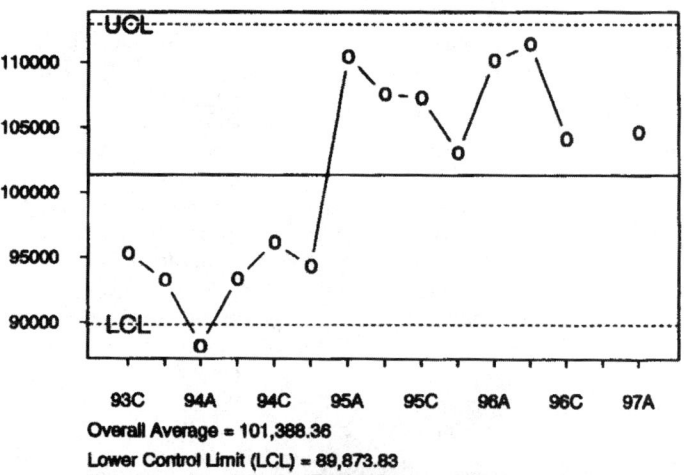

Overall Average = 101,388.36
Lower Control Limit (LCL) = 89,873.83
Upper Control Limit (UCL) = 112,902.88

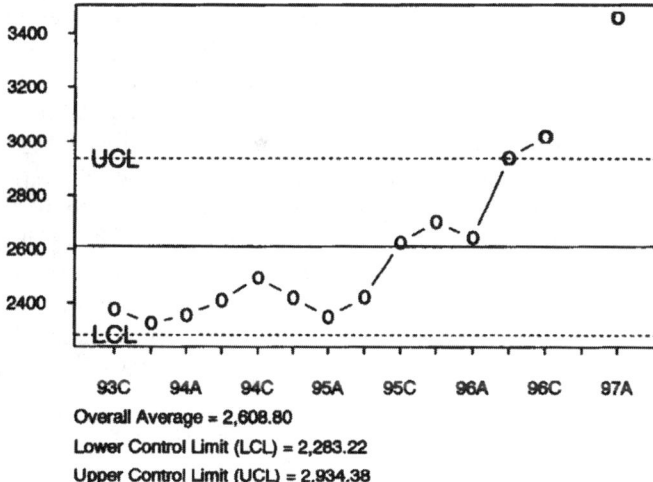

Figure 43.3 Control chart for internal benchmarking. The parameter depicted in this chart, billable tests per FTE, is the product of the changes depicted in Fig. 43.1 and 43.2. Despite the dramatic increase in FTE in the first quarter of 1995, the productivity of the laboratory steadily increased. Plotting the ratio tells a more complete picture than viewing only the components would allow. Data adapted from a report provided to a participant in the LMIP of the CAP.

CEO: That is Superstar Medical Center, which is always ranked in the top 10 in the national polls.

Act II, One Month Later *(Office of the CEO)*

Laboratory Director: Thank you for agreeing to see us. After our last meeting the laboratory financial manager and I talked in detail to our counterparts at Superstar Medical Center. They confirmed that their productivity goal, which they regularly meet, is 0.2 h per test. It turns out, however, that they are a very dispersed academic medical center. Many of the units that are part of our laboratory are separate administrative units at Superstar. Examples include anatomic pathology, cytogenetics, and electron microscopy, which are among the most manual and most labor-intensive divisions. If one drops out those units from our mix, we are meeting the 0.2 h per test standard already. I hope that makes you feel better about our performance.

CEO: Well now, actually, Superstar Medical Center was only one of the institutions I had in mind. There are a number of others that are even more productive.

Act III, Scene One, Two Years Later *(Office of the Laboratory Director)*

Laboratory Director: Isn't it a shame that the Board fired the CEO?

Laboratory Financial Manager: I'm crying buckets.

Act III, Scene Two, One Year Later *(Office of the CEO)*

CEO: I have been reviewing the records of the previous administration and I have now visited with each of the major divisions. What is your assessment?

Chief Operating Officer: (a holdover from the previous administration): Well, it seems clear that the laboratory is still a problem. I am not at all sure that I trust their assessment of productivity and competitiveness.

CEO: That may be true, but we have the regulators breathing down our necks. The nurses want to unionize. The Board has been chastened and is getting too darned active for their own (read "our own") good. It does appear that the laboratory is making money from their active outreach program, so I think we are better off letting sleeping dogs lie.

CURTAIN

2. Comparisons with peers: All external benchmarking programs seek to form comparison groups of peers, who are as like each other in critical characteristics as possible. It seems intuitively obvious that a voluntary comparison should be constructed similarly. If you set a goal to reduce cost per test year after year (a form of competitive benchmarking), you could, for example, compare local performance with that of other laboratories by following the change in cost per test from period to period. The velocity, rate, or percentage change in local costs compared to similar laboratories, rather than the absolute cost per test, would be the benchmark against which performance is then measured. If you succeed in reducing cost per test at

Table 43.4 Internal benchmarking with "homemade" standard by reference to published information on publicly traded commercial laboratories[a]

Parameter	Commercial laboratory A	Commercial laboratory B	Combined total for 20 independent laboratories	University hospital laboratory
Annual billable tests	306,020,000	205,660,000	26,344,792	2,271,772
FTEs	33,200	24,000	3,037	255
Annual billable tests per FTE	9,217	8,569	8,675	8,897
Daily billable tests per FTE	35.5	33.0	33.4	34.2
Hours per billable test	0.226	0.243	0.240	0.234

[a]Data courtesy of Thomas Wadsworth.

a faster rate than peers, you will eventually achieve a lower cost per test, no matter what the starting point.

3. The counterintuitive approach of comparing oneself with a competitor who should be much more productive and efficient than oneself, however, also has some advantages and attractions. Managers in their right minds would not perform such a comparison publicly or make the results known unless they were favorable. If the expected unfavorable results materialize, they could be used inappropriately against the laboratory by institutional managers who do not understand the nature of the exercise. Such a comparison between an academic medical center (local data) and publicly traded laboratory companies (data from company reports, available on the Internet) is summarized in Table 43.4.

External Benchmarking

All things being equal, the value added of external benchmarking should make it the evaluation method of choice (Table 43.3). You could then track performance internally to observe temporal changes, but you could also measure local performance against the best in the field. To use a sports analogy, internal benchmarking would be similar to a sprinter measuring performance only by comparison to previous efforts without ever testing that performance against the best in the field, representing external benchmarking. It is certainly true that it is possible to get better continuously without ever actually being very good. On the other hand, a healthy athlete who competed only against handicapped performers could look great on paper without actually being very good. In the best of all worlds, of course, you would do both internal and external comparisons, but financial and workforce constraints may make it difficult to live in Camelot (and remember there was hanky-panky going on even there).

There are two types of formal external benchmarking approaches (exclusive of the kinds of informal comparisons described under internal benchmarking). In each, an external organization, which may be a for-profit entity or a not-for-profit group, provides a service. In one case the benchmarking program for the laboratory is part of a comprehensive system that covers the whole institution, usually a hospital or medical center. In the other case, the program is focused on laboratories and does not address issues outside of the laboratory. Two such programs have been described in published reports (3, 6).

The advantages and disadvantages of these two external benchmarking alternatives are summarized in Table 43.3. Both alternatives suffer from a common defect, which will vary in severity from program to program—the comparison group will be constructed of participants who have volunteered to be a part of the process. Admittedly, for the hospital-wide programs, the "voluntary" aspect may be on the part of the institutional rather than the laboratory administration. That selectivity means that the comparison groups are not random; careful attention to this difficulty

by statisticians can ameliorate the problem, but cannot eliminate it. It has been documented by the organizers of some programs that participants who withdraw or do not continue participation have performed less well than those who remain in the program. Such a result is not surprising because no one wants to look bad (especially if the results may be seen by superiors), and it is easy to argue that the program was simply inadequate and the results, therefore, invalid (an argument that could either be true or a rationalization). Whatever the reason for withdrawal, the result is to tighten the comparison group and skew the results by trimming off only one end (the lower one) of the curve.

Those who participate in an external benchmarking program should assure themselves that:

- The comparison group is comparable to the local institution and there are enough members of the group to make statistical comparisons reasonable.

- There is adequate and sophisticated statistical analysis of data. The purveyors should be able to document the validity of their criteria for comparison and the adequacy of their comparison groups.

- Data are analyzed and the results are returned in a timely fashion. It should be noted that the goal of external benchmarking is not fine-tuning of operating issues, so it is better to accept a somewhat extended time for analysis in return for sophisticated, useful information. There is no need for external benchmarking more frequently than quarterly. Semiannual or even annual evaluation is adequate and probably preferable because the volume of data will be larger and the extra work required to access information for external providers will be limited to once or twice a year.

- The data required by the external agency are reasonable and that the laboratory is comfortable with the accuracy of the data. You should direct particular skepticism at data that are generated by hospital financial analysts without review and acceptance by knowledgeable departmental managers, including those in the laboratory.

- There is an understanding by administrators and managers both in the laboratory and in the institution that the results will be evaluated honestly and without prejudice. The goal should be to understand the data, accept or reject the apparent "messages," and improve performance. A program that is used only to punish or denigrate people or departments will be circumvented and cannot succeed.

If a hospital-wide benchmarking program is mandated by the leadership of the institution, the managers of the laboratory should also consider participating in a program that is focused specifically on the laboratory. Wilkinson and Reynolds provided a dramatic illustration of the use of data from a laboratory-focused program (LMIP of the

CAP) to identify problems that were produced by a less finely tuned hospital-wide program (Healthcare Benchmarking Systems International) (7).

Interpretation of Internal Benchmarking Data

"Team" Benchmarking

Using a simple number such as average cost per test as the main financial benchmark can provide insights into your own operations as well as those of other laboratories. Most laboratories can derive a number such as overall cost per test with relatively little effort.

Using a measure such as overall cost per test means that the accumulation of each small decision made in every section of the laboratory must, on average, move the laboratory towards the goal of reducing cost per test. This approach might be designated "team benchmarking." A focus on a global goal, rather than on multiple smaller departmental goals, allows you the opportunity to make an upfront investment in one area with the aim of achieving eventually much lower overall costs. This approach may be viewed as a team investment in the future, whereas a department-by-department approach inhibits development of a team spirit and such future investment. Use of an overall number such as cost per test may also enhance your ability to invest in changes that may not yield results within 1 or 2 years. If a particular investment for the future raises costs in a certain area, such a consequence may not matter as long as overall performance measured for the total laboratory demonstrates a continuing reduction in costs that meets or exceeds targets. In this case, all savings possible may not be captured in any given year because an investment has been made for even greater savings in the future. Managers experience this sort of future investment when they purchase a newer, more productive laboratory instrument but must pay the up-front costs in 1 year to achieve savings over the following years.

Qualities Needed for "Team Benchmarking"

For a team benchmarking system to work, the leadership of the laboratory and/or the institution must exhibit a number of qualities. Honesty requires us to admit that the scenario we envision may be utopian. Some of these characteristics and approaches are:

- Management must not depend on numbers alone but must use all senses to sort out where the problems are and where attention must be directed. We suspect that everyone in many laboratories knows where the problems, challenges, and opportunities are, although they may not be identified openly and honestly.

- Management must treat all members of the laboratory as if they are truly members of a team. Such an approach requires an honest understanding of barriers and challenges combined with a willingness to face

them together. If resolution of issues is difficult or impossible for a supervisor who is trying, support rather than recrimination is essential. If sacrifices must be made in a certain division or if that division must do without until its time comes, that sacrifice must be appreciated and a good faith effort must be made to ensure that the time does indeed come for that division in a realistic time frame.

- All members of the laboratory must truly believe that they are part of a team, that their efforts are recognized and appreciated, and that they will not be penalized for sacrifices made for the greater good.

Whether the team is the laboratory as a whole or a subunit, when the internal benchmarking approach is used, analysis consists of directing constant attention to improving all relevant ratios and following the improvement or lack of improvement in each ratio. Attention can then be directed to any indicators (ratios) that are not improving with time.

If there is an informal and/or arbitrary standard against which the laboratory is to be measured, such as the directive of the CEO in the drama above, analysis must focus on attempting to understand deviations from the goal.

Interpretation of External Benchmark Data

When the external benchmarking approach has been chosen, the analysis can be more sophisticated and potentially more instructive, but the process is also more complicated. When the external benchmarking is through a contracted service, the analysis is both assisted by and limited by the

Figure 43.4 Percentile graph of billable tests for an institution for a single time period. The results of the participant laboratory can be compared with (i) all the laboratories in the database, (ii) all participating laboratories in the same region, (iii) a group of laboratories selected (from a list of participating laboratories) by the participant, (iv) a "fingerprint cluster" of laboratories that were closest to the participant by statistical analysis (performed by the program), and (v) the two closest matches to the participant. Notice that the participant laboratory is an outlier when compared to other laboratories in the program as a whole and in the region, but it falls into a similar range with more closely matched laboratories, whether they were self-selected or chosen by the program. There are obvious advantages to having multiple comparison groups from which to draw conclusions. Data adapted from a report provided to a participant in the LMIP of the CAP.

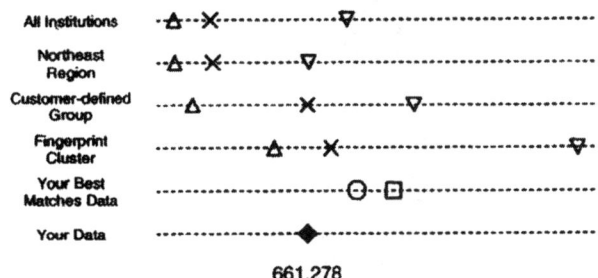

661,278

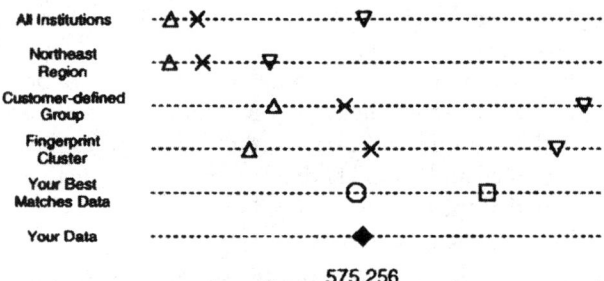

575,256

Figure 43.5 Percentile graph of blood expense for an institution for a single time period. Comparisons are as described in Fig. 43.4. The expenses for the participant institution are considerably higher than those for the program as a whole and for the laboratories in the region, but they are in line with the laboratories in the comparison groups that are better matched. The importance of multiple comparisons and valid comparison groups are, once again, demonstrated. Data adapted from a report provided to a participant in the LMIP of the CAP.

way the data are massaged and presented by the benchmarking service. It is obvious that one limitation is the choice of items that is presented by the program and the statistical rigor of the presentation. The simplest presentation is depiction of institutional data on a continuous scale with other participants, usually divided into quartiles or deciles (Fig. 43.4 and 43.5). The drawback of percentile analysis is that 25% of participants will always be in the bottom quarter, even if everyone is performing adequately on an absolute scale. Conversely, the top 25% of participants will always be in the top quartile, although the per-

formance of the group as a whole may be lackluster in absolute terms. Additionally, each item will be viewed in isolation, unrelated to other important parameters.

More sophisticated analytical schemes may present several relevant indicators as a single graphical summary; for example, a productivity ratio on one axis and a cost ratio on the other axis. The best performers will have high productivity and low cost; the worst performers will conversely have high cost and low productivity. An example from the LMIP of the CAP is shown in Fig. 43.6.

When data are available for each indicator, it is possible to dissect the information and construct possible explanations for the observations. It may be impossible to discover *the* explanation, but at least the laboratory manager has the data to supplement direct observation of laboratory performance. It must be mentioned once again that no analytical program can substitute for astute management, careful study of daily events in the laboratory, and, most importantly, listening to peers and subordinates.

Given the complexity of laboratory function and the variability of available benchmarking programs, it is not possible to provide an exhaustive catalogue of all possible analytical permutations. In Appendix 43.2, the benchmarking data from four laboratories during one time period are compared and analyzed. Two of the laboratories (A and B) are similar, and these comparisons are closest to the paragon of "apples to apples." The other two laboratories differ in enough parameters from each other and from the first two to make comparisons more problematic. In each instance, the benchmarking data should be viewed

Figure 43.6 Graphical depiction of laboratory performance. Cost is plotted on the *Y*-axis (manageable expense per billable test); productivity is plotted on the *X*-axis (billable test per FTE). The position of the "best performing" laboratory in the group is in the lower right corner (greatest productivity and lowest cost). The upper left corner (lowest productivity and highest cost) is the least desirable position. The center of the graph is "middle of the road." The participant laboratory is represented by a black diamond, which is positioned in the lower right quadrant but relatively close to the center point. Thus, the performance is respectable, but there is room for improvement. Such a graphical depiction of complex data takes a morass of data that are potentially confusing and makes it much easier to see the big picture. Data adapted from a report provided to a participant in the LMIP of the CAP.

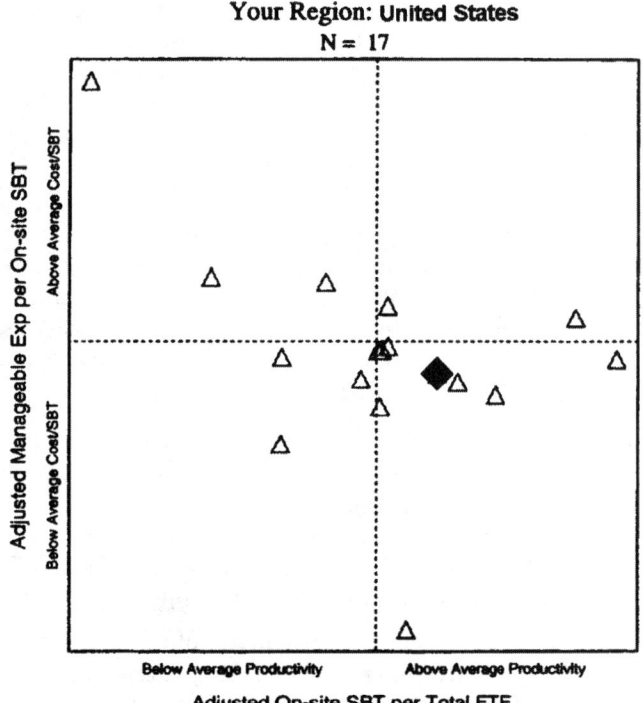

only as a starting point from which to work. The most useful purpose served by the comparisons is that they may point the way to useful lessons about your own business and the road to improvement.

Summary

Determining which improvements in technology, which computer systems, and what test mix will improve patient outcomes, provide the best quality, and meet financial objectives is an overwhelming task. With benchmarking, we have a method to measure performance and improve our ability to meet our goals, which typically include improved health, high quality, and an overall increase in efficiency. Accreditation and licensure focus primarily on improving health and increasing quality without much focus on efficiency. Most hospital laboratories operate on a 24-h, 7-day-per-week schedule, resulting in a high fixed-cost structure in an environment of declining reimbursements and continuing shortages of personnel. Continuous and significant gains in productivity and efficiency are required to do more with less each year.

KEY POINTS

- A creative approach to benchmarking allows you to find measures of industry-leading performance in almost any area.

- The most effective benchmarks either address a specific concern (such as the Q-Probes and Q-Tracks) or overall concerns reflecting performance of most of the laboratory in a single index.

- Validation of high-level benchmarks often yields more information about overall performance.

- If the resources are available, it is optimal to participate in both internal and external benchmarking activities.

- Review of performance against the benchmark frequently identifies areas in which additional interventions could yield additional improvements in performance.

- Networking and membership in leading laboratory organizations is an excellent way to find relevant benchmarks. A number of the programs for laboratory managers at the 2003 CLMA national meeting included the word "benchmark" in their title, and many other programs referenced benchmarks even though the word was not in the title of the program.

GLOSSARY

Accreditation Approval, generally for a limited time, of an institution or program based on a review of the institution or program by one or more independent examiner(s) who determine that specific requirements or standards have been met.

Accrediting agencies Organizations that validate the ability of a laboratory to perform laboratory testing. In the United States,

the federal government is charged by statute (CLIA '67 and CLIA '88) with the task of regulating diagnostic laboratory testing on human subjects. CMS (formerly Health Care and Finance Administration) is charged by Congress with the task of developing and implementing regulations. CMS can "deem" other organizations to issue accreditation if their standards substantially meet or exceed those of CMS. Testing of animals and research subjects is not covered by these regulations.

Benchmark A standard against which performance is measured. The standard typically represents performance that is considered the best in the field or the gold standard of possible performance. Various internal, external, industry-wide, and non-industry performance measures may all be used as benchmarks.

Benchmarking Comparing your own performance against a standard usually representing the gold standard or best performance for similar activities and engaging in processes to improve performance against the chosen standard.

Billable test Usually defined in benchmarking parlance as a test for which there is a CPT-4 code and that could, therefore, be billed to Medicare (and most other insurers).

Billed test A test that is actually billed to an insurer or client. Billable test is the parameter usually preferred by benchmarking programs because institutions vary in what they actually bill.

Clinical Laboratory Improvement Act of 1967 (CLIA '67) Established the initial authority to regulate laboratories in the United States. It was superseded by CLIA '88.

Clinical Laboratory Improvement Amendments of 1988 (CLIA '88) Currently the governing authority for regulations regarding function of all laboratories that perform testing on human specimens in the United States.

Clinical Laboratory Management Association (CLMA) Professional organization concerned with all aspects of laboratory management. Many local chapters have been organized.

Competitive benchmarking Comparing your own performance against competitors in the same industry or market rather than focusing primarily on gold standards or best practices as standards for performance.

Deemed authority The approval by CMS, as agent for the federal government, of another organization to represent the government in accrediting clinical laboratories that evaluate human specimens, whether they be hospital laboratories, commercial laboratories, or physician office laboratories. Deemed status is time-limited, so each deemed organization must document that it holds a valid certificate of certification. The standards of each deemed organization must be reviewed and accepted by CMS.

External benchmarking Benchmarking activities that include comparison of the performance of one laboratory with that of its peers. The comparisons may be made through the intermediary of an external organization or by informal arrangement among laboratories.

Full-time employee (FTE) A measure of the workforce. Part-time employees are counted as fractions of an FTE. Generally, FTEs are calculated by dividing total paid hours by 2,080 (52 weeks of 40 h each).

Internal benchmarking Benchmarking activities within an organization, usually by tracking the performance of a laboratory over time.

Nonproductive FTE Commonly used to describe those personnel who are not involved directly in generation of test results. This category includes supervisory personnel, support personnel (marketing, customer service, washroom, etc.), and the portion of line personnel devoted to activities such as quality control and maintenance.

Paid hours The number of employee hours actually paid by the laboratory. It includes those hours that were worked and those that are due the employee as part of a benefit package (sick leave, vacations, etc.).

Productive FTE Usually employed to define those laboratory workers who actually produce test results. In practice, defining who these individuals (or parts of individuals) are becomes very difficult, and even more difficult to calculate. For instance, do you count those people who enter the specimen into the system or enter results into the information system?

Quality assurance A process to ensure that all services involved in the delivery of patient care have been accomplished in the appropriate manner that will maintain excellence in medical care. The U.S. Food and Drug Administration defines quality assurance as planned and systematic activities to ensure that a laboratory will meet certain requirements for quality (from the FDA website, http://www.fda.gov).

Quality improvement Involves outcomes, results, ends, and information rather than just concerns with specific processes. Whereas quality assurance is focused on providing a quality test result, QI is concerned with improving the entire process so that the results are more accurate, more timely, and presented in a more useful and informative manner to the clinician. Thus, QI is concerned with all aspects of testing, including the preanalytic, analytic, and postanalytic phases.

Six Sigma An approach to improving quality that involves measuring defects or adverse events against "sigma," a common measure of variation. The goal is to reduce sigma to a minimum. This approach could be viewed as a variation on internal benchmarking.

Skill mix The mixture of personnel with varying degrees of training, education, and certification. Examples include laboratory technicians, medical laboratory technicians, and medical laboratory technologists.

Testing FTE *See* Productive FTE.

Total FTE The total number of FTEs employed in the laboratory, regardless of their duties.

Total quality management An approach to integrating multiple activities revolving around QI.

Unit of service (UOS) The denominator in ratios used to analyze cost or productivity. The most commonly used UOS is the billable test.

Worked hours The number of hours actually worked by employees (compare "paid hours").

Workload recording A means of measuring laboratory output and consequently productivity by tallying individual components of laboratory tests quantitatively. The most prominent national program that provided norms for quantifying effort was eventually abandoned because of the difficulty in maintaining a viable system.

REFERENCES

1. American Medical Association. 2003. *Current Procedural Terminology.* CPT 2003. AMA Press, Chicago, Ill.

2. Galloway, M., and L. Nadin. 2001. Benchmarking and the laboratory. *J. Clin. Pathol.* **54:**590–597.

3. Heatherley, S. S. 1997. Key performance indicators to assess laboratory operations. Benchmarking for survival. *Clin. Lab Manage. Rev.* **11:**164–170.

4. Lawson, N. S., and P. J. Howanitz. 1997. The College of American Pathologists, 1946–1996. Quality Assurance Service. *Arch. Pathol. Lab. Med.* **121:**1000–1008.

5. Nevalainen, D., L. Berte, C. Kraft, E. Leigh, L. Picaso, and T. Morgan. 2000. Evaluating laboratory performance on quality indicators with the six sigma scale. *Arch. Pathol. Lab. Med.* **124:**516–519.

6. Portugal, B. 1993. Benchmarking hospital laboratory financial and operational performance. *Hosp. Technol. Ser.* **12:**1–21.

7. Wilkinson, D. S., and D. D. Reynolds. 2003. Using benchmarking to manage your laboratory. *Clin. Leadersh. Manage. Rev.* **17:**5–8.

8. Zarbo, R. J., B. A. Jones, R. C. Friedberg, P. N. Valenstein, S. W. Renner, R. B. Schifman, M. K. Walsh, and P. J. Howanitz. 2002. Q-tracks: a College of American Pathologists program of continuous laboratory monitoring and longitudinal tracking. *Arch. Pathol. Lab. Med.* **126:**1036–1044.

APPENDIX 43.1 Internal Benchmarking by Monitoring Financial and Productivity Data on a Sequential Basis, Using Ratios[a]

Appendix 1. Internal benchmarking by monitoring financial and productivity data on a sequential basis, using ratios.

	FY 2003 Total Operating Budget	FY 2003 Operating Budget Year to Date	October	November	December	January	February	March	April	May	June	Year to Date Actual	Year to Date Variance	Year to Date Variance (%)
VOLUMES														
Unit Of Service														
Inpatient Volume	47,283	35,462	4,117	4,002	4,154	4,204	3,820	3,783	4,258	3,854	3,376	35,568	106	0.30
Outpatient Volume	100,476	75,357	9,291	8,346	8,202	8,999	9,280	9,060	9,604	9,766	8,801	81,349	5,992	7.95
Total Volume	147,759	110,819	13,408	12,348	12,356	13,203	13,100	12,843	13,862	13,620	12,177	116,917	6,098	5.50
EXPENSES														
LABOR EXPENSE														
NON PRODUCTIVE REG SAL	104,768	78,576	5,014	6,352	13,724	8,014	10,000	8,577	12,443	9,482	12,386	85,990	(7,414)	(9.44)
PRODUCTIVE REG SAL	847,665	635,749	70,081	69,251	65,022	69,482	61,895	72,066	64,387	69,622	62,193	603,999	31,750	4.99
PRODUCTIVE OT SAL	4,685	3,514	625	3	84	557	602	(103)	107	1,226	117	3,217	297	8.45
Staff Salaries	957,117	717,838	75,720	75,606	78,829	78,054	72,496	80,539	76,936	80,330	74,696	693,205	24,633	3.43
EMPLOYEE APPRECIATION	2,070	1,552	0	0	0	0	15	685	150	100	125	1,075	478	30.78
Other Personnel Expense	2,070	1,552	0	0	0	0	15	685	150	100	125	**1,075**	478	30.78
Total Salaries	959,187	719,390	75,720	75,606	78,829	78,054	72,511	81,224	77,086	80,430	74,821	694,279	25,111	3.49
Allocated Fringe Benefits	259,857	194,893	20,558	20,527	21,402	21,192	19,683	21,866	20,888	21,809	20,280	188,205	6,688	3.43
Total Salaries & Fringe Benefits	1,219,044	914,283	96,278	96,133	100,231	99,246	92,193	103,090	97,974	102,239	95,101	882,485	31,798	3.48
CONSUMABLE EXPENSES														
MEDICAL SURGICAL	5,130	3,848	126	94	277	39	129	295	86	201	119	1,367	2,480	64.46
LAB SUPPLIES	589,658	442,243	29,178	44,099	57,780	103,427	61,828	93,519	64,662	38,125	54,661	547,280	(105,037)	(23.75)
OXYGEN	5,130	3,848	233	359	233	233	277	204	175	550	303	2,567	1,281	33.29
INSTRUMENTS AND NEEDLES	667	500	36	36	61	36	73	36	36	0	61	376	124	24.82
Med/Surg Supplies	600,584	450,438	29,574	44,589	58,350	103,736	62,307	94,054	64,960	38,876	55,144	551,590	(101,151)	(22.46)
PHARMACEUTICALS	156	117	16	0	5	0	1	5	8	20	0	55	62	52.80
IV-IRRIGATING SOLUTIONS	52	39	0	11	0	0	11	0	11	0	0	32	7	18.15
Pharmaceuticals	207	156	**16**	**11**	**5**	**0**	**12**	**5**	**18**	**20**	**0**	**87**	69	44.14
OFFICE SUPPLIES	0	0	1	7	0	0	0	0	0	0	333	341	(341)	--
SUPPLIES OFFICE-PRINTED	0	0	0	50	3	2	0	863	0	0	288	1,205	(1,205)	--
SUPPLIES OFFICE-GENERAL	0	0	0	0	0	0	0	4	0	2	4	10	(10)	--
CHINA GLASS AND FLATWARE	100	75	0	0	0	0	0	0	0	0	0	0	75	100.00
Supplies Other	100	75	1	57	3	2	0	867	0	2	624	**1,556**	(1,481)	(1,974.93)
MAIL & PRODUCTION	0	0	70	(65)	0	1	0	0	0	0	0	6	(6)	--
Utilities	0	0	**70**	**(65)**	**0**	**1**	**0**	**0**	**0**	**0**	**0**	**6**	(6)	--

(continued)

APPENDIX 43.1 Internal Benchmarking by Monitoring Financial and Productivity Data on a Sequential Basis, Using Ratios[a] *(continued)*

	FY 2003 Total Operating Budget	FY 2003 Operating Budget Year to Date	October	November	December	January	February	March	April	May	June	Year to Date Actual	Year to Date Variance	Year to Date Variance (%)
BOOKS/SUBS/DUES NONMD	150	113	81	0	60	0	0	320	129	0	0	590	(478)	(424.54)
TRAVEL/MEET/DUES-GENERAL	1,599	1,199	0	0	0	0	0	0	0	0	0	0	1,199	100.00
UVM MAINT/REPAIR OFFICE	0	0	0	0	500	395	0	0	0	0	0	895	(895)	--
MAINTENANCE-NONCONTRACT	1,261	946	0	0	15	3,535	0	50	0	0	0	3,600	(2,654)	(280.63)
CAFETERIA	250	188	0	0	44	0	0	0	0	0	0	44	144	76.66
CELEBRATION FUNDS	418	314	0	0	0	69	0	0	0	0	0	69	245	78.09
PROFESSIONAL DEVELOP NON	303	227	0	0	0	0	0	0	0	0	0	0	227	100.00
SMALL EQUIPMENT	550	413	0	0	0	0	0	0	0	0	0	0	413	100.00
Other Expenses	4,531	3,398	81	0	619	3,999	0	370	129	0	0	5,198	(1,799)	(52.94)
Total Consumable Expense	605,423	454,067	29,742	44,591	58,977	107,737	62,318	95,295	65,107	38,899	55,769	558,436	(104,369)	(22.99)
TOTAL EXPENSE	1,824,467	1,368,350	126,019	140,724	159,208	206,983	154,512	198,387	163,081	141,138	150,869	1,440,921	(72,570)	(5.30)
LABOR														
Staffing FTEs														
Productive-Regular FTEs	18.36	18.36	17.32	18.85	15.72	17.12	17.83	18.13	16.83	17.92	15.96	17.30	1.06	5.77
Productive-Overtime FTEs	0.07	0.07	0.10	0.00	0.02	0.10	0.08	0.00	0.03	0.22	0.04	0.07	0.01	10.72
Subtotal Productive FTEs	18.43	18.43	17.43	18.85	15.73	17.22	17.92	18.14	16.86	18.14	15.99	17.36	1.07	5.79
Non-Productive FTEs	2.27	2.27	1.62	0.93	4.21	2.51	2.77	2.35	3.52	2.29	3.80	2.67	(0.40)	(17.61)
Total FTEs	**20.70**	**20.70**	**19.05**	**19.78**	**19.94**	**19.73**	**20.68**	**20.49**	**20.38**	**20.43**	**19.80**	**20.03**	**0.67**	**3.22**
Productivity Labor Hours														
Productive-Regular Hours	38,181.00	28,635.75	3,059.93	3,221.98	2,776.22	3,024.66	2,845.17	3,203.11	2,877.70	3,165.51	2,728.42	26,903	1,733	6.05
Productive-Overtime Hours	153.00	114.75	18.50	0.14	3.36	16.82	13.39	0.79	4.75	38.78	6.08	103	12	10.58
Subtotal Productive Hours	38,334.00	28,750.50	3,078.43	3,222.12	2,779.58	3,041.48	2,858.56	3,203.50	2,882.45	3,204.29	2,734.50	27,005	1,745	6.07
Non-Productive Hours	4,719.00	3,539.25	286.81	159.76	743.31	444.11	441.35	415.8:	601.79	404.67	650.30	4,148	(609)	(17.20)
Total Hours	**43,053.00**	**32,289.75**	**3,365.24**	**3,381.88**	**3,522.89**	**3,485.59**	**3,299.91**	**3,619.71**	**3,484.24**	**3,608.96**	**3,384.80**	**31,153**	**1,137**	**3.52**
Per Unit of Service (UOS) Statistics														
Total Salaries & Fringe Benefits/UOS	8.25	8.25	7.18	7.79	8.11	7.52	7.04	8.03	7.07	7.51	7.81	7.61	0.64	7.77
Med/Surg Supplies/UOS	4.06	4.06	2.21	3.61	4.72	7.86	4.76	7.32	4.69	2.85	4.53	4.68	(0.61)	(15.03)
Other Expense/UOS	4.10	4.10	2.22	3.61	4.77	8.16	4.76	7.42	4.70	2.86	4.58	4.73	(0.63)	(15.49)
Total Expense/UOS	**12.35**	**12.35**	**9.40**	**11.40**	**12.89**	**15.68**	**11.79**	**15.45**	**11.76**	**10.36**	**12.39**	**12.34**	**0.01**	**0.05**
Productive Hours/UOS	0.26	0.26	0.23	0.26	0.22	0.23	0.22	0.25	0.21	0.24	0.22	0.24	0.02	9.37
Total Hours/UOS	**0.29**	**0.29**	**0.25**	**0.27**	**0.29**	**0.26**	**0.25**	**0.28**	**0.25**	**0.26**	**0.28**	**0.27**	**0.02**	**7.89**
Productive to Total Hrs Ratio	89.04	89.04	91.48	95.28	78.90	87.26	86.63	88.51	82.73	88.79	80.79	87.62	1.42	1.59

(continued)

APPENDIX 43.1 Internal Benchmarking by Monitoring Financial and Productivity Data on a Sequential Basis, Using Ratios[a] *(continued)*

NOTES

1. Test volume (measured as billable tests), labor expense, consumable expense, other expense, and staffing are displayed as absolute numbers. The budgeted amount is adjusted for a 9-month time period. Deviations of actual data from budgeted projections are depicted as a variance and percent variance.

2. FTEs are calculated as paid hours divided by the appropriate number of hours. On a yearly basis, that calculation is paid hours divided by 2,080. The denominator varies from month to month because of the varying length of the months, so a simple conversion is not easy.

3. Ratios are displayed with financial (or labor) data as numerator and test volume (billable tests) as denominator. The actual data for year-to-date is compared to the budgeted number to obtain the variance.

4. Fringe benefits are driven by a formula that will vary by institution, depending on organizational policies.

5. When finances are tracked monthly, there will be large swings from month to month, especially in categories with small budgets. The manager must recognize the variation and not overreact to an outlier. For instance, in January, there was a large expense for noncontract maintenance (cell G52) that stands out among the other months and actually puts the category over budget. It is likely that in the long term (multiple years) maintenance expenses are well controlled.

6. For those who believe in operations budgets, it is important to recognize that they represent projections and even "best guesses." When there is a deviation from the budget (variance), it is most important that the manager(s) understand the reason(s) for the discrepancies.

OBSERVATIONS

1. Test volume has a positive variance, most of which is caused by an increase in outpatient tests (row 7). Budgeted volume data are projections that are based on past experience and estimates of the local market. The figure should have input from both financial and scientific personnel. If the budget is adjusted for volume, a shortfall in tests can obviously cause headaches for the manager. Conversely, greater than predicted volumes can improve the perception of performance but can cause significant problems for staff if sustained.

2. Despite the variance in test volume, there is a positive variance in labor expense, both as an absolute number (rows 17 and 21) and per UOS (row 81). Total FTEs are close to budget (row 70), so the explanation is probably that some budgeted employees are not being paid. Possible reasons include employees who have exhausted allotted time for illness or family leave or have taken a temporary leave of absence for other personal reasons. Such shortfalls can be tolerated for brief periods but may produce difficulties for remaining workers if sustained. If the combination of increased volume and decreased staffing continues, a manager could question whether the staffing levels are too high. The unit manager must make every effort to limit the duration of the staff shortage if it is causing problems but must be forthright if the staffing level is, in fact, greater than necessary.

3. It is very difficult to hit budget targets on the head. Policies on variances may vary among institutions. A common recommendation is to investigate variances that exceed 5% or $1,000. The variances in test volume and labor expense have been noted. In addition, there is a considerable variance in consumable expense (row 59). That variance is almost completely determined by an overage in lab supplies (row 30) and consequent negative variance in Med/surg supplies (row 33). After careful analysis of consumable expenses, the manager determined that the negative variance was entirely related to a change in the methodology for a small number of tests from a nucleic acid probe (lower cost for reagents) to amplified molecular testing (more expensive reagents). The switch had been justified by improved quality of results and service for clients. The administrative managers of the laboratory and of the institution approved the switch but a change in the middle of the year after budgets had been established resulted in an ongoing variance.

The negative variance in consumable expense is sufficiently great that the positive variance in salary expense cannot compensate. As a result, there is a small negative variance in total expense (row 61). Because of the increased volume in outpatient testing, however, there is actually a very small positive variance when expenses are calculated as a ratio against UOS (row 84). The power of increasing test volume in a volume-adjusted budget is very apparent.

[a]The spreadsheet illustrates the data from a microbiology laboratory for a portion of a fiscal year (October 2002 through June 2003).

APPENDIX 43.2   Performance Characteristics of Four Laboratories

	A	B	C	D	E
3	**PARAMETER**	**LABORATORY A**	**LABORATORY B**	**LABORATORY C**	**LABORATORY D**
4	Total Billable Tests (BT)	788,674	1,014,980	878,932	956,873
5	On-Site Billable Tests	777,448	1,009,087	786,453	954,417
6	Referred Tests	11,226	5,893	92,479	2,456
7	Inpatient Billable Tests	257,896	573,217	784,921	0
8	Outpatient Billable Tests	466,916	389,529	94,011	750,275
9	Nonpatient Billable Tests	63,862	52,234	0	204,142
10	Hospital Inpatient Days	28,656	47,504	62,879	NA
11	Hospital Inpatient Discharges	5,037	8,023	7,543	NA
12	Outpatient Visits	57,233	74,167	18,802	NA
13	Productive Paid Hours	61,269	75,421	60,720	63,191
14	Total Laboratory Worked Hours	90,357	116,902	82,406	77,409
15	Total Laboratory Paid Hours	100,662	125,701	86,743	78,989
16	Calculated Productive FTEs	117.83	145.04	116.77	121.52
17	Calculated Total FTEs	193.58	241.73	166.81	151.90
18	Productive Labor Expense ($)	1,569,131	1,552,929	971,522	884,677
19	Total Labor Expense ($)	2,348,641	2,352,923	1,387,888	1,105,846
20	Consumable Expense ($)	1,074,239	1,418,697	983,066	1,049,859
21	Equipment Maintenance and Repair ($)	68,429	67,707	54,987	32,343
22	Equipment Depreciation ($)	96,952	121,494	76,354	54,985
23	Referred Test Expense ($)	154,406	136,750	801,793	12,771
24	Blood Expense ($)	604,654	926,001	345,890	0
25					
26	**RATIOS**				
27	On-Site BT as % of Total BT	98.58	99.42	77.48	94.03
28	Referred Tests as % of Total BT	1.42	0.58	9.11	0.24
29	Inpatient BT as % of Total BT	32.70	56.48	77.33	0.00
30	Outpatient BT as % of Total BT	59.20	38.38	9.26	73.92
31	Nonpatient BT as % of Total BT	8.10	5.15	0.00	20.11
32	On-Site BT/Productive FTE	6,598	6,957	6,735	7,854
33	On-Site BT/Total FTE	4,016	4,174	4,715	6,283
34	Productive FTE/Total FTE	0.61	0.60	0.70	0.80
35	On-Site BT/Total Worked Hour	8.60	8.63	9.54	12.33
36	On-Site BT/Total Paid Hour	7.72	8.03	9.07	12.08
37	Total Worked Hours/Total Paid Hours	0.90	0.93	0.95	0.98
38	On-Site BT/Total BT	0.99	0.99	0.89	>0.99
39	Inpatient BT/Day	9.00	12.07	12.48	NA
40	Inpatient BT/Discharge	51.20	71.45	104.06	NA
41	Outpatient BT/Outpatient Visit	8.16	5.25	5.00	NA
42	Productive Labor Expense/On-Site BT ($)	2.02	1.54	1.24	0.93
43	Total Labor Expense/On-Site BT ($)	3.02	2.33	1.76	1.16
44	Consumable Expense/On-Site BT ($)	1.38	1.41	1.25	1.10
45	Referred Test Expense/ Referred BT ($)	13.75	23.21	8.67	5.20
46	Testing Paid Hours/On-site BT	0.08	0.07	0.08	0.07
47	Worked Hours/On-site BT	0.12	0.12	0.10	0.08
48	Paid Hours/On-site BT	0.13	0.12	0.11	0.08
49	Worked Hours/On-Site Billable Test	0.12	0.12	0.10	0.08
50	Paid Hours/On-Site Billable Test	0.13	0.12	0.11	0.08
51					
52	**LABORATORY CHARACTERISTICS**				
53	University Affiliated Laboratory	Yes	Yes	Yes	No
54	Primary University Laboratory	Yes	Yes	No	No
55	Pathology Residency Program	Yes	Yes	Yes	No
56	Number of Pathology Residents	14	25	4	0
57	Surgical Pathology	Yes	Yes	Yes	No
58	Cytopathology	Yes	Yes	Yes	No
59	Cytogenetics	Yes	Yes	No	No
60	Autopsy	Yes	Yes	Yes	No
61	Electron Microscopy	Yes	Yes	No	No
62	Molecular Diagnostics Laboratory	No	Yes	No	No
63	Courier Service	Yes	Yes	No	Yes
64	Marketing Personnel	Yes	Yes	No	Yes
65	Customer Service Personnel	Yes	Yes	Yes	Yes
66	Dedicated Compliance Personnel	Yes	Yes	Yes	Yes

(continued)

APPENDIX 43.2   Performance Characteristics of Four Laboratories (*continued*)

NOTES

First examine the characteristics of the four laboratories. Note that the "numbers" serve only as clues as to which issues require deeper analysis. Laboratories A and B represent those for which comparisons are most legitimate. It is more difficult to compare either of them to laboratory C, and laboratory D is in quite a different category from the other three.

1. The test volume of all four laboratories is similar (laboratory B>D>C>A).
2. Laboratories A and B are the most complex of the group. Both are primary university-affiliated laboratories with large pathology residency programs, a full range of services, and a relatively small number of referred tests. Blood expense is correspondingly high. Laboratory B appears to be the most complex of the group.
3. Laboratory C is also a hospital laboratory but with a more restricted range of services. It is a teaching hospital but is an affiliate with a small number of pathology residents.
4. Laboratory D is an independent laboratory with a clientele that consists entirely of outpatients and nonpatients. The menu of offered services appears to consist of simple tests because a very small percentage of tests are referred and the laboratory does not contain scientifically complex divisions. The nonpatient tests could represent work done for physicians who bill as a group or could represent work from other institutions, such as nursing homes and other chronic care facilities.
5. Compare laboratories A and B (Columns B–C), the two primary university laboratories.

   a. They are similar in most parameters (columns B–C; rows 53–66), but laboratory B performs a larger volume of tests (row 4).
   b. Both laboratories do most of their testing on-site (columns B–C; row 27) and send only a small fraction of tests to a referral laboratory (columns B–C; row 28).
   c. The two laboratories differ in the origin of their testing (columns B–C; rows 29–30); the majority of business for laboratory A is from their outpatient population, whereas the situation is reversed for laboratory B. Nonpatient tests account for a minority of business for both laboratories but a slightly higher percentage for laboratory A.
   d. Productivity for the two laboratories is similar, whether measured by productive paid hours, total paid hours, or FTEs (columns B–C; rows 32–36, 46–50).
   e. Consumable expenses are similar in the two laboratories (columns B–C; row 44).
   f. Referred test expense is greater for laboratory B than for laboratory A (columns B–C; row 45), suggesting that the tests sent out by Laboratory B are more time-consuming, use more expensive reagents, or are less susceptible to competition in the marketplace. Alternatively, laboratory A may use a less expensive reference laboratory or have negotiated a better contract than did laboratory B.
   g. Although productivity, as measured by hours, is similar between the two laboratories, labor expenses are very different (columns B–C; rows 42–43). There are several possible

explanations for the difference; the explanation may be due to a single factor or a combination of the following:

- The ratio of worked hours to paid hours is higher for laboratory B (columns B–C; row 37), suggesting that the benefits are more generous in laboratory A than in laboratory B. Alternatively, personnel in laboratory A may have achieved better benefits because of a longer average length of service (turnover of personnel).
- The salaries in laboratory A may be higher than in laboratory B because of regional differences, competitive factors in the local marketplace, or better negotiated contracts if the workforce is unionized. Once again, if the workers in laboratory A have greater length of service, their salaries may be higher on average than those in laboratory B.
- The skill mix utilized in the two laboratories may be different. If laboratory B uses more technical assistants and medical technicians, whereas laboratory A uses more medical technologists, labor costs would be higher in laboratory A. Ultimately, all of the possible differences in labor costs might be acceptable to the management of each laboratory because of other perceived advantages.

   h. The utilization of tests for inpatients is more efficient in laboratory A than in laboratory B (columns B–C; rows 39–40). Once again, there are several possible explanations:

- Laboratory A may have better control over the utilization of laboratory services than does laboratory B.
- There may be more chronic care patients, who require less intensive laboratory support, in the institution served by laboratory A (less likely as an explanation because the phenomenon is observed whether the denominator is inpatient days or discharges).
- The acuity of illness of patients served by laboratory B may be greater than that of patients covered by laboratory A (more trauma, more transplants, etc.). To some extent, this variable could be analyzed by including objective characterizations of the patient population, such as the Medicare acuity index.

   i. The reverse situation occurs with outpatient tests, where laboratory B appears to function better. This parameter is more difficult to assess because of the difficulties involved in determining outpatient visits objectively and comparatively.
6. Compare laboratory C with laboratories A and B (columns B–D).

   a. Laboratory C is a university-affiliated laboratory with a pathology residency program but only a small number of residents (column D; rows 53–66).
   b. Laboratory C serves inpatients primarily (column D; rows 7–9; 29–31); notably, there are no nonpatient tests.

(*continued*)

APPENDIX 43.2 Performance Characteristics of Four Laboratories *(continued)*

c. Laboratory C sends a relatively large percentage of its tests to a reference laboratory (column D; rows 5–6, 27–28), compatible with a general hospital laboratory.

d. Productivity for laboratory C is, not surprisingly for a less complicated laboratory, better than for laboratories A and B (columns B–D; rows 32–33, 35–36). Interestingly, productivity looks less different when only productive labor is compared (columns B–D, row 32) because laboratory C has relatively few nonproductive personnel (more of the employees in that laboratory are actually involved in turning out results; fewer are in managerial or support services) (columns B–D; row 34).

e. All costs are less for laboratory C than for laboratories A or B (columns B–D; rows 42–44). The fact that testing (productive) costs are also less suggests that salaries and/or benefits may be lower in this laboratory (column B–D; row 42). This interpretation is compatible with the observation that the ratio of productive to total personnel is higher in laboratory C than in either laboratory A or B (columns B–D; row 34).

f. Although the number of tests sent to a reference laboratory from laboratory C is higher than for either laboratory A or B (columns B–D; rows 6 and 28), the cost of referral testing is less on a unit basis (columns B–D; row 45). The explanation for this phenomenon may be that laboratory C is performing less complicated or sophisticated testing in general and is also sending less complicated tests to the referral laboratory than are laboratories A and B. In fact, laboratory A or B could be the referral laboratory for laboratory C.

g. Utilization of laboratory resources for inpatients is actually higher in laboratory C than in the two primary university laboratories (columns B–D; rows 39–40). The difference is greater when test per discharge is compared than when the comparison is with test per inpatient day. This situation suggests a greater proportion of chronic care patients in the institution served by laboratory C and provides a potential target for improvement of laboratory utilization and costs. Outpatient utilization appears similar in the three institutions (columns B–D, row 41).

7. Comparison of laboratory D with laboratories A, B, and C (columns B–E).

a. Laboratory D is very different from any of the other three laboratories (columns B–E; rows 53–66). It serves outpatients and nonpatients exclusively (column E; rows 7–9, 29–31). The nonpatients may represent patients of physicians with whom the laboratory has a contract or patients in chronic care facilities such as nursing homes. Data for outpatient visits are not given (column E; row 12), suggesting that the laboratory does not have access to the records of those patients who are classified as outpatients. Not surprisingly, there is no blood expense (column E; row 24). If the data were broken out in more detail, you might expect to find a high percentage of simple automated chemistry and hematology tests in the workload of laboratory D.

b. Despite the large volume of tests, very few of laboratory D's tests are sent to a reference laboratory (column E; rows 6 and 28). The cost of these referral tests is low (column E; row 45), suggesting that they are relatively uncomplicated.

c. All major costs are less for laboratory D than the other three (columns B–E; rows 18–22, 42–44), again reflecting the outpatient nature of the laboratory.

d. Some clues as to the reasons for lower labor costs can be found in the high ratios of worked to paid hours and of productive to total FTEs (columns B–E; rows 34 and 37).

APPENDIX 43.3   Organizations and Websites

The American Association of Blood Banks (AABB)
(http://www.aabb.org)

AABB is an international association of blood banks and related services dedicated to promoting the highest standard of care for patients and donors in all aspects of blood banking, transfusion medicine, cellular and gene therapies, and tissue transplantation. AABB accredits transfusion services, blood banks, parentage testing laboratories, hematopoietic progenitor cell services, and cord blood services.

The American Association for Clinical Chemistry (AACC)
(http://www.aacc.org)

AACC is an international scientific/medical society of clinical laboratory professionals, physicians, scientists, and others advancing the practice and profession of clinical laboratory science and its application to healthcare.

The American College of Medical Genetics (ACMG)
(http://www.acmg.net)

ACMG provides resources and a voice to the medical genetics profession and promotes the development and implementation of methods to diagnose, treat, and prevent genetic disease. The ACMG provides a publication, *Standards and Guidelines for Clinical Genetics Laboratories*, used to improve genetic testing.

The American Society for Microbiology (ASM)
(http://asm.org)

ASM is a worldwide professional organization that is open to all practicing microbiologists, including those who are active in the clinical laboratory. ASM Press publishes books and materials in all fields of microbiology; this book is just one indication of the interest of this organization in laboratory improvement.

The American Society for Reproductive Medicine (ASRM)
(http://asrm.org)

ASRM is devoted to advancing knowledge and expertise in infertility and maintains a joint program for accreditation of fertility laboratories with the College of American Pathologists.

The Center for Medicare and Medicaid Services (CMS)
(http://www.cms.gov)

CMS is a United States government agency with responsibility for administering the Medicare and Medicaid programs in the United States and therefore responsible for monitoring laboratories which bill for services to Medicare and Medicaid recipients.

The Centers for Disease Control and Prevention (CDC)
(http://www.cdc.gov)

CDC is a United States government agency protecting the health and safety of people through applying disease prevention and control, environmental health, and health promotion and education.

COLA
(http://www.cola.org)

Formerly the Commission on Office Laboratory Accreditation, COLA is a nonprofit organization providing programs of voluntary education, consultation, and accreditation including laboratory accreditation.

The College of American Pathologists (CAP)
(http://www.cap.org)

CAP is a medical society in the United States serving more than 15,000 pathologist members and is considered a leader in providing laboratory quality improvement programs and also laboratory accreditation programs.

U.S. Food and Drug Administration (FDA)
(http://www.fda.gov)

The FDA defines quality assurance as planned and systematic activities to ensure that a laboratory will meet certain requirements for quality.

The Joint Commission on Accreditation of Healthcare Organizations (JCAHO)
(http://www.jcaho.org)

JCAHO sets standards by which healthcare is measured and accredits institutions and laboratories worldwide.

Controlling Test Utilization and Relevancy

Michael L. Wilson, Gary W. Procop, and L. Barth Reller

OBJECTIVES

To become familiar with the concepts of clinical relevance and cost effectiveness and how they are related

To learn how to document the extent of the problem of laboratory test utilization, including relevant sources of information

To learn laboratory-based approaches to the control of laboratory test utilization

To learn institutional-based approaches to the control of laboratory test utilization

To learn one approach for the implementation of change in a patient care setting (McLaughlin's approach)

To learn one approach for integrating evidence-based medicine with computer-based systems for controlling laboratory test utilization

The truth is always the strongest argument.

SOPHOCLES

CLINICAL MICROBIOLOGY LABORATORIES perform tests to aid in the diagnosis of infectious diseases, to help guide therapy for those diseases, to help control and prevent infection in healthcare settings, and to educate and train professionals. This is a broad and challenging mission. To accomplish this mission, a clinical microbiology laboratory must provide a wide variety of tests that span a number of different disciplines, from virology to parasitology to antimicrobial susceptibility testing. This mission has become even more challenging in recent years because of the emphasis on cost control in healthcare, the introduction of new (and often more expensive) diagnostic technologies, and increasing regulations. Thus, to meet their mission, laboratories must maintain or expand their services with fewer resources. One of many approaches to this dilemma is for laboratories to focus and limit testing to those tests that are both clinically relevant and cost-effective.

In the past, laboratories could control costs by use of traditional management techniques, yet most laboratories exploited this technique to its fullest many years ago (40). For most of the recent past, there has been little reason or incentive to control the clinical relevance of tests, as there were more—or stronger—reasons to perform tests than there were to limit their utilization. Only in the past few years have economic incentives for limiting utilization coincided with medical incentives for improving clinical relevancy. Because these incentives are now aligned, clinical laboratories should take advantage of this opportunity to eliminate useless tests, to offer tests that are known to be clinically relevant, and to begin using information technology to disseminate information that will facilitate implementation of these changes.

The purpose of this chapter is to provide the reader with a strategy for making changes in laboratory utilization that are based on the clinical relevance of the tests. The information contained herein is not meant to be a theoretical approach to making change. Rather, it specifically addresses strategies for dealing with political realities and other impediments to making change. Although this book covers clinical laboratory management in general, the information that has been selected for this chapter deals primarily with clinical microbiology. This information was selected because some of the information and tactics were developed first and specifically for clinical microbiology laboratories. Another reason for using clinical microbiology as a paradigm for change was that attempts at changing utilization of microbiology services can be more controversial than in other areas of the laboratory. This is because clinical microbiology tests (i) are more interpretive in nature compared with most other clinical laboratory tests, (ii) are less standardized than are many other clinical laboratory tests, (iii) deal with living microorganisms that have variable phenotypic characteristics, and (iv) are often made more complicated by the presence of contaminating flora.

Evaluating Potential and Real Problems

Attempts to improve laboratory utilization must begin with an assessment of current and potential problems with laboratory utilization. The question of "Where to start?" is easier to answer than is the question "When to start?" One can approach the issue of laboratory utilization from a number of perspectives, including those that are based on financial models, staffing ratios, productivity or other benchmarks, treatment and evaluation guidelines, and so on. To some extent, the approach that is selected should be the one that prompted the assessment. For example, if a laboratory is being reorganized to meet financial constraints, then financial models and productivity benchmarks should be guides for the assessment. If the assessment is being done because of the introduction of new diagnostic technology or the expansion of services to meet new clinical needs, then the assessment should be based on treatment and evaluation guidelines, clinical protocols, or other clinically driven considerations. Regardless of the approach that is taken, the one principle that must play a role in any assessment of laboratory utilization is that of clinical relevancy; no test can be cost-effective, no laboratory can be efficient and productive, and no organization can provide good patient care unless laboratory testing is clinically relevant.

Most laboratorians and providers have an idea of what is meant by the term "clinical relevance" (or the roughly synonymous terms of "clinical significance" and "clinical importance"). The term is not used consistently, however, because there is no standard definition nor is there yet a quantifiable way to measure clinical relevance. This lack of objectivity should not impede assessments of clinical relevance or lead to inaction. As shown in Table 44.1, clinically relevant tests share certain characteristics that can be used in an assessment.

Documenting the Extent of the Problem

Effective laboratory management requires continuous evaluation of the tests performed in the laboratory in terms of their clinical relevance, cost effectiveness, and whether new diagnostic methods should be used, either to replace methods currently in use or as new tests. This type of evaluation requires an unbiased assessment of the test in light of published information, including a review of the literature, use of centralized studies that yield benchmark information, and, if necessary, use of local data.

Literature Review

The published data regarding appropriate laboratory utilization has, until recently, focused on the issues of the relative accuracy of diagnostic methods, clinical relevance of tests, or the cost-effectiveness of different diagnostic methods. These issues first received emphasis in the early 1970s, when controlled clinical comparisons of diagnostic laboratory methods became more common, investigators began looking at the clinical relevance of diagnostic tests, and the issue of cost control became increasingly important. As noted by van Walraven and Naylor (38) and commented on by Lundberg (16), much of the published literature about clinical relevance and cost-effectiveness lacks the scientific rigor that characterizes evaluations of other diagnostic modalities and therapies.

These criticisms almost certainly are valid, but holding laboratory tests to the same standards as other diagnostic procedures or methods may be unrealistic. There are two reasons for this. First, laboratory methods usually are used to confirm clinical impressions or to supplement clinical, radiographic, or other laboratory data. This is different from, for example, a biopsy that by itself may provide definitive diagnostic information. In other words, many laboratory tests do not stand alone for the purposes of making

Table 44.1 Characteristics of clinically relevant laboratory tests

Test results can be used to initiate, modify, or terminate therapy.
Test results are available in an acceptable time frame.
Test sensitivity and specificity are acceptable to users.
Test positive and negative predictive values are acceptable to users.
Test results are easily reported to and interpreted by users.

diagnoses, whereas many other types of diagnostic methods or therapies do. Second, the clinical impression of the provider has an important effect on the interpretation of the test result. This is because the pretest probability of a disease affects the posttest probability of a laboratory test result. (For an example and further statistical explanation, the reader is referred to Aronson and Bor's (3) discussion of blood cultures, specifically the section on the influence of pretest probability on posttest probability). Thus, while it often is possible to design controlled clinical trials of novel diagnostic methods or therapies, evaluating laboratory methods is not as straightforward because other factors affect the interpretation of the laboratory test. This is not true of many other types of clinical evaluations, in which the process of blinding the study can remove clinical impressions as a factor in test interpretation.

Despite these limitations, some issues regarding laboratory tests can be studied adequately via controlled clinical trials, including product comparisons, comparison of new diagnostic tests with older methods, evaluations of the relative cost effectiveness of different tests, and even some evaluations of clinical relevance. Some aspects of the clinical effects of laboratory testing also can be studied adequately, such as the impact of the timeliness of result reporting (7, 10).

Centralized Studies

A second type of study exists that can be useful in comparing laboratory practices with those of peer groups. These studies can be broadly categorized as benchmarking studies. These studies differ from scientific studies in that the purpose is not to test a hypothesis but rather to document or characterize different laboratory practices. By their design they do not test clinical outcomes, so they cannot be used to determine clinical efficacy. Nonetheless, because these studies tend to involve many hospitals and laboratories, they can be used to collect large amounts of data about laboratory practices. These data, in turn, can be compared with local practices.

Examples of centralized studies include the College of American Pathologists (CAP) Q-Probes and Q-Tracks programs (36). In these studies, laboratories provide data about specific laboratory practices, which are then collated and analyzed. The Q-Probe is based on a single observation, such as turnaround times for certain tests sent from emergency departments, used to establish benchmarks for specific tests. In contrast, the Q-Track is based on a series of observations taken during specific times to determine trends for specific tests. These studies typically involve collecting data from hundreds of hospitals for hundreds of thousands of tests. As a result, they are of a scale that is unique in the United States, matched only by reporting to the Centers for Disease Control and Prevention (e.g., the National Nosocomial Infections Study) and other data collected by the federal government. When the data are sorted and analyzed by hospital type, size, geographic region, and other parameters, they provide laboratory directors with a powerful benchmark tool.

Large data sets also are collected as part of the CAP Proficiency Testing program. These data are not collected for the purpose of evaluating specific laboratory tests, but some of the results can be pooled to yield information regarding laboratory practices. As an example, the CAP Microbiology Resource Committee recently evaluated data regarding the utility of user-based quality control (QC) for commercial microbiological media (14a). The data show that, for a number of types of commerical media, user QC adds little to manufacturer QC and therefore can be eliminated without adversely affecting quality (14a). Eliminating superfluous QC not only saves money but also allows technologists to focus their time and efforts on tasks that are more beneficial to patient care.

Local Data

Making a change often requires convincing users that the change is necessary and that the decision to make the change was based on data. For the most part, data should be from published clinical trials, particularly those that meet the requirements of evidence-based medicine. In specific circumstances, as noted by McLaughlin, it helps to supplement published data with data collected locally (18). The reason for this is that many providers believe that their patients are in some way different from those elsewhere. While this may be true if one is dealing with patient populations that are specific in terms of age, gender, or ethnicity, it is not true when applied to the general population. Nonetheless, many providers do believe that their patients are different, and collecting local data can help to convince them that the observations made elsewhere do apply to their patients.

While collecting local data may be necessary for specific purposes, studies performed locally are unlikely to meet the requirements of evidence-based medicine. They are expensive, and performing them delays implementation of necessary changes. Moreover, even though there has not been a systematic study of this issue, it is unlikely that the results of local studies (if performed correctly) will differ from those performed on broader populations. Most clinical studies published in peer-reviewed publications are of a magnitude and cost that cannot be duplicated locally. Additionally, if a local study yields findings that are different from those of larger studies, the investigator will be in the position of needing to explain why the results differed and were not just wrong. If the results are valid, the investigator should publish the findings in a peer-reviewed journal so that others can benefit from the observations. As an example, in 1990, Siegel, Edelstein, and Nachamkin published a study showing that there was no yield in performing stool cultures or tests for ova and parasites after patients had been hospitalized for three or more days (28). This study was repeated in a number of hospitals during the next few years, culminating with a CAP Q-Probe study that was published in 1996 (11, 22, 36). Each of these studies yielded almost identical results as the Siegel study. In one author's experience (MLW), the local data were found to be more persuasive than were the original data in convincing physicians to accept the recommended changes, which initially were met with some skepticism by providers. Subsequent studies have indicated some exceptions to the initial findings, but for the most part the "three-day rule" is now standard practice in clinical microbiology laboratories.

Other examples of local data that were published and that have resulted in widespread changes in laboratory practice include screening of cerebrospinal fluid specimens before performing cerebrospinal fluid Venereal Disease Research Laboratory tests or mycobacterial smears and cultures (1, 2); performing nucleic acid amplification tests for the etiologic agents of viral meningoencephalitis (29, 32); eliminating bacterial antigen tests for the diagnosis of bacterial meningitis (12, 19, 24); and eliminating broth "back up" cultures for most tissue and fluid specimens (21). Morris et al. reviewed the cost and time savings that resulted when several of these changes were made in one laboratory; the time savings in particular were substantial (20).

Laboratory-Based Approaches to Control

In many ways, the laboratory is the best place to control (limit) test utilization. Not only is the laboratory the site where specimens are processed and testing is performed, in many hospitals the laboratory is responsible for the phlebotomy service. In addition, laboratories are ultimately responsible for specimen collection. A number of laboratory-based approaches to control laboratory test utilization have been described (Table 44.2).

Newsletters

Newsletters, like all written materials, often are ineffective as a means of communication for the obvious reason that busy providers are unlikely to read them. This is particularly true if they are not written well, are not timely, or contain a lot of trivial information. On the other hand, they have the advantage of being a dispassionate means of disseminating information. This can be a strategic advantage when introducing contentious changes. They also have the advantage of being impersonal, which again can be advantageous when introducing contentious or unpopular changes.

Table 44.2 Laboratory-based approaches to control

Newsletters

Policy changes

Personal and ad hoc communication

LIS-based controls on test ordering

LIS-based feedback in reports

Although one should never dodge the responsibility of explaining and defending proposed changes to those who will be affected the most, there is only a finite amount of time for doing so, and it is unrealistic to meet with every provider or stakeholder, particularly in large organizations. Moreover, some individuals will not agree to proposed changes no matter how rational the change is, so there is little point in trying to persuade them. When this occurs, it is better simply to announce the change as a *fait accompli*, usually as a policy change, and move on to other issues.

Policy Changes

As with newsletters, policy changes have the advantages of being impersonal and dispassionate. They have the additional advantage of having an air of authority about them, an attribute that can be advantageous when it can be anticipated that the policy will face some opposition.

Personal and Ad Hoc Communication

The preceding paragraphs emphasize the use of dispassionate and impersonal written communication as a mechanism of reducing any potential opposition to making changes in laboratory practices. This is not intended to be a substitute for direct personal communication with providers as a means of explaining why changes are necessary, for receiving input from those who will be affected by the changes, and for monitoring the effect of the changes. One of the first steps in making change is to discuss the changes at length with those who will be affected. These discussions may not reverse the decision to make the change, but merely having the discussions often ameliorates the emotional impact of the changes. On the other hand, approaching changes from the perspective of the provider can affect the way that the change is implemented.

LIS-Based Controls on Test Ordering

Modifying the test ordering process has been shown to be an effective approach to changing test utilization behavior. Tierney et al. showed that the computerized display of test charges for outpatients resulted in a significant decrease in test utilization (33). Although Bates et al. showed that a similar effect did not occur with inpatients, there were trends in that direction (5). The same authors, in a similar study, showed that computerized display of redundant tests was an effective intervention, but that the effect was limited (6). In another similar study, Solomon et al. showed that a computer-based intervention was effective in reducing unnecessary serologic testing in an inpatient setting (31). Despite the limited effect associated with some of these interventions, there appears to be increasing evidence that computer-based interventions can be effective for changing test utilization behavior.

Most commercial laboratory information systems (LIS) have the capability to identify duplicate orders, to flag orders that meet specific criteria (e.g., the number of blood cultures ordered within a defined period), to document test changes or cancellations, and to notify providers of changes to an order. These rudimentary capabilities allow laboratories to improve test utilization substantially, as duplicate or redundant tests are by any definition clinically irrelevant and wasteful. This is particularly important in settings where more than one provider may be ordering tests for patients, a circumstance that results in increased duplicate testing (9, 35). The ability to determine test utilization by provider also is within the capability of most commercial LIS, information that can be used to track test ordering patterns and to provide feedback to the provider.

As useful as these capabilities may be, by no means are they a feature of all commercial LIS. Moreover, many LIS cannot be used to modify test ordering at the time orders are placed. This capability is a feature of LIS that can be used for computerized physician order entry (CPOE). These LIS are integrated with the hospital or organization information system; the more sophisticated CPOE systems are integrated with software that allows for the analysis of information regarding other laboratory tests, drug allergies and other adverse drug reactions, nutrition, radiographic findings, and clinical findings. The LIS that have some CPOE capability vary considerably in their ability to integrate this information so that orders can be modified either by alerting the provider at the time of entry or by the CPOE system directly. A fully functional and robust CPOE system would have all of these features and would have the potential to reduce errors and to change orders so that practice standards, clinical pathways, and other efforts to improve care would be realized (25, 26, 30).

LIS-Based Feedback in Reports

Even without a rules-based CPOE system, many LIS can be programmed to provide information about the cost of laboratory tests, information regarding the clinical utility of tests, and warnings about the use of certain drugs in patients with specific laboratory findings (such as renal failure). Many LIS have the ability to show specific comments either automatically (based on rules within the system) or by manual ad hoc request. These systems can be an inexpensive and effective way to disseminate information to providers.

There are a number of types of feedback that can be given to providers. In clinical microbiology, one of the most commonly used types of feedback is the selective reporting of antimicrobial susceptibility test results, with or without comments to help guide interpretation of the results. Even without comments, the provider receives test results only for those antimicrobial agents that are likely to be clinically relevant, information that should improve patient care. Another common type of feedback is the average daily cost of drugs that are reported for antimicrobial

susceptibility test results. Other common types of feedback for microbiology tests include comments regarding the presence of contaminating flora, the lack of clinical relevance for some types of testing (e.g., microorganisms recovered only from broth cultures), specimen adequacy (e.g., the evaluation of sputum specimens for neutrophils and epithelial cells), the types and numbers of microorganisms recovered from midstream urine specimens and their likely clinical relevance, and the number and adequacy of specimens received for blood culture. Given adequate laboratory and computer resources, comments can be developed to help guide the interpretation of most laboratory tests.

Institutional-Based Approaches to Control

As with laboratory-based approaches to control, a number of institutional-based approaches to control laboratory test utilization have been described (Table 44.3). The two types of approaches are not exclusive: each complements the other, and used together, they might be more effective than either type of approach used alone.

Working with the Medical Staff

In most organizations, the medical staff is in a leadership position regarding patient care. There are several reasons for this. First, most hospital-based medical care continues to be provided by physicians, and hospital care is much more expensive than is outpatient primary care. Second, physicians provide most outpatient specialty care, and specialty care often is the most expensive and cutting edge and therefore requires the most immediate oversight of cost control. Third, the Joint Commission for the Accreditation of Healthcare Organizations (JCAHO) requires that the medical staff fulfill specific roles within organizations, including overseeing the quality of medical care in the organization, participating in committees that affect patient care (e.g., the pharmacy and therapeutics committee), and in overseeing graduate medical education (resident training). Fourth, although nonphysician providers such as nurse practitioners and physician assistants provide a great deal of primary (and some specialty) care, in many states these providers work under the supervision of a physician. Last, physicians generally are the most outspoken group when changes in patient care are proposed, and some changes are unlikely to occur without their concurrence.

Table 44.3 Institutional-based approaches to control

Working with the medical staff
Formal protocols validated by medical staff
Working with the nursing staff
Institutional protocols
Using major problems to effect change

One can approach the medical staff in a number of ways when a change is needed. One effective strategy is to first meet with the medical staff leadership and senior physicians before meeting with the general membership. This is because (1) medical staff leaders typically have a better understanding of issues that necessitate changes; (2) leaders are selected because of their experience and the respect that physicians have for them; (3) most leaders have been through a number of changes and thus are less resistant to change; and (4) obtaining leader support facilitates changing the way medicine is practiced. The leadership can also serve as a liaison with the general membership. It is difficult to overstate the importance of having their support when contentious or unpopular changes must be made.

Formal Protocols Validated by Medical Staff

A particularly effective means of implementing changes is the use of clinical protocols that have been reviewed and validated by the medical staff. These protocols have a number of synonyms, including care protocols, clinical pathways, and key clinical pathways. When done correctly, these protocols incorporate findings and guidelines from evidence-based medicine, as well as specific guidelines from organizations such as the Centers for Disease Control and Prevention, with the practices and workflow for an organization. The end result should be the application of state-of-the-art medical knowledge to a specific patient population in a specific setting. Such protocols not only provide the best patient care, they also improve medical training and education and should help providers use the most cost-effective approach to healthcare. For obvious reasons, these protocols should specify the use of the most appropriate laboratory testing and radiologic tests and procedures.

Working with the Nursing Staff

In the hospital and the outpatient clinic settings, there is no other group than the nursing staff that can be of more support in making changes. Nurses provide almost all of the immediate patient care in hospitals. They provide a large amount of primary care, they are responsible for most specimen collection in both inpatient and outpatient settings, and they play an important role in medical training and education. Moreover, nurses have a different training and insight to patient care that is just as important as that of physicians. Thus, having the informed support of nursing staff is crucial for implementing changes. It is of particular importance to discuss proposed changes with nurses, as they know best the practical side of implementing changes and how each setting functions throughout the day and the week.

One of the current challenges in working with the nursing staff is the shortage of trained nurses in the United States. To maintain appropriate nurse-to-patient ratios, hospitals have opted to use nurses from companies that provide nurses for varying periods, from one shift to several months. Another change, particularly in hospitals, is to assign nurses to different units depending upon the number of patients on those units at a given time. Although these staffing approaches are necessary for purposes of patient care, one consequence is that it is more difficult to train nurses adequately and to work with them to implement changes smoothly. It is unlikely that this will change in the immediate future. In light of that, the best approach at this time is to work with the nursing leadership in the organization and to take the extra steps necessary to work with the nurses who are temporarily assigned to a given setting.

Institutional Protocols (e.g., Clinical Protocols)

Institutional protocols, like clinical protocols that are validated by the medical staff, are a method for implementing guidelines that are based on objective data tailored to a specific setting. The difference between these guidelines and the clinical protocols is that institutional protocols are used to implement policies as set forth by the governing body or administration of the organization. Typically, these concern issues such as access to healthcare, use of screening tests or procedures on populations, and other issues that apply more broadly. In some instances, institutional protocols can be an effective means of implementing change, if for no reason other than that providers within an organization have no choice but to follow them. However, for the most part, they cannot be used to implement changes because most changes are not of sufficient magnitude to warrant the time and attention of the governing body or of the senior administration.

Using Major Events To Effect Change (e.g., Institutional QA Office, Root Cause Analysis)

Major events in healthcare provide opportunities to make changes that otherwise may not be possible. This is neither a cynical observation nor opportunistic management. Rather, it is recognition of the fact that some issues cannot be dealt with under normal circumstances because of political, financial, or other constraints. During major events, however, these constraints may diminish or disappear, providing an opportunity to bypass them. Change occurs more easily during major events because there typically is an acknowledgment that the status quo no longer can be preserved, individuals may need to take a different view of circumstances, and many departments may be involved. A particularly opportune time to eliminate procedures or tests that are of marginal utility, or that providers are unwilling to give up at other times, may be during a reduction in operating budgets. Other events that provide unique opportunities for change include changes in organizational management, changes in ownership, relocation of laboratory facilities within the building or complex, construction of new facilities, implementation of computerized order entry systems (particularly when rules-based orders will be implemented), and changes in academic or other types of affiliations. Although these changes may not afford equal opportunity for change, or for the same types of change, laboratory directors should look for opportunities that accompany what otherwise are challenging circumstances.

Important allies for implementing changes include the Quality Assurance (QA) Office and the Compliance Office. The QA office plays a number of important roles within organizations, including ensuring compliance with accreditation standards, investigating adverse events, performing root cause analyses, and developing organizational policies and procedures. The compliance office deals primarily with ethics, business practices, and compliance issues related to financial matters. The QA office, by its broader role within the organization, can assist with change by helping develop clinical protocols, particularly those that involve changing organizational policies and procedures. It can also assist with change when an adverse event or the findings from a root cause analysis indicate that a change is necessary. Obviously, either office can assist with change when the change is necessary for compliance reasons. In some cases, this type of assistance can be invaluable for making changes that are contentious but necessary.

What Works and Doesn't Work: How To Take the First Steps

There is a substantial body of literature regarding the effectiveness of different methods for changing laboratory test utilization. Most of this literature reflects the notion that "changing" test utilization usually means limiting test utilization. This undoubtedly is an oversimplification of the issue, as there are good examples of how laboratory tests can be underutilized as well as overutilized. Nonetheless, the problem of overutilization receives more emphasis because it probably is more pervasive in modern medicine than is underutilization and decreasing overutilization can yield substantial cost savings. It is true that increasing the use of tests that are underutilized can decrease costs in the healthcare system as a whole, but until recently, few systems have taken the broader approach to cost control, instead focusing cost control efforts on specific issues.

Changing/controlling laboratory test utilization means changing/controlling provider (usually physician) behavior. This has proven to be a complex and difficult issue for healthcare systems to address, as most interventions intended to change physician behavior have been ineffective or have had only a temporary effect (4, 34). As reviewed by Valenstein, physician education has been shown to be an ineffective approach to changing test utilization (despite being the most commonly used intervention), and both clinical and financial feedback has been shown to have

variable effectiveness (34). In the same review, Valenstein noted that administrative interventions have been shown to be effective in changing test utilization (34). These include requiring justification for certain tests, changing the test request process, and changing "informal testing rituals" (23, 34). The first of these, requiring justification for certain tests, may be an effective intervention, but it is impractical to implement in many settings and almost certainly will be unpopular with physicians. The second, changing the test request process, may ultimately be the most practical and effective intervention, particularly when it involves the use of computerized order entry systems. Hindmarsh and Lyon report a similar observation (13). The third, changing testing "rituals," usually falls under the penumbra of clinical pathways, and in settings where physicians adhere to the pathways it can be an effective intervention (8).

In their review, Axt-Adam et al. noted that one explanation for the lack of effectiveness of many interventions is that physician behavior depends upon the physician's personality, education, training, specialty, location of practice, years of clinical experience, estimated test charges, and expectations (4). Malcolm et al. also reported that "personal factors" affect the way physicians use laboratory tests (17). The effect of clinical experience on test utilization has been reported in a number of studies, one recent example being the increased use of ancillary tests by inexperienced physicians in the evaluation of acute febrile illness (27). In his review, Valenstein reported that risk-taking attitudes might affect test-ordering behavior, although some investigators have not found a relationship between personality and test utilization (34). Given the number of factors that may affect test-ordering behavior, it comes as no surprise that many specific interventions have been found to be ineffective in changing behavior. It may be that at any time and in any place only a subset of physicians is amenable to a particular intervention, and that over time no static intervention will result in sustained changes in test utilization behavior. As Valenstein noted in his review, ". . . To the extent that differences in the test-ordering behavior of physicians reflect ingrained and immutable psychological traits, one would expect little success in modulating test utilization by trying to influence individual providers. . . ." (34). This may well be the most realistic assessment of the effect of personality on test utilization behavior and the lack of effect of educational interventions on changing that behavior.

Despite the reported variable success in changing test utilization behavior and the difficulty in sustaining changes, there is cause for optimism. First, there has been for many years little or no doubt among laboratorians—and many clinicians—that more laboratory tests are performed than are needed for patient care and that many laboratory tests are used incorrectly (14, 15). Second, there is a growing awareness among providers that healthcare resources are limited and should be allocated so as to maximize their benefit to patients. Third, improvements in information systems have resulted in computerized order entry systems that have the capability to affect test utilization via immediate feedback to providers as well as by use of artificial intelligence. Last, the growing body of literature on evidence-based medicine makes it much easier for healthcare systems to develop rational clinical pathways and for laboratorians to use those pathways as part of their strategy to change test utilization.

From a purely pragmatic standpoint of making changes in diagnostic microbiology testing, McLaughlin has published a step-by-step approach that is rational, practical, and (by anecdotal experience) effective (18). A modified version of this approach is shown in Table 44.4. As emphasized in McLaughlin's approach, building support for changes is crucial (18). Many changes that are needed to make a laboratory more cost-effective or clinically relevant are contentious, even when they are not costly. There are several reasons for this. The first is that making changes can mean taking something away from providers, and it is axiomatic that it is more difficult to take something away than it is to not give it in the first place. The second reason is that making changes shifts control from the provider to the laboratory, and providers may perceive that this affects their clinical autonomy and/or their ability to act on behalf of their patients. The backlash against managed care by providers illustrates this principle. Last, making changes is difficult under most circumstances, even when it is perceived to be in ones' best interests. To facilitate changes, having the support of departmental and organizational leadership is crucial. By support, one hopes for an understanding and analysis of the recommended changes, including an understanding of the impact on services as well as of benefits, costs, and alternatives. In all circumstances, one should avoid presenting support as an edict, as this approach may result in the opposite response than was hoped for.

Perhaps the single most effective argument that can be presented to providers is to emphasize that the change will result in the best care for the patient. That may mean that the change is supported by evidence-based medicine, a topic that has received much emphasis recently. This concept is a process by which evaluation and treatment guidelines are based on published evidence regarding their effectiveness.

Putting It All Together

Base Policy Approaches and LIS-Based Controls on Evidence-Based Medicine

The published data about changing physician behavior indicate that most approaches achieve only a temporary effect or are ineffective altogether. Of the described methods that have been shown to be effective, use of LIS-based controls may be one of the more effective methods. Data regarding the effectiveness of evidence-based medicine as a tool for limiting test utilization are available for only a limited number of tests, but the data that are available (as well as anecdotal experience) suggest that physicians may be more accepting of changes that are derived from evidence-based medicine (39). There are at least two reasons why this observation may be true. First, by the nature of their education and training, physicians are more receptive to information based on sound scientific or medical research. Second, information that is scientifically persuasive is likely to be adopted as the standard of care, and physicians by and large adhere to what is perceived to be the standard of care within their community. Thus, one approach to increase the likelihood that physicians will accept change is to use LIS-based controls on physician ordering and to base the changes on evidence-based medicine. As stated previously, one of the advantages to the use of LIS-based controls is that test-ordering patterns can be tracked automatically, thereby generating physician-specific utilization data.

Track Results

As with any type of decision to make changes within an organization, the effectiveness of changes in laboratory test utilization is determined by (i) the quality of the decision to make the change; (ii) the success of the implementation; (iii) the likelihood that the intervention can be sustained; (iv) the willingness to modify the change as needed; and (v) whether the change improves patient care and/or outcomes. Documenting the effectiveness of the change requires the collection of data prior to implementation of the change followed by tracking the results of the change. For some changes, this is simple. Changes made to decrease or increase utilization of a specific test can be tracked simply by auditing test utilization over specific intervals. On the other hand, changes intended to improve patient care or outcomes require the collection of large amounts of data, often over long periods of time and interpretation of the data in light of other clinical, radiographic, and laboratory findings. In some instances, they require formal study of the issue via randomized clinical trials.

Table 44.4 Implementation of diagnostic microbiology policies[a]

Base proposed changes on published data.

Supplement these data with in-house data.

Gain the support of the infectious diseases service.

Discuss proposed changes in advance with influential providers.

Educate providers who will be affected by the changes.

Announce changes by effective means of communication.

Educate laboratory staff who will implement the changes.

Revise laboratory manuals accordingly.

Initially give providers an "override" mechanism.

Provide necessary explanations and follow-up to users.

[a]Modified from reference 18.

Plan, Do, Study, Act Model

Once the effects of a change have been tracked for some time, a decision can be made to either continue the change without modification, to modify it, or to discontinue the change. This approach parallels what JCAHO refers to as the plan, do, study, act approach for making change. The approach is self-explanatory, is simple, and can be used to address many types of issues. For this approach to be used effectively, the study and act stages of the process require the use of quantifiable data that can be tracked through time. Nardella et al. described a model system that incorporates many of the issues discussed in this chapter (23). The model is a good example, without use of the specific terms, of the plan, do, study, act model for creating an effective intervention.

Summary

The principle that guides changes in laboratory test utilization must be that of clinical relevance. Clinically relevant tests may or may not be cost-effective, but tests that are not clinically relevant cannot be cost-effective, regardless of how inexpensive they may be. Although the tools for assessing clinical relevance are imperfect, efforts are being made to improve the way that clinical evaluations of laboratory tests are performed so that assessments of clinical relevance, the impact on patient outcomes, and cost effectiveness can be standardized and quantified. Until those assessment tools are available, however, laboratorians should make use of the characteristics of clinically relevant tests presented in Table 44.1.

There is now good evidence that any effective and sustainable approach must include a combination of interventions (37). Based on the available evidence and on the experience of the authors and others, changing laboratory test utilization requires (i) careful planning and preparation; (ii) the establishment of guidelines (clinical pathways or other types) that are derived from evidence-based medicine; (iii) a detailed plan for introducing and implementing the changes (McLaughlin's approach is one example); (iv) use of informatics to disseminate guidelines, to automatically perform some tasks (e.g., elimination of duplicate tests), and to track data regarding utilization; (v) continuous monitoring of the effectiveness (and the effects of) the change; and (vi) continuous modifications as they become necessary.

KEY POINTS

- A number of laboratory-based approaches to controlling laboratory test utilization are described, including newsletters, policy changes, personal and ad hoc communication, LIS-based controls, and LIS-based feedback in reports.
- A number of institution-based approaches to controlling laboratory test utilization are described, including approaches to working with the medical and nursing staff and using formal protocols that have been validated by the medical staff, institutional protocols such as clinical pathways, and major events to effect change.

- Effective control of laboratory test utilization requires use of more than one approach or intervention. Of the different types of interventions that have been evaluated, education appears to be the least effective. Feedback to providers appears to be the most effective intervention, particularly when it is computer-based and when it is linked to evidence-based medicine.

- Effective interventions require tracking of results, modification as indicated by data, and sustained effort.

GLOSSARY

Cerebrospinal fluid Venereal Disease Research Laboratory (CSF-VDRL) test A serologic test for neurosyphilis that is performed on a cerebrospinal fluid specimen rather than on a peripheral blood specimen.

College of American Pathologists (CAP) One of the professional societies for pathologists. One of the organizations that accredits laboratories and provides a service for proficiency testing. CAP also provides services such as Q-Probes and Q-Tracks (see below).

Computerized physician order entry (CPOE) A computer-based system for placing clinical orders. Some systems have the ability to integrate orders with pharmacy and laboratory data, to make recommendations for drug dosage and timing, and to alert the ordering physician of issues such as drug allergy.

Evidence-based medicine The application of medical data (evidence) that have been analyzed using rigorous criteria to clinical decision making.

Joint Commission for the Accreditation of Healthcare Organizations (JCAHO) An organization that accredits most hospitals and healthcare organizations in the United States. JCAHO can also be used to accredit clinical laboratories.

Laboratory information system (LIS) A computer system used to report laboratory test results. A large number of commercial systems are available. Most can be interfaced directly with instruments to facilitate test result reporting and to minimize the need for manual data entry. Some systems have added functionality such as order entry.

Quality assurance (QA) Systematic approaches to assessing and improving the quality of care within a specific healthcare setting (e.g., a hospital or clinic) or healthcare program.

Q-Probes A program provided by the CAP that allows laboratories to collect data regarding laboratory processes and to compare their data with data collected from peer organizations. The data are collected for one time only.

Q-Tracks A program provided by the CAP that allows laboratories to collect data *through time* regarding laboratory processes and to compare their data with data collected from peer organizations on a quarterly basis.

REFERENCES

1. Albright, R. E., R. H. Christenson, J. L. Emlet, C. B. Graham, E. G. Estevez, M. L. Wilson, L. B. Reller, and K. A. Schneider. 1991. Issues in cerebrospinal fluid management. CSF Venereal Disease Research Laboratory testing. *Am. J. Clin. Pathol.* **95:**397–401.

2. Albright, R. E., C. B. Graham, R. H. Christenson, W. A. Schell, M. C. Bledsoe, J. L. Emlet, T. P. Mears, L. B. Reller, and K. A. Schneider. 1991. Issues in cerebrospinal fluid management. Acid-fast bacillus smear and culture. *Am. J. Clin. Pathol.* **95:**418–423.

3. Aronson, M. D., and D. H. Bor. 1987. Blood cultures. *Ann. Intern. Med.* **106:**246–253.

4. Axt-Adam, P., J. C. van der Wouden, and E. van der Does. 1993. Influencing behavior of physicians ordering laboratory tests: a literature study. *Med. Care* **31:**784–794.

5. Bates, D. W., G. J. Kuperman, A. Jha, J. M. Teich, E. J. Orav, N. Ma'luf, A. Onderdonk, R. Pugatch, D. Wybenga, J. Winkelman, T. A. Brennan, A. L. Komaroff, and M. J. Tanasijevic. 1997. Does the computerized display of charges affect inpatient ancillary test utilization? *Arch. Intern. Med.* **157:**2501–2508.

6. Bates, D. W., G. J. Kuperman, E. Rittenberg, J. M. Teich, J. Fiskio, N. Ma'luf, A. Onderdonk, D. Wybenga, J. Winkelman, T. A. Brennan, A. L. Komaroff, and M. J. Tanasijevic. 1999. A randomized trial of a computer-based intervention to reduce utilization of redundant laboratory tests. *Am. J. Med.* **106:**144–150.

7. Beekmann, S. E., D. J. Diekema, K. C. Chapin, and G. V. Doern. 2003. Effects of rapid detection of bloodstream infections on length of hospitalization and hospital charges. *J. Clin. Microbiol.* **41:**3119–3125.

8. Board, N., N. Brennan, and G. Caplan. 2000. Use of pathology services in re-engineered clinical pathways. *J. Qual. Clin. Pract.* **20:**24–29.

9. Branger, P. J., R. J. M. Van Oers, J. C. Van Der Wouden, and J. van der Lei. 1995. Laboratory services utilization: a survey of repeat investigations in ambulatory care. *Neth. J. Med.* **47:**208–213.

10. Doern, G. V., R. Vautour, M. Gaudet, and B. Levy. 1994. Clinical impact of rapid in vitro susceptibility testing and bacterial identification. *J. Clin. Microbiol.* **32:**1757–1762.

11. Fan, K., A. J. Morris, and L. B. Reller. 1993. Application of rejection criteria for stool cultures for bacterial enteric pathogens. *J. Clin. Microbiol.* **31:**2233–2235.

12. Hayden, R. T., and L. D. Frenkel. 2000. More laboratory testing: greater cost but not necessarily better. *Pediatr. Infect. Dis. J.* **19:**290–292.

13. Hindmarsh, J. T., and A. W. Lyon. 1996. Strategies to promote rational clinical chemistry test utilization. *Clin. Biochem.* **29:**291–299.

14. Johnson, H. A. 1991. Diminishing returns on the road to diagnostic certainty. *JAMA* **265:**2229–2231.

14a. Jones, R. N., K. Krisher, and D. S. Bird, for the College of American Pathologists Microbiology Resource Committee. 2003. Results of the Survey of the Quality Assurance for Commercially Prepared Microbiology Media. Update from the College of American Pathologists Microbiology Surveys Program (2001). *Arch. Pathol. Lab. Med.* **127:**661–665.

15. Kassirer, J. P. 1989. Our stubborn quest for diagnostic certainty. A cause of excessive testing. *N. Engl. J. Med.* **320:**1489–1491.

16. Lundberg, G. D. 1998. The need for an outcomes research agenda for clinical laboratory testing. *JAMA* **280:**565–566.

17. Malcolm, L., L. Wright, M. Seers, L. Davies, and J. Guthrie. 2000. Laboratory expenditure in Pegasus Medical Group: a comparison of high and low users of laboratory tests with academics. *N. Z. Med. J.* **113:**79–81.

18. McLaughlin, J. 1995. The implementation of cost-effective, clinically relevant diagnostic microbiology policies: the approach. *Clin. Microbiol. Newsl.* **17:**70–71.

19. Mein, J., and G. Lum. 1999. CSF bacterial antigen detection tests offer no advantage over Gram's stain in the diagnosis of bacterial meningitis. *Pathol.* **31:**67–69.

20. Morris, A. J., L. K. Smith, S. Mirrett, and L. B. Reller. 1996. Cost and time savings following introduction of rejection criteria for clinical specimens. *J. Clin. Microbiol.* **34:**355–357.

21. Morris, A. J., S. J. Wilson, C. E. Marx, M. L. Wilson, S. Mirrett, and L. B. Reller. 1995. Clinical impact of bacteria and fungi recovered only from broth cultures. *J. Clin. Microbiol.* **33:**161–165.

22. Morris, A. J., M. L. Wilson, and L. B. Reller. 1992. Application of rejection criteria for stool ovum and parasite examinations. *J. Clin. Microbiol.* **30:**3213–3216.

23. Nardella, A., M. Farrell, L. Pechet, and L. M. Snyder. 1994. Continuous improvement, quality control, and cost containment in clinical laboratory testing. Enhancement of physicians' laboratory-ordering practices. *Arch. Pathol. Lab. Med.* **118:**965–968.

24. Perkins, M. D., S. Mirrett, and L. B. Reller. 1995. Rapid bacterial antigen detection is not clinically useful. *J. Clin. Microbiol.* **33:**1486–1491.

25. Peters, M. 1995. Managing test demand by clinicians: computer assisted guidelines. *J. Clin. Pathol.* **48:**98–100.

26. Peters, M., and P. M. G. Broughton. 1993. The role of expert systems in improving the test requesting patterns of clinicians. *Ann. Clin. Biochem.* **30:**52–59.

27. Procop, G. W., J. S. Hartman, and F. Sedor. 1997. Laboratory tests in evaluation of acute febrile illness in pediatric emergency room patients. *Am. J. Clin. Pathol.* **107:**114–121.

28. Siegel, D. L., P. H. Edelstein, and I. Nachamkin. 1990. Inappropriate testing for diarrheal diseases in the hospital. *JAMA* **263:**979–982.

29. Simko, J. P., A. M. Caliendo, K. Hogle, and J. Versalovic. 2002. Differences in laboratory findings for cerebrospinal fluid specimens obtained from patients with meningitis or encephalitis due to herpes simplex virus (HSV) documented by detection of HSV DNA. *Clin. Infect. Dis.* **35:**414–419.

30. Smith, B. J., and M. D. D. McNeely. 1999. The influence of an expert system for test ordering and interpretation on laboratory investigations. *Clin. Chem.* **45:**1168–1175.

31. Solomon, D. H., R. H. Shmerling, P. H. Schur, R. Lew, J. Fiskio, and D. W. Bates. 1999. A computer based intervention to reduce unnecessary serologic testing. *J. Rheumatol.* **26:**2578–2584.

32. Tang, Y. W., J. R. Hibbs, K. R. Tau, Q. Qian, H. A. Skarhus, T. F. Smith, and D. H. Persing. 1999. Effective use of polymerase chain reaction for diagnosis of central nervous system infections. *Clin. Infect. Dis.* **29:**803–806.

33. Tierney, W. M., M. E. Miller, and C. J. McDonald. 1990. The effect on test ordering of informing physicians of the charges for outpatient diagnostic tests. *N. Engl. J. Med.* **322:**1499–1504.

34. Valenstein, P. 1996. Managing physician use of laboratory tests. *Clin. Lab. Med.* **16:**749–771.

35. Valenstein, P., A. Leiken, and C. Lehmann. 1988. Test-ordering by multiple physicians increases unnecessary laboratory examinations. *Arch. Pathol. Lab. Med.* **112:**238–241.

36. Valenstein, P., M. Pfaller, and M. Yungbluth. 1996. The use and abuse of routine stool microbiology. A College of American Pathologists Q-Probes study of 601 institutions. *Arch. Pathol. Lab. Med.* **120:**206–211.

37. van Walraven, C., V. Goel, and B. Chan. 1998. Effect of population–based interventions on laboratory utilization. A time-series analysis. *JAMA* **280:**2028–2033.

38. van Walraven, C., and C. D. Naylor. 1998. Do we know what inappropriate laboratory utilization is? A systematic review of laboratory clinical audits. *JAMA* **280:**550–558.

39. van Wijk, M. A. M., J. van der Lei, M. Mosseveld, A. M. Bohnen, and J. H. van Bemmel. 2001. Assessment of decision support for blood test ordering in primary care. A randomized trial. *Ann. Intern. Med.* **134:**274–281.

40. Wilson, M. L. 1997. Clinically relevant, cost-effective clinical microbiology. Strategies to decrease unnecessary testing. *Am. J. Clin. Pathol.* **107:**154–167.

APPENDIX 44.1   Websites

The Cochrane Collaboration
(http://www.cochrane.org/)
A nonprofit organization that studies the effects of healthcare interventions. One of the leading organizations for evidence-based medicine.

PubMed
(http://www.ncbi.nlm.nih.gov/PubMed/)
One of the easiest ways to search the medical literature. This website is supported by the National Library of Medicine. Provides access to the published results of controlled clinical trials conducted during the recent past.

U.S. Food and Drug Administration Center for Devices and Radiological Health
(http://www.fda.gov/cdrh/)
Provides access to a wide variety of information regarding laboratory devices that are regulated by the FDA.

EBM Online
(http://ebm.bmjjournals.com/)
The web site for the electronic version of the journal *Evidence-Based Medicine.*

45

Benchmarking for Your Laboratory: What's Appropriate?

Washington C. Winn, Jr.

> *there is always*
> *something to be thankful*
> *for you would not*
> *think that a cockroach*
> *had much ground*
> *for optimism*
> *but as the fishing season*
> *opens up I grow*
> *more and more*
> *cheerful at the thought*
> *that nobody ever got*
> *the notion of using*
> *cockroaches for bait.*
>
> DON MARQUIS, "CERTAIN MAXIMS OF ARCHY" IN *ARCHY AND MEHITABEL,* 1927

EVERY LABORATORY MANAGER has a vested interest in benchmarking. The drive to achieve superior performance is part of our culture. Comparing yourself to your peers is a way of testing yourself, documenting excellent performance, and finding ways to improve. If the internal drive were not enough, there are plenty of forces, be they from within the institution or external, for example, requirements of government regulators, that ensure the importance of monitoring performance, another name for benchmarking.

Many of the critical aspects of self-evaluation have been discussed in this section. The next step for a laboratory manager is to decide which of those tools is applicable locally and how to proceed with the implementation. The goal of this chapter is to provide guidance in that task.

The general approaches needed to decide on a strategy for the laboratory are applicable to the major types of benchmarking: finances, quality, and productivity. If all politics are local, so all business applications are ultimately local.

Variables To Be Considered When Deciding on an Approach

The first considerations will be local resources, the local competitive market, and the nature of the laboratory and the institution. Approaches that work for a large and/or academic medical center will be neither appropriate nor workable for a small local laboratory. In this chapter the assumption will be that, although there may be regulatory requirements for many activities, there is sufficient value to make the tasks worthwhile in their own right. That assumption may not be universally valid, but it is generally defensible. A British perspective from within the National Health Service is provided by Galloway and Nadin (1).

Scientific Resources

If the medical resources available to a laboratory are very limited, it may be both reasonable and necessary to rely on outside assistance for studies of test utilization and test appropriateness (Table 45.1). The Q-Probes and Q-Tracks programs provided by the College of American Pathologists (CAP) (3, 5) are an excellent way for a small laboratory with limited medical resources to monitor services for medical relevance and enhance appropriate utilization of services (chapter 44).

A single laboratory director will have difficulty providing all the expertise needed to cover the scientific waterfront. It may be possible to elicit support from other members of the medical staff, from specialists in surrounding institutions, or from specialists in a major reference laboratory used by the local institution. Such scientific backup may be part of the negotiations for the referral contract. Resources such as video- or audiotaped conferences and written educational material may be available from the referral laboratory; from professional organizations such as CAP, the American Society of Clinical Pathologists, the American Association for Clinical Chemistry, or the American Society for Microbiology; or from governmental agencies, such as the Centers for Disease Control and Prevention.

For larger institutions with medical expertise in each scientific division, it may be possible to do most or all of the analysis, recommendations, and communication locally. As mentioned by Wilson and colleagues (chapter 44), locally generated data are often more persuasive than more impersonal national recommendations from distant gurus and even more remote reports from the medical literature. A combination of local and national expertise is ideal.

No matter what the size and resources of the laboratory, every hospital-based laboratory must develop a working relationship with the medical and nursing staffs.

When implementing recommendations for optimum utilization of services, nothing is as critical as the reputation of the director(s) of the laboratory with clinical colleagues. A useful strategy is to enlist the help and support—before implementation is attempted—of the clinical leaders in whatever specialty or subspecialty will be affected. There are almost always a small number of individuals who have the stature among their peers to carry the day when approaching even the most thorny of clinical problems.

Technical as well as medical sophistication must also be considered. With appropriate information technology—and the expertise to take advantage of it—analysis of laboratory utilization may achieve great depth. This exercise is sometimes referred to as "data mining." In essence, such an approach is benchmarking clinical performance. As such, it is subject to all the vagaries of laboratory benchmarking (are all the parameters being considered, are the patients of the physicians in the group truly comparable, etc.), but the implications of providing unflattering characterizations of clients are potentially much greater, so extreme caution is advised. Data mining may strike a new vein of precious metal, but it may also strike an underground river that will flood the mine.

Financial Resources

There are two components to be considered when deciding how to approach financial benchmarking (Table 45.2). Each will have a major impact on the type of program that is feasible. The first is the source and accessibility of financial data. Where are the data kept? Under whose control are they maintained? How detailed are the data and are they in a form that is useful for laboratory use? If not, are the keepers of the data willing and able to massage the information into a usable format? The second issue is the sophistication of financial analyzers in the laboratory or accessible to the laboratory. The optimal condition is to have a financial analyst—either in the laboratory or assigned to the laboratory—who is either familiar with laboratory science or who can communicate effectively with those who are.

Table 45.1 Assessing the variables in choosing the appropriate strategy for test utilization[a]

Option	Internal medical expertise	Institutional medical expertise	Consultant medical expertise	Examples
Local utilization programs	High	+/−	+/−	Internal utilization studies and/or expert opinion
Literature review and documentation	High	+/−	±/−	
Clinical specialists	Low or moderate	High	+/−	Internal utilization studies and/or expert opinion
External specialists	Low or moderate	Low or moderate	+	Literature review and/or expert opinion
Prepackaged programs	Low or moderate	Low or moderate	+/−	Q-tracks Q-probes

[a]+/−, present or absent.

Table 45.2 Assessing the variables in choosing a benchmarking program[a]

Financial and personnel resources	Competitive environment	Internal benchmarking	External benchmarking	Both internal and external benchmarking
High	High	Yes	Yes	Yes, if possible
High	Low	Yes	Not essential	Not essential
Low	High	Yes, to the fullest extent possible	If at all possible	If at all possible
Low	Low	Yes, to the fullest extent possible	No	No

[a]It is assumed that there is a "trusting relationship" between the administrations of the laboratory and the hospital.

If a competent analyst is available to the laboratory and the data are sufficient to generate the desired reports, all options are open to the laboratory. If not, the laboratory manager will have to decide what analyses are possible under the extant limitations. It may be difficult or impossible to participate in external benchmarking if the required data either are not available or are so difficult to generate that they are effectively unavailable.

The data needed for financial analysis will also cover productivity analysis in most cases. Thus, the comments will usually apply to both activities, although it is possible that sufficient information is available in a human resources department to make up for holes in a financial department.

Nature of Institutional Administration and Relationship with the Laboratory

Obviously issues related to the type of institutional administration and its relationship with the laboratory will not apply if the management of the laboratory and the institution are one and the same, as may be found in a commercial laboratory or a physician's office laboratory. In laboratories that are based in hospitals, the important individual may be the Chief Executive Officer, the Chief Operating Officer (or deputy), the Chief Financial Officer, or a combination of them (subsumed under the name "administration" in this chapter).

It is a maxim of life that the ideal situation is when your boss (1) doesn't understand what you do, and (2) thinks what you do is very important—or even better, essential. Fulfillment of only one parameter may be adequate, but is not a guarantee of impunity. If both conditions are met, then the laboratory manager can proceed to Boardwalk without passing Go and collect $200. All options will be open and a summary statement of good performance may be all that is needed for output from the various analyses. A second maxim (at least for life in medical institutions) is that if you have the medical staff behind you, you can accomplish many things that would be otherwise impossible. The converse is that you will have an (very) uphill battle if there is an adversarial relationship between the laboratory and the medical staff.

If the relationships between the laboratory and administration are not optimal, accommodations may be required. A good bit of ingenuity and creativity may also be necessary.

It may be necessary to use an external benchmarking program with which the administration is comfortable—often one of the hospital-wide programs. As mentioned in chapter 43 the gain in breadth from covering the whole hospital is sometimes accompanied by a loss of detail within each section. One approach to minimize damage is to generate relevant data using another source. The other source may be a voluntary agreement with another institution(s) (2) or, as discussed by Wilkinson and Reynolds (4), use of a laboratory-specific monitoring program.

If the administration has a specific benchmark target in mind, it is important to ensure that the target is appropriate for your laboratory. If possible, it is worth validating the appropriateness of the proffered "gold standard," as discussed in chapter 43.

Decision-Making Steps

The following steps will help you choose an appropriate benchmarking system(s) (5).

1. Assemble the critical participants within the laboratory (face-to-face, by phone, by memorandum, or by e-mail; or by a combination of these methods).
2. Characterize the important variables in terms of the specific institution.
3. Assess the capabilities of systems and personnel, both inside and outside the laboratory. Frankness and honesty are very important.
4. Consider each type of benchmarking activity separately.
5. Evaluate the advantages and disadvantages of adopting multiple systems or multiple approaches.
6. Assess (once again with frankness and honesty) the capability of systems and personnel for institution of the chosen approaches.

Evaluation of Data

All benchmarking data, whether internal or external, must be evaluated critically in the crucible of local experience (Table 45.3). If an implication from the benchmarking

Table 45.3 Evaluation of data from benchmarking programs

Condition	Action	Qualifiers
Internal benchmarking indicates continuous improvement	Encourage managers to continue on track	Be certain that unrecognized factors do not permit even better performance
Internal benchmarking indicates static or deteriorating results	Analyze the component(s) that appear to be responsible and initiate appropriate action	Be sure to involve the relevant manager(s) in the process and view performance as a systems issue, not a performance issue
External benchmarking indicates good performance relative to peers	Compliment managers on their excellent performance	Ensure that comparisons are legitimate and that even better improvement is not possible
External benchmarking indicates suboptimal performance	Examine comparisons to be sure they are legitimate; analyze component(s) to determine if the explanations can be pinpointed	Be sure to involve the relevant manager(s) in the process and view performance as a systems issue, not a performance issue

doesn't ring true, it may be because it is not true. The example described by Wilkinson and Reynolds illustrates critical examination of a benchmarking program combined with appropriate action to evaluate the accuracy of the data (4). It is, however, most important that unpleasant or potentially embarrassing implications not be "blown off" by laboratory management. Before dismissing a finding as a defect in a benchmarking activity, whether internal or external, it is essential to be sure that the identified problem isn't real.

If both internal and external benchmarking methods are employed, the two approaches can sometimes be used as a check on each other. Similarly, if more than one external benchmarking program is utilized—out of choice or compulsion—it is often possible to derive useful information from comparison of the two. Finally, it is sometimes instructive to compare results with a similar institution. Some external benchmarking programs will make the names and contacts of similar institutions available, if they have agreed in advance to be contacted. Alternatively, there may be a network of contacts, either formal or informal, that can be tapped.

It is often possible to enrich the interpretation of benchmarking data by evaluating the interplay among parameters. For instance, if a laboratory is competitive in worked hours per billable tests, but not in paid hours per billable test, the apparent inefficiency may reside in regional salary ranges or in the institutional policies on vacation, sick leave, or attendance at scientific or management meetings. These factors may or may not be under the control of laboratory management. The "less efficient" position may even be desirable for an enlightened institution if it results in greater employee loyalty and consequently increased retention of skilled personnel in a competitive marketplace. Once again, the final interpretation must be based on an assessment of all factors, not just the numbers (although the numbers must result in a positive bottom line for the institution).

If the laboratory has sufficiently sophisticated resources to analyze utilization data by provider, it may be possible to generate some very useful information that physician clients can use to manage their own businesses. These kinds of complicated analyses are very difficult to do correctly. Managers must be confident in their ability to provide useful information; otherwise, they risk alienating clients instead of helping them.

Summary

There is no universally correct answer for optimizing utilization of the laboratory, for benchmarking financial performance, or for measuring laboratory productivity. Each laboratory is different, although it will share certain challenges and opportunities with other similar laboratories. There are several variables to consider in choosing an approach to benchmarking. It is essential that decision makers evaluate the choices honestly, considering carefully the resources at their disposal. The best-designed program will founder if there is insufficient expertise or available time to implement it properly. Finally, interpretation of data generated must also be evaluated carefully in light of local conditions.

KEY POINTS

- Be sure that all the critical participants are involved in the decisions about which benchmarking programs to undertake.

- Evaluate the important variables in the laboratory, in the institution, and in the local competitive market before deciding on an approach.

- Use a similar process when evaluating the results of a chosen method. Do not assume that a choice, once made, is irrevocable. If it does not seem to be working, don't hesitate to try another approach.

GLOSSARY

Benchmarking A management tool that involves comparing one's performance with peers. The goal is to identify a "best performer" and understand how one deviates from the ideal.

Data mining A term used to describe the detailed analysis of data by looking at progressively increasing detail in the data ("drilling down").

REFERENCES

1. **Galloway, M., and L. Nadin.** 2001. Benchmarking and the laboratory. *J. Clin. Pathol.* **54:**590–597.

2. **Kelley, L. A., and B. S. Street.** 1996. Seeking improvement through laboratory benchmarking. The Western North Carolina Collaborative Group. *Clin. Lab. Manage. Rev.* **10:**244–248, 250–251.

3. **Lawson, N. S., and P. J. Howanitz.** 1997. The College of American Pathologists, 1946–1996. Quality Assurance Service. *Arch. Pathol. Lab. Med.* **121:**1000–1008.

4. **Wilkinson, D. S., and D. D. Reynolds.** 2003. Using benchmarking to manage your laboratory. *Clin. Leadersh. Manag. Rev.* **17:**5–8.

5. **Zarbo, R. J., B. A. Jones, R. C. Friedberg, P. N. Valenstein, S. W. Renner, R. B. Schifman, M. K. Walsh, and P. J. Howanitz.** 2002. Q-tracks: a College of American Pathologists program of continuous laboratory monitoring and longitudinal tracking. *Arch. Pathol. Lab. Med.* **126:**1036–1044.

APPENDIX 45.1   Websites

American Society for Microbiology
(http://www.asm.org)
A professional organization open to any individual who is interested in any aspect of the science of microbiology.

American Association for Clinical Chemistry
(http://aacc.org)
A professional organization devoted to the science of diagnostic (clinical) biochemistry.

American Society of Clinical Pathologists
(http://www.ascp.org)
A professional organization of individuals who are involved in the practice of pathology.

Centers for Disease Control and Prevention
(http://cdc.gov)
A government agency responsible for a wide variety of health-related services.

College of American Pathologists
(http://www.cap.org)
A professional organization of individuals with training in approved pathology residency programs.

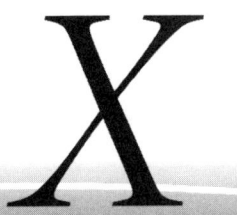

The Future of Clinical Laboratories

(Section Editor, *M. Desmond Burke*)

46

Future Political, Social, Economic, and Regulatory Impacts on Pathology and Laboratory Medicine

Paul Bachner

OBJECTIVES

To discuss major features of the current healthcare environment

To describe current regulations affecting laboratory practice

To identify likely future regulations and political and economic events impacting pathology and laboratory practice

All predictions are wrong, that's one of the few certainties granted to mankind. But, though predictions may be wrong, they are right about the people who voice them, not about their future but about their experience of the present moment.

M. KUNDERA (4)

IT IS ALLEGED that Henry Ford observed, "History is bunk." If he was correct, predictions about future events are even more suspect. Given the volatility of current political, economic, and social events and the enormous changes that we have witnessed in the science, technology, and practices of healthcare during the last half of the 20th century, any attempt at predicting the future is undertaken with considerable temerity and only because it is extremely unlikely that the inhabitants of that future will remember the accuracy of prior predictions. It is my intention to examine the current environment of healthcare with particular attention to political, social, economic, and regulatory factors and to attempt to identify trends within and external to that environment which are likely to influence future developments. I will restrict myself to trends that I believe will emerge during the next decade; any attempt to try to "see" farther into the future would be foolhardy since I believe the axiom that prediction is very difficult, especially about the future! Rather than making explicit predictions, I will emphasize emerging and at times conflicting trends and suggest what I believe to be likely options and directions that may arise in response to those trends. My summary of regulatory requirements is meant to be illustrative only. Readers are referred to the references and to Appendix 1 for websites that provide greater detail and additional information. Readers are also strongly urged to seek legal and other professional advice for specific issues related to their own laboratory practice and environment.

The Current Environment of Healthcare

A high level of volatility and uncertainty that reflects the political, economic, and social instability of our current environment characterizes healthcare in the United States in the opening years of the 21st century. Our country, which has enjoyed a prolonged period of political stability, economic growth, and prosperity, is now enmeshed in economic uncertainty and unprecedented concerns about national security. Funding and support for healthcare are uncertain, and the economic future of healthcare is hostage to the following identifiable trends and concerns:

- A growing federal deficit and concerns about the future viability of Medicare

- The increasing inability of state budgets to fund rising Medicaid expenditures

- An aging population that will generate increasing demands on healthcare resources

- The expanding potential of molecularly based technologies to identify disease at the genotypic level prior to the onset of detectable phenotypic changes

- The proliferation of costly technological and pharmacological advances in the ability to diagnose and treat disease

- A healthcare insurance and delivery system unable to provide insurance and predictable access to care for approximately 40 million Americans

- An insurance, payment, and delivery system for healthcare, loosely described as "managed care," that is increasingly viewed as dysfunctional by consumers (also known as "patients"), providers, and employers, the last constituting the primary source of funding for health insurance for the employed sector of the population

- Renewed major increases in healthcare costs no longer contained by the temporary cost-saving effects of the managed-care system

- A climate of blame in which the various players in the healthcare arena—insurers, drug companies, providers, lawyers, and economists—all reproach each other and advance conflicting solutions. Although the "demise" or significant modification of the managed-care system is widely predicted, there is a notable absence of any consensus about the contours of politically or economically viable alternatives. Nonetheless, it appears that "something else" will emerge—a return of the "managed competition" plan proposed in the early years of the Clinton presidency, a national health model resembling the Canadian system, implicit and explicit rationing of resources, or other combinations and approaches.

Current Regulations

Historically, regulations concerning the public health and healthcare in general, as well as those affecting laboratory medicine specifically, have tended to reflect social and political concerns. They have also reflected the periodicity of alternating cycles of regulatory enthusiasm for consumer protection versus traditional American reluctance to restrict and regulate commerce. The locus of regulations concerning public health and the laboratory community has traditionally been at the state level, reflecting a constitutional and judicial preference to default health and welfare issues to the states. The initiatives to establish and regulate public health and safety testing that took place in the middle-years of the 20th century were largely at the level of municipal and state health departments and were concerned primarily with environmental issues such as safe water and food and sanitation on the one hand and infectious disease prevention on the other. More recently, Congress has turned its attention to legislation and regulation in healthcare, perhaps the two most striking examples of which are the Clinical Laboratory Improvement Amendments of 1988 (CLIA '88) and the Health Insurance Portability and Accountability Act (HIPAA). A partial listing of four federal laws and regulations that are particularly pertinent to pathology and laboratory medicine services includes CLIA '88, HIPAA, the Occupational Safety and Health Administration (OSHA) standards for occupational exposure to blood-borne pathogens, and the Stark regulations.

CLIA '88

CLIA '88 represents the foundation of regulation and accreditation of laboratory testing in the United States. (1, 2) Subsequent to a series of Pulitzer Prize-winning newspaper articles appearing in the *Wall Street Journal* in 1988 and depicting major flaws in cytopathology testing and laboratory testing practices in physicians' offices, a series of Congressional hearings resulted in the very rapid passage by Congress and the signing into law of the amendments by the President. Although the law was enacted in 1988, the regulations were not implemented until 1992, in part because of a prolonged and contentious rule-making process involving two federal agencies (the Health Care Financing Administration [now called the Centers for Medicare and Medicaid Services] and the Centers for Disease Control and Prevention [CDC]) and extended commentary periods characterized by lobbying efforts by organized medicine, by the laboratory equipment manufacturing industry, by groups representing hospitals to make the regulations less stringent, and by organizations representing laboratory professionals to maintain personnel and quality control standards. Although changes to the regulations continue to be made, the amendments in their current form have been well established for many years and are applicable to all testing performed on humans, with few exceptions and without regard to venue of testing (site neutrality). The regulations encompass personnel standards, patient test management, quality assurance, proficiency testing, provisions for inspection and certification, and both civil and criminal penalties for noncompliance. Inspection and accreditation options are multiple and include government and private-sector organizations such as the College of American Pathologists and the Joint Commission on Accreditation of Healthcare Organizations.

HIPAA

Congress enacted HIPAA partially in response to public concerns about problems in transferability of employer-provided health insurance for workers changing jobs as well as similar concerns about denial of insurance coverage for preexisting medical conditions. The administrative simplification components of the law—which were enacted very much below the radar screens of major insurance industry, hospital, and healthcare professional organizations—contain far-reaching standards concerning simplification of electronic transactions and the privacy and security of protected health information (PHI). The privacy standards do the following:

- Limit the use and disclosure of health information
- Provide patients the right to access their medical records, to know who has accessed their records, and to request amendments to their records and restrict access to their records
- Restrict disclosure to "minimum necessary" purposes
- Establish criminal and civil penalties for improper use and disclosure and restrict access to records for research purposes

The regulations permit the use and disclosure of PHI for treatment, payment, or healthcare operations (e.g., quality assurance, accreditation, certification, credentialing, medical review) without consent or authorization and also allow for disclosure of PHI for treatment activities of another healthcare provider.

Standards for Occupational Exposure to Blood-Borne Pathogens

The standards for exposure to blood-borne pathogens were promulgated in 1991 by OSHA of the Department of Labor in response to widespread concerns by organized labor—particularly unions representing health and hospital workers—about the inadequacy of protective practices, equipment, and other safeguards for employees with regular and predictable exposure to body fluids and substances with the potential to transmit human immunodeficiency virus and hepatitis B virus. Information is available on the OSHA website at http://www.osha.gov/SLTC/bloodborne-pathogens/index.html.

The Stark Regulations

The Stark regulations constitute a series of congressional actions enacted over a period of several years that severely limit referral of a wide variety of services—including laboratory testing—to entities in which the referring provider has a financial stake. The regulations are named for Rep. Fortney "Pete" Stark (D. - Calif.), who was the legislative sponsor of the initial regulations, enacted in 1992 (Stark I), that prohibited a physician from making Medicare referrals for clinical laboratory services if the physician or an immediate family member had any financial relationship with the laboratory. The Stark II legislation, enacted in 1993, extended the regulations to Medicaid and broadened coverage to 10 additional health services, including, among others, occupational and physical therapy, durable medical equipment, radiology, and radiation therapy. The regulations—which are very complex and difficult to interpret—are often regarded as inhibiting innovative and potentially beneficial restructuring of the relationships between healthcare providers and entities. Enforcement by the government—particularly the Justice Department—is closely linked to other "fraud and abuse" enforcements under a variety of federal anti-kickback statutes.

Liability Considerations

Although the scope of this chapter and space considerations preclude a discussion in detail, a presentation of legislative and regulatory influences on the practice of medicine and laboratory medicine is incomplete without mention of the enormous impact of the judicial system and medical liability concerns on laboratory practice. Decisions by juries and judges at primary and appellate levels—particularly the increasingly high monetary awards for noneconomic damages ("pain and suffering")—are increasingly having an impact on decisions by hospitals and physicians concerning services to be offered and the circumstances under which services should be made available. This impact may also play a role in decisions concerning how laboratory medicine and pathology are practiced. (3) Specific examples include concerns about the reporting of results from non-Food and Drug Administration-approved tests or decisions by blood transfusion services to not implement available screening tests for infectious markers absent clear mandates or regulatory requirements. Although neither of these practices are violations of existing law or regulations, concerns about possible future civil law claims of failure to follow "standards" may determine decisions by laboratory services.

The Future Regulatory Climate under CLIA '88

CLIA '88 was conceived as an attempt by Congress to protect consumers against shoddy and poor-quality laboratory testing, particularly in physician office laboratories and "Pap mills" in which cytotechnologists were paid "by the slide." Although widely viewed by the organized physician community as a regulatory overreach by the federal government and by major segments of the professional laboratory community as a dangerous lessening of federal standards for testing personnel, CLIA '88 has by now been generally accepted—albeit with some reluctance—by most interested parties as the law of the land, and it is unlikely that in the foreseeable future there will be serious legislative initiatives to repeal or significantly modify CLIA '88. The broad outlines of laboratory practice under CLIA '88 will continue to include the following features.

Personnel Standards and Quality Control Standards

Personnel standards, quality control standards, and inspection requirements will vary with the complexity of testing categories. Some modification in quality control requirements will reflect changes in technology, particularly the advent of unitized, self-contained testing platforms. Recent changes have included the promulgation of a single set of quality control standards for all nonwaived testing (moderate and high complexity) as well as a reduction in frequency requirements for most specialties and subspecialties of testing.

Complexity Categories

Complexity categories are based upon analyst training and experience as well as operational characteristics of testing that is performed. The complexity categories may remain as (i) high complexity, e.g., histopathology, cytopathology, cytogenetics, blood banking, histocompatibility, and complicated chemistry, hematology, and microbiology procedures; (ii) moderate complexity, for the bulk of routine hematology, and chemistry procedures; (iii) provider-performed microscopy, encompassing a limited number of procedures (e.g., microscopic urinalysis) commonly performed in physician offices in conjunction with patient visits; and (iv) waived testing, performed in any location with minimal quality control and personnel requirements and without any inspection requirement. It is also possible that complexity categories will be simplified and will consist of waived and nonwaived categories only.

Waived Testing

In the decade since the regulations were implemented, the category of waived testing has undergone the most change, with a striking expansion of the original list of 8 waived tests to the current count in excess of 800 procedures! Although many of these tests represent competing analytic versions of common tests such as hemoglobin, occult blood, and cholesterol, more "exotic" procedures have been approved in recent years (e.g., influenza virus testing). Undoubtedly there will be continuing efforts at the regulatory level to increase the scope and breadth of waived testing and continuing debate as to the relative allocation of the responsibility for guaranteeing quality testing standards between the laboratories and the manufacturers of diagnostic systems.

The Impact of HIPAA

In the opinion of many knowledgeable observers, HIPAA will be the most important legislative and regulatory event of the first decade of the 21st century. The final privacy rule regulations specified that by 14 April 2003, laboratories that transmit data electronically must implement policies and procedures safeguarding against unauthorized use of or disclosure of identifiable patient information.

Laboratory Requirements

To comply with the regulations, a laboratory is required to do the following.

- Designate a "privacy official" to assume responsibility for developing and implementing privacy rules and procedures. This individual may have other responsibilities.
- Develop specific policies and procedures stating how PHI may be used and disclosed by its employees and agents and state how the laboratory intends to comply with the HIPAA rules.
- Train all personnel on understanding and enforcing privacy policies and procedures. Documentation of training must be available.
- Prepare a notice of privacy practices explaining how the laboratory will protect, use, and disclose PHI. While direct treatment providers must make a good-faith effort to obtain written acknowledgment from the patient of provision of the notice of privacy, pathologists and laboratories as indirect providers are exempt from this requirement.
- Establish administrative, technical, and physical safeguards for PHI. These may include periodic audits, password protection schemes, and physical safeguards, such as secured backup copies of patient data.

Regulations concerning electronic data transmission standards are pending. Information about the final privacy rule can be found on the College of American Pathologists website http://www.cap.org/practicing_pathology/hipaa/hipaa_resources.cfm.

The Future of HIPAA

In view of these mandates, it is now obvious that HIPAA will have enormous operational and economic impacts upon the entire healthcare enterprise. The scope and extent of this impact and efforts to respond to the regulations are likely to require the expenditure of significant economic and human resources. Although the societal benefits of HIPAA in safeguarding patient privacy are obvious, the law and the implementing regulations clearly constitute another unfunded mandate for an already heavily burdened healthcare system. Since the regulations have only recently been announced, there is no body of experience concerning implementation, and it is too soon to speculate about the stringency of enforcement and what mechanisms and agencies will play the major role in developing enforcement policies. Most informed observers believe that many changes in the regulations are to be expected.

Bioterrorism

Recent History

In the wake of the events of 11 September 2001, credible threats of terrorism that include the potential for use of nuclear, chemical, and biological agents will have—and are already having—significant impacts on the funding and costs of providing laboratory services. The identification of clinical cases and environmental contamination attributable to deliberate dissemination of *Bacillus anthracis* through the mail system during the early part of 2002 brought this lesson home to a number of microbiology laboratories. These events and the fear of additional terroristic use of other infectious agents—not to mention the concurrent emergence of other "natural" biological threats to public health such as severe acute respiratory syndrome and West Nile virus—have not only alarmed the public, the government, and the medical and microbiological community but also focused attention on technical capabilities and staff preparation.

Future Impact

Public anxiety and governmental action in response to these threats are likely to have significant budgetary impacts on a wide variety of healthcare facilities, including laboratories. These budget impacts will reflect training costs, acquisition and deployment of equipment, facility modification, and other unfunded mandates, such as the recent CDC-issued rules (August 2002) requiring all laboratories to report to the government whether they are in possession of "select agents" that could be used in a bioterroristic attack. The rule is available on the CDC website at http://www.cdc.gov/od/ohs/1rsat/possess.htm.

Increased federal concerns about laboratory preparedness may generate some increased funding for specific areas of the laboratory; it is more likely that in the event of actual or suspected biological attacks, the impact on all areas of the laboratory will be to significantly increase utilization of laboratory services not only for unusual diagnostic challenges but also because of potentially massive increases in demand for routine laboratory services required for the care of large numbers of acutely ill patients.

Long-Term Effects: Legislation, Regulation, Accreditation

It is important to remember that legislative and regulatory mandates—both of which are closely intertwined with the requirements of accreditation and certification organizations—play a significant role in the delivery of healthcare services and the conditions of access to those services. In general, in addition to other economic imperatives, increases in the often fixed "overhead" costs of regulations tend to be more easily absorbed by larger entities, particularly in an industry in which prices and payments are often fixed by regulatory authority or subject to market force constraints. Thus, any increase in regulatory burdens can be expected to accelerate the trend of aggregation of laboratory services into larger and larger entities.

The Leapfrog Group

As the societal, market-driven, and political pressures for increased standardization in healthcare increase, partially in response to demands for improved patient safety by powerful private-sector and government entities, demands for external standards will become more prevalent in all dimensions of medical and laboratory practice—scientific, operational, fiscal, and legal. A potent example of this movement is the Leapfrog Group—an influential coalition of more than 100 public and private organizations that includes a large number of Fortune 500 companies that provide healthcare benefits—that was created "to help save lives and reduce preventable medical mistakes by mobilizing employer purchasing power to initiate breakthrough improvements in the safety of health care and by giving consumers information to make more informed hospital choices." The Leapfrog Group works with medical experts to identify problems and solutions relevant to quality of care in hospitals. Employers are encouraged to commit to the Leapfrog Group's healthcare purchasing principles, which can be found at the Leapfrog Group website, http://www.leapfroggroup.org/about.htm. This website provides survey-based reports concerning adherence to safety standards of geographically proximate hospitals. Efforts such as this—grounded in the belief that practice improvement can be achieved through benchmarking and performance-based ratings—are at present not well developed for pathology and laboratory medicine save for a few indicators, such as frequency of Pap smears, diabetes screening and monitoring, cholesterol screening, and screening for colon cancer. Furthermore, these indicators generally address whether patients are provided access to these measures rather than specific performance by laboratories.

Improved Patient Safety Outcomes

The interactions between the above-described initiatives for standardization, patient safety, and error prevention with the movement for evidence-based medicine will be considerable and important. It is already evident that the prevention of adverse events (i.e., error) has been confounded with other aspects of provision of optimal care (5). It may be reasonable to predict that standardization of laboratory practice arising from multiple sources, such as consolidation of laboratories and laboratory testing platforms, automation, bar coding, and other "fail-safe" patient and specimen identification systems, including standardized nomenclatures and languages (6), will have a positive impact on improved patient safety outcomes. The availability of standardized nomenclatures and languages that will allow for coded capture, aggregation, and retrieval of granular (detailed) data expressed in a variety of terminologies and across a variety of information systems will become increasingly important in patient safety and quality improvement efforts as well as for more mundane operational applications. The efforts of public and private sector organizations to promote increased standardization and improvement in educational practices will also play a positive role (7).

Issues Affecting Research and Academic Laboratories

The future of academic laboratories—the traditional source for much of the innovation and new knowledge that has infused American medicine—remains cloudy. This uncertainty reflects many realities, including the fiscal perils facing academic health centers as they attempt to fulfill their traditional missions of patient care, education, and research in the face of decreasing clinical revenues, flat or diminished support for teaching activities, and heightened competition for research funding.

Stem Cell Research

An area of research and laboratory practice that will be critically impacted by political developments, and therefore by complex and interrelated legislative, regulatory, and administrative events, is stem cell research and, eventually, the application of so-called cloning technology to medical practice in two broad areas: tissue and organ transplantation and reproductive technology. At the time of this writing, President Bush's Council on Bioethics has been unable to reach a consensus on whether to recommend a ban on reproductive cloning and impose a moratorium on therapeutic cloning (somatic cell nuclear transfer). The cloning research issue is closely tied to the highly emotional controversy over abortion and genetic manipulation and has elicited strong and conflicting opinions from various constituencies, including the research and medical community, religious groups, and organizations committed to research and treatment of specific diseases. Pending some resolution of this controversy—an unlikely event because of the enormous social and political implications of this debate—the continuing uncertainty of funding and the threat of federal and state restrictions on research in both reproductive and stem cell cloning will impede research into stem cell technology and may drive investigators to other countries that are more supportive of stem cell research.

Restrictive Patents and Restraints on Use of Human Tissues

Two other areas of potential threat to research and laboratory practice are restrictive patents and excessive restraints on the use of human tissue and data for research purposes. In general, the laboratory community has opposed attempts to patent life forms and has argued that attempts to do so will impede scientific progress and lead to high laboratory testing costs. This view is strongly supported by public and political groups in the United States, Canada, and Europe, but industry and portions of the academic research community argue that to eliminate genetic patenting will impede research. Legislation is currently pending in Congress to provide medical researchers and physicians with access to patented genes for use in clinical testing and noncommercial genetic research, but the outcome of this and related legislative initiatives remains unknown at this time.

Summary

Political, social, and economic trends and events are inextricably intertwined and often interact with the legislative and regulatory arena in unpredictable ways. The economic future of healthcare funding in the United States is uncertain and subject to continuing competition for resources within and external to the healthcare industry. The National Priorities Project data website at http://www.nationalpriorities.org/taxes/IncomeTaxChart.html shows that healthcare is responsible for 18% of income tax revenues disbursed by government, exceeded only by interest on debt (26%) and military expenditures (23%). As U.S. healthcare spending is projected to climb to $2.8 trillion by 2011, an average annual rate of increase of 7.3%, it is more than reasonable to predict that legislative and regulatory mandates as well as market forces will constrain that rate of growth. The recently enacted $350 billion federal tax cut may, as a result of decreased federal revenues, result in further diminution of federal and state funds for healthcare and research. As part of the response to these events, enhanced deployment of automation, robotic technologies, and miniaturization will be inevitably accompanied by increasing concentration within the healthcare delivery and laboratory industry. Parallel phenomena will include increasing "commoditization" of the laboratory product, the growth of alternate-site testing, "consumerism," and self-directed healthcare, including direct-access testing. All of these phenomena will occur in the context of the globalization of communication and other components of healthcare and laboratory practice.

In tandem with those mandates, the medical model will shift to one dominated by a medical effectiveness and "a need to know" logic that will compel a linkage between the gathering of patient data (testing), available therapeutic and management options, and positive outcomes (clinical relevance). Although the progression may be less rapid than predicted by some, I believe that the database of pathology and laboratory medicine—currently characterized by static and discontinuous phenotypic, quantitative, and morphological observations—will be superceded by an augmented and integrated continuum of morphological, immunophenotypic, genetic-proteomic, and clinical information. Thus, the paradigm will shift from morphological and other classification schemata based on laboratory data to classification hierarchies that emphasize biological homogeneity and clinical relevance with an increased emphasis on specific disease entities susceptible to targeted therapies. An interesting—and important—side effect of this emphasis for the pathology community will be the blurring of the traditional distinction between anatomic and clinical pathology.

The time frame in which these predictions will take place will be influenced by the rate of development of technology, by the extent to which healthcare will remain as a social contract or will be replaced by a marketplace ethic, and to an unpredictable extent by external events totally unrelated to healthcare.

KEY POINTS

- Laboratory practice is currently constrained and will be increasingly so in the coming years by political, social, economic, and regulatory considerations.

- The most important of the regulatory controls will be CLIA '88, HIPAA, OSHA, and enforcement under the Stark regulations and related fraud and abuse statutes.

- Funding and payment restrictions, concerns about legal liability, and a changing medical model emphasizing effectiveness and evidence-based care will also significantly impact how laboratory services will be delivered.

GLOSSARY

Centers for Disease Control and Prevention (CDC) The federal agency within the Department of Health and Human Services with broad responsibility for disease monitoring and prevention, epidemiology and statistics, and laboratory practice.

Clinical Laboratory Improvement Amendments (CLIA) Complexity categories based upon analyst training and experience as well as operational characteristics of testing that is performed. They include (i) high complexity, e.g., histopathology, cytopathology, cytogenetics, blood banking, histocompatibility, and complicated chemistry, hematology, and microbiology procedures; (ii) moderate complexity, for the bulk of routine hematology and chemistry procedures; (iii) provider-performed microscopy, encompassing a limited number of procedures (e.g., microscopic urinalysis) commonly performed in physician offices in conjunction with patient visits; and (iv) waived testing, performed in any location with minimal quality control and personnel requirements and without any inspection requirement. In 2003, a final rule was issued in the *Federal Register* that defined some new regulations and changed the categorization of tests into two categories (waived and nonwaived tests).

Clinical Laboratory Improvement Amendments of 1988 (CLIA '88) Federal law and regulations constituting the foundation of regulation and accreditation of all laboratory testing in the United States. The amendments are applicable to all testing performed on humans in all locations.

Evidence-based medicine An approach to the teaching and practice of medicine that utilizes literature review and outcome-based studies of effectiveness and possible harm to patients, rather than tradition or anecdotal experience, to guide diagnostic and treatment interventions.

Health Care Financing Administration Now renamed Centers for Medicare and Medicaid Services; the federal agency within the Department of Health and Human Services with primary responsibility for payment and payment standards for the Medicare and Medicaid programs.

Health Insurance Portability and Accountability Act of 1996 (HIPAA) Federal regulations establishing conditions for eligibility and transferability of health insurance and provisions for "administrative simplification" that promulgate far-reaching standards concerning electronic transactions of health data and the privacy and security of protected health information.

Indirect provider Under the HIPAA regulations, an indirect provider is an entity or individual (e.g., laboratory or pathologist) without a direct treatment relationship to a patient. The indirect provider delivers healthcare based on the orders of another provider and typically provides services or reports the diagnosis or results to another provider.

Stark regulations Federal regulations prohibiting referral of laboratory and other health services to entities in which the referring provider has a financial interest.

REFERENCES

1. Bachner, P., and W. B. Hamlin. 1993. Federal regulation of clinical laboratories and the Clinical Laboratory Improvement Amendments of 1988—Part I. *Clin. Lab. Med.* **13:**739–752.

2. Bachner, P., and W. B. Hamlin. 1993. Federal regulation of clinical laboratories and the Clinical Laboratory Improvement Amendments of 1988—Part II. *Clin. Lab. Med.* **13:**987–994.

3. Bierig, J. R. 2002. Liability and payment issues in the selection of pathology assays. *Arch. Pathol. Lab. Med.* **126:**652–657.

4. Kundera, M. 2002. The great return. *The New Yorker,* 20 May 2002.

5. Leape, L. L., D. M. Berwick, and D. W. Bates. 2002. What practices will most improve safety? Evidence-based medicine meets patient safety. *JAMA* **288:**501–507.

6. Spackman, K. 2002. SNOMED CT unlocks the power of clinical data for pathologists. *Lab. Med.* **33:**(3), Special Report, p. 1–4.

7. Wilson, M. L. 2002. Education and training: practice makes perfect. *Am. J. Clin. Pathol.* **118:**167–169.

APPENDIX 46.1   Websites

College of American Pathologists
(http://www.cap.org/apps/docs/statline/HIPAA_Special_Report.html)
Information concerning the final privacy rule.

Centers for Disease Control "select agents" rules
(http://www.cdc.gov/od/sap)
The CDC rules issued in August 2002 require all laboratories to report to the government whether they are in possession of "select agents" that could be used in a bioterrorism attack.

The Leapfrog Group
(http://www.leapfroggroup.org/about)
The website of an influential coalition of more than 100 public and private organizations that provide health care benefits committed to

helping to "save lives and reduce preventable medical mistakes by mobilizing employer purchasing power to initiate breakthrough improvements in the safety of health care and by giving consumers information to make more informed hospital choices."

The National Priorities Project
(http://www.nationalpriorities.org/taxes/IncomeTaxChart.html)
The National Priorities Project data website provides data on allocation and disbursement of federal tax revenues.

Occupational Safety and Health Administration (OSHA)
(http://www.osha.gov/SLTC/bloodbornepathogens/index.html)
Federal Government website for current information about OSHA regulations on blood-borne pathogens and needlestick prevention.

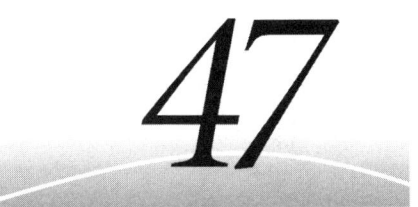

The Future of the Clinical Scientist Workforce

Diana Mass and John R. Snyder

OBJECTIVES

To describe laboratory practices that provide value-added services

To discuss the information society as it relates to clinical laboratory services and patient safety needs

To define the "knowledge worker" and advocate the benefits of clinical scientists who perform this role

To compare and contrast the old laboratory and new laboratory paradigms and determine the value of the new laboratory as it improves patient safety

To describe conditions of good work, which can have a positive impact on current clinical laboratory vacancy rates

To explain the consultation process and determine the benefits in clinical laboratory practice as it relates to patient safety

To characterize four interactive skills that contribute to the effectiveness of consulting practice

To describe the various competencies of successful consultants

To assess the benefits to the healthcare delivery system when clinical scientists act as consultants

---

The task is not so much to see what no one yet has seen, but to think what nobody yet has thought about that which everybody sees.

ARTHUR SCHOPENHAUER, 1788–1860

TODAY'S LABORATORY MANAGER faces a unique set of challenges in a healthcare environment shaped by financial constraints and increasing federal regulation. An imperative exists to ensure quality while exercising prudent fiscal responsibility, and this within the context of a dramatically changing workforce (7, 29) that must better serve patients in an era of expanding knowledge and rapid change. Further, "value-added" laboratory services has become today's watchword because customer satisfaction is necessary to achieve the goal of long-term sustainability and economic success for the laboratory (15, 29). The focus of this chapter is the discussion of this value-added service, that is, service which addresses effectiveness as well as cost and efficiency. This can only be accomplished if the right test is ordered and interpreted properly: regardless of how accurate and precise the result is, it is of no value unless it contributes to appropriate and timely diagnosis and treatment (3). Thus, the future workforce not only must provide accurate and reliable laboratory results but also must be prepared to interact with healthcare providers in a consultative manner regarding appropriate test utilization (13, 15, 22, 29).

Essential Role in Healthcare

Traditionally the service provided by the clinical scientist (clinical laboratory scientist/medical technologist) workforce has been essential in the diagnosis and treatment of patients. There is no doubt that their expertise has provided information that physicians require to make critical decisions regarding their patient care responsibilities (3). In 1985, Strandjord estimated that 45% of medical decision making relied on information generated by laboratory tests (39). Today this number is estimated to be 70% (14). The Mayo Health System demonstrated that the laboratory contributes as much as 94% of the objective data in a clinical record. Furthermore, this information is accessed as often as 200,000 times per day as evidenced by retrievals from an electronic medical record (15). Thus, there can be no doubt that the laboratory services are essential to the delivery of healthcare. Additionally, a knowledgeable and committed workforce that provides clinical laboratory consultative services by communicating directly to healthcare providers regarding appropriate testing protocols is now a mandate (18). This was a recurring theme at the CDC Quality Institute held in Atlanta, Ga., in April 2003, that is, the need to improve laboratory services in the preanalytical and postanalytical phases of the laboratory service continuum (2).

Engagement in preanalytical and postanalytical phases of laboratory service signals a fundamental shift in the nature of laboratory work. The shift is *away from* a focus on technology and the performance of procedures *toward* the generation of laboratory information, an "information revolution" in laboratory medicine. Inherent in this information revolution are new tasks related to gathering, distributing, and adding value to the information provided by clinical laboratories.

More than 20 years ago, Peter Drucker foresaw the transformation from an industrial society to an information society (9, 10). He noted a new era in information technology, one in which information concepts would take the place of a focus on data collection, storage, transmission, and presentation. Drucker proposed that the question, "What is the *meaning* of information and its *purpose*?" would help define a hierarchy of information. Indeed, data as simply raw descriptors may help diagnostic efficacy. Data in context become information improving diagnostic effectiveness. Information in light of experiences and judgment becomes knowledge, improving therapeutic efficacy and effectiveness. Outcome-based testing protocols support enhanced service and aggregate cost savings but do require workers with expanded roles.

Drucker coined the term "knowledge worker" for those fulfilling these expanded roles by gathering, distributing, and adding value to information. Throughout this chapter,

the imperative for an information revolution in laboratory medicine practice will be described with corresponding implications for a future workforce comprised of clinical scientists as knowledge workers.

Other Emerging Imperatives

In 1995, the Pew Health Professions Commission Report described an emerging transformation of traditional healthcare practice into "systems of integrated care that combine primary, specialty, and hospital services" that require extraordinary collaboration skills across all levels and types of healthcare professions (22). Nowhere is the change more urgent than in the clinical laboratory, where institutional goals can be achieved only by effectively collaborating with other healthcare practitioners to enhance the quality of diagnostic and therapeutic decisions.

Subsequent to the Pew Report, the 1999 Institute of Medicine report "To Err Is Human: Building a Safer Health System" (18) was published indicating that as many as 98,000 people die annually in U.S. hospitals as a result of medical errors. This stunning statistic does not even represent the additional deaths associated with missing a diagnosis from failing to order a laboratory test or incorrectly interpreting test results (20). The need for educating physicians to utilize the appropriate tests and understand their clinical significance may never have been greater than it is now. This is not a new issue. The call for the laboratory to accept the responsibility to directly communicate to physicians regarding proper test utilization has been discussed for over 20 years (8). Unfortunately, the will and courage in laboratory management to do so have been lacking. The parochial view of providing only test results and algorithms will not lead to optimal patient care or financial success. In the final analysis, it is only by appropriately utilizing the clinical scientist workforce that patient safety can be enhanced and fiscal objectives met (7).

Clinical laboratory scientists/medical technologists have for decades been taught clinical correlation with disease status but have only recently been expected to apply this knowledge in practice lest they tread on turf sacred to the practice of medicine. Consequently, an underutilized laboratory workforce has contributed directly to some of the safety, efficiency, and effectiveness problems plaguing healthcare.

Engaging laboratory scientists in the pre- and postanalytical phases of testing requires a fundamental shift in operations. Few scientists are engaged in the input subsystem (physician order and requisition) despite their unique understanding of the subtle differences of testing procedures. Similarly, few scientists are consulted on the output subsystem (physician review, interpretation, and appropriate action) despite their knowledge of predictive value and potential limitations of laboratory results (19).

To prepare and deploy a knowledge worker laboratory workforce, and indeed legitimize the clinical scientist worker title, laboratorians must be engaged in the testing process as a scientific process, from posing hypothetical answers, through generation and analysis of information to illuminate those answers, to considering the patient care outcome of those answers.

If the clinical scientist staff is more appropriately deployed in an interactive, consultative role in improving test utilization, it is expected that unnecessary testing will diminish, which will have a positive impact on the laboratory's budget in some extraordinary ways. Additionally, a laboratory is cost-effective only if the staff is used at the highest level of capability, not their lowest; thus, in a cost-effective operation you use people at their highest potential (22).

A New Workforce

The emergence of clinical scientists as consultants represents a natural evolutionary growth in the role of the clinical laboratory profession as it adapts to a changing environment. This emerging role is being fostered not only by the need to improve laboratory test utilization (25), as already discussed, but also by the extraordinary growth of decentralized testing (37). The increasing complexity of the clinical laboratory sciences is causing many physicians to seek information and interpretive guidelines necessary to make optimal and cost-effective use of the laboratory. This was first evidenced following the diagnosis-related group initiatives (40). Similarly, rapid advances in clinical laboratory technology and diagnostics have made it nearly impossible for physicians and other healthcare providers to stay abreast of available tests and their implications for diagnosis and treatment (41).

Fueling this process are the medical-necessity guidelines released by the Centers for Medicare and Medicaid Services, formerly known as the Health Care Financing Administration, which prohibit Medicare and Medicaid from reimbursing for Part B services that are not medically necessary and reasonable for the diagnosis and/or treatment of the disease suspected (1). The clinical scientist is a natural link between the clinical laboratory and other providers or patients on matters of test selection, specimen collection, interpretation of test results in light of specimen quality and sources of interference, and patient education. Laboratory professionals are expected to provide information, solve problems, analyze situations, and implement decisions related to laboratory testing (20).

The second development, decentralized testing, is due to a variety of incentives which have caused a shift of various diagnostic testing outside of hospital and private laboratories. Decentralized testing continues to grow with respect to types and numbers of tests because technology has developed less labor-intensive, more compact, and inexpensive equipment as well as reliable diagnostic kits which offer a wide range of testing. At these sites physicians and other healthcare providers require advice and instruction on clinical laboratory practice and management (26).

This new consultative role will enrich the work of clinical scientists who desire new responsibilities that are beyond the process of producing a test result. Now an additional set of skills is also valued: skills to determine whether a test should be done at all and that assist physicians and other healthcare professionals to use the laboratory appropriately. Clinical scientists are well practiced in the science of problem solving. Now we need to take these skills outside of the laboratory to the source of potential problems and begin to prevent problems by interacting with physicians and other healthcare providers to ensure patient safety (22, 27).

It is important to recognize that clinical scientist knowledge workers do both knowledge work and "manual work" (10). Performance of a laboratory procedure constitutes manual work. Knowledge work related to the laboratory procedure begins with data analysis and the use of personal intellectual capital (experience). Knowledge work also includes consultation with other clinical service providers (pooled intellectual capital) and electronically available intellectual capital.

This new workforce of clinical scientist knowledge workers has some unique characteristics, which managers will need to recognize and support (9, 38):

- Knowledge workers are *specialized*.
- They are able to *acquire and supply* theoretical and analytical knowledge.
- They are learning based, prepared through *formal education*.
- They exhibit the habit of *lifelong learning*.
- They are effective in *teams*.
- They seek *meaning* in their work and *advancement opportunities*.
- They require flexible, fully *networked and connected* environments.
- They reach *decisions by consensus*, not command.

Obviously, development and retention of knowledge workers in laboratory medicine pose a challenge.

Laboratory Paradigms

Before describing specific consultative roles, it is useful to discuss the new interactive laboratory and compare it to the old, or traditional, laboratory. The concept of the new interactive laboratory was formulated (3) prior to the Clinical Laboratory Improvement Amendments of 1988 (CLIA '88) (12); however, regulations promulgated under this law defined a total testing process as a continuum in laboratory practice that has been universally accepted by the laboratory community. The CLIA '88 concepts of preanalytical, analytical, and postanalytical activities serve as

Figure 47.1 The new interactive laboratory model. (Adapted from reference 3.)

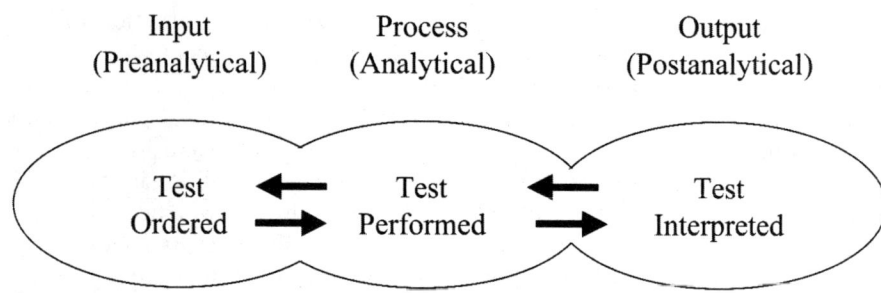

benchmarks for laboratory practice. These three phases as they occur in the new laboratory are described by Barr's (3) model of laboratory utilization (Fig. 47.1) as input, process, and output.

The Old Laboratory

Today, many clinical laboratories still operate according to the traditional laboratory model (Fig. 47.2), which is a linear, unidirectional flow process of one activity preceding the next activity. The major concern in this model is the quality of the test performance and the production features and internal organization of the laboratory (analytical phase). In the traditional model, the focus is on the science and technology and quality of test performance, and communication is almost nonexistent prior to the test request or after the result is released. In this model, the clinical laboratory is not concerned with clinical appropriateness or interpretation of test results (3).

The New Laboratory

The new laboratory model (Fig. 47.3) is an interactive process, and the scope of laboratory services is broader. In this model, the focus is not only on the quality of test data generated (process/analytical) but also on the clinical appropriateness of test requests (input/preanalytical) and the correct interpretation of and response to laboratory information (output/postanalytical). The laboratory's involvement in the entire total testing process will have a positive impact on patient outcomes, improve the clinical relevance and value of the laboratory's service, and greatly enhance the cost-effectiveness of the laboratory operation (3).

To demonstrate how appropriate test utilization will promote a better integration of laboratory services into the patient care process, Barr's model is briefly described. In the input phase, one must question if the test is appropriate for the stage of the clinical condition and if the time of specimen collection is correct. During the process phase, one must determine if, within clinically relevant guidelines, the test result is accurate and precise and timely with respect to the turnaround time needs of physicians. Finally, in the output phase, one must evaluate if the results are properly interpreted and integrated into patient care or if data overload is confusing or misleading physicians.

Barr's model identifies the factors that affect the clinician's decisions or actions at each step of the laboratory use process. It also demonstrates any appropriate roles for the clinical scientist at each step of this process. Starting with the clinician's assessment of the patient's condition, the laboratory utilization process proceeds in seven steps, which results in the application and integration of the test results into patient care.

All three phases are critical. If a test is not clinically indicated, or the laboratory's precision is beyond that needed for clinical judgments, or if the result is misinterpreted, then an accurate and precise laboratory result is of no value. It must be acknowledged that such tests are of no value because they unnecessarily consume the limited healthcare resources and may lead to diagnostic and therapeutic delay and patient harm (3, 22).

Clinical laboratory sciences/medical technology educational programs have historically included pathophysiology, clinical correlation, algorithms, and more recently

Figure 47.2 Traditional laboratory model. (Adapted from reference 3.)

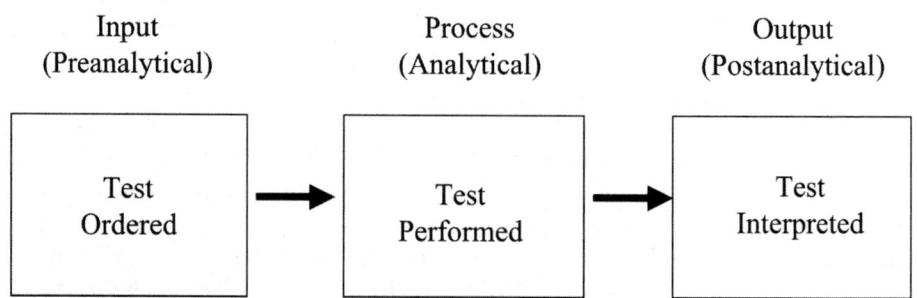

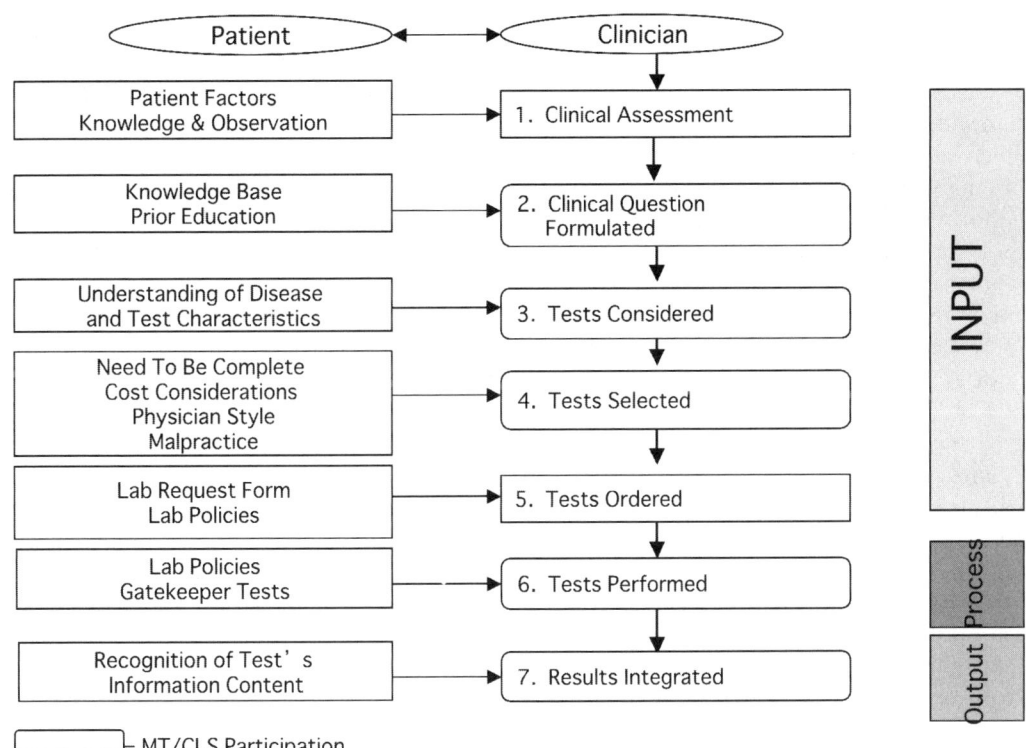

Figure 47.3 Model of laboratory utilization. MT/CLS, Medical Technologist/Clinical Laboratory Scientists. (Adapted from B. Davis, D. Mass, and M. Bishop [ed.], *Principles of Laboratory Utilization and Consultation*, W. B. Saunders, Philadelphia, Pa., 1999.)

clinical pathways in the curriculum (25). This clinical knowledge was always a part of the graduates' knowledge/skill mix, but they have not been called upon to use it due to the laboratory management's lack of vision regarding the role of this knowledge in the total testing process.

The Changing Workforce

The clinical laboratory profession is experiencing unprecedented vacancy rates that will not be resolved in the near future (43). Statistical projections show that an overall expanding population that includes a large elderly group with chronic health problems will require a greater supply of healthcare professionals that currently are in short supply (6). Meeting staffing needs has become the laboratory manager's most pressing problem on a daily basis. As the shortage of certified medical technologists/clinical laboratory scientists continues to grow due to fewer graduates entering the workforce and baby boomers beginning to retire, laboratory managers are evaluating staffing patterns needed for various testing methodologies. While laboratory managers prefer to hire the most highly educated personnel, the fact that these personnel are dwindling is causing managers to assess the requisite skills necessary to perform more routine procedures and hire less educated personnel to fill this need (4).

The appropriate role of the various levels of clinical laboratory personnel is the focus of much discussion and contention today. While the crisis of the shortage of staffing is creating much debate as to the appropriate levels needed to perform various types of testing, the crisis of patient safety needs is unveiling a major contribution that must be provided to improve patient outcomes, that is, better utilization. These two concurrent challenges must be faced with creativity, innovation, and courage by laboratory management in order to provide laboratory services that not only are reliable but also add value to patient care.

Pontius interviewed the chief executive officers of the major laboratory manufacturers in a series of published articles. It is not surprising that most chief executive officers believe that technology, automation, and robotics will substitute for large numbers of personnel (30–36). Indeed, this has been industry's mantra for 30 years (25). Many laboratories have moved to increasingly automated operations. This direction, however, has proved inadequate, as the declining workforce has deprived the operation of the cognitive abilities necessary to provide accurate laboratory information in direct patient care. It is now evident that technology and automation cannot substitute for qualified personnel in the numbers originally suggested (28).

In the absence of state personnel licensure for clinical laboratories, the mix of people with various levels of training and credentialing has created a nightmare for laboratory management. In a profession dictated by stringent rules regarding test performance, it is ironic that rules regarding personnel are so ambiguous and inconsistent.

The implementation of CLIA '88 in 1992 forever changed laboratory management's perception of the laboratory workforce. In essence, CLIA '88 regulations gave many laboratory managers permission to use less qualified personnel to perform moderate-complexity tests. This option allowed these managers to hire less trained individuals. In some laboratories, such as large reference laboratories, this option may work well if there is sufficient oversight. In other laboratories, particularly community hospital laboratories, this experiment may have proven to be disastrous (28).

Forecasting or speculation regarding workforce needs has almost become sport in various circles. Laboratory financial officers claim that they can effectively operate a laboratory with individuals who can simply function routinely. It is a fact that workforce needs can vary according to laboratory function and tasks. For example, a high-volume chemistry department in an urban reference laboratory with highly automated, sophisticated instrumentation may use supportive-level personnel to operate the equipment. However, if the instrumentation is highly sophisticated and complicated, supervisory oversight is even more necessary. Every laboratory operation will need to determine the appropriate staffing pattern for their unique analytical processes (4). Assuming that test information is reliable and accurate, the more important question with regard to service to the physician, and thus the patient, will be, what does this result mean with respect to patient safety (20)?

Creating Conditions of Good Work

Contributing to the unprecedented vacancy rates in the clinical laboratory is not only the lack of graduates and predictable retirements but also the purposeful defection of qualified people for other opportunities which grant them respect, value their intellectual worth, and financially reward their contributions (29). In the search for profit, clinical laboratories have neglected to provide meaningful and challenging opportunities for their workforce, who are being underutilized.

In the global economy and now within the broader scope of laboratory practice as described above, knowledge workers are identified as the route to success (38). Using the clinical scientist workforce as the knowledge workers in ensuring patient safety will lead to clinical scientist careers that are viewed as meaningful, challenging, and rewarding (15). In addition, the fulfillment of good work leads to personnel recruitment and retention, which contribute to a much-needed stable workforce that will improve the budget's bottom line (29).

By the same token, supportive personnel with appropriate oversight can perform the more routine analytical processes in the laboratory. However, it should be kept in mind that there are analytical processes that require a more educated scientist because of the requirements for problem solving and diagnostic interpretation. Best conducted a task analysis to determine the appropriate staffing levels for various types of tests. It was found that in the laboratory environment, there does exist a need for clinical scientists to perform various functions that are scientific and technical in nature as well as a myriad of roles in a supervisory and administrative capacity (4). The idea here is that many talented scientists prefer work that typically exists in the traditional laboratory (internal operations and sophisticated technical analytical processes), while others prefer to be involved with patient care in a consultative capacity. All functions are necessary, however, and the latter needs to be cultivated and encouraged (15).

Limiting laboratory work to the application of technology to produce patient care information, devoid of the connection to why the information is requested or how the information is used has led to more than just underutilization; it has led to a sense of "invisibility," to a lack of recognition, and ultimately to declining self-worth and the search for more challenging work. For work to be intrinsically rewarding to individuals, there must be a link between behavior and reward with the following psychological conditions (17):

- Experienced meaningfulness
- Experienced responsibility
- Knowledge of results

Unfortunately, job design for laboratory personnel has traditionally been accomplished using a technical approach based in scientific management rather than a psychological approach. The technical approach extracts "maximum efficiency from workers by designing narrow, repetitive jobs" (5). By contrast, a psychological approach to job design seeks to motivate workers with responsibilities which are broad and relatively autonomous from supervisors. Proponents of the technical approach advocate that simplifying work enables the worker to develop proficiency through repetition of tasks, making a highly skilled worker who is productive. Advocates of the psychological approach argue that repetitive tasks are not rewarding to individuals and that work should represent whole tasks with which the worker can identify, e.g., the preanalytical through postanalytical process in laboratory testing.

Additional insight about creating conditions for good work is found in the *motivating potential* of a job. Hackman et al. (17) expressed a job's motivating potential score (MPS) as follows:

$$\text{MPS} = 1/3 \ (\text{skill variety} + \text{task identity} + \text{task significance}) \times \text{autonomy} \times \text{feedback}$$

The higher the MPS, the higher the motivation for the employee.

Knowledge workers with a strong need for achievement and personal development will be most motivated if they are given full opportunity to use their education and potential through consultative activities and have a sense of accomplishment in how patient care was affected by laboratory information rather than simple accomplishment of a procedure.

The Changing Nature of Work

The Consultation Role and Process

Consultants are individuals with recognized expertise who are asked by a client, in this case a healthcare provider, to apply their knowledge and skills to a given situation. A consultant is a facilitator and a specialist in determining needs and identifying resources. The primary value of a consultant lies in the expertise to accurately identify, analyze, and resolve the problems and needs of the client.

Consultants can be categorized as either internal or external. Internal consultants are employees of the organization for which they consult, and many clinical scientists have been serving in this capacity without being formally identified as such in a job description. External consultants are proprietors of private consulting businesses. These individuals have total responsibility, authority, and accountability for their professional practices (24). The acceptance and legitimization of clinical scientists as consultants have been demonstrated by the federal regulatory authority of CLIA '88, which specifies the position of a "technical consultant" who is responsible for the technical and scientific oversight of laboratory testing in moderate-complexity laboratories (12). In the last 10 years, clinical scientists have performed the functions as outlined in the regulations and have proven their abilities to occupy this role. Now, this role must be internalized in the clinical setting, where test utilization questions require clinical scientist input to ensure patient safety.

The consultation process can involve the following general functions: evaluation of a problem, research, advising, planning, implementation, supervising, training, and evaluation of problem resolution. Consulting is aimed at helping a person or a group deal with confrontation of problems and efforts to change. "Change" is the operative word, because consultants deal primarily with the effect of change on an organization and on its staff.

Consulting involves people dealing with people, as opposed to people dealing with machines or mathematical solutions. Successful consultants understand organizational dynamics and the unique functions and boundaries of the consultant role. They are aware of the effects and conflicts of using new technologies. They understand change processes and the powerful influence of individual and organizational resistance. They are clear about the boundaries of their role, and they do not become involved in unproductive conflicts over authority and responsibility.

They avoid using a narrow set of techniques without evaluating their relevance to a particular situation. The inability to understand these concepts and to apply these skills can produce barriers to positive outcomes, resulting in consultant services that are ineffectual (11, 16, 21, 24, 42).

Consultant Skills

The consultant's potential to affect the quality of laboratory testing depends on the effectiveness of the consulting practice. A combination of four interactive skills makes a successful consultant. A consultant must excel in the area of *technical knowledge and skill*. The successful consultant translates expert knowledge into useful application. The consultant's knowledge must encompass the leading edge of the client's technology; he or she should be aware of emerging technologies and should evaluate their application. If consultants have the best information and approach, or the most effective solution to a problem, but they do not have the ability to work with the client, then the result is negative and failure is inevitable. Therefore, a consultant must excel in *interpersonal skills*, the second area, which includes skills in leadership, communication, understanding value structures, conflict resolution, and teamwork. Good *conceptual skills* are another important requirement. A consultant must be able to see beyond the immediate problem, relate all of the pieces, and integrate them into a conceptual working whole (24). And finally, *empowerment skills* enable the consultant to demonstrate the confidence necessary to influence others (29).

Consultative competencies have been identified and grouped according to the knowledge, skills, and attitudes necessary for success. These competencies are identified in Table 47.1 (21, 27). If we examine these competencies and relate them to a similar set for clinical laboratory sciences, we will find a great disparity. Since the traditional role and environment of clinical laboratory personnel are remarkably different from those of a consultant, this should be expected. Consulting is based on the behavioral sciences, an area that has not been stressed in the highly technical education of clinical laboratory personnel.

The Internal Consultant

Internal consultants include clinical scientists who attend patient rounds in teaching hospitals and advise physicians on the selection of laboratory tests, or those who work for reference laboratories as sales or client representatives and advise physicians on proper screening methods with appropriate reflex (follow-up) testing. The internal consultant role is one that usually does not require the establishment of a formal consultant-client relationship each time service is provided. When clinical scientists who are internal consultants earn the respect of their colleagues in the organization, they often become essential participants on the healthcare team.

Table 47.1 Consultant competencies

Knowledge areas

Foundation in administrative philosophies, policies, and practices

Knowledge of educational and training methods

An understanding of the stages in the growth of individuals, groups, and organizations

Knowledge of how to design and help a change process

Knowledge and understanding of human personality, attitude formation, and change

Knowledge of oneself: motivations, strengths, weaknesses, and biases

Skill areas

Communication skills: listening, observing, identifying, and reporting

Teaching and persuasion skills: ability to impart new ideas and insights effectively

Counseling skills to help others reach meaningful decisions

Skill in designing surveys, interviewing, and other data-collecting methods

Skill in using problem solving techniques and in assisting others in problem solving

Ability to work with groups and teams in planning and implementing change

Ability to be flexible in dealing with all types of situations

Ability to form relationships based on trust

Attitude areas

Attitude of a professional: competence, integrity, feeling of responsibility

Maturity: self-confidence, willingness to take necessary risks, ability to cope with rejection, hostility, and suspicion

Open-mindedness, honesty, intelligence

Possession of a humanistic value system

Table 47.2 Laboratory resource consultant tasks[a]

Monitor utilization reports of high-volume test usage patients

Communicate opportunities for improved utilization to case managers, physicians, and service line administrators

Assess need for involvement of pathologists/administrators in utilization issues

Review care paths to affirm appropriate laboratory utilization

Consult with physicians, nurses, and laboratory professionals on current guidelines and protocols for proper test ordering

Educate physicians and nursing groups on current and new policies and procedures regarding laboratory utilization, medical-necessity, and compliance issues

Consult with laboratory administrators and practitioners about current laboratory utilization practices

[a]Adapted from reference 22.

The consultant within the hospital environment can function in a variety of ways to improve patient care and enhance the efficiency of the facility. Too often the role of the laboratory has been perceived to begin with receipt of a specimen and end with reporting of a result. On the contrary, there are numerous opportunities in the preanalytical and postanalytical phases of the testing process that require consultation in addition to clarification regarding the various aspects of the analytical phase. One important utilization activity that should be increased is the clinical scientist's involvement in interpreting and integrating laboratory information in the management of the patient's condition. Recent studies conducted at the Center for Quality Improvement and Patient Safety confirm this need (44). A successful program to improve laboratory utilization described by Luckey and Davis uses clinical scientists as "laboratory resource consultants." Initially the program focused on the more frequently ordered tests and diagnosis-related groups. With time, the program expanded and provided other needed services. Refer to Table 47.2 for an example of internal consultant functions conducted by the laboratory resource consultant (22).

Clinical scientists should be involved in ordering tests. What test will provide the most information? What type of specimen should be obtained? Under what conditions should the specimen be collected? When and how often? Involvement in discussions with physicians about the patient's situation could avoid delays and inadequate or inappropriate samples, reduce the patient's trauma due to unnecessary venipunctures, and improve the cost-effectiveness of patient care.

The laboratory's responsibility does not end when an accurate test value is obtained. The clinical scientist must ensure that the physician, nurse, therapist, pharmacist, or other healthcare provider understands the *meaning* of the results. The care these persons give depends on such understanding. Whether the test results are inconclusive or appropriate, subsequent steps are indicated; the clinical scientist should discuss these steps with the physician or follow up with institutionally sanctioned protocols (3, 22, 23).

Summary

It is clear that today both the nature of work in laboratory medicine and the workforce to perform testing and provide relevant information are in transition. Spurred by continued demands for efficiency and effectiveness and new demands for safety and better utilization, managers are challenged to rethink the development of clinical scientists.

The broadened role of clinical scientists, engaged with other healthcare providers in an interactive process about the supportiveness of clinical tests (input/preanalytical), the generation of value-added test data and information (process/analytical), and the correct interpretation of and response to laboratory information (output/postanalytical), begs the advent of laboratory knowledge workers.

The laboratory manager of the 21st century has the obligation not only to introduce a new laboratory paradigm but also to create, foster, and nourish a new workforce to bring about substantive change.

KEY POINTS

- Work and the workforce in laboratory medicine are in transition.

- The broadened role of clinical scientists will require those who can gather and distribute information with a value-added component.

- The total testing process will become very interactive; the focus will encompass the preanalytical (appropriateness of test requests), analytical (generation of test data), and postanalytical (correct interpretation of and response to laboratory information) aspects of testing.

- Only clinical laboratory personnel effectively collaborating with other healthcare practitioners to enhance the quality of diagnostic and therapeutic decisions can achieve institutional goals.

- In the global economy and now within the broader scope of laboratory practice, knowledge workers (those who are specialized, acquire and supply theoretical and analytical knowledge, possess learning based through formal education, engage in lifelong learning, are effective team players, seek meaning in their work, are fully networked and connected, and reach decisions by consensus) are identified as the route to success.

GLOSSARY

Barr's model of laboratory utilization A model that identifies the factors that affect the clinician's decisions or actions at each step of the laboratory utilization process.

Clinical laboratory consultative services Services that provide direct communications to healthcare providers regarding appropriate testing protocols.

Clinical Laboratory Improvement Amendments of 1988 (CLIA '88) technical consultant One who is responsible for the technical and scientific oversight of laboratory testing in moderate-complexity laboratories.

Clinical scientist A title that currently represents the clinical laboratory scientist/medical technologist.

Consultants Individuals with recognized expertise who are asked by a client, in this case a healthcare provider, to apply their knowledge and skills to a given situation.

Information revolution in laboratory medicine A change in laboratory services that includes tasks related to gathering, distributing, and adding value to the information provided by clinical laboratories.

Knowledge work Work that begins with data analysis and the use of personal intellectual capital and includes consultation with other clinical service providers.

Knowledge workers Those who fulfill expanded roles by gathering, distributing, and adding value to information.

New laboratory model A model that describes the total testing process as an interactive process; the focus is not only on the quality of test data generated (process/analytical) but also on the clinical appropriateness of test requests (input/preanalytical) and the correct interpretation of and response to laboratory information (output/postanalytical).

Value-added service Laboratory service which addresses effectiveness as well as cost and efficiency.

REFERENCES

1. **Auxter, S.** 1969. What to expect from HCFA's medical necessity policy. *Clin. Lab. Newsl.* **22:**1–3.

2. **Auxter, S.** 2003. Partnering with others to ensure patient safety: will the quality institute lead the way for lab services? *Clin. Lab. Newsl.* **29:**6.

3. **Barr, J. T.** 1999. Clinical laboratory utilization: rationale, p. 3–16. *In* B. Davis, D. Mass, and M. Bishop (ed.), *Principles of Laboratory Utilization and Consultation.* W. B. Saunders, Philadelphia, Pa.

4. **Best, M. L.** 2002. Avoiding crisis: right-sizing staffing for the future. *Clin. Leadersh. Manag. Rev.* **16:**428–432.

5. **Charns, M. P, and J. H. Janson.** 2000. Work design, p. 191–209. *In* S. M. Shonfell, and A. D. Kaluzny (ed.), *Health Care Management: Organization Design and Behavior,* 4th ed. Delmar Thomson Learning, Albany, N.Y.

6. **Davidson, J. D., and O. M. Kimball.** 2002. Educating laboratory staff for the future. *Clin. Leadersh. Manag. Rev.* **16:**374–379.

7. **Davis, B.** 2000. *Lab Utilization: CLMA Guide to Managing a Clinical Laboratory,* 3rd ed., p. 167–178. Clinical Laboratory Management Association, Wayne, Pa.

8. **Davis, B. G., M. L. Bishop, and D. Mass (ed.).** 1989. *Clinical Laboratory Science: Strategies for Practice.* J. B. Lippincott, Philadelphia, Pa.

9. **Drucker, P. F.** 1992. *Managing for the Future. The 1990s and Beyond.* Truman Talley Books, New York, N.Y.

10. **Drucker, P. F.** 1999. *Management Challenges for the 21st Century.* HarperCollins Publishers, Inc., New York, N.Y.

11. **Ellis, J., and S. Helbig.** 1981. *The Health Care Consultant as a Change Agent.* American Medical Record Association, Chicago, Ill.

12. *Federal Register.* 1992. Medicare, Medicaid, and CLIA programs; regulations implementing the Clinical Laboratory Improvement Amendments of 1988 (CLIA)—HCFA. Final rule with comment period. *Fed. Regist.* **57:**7002–7186.

13. **Finn, A F., Jr., P. N. Valenstein, and M. D. Burk.** 1988. Alteration of physicians' orders by nonphysicians. *JAMA* **259:**2549–2552.

14. **Forsman, R. W.** 1996. Why is the laboratory an afterthought for managed care organizations. *Clin. Chem.* **42:**813–816.

15. **Forsman, R. W.** 2002. The value of the laboratory professional in the continuum of care. *Clin. Leadersh. Manag. Rev.* **16:**370–373.

16. **Gallessich, J.** 1982. *The Profession and Practice of Consultation,* p. 1–85. Jossey-Bass, San Francisco, Calif.

17. **Hackman, J. R., R. Janson, G. R. Oldham, and K. Purdy.** 1975. A new strategy for job enrichment. *Calif. Manag. Rev.* **17**(4):57–71.

18. **Institute of Medicine.** 1999. *To Err Is Human: Building a Safer Health Care System.* National Academy Press, Washington, D.C.

19. Krieg, A. F. 1978. *Laboratory Communication,* p. 25–33. Medical Economics Company Book Division, Orsdell, N.J.

20. Laposata, M. 2002. *Laboratory Medicine.* American Society for Clinical Pathology Press, Chicago, Ill.

21. Lippitt, G., and R. Lippitt. 1978. *The Consulting Process in Action.* University Associates, La Jolla, Calif.

22. Luckey, L., and B. Davis. 1999. Clinical laboratory utilization: implementation, p. 17–36. *In* B. Davis, D. Mass, and M. Bishop (ed.), *Principles of Laboratory Utilization and Consultation.* W. B. Saunders, Philadelphia, Pa.

23. Lundberg, G. D. 1998. Changing physician behavior in ordering diagnostic tests. *JAMA* **280:**2036.

24. Mass, D. 1988. The clinical laboratory scientist's transition to consulting, p. 1–16. *In* J. R. Crowley (ed.), *A Manual for the Clinical Laboratory Scientist Consultant.* American Society for Medical Technology, Washington, D. C.

25. Mass, D. 1993. Medical technologists of the future: new practice, new service, new functions. *Lab. Med.* **24:**402–406.

26. Mass, D. 1997. Consulting in physician office laboratories, p. 443–450. *In* J. R. Snyder and D. S. Wilkinson (ed.), *Management in Laboratory Medicine,* 3rd ed. J. B. Lippincott, Philadelphia, Pa.

27. Mass, D. 1999. Consulting as a professional role for the clinical laboratory scientist, p. 37–45. *In* B. Davis, D. Mass, and M. Bishop (ed.), *Principles of Laboratory Utilization and Consultation.* W. B. Saunders, Philadelphia, Pa.

28. Mass, D. 2002. The manpower shortage: what next? *Lab. Med.* **33**(7):505–510.

29. Mass, D. 2002. Staff retention and empowerment: functions of leadership. *Clin. Leadersh. Manag. Rev.* **16:**391–398.

30. Pontius, A. 2002. Talking with Albert Ziegler of Beckman Coulter. *MLO Med. Lab. Obs.* **34**(1):34–37.

31. Pontius, A. 2002. Talking with Mark Smits of Abbott Diagnostics. *MLO Med. Lab. Obs.* **34**(3):10–11.

32. Pontius, A. 2002. Talking with Richard Aderman of Roche Laboratory Systems. *MLO Med. Lab. Obs.* **34**(4):20–21.

33. Pontius, A. 2002. Talking with Rudy Mareel of BD Biosciences Immunocytometry Systems. *MLO Med. Lab. Obs.* **34**(5):22–23.

34. Pontius, A. 2002. Talking with Lee Shuett of Nikon Instruments Inc. *MLO Med. Lab. Obs.* **34**(7):24, 26.

35. Pontius, A. 2002. Talking with Rob Bush, president of Orchard Software Corporation. *MLO Med. Lab. Obs.* **34**(8):16, 19.

36. Pontius, A. 2002. Rolf Classon, president of Bayer Diagnostics, shares his views. *MLO Med. Lab. Obs.* **34**(9):22–23.

37. Rock, R. C. 1991. Why testing is being moved to the site of patient care. *MLO Med. Lab. Obs.* **23**(9S):2–5.

38. Snyder, J. R. 2001. Managing knowledge workers in clinical systems. *Clin. Leadersh. Manag. Rev.* **15:**120–123.

39. Strandjord, P. 1985. Laboratory medicine—excellence must be maintained, p. 214–225. *In* E. Bermes, Jr. (ed.), *The Clinical Laboratory in the New Era: Quality, Cost, and Diagnostic Demands.* AACC Press, Washington, D.C.

40. Title VI, Section 1886(d). 1983. Prospective Payment of Inpatient Hospital Services. Social Security Amendments of 1983 (P.L. 98-369) (enacted 20 April 1983).

41. Title III, Division B. 1984. Deficit Reduction Act of 1984. The Medicare and Medicaid Budget Reconciliation Amendments of 1984 (P.L. 98-369) (enacted 18 July 1984).

42. Turner, A. 1982. Consulting is more than giving advice. *Harv. Bus. Rev.* **60**(5):120–129.

43. Ward-Cook, K. 2002. Medical laboratory workforce trends and projections: what is past is prologue. *Clin. Leadersh. Manag. Rev.* **16:**364–369.

44. Zhan, C., and M. R. Miller. 2003. Excess length of stay, charges, and mortality attributable to medical injuries during hospitalization. *JAMA* **290:**1868–1874.

48

Computers, Utilization, and Knowledge Support

Michael D. D. McNeely

OBJECTIVES

To introduce the concept of knowledge support

To explain why knowledge support will be necessary to control utilization and standardize care

To present some current examples of knowledge support for laboratory ordering and interpretation

To introduce the information complexity that will come with molecular genetic testing

We are entering an "era of knowledge" where there will be no possible way to employ laboratory testing without the assistance of a computer.

CLINICAL PATHOLOGY PRACTICE has emphasized the accuracy, precision, convenience, turnaround time, and cost of performing tests. Having achieved many of these goals, it is entering a new era where correct test selection and result interpretation will become the dominant challenge.

This "era of knowledge" will emerge because of concerns over test utilization (i.e., cost), the need to standardize medical care in order to optimize outcomes, and the availability of emerging "knowledge-hungry" molecular diagnostic techniques, which will coalesce with developments in electronic data handling and communication. We will see test orders driven by thousands of highly prescribed and often complex clinical strategies. Interpretation will require access to vast data banks of information that will change by the hour. There will be no possible way to employ laboratory testing without the assistance of computers.

The fundamental technology that will be used is known as knowledge support (or clinical decision support). Electronic knowledge support is computer software that is able to present key factual information in such a way that it speeds or enhances the accuracy of a clinical decision. It is more than simply presenting neatly tabulated laboratory test results, even though such a service will certainly aid clinical decision making. What must also be provided is advice regarding what to do and, when appropriate, additional pertinent information about risk, cost, prevalence, treatment, etiology, and where to find published review articles on related subjects.

Knowledge Support: Static and Context-Appropriate Real-Time

Knowledge support takes two forms: static (encyclopedic) and context-appropriate real-time (also known as "just in time").

Encyclopedic knowledge support is what is generally available today. Using powerful Internet search engines (e.g., Google [http://www.google.ca/]), web portals (e.g., Medical Matrix [http://www.medmatrix.org/reg/login.asp]), specified websites (e.g., National Guidelines Clearinghouse [http://www.guideline.gov/index.asp]), test dictionaries (e.g., Lab Tests Online [http://www.labtestsonline.org/]), or literature search services (e.g., PubMed Search [http://www.ncbi.nlm.nih.gov/entrez/query.fcgi]), a practitioner can discover almost all the information he or she needs to address a given problem. But such activity cannot routinely be carried out during a patient encounter.

The other form of knowledge support (context-appropriate real-time knowledge support [CARTKS]) (30) has the ability to provide the information that is needed to solve a problem at the time the problem arises, using a technique that blends conveniently into the normal flow of work. There are only a few examples of CARTKS in routine use because of physician culture, technical constraints, and poor availability of extremely useful and rapidly functioning applications. As the *New England Journal of Medicine* has stated, "To be widely accepted by practicing clinicians, computerized support systems for decision making must be integrated into the clinical work flow. They must present the right information, in the right format, at the right time, without requiring special effort" (21).

Today, the hardware and software platforms that will support CARTKS are beginning to appear. The most powerful tool for the introduction of CARTKS is the emerging generation of portable computing devices such as personal digital assistants (PDAs) (e.g., Palm Pilot [Palm Inc., Milpitas, Calif.] and Blackberry [Research In Motion, Waterloo, Ontario, Canada]). "Today, the personal digital assistant (PDA) is taking the place of the fat little notebook in the coat pocket of many clinicians" (21). Decision support software, much of it free, is evolving rapidly. Drug information is the first significant application (e.g., ePocrates [http://www.epocrates.com]), and this alone is encouraging the use of PDAs on the ward and in the clinic.

Internet technology will provide the conduit for either updating handheld devices or allowing continuous linkage to the World Wide Web or to an institution's intranet. The progress being made in these devices and the networks that link them is so rapid that no physician will be without one of these devices in 3 years. Tablet terminals that look like conventional clipboards will probably be the most popular format for the clinic because they are easy to use and less intrusive on the interaction between patient and physician.

Laboratory results are becoming widely available online, which is another factor that is bringing the computer terminal into the clinical encounter (examining room) (6). In certain jurisdictions, health maintenance organizations and medical centers, all medical personnel have electronic access to laboratory reports. It is not a major step to see how knowledge support will be added to such software platforms.

Practice management systems are used in real time by fewer than 20% of practicing physicians even though computers per se are found in virtually every physician's office. Data entry has been one of the major obstacles to the development of full practice management systems, but this impediment is rapidly dissolving with handwriting recognition, voice recognition, and clearly designed, menu-driven touch screens that will allow physicians to communicate with the computer throughout the patient encounter.

The future of laboratory medicine will evolve because of knowledge support software that will control costs, standardize care, and assist physicians with extraordinarily complex decision making.

Rationale

Utilization Control

Laboratory testing has continued to increase in volume. There are a number of reasons for this trend, including defensive action, rapid office throughput, availability of testing, marketing, patient demand, new tests, introduction of highly valuable tests, deficiencies in physician education, and an aging population.

There is continued evidence that many investigations are not necessary (50), and there are numerous examples of wide variation in laboratory practice without related differences in patient outcomes. For example, the Canadian province of British Columbia has witnessed short-term test reductions of up to 10% on several occasions following fee negotiations between the government and doctors whose reimbursement was linked to lab utilization. No untoward clinical effects were reported as a result (31). In my outpatient laboratory, a great variation in test usage among physicians has been observed. For example, 5% of physicians account for 17% of all outpatient test requests, without a discernible difference in clinical outcome between those who order numerous tests and those physicians whose laboratory use is close to the mean (31). The variability issue has been well studied, and the simple inference is that if patient care and outcomes are independent of extremes in laboratory test ordering, then there is no reason why test ordering cannot be reduced (19, 35).

Excess ordering is the main target, but it is also recognized that an insufficient number of tests are ordered in some circumstances. For example, we examined the monitoring of diabetes in a community of 300,000, and found that among the known diabetics, only 68% receive HbA1c monitoring at the recommended interval of 3 to 4 months and only 25% receive the recommended annual urine microalbumin test. Another study, from Nottingham, England, focused on liver disease and discovered that up to

10% of patients with hepatic disorders did not receive adequate follow-up (41).

Controlling utilization has been the subject of many studies and administrative projects. Initiatives to influence ordering have included feedback, education, financial incentives, administrative change, and protocols (Table 48.1) (18, 49).

Feedback involves informing physicians about the number of tests and/or costs per patient. Such programs have had variable success (50), but the consensus is that they must be specific to the individual physician, who must be compared fairly and nonpunitively with an appropriate peer group. To be effective, feedback must occur in a timely fashion. Electronic test ordering and result presentation afford the possibility of providing this information (feedback) at the moment the test is being ordered. A simple and effective approach has been to display the cost of the tests to the clinician at the time of ordering (45). In some instances, feedback results in an increase in utilization among physicians who have been conservative.

Educational programs involving lectures, manuals, bulletins, and other conventional teaching approaches have had a variable effect on utilization, and they often show a rebound effect by increasing utilization. It is generally accepted that educational programs alone have limited influence, but they play an invaluable and necessary adjunct role for other utilization control measures. Education can be directed toward the scientific basis for rational test use or may cover the budgetary aspects of laboratory testing. If successful, educational efforts will help to create a cultural change wherein concern about appropriate test selection becomes a high priority (14).

Financial incentives given directly to the ordering physician have been shown to have no effect (25). Physician participation in budgeting has been more successful (16). More significant incentives (known as risk sharing) have had some overall influence. As mentioned above, in British Columbia, the amount paid to physicians by the government-run medical system has been "clawed back" by reduced fees if the budget for physician payments is exceeded. The cost of diagnostic testing is included in the same budget as physicians' services, thereby providing a

clear inducement for careful ordering practices (32). However, the reality is that this form of risk sharing has a minimal (1 to 4%) effect on utilization while causing maximal ill will.

Administrative changes usually involve some form of barrier or prescribed ordering process. A simple administrative approach is to ensure that ordering forms do not encourage testing (12). A requisition with a huge list of every possible test encourages ordering and therefore possible overuse. However, a request form that is too spare may be difficult for the laboratory to decipher, and it limits novel approaches to ordering. Lundberg (23) demonstrated that a carefully crafted request form could be used to guide and teach. Experience has shown that form control must allow changes to be made to reflect advances in medical science and that the format should be coordinated with the introduction of ordering protocols and guidelines. A related study by Finn et al. (15) showed that clerical staff, following carefully prescribed rules, could alter laboratory requests in a positive way.

Rationing is another form of administrative control. In one program, physicians were limited to eight tests per day per patient. While laboratory volume fell by 25%, the system was abandoned as being too difficult to administer (9). Draconian methods of this nature are generally not sustainable (17).

One of the most effective approaches is the use of ordering protocols. For example, in British Columbia the Pathology Association introduced this device in 1981 with a thyroid protocol that permitted only a single thyroid function test as a routine starting point in thyroid investigations. Additional thyroid function tests were provided upon request after the initial test was completed. This protocol was successful in reducing overall thyroid testing by 15% and charges by 12% over a 2-year period. Thyroid testing continued to increase subsequently, but the one-time reduction was successfully maintained (18). Additional early protocols for serum electrolytes and the hematology profile (complete blood count) were equally successful and demonstrated the power of protocol-driven utilization reduction, the importance of gaining widespread professional agreement, the need for targeting

Table 48.1 Summary of utilization measures

Strategy	Description	Effect
Feedback	Informs physicians about the number of tests and/or costs per patient	Variable
Education	Lectures, manuals, bulletins, and other conventional teaching approaches	Variable
Financial incentives	Incentives given directly to the ordering physician	No effect
	Physician participation in budgeting	Successful
Administrative change	Requisition form	Successful
	Rationing	Initial but unsustainable success
Protocols	Prescribed, enforced ordering pattern	Limited success
Knowledge support	Computer guidance	20% reduction, but infrastructure required

high-volume areas, and the need for converting physicians to the culture of protocol use.

Carl van Walraven et al. (47) studied the effect of guidelines and requisition form changes on all laboratories in Ontario for a 6-year period from July 1991 to April 1997. Specific guidelines for appropriate use combined with removal of certain tests from the requisition form decreased utilization by 58% for erythrocyte sedimentation rate and 57% for urea. The guideline that recommended screening urinalysis by dipstick only caused urine microscopy to decrease by 14% and dipstick-only urinalysis to increase by 1,700%. Serum iron measurements decreased by 80% and ferritin measurements increased by 34%. Total thyroxine testing declined by 96% when provincial Medicare discontinued reimbursement for the assay. When thyroid-stimulating hormone was removed from the requisition form, an additional 12% decline was seen. The study by van Walraven et al. shows that ordering protocols do actually work to decrease utilization across an entire population area.

Although substantial utilization savings can be realized, it is clear that there is a practical upper limit to the number of protocols that can be introduced. The need to reduce protocols to a few (one to two) simple rules that can be easily implemented while upholding good medical practice severely limits the number of feasible applications.

Greater complexity is possible if the protocols and guidelines are handled by a computer (32). It has even been suggested that this development cease until appropriate methods of implementation become available (8).

CPGs

Laboratory ordering protocols are a specific, and rather rigid, instance of clinical practice guidelines (CPGs) that can be described as evidence-based, consensus-approved pathways for quality medical care in selected situations. CPGs address specific instances, such as the diagnosis of hyperthyroidism, whether to X ray an injured ankle, or when and if to initiate penicillin therapy for a sore throat. The development of CPGs has been stimulated by the observation that there is a great diversity in the way physicians deal with the same common conditions and not every physician can therefore be correct.

Recently, it has been recognized that preventable errors are a more common cause of patient harm than previously thought, and each year in the United States more than 1,000,000 injuries and as many as 98,000 deaths can be attributed to medical errors (7). A 2001 editorial in the *New England Journal of Medicine* makes the statement that ". . . clinical performance in the United States still falls far short of its theoretical potentials" (21). Moreover, clinical performance of otherwise competent physicians will lapse under conditions of time pressure and distractions (11).

Unfortunately, CPGs have not had the overall impact on medical care that specific studies of individual CPGs would have us believe. There are many reasons why physicians do not adhere to guidelines, and these have been reviewed and summarized in 10 points by Cabana et al. (3).

1. Lack of awareness due to the rapid growth in numbers of CPGs. (Note: a computerized system can provide access to appropriate CPGs by using a search engine or an automated linkage based upon clinical symptoms.)
2. Lack of familiarity with guideline details prevents appropriate initiation and leads to noncompliance when the guideline is initiated. (Note: a computerized system would direct the physician and patient through each step of the guideline.)
3. Lack of agreement. (Note: lack of agreement with a guideline can be caused by a failure to keep the guideline up-to-date. This will also affect computerized systems. The other cause of lack of agreement is that several legitimate approaches may coexist. In a traditional CPG only one of these approaches can be selected. In a computerized CPG, all reasonable pathways can be provided. Moreover, with use, the computerized system will assist with the review of the options.)
4. Lack of self-efficacy (or the belief that one can actually perform a behavior). This is due to lack of confidence or preparation. (Note: a computerized system, with options, can provide greater confidence if properly maintained.)
5. Lack of outcome expectancy: in other words, a lack of confidence that following the guideline will result in a positive outcome. (Note: this will be an equal concern with computerized systems.)
6. Inertia of previous practice. (Note: this will be an equal concern with computerized systems.)
7. External barriers (time limitations, lack of reminder system). (Note: CARTKS should be optimized to enhance efficiency and will have built-in reminders.)
8. Guideline-related barriers—how easy and convenient the guideline is to use. (Note: this will be an equal concern with computerized systems.)
9. Patient-related barriers—patients may not adhere or may prefer a different treatment option. (Note: options can be made part of a computerized guideline, and patient instructions should be available.)
10. Environmentally related barriers—acquisition of new resources or facilities, lack of counseling materials, insufficient staff, poor reimbursement, increased costs, liability. (Note: this will be an equal concern with computerized systems.)

Certainly one reason why CPGs have not been widely adopted is that there are so many of them and some even give conflicting advice. Consider that there are now over 2,000 CPGs posted on the National Guideline Clearinghouse website (http://www.guidelines.gov/index.asp). Just as with protocol development, CPGs must employ a simple set of rules that can be easily remembered or depicted on a reference guide. At the same time, the CPGs must ensure sound medical practice for the vast majority of patients and above all must do no harm. The reality of medical practice is that patients often have more than one disorder, must be permitted their own choice, and may not all react in the same way. CPGs generally fail to cover all possibilities.

Knowledge-based computer systems capable of administering or guiding a patient and doctor through multiple variations of a clinical problem will be the answer to making CPGs a standard reality. Indeed, Elson and Connelly have noted that the improvement that results from computerized knowledge support is so well proven that it may be unethical to continue to undertake trials (11).

A further drawback to the use of guidelines for utilization control is that guideline dissemination alone does not sustain clinician behavior change even when clinicians are in agreement. Guideline implementation is more likely to succeed when accompanied by changes in the practice environment that make it easier for physicians to maintain a new desired behavior (43). The work environment must provide opportunities to practice the new behavior and provide continuing reinforcement and feedback. "Physicians' behavior cannot be systematically corrected merely by changing knowledge, attitudes and/or motivation . . . they need new tools that will make it easier for them to do the right thing" (19). An example of this is a recent study investigating the laboratory testing of 969 newly diagnosed cases of essential hypertension (26). It was found that 24% of the patients did not receive the laboratory testing recommended by the guidelines of the Canadian Hypertension Society, while over 50% received tests that were not specifically recommended. The Canadian Hypertension Society guidelines were widely disseminated: mailed to every licensed physician in the country and published in the *Canadian Medical Association Journal*. The authors noted, "It is unlikely that any guideline could be more widely disseminated without extraordinary expense."

The future of CPGs will be realized only when they can be introduced into routine clinical practice with the aid of computers.

Disease Management

Beyond CPGs, what is now emerging is disease management. This may be as simple as a series of CPGs brought together into a set of guidelines for a single disease entity or can be an entire life plan involving the patient with a coordinated team of healthcare professionals. The Disease Management Association of America (http://www.dmaa.org) defines this practice as ". . . a system of coordinated healthcare interventions and communications for populations with conditions in which patient self-care efforts are significant."

Diabetes is the prototype for disease management programs. Diabetes affects 6% of the population and is the seventh leading cause of death in the United States. It can be clearly defined and has readily available, standardized tests that can be used to monitor the progression of the disease and efficacy of treatment. Diabetes leads to a number of devastating (and costly) medical complications, including chronic renal failure, amputations, blindness, coronary artery disease, stroke, and infections. The general compliance with evidence-based care is poor, but complications can be prevented in type II diabetics and delayed in type I diabetics if normal glycemia can be achieved. There are over 200 CPGs related to diabetic care, including diagnosis, monitoring with HbA1c and microalbumin, referral, pregnancy, nephropathy, nutrition, foot care, hypertension, and many others.

Another similar area is chronic renal failure, a disease for which 15 guidelines with full evidence-based documentation were published in 2002 by the National Kidney Foundation (http://www.kidney.org/professionals/doqi/index.cfm) (22). Clearly, the care of diabetics and patients with chronic renal failure is becoming highly structured. As noted by McDonald et al., much medical activity requires compulsive attention to protocol rather than intellectual brilliance (27). This is why knowledge support used to provide the compulsive attention is so essential.

Wellness

Just as there are now CPGs for specific disease entities, there are an emerging number of tests and test "packages" designed to detect disease risk factors so they can be monitored and modified or to identify diseases early enough to take preventative action. Many of these tests can be supported by sound medical evidence; others cannot. However, the reality is that screening and risk identification are here to stay. Adding to this area will be an ever-increasing number of molecular genetic tests that will cover a wide spectrum of disease entities but will become increasingly difficult to interpret. Moreover, patient access to test results and direct patient ordering of tests will open major areas for information provision that will require computer support.

Regrettably, numerous studies have shown a general failure of physicians to offer standard, widely accepted preventative services (20). Electronic reminder systems will be useful in correcting this defect.

Data Mining

Data mining is the practice wherein large organized repositories of information (databases) are examined to extract knowledge. These can be structured searches, such as epidemiological reviews or an investigation into the number of HbA1c tests ordered per patient each year, or they can be exploratory searches wherein trends and associations not previously known are discovered.

Structured data mining is necessary to determine whether protocols and guidelines are being used and whether they are being used properly, to track deviations from the guidelines in order to improve them and to provide education and feedback. Such searches are necessary to determine areas where protocols and guidelines may have an impact. For example, a review of antinuclear antibody tests might demonstrate that only 10% of patients being investigated have positive results. Such a discovery would indicate that insufficient patient selection is being applied to this test's orders and a guideline may be warranted. As more laboratory information systems provide relational database capability and linkage to SQL (system query language) and other extraction tools (e.g., Cognos Query; Cognos Inc., Ottawa, Ontario, Canada [http://www.cognos.com/index.html]), the laboratory will be relied upon to provide unique knowledge.

Example Systems

A number of experimental systems and a smaller number of actual applications of CARTKS have been studied and described.

Software

Experimental systems have employed a number of software approaches. The most direct is to make code changes in the system (laboratory information system [LIS], practice management system, hospital information system). This may be practical for those few settings which maintain their own information technology departments with programming staff and access to their system's code. However, this type of knowledge support is difficult to change, must remain relatively simple, and may be rendered obsolete by major system upgrades.

Web technology (the World Wide Web or institution-based intranet) offers exciting possibilities in providing real-time knowledge using hyperlinks. Even two-way information flow is possible with web technology. This is the most realistic form of knowledge support to offer at the present time.

For sophisticated applications involving multiple possibilities and decision making that may rely on scores, statistics, or weighting, an artificial-intelligence expert system is required. An expert system is a computer program that emulates the decision-making capability of an expert human in a limited area. There are a variety of platforms for expert systems, including deterministic models, production rule-based systems, and neural networks.

The advantages of expert systems in the clinical laboratory have been enumerated (5, 36). Expert systems provide consistent advice 24 h per day and 7 days per week without suffering fatigue. They have the ability to automatically monitor high volumes of data quickly, efficiently, and reliably. Unlike humans, they tolerate repetition and uncertainty, and they can be modified to deal with local clinical and laboratory operational needs.

Automated Result Interpretation

The first application of knowledge support in laboratory testing was automated interpretive reporting. The earliest systems used in routine practice were those of Reece and Hobbie (40), Pribor (38), and McNeely (28, 29).

Reece and Hobbie (40) developed a program 30 years ago at Lufkin Medical Laboratory in Minnesota that provided interpretations of routine complete blood count and chemistry panels. While providing a reasonable reminder list of possible disease entities, the system lacked specificity because the underlying clinical problem was not known. A review of this system (2) confirmed the validity of the approach and demonstrated that it was more useful for outpatient practice than a hospital setting. This points out that the usefulness of such systems is highly dependent on the environment in which they are used and therefore should be locally modifiable.

The very nature of a specialized test usually defines the clinical problem under consideration. For example, the reason for ordering an alpha-fetoprotein test for a 50-year-old man is more apparent than the reason for ordering a serum sodium or alkaline phosphatase test. Both the Pribor and McNeely systems were applied to specialized tests and were well accepted and appreciated by clinicians in over 20 years of use.

Subsequently, many different systems for providing interpretive reports have been developed and proven for general and special hematology, thyroid problems, connective tissue disease, anticoagulation, drug therapy, tumor markers, pheochromocytoma, antibiotic selection, anemia, acid-base, liver disorders, and protein electrophoresis, to name only a few applications. A number of these programs have been prospectively evaluated. For example, the microbiology interpretive program developed at the LDS Hospital combines laboratory findings and epidemiological evidence to suggest the most appropriate antibiotic therapy. There were fewer drug-related adverse reactions, drug costs were more than two-thirds lower, and patient stay was 20% shorter than in the preprogram phase (13).

Today, the ability to provide automated interpretive comments is a commonly provided feature of LISs. Simple automated interpretations have entered the mainstream.

Another approach is background monitoring, wherein a report is issued only when a risk situation is discovered. This is a standard feature of LISs for "critical value" reporting. In a system developed by Bronzino et al. (1), records were examined for all patients receiving selected drugs to ensure that appropriate laboratory monitoring was being undertaken and that drug concentrations were within the accepted therapeutic ranges. Only when a lapse in treatment was noted was a warning issued. Background monitoring of laboratory tests during drug therapy has been successfully employed by the HELP system (LDS Hospital) for many years (39). Another background application for expert systems is autoverification of results so that they can be reported moments after being analyzed without the need for human visual scrutiny. This is very effective, and the College of American Pathologists now recognizes this practice in its inspections. Expert systems are also used in controlling reflexive testing. In this process, the next test in a diagnostic sequence is automatically added only if specified test results are obtained. For example, a free T4 test is performed only when a thyroid-stimulating hormone result is outside the reference range (46).

Expert systems have also been employed at the "back end" of the laboratory testing process to assist laboratory professionals in rendering expert opinions (34).

Ordering

Computer-assisted laboratory test ordering was first suggested in 1984 by Chang et al. (4). The design of an expert system to assist with ordering is more complex than developing one to provide interpretation. Benefiting from knowledge support during ordering requires the physician to work interactively with the expert system during the clinical encounter, and this factor is a major impediment to the introduction of ordering modules. On the other hand, an ordering system allows the collection of key clinical information that allows highly specific interpretations of the test results.

Two systems employing ordering demonstrate the power of knowledge support. These are the BloodLink system of van Wijk et al. (48) and the Laboratory Advisory System (LAS) developed by Smith and McNeely (43).

BloodLink

The most important study to demonstrate the effectiveness of computerized guidelines was undertaken by Marc van Wijk et al. (48). In Holland, the College of General Practice has developed 54 clinical practice guidelines that cover over 90% of office visits to family doctors. In addition, over 90% of Dutch practitioners use a practice management system that has been provided without charge by the Dutch government. Twenty-three of the guidelines employ laboratory testing, and these requirements were incorporated into a program (called BloodLink) that acts as a laboratory test ordering tool. To use it, the physician identifies the patient's clinical problem. If a guideline is available, the system quickly presents the recommended tests. For example, the practitioner is confronted with a patient with liver disease. She activates the "guideline" window and picks "liver disorders" from a list of 18 guideline categories. A second window appears with 8 categories of liver disease. The practitioner then selects "hepatitis B," and a third window appears with four possible hepatitis B scenarios ("control course," "exclusion of carrier," "exclusion of chronic hepatitis," and "recent infection hepatitis B"). The practitioner selects "recent infection," and a set of tests (i.e., alanine aminotransferase, anti-HBc, HBsAg) is displayed; the practitioner also has the opportunity to add additional tests.

Van Wijk installed the system in the offices of 25 practitioners, who then used it for an entire year. As a control he provided another system to a matched set of 25 doctors. The control software (BloodLink-Restricted) offered no knowledge support but merely provided a short list of commonly used tests and the ability to order anything else by typing. At the end of the trial period several conclusions were made:

- Physicians easily adapted to the use of such a system.
- Adherence to the CPGs was greatly improved, and the only significant deviation was in areas where the CPGs had not been kept up-to-date.
- BloodLink-Guidelines handled 12,700 patients, and 70,479 tests were ordered. The control group using BloodLink-Restricted handled an almost identical 12,786 patients with 87,654 tests. In other words, a test reduction of 19.6% was achieved.

LAS

The LAS (Acquired Intelligence Inc., Victoria, Canada [http://www.aiinc.com]) is a deterministic expert system that guides physicians through the ordering of laboratory tests, interprets the results of the tests, and suggests and assists with further action.

Figures 48.1 to 48.3 show actual screens from the system being run on a PDA emulator. In Fig. 48.1 is the menu that provides access to the four modes of operation. In "Requisition" are contained the programs that

Figure 48.1 PDA menu for the LAS system showing the four program options.

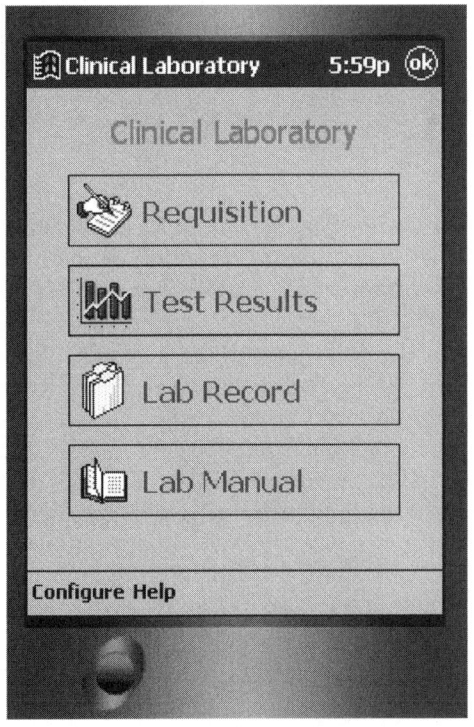

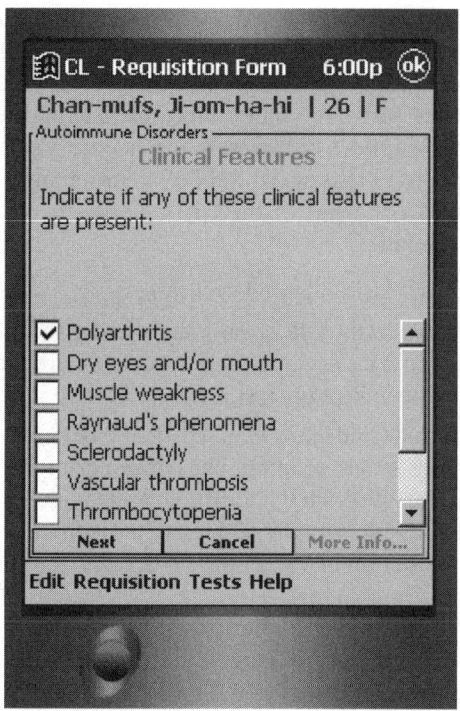

Figure 48.2 An example ordering screen from the LAS system that shows how clinical features are collected prior to ordering tests to investigate a possible autoimmune disorder.

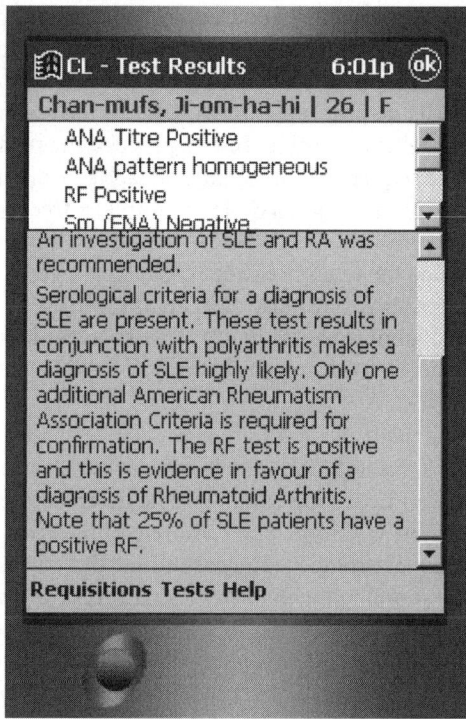

Figure 48.3 An example LAS result presentation. The test results are in the upper window. The interpretation is in the lower window. Both windows can be scrolled.

assist with ordering. "Test Results" presents the completed reports as they are delivered electronically from the laboratory. These reports are automatically interpreted by the system, and the ability to add additional tests is provided at the same time. "Lab Record" is a set of tools that allows a historical review of patient's records. "Lab Manual" is an encyclopedia of laboratory test information.

To use the system, the physician touches the requisition icon. A new screen appears that presents a list of clinical problems. The clinician selects the appropriate one. (There is also the provision to order tests directly in the traditional fashion.) As an example, let us assume that the clinician is considering an autoimmune-based connective tissue disorder. Figure 48.2 shows a presentation of several clinical features whose presence can be indicated by touching the open boxes with a stylus. When the clinical features are entered, the system proposes a testing strategy for approval by the doctor. The laboratory then carries out the tests, and once they are run, the results can be presented as shown in Fig. 48.3. Here the test results are shown in the upper window, while the interpretation is given in the lower window (both windows can be scrolled).

In some situations, the system may suggest an additional test (or tests) that will further clarify the diagnosis. The opportunity is then provided to perform these tests on the sample being held in the laboratory. Using this feature, the

diagnosis can be refined without the expense, inconvenience, and time delay of an additional venipuncture.

At any time during the process of ordering or reviewing the results, the clinician may consult the electronic textbook, which provides in-depth interpretive information. Another feature is the ability to contact a clinical pathologist via e-mail and request a reply by either e-mail or telephone.

A clinical trial of the system was carried out (43) with six clinicians who were given vignette clinical cases and asked to work through them using the conventional (paper-based) system or the LAS (mixed in a randomized fashion). This trial showed that the expert system was more accurate and solved the cases using about half the number of tests, with 16% overall cost savings, improved turnaround time for the complete investigation, and a significantly reduced number of referrals to specialists.

In addition, because the LAS relational database contains clinical features, test results, and responses to various questions and decisions, it allows the laboratory to evaluate the validity and efficiency of the expert system modules. For example, in the autoimmune screening module it would be possible to add the clinical condition "fatigue." It would then be possible to evaluate how often an antinuclear antibody test was positive when the only clinical symptom or sign was fatigue. It would also be possible to use the clinical information that is gathered as a way of scientifically conducting billing compliance.

Other Ordering Systems

Early work by Myers led to the development of the expert system known as INTERNIST-1 (Caduceus), which was intended to encompass all of internal medicine. After applying INTERNIST-1 to case records published in the *New England Journal of Medicine*, Myers concluded that expert systems would be useful in guiding laboratory workups (33).

The literature now has a number of examples of knowledge support systems for test ordering in a variety of settings. There is a very consistent reduction in test ordering of 17 to 30%, with up to a 50% reduction in selected circumstances. For example, a 30% test reduction and enhanced standardization were observed at Vanderbilt University with the development of a system known as Wiz Order as a way of decreasing the variability in medical practice (44).

Thus, the case is clearly proven that expert systems applied to the ordering and interpretation of laboratory testing can improve standardization of practice, reduce costs, enhance diagnosis, and improve efficiency. However, such systems require a sophisticated communication infrastructure, specialized expert system software, a behavioral change by physicians, and some method of keeping the systems current.

Future State

The biggest impact on laboratory testing will be created by developments in molecular diagnostics. Such testing is now available for most known genetic disorders. Soon it will also be possible to reclassify many diseases based upon the multigenetic influences on them. When such testing is carried out routinely, we will need sophisticated expert system software to "decode" the genetic sequences and map them to huge databases. We will also need other knowledge support systems to suggest appropriate testing and translate the findings and integrate them into the patient's specific clinical situation. Knowledge support systems will be necessary because it will be beyond the capability of any physician to encompass the required detail. Even with the relatively well-understood single-gene disorders, not all the culpable genes have been discovered, nor have all the possible mutations been identified. For example, cystic fibrosis is known to involve almost 1,000 mutations. Even if known, the mutations may not have been tested. Routine genetic testing may fail to identify mutations in up to 40% of subjects undergoing testing. Adding further to the complexity is the emerging recognition that single-gene disorders vary in presentation through interaction with other genes (42).

This complexity expands combinatorially with multigene disorders. After the known genetic information has been deciphered, there must be mechanisms in place to revise the interpretation or recall the patient or to retest the sample as additional knowledge is discovered.

Knowledge of the gene complement is only "raw data," and each patient study must be interpreted in the clinical context of the patient. Thus, information for patients will also be required that will provide easily understood explanations of disease risk and/or treatment options. Knowledge support will assist physicians and patients as they make future health plans. This will become a standard activity for a family physician using knowledge support tools. Formal genetic counseling will be reserved for selected situations involving fertility and serious preventative options such as mastectomy.

The main ongoing challenge for knowledge support systems will be their maintenance. As such systems grow and encompass a greater breadth of medical practice, the requirement to keep them current will be daunting. The critical usefulness and currency of a knowledge support system may become the most distinguishing feature of a laboratory's product. Sharing knowledge will become desirable, and standards such as the ARDEN Syntax will facilitate this by allowing clinical information to be structured within electronic medical records (37). It is also likely that peer-reviewed research articles will be published with editorially approved "knowledge statements" suitable for incorporation directly into expert system knowledge bases or knowledge search engines.

Because knowledge support will be such an important component of laboratory services, the knowledge presentation will need to be under quality assurance scrutiny. It will no doubt be a component of accreditation inspections. Such a scheme has been developed for nonautomated interpretations in the United Kingdom (24) and Australia (49).

Ebell and coworkers studied features of software and hardware that are required for the success of computerized clinical decision support (10). Such systems should do the following:

- Be available for handheld as well as networked computers
- Include drug information
- Include overviews of treatment recommendations
- Include patient educational material
- Have a uniform user interface and be updated at least annually

Summary

As laboratory medicine evolves over the next decade, there will be increasing demand for knowledge support to facilitate optimal test selection and result interpretation. This will be driven by the need to minimize costs, standardize medical practice, and cope with the complexity of evolving molecular diagnostic testing.

A number of prototype and functional systems have been developed and evaluated. It is clear that such systems routinely reduce test utilization from 10 to 30%, improve patient care, and enhance conformity to evidence-based clinical practice guidelines. Such systems will be an absolute necessity to handle the knowledge-intensive era of molecular diagnostics. Knowledge support will be provided to patients who will be in a position to order, interpret, and act on the results of laboratory tests.

Communication systems and software and hardware development have evolved to the point where CARTKS is both technically and medically feasible. It will no doubt be a significant aspect of laboratory medicine service delivery in the future.

KEY POINTS

- Laboratory testing volume continues to increase, and attempts to control utilization have had limited success.

- Medical practice is variable, and CPGs that have been designed to standardize care have not been as successful as anticipated.

- Computerized knowledge support has been demonstrated in many studies to consistently reduce utilization by 10 to 30% while improving standardization of practice.

- Rapidly emerging electronic technology will facilitate the introduction of knowledge support systems.

- As molecular diagnostic testing becomes more common and more complex, it will be absolutely necessary to employ knowledge support tools to order and interpret results.

GLOSSARY

Clinical practice guideline (CPG) A set of recommendations for addressing selected clinical problems.

Context-appropriate real-time knowledge support (CARTKS) Knowledge support that is directed specifically to the clinical problem at hand and is presented in such a way that it does not interrupt the normal flow of work.

Data mining A practice in which large organized repositories of information (databases) are examined to extract knowledge.

Disease management A system of coordinated interventions and communications for populations with conditions in which patient self-care efforts are significant.

Expert system A computer program that emulates the decision-making capability of an expert human in a limited area.

Knowledge support (clinical decision support) Computer software that is able to present key factual information in such a way that it speeds or enhances the accuracy of a clinical decision.

Personal digital assistant (PDA) A small computer that fits into a shirt pocket.

Practice management systems Computer systems that handle all the paperwork (both medical charts and organization aspects) in a physician's office.

Protocols A set of prescribed actions that control the way an activity is performed.

REFERENCES

1. **Bronzino, J. D., R. A. Morelli, and J. W. Goethe.** 1989. OVERSEER: a prototype expert system for monitoring drug treatment in the psychiatric clinic. *IEEE Trans. Biomed. Eng.* **36:**533–540.

2. **Button, K. F., and S. R. Gambino.** 1973. Laboratory diagnosis by computer. *Comput. Biol. Med.* **3:**131–136.

3. **Cabana, M. D., C. S. Rand, N. R. Powe, A. W. Wu, M. H. Wilson, P.-A. C. Abboud, and H. R. Rubin.** 1999. Why don't physicians follow clinical practice guidelines: a framework for improvement. *JAMA* **282:**1458–1465.

4. **Chang, E., M. McNeely, and K. Gamble.** 1984. Strategies for choosing the next test in an expert system. *Proc. AAMSI Congr.* **1984:**198–202.

5. **Connelly, D. P., K. E. Willard, and J. H. Hallgren.** 1996. Closing the clinical laboratory testing loop with information technology. *Am. J. Clin. Pathol.* **105**(4 Suppl. 1):S40–S47.

6. **Dark, R. L.** 2001. New products for lab test results reporting via Web. *Dark Rep.* Feb. 26 **8**(3):6–10.

7. **Davenport, T. H., and J. Glaser.** 2002. Just-in-time delivery comes to knowledge management. *Harv. Bus. Rev.* **80:**107–111.

8. **Delamothe, T.** 1993. Wanted: guidelines that doctors will follow. *Br. Med. J.* **307:**218.

9. **Dixon, R. H., and J. Laszlo.** 1974. Utilisation of clinical chemistry services by medical house staff. *Arch. Intern. Med.* **134:**1064–1067.

10. **Ebell, M. H., D. L. Gaspar, and S. Khurana.** 1997. Family physicians' preferences for computerized decision-support hardware and software. *J. Fam. Pract.* **45:**137–141.

11. **Elson, R., and D. T. Connelly.** 1998. Applications of computer-based clinical guidelines. *JAMA* **279:**989–990.

12. **Emerson, J. F., and S. S. Emerson.** 2002. The impact of requisition design on laboratory utilization. *Am. J. Clin. Pathol.* **116:**879–884.

13. **Evans, R. S., D. C. Classen, S. L. Pestotnik, H. P. Lundsgaarde, and J. P. Burke.** 1994. Improving empiric antibiotic selection using computer decision support. *Arch. Intern. Med.* **154:**878–884.

14. **Everett, G. D., S. de Blois, P. F. Chang, and T. Holets.** 1983. Effect of cost education, cost audits and faculty chart review on the use of laboratory services. *Arch. Intern. Med.* **143:**942–944.

15. **Finn, A. F., T. N. Valenstein, and M. D. Burke.** 1988. Alteration of physician's test orders by non-physicians. *JAMA* **259:**2549–2552.

16. **Fowkes, F. G. R.** 1985. Containing the use of diagnostic tests. *BMJ* **290:**488–489.

17. **Fraser, C. G., and F. P. Woodford.** 1987. Strategies to modify the test-requesting patterns of clinicians. *Ann. Clin. Biochem.* **24:**223–231.

18. **Hardwick, D. F., J. L. Morrison, J. Tydeman, P. A. Cassidy, and W. H. Chase.** 1982. Structuring complexity of testing: a process oriented approach to limiting unnecessary laboratory use. *Am. J. Med. Technol.* **48:**605–608.

19. **Hartley, R. M., A. M. Epstein, C. M. Harris, and B. J. McNeil.** 1987. Differences in ambulatory test ordering in England and America: role of doctors' beliefs and attitudes. *Am. J. Med.* **82:**513–517.

20. **Hutchinson, B., C. A. Woodward, G. R. Norman, J. Abelson, and J. A. Brown.** 1998. Provision of preventive care to unannounced standardized patients. *Can. Med. Assoc. J.* **158:**185–193.

21. **James, B. C.** 2001. Making it easy to do right. *N. Engl. J. Med.* **345:**991–993.

22. **K/DOQI Working Group.** 2002. K/DOQI clinical practice guidelines for chronic kidney disease: evaluation, classification, and stratification. Kidney Disease Outcome Quality Initiative. *Am. J. Kidney Dis.* **39**(2 Suppl. 2)**:**S1–S246.

23. **Lundberg, G. D.** 1983. Laboratory request forms (menus) that guide and teach. *JAMA* **249:**3075.

24. **Marshall, W. J., and G. S. Challand.** 2000. Provision of interpretative comments on biochemical report forms. *Ann. Clin. Biochem.* **37:**758–763.

25. **Martin, A. R., W. A. Wolf, L. A. Thibodeau, V. Dzau, and E. Braunwald.** 1980. A trial of two strategies to modify the test-ordering behavior of medical residents. *N. Engl. J. Med.* **303:**1330–1336.

26. **McAlister, F. A., K. T. Koon, R. Z. Lewanczuk, G. Wells, and T. J. Montague.** 1997. Contemporary practice patterns in the management of newly diagnosed hypertension. *Can. Med. Assoc. J.* **157:**23–30.

27. **McDonald, C. J., S. L. Hui, and D. M. Smith.** 1976. Use of a computer to detect and respond to clinical events: its effect on clinician behavior. *Ann. Intern. Med.* **84:**162–167.

28. **McNeely, M. D. D.** 1982. LABDOC: a microcomputer-based system for providing interpretations of clinical laboratory tests, p. 316–320. *In* B. I. Blum (ed.), Proceedings of the Sixth Symposium on Computer Applications in Medical Care. IEEE Computer Society Press, Los Alamitos, Calif.

29. **McNeely, M. D. D.** 1983. Computerized interpretation of laboratory tests: an overview of systems, basic principles and techniques. *Clin. Biochem.* **16:**141–146.

30. **McNeely, M. D. D., D. P. Connelly, and M. A. M. van Wijk.** 2001. Assisting clinicians with ordering and interpretation of laboratory investigations. *Clin. Chem.* **47**(Suppl.)**:**S33–S34.

31. **McNeely, M. D. D.** 2002. The use of ordering protocols and other maneuvers: the Canadian experience. *Clin. Lab. Med.* **22:**505–514.

32. **Mutimer, D., B. McCauley, P. Nightingale, M. Ryan, M. Peters, and J. Neuberger.** 1992. Computerized protocols for laboratory investigations and their effect on use of medical time and resources. *J. Clin. Pathol.* **45:**572–574.

33. **Myers, J. D.** 1986. The computer as a diagnostic consultant with emphasis on use of laboratory data. *Clin. Chem.* **32:**1714–1718.

34. **Nguyen D. T., L. W. Diamond, J. D. Cavenagh, R. Parameswaran, and J. A. Amess.** 1997. Haematological validation of a computer-based bone marrow reporting system. *J. Clin. Pathol.* **50:**375–378.

35. **Peters, M., P. M. G. Broughton, and P. G. Nightingale.** 1991. Use of information technology for auditing effective use of laboratory services. *J. Clin. Pathol.* **41:**539–542.

36. **Peters, M., and P. M. G. Broughton.** 1993. The role of expert systems in improving the test requesting patterns of clinicians. *Ann. Clin. Biochem.* **30:**52–59.

37. **Poikonen, J.** 1997. Arden Syntax: the emerging standard language for representing medical knowledge in computer systems. *Am. J. Health Syst. Pharm.* **54:**281–284.

38. **Pribor, H. C.** 1989. Expert systems in laboratory medicine: a practical consultative application. *J. Med. Syst.* **13:**103–109.

39. **Pryor, T. A.** 1994. The use of medical logic modules at LDS hospital. *Comput. Biol. Med.* **24:**391–395.

40. **Reece, R. L., and R. K. Hobbie.** 1972. Computer evaluation of chemistry values: a reporting and diagnostic aid. *Am. J. Clin. Pathol.* **57:**664–675.

41. **Sherwood, P., I. Lyburn, S. Brown, and S. Ryder.** 2001. How are abnormal results for liver function tests dealt with in primary care? Audit of yield and impact. *BMJ* **322:**276–278.

42. **Sinclair, A.** 2002. Genetics 101: detecting mutations in human genes. *Can. Med. Assoc. J.* **167:**275–279.

43. **Smith, B. J., and M. D. McNeely.** 1999. The influence of an expert system for test ordering and interpretation on laboratory investigations. *Clin. Chem.* **45:**1168–1175.

44. **Stead, W. W., A. J. Olsen, S. A. Benner, M. Blackwelder, L. Cooperstock, J. A. Paton, F. K. Russell, and P. Van Hine.** 1997. The IAIMS—an essential infrastructure for increasing the competitiveness of health care practices. *J. Am. Med. Inf. Assoc.* **4**(2 Suppl.)**:** S73–S76.

45. **Tierney, W. M., M. E. Miller, and C. J. McDonald.** 1990. The effect on test ordering of informing physicians of the charges for outpatient diagnostic tests. *N. Engl. J. Med.* **322:**1499–1504.

46. **Van Lente, F., W. Castellani, D. Chou, R. N. Matzen, and R. S. Galen.** 1986. Application of an EXPERT consultation system to accelerated laboratory testing and interpretation. *Clin. Chem.* **32:** 1719–1725.

47. **van Walraven, C., V. Goel, and B. Chan.** 1998. Effect of population-based interventions on laboratory utilization: a time-series analysis. *JAMA* **280:**2028–2033.

48. **Van Wijk, M. A. M., J. van der Lei, M. Mosseveld, A. M. Bohnen, and J. H. van Bemmel.** 2002. Compliance of general practitioners with a guideline-based decision support system for ordering blood tests. *Clin. Chem.* **48:**55–60.

49. **Vasikaran, S. D., L. Penberthy, J. Gill, S. Scott, and K. A. Sikaris.** 2002. Review of a pilot quality-assessment program for interpretative comments. *Ann. Clin. Biochem.* **39**(Pt. 3)**:**250–260.

50. **Young, D. W.** 1988. Improving laboratory usage: a review. *Postgrad. Med. J.* **64:**283–289.

49

Current Trends in Instrumentation and Technology: Outlook for the Future

Sheshadri Narayanan

OBJECTIVES

To provide the reader an overview of current trends in instrumentation and technology in the clinical laboratory (chemistry, hematology, coagulation, microbiology, and molecular, point-of-care, and noninvasive testing)

To acquaint the reader with current trends in miniaturization and micro- and nanofluidic technology and their impact on microarray and chip technology in a lab-on-a-chip format

To provide a perspective on how these developments and other new ultrasensitive technologies will shape the laboratory of the future

As in life, so in science; our incredibly wild prophecies of today become the routine realities of tomorrow.

ANONYMOUS

THIS CHAPTER EXAMINES current trends in instrumentation and technology in key disciplines in the clinical laboratory. It also provides an outlook for the future based on the driving forces toward technology for miniaturization and microfluidics, with applications ranging from bedside analysis geared toward instituting prompt and optimal therapy to molecular analysis of pathogens and the study of mechanisms of malignancy. Before beginning a discussion of current trends in instrumentation and technology in each key laboratory discipline, it is appropriate to briefly touch upon the physical organization of the clinical laboratory. The Japanese model of clustering automated chemistry and hematology instruments around a belt line is the model that has been generally emulated by some of the highly mechanized large-volume core and reference laboratories without walls. Depending on the turnaround time and the throughput needed, automation extends also to the preanalytical process. However, unlike in Japan, where a shortage of medical technologists made it necessary to innovate in the direction of total automation including the preanalytical process, in the United States, total laboratory automation (TLA) has been limited to a few of the large medical centers and corporate reference laboratories. A recent College of American Pathologists survey listed fewer than 200 sites where TLA including automated centrifugation was in place (4). Daunted by the huge costs of TLA and the long time frame needed to achieve returns on investments, there has been a focus on the front end of automation confined to specimen sorting, decapping, aliquoting, and even centrifugation steps. As needed, instruments can be added to the automated line in a modular approach.

There are, however, some who question the economics of this piecemeal approach and favor TLA. Without going into the merits of the modular approach versus TLA, suffice it to say that while the extent of automation varies depending on the needs and cost constraints of specific laboratory operations, the trend is toward integration of compact instruments with laboratory information system (LIS) functions under one roof. Thus, typically even a rapid-response laboratory would be expected to be configured in one room with blood gas instruments, chemistry, hematology, coagulation, and urinalysis instruments nestled side by side.

The synergy between the LIS and the intelligent computerized instruments contributes to the efficiency of total automation from the time of accessioning and receipt of specimen to analysis and reporting of the results to the physician's workstation. Indeed, the computerized instruments are able to perform many tasks, like the application of quality control rules, delta checking, and reflex testing, on their own without the aid of the LIS. As laboratory automation evolves, the challenging task would be not only to closely integrate the functions of the LIS and the highly intelligent automated instruments that it serves, thereby eliminating redundancy by ensuring minimal overlap of functions, but also to bring under its umbrella a variety of analyzers currently ensconced in separate locations.

The level of sophistication in the clinical laboratory has been made possible with advances in instrumentation and technology, going hand in hand with great expectations for doing "more for less" in a cost-conscious healthcare environment. With this introductory background, let us now turn to the exploration of the current trends in instrumentation and technology in key laboratory disciplines and how these trends can forebode the future.

Chemistry

Core Laboratory

Although we are not there yet, we are rapidly progressing toward a single analyzer incorporating multiple measurement principles ranging from spectrophotometric, potentiometric, fluorometric, nephelometric, turbidimetric, to chemiluminometric, to list a few.

While the bulk of routinely assayed clinical chemistry analytes are still traditionally measured on a single analyzer with spectrophotometric, fluorometric, and potentiometric (ion-selective electrodes) detection capabilities, the technology for immunoassay detection has proliferated. While hitherto-dedicated immunoassay instruments measured a limited profile of analytes, it is now possible by incorporating multiple detection technologies in a single instrument to be able to measure a wide selection of analytes ranging from therapeutic drugs, hormones, to tumor, cardiac, hematological, and infectious disease markers and to detect autoimmune disease (1). Just as homogeneous enzyme and fluorometric immunoassays and fluorescence polarization immunoassays revolutionized the measurement of therapeutic drugs and drugs of abuse over the last two decades, chemiluminescence and other ultrasensitive immunoassays have expanded the scope of detection to a wide range of diagnostically relevant analytes. Indeed, hormones such as thyrotrophin can be measured down to 0.001 μIU/ml with chemiluminescent labels.

Evolution of ultrasensitive immunoassay technologies. As ultrasensitive technologies have been introduced, their limitations have also been uncovered, thus leading to a refinement of the original assays. Using chemiluminescence technology as an example, it is appropriate to review some of the problems associated with chemiluminescent labels. Conventional acridinium esters, which are widely used as chemiluminescent labels, when attached to small molecules in a competitive assay result in the formation of poorly chemiluminescent products with very short half-lives. In addition, at alkaline pH, nonchemiluminescent products called "pseudobases" are formed which can affect the sensitivity of the assay. However, since chemiluminescence can only be initiated at strong alkaline pH (12.0 to 13.0) in the presence of hydrogen peroxide, it is necessary to preincubate the acridinium esters with hydrogen peroxide at a pH range of 5 to 7 to ensure the reconversion of any preformed pseudobase back to the acridinium ester prior to rapidly increasing the pH with strong alkali (sodium hydroxide) to initiate the chemiluminescent reaction (30, 35, 37).

Problems have also been encountered with other chemiluminescent labels. For instance, luminol, as a chemiluminescent label, when attached to antibodies and small molecules can reduce the amount of chemiluminescence and hence decrease the sensitivity of the assay. The reagent blank itself can contribute to nonspecific light emission. The water used in the preparation of buffer should be free from contaminants, as otherwise the background signal generated can be high. Even the type of buffer should be chosen with care to ensure that it does not contribute to a high background signal or noise. Some of the problems associated with luminol have been partially circumvented by labeling the antibody with an enzyme such as horseradish peroxidase. Luminol is then used as a chemiluminescent substrate, which is oxidized by hydrogen peroxide and alkali in the presence of peroxidase label to generate chemiluminescence.

The efficiency of chemiluminescence generated with adamantyl dioxetane phenyl phosphate and alkaline phosphatase to cleave the phosphate group can be enhanced by energy transfer from the resulting chemiluminescent meta-oxy-benzoate anion to fluorescent surfactants, such as micelles formed from cetyltrimethylammonium bromide and 5-(*N*-tetradecanoyl) amino fluorescein (35). The implication for an assay that does not use such surfactants for enhancing chemiluminescence is the possibility of contamination with extraneous surfactants to overestimate a constituent that is measured due to the apparently increased intensity of chemiluminescence that is generated. The type of solid matrix that is used in immunoassays, such as antibody-coated magnetic beads versus antibody-coated wells, is also a consideration in the assessment of interference in ultrasensitive immunoassays. In general, the larger the sample volume, the greater the likelihood of interference. The efficiency of the washing step in the assay is critical to the elimination of specimen matrix effects (39).

Another limitation with conventional chemiluminescent labels is their insolubility in aqueous buffers, which makes the labeling of antibodies or proteins complicated. These labels have a limited shelf life due to their instability and contribute to inconsistent background signal and noise.

Recognizing the above problems, attempts have been made to increase the stability and water solubility of acridinium derivatives. The choice of acridinium (*N*-sulfonyl) carboxamides, which provides increased quantum yield of chemiluminescence, has increased the sensitivity of the assay. The sulfopropyl substituent has the advantage of reducing background interference while also increasing water solubility and shelf life (45).

Besides chemiluminescence, the resolving power of time-resolved fluorescence coupled with the relative absence of competing fluorescent interfering substances has provided the impetus for the development of time-resolved fluorescence immunoassay instrumentation. The basis for this specificity lies in the wide separation, nearly 250 nm, between the excitation and fluorescence emission wavelengths of the rare-earth lanthanide chelates such as europium and terbium, compared to a mere 25-nm separation of the two wavelengths for fluorescein. Furthermore, these rare-earth labels have long fluorescence lifetimes on the order of 10 to 1,000 μs, as opposed to nanoseconds for conventional fluorescence labels. Additionally, the fact that the fluorescence emission wavelengths of europium (excitation, 308 nm; emission, 614 nm) and terbium (excitation, 307 nm; emission, 544 nm) are different makes them attractive for use as dual-label probes for the simultaneous immunoassay measurement of two constituents in the same sample. However, of the two labels, europium has a clear advantage over terbium in terms of long fluorescence decay times (1,020 μs for europium versus 148 μs for terbium), low background signal (420 counts/s for europium versus 4,490 counts/s for terbium), and detection limit (1 pmol/liter for europium versus 40 pmol/liter for terbium). Table 49.1 presents a listing of representative ultrasensitive immunoassay techniques.

Automation of time-consuming heterogeneous immunoassays with multiple steps, such as enzyme-linked

Table 49.1 Ultrasensitive immunoassay techniques

Chemiluminescence: labels used
   Acridinium esters
   Acridinium (*N*-sulfonyl) carboxamides
   Luminol
   Adamantyl dioxetane phenyl phosphate
   Ruthenium (II)-tris(bipyridyl) complex (electrochemiluminescence)
Time-resolved fluorescence: labels used
   Lanthanide chelates: europium and terbium

immunosorbent assay, and refinement of immunoassay formats have improved the quality of immunoassays. However, potential problems from either hemolyzed samples or fibrin can still be encountered. For instance, some assays capture the antibody-analyte-label antibody complex on a fiber matrix. Theoretically this step should permit washing away of the unbound label, so that in the next step when the substrate is added, the signal produced due to the formation of product can be directly related to the concentration of analyte in the sample. However, erythrocyte membrane fragments produced during hemolysis could cause nonspecific absorption of labeled antibody to the fiber matrix, thus artifactually overestimating the concentration of analyte, as was reported with troponin I (TnI) (38a). In such cases, filtration of hemolysed samples could eliminate the interference. A similar artifactual increase in TnI has been reported to be due to residual fibrin strands becoming trapped on a fiber matrix containing the immobilized monoclonal antibody (50).

A major problem with immunoassays using mouse (murine) monoclonal antibodies is the interference due to the presence of human anti-mouse antibodies (HAMA) in patients' sera. Patients who either are receiving radio-immunotherapy with mouse monoclonal antibodies, are exposed to imaging techniques, or handle experimental animals such as mice are apt to develop HAMA. While many strategies are available to overcome interference due to HAMA, one attractive strategy that may gain wider acceptance is the substitution of a chimeric antibody for the commonly used murine monoclonal antibody as the assay reagent. This strategy is based on the premise that most of the circulating HAMA is directed to the Fc portion of mouse immunoglobulin G (IgG). Thus, the use of chimeric antibody where the Fc portion is of human origin can overcome the interfering effect of HAMA, which is a serious problem associated with the widely used murine monoclonal-based two-site immunoassays in the clinical laboratory (27, 37).

Refining manual assays: protein electrophoresis and urinalysis.

Protein electrophoresis. Protein electrophoresis is one area in the core laboratory that could benefit from the elimination of staining steps. This can be achieved by the technique of capillary electrophoresis on fused silica columns. In this technique the separated protein fractions are monitored by the measurement of absorbance in the UV region at 254 nm as they are eluted from the column. This technique can also be used to monitor monoclonal gammopathies by using a technique called antibody subtraction, which eliminates the UV absorbance of the specific antiserum-adsorbed monoclonal species (either IgG, IgA, or IgM, kappa or lambda).

Urinalysis. It is an irony that the screening, diagnostic, and monitoring potential of urinalysis has not received the same degree of attention as serum, plasma, or whole-blood analysis. To paraphrase the famous comedian Rodney Dangerfield, it is as if urinalysis "don't get no respect," a situation that, however, is slowly changing. Indeed, we have progressed from the automation of urine dipstick analysis by reflectance measurements to total automation of urinalysis, including video camera detection of formed elements and elegant detection of specific gravity by harmonic oscillation. Flow cytometric principles have been adapted to automated urine cell analysis of formed elements. Thus, particles are double stained for DNA and membranes and identified by the measurement of fluorescent light intensity, forward light scatter, and the widths of these signals. Quantitative enumeration of formed elements as red blood cells (RBC), white blood cells (WBC), large epithelial cells, bacteria, and casts is possible by this elegant approach (26).

Rapid-Response Laboratory

Even the instruments in a rapid-response laboratory dedicated to critical care testing, such as blood gas analyzers, are undergoing considerable refinement in terms of ease of use, quality control functions, and options to display and print out nomograms of acid-base status. Besides being able to perform pulse oximetry measurements, these analyzers also have the ability to measure electrolytes, lactate, glucose, and bilirubin all from the same whole-blood sample.

Sophistication in technology for blood gas analysis ranges from the use of disposable-cartridge-based systems complete with sensors (potentiometric, amperometric), calibrants, and sealed waste containers to the use of fluorescent indicators to measure pH, pCO_2, and pO_2. Some blood gas analyzers provide conductivity-based hematocrit measurements.

Dedicated bench top instruments with a comprehensive test menu that ranges from stat analytes, therapeutic drugs, nutritional and anemia markers, glycated hemoglobin (HbA_{1c}), and specific proteins, to hormones bring the capability to perform most of the tests needed in a rapid-response laboratory. Some of these instruments have positive sample identification capability and the ability to transmit results to the LIS (2). The varied menu offered by some of the bench top analyzers is made possible by the use of photometric, potentiometric, and turbidimetric techniques and measurement techniques based on a variety of immunoassay principles.

Many rapid-response laboratories also have introduced cartridge-based immunoassays to perform whole-blood analysis of cardiac markers (TnI, creatine kinase [CK]-MB isozyme, and myoglobin) and analysis of drugs of abuse in urine.

A recent innovation is the use of automated biochip array immunoassay technology with chemiluminescence detection for the measurement of a panel of specific markers, such as fertility and other hormones, tumor markers, cardiovascular disease markers, cytokines, and drugs of abuse. Signal from each region of the biochip containing immobilized reagent (antibody) and applied sample is captured by a charge-coupled device (CCD) camera, and the image processing software relates the signal to the concentration of the analyte in the sample applied to each discrete region of the biochip. Such a technology with its miniaturization offers potential for rapid testing at the bedside with no more than a drop of blood or body fluid (33).

Noninvasive Testing

Noninvasive testing can be accomplished either with an ex vivo monitoring device or through implantable in vivo monitoring sensors. Ex vivo monitoring sensors are ideal for use in the critical care monitoring of blood gases at the bedside. Fiber optic technology (fiber optic chemical sensors or optodes) with either absorption (color indicators) or fluorescence intensity (fluorescent indicator) sensors lends itself readily for use in a tubing set that can be connected to the patient's arterial line. In this arrangement, blood can be withdrawn from the patient over the sensors to obtain pH, pCO_2, and pO_2 measurements, following which blood is returned to the patient. Use of such devices permits a nearly continuous monitoring of blood gases in a patient at, in some cases, 2-min intervals, while also conserving blood, which is returned to the patient (31). The sensors, however, have a limited lifetime and need to be replaced after a set number of determinations or hours of use.

Ex vivo sensors can also be used in the extracorporeal circuit, thus permitting continuous monitoring of blood gases and, with appropriate sensors, also electrolytes, including ionic calcium and magnesium, glucose, lactate, and hematocrit, during a cardiopulmonary bypass procedure.

Instead of blood, ex vivo monitoring sensors can be used to measure a sample of dialysate when the sensors are connected to the extracorporeal loop of hemodialysis machines.

In recent years, considerable efforts have been made to achieve a noninvasive measurement of glucose by monitoring its near-infrared spectrum. However, such a device for routine use remains yet to be perfected.

In contrast to ex vivo monitoring, in vivo monitoring through implantation of a device, such as a glucose-oxidase sensor in the abdominal area for continuous subcutaneous monitoring of glucose, has been problematic. Problems such as sensor stability, drift, and particularly the lack of correlation between extracellular and blood glucose levels are some of the issues with in vivo subcutaneous glucose monitoring (52).

In spite of the potential hurdles associated with in vivo monitoring, instruments for in vivo intravascular monitoring of blood gases requiring insertion through a catheter of a probe containing sensors (pH, pCO_2, and pO_2) in the radial artery have been made commercially available (56).

Given the potential benefits of noninvasive testing at the patient's bedside, progress in this area continues, and with refinements in technology, noninvasive testing is expected to gain greater acceptance in the future.

Hematology

Automation in the Routine Laboratory

According to the so-called "Coulter principle" enunciated by Wally and Joseph Coulter in the early 1950s, cells suspended in an electrolyte when passed through an aperture offer resistance to current flow. Also, the amount of resistance can be related to the number of cells, while the amplitude of signal can be related to the cell volume; these facts paved the way for automated cell counting by the impedance method.

In the decades that have followed, technology has progressed in steps from cell counting and enumeration of red cell indices to first a three-part WBC differential count and later a five-part WBC differential count. Today, the hematology analyzer has incorporated flow cytometric principles, and the scope of its measurement is expanding year by year.

One of the features of flow cytometry instrumentation adopted by these analyzers is the ability to analyze cells in a single file by the hydrodynamic focusing principle. Essentially this involves injecting cells into the center of the flow stream using a sheath fluid, so that the cells pass into the instrument one behind the other in a single file. This feature also prevents two cells from passing together through an aperture and being counted as one, which would introduce "coincidence error" and, in turn, result in an underestimation of the cell count.

The major automated instruments in today's hematology laboratory have some subtle differences in the way they generate a five-part WBC differential count, which is worth noting. These differences become apparent in the process of surveying the design of some of the currently widely used hematology instruments (58).

One of these analyzers relies on volume (impedance), conductivity, and laser light scatter measurements. The familiar impedance measurement estimates cell volume. Conductivity measurements involve probing the internal structure of the cell with high-frequency current so that WBC can be classified based on their cytoplasmic and nuclear content. Laser light scatter at 10 to 70° angles per-

mits the differentiation of the granulocyte populations, since the extent of light scatter is related to granularity. This enables the differentiation of coarsely granular cells, which scatter more light, from finely granular cells.

Another analyzer uses a combination of direct current and radio frequency measurements to arrive at a WBC differential count. Direct current (impedance) measurements provide an estimate of cell size. Radio frequency measurements reflect nuclear size and density. Actually, this analyzer produces initially a three-part differential count (lymphocytes, monocytes, and granulocytes). Eosinophils and basophils in the granulocyte population are subsequently resolved from the neutrophils by differential temperature treatment using two different buffers. A further refinement of this technology made possible by exploiting the use of radio frequency and direct current to detect chemical and electrical differences between immature and normal WBC allows estimation of WBC immaturity.

Multiangle polarized scatter separation is another approach to automated WBC differential analysis. An analyzer based on this principle uses a combination of small-angle forward light scatter and 90° (orthogonal) light scatter to differentiate the granulocyte populations. Neutrophils are differentiated from eosinophils since the latter depolarize the 90° light scatter, while 10° light scatter allows discrimination of basophils. An instrument principle different from the ones discussed so far is the basis of an analyzer that utilizes cytochemical staining in combination with forward-angle light scatter measurements. In contrast to the impedance method, the RBC and platelets are isovolumetrically sphered and fixed. The size or volume of the RBC is determined at low-angle light scatter (2 to 3°), while the hemoglobin concentration within each RBC is determined by the absorbance at high-angle light scatter (5 to 15°). Various red cell indices are subsequently calculated. Platelets and their volume (mean platelet volume) are computed from a plot of low-angle versus high-angle light scatter. After lysis of the RBC, a separate hemoglobin measurement is made by spectrophotometry as the released heme is reacted with cyanide to produce cyanomethoglobin. Thus, the instrument provides both a total hemoglobin value and an estimate of the amount of hemoglobin within each RBC.

WBC are fixed with formalin after the lysis of RBC and stained for peroxidase. The intensity of staining will vary since neutrophils, eosinophils, and monocytes contain various amounts of peroxidase. These cells are then classified based on their degree of light scatter and absorption (staining intensity). Lymphocytes and large cells without peroxidase are not stained. In a separate channel called the basophil/lobularity channel, basophils are counted after the cell membrane and cytoplasm of neutrophils, eosinophils, lymphocytes, and monocytes are stripped off at low pH, leaving only the bare nuclei of these cells. The degree of nuclear segmentation is computed by a combination of low-angle light scatter, which estimates size, and high-angle light scatter, which estimates nuclear segmentation or lobularity. The ratio of segmented or polymorphonuclear nuclei to mononuclear nuclei estimates the degree of nuclear segmentation, which can be of diagnostic value, such as a shift to the left. Data presentation both numerical and in the form of histograms and scatter plots is a common feature of the various hematology analyzers.

Furthermore, today, virtually all of the major hematology analyzers are able to stain residual RNA within the reticulocytes with fluorescent dyes and not only provide a reticulocyte count but also classify the reticulocyte population based on differences in maturity, thereby providing an assessment of the immature reticulocyte fraction.

Hematology analyzers exploiting the unique design features of each of their instrumentations are constantly adding more tests. Thus, the ability of a fluorescent dye to bind DNA within the nucleated RBC (NRBC) has been exploited to enumerate NRBC (17).

The ability of live cells with intact membranes to exclude a fluorescent dye such as propidium iodide is the basis of enumeration of nonviable (or dead) WBC, which are stained by the dye, thus providing a measurement of percent nonviable WBC.

Enumeration of reticulated platelets has also been introduced. Simultaneous measurement of the volume and the refractive index of platelets using two angles of laser light scatter has significantly improved platelet counting. By this two-dimensional analysis, platelet counts of less than 50×10^9/liter can be measured, allowing discrimination between platelets and interfering nonplatelet particles (11). Automated peripheral blood smear preparation is also a current option available on several hematology analyzers.

Advances in image analysis have permitted capturing the microscopic images of stained WBC on a screen prior to review and acceptance by medical technologists. If intelligent microscopy of stained WBC can be performed rapidly, it could conceivably replace the way a five-part WBC differential count is currently performed on automated analyzers.

Given the flow cytometry capabilities of hematology analyzers, the measurement of cell surface markers using monoclonal antibodies is a logical extension. Indeed, a study of platelet activation markers such as p-selectin (CD62-p), which is not found on the surface of the resting platelet, and the measurement of the decrease in the platelet surface expression of glycoprotein Ib-V-IX complex (CD42) upon platelet activation could conceivably be added to the capabilities of current hematology analyzers (40).

We should expect the hematology instrument of the future to possess software that would be able to correlate traditional hematology results to a flow cytometry panel of leukemia/lymphoma markers that was also analyzed on the same instrument. Indeed, the hematology instrument of the future would also serve the special hematology laboratory by being able to assess neutrophil and monocyte function, thus providing the clinician valuable information for the assessment of neutrophil and monocyte defects. Table 49.2 summarizes some of the features of automated hematology analyzers.

Coagulation

Routine

The mainstay of many routine coagulation laboratories is still the global tests, such as the prothrombin time (PT) and activated partial thromboplastin time (aPTT). With the instrumentation being able to perform these tests rapidly, in addition to tests such as fibrinogen and thrombin time, the menu of automated tests is constantly increasing. Currently we have instruments that have the capability to perform chromogenic substrate tests for antithrombin III, factor Xa inhibition (to monitor heparin), protein C, and factor VIII activity, to list a few. Adding to this list, the capability to measure other key parameters, such as D-dimer by enzyme-linked immunosorbent assay, factor V Leiden (activated protein C resistance), antiphospholipid antibodies, protein S, and among fibrinolytic assays tPA and PAI-1, enables the coagulation analyzer to provide a full coagulation and fibrinolytic profile on a patient. Indeed, we may expect a multipurpose coagulation analyzer to offer a broad menu of tests and add to the existing menu of coagulation and fibrinolytic profiles the ability to monitor newer anticoagulants, such as direct thrombin inhibitors like hirudin and argatroban and markers such as tissue factor pathway inhibitor.

POC

Considerable progress has been made in recent years in conducting at the bedside tests to measure such parameters as activated clotting time (ACT), PT, and aPTT.

Table 49.2 Principles and features of automated hematology analyzers

Volume (impedance), conductivity, and laser light scatter
Direct current (impedance), radio frequency (nuclear size, cell density): allows detection of chemical and electrical differences between immature and normal WBC. Permits estimation of WBC immaturity. Can be used to enumerate NRBC by dye binding of DNA.
Multiangle polarized light scatter: measures % nonviable WBC by ability of live cells to exclude a fluorescent dye. Can be used to enumerate NRBC by fluorescent dye binding of DNA.
Isovolumetric sphering, low- and high-angle light scatter, and cytochemical staining: two-dimensional platelet counting by simultaneous measurement of volume and refractive index of platelets at two angles of laser light scatter. Can be used to enumerate reticulated platelets.
Virtually all of the hematology analyzers can count and classify reticulocytes according to maturity.
Automated slide (peripheral blood smear) is also an optional feature.

Instruments first developed for point-of-care (POC) testing utilized tubes containing reagents specific for a test together with a magnet into which blood is drawn. Subsequent to blood collection, these tubes were inserted in a magnetic sensing, temperature-controlled (37°C) testing well which sensed clot formation, and hence the clotting time, as the motion of the rotating magnet in the tube slowed down upon clot formation and moved out of alignment with the magnetic sensing device. A refinement of this system uses only 50 μl of whole blood, in contrast to 2 ml with the earlier system. It also utilizes cuvettes containing reagents specific for a test and uses optical sensors to monitor clot formation to signal the clotting time (6).

In addition to the type of instrument described above, instruments using test cards and test strips for specific tests are also currently available. These devices generally contain iron oxide particles and reagents specific for a test. When blood (citrated or noncitrated) is added to the cards or strips and inserted into the instrument, coagulation is initiated upon contact of blood with the reagent. As the clot forms, the motion of the iron oxide particles slows, which is monitored optically as a decrease in reflectance (44). The measurement of ACT permits monitoring of heparin therapy during cardiopulmonary bypass and hemodialysis. Low-range heparin concentrations (0.05 to 0.70 kIU/liter) typically found in extracorporeal membrane oxygenation, a modified form of heart-lung bypass used for treating critically ill infants, can also be measured by variations of ACT, such as in the low-range heparin management test. However, a poor correlation between absolute clotting times and heparin concentrations has been reported in addition to patient-to-patient variability (5). Some patients, however, showed a good correlation between absolute clotting time and heparin concentration across instruments. These POC instruments, however, do have utility for monitoring changes in clotting time with changes in heparin dosage.

While aPTT is not quite optimal as a test for monitoring heparin therapy even on laboratory-based instruments, which incidentally evidenced just an 82% agreement between lab-based aPTT and heparin concentrations, the agreement between POC instruments and heparin concentrations was reduced further, to between 64 and 65% (53). POC instruments for monitoring PT differ in the type of thromboplastin used and algorithms employed to display the results. Thus, one instrument displays results that would have been obtained with a traditional, less sensitive high-international-sensitivity-index thromboplastin. Another instrument displays a PT result that would have been obtained on a laboratory instrument, even though the actual clotting time obtained on the POC instrument was longer.

While failing to meet the current World Health Organization-recommended limit of 3% for coefficient of variation for slope set for conventional PT testing, PT-testing POC instruments are able to meet a coefficient of variation of <5% (44).

A current listing of coagulation analyzers intended for POC and self-monitoring has been published (3). Table 49.3 summarizes the features of representative coagulation analyzers intended for POC testing.

Among other tests that have been developed for POC testing, a rapid bedside measurement of D-dimer deserves mention.

An elegant approach to the assessment of platelet function has been addressed in an instrument that uses disposable cartridges containing either collagen and epinephrine or collagen and ADP. The former is sensitive to qualitative platelet defects, including aspirin (acetylsalicylic acid)-induced abnormalities, while the latter is insensitive to aspirin and detects only thrombocytopathies and von Willebrand's disease.

The procedure involves aspirating citrated whole blood into an aperture in the membrane of the cartridge, which is coated with specific reagents. The time in seconds that is required for blood to occlude the aperture (no more than 300 s) is the test endpoint and is reported as closure time (32). If this screening test for platelet function is abnormal, the patient can be monitored further with tests such as platelet aggregometry in order to establish a diagnosis.

Molecular Testing

Molecular methods lend themselves to the detection of specific mutations. Thus, a mutation in the factor V gene (factor V Leiden: G 1691 A) which results in the substitution of arginine (R) for glutamine (Q) at position 506 (R506Q), as a result of the replacement of guanine for adenine in the mutated factor V gene, can be detected by both PCR- and non-PCR-based methods.

Methods involving multiple steps have all been simplified, including PCR amplification, restriction enzyme digestion that cleaves only the nonmutated (wild-type) sequence, and electrophoresis to visualize the electrophoretic bands revealing the presence or absence of mutations that require a minimum of 4 to 6 h.

Thus, real-time fluorescence genotyping of the G 1691 A mutation can be accomplished by rapid-cycle PCR amplification in closed tubes in approximately 30 min by analysis of melting curves to distinguish between mutant (homozygous, heterozygous) and wild-type sequences. Steps such as restriction enzyme digestion and electrophoresis are eliminated (28).

Table 49.3 Features of POC coagulation analyzers

Magnetic sensing of clot formation
Optical sensors to detect clot formation
Test cards and test strips containing iron oxide particles: clot sensing by the decrease in reflectance with the slowing of motion of iron oxide particles

A non-PCR method for the detection of factor V Leiden is performed isothermally in a microtiter plate and relies on cleavage by a thermostable endonuclease (cleavase), which cleaves only the mutant oligonucleotide probe and not the wild-type probe. In a subsequent reaction, the cleaved probe cleaves in turn a fluorescently labeled secondary signal probe, which fluoresces only upon cleavage, since in the intact form the fluorescence is quenched by a dye that is in close proximity. The high temperature used in the reaction promotes primary probe turnover, and by maintaining an excess of signal probes, multiple probes are cleaved for each target sequence that is present, thus producing a linear increase of signal over time. The ratio of wild-type to mutant fluorescence is used to establish the genotype (23).

Patients with mutations in the prothrombin gene (G 20210 A) together with factor V Leiden and possibly the mutation in the methylene tetrahydrofolate reductase (MTHFR) gene C 677 T mutation, which leads to an increase in homocysteine, a risk factor for coronary artery disease) are at much greater risk for thrombosis than those having an isolated factor V Leiden mutation. Both multiplex PCR and non-PCR methods described above for the study of factor V Leiden mutation are suited to the study of mutations in both the prothrombin and MTHFR genes.

Depending on the need, molecular testing in the coagulation laboratory can also extend to the study of other mutations, such as, for instance, protein C and protein S, which are also risk factors for thrombophilia (40).

Microbiology

Automation

There has been an evolution in the development of automated blood culture systems. Radiometric systems designed to detect $^{14}CO_2$ released from ^{14}C-labeled substrates into the headspace of the sealed blood culture bottle as a result of microbial metabolism have given way to less hazardous nonradiometric detection instruments where the infrared spectra of CO_2 released from nonradiolabeled substrates are measured (7, 16, 43, 47). Aspiration of headspace CO_2 for measurement is obviated in an instrument that uses a colorimetric indicator embedded at the bottom of the culture bottle (7). The indicator is sequestered from the growth medium by a gas-permeable membrane. This arrangement permits the instrument to continuously monitor cultures by taking reflectance measurements as color changes occur due to bacterial growth.

Blood culture systems that use fluorescence sensors for CO_2 detection and instruments that detect the consumption and/or production of gases by microbes growing in the culture broth are other approaches for detection of microbial growth. A variety of automated instruments are available for identification and antibiotic susceptibility testing. One instrument relies on plastic cards each of which has 30 wells containing either substrates for microbial identification or antimicrobials for susceptibility testing. Depending on the type of organism to be detected, a variety of cards are available. The turbidity that results as microorganisms grow is monitored by the resulting decrease in light transmittance. Cards used for anaerobic identification and for *Neisseria* and *Haemophilus* identification, which contain chromogenic substrates, are monitored by increases in color (absorbance) as bacteria cleave the substrates.

For antibiotic susceptibility testing, cards containing a variety of antibiotics to test against either gram-positive or gram-negative organisms are included. The turbidity from bacterial growth is related to the decrease in light transmittance. The growth in each well is compared to the growth in the positive control well. Slopes are computed for each well ranging from zero for no growth, indicating that the organism is susceptible, to 1, indicating growth equivalent to that obtained in the positive control well. Regression analysis is used to compute the MIC of a particular antibiotic for the test organism. A newer version of the above instrument uses fluorescence-based technology with cards being monitored by kinetic fluorescence measurements every 15 min (29). Identification data are available in 3 h, while susceptibility testing takes 8 h to complete. Instrument software allows data analysis and automated reporting of results. Contamination is avoided in this closed system.

Fully automated instruments for identification and susceptibility testing that use 96-well microtiter plates containing a wide range of fluorescence-quenched biochemical substrates and antibiotics are available. Fluorescence generated as microbial enzymes resulting from growth cleave the fluorogenic substrate is monitored, thus identifying the organism. Antibiotic susceptibility is determined by comparison of fluorescence in the well containing the mixture of antibiotic, inoculum, and fluorogenic substrate with that in the well containing only the bacterial suspension and fluorogenic substrate. With this instrument, identification results can be obtained in 2 h, while the susceptibility testing results are completed in 3.5 to 15 h (49). Table 49.4 summarizes the features of automated microbiology instruments.

Other automated instruments, each with its own unique features, have been introduced in the clinical laboratory. A novel approach used by one instrument is the interpretation of reaction in each well with the aid of a video camera.

With automation tremendously improving the efficiency of the microbiology laboratory, and thus advancing the quality of patient care, the trend toward more novel approaches to optimized automated detection, identification, and susceptibility testing is bound to continue in the future.

Molecular Testing

The potential of molecular methods for the rapid diagnosis of bacterial and viral infections has been successfully exploited in the microbiology laboratory. Indeed, instruments

Table 49.4 Features of automated microbiology instruments

Automated blood culture systems: types of CO_2 detection
- Radiometric
- Infrared
- Colorimetric (reflectance)
- Fluorescence

Identification and antibiotic susceptibility testing

Plastic cards with wells containing substrates for microbial identification or antimicrobials for susceptibility testing: turbidity due to microbial growth monitored by decrease in light transmittance. Antibiotic susceptibility monitored by decrease in turbidity (increase in light transmittance). Chromogenic substrates used for anaerobic identification.

Fluorescence-based technology: kinetic fluorescence measurements every 15 min

Ninety-six-well microtiter plates containing fluorescence-quenched biochemical substrates and antibiotics: fluorescence measurements to monitor growth. Antibiotic susceptibility computed by comparison of fluorescence in well containing antibiotic, fluorogenic substrate, and bacteria to fluorescence in well containing only bacteria and fluorogenic substrate.

dedicated to specific nucleic acid amplification technologies, such as PCR, ligase chain reaction, nucleic acid sequence-based amplification, and branched-chain DNA assay, have been used to measure both human immunodeficiency virus and hepatitis C virus viral load (35, 36). Other amplification assays that have found application in infectious disease detection include transcription-mediated amplification and strand displacement assay (60).

Nucleic acid amplification methods have been used to detect *Mycobacterium tuberculosis* in respiratory specimens and *Chlamydia trachomatis* and *Neisseria gonorrhoeae* in urethral swabs. Table 49.5 provides a listing of some of the currently used molecular methods for bacterial and viral detection.

The amplification of the 16S rRNA gene, which is found in multiple copies in the genomes of human bacterial pathogens, has been used for the detection of various organisms, such as *M. tuberculosis*, *Neisseria meningitidis*, *Escherichia coli*, *Haemophilus influenzae*, *Streptococcus pneumoniae*, and *Listeria monocytogenes*. Since the 16S rRNA gene is present in multiple copies, with many bacterial species possessing up to seven copies of the gene, the

Table 49.5 Molecular methods for bacterial and viral detection

PCR
Ligase chain reaction
Nucleic acid sequence-based amplification
Branched-chain DNA assay
Transcription-mediated amplification
Strand displacement assay
Pulsed-field gel electrophoresis for DNA typing of microorganisms

detection of a very small number of causative microorganisms is facilitated compared to an assay for the detection of a single-copy gene. Another advantage is that there is sufficient variation within the 16S rRNA gene to allow for species-specific distinction among various organisms (46). However, contamination with DNA from bacterial sources, such as the polymerase enzyme (*Taq* polymerase) used in PCR and other reagents and plasticware, can cause sensitivity problems with 16S rRNA gene PCR amplification procedures (13). Indeed, such assays for the detection of *M. tuberculosis* have been restricted by the Food and Drug Administration for use with only sputum specimens positive by acid-fast bacterium smear. Furthermore, since amplification tests amplify both dead and live organisms, such tests have limitations in monitoring therapy.

An application of molecular technology that is ideally suited to the simultaneous detection of various drug resistance mycobacterial genes is the use of DNA microarrays. In a typical assay, fluorescently labeled amplicons derived from the patient's sample positive for mycobacteria are applied to a DNA array containing nucleic acid probes based on 82 unique 16S rRNA sequences. The assay can provide discrimination among 54 mycobacterial species and 51 sequences containing unique *rpoB* gene mutations. The *rpoB* gene codes for the β subunit of RNA polymerase, to which the antibiotic rifamycin binds and inhibits transcription. Mutation in the *rpoB* gene confers resistance to rifamycin (20, 55).

The molecular methods available for the typing of microbial organisms are legion. At least five variations of PCR have been used for DNA typing of microbial organisms (41). Some of the PCR-based methods are easy to use, while others are of moderate complexity. In contrast, while DNA sequencing is considered a "gold standard" for viral typing, for typing of bacteria and fungi, the size of DNA that needs to be sequenced becomes a limiting factor. The prohibitive costs associated with automated DNA sequencers, and the high degree of technical skill needed to perform gel-based DNA sequencing, also make this approach limiting. However, these limitations can be circumvented by the use of non-gel-based sequencing methods that are applied to amplicons hybridized to gene-specific DNA chips (55).

An electrophoretic method that has been used to separate DNA fragments exceeding 20,000 bp resulting from restriction fragment length polymorphism analysis has also been used for DNA typing of microorganisms. The method is called pulsed-field gel electrophoresis. While this method is of moderate complexity, is easy to interpret, and has because of its high discriminating power also come to be considered a gold standard, the procedure is time-consuming, requiring 2 to 3 days for completion (41). The applications for molecular methods in the microbiology laboratory are constantly expanding, with such testing increasingly in the future expected to take place at the bedside upon admission in order to permit prompt identification of the causative microorganism, determine antibiotic resistance, and institute appropriate therapy.

Outlook for the Future

Driving Forces

The gigantic hurdles facing today's healthcare environment may veritably lead us to seek out the emerging developments in the miniaturization of ultrasensitive technologies to forge a brighter future for diagnostic medicine and the quality of patient care. These hurdles manifest themselves as spiraling costs of hospital stays and unbelievably high costs of billed laboratory tests, in the face of shrinking reimbursements and ever-rising health insurance costs.

In this environment we have no alternative but to do much more with less and yet achieve efficiency and excellence in patient care. This can be done only if we can reduce the length of hospital stays by diagnosing and treating disease rapidly. Clearly, innovative strategies are waiting to be devised to make laboratory testing simplified and user-friendly to the point where the patient can perform self-testing and electronically seek consultation from the physician for proper treatment. To visualize how the practice of laboratory medicine a decade or two hence will appear totally different, one has only to review sweeping changes that are taking place in the miniaturization of technologies.

Miniaturization and Microfluidics

Miniaturization has been at the heart of many developments in both computers and diagnostic devices patterned on microfluidics. Indeed, we are at the threshold of a next generation of chemically assembled electronic nanocomputers with molecular switches created from a class of organic molecules called rotaxanes (12, 38). Sandwiching a monolayer of rotaxane molecules between two perpendicular electrodes creates the molecular switch. Thus, the next generation of chemically assembled electronic-nanocomputers patterned on molecular switches and infinitesimally small tube wires can lead to the development of superfast computers. Such miniaturization in computerization, in turn, can lead to the miniaturization of implantable or ex vivo noninvasive devices intended for diagnostic testing of the patient.

Microfluidic systems etched on disposable plastic cards or chips are expected in the future to make a transition from prototype diagnostic devices to devices in routine use. These microfluidic systems consist of fluid channels and chambers of micrometer dimensions. In these microchannels or capillaries fabricated on an electronic chip, reactions are carried out. Fluid flow in microchannels is laminar, providing an environment for controlled mixing. Thus, fluids flow in these microchannels with no turbulent or random mixing (34). This property permits two or more miscible nonreacting fluids to flow past each other without mixing.

A T- or Y-shaped capillary (T-sensor) microfluidic device utilizing laminar flow allows introduction of a sample (whole blood), a standard or reference solution, and an indicating or signaling reagent (fluorescence or absorption indicator) into it. These three streams flow in parallel in a single microfluidic channel, with each fluid maintaining distinct boundaries as it flows past another without mixing. Diffusion of constituents in the sample into the reagent stream occurs according to size. Small molecules and ions diffuse rapidly and form diffusion interaction zones, which can be either visualized or quantified. Large molecules, however, diffuse slowly and thus do not overlap with the diffusion interaction zones of small molecules of interest. Precise quantification of the reaction is possible by continuous monitoring of the signal either with a CCD camera or by the use of linear diode arrays or scanning lasers. By determining the ratio of the signal from the sample analyte to the reference or standard, quantitative analysis can be accomplished. Alternatively, visual comparison of the characteristics of the diffusion zone, such as color intensity, with a standard chart allows for qualitative or semiquantitative analysis. Centrifugation of blood to separate plasma from cells is eliminated with the microfluidic device, since cells in blood, because of their large size, do not diffuse sufficiently and hence do not interfere within the short time span of the analysis (38, 59).

Instead of using a reaction reagent stream, microfluidic devices can be designed such that the affinity of a diffusing molecule in the sample stream to an immobilized ligand, such as antibody, can be exploited by using the ligand to coat the surface of the capillary wall. This allows for the design of immunoassays for small molecules, such as drug molecules. This microfluidic, diffusion-based separation and quantification principle can be exploited to design tests for a wide range of clinical analytes.

Lab-on-a-chip. Microfluidic devices to which pumps, valves, and detectors have been added constitute micrototal analysis systems, which are also referred to as "lab-on-a-chip" (48). Microfluidic-based PCR analysis is an example of a lab-on-a-chip. In one such system, the components needed to handle nanoliter quantities of DNA samples and reagents for effecting mixing and PCR amplification are microfabricated on a chip. The amplified DNA is digested with restriction enzymes, and the resulting products are separated by electrophoresis (8, 38).

Microfluidic-based PCR devices utilize electrophoresis to rapidly separate DNA fragments in a time frame measured in seconds. These devices also provide excellent separation using picoliter-sized samples.

Control of fluid flow in chip-based microfluidic systems can also be affected by techniques that utilize pressure-controlled air bubbles, surface tension, and gravity or by the mere application of electrical potential. An elegant approach to the control of microfluidic flow is the use of colloidal microspheres to create micrometer scale fluid pumps and particulate valves (54). Since colloids can be manipulated by the application of electric or magnetic fields, colloid-based control of microfluidic flow offers potential for the design of complex lab-on-a-chip systems.

The obvious applications of lab-on-a-chip microfluidic-based nucleic acid amplification systems are rapid detection of an organism at a patient's bedside, assessment of a drug's effectiveness by monitoring expression of a specific gene, and determination of antibiotic susceptibility. Indeed, continuous-flow PCR on a chip has been used to amplify a 176-bp fragment of a gene for *N. gonorrhoeae* in a time frame ranging from 90 s to 18.7 min depending on the fluid flow rate (25). Real-time PCR analysis adapted to microfluidic lab-on-a-chip technology can allow for self-testing of infectious disease pathogens. Cell separation and sorting have been made possible by fabricating a fluorescence-activated cell sorter on a silicone elastomer chip (19). Indeed, cartridges can be devised to perform hematology analysis including a WBC differential count by the use of flow cytometer principles and light scattering.

Microfluidic diffusion-based separation and quantification of chemical analytes. Microfluidic diffusion-based separation using a T-sensor, discussed earlier, is ideal for the design of immunoassay methods for small molecules, such as drug molecules. A rapid diffusion-based homogeneous immunoassay for phenytoin using a T-sensor has been described that takes less than 1 min to perform. The assay can measure nanomolar concentrations requiring less than 1 μl of reagents and sample (22). In this procedure, antibody to phenytoin and a sample mixed with a fixed concentration of fluorescein-labeled phenytoin are pumped through the two inlets of the T-sensor. As the two streams meet at the main channel they flow past each other, with mixing occurring only by diffusion. When phenytoin molecules, both labeled and unlabeled, diffuse and bind to the antibody, their diffusion profile changes relative to the freely diffusing unbound antigen. In effect, bound antigen accumulates at a point in the channel where antigen and antibody interdiffuse. The diffusion profile of labeled phenytoin is dependent on the concentration of phenytoin in the sample. The fluorescent intensity signals captured on a CCD camera are used to compute the concentration of phenytoin in the sample. Concepts such as these can be applied to POC testing by using miniaturized systems that are coupled to laser-induced fluorescence and detection with a CCD chip.

T-sensor microfluidic devices can be used to sequentially analyze different analytes through a single channel. Alternatively, the differences in diffusion characteristics of small to medium-sized analytes based on differences in

molecular weight can be exploited to perform simultaneous analysis of multiple analytes from a single sample.

Biochips

Biochips are microarrays intended for a variety of research and diagnostic applications. Microarray chips that are intended for DNA studies are referred to as DNA arrays. These chips may contain either oligonucleotides or cDNA probes. Current techniques, such as direct-writedip-pen nanolithography, are capable of anchoring 100,000 oligonucleotide spots in an area of 100 by 100 μm, literally driving miniaturization to its limits (15). To detect a DNA sequence of interest, labeled amplified DNA can be added to the oligonucleotide microarray. The sequence of interest will bind to the complementary oligonucleotide arrayed on the microchip and thus can be detected. cDNA probes are prepared by reverse transcribing mRNA and are then arrayed on the microchip. cDNA probe chips are used for expression profiling, where monitoring the amount of mRNA the cell is synthesizing assesses cellular expression.

Protein chips are designed to measure interaction of proteins with related molecules, such as antibodies and receptors arrayed on the protein chip. Proteins that bind to the array can be labeled and identified. Dip-pin nanolithography techniques that are used for arraying oligonucleotides can also be used to construct protein arrays in sizes ranging from 100 to 350 nm.

Applications.

Microorganism identification and determination of drug resistance. Microarrays can be used to identify to the species level organisms in culture-positive specimens. Typically, fluorescently labeled amplicons derived from bacterial colonies are applied to a microarray containing bacterial species sequence-specific oligonucleotides. Fluorescence generated upon binding of the amplified bacterial sequence to the complementary oligonucleotide on the microarray provides an identification of the organism.

Mutations in the bacterial genome can lead to drug resistance. Microarrays can be used to screen for drug resistance genes. As discussed earlier under "Molecular Testing," an example of the use of microarray technology in the detection of drug resistance genes is the detection of *rpoB* gene mutations that confer on *Mycobacteria* resistance to the drug rifamycin. Indeed, a variety of drug resistance mutations in the *M. tuberculosis* genome can be identified using microarray technology (20).

Although the identification of drug resistance genes is useful in designing appropriate drug therapy, the absence of drug resistance genes does not necessarily imply that the organism is susceptible to a specific drug. Conventional antibiotic susceptibility testing would in such cases be needed to establish susceptibility to a specific drug.

Activation of gene expression. DNA microarrays containing gene-specific polynucleotides so selected, for example, to represent genes expressed preferentially in lymphoid cells and genes of importance to cancer can be used to classify cancer based on gene expression. To such an arrayed chip is hybridized a mixture of fluorescent cDNA probes from sample mRNA and reference mRNA prepared from a pool of specific cancer cell lines. Since the sample and reference are labeled with different fluorophores, it is possible to estimate by the measurement of the fluorescence ratio the relative abundance of genes expressed in each sample compared with the reference (18). This approach has been used for the molecular classification of tumors based on gene expression and to detect new subtypes of tumors (21). Thus, DNA microarray profiling has great potential for assisting in the optimization of cancer therapy and predicting clinical outcome. It is now possible to examine a single cell from tumor tissue using a microscope-guided technique called laser capture microdissection. Gene expression can be studied using laser capture microdissection-derived samples subsequent to an amplification step to obtain sufficient cDNA for DNA microarray analysis (51).

Alternatively, the cell lysate from the sample can be added to a protein array containing immobilized affinity ligands, such as antibodies or receptors, to generate a tumor protein profile, after subjecting the protein-bound array to ionization by laser and detection according to molecular mass by mass spectrometry.

DNA Sensors

The electrical signals generated by DNA as it hybridizes to an immobilized target probe form the basis of DNA sensors. The capture probe in a DNA sensor can be attached to a gold microelectrode through a molecular phenylacetylene wire, which enables electrical contact to be made between the probe and the surface of the electrode. As sample is added to the DNA sensor, the sample DNA, which is released by appropriate chemical or physical treatment, binds to the capture probe, provided its sequence is complementary to the probe sequence. Another probe labeled with an organometallic complex, such as ferrocene, is added to bind DNA that is already bound to the capture probe. After DNA has bound to both the capture and labeled probes, an electrical potential in millivolts is applied, leading to the release of electrons from the labeled probe which are detected as an electrical signal and amplified to identify the target DNA in the sample (14, 38). Target DNA concentrations as low as 500 fM have been detected with gold nanoparticle probes and short capture strands positioned between two electrodes. As sample DNA binds to the capture strand and the gold nanoparticle probe, the gold nanoparticle probe bridges the gap between the two electrodes. The deposition of silver enhancer solution on the gold nanoparticle probe

causes current to flow in proportion to the amount of sample DNA that is captured (42). Such techniques may well be incorporated into the DNA sensors of the future.

DNA sensing can be driven down to the level of a single base. The basis for such detection is the ability to measure changes in ionic conductivity when a DNA or RNA molecule is threaded through a nanopore or membrane channel. In one prototype of a membrane channel, the nanopore was created by inserting α-hemolysin into a lipid bilayer (57). A steady current is produced when the nanopore is filled with an electrolyte and a voltage potential is applied. As single- or double-stranded oligonucleotides are drawn through the nanopore, the current is reduced. Since the reduction in current is correlated with the influx of the four different bases of the DNA strand through the nanopore, single base mutations can be detected.

Indeed, it has been estimated that DNA can be threaded through a 10^{-9} m pore at a rate of 2 million bases per second. Thus, nanopore sequencers that are being developed could conceivably sequence the entire genome in less than 2 h (34).

Applications.

Handheld devices for bedside screening. Handheld DNA sensors based merely on the detection of electrical signal constitute a simplified cost-effective approach to a variety of diagnostic applications. Devices with femtomolar detection limits could be used not only for screening of infectious disease organisms but also to screen for clinically important mutations, such as the factor V Leiden and prothrombin genes, which are risk factors for thrombophilia, and MTHFR deficiency, a risk factor for cardiovascular disease.

Nanofluidic systems utilizing nanopore technology offer potential for screening of bacterial or viral drug resistance mutations (24).

Finally, nanoparticles referred to earlier in the discussion on DNA sensors might well be the basis of the next generation of labeling technology for diagnostic applications. Gold nanoparticles labeled with oligonucleotides and Raman active dyes can be used to detect multiple oligonucleotide targets. The assay can be performed in a microarray chip format. The gold nanoparticle probe, when treated with a silver enhancement solution, facilitates the formation of a silver coating that acts as a surface-enhanced Raman scattering promoter when the dye-labeled nanoparticle probe binds to the sample target DNA sequence that has been captured by a complementary sequence immobilized on the chip. The Raman spectrum of the labeled dye identifies the sample target DNA. By using six different Raman labels and oligonucleotide-modified gold nanoparticles specific for sequences of the hepatitis A virus gene, hepatitis B virus surface antigen gene, human immunodeficiency virus gene, Ebola virus gene, variola virus (smallpox) gene, and *Bacillus anthracis* protective antigen gene, a simultaneous

Table 49.6 Next-generation technologies for clinical laboratory diagnostic applications

Microfluidic systems etched on plastic cards or chips: T-sensor microfluidic device for immunoassay of drugs without cell separation

Micro-total analysis systems or lab-on-a-chip
  Continuous-flow PCR on a chip for microbial detection
  Fluorescence-activated cell sorter on a chip
  Hematology analyzer on a cartridge based on flow cytometric and light scattering principles

Biochips (microarray chips): DNA and protein assays
  Microarray chips for microbial identification and to screen for drug resistance
  DNA microarrays to classify tumors based on gene expression

DNA sensors based on electrical detection: nanopore DNA sequencers to study mutations and sequence entire genomes

Nanofluidic systems utilizing nanopore technology for bacterial and viral screening and determination of drug resistance

Nanoparticles: next generation of labeling technology. Gold particles labeled with oligonucleotides and Raman active dyes for detection of multiple organisms in microchip format using 20 fM sensitive surface-enhanced Raman spectroscopy technique

detection of multiple pathogens has been demonstrated with this surface-enhanced Raman spectroscopy technique (9). The current unoptimized detection limit of this technique is 20 fM. Table 49.6 provides a selected listing of next-generation technology for clinical laboratory diagnosis.

Obsolete tests: Gram stain versus porous silicon biosensors. As new DNA sensing technology evolves and matures, older tests for bacterial identification and classification might well become relics of a bygone era.

Indeed, a porous silicon biosensor has been developed which encases in the porous silicon microcavity an organic receptor that specifically binds to the lipid A component of the cell membrane of gram-negative bacteria. The color of the biosensor shifts to the red region of the spectrum when the sensor binds only to gram-negative bacteria. Thus, a differentiation of gram-negative from gram-positive bacteria can be made with this stainless technique (10).

Summary

In this chapter I have provided an overview of current technology in the clinical laboratory and also discussed emerging technology that will transform the clinical laboratory and testing of the future. The writing on the wall is miniaturization, miniaturization, and more miniaturization. Devices and clinical samples handled by miniaturized devices will be infinitesimally small. Centrifuges will become obsolete with the introduction of micro- and nanofluidic devices.

We are approaching an era when testing will be simplified and rapid, and therapy will be tailored immediately upon completion of testing. In effect, we may expect in the coming decades the entire dynamics of diagnostic testing to change in the Lilliputian new world of miniaturized devices and incredibly sensitive technologies. Conceivably the laboratory of the future will be configured in a tiny lab-on-a-chip.

While it is difficult to predict the future, the promise of new miniaturized technology is compelling. It is reasonable to expect that mass production of miniaturized chips will bring their costs down. Potential savings in terms of labor translated in terms of full-time equivalents can be anticipated by replacement of conventional phlebotomy by a device integrated with a chip that will draw a nanoliter-size sample from the patient. Elimination of conventional blood collection tubes and supplies for collection of blood and elimination of centrifuges ought to result in substantial reduction in material costs. The ability to perform tests at the bedside, rapidly diagnose an infection, and determine appropriate therapy based on the antibiotic susceptibility testing and gene expression profile has the potential to dramatically bring down the need for hospital stays and thus significantly reduce healthcare costs. With space requirements for the futuristic lab-on-a-chip being infinitesimally small, overhead costs can likewise be expected to shrink dramatically. In a nutshell, we may expect that miniaturization of laboratory functions in the coming decades through such new technology ought to result in improved patient care at a cost considerably lower than it is today.

KEY POINTS

■ The trend in the clinical laboratory is toward miniaturization and nanoscale analysis. This trend will provide a tremendous impetus for POC testing and self-testing.

■ Amplification technologies like PCR will give way to simplified DNA or RNA detection techniques without the need for a prior amplification step.

■ A literally card-sized analytical platform designed around a nanofluidic or chip-based device with computer links to the physician is expected to usher in a new era in diagnostic testing.

GLOSSARY

Amperometry Measurement of current produced upon application of voltage potential.

Charge-coupled device (CCD) camera A video camera that uses a silicon detector as sensor.

Chemiluminescence Luminescence or a flash of light resulting from a chemical reaction.

Delta check A delta check is used to check patient results obtained at previous testing in order to ascertain if any of the results have changed significantly. It is also used to compare results of two or more analytes reflecting a particular pathology or organ dysfunction, such as blood urea nitrogen and creatinine, which are both expected to be elevated in renal disease. If only one of the analytes, such as creatinine, is elevated, the elevation would be suggestive of drug interference. On the other hand, an elevation of blood urea nitrogen alone would rule out renal involvement.

Electrochemiluminescence Luminescence that is produced when a chemical reaction occurs at the surface of an electrode upon application of a voltage potential.

Heterogeneous immunoassays Immunoassays with multiple separation or washing steps, in contrast to homogeneous immunoassays, where no separation steps are involved.

Impedance The resistance offered by nonconducting cells in blood suspended in an electrolyte as they pass through the aperture of a hematology analyzer.

Modular automation A process where only certain components of laboratory work flow or laboratory functions are automated. This process allows the flexibility to add additional automated modules as workload requirements increase and future automation can be cost justified.

Potentiometry Measurement of potential that develops at the surface of an electrode, which is measured against a standard reference potential. This principle is the basis for the measurement of hydrogen ion concentration (pH) and pCO_2.

Pulse oximetry A portable spectrophotometric device that is applied to a heel or fingertip to obtain a continuous measurement of oxygen saturation. In principle, two specific wavelengths in the near-infrared region are used, with one wavelength dedicated to the measurement of deoxyhemoglobin while the other wavelength measures all forms of hemoglobin.

Reflex testing A process in which a primary test reflective of organ dysfunction or pathology is chosen, and only if that test result is abnormal are additional tests performed to confirm or rule out a diagnosis. A typical example is the use of thyroid-stimulating hormone as a primary thyroid function test. If thyroid-stimulating hormone is abnormal, additional laboratory tests are performed to establish diagnosis.

Restriction fragment length polymorphism (RFLP) Variations in the base sequence of a short DNA segment are the basis for the formation of RFLPs. Restriction enzymes that cleave DNA at a specific sequence can be used to uncover RFLPs. The name RFLP derives from the fact that fragments of various lengths are obtained on electrophoresis depending on whether the polymorphism was within or outside the restriction enzyme cleavage site. RFLPs can be used to type microbial organisms.

Time-resolved fluorescence Fluorescence is energy released at a longer wavelength upon excitation of a molecule at a relatively shorter wavelength. In time-resolved fluorescence, the lifetime of fluorescence is longer and there is a wide separation (in nanometers) between the excitation and fluorescence emission wavelengths (nearly 250 nm) compared to that in conventional fluorescence labels.

Total automation The process of automating all the functions of the laboratory (preanalytical, analytical, and postanalytical data reporting steps) at one time.

REFERENCES

1. Aller, R. D. 2002. Survey of automated immunoassay analyzers. *CAP Today* **16**(4):60–92.

2. Aller, R. D. 2002. Survey of chemistry analyzers (for low-volume laboratories). *CAP Today* **16**(6):60–84.

3. Aller, R. D. 2002. Survey of coagulation analyzers (point-of-care and self monitoring). *CAP Today* **16**(8):52–58.

4. Aller, R. D. 2002. Survey of laboratory automation systems and work cells. *CAP Today* **16**(5):90–100.

5. Ambrose, T. M., C. A. Parvin, E. Mendeloff, and L. Luchtman-Jones. 2001. Evaluation of the TAS analyzer and the low-range heparin management test in patients undergoing extracorporeal membrane oxygenation. *Clin. Chem.* **47**:858–866.

6. Andrew, M., V. Marzinotto, M. Adams, C. Cimini, and F. LaDuca. 1995. Monitoring of oral anticoagulant therapy in pediatric patients using a new microsample PT device. *Blood* **86**(Suppl.):863.

7. Bourbeau, P. P., and J. K. Polman. 2001. Three days of incubation may be sufficient for routine blood cultures with BacT/Alert FAN blood culture bottles. *J. Clin. Microbiol.* **39**:2079–2082.

8. Burns, M. A., B. N. Johnson, S. N. Brahmasandra, K. Handique, J. R. Webster, M. Krishnan, T. S. Sammarco, P. M. Man, D. Jones, D. Heldsinger, C. H. Mastrangelo, and D. T. Burke. 1998. An integrated nanoliter DNA analysis device. *Science* **282**:484–487.

9. Cao, Y. C., R. Jin, and C. A. Mirkin. 2002. Nanoparticles with Raman spectroscopic fingerprints for DNA and RNA detection. *Science* **297**:1536–1540.

10. Chan, S., S. R. Horner, P. M. Fauchet, and B. L. Miller. 2001. Identification of Gram negative bacteria using nano scale silicon microcavities. *J. Am. Chem. Soc.* **123**:11797–11798.

11. Chapman, D. H., J. A. Hardin, M. Miers, S. Moyle, and M. C. Kinney. 2001. Reduction of the platelet review rate using the two-dimensional platelet method. *Am. J. Clin. Pathol.* **115**:894–898.

12. Collier, C. P., E. W. Wong, M. Belohradsky, F. M. Raymo, J. F. Stoddart, P. J. Kuekes, R. S. Williams, and J. R. Heath. 1999. Electronically configurable molecular-based logic gates. *Science* **285**:391–394.

13. Corless, C. E., M. Guiver, R. Borrow, V. Edwards-Jones, E. B. Kaczmarski, and A. J. Fox. 2000. Contamination and sensitivity issues with a real-time universal 16S rRNA PCR. *J. Clin. Microbiol.* **38**:1747–1752.

14. Creager, S., C. J. Yu, C. Bamdad, S. O'Conner, T. MacLean, E. Lam, Y. Chong, G. T. Olsen, J. Luo, M. Gozin, and J. F. Kayyem. 1999. Electron transfer at electrodes through conjugated "molecular wire" bridges. *J. Am. Chem. Soc.* **121**:1059–1064.

15. Demers, L. M., D. S. Ginger, S. J. Park, Z. Li, S. W. Chung, and C. A. Mirkin. 2002. Direct patterning of modified oligonucleotides on metals and insulators by dip-pen nanolithography. *Science* **296**:1836–1838.

16. Doern, G. V., A. B. Brueggemann, W. M. Dunne, S. G. Jenkins, D. C. Halstead, and J. C. McLaughlin. 1997. Four-day incubation period for blood culture bottles processed with the Difco ESP blood culture system. *J. Clin. Microbiol.* **35**:1290–1292.

17. D'Onofrio, G., G. Zini, M. Tommasi, and L. Van Hove. 1996. Integration of fluorescence and hemocytometry in the CELL-DYN 4000: reticulocyte, nucleated red blood cell, and white blood cell viability study. *Lab. Hematol.* **2**:131–138.

18. **Duggan, D. J., M. Bittner, Y. Chen, P. Meltzer, and J. M. Trent.** 1999. Expression profiling using cDNA microarrays. *Nat. Genet.* **21**(1 Suppl.):10–14.

19. **Fu, A. Y., C. Spence, A. Scherer, F. H. Arnold, and S. R. Quake.** 1999. A microfabricated fluorescence-activated cell sorter. *Nat. Biotechnol.* **17**:1109–1111.

20. **Gingeras, T. R., G. Ghandour, E. Wang, A. Berno, P. M. Small, F. Drobniewski, D. Alland, D. Desmond, E. Holodniy, and M. Drenkow.** 1998. Simultaneous genotyping and species identification using hybridization pattern recognition analysis of generic *Mycobacterium* DNA arrays. *Genome Res.* **8**:435–448.

21. **Golub, T. R., D. K. Slonim, P. Tamayo, C. Huard, M. Gaasenbeek, J. P. Mesirov, H. Coller, M. L. Loh, J. R. Downing, M. A. Caligiuri, C. D. Bloomfield, and E. S. Lander.** 1999. Molecular classification of cancer: class discovery and class prediction by gene expression monitoring. *Science* **286**:531–537.

22. **Hatch, A., A. E. Kamholz, K. R. Hawkins, M. S. Munson, E. A. Schilling, B. H. Weigl, and P. Yager.** 2001. A rapid diffusion immunoassay in a T-Sensor. *Nat. Biotechnol.* **19**:461–465.

23. **Hessner, M. J., M. A. Budish, and K. D. Freidman.** 2000. Genotyping of factor V G1691A (Leiden) without the use of PCR by invasive cleavage of oligonucleotide probes. *Clin. Chem.* **46**:1051–1056.

24. **Howorka, S., S. Cheley, and H. Bayley.** 2001. Sequence-specific detection of individual DNA strands using engineered nanopores. *Nat. Biotechnol.* **19**:636–639.

25. **Kopp, M. U., A. J. de Mello, and A. Manz.** 1998. Chemical amplification: continuous flow PCR on a chip. *Science* **280**:1046–1048.

26. **Kouri, T. T., U. Kahkonen, K. Malminiemi, R. Vuento, and R. M. Rowan.** 1999. Evaluation of Sysmex UF-100 urine flow cytometer vs. chamber counting of supravitally stained specimens and conventional bacterial cultures. *Am. J. Clin. Pathol.* **112**:25–35.

27. **Kuroki, M., Y. Matsumoto, F. Arakawa, M. Haruno, M. Murakami, M. Kuwahara, H. Ozaki, T. Senba, and Y. Matsuoka.** 1995. Reducing interference from heterophilic antibodies in a two-site immunoassay for carcinoembryonic antigen (CEA) by using a human/mouse chimeric antibody to CEA as a tracer. *J. Immunol. Methods* **180**:81–91.

28. **Lay, M. J., and C. T. Wittewer.** 1997. Real-time fluorescence genotyping of factor V Leiden during rapid-cycle PCR. *Clin. Chem.* **43**:2262–2267.

29. **Ling, T. K. W., P. C. Tam, Z. K. Liu, and A. F. B. Cheng.** 2001. Evaluation of Vitek 2 rapid identification and susceptibility testing system against gram-negative clinical isolates. *J. Clin. Microbiol.* **39**:2964–2966.

30. **Littig, J. S., and T. A. Nieman.** 1992. Quantitation of acridinium esters using electrogenerated chemiluminescence and flow injection. *Anal. Chem.* **64**:1140–1144.

31. **Mahutte, C. K.** 1994. Continuous intra-arterial blood gas monitoring. *Intensive Care Med.* **20**:85–86.

32. **Mammen, E. F., P. C. Comp, R. Gosselin, C. Greenberg, W. K. Hoots, C. M. Kessler, E. C. Larkin, D. Liles, and D. J. Nugent.** 1998. PFA-100 system: a new method for assessment of platelet dysfunction. *Semin. Thromb. Hemost.* **24**:195–202.

33. **McCusker, M. D., I. McConnell, J. V. Lamont, and S. P. Fitzgerald.** 2002. Simultaneous multi-analyte analysis by biochip array technology. Poster 1. [Online.] http://www.randox.com.

34. **Meldrum, D. R., and M. R. Holl.** 2002. Microscale bioanalytical systems. *Science* **297**:1197–1198.

35. **Narayanan, S.** 1996. Concepts, principles and applications of selected molecular biology techniques in clinical biochemistry. *Adv. Clin. Chem.* **32**:1–38.

36. **Narayanan, S.** 1997. Preanalytical and analytical pitfalls in molecular biology techniques. *J. Clin. Ligand Assay* **20**:200–205.

37. **Narayanan, S.** 1998. Quality control in tumor marker analysis: preanalytical, analytical and postanalytical issues. *J. Clin. Ligand Assay* **21**:11–17.

38. **Narayanan, S.** 2000. Technology and laboratory instrumentation in the next decade. *MLO Med. Lab. Obs.* **32**:24–31.

38a. **Narayanan, S.** 2000. Current perspectives on laboratory markers for the assessment of cardiovascular disease and myocardial damage. *Indian J. Clin. Biochem.* **14**:117–128.

39. **Narayanan, S.** 2001. Impact of ultra-sensitive technology and contemporary therapy on laboratory results. *Indian J. Clin. Biochem.* **16**:15–21.

40. **Narayanan, S., and N. Hamasaki.** 1998. Current concepts of coagulation and fibrinolysis. *Adv. Clin. Chem.* **33**:133–168.

41. **Olive, D. M., and P. Bean.** 1999. Principles and applications of methods for DNA-based typing of microbial organisms. *J. Clin. Microbiol.* **37**:1661–1669.

42. **Park, S.-J., T. A. Taton, and C. A. Mirkin.** 2002. Array-based electrical detection of DNA with nanoparticle probes. *Science* **295**:1503–1506.

43. **Piersimoni, C., C. Scarparo, A. Callegaro, C. P. Tosi, D. Nista, S. Bornigia, M. Scagnelli, A. Rigon, G. Ruggiero, and A. Goglio.** 2001. Comparison of MB/BacT ALERT 3D system with radiometric BACTEC system and Löwenstein-Jensen medium for recovery and identification of mycobacteria from clinical specimens: a multicenter study. *J. Clin. Microbiol.* **39**:651–657.

44. **Poller, L., M. Keown, N. Chauhan, A. M. H. P. Van Den Besselaar, A. Tripodi, J. Jespersen, C. Schiach, M. H. Horellou, D. Dias, N. Egberg, J. A. Iriarte, I. Kontopoulou-Griva, and B. Otridge.** 2002. European concerted action on anticoagulation (ECAA): multicentre international sensitivity index calibration of two types of point-of-care prothrombin time monitor systems. *Br. J. Haematol.* **116**:844–850.

45. **Pringle, M. J.** 1999. Acridinium ester labels: esters, sulfonamides and their applications. *J. Clin. Ligand Assay* **22**:105–122.

46. **Radstrom, P., A. Backman, N. Qian, P. Kragsbjerg, C. Pahlson, and P. Olcen.** 1994. Detection of bacterial DNA in cerebrospinal fluid by an assay for simultaneous detection of *Neisseria meningitidis, Haemophilus influenzae,* and streptococci using a seminested PCR strategy. *J. Clin. Microbiol.* **32**:2738–2744.

47. **Reisner, B. S., and G. L. Woods.** 1999. Times to detection of bacteria and yeasts in BACTEC 9240 blood culture bottles. *J. Clin. Microbiol.* **37**:2024–2026.

48. **Reyes, D. R., D. Iossifidis, P.-A. Auroux, and A. Manz.** 2002. Micrototal analysis systems. 1. Introduction, theory and technology. *Anal. Chem.* **74**:2623–2636.

49. **Rhoads, S., L. Marinelli, C. A. Imperatrice, and I. Nachamkin.** 1995. Comparison of Microscan WalkAway system and Vitek system for identification of gram-negative bacteria. *J. Clin. Microbiol.* **33**:3044–3046.

50. Roberts, W. L., C. B. Calcote, B. K. De, V. Holmstrom, C. Narlock, and F. S. Apple. 1997. Prevention of analytical false-positive increases in troponin I on the Stratus II analyzer. *Clin. Chem.* **43:**860–861. (Letter to the editor.)

51. Rubin, M. A. 2002. Understanding disease cell by cell. *Science* **296:**1329–1330.

52. Schmidt, F. J., W. J. Sluiter, and A. J. M. Schoonen. 1993. Glucose concentration in subcutaneous extracellular space. *Diabetes Care* **16:**695–700.

53. Smythe, M. A., J. M. Koerber, S. J. Westley, S. N. Nowak, R. L. Begle, M. Balasubramaniam, and J. C. Mattson. 2001. Use of the activated partial thromboplastin time for heparin monitoring. *Am. J. Clin. Pathol.* **115:**148–155.

54. Terray, A., J. Oakey, and D. W. M. Marr. 2002. Microfluidic control using colloidal devices. *Science* **296:**1841–1844.

55. Troesch, A., H. Nguyen, C. G. Miyada, S. Desvarenne, T. R. Gingeras, P. M. Kaplan, P. Cros, and C. Mabilat. 1999. *Mycobacterium* species identification and rifampin resistance testing with high-density DNA probe arrays. *J. Clin. Microbiol.* **37:**49–55.

56. Venkatesh, B., T. H. Clutton-Brock, and S. P. Hendry. 1994. A multiparameter sensor for continuous intra-arterial blood gas monitoring: a prospective evaluation. *Crit. Care Med.* **22:**588–594.

57. Vercoutere, W., S. Winters-Hilt, H. Olsen, D. Deamer, D. Haussler, and M. Akeson. 2001. Rapid discrimination among individual DNA hairpin molecules at single-nucleotide resolution using an ion channel. *Nat. Biotechnol.* **19:**248–252.

58. Ward, P. C. J. 2000. The CBC at the turn of the millennium: an overview. *Clin. Chem.* **46:**1215–1220.

59. Weigl, B. H., and P. Yager. 1999. Microfluidic diffusion-based separation and detection. *Science* **283:**346–347.

60. Winn-Deen, E. S. 1996. Automation of molecular genetic methods—part 2: DNA amplification techniques. *J. Clin. Ligand Assay* **19:**21–26.

APPENDIX 49.1 **Brief Synopsis of Major Molecular Methods Used in the Clinical Laboratory**

PCR

PCR is the most widely used amplification reaction for molecular biology applications. In its simplest form, the reaction involves denaturation of DNA to obtain single strands by heating to a high temperature (approximately 94°C), cooling the DNA (approximately to 55°C) to anneal to two primers, one for each strand, and raising the temperature (approximately 72°C) to synthesize DNA complementary to the strand template. At each cycle of heating, cooling, and reheating, the number of strands is doubled. At the end of 20 cycles, the two original strands of DNA will have been amplified a million times. PCR has undergone considerable refinement since its inception with the introduction of DNA polymerase enzyme of high fidelity to prevent nonspecific priming and the introduction of other strategies to minimize interferences. RNA amplification is achieved by first transcribing RNA to cDNA, which in turn is amplified. This process is achieved by using a single enzyme that at different temperatures can convert RNA to DNA (function as a reverse transcriptase enzyme) and subsequently amplify cDNA (function as DNA polymerase). This technique for the conversion of RNA to DNA is called reverse transcriptase PCR (RT-PCR). There are many variations of PCR. One technique that allows monitoring of DNA amplification during the reaction in closed tubes is called real-time PCR and because of its importance deserves discussion.

REAL-TIME PCR

Although there are different strategies to perform real-time PCR, such as the use of a dye that binds directly to amplified DNA or the use of a fluorescence-quenched probe together with the primers used to amplify DNA, in principle, the fluorescence generated at each cycle is monitored. The cycle at which the intensity of fluorescence becomes significant is called the threshold cycle (C_T), which is inversely related to the amount of DNA in the original sample. Thus, one does not have to wait for 20 cycles for amplification to be completed. In addition, time-consuming steps, like electrophoresis to visualize the amplified DNA, are eliminated. Real-time PCR coupled to microfluidic technology in disposable devices is expected to revolutionize diagnostic POC testing and self-testing for infectious pathogens.

LIGASE CHAIN REACTION

The basis of the ligase chain reaction is the use of four single-stranded probes, with one pair of probes targeting the 3′ and 5′ regions of one strand while the second pair of probes targets the other strand. After each amplification cycle performed in the presence of DNA polymerase, the newly synthesized strands left with a gap between the probe pair are bridged or ligated in the presence of an enzyme called DNA ligase to form amplicons. These amplicons are captured by a solid phase and detected. This reaction also requires 20 or more cycles of amplification.

BRANCHED-CHAIN DNA ASSAY

In the branched-chain DNA assay, target DNA is hybridized to a capture probe attached to a solid phase. Synthetic branched-chain-DNA-bearing multiple alkaline phosphatase-labeled probes are added to hybridize to target DNA. Finally, when a chemiluminescent substrate, such as dioxetane phenyl phosphate, is added, alkaline phosphatase cleaves the substrate to yield a chemiluminescent signal, the intensity of which is related to the amount of target DNA in the sample.

PULSED-FIELD GEL ELECTROPHORESIS

Pulsed-field gel electrophoresis is used to separate large DNA fragments exceeding 20,000 bp that result upon treatment with restriction enzymes. In this technique, electrical current is switched alternately between two sets of directional electrodes. DNA molecules exposed to alternating electrical fields are separated on an agarose gel, based on the rate at which they change their configuration inside the gel. This technique allows uncovering restriction fragment length polymorphisms and therefore is used in DNA typing. This technique has applications in the subtyping of bacteria and fungi.

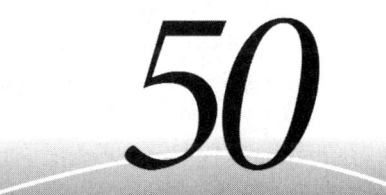

50

The Future Practice of Laboratory Medicine

M. Desmond Burke

OBJECTIVES

To familiarize the reader with the historic development of clinical pathology and laboratory medicine in the United States

To encourage an appreciation for the changes taking place in the healthcare environment that influence the future practice of laboratory medicine

The future isn't what it used to be.

R. M. SATAVA (27)

HISTORICALLY, the provision of clinical laboratory services in the United States can be traced to two distinct traditions: clinical pathology originating in the community hospital and laboratory medicine in the academic medical center (1). The term laboratory medicine is more commonly used worldwide (5). In the years following World War II, clinical pathology grew in strength and community hospital clinical pathologists became adept at helping primary care physicians to choose appropriate laboratory tests and to interpret results (2). This ability never developed to the same extent in academic medical centers and is reflected in inadequacies in residency training (2). Now as we begin a new century, there is an increasing need to contain costs and at the same time provide quality error-free laboratory testing (4–6). In this chapter, the future practice of laboratory medicine is explored against the background of a rapidly changing healthcare environment.

Laboratory Medicine: Origins and Historic Development

"Laboratory medicine" is the term used in most countries to describe the use of laboratory tests as aids to clinical decision making. The United States is an exception in that the terms "clinical pathology" and "laboratory medicine" are often used interchangeably. Both terms are used to indicate those areas of the hospital laboratory distinct from anatomic pathology. They derive, however, from two distinct traditions. Clinical pathology may well be unique in that it developed not in the academic medical centers but in the community hospitals of the United States. Laboratory medicine, on the other hand, developed in the academic setting (1).

Clinical Pathology

With the discovery of blood groups and the development of chemical analyses of body fluids that occurred in the 1920s, the demand for laboratory tests grew to the extent that hospitals needed full-time laboratory physicians. Since pathologists were needed to perform autopsies, they became the obvious choice to assume responsibility for community hospital laboratory services, hence the term clinical pathology. Initially, laboratory procedures were entirely manual and were performed by pathologists themselves. Pathologists also interpreted results and communicated directly with clinicians. With the increasing reliance on laboratory testing that began after World War II followed by developments in automation beginning in the 1960s, clinical pathology grew in importance, and clinical pathologists developed strengths primarily in clinical consultation and management of laboratory resources. Since the 1960s, the use of laboratory tests continued to increase, and by the end of the 20th century, technology in general and laboratory tests in particular had come to dominate the practice of medicine (2–6). Despite this increasing dominance, however, the role of the clinical pathologist as a consultant has diminished considerably in recent years. Three reasons have been offered to account for this. (i) Payors no longer consider clinical pathology to be a professional reimbursable service. (ii) Clinical pathologists are no longer deemed effective laboratory consultants and in this regard are considered inferior to specialists in clinical medicine. (iii) The increasing numbers of tests performed by technologists together with the growth of automation have removed pathologists from hands-on control of laboratory operations (5). Now, as we enter the 21st century, the role of the community hospital pathologist as a consultant to the clinician on the selection and interpretation of laboratory tests appears to have diminished considerably (15, 16).

Laboratory Medicine

The development of laboratory services in university hospital settings was quite different. Here, clinical laboratories developed as service components of research laboratories, mostly in departments of medicine and pediatrics (1). This resulted, in many instances, in a multiplicity of disconnected laboratories, each devoted to a test menu confined to the areas of interest and expertise of the particular clinical specialist concerned. Because of the greater numbers of clinical specialists in academic medical centers than in community hospitals, demands for the interpretative skills of the clinical pathologist never developed to the same extent as in the community hospital. Instead, the emphasis was more on the analytical aspects of the discipline, as carried out for the most part by clinical laboratory scientists rather than clinical pathologists (2). In recent years, primarily in the interest of cost-effectiveness, most academic medical center clinical laboratories have been consolidated into a central laboratory facility, usually within a department of pathology. The tendency in recent years has been to designate university hospital clinical laboratories "laboratory medicine divisions" of pathology departments. They remain, however, primarily service oriented. The result of

these events at the community hospital and academic medical center levels has been a failure of clinical pathology to develop an academic base, little or no teaching of clinical pathology in the U.S. medical school curriculum, and no clinical pathology consultant role models in academic medical centers (1).

The term "laboratory medicine" may be more appropriately applied to a tradition that originated relatively recently—in the 1950s—in departments of medicine and pediatrics. It grew out of the realization that the needs of the discipline as they related to practice, teaching, and research were not being met by clinical pathology. Departments of laboratory medicine, separate from pathology, were developed first at the University of Minnesota and later at Yale, the University of California at San Francisco, the University of Washington, Washington University, and the University of Pennsylvania (1). In these departments, emphasis was placed on a balance among research, teaching, and practice. Since 1973, when the University of Minnesota's departments of pathology and laboratory medicine merged, the trend has been away from separate departments of laboratory medicine and toward integration with departments of pathology (1). This has come about not only as a result of economic and political considerations but also because of the increasing overlap between the clinical laboratory disciplines and anatomic pathology. Despite the decline in the number of separate laboratory medicine departments, the laboratory medicine tradition of serious attention to the research and teaching aspects of the discipline continues in several combined departments. Moreover, in some, increasing emphasis is being placed on developing expertise in clinical laboratory consultation (7, 11, 19, 21).

Recent Trends in Clinical Practice

Although history taking and physical examination are still the mainstay of clinical practice, practicing physicians rely more and more on the use of technology, in particular laboratory testing, to solve clinical problems. The trends are in the direction of increasingly complex and costly laboratory molecular techniques designed to aid the diagnosis and management of equally complex and costly clinical problems (9, 33). This increasing reliance on technology is regarded as a major contributor to the increasing costs of medical care. The difficulty is that there must be a limit to how much any society is willing to pay for medical care. It appears likely, therefore, that at some point limits will have to be placed on utilization—including laboratory utilization. To date, efforts to limit overuse and misuse of laboratory testing have not been uniformly successful (23, 24). Success in this regard may prove doubly difficult because of demands for the highest-quality care from an increasingly sophisticated and consumer-oriented public (34). These developments, together with increasing application of point-of-care and patient-directed testing as well as the influence of the current electronic revolution, are likely to create a demand for laboratory consultants capable of interpreting laboratory results (5, 6, 11, 13, 19, 21).

Increasing Utilization of Laboratory Services

The number of laboratory tests performed annually has been increasing steadily for the past 40 years (32). It has been suggested that as many as one-half of the tests performed may be unnecessary or inappropriate (3). The clinical laboratory itself has been to some extent responsible by providing rapid turnaround of accurate and precise automated test results essentially on demand. Other factors accounting for overuse or inappropriate test use are societal influences, e.g., the demands of patients or their relatives and the avoidance of malpractice (3).

Physicians are also responsible. They may not always be aware of test limitations and often have a limited understanding of the analytical principles and diagnostic characteristics that underlie appropriate test use. In this regard, it is noteworthy that despite the emphasis placed on laboratory testing as adjuncts to clinical problem solving, formal teaching of laboratory medicine is a relatively neglected component of the medical school curriculum. Educational efforts to promote more appropriate utilization have not, however, had much success. Neither have other approaches, e.g., feedback of utilization and charge data, rationing, or penalties and rewards. Recently, the institution of formal laboratory consultation has been advocated as possibly the best means of ensuring appropriate use (3, 5, 11, 20, 22). Ultimately, computerized decision support systems may be more effective (8, 12, 23, 24).

Growth of Point-of-Care Testing

The practicing physician at the point of care performed the earliest laboratory tests, e.g., urinalysis. This took place at the bedside, in the clinic, or at the doctor's office. As tests became more complex, laboratory services were centralized. Centralization provides distinct advantages. The availability of trained technical personnel and developments in automation allow for improved accuracy and precision. Notable disadvantages of centralized testing, however, are delays in specimen transport and reporting of results. Increasing emphasis on rapid test turnaround times as a means of facilitating expeditious diagnosis and management and timely patient discharge has been mainly responsible for the recent growth in point-of-care testing (6). There are, however, disadvantages: tests are performed by nontechnical personnel, raising concerns about the accuracy of test results, and difficulties arise in integrating test results with hospital or laboratory information systems. These problems have been solved to a considerable extent, and the likelihood is that over the next several years many of the routine hematological and chemistry tests performed in central laboratories today will be available at the point of care.

Increasing Autonomy of Nonphysician Healthcare Providers

In recent years, state legislatures have broadened the authority of nurse practitioners. Several states now authorize nurse practitioners to write prescriptions and order laboratory tests independently of physicians. Although for the most part nurse practitioners operate in collaboration with physicians, some practice independently, and their services are reimbursed by private insurance companies and managed-care organizations (5, 6, 25). Physicians have become more interested in specialty and subspecialty medicine than in primary care (25). Moreover, this trend is likely to intensify in the future. Nurse practitioners, on the other hand, are becoming increasingly interested in primary care. As a result, it may be that much of the primary care of the future will be in the hands of nurse practitioners and other allied healthcare personnel.

The Electronic Revolution and Clinical Practice

The last years of the 20th century witnessed one of history's most remarkable advances and one that has affected and will continue to affect all our lives. The effect on medical practice is already evident, and this advance is likely to profoundly affect the way physicians, patients, and support systems such as clinical laboratories communicate with each other (18). Prior to the invention of the telephone, physicians and patients communicated directly or through an intermediary or by letter. At this point, the telephone has become almost indispensable as a means of communication to the extent that physicians and other healthcare workers feel obligated to be available by telephone. E-mail and Internet communications are now replacing the telephone (30). Already, the Internet is the major source of information—including healthcare information—for an increasing number of people around the world. Increasingly, patient-clinician-laboratory interaction will be Web based. This, coupled with increasing "consumerism" and the "informed patient," will change the relationship patients have with their physicians (34). Patients will be more likely to regard physicians as healthcare advisors, and as a result, they will be more inclined to consult directly with laboratory professionals and bypass the physician in the ordering of laboratory tests.

Reaction to Recent Trends

The reaction to the changes that have occurred in the healthcare environment in recent years is essentially twofold: increased efforts to contain costs and increased public demand for appropriate and error-free medical care (6, 34). Although total elimination of error is unrealistic, decreases in error comparable to those in many industries are now being viewed as within the range of a number of medical services, including laboratory medicine. The indications are that in the future, greater efforts will be made to ensure cost-effective error-free laboratory services. In this regard, interest is increasing in further efforts to teach test strategy and interpretation to pathology residents and to promote clinical laboratory consultative services with increasing reliance on the use of evidence-based medicine and medical informatics (5).

Clinical Laboratory Consultation

Consultation is the traditional approach to the solution of clinical problems that are beyond the competence of the referring clinician (3). As mentioned previously, clinical laboratory consultation was common in the past, when such consultations were reimbursable and when clinical specialists were less numerous than they are today. Recently, however, there has been a renewed interest in clinical laboratory consultation as a means of containing costs while ensuring quality. There are several reasons for this development, not the least of which is the failure of other approaches, e.g., formal educational strategies, in dealing with overuse and misuse of laboratory tests. There is also the awareness that advances in science and technology continue to account for the introduction of complex and costly new treatments, the application of which frequently requires equally complex and costly laboratory test support (5). This support requires more than the reporting of raw data, which unless accompanied by explanation may be in many instances meaningless to the requesting physician. When one considers the recent trends already alluded to, i.e., growth in point-of-care testing, increasing autonomy of nurse practitioners, and a well-informed consumer-oriented public with direct access to clinical laboratory tests, it is hard to imagine a future without the clinical laboratory taking responsibility for explaining the meaning of test results. Moreover, there is some evidence that primary care physicians believe that the scope of care they are expected to provide is greater than it should be and that they would welcome the addition of interpretative comments to laboratory test reports (11). When a group of hospital physicians were asked their opinion of interpretative comments, 98% indicated that they were useful and informative and 72% indicated that they shortened the time to diagnosis and helped to avoid misdiagnosis (11). Despite several published recommendations advocating that pathologists become more active clinically by providing clinical laboratory consultative services, few institutions do so to any significant extent. A notable exception is Massachusetts General Hospital. Clinical pathologists at this institution conduct "interpretative rounds" in several clinical laboratory areas, e.g., coagulation, autoimmune disorders, serum protein analyses, toxicology, molecular diagnostics, and transfusion medicine. These rounds, conducted in a laboratory setting, generate

formal interpretative comments and are analogous to "sign-out" in surgical pathology settings (11, 19). These comments are billable provided certain requirements are met (21). The most important requirement is that the interpretation must be requested formally by a practicing physician. There are exceptions. Under current (2003) Medicare rules, certain tests (designated by a -26 modifier to the applicable Current Procedural Terminology codes)—immunofixation, nucleic acid probes, Western blotting, and platelet aggregation studies, among others— are billable without specific requests provided the medical board of the institution has issued prior approval (21). There is, however, the additional requirement that interpretative comments be patient specific, require medical judgment, be signed by a physician by hand or electronically, and be filed in the patient record. Although it seems likely that interpretative reporting will become the norm in the future, particularly in the case of more complex laboratory procedures, in the near term, several barriers limit more widespread application. One is a scarcity of laboratory physicians sufficiently expert to be capable of providing credible clinically useful advice on appropriate test strategy and interpretation of results. Other potential barriers include lack of acceptance by practicing physicians, who may view interpretative reporting by the laboratory as an intrusion into an area that traditionally has been the province of the practicing physician, and reluctance on the part of hospital administrations to hire additional clinical pathologists and on the part of healthcare insurers to pay laboratory consultants (5). Many laboratory directors would agree with the argument that clinical laboratory consultation with provision of interpretative comments is the intervention most likely to contribute to cost containment and at the same time provide assurance of quality. The difficulty is that as yet there are no formal scientific studies published to support the argument (3). As a result, promotion and eventual institution of such services depend primarily on the efforts of too small a number of credible, interested, and enthusiastic clinical pathologists.

Teaching Test Strategy and Interpretation of Results

In the early 1990s, the growing concern that clinical pathology residents were not being adequately prepared for a future dominated by increasingly complex and difficult-to-interpret laboratory procedures led to a series of national meetings designed to deal with the problem. These meetings resulted in 1995 in publication of the Graylyn Conference Report, which stated that clinical pathologists should be capable of serving as consultants to other physicians, of developing and managing a variety of widely distributed technologies, and of playing leadership roles in an increasingly complex healthcare delivery system (7). The report emphasized that if residency programs were to be successful in training residents to serve as credible and useful consultants to clinicians, clinical pathology faculty would have to devise effective ways of teaching test strategy and interpretation. These concerns expressed in the Graylyn Conference Report were mentioned in a commentary on community hospital pathology reported in 1993 and borne out by the results of a survey of practicing physicians in conducted in 1996 (15, 16). In the reported commentary, Richard Horowitz, a practicing pathologist in California, said, "The current product of our clinical pathology training programs is not very useful to the community hospital or its laboratory" (15). When 75 California community hospital pathologists were surveyed about the skills and knowledge required for successful community pathology practice, knowledge of test interpretation and test strategies was considered essential or useful by all respondents, with 60% considering it essential and 40% useful (16).

Education and training requirements. When it comes to the abilities required to function effectively as a consultant, it appears that the clinical pathologist is at a disadvantage compared with the clinician subspecialist. The abilities needed are as follows: an understanding of analytical error, knowledge of sensitivity, specificity, and predictive value, knowledge of pathophysiology, appreciation of the probabilistic relationship between disease and test results, and—most importantly—an identification with clinical problems (3, 5). The last item poses the greatest difficulty for training programs in pathology. Most pathology residents have no direct exposure to patient care beyond medical school, and consequently the only way they can become familiar with clinical problems is by actively consulting. The Accreditation Council on Graduate Medical Education, through its residency review process, now requires programs to provide consultative experiences. The result is that in recent years, residency programs have adopted a variety of service responsibilities to be undertaken by residents in clinical pathology. Among the more common approaches are the following: carrying a pager, faculty review of pager calls, calling physicians with unusual and critical test results, preparation of formal interpretative reports, participation in the "morning report" conducted by clinical services, and attendance at clinical specialty conferences (5). No data are as yet available to indicate whether this greater emphasis on learning how to consult has had an appreciable effect on the prevalence and scope of laboratory consultation services in pathology practices. The impression is, however, that departments of pathology in academic medical centers are becoming increasingly interested in developing such services.

Evidence-Based Medicine and Medical Informatics
Historically, the practice of medicine has relied for the most part on the accumulation of individual clinical experiences (31). In recent years, individual case reports and series of cases have given way to more scientifically rigorous clinical trials providing the most recent and reliable information,

thereby providing the physician with the tools to practice evidence-based medicine. Evidence-based medicine has been defined as " the conscientious, explicit, and judicious use of current best evidence in making decisions about the care of individual patients"(31). The information available is growing at an enormous rate, making it increasingly difficult for the practicing physician to stay current. Moreover, recent reports from the Institute of Medicine indicate unacceptable levels of medical error, raising concerns that information is not being used as effectively as possible in the care of patients (14). Increasingly, the tendency is to look to the field of medical informatics, specifically to computerized methods of information retrieval and decision support systems. In the case of information retrieval, a large variety of online resources are now available, including the bibliographic database MEDLINE, several standard texts, and clinical practice guidelines. Realizing that few clinicians have the time to spend searching online, the focus is changing to the provision of concise information directed to the solution of individual clinical problems (14). In the 1970s and '80s, computerized support of clinical decision making took the form of comprehensive diagnostic systems that attempted to create an electronic diagnostician. These efforts were largely unsuccessful. Decision support systems in the form of optimal test strategies directed to individual clinical presentations as well as interpretations of test results are now in the process of development. These support systems are embedded in electronic medical records and are accessible via the Web (8, 12, 23, 24, 26, 28).

Predictions for the 21st Century
- Advances in science and technology will continue to fuel a procedure-dominated medical practice.
- Increasingly complex and expensive treatments will require equally complex and expensive diagnostic testing.
- The economic imperative to contain costs will intensify.
- Evidence-based medicine will be the norm and will be supported by computer-based decision support systems in an environment with the patient at the center of an electronic communication system that will include the hospital, the pharmacy, the primary care physician or nurse practitioner, the laboratory, and the laboratory consultant.
- Patients will be better informed and increasingly intolerant of medical error.
- Patients will have direct access to clinical laboratories and will play a much larger role in clinical decisions (10, 29).
- Comprehensive laboratory consultation services will be provided by both physicians and laboratory scientists to support the patient, the primary care physician,

the nurse practitioner, and the medical specialist who requests laboratory tests outside the realm of his or her own practice.

- The era of the generalist in pathology will end, and all pathologists and laboratory scientists will specialize.
- The distinction between anatomic and clinical pathology will eventually disappear, and the specialty will be called either pathology or laboratory medicine.

Summary

The role of laboratory testing in clinical decision making, which increased throughout the second half of the 20th century, will continue to increase and will dominate the practice of medicine in the 21st century. This will be the result of continued advances in science and technology and will occur against a background of further developments in informatics and electronic communications. Laboratory professionals, pathologists, and Ph.D. scientists will be primarily responsible for integrating disparate laboratory information and providing consultation services to physicians, nurse practitioners, and patients. Laboratory consultation services will be institutionalized and will be conducted by both physicians and laboratory scientists. The distinction between anatomic and clinical pathology will disappear.

KEY POINTS

- Medical technology will continue to dominate the practice of medicine.
- Future laboratory tests will be so complex that interpretation by laboratory physicians or scientists will be required.
- The patient of the future will play a more active role in his or her medical decisions.

GLOSSARY

Academic medical centers Hospitals associated with medical schools

Clinical laboratory consultation Providing advice on test strategy and interpretation of test results

Clinical pathology That branch of pathology which deals with laboratory testing, as opposed to anatomic pathology, which deals with gross and microscopic diagnosis of surgical and autopsy tissues

Current Procedural Terminology codes Systematic five-digit codes defining medical procedures or services and required for billing purposes

Laboratory medicine Virtually synonymous with "clinical pathology," with the exception that the term is more used when referring to academic medical centers as opposed to community hospitals

Laboratory utilization The frequency with which laboratory tests are ordered and performed

Point-of-care testing Testing usually conducted by nontechnical personnel at the bedside, in the clinic, or in the home

REFERENCES

1. Benson, E. S. 1981. Laboratory medicine in the United States—the dream and the reality. *Am. J. Clin. Pathol.* **76:**1–7.

2. Burke, M. D. 1994. Clinical pathology residency training: the need for reform. *Arch. Pathol. Lab. Med.* **118:**489–490.

3. Burke, M. D. 1995. Clinical laboratory consultation. *Clin. Chem.* **41:**1237–1240.

4. Burke, M. D. 1995. The future of clinical pathology. *Am. J. Clin. Pathol.* **103:**121–122.

5. Burke, M. D. 2003. Clinical laboratory consultation: appropriateness to laboratory medicine. *Clin. Chim. Acta* **333:**125–129.

6. Burke, M. D. 2000. Laboratory medicine in the 21st century. *Am. J. Clin. Pathol.* **114:**841–846.

7. Conjoint Task Force of Clinical Pathology Residency Training Writing Committee. 1995. Graylyn Conference Report. Recommendations for reform of clinical pathology residency training. *Am. J. Clin. Pathol.* **103:**127–129.

8. Connelly, D. 2002. Using web technologies for implementing testing strategies. *Clin. Lab. Med.* **22:**529–545.

9. The Dark Report. 2002. Newsmaker interview **9**(6):9–14.

10. The Dark Report. 2002. Pathology trends for 2002 show future direction. **9**(1):2–8.

11. Dighe, A. S., B. L. Soderberg, and M. Laposata. 2001. Narrative interpretations for clinical laboratory evaluations. *Am. J. Clin. Pathol.* **116**(Suppl. 1):S123–S128.

12. Elson, R. B., and D. T. Connelly. 1998. Applications of computer-based clinical guidelines. *JAMA* **279:**989–990.

13. Hallworth, M., K. Hyde, A. Cumming, and I. Peake. 2002. The future for clinical scientists in laboratory medicine. *Clin. Lab. Haematol.* **24:**197–204.

14. Hersh, W. R. 2002. Medical informatics: improving health care through information. *JAMA* **288:**1955–1958.

15. Horowitz, R. E. 1993. Clinical pathology in the community hospital. *Am. J. Clin. Pathol.* **100**(Suppl. 1):S24–S25.

16. Horowitz, R. E. 1998. The successful community hospital pathologist—what it takes. *Hum. Pathol.* **29:**211–214.

17. Hunt, D. L., B. Haynes, S. E. Hanna, and K. Smith. 1998. Effect of computer-based decision support systems on physician performance and patient outcomes. *JAMA* **280:**1339–1346.

18. Kassirer, J. P. 2000. Patients, physicians, and the internet. *Health Aff.* **19:**115–123.

19. Kratz, A., B. L. Soderberg, Z. M. Szczepiorkowski, A. S. Dighe, J. Versalovic, and M. Laposata. 2001. The generation of narrative interpretations in laboratory medicine: a description of service-specific sign-out rounds. *Am. J. Clin. Pathol.* **116**(Suppl. 1):S133–S140.

20. Linsell, W. D. 1982. Clinical pathologists—a threatened species? *J. Clin. Pathol.* **35:**249–256.

21. MacMillan, D. H., B. L. Soderberg, and M. Laposata. 2001. Regulations regarding reflexive testing and narrative interpretations in laboratory medicine. *Am. J. Clin. Pathol.* **116**(Suppl. 1):S129–S132.

22. Marshall, W. J., and G. S. Challand. 2000. Provision of interpretative comments on biochemical report forms. *Ann. Clin. Biochem.* **37:**758–763.

23. McNeely, M. D. D. 2002. The use of expert systems for improving test use and enhancing the accuracy of diagnosis. *Clin. Lab. Med.* **22:**515–528.

24. McNeely, M. D. D. 2002. The use of ordering protocols and other maneuvers: the Canadian experience. *Clin. Lab. Med.* **22:**505–514.

25. Mundinger, M. O. 1994. Advanced practice nursing—good medicine for physicians. *N. Engl. J. Med.* **330:**211–214.

26. Sackett, D. L., and S. E. Straus. 1998. Finding and applying evidence during clinical rounds: the "evidence cart." *JAMA* **280:**1336–1338.

27. Satava, R. M. 1999. Telemedicine and virtual reality, p. 17–21. *Proc. Am. Telemed. Assoc. Meet.*

28. Smith, B. J., and M. D. D. McNeely. 1999. The influence of an expert system for test ordering and interpretation on laboratory investigations. *Clin. Chem.* **45:**1168–1175.

29. Soloway, H. B. 1990. Patient-initiated laboratory testing: applauding the inevitable. *JAMA* **264:**718.

30. Spielberg, A. R. 1998. Sociohistorical, legal, and ethical implications of E-mail for the patient physician relationship. *JAMA* **280:**1353–1359.

31. Stewart, A. 1999. Evidence-based medicine: a new paradigm for the teaching and practice of medicine. *Ann. Saudi Med.* **19:**32–36.

32. Van Walraven, C., and C. D. Naylor. 1998. Do we know what inappropriate laboratory utilization is? *JAMA* **280:**550–558.

33. Wildsmith, S. E. 2001. Microarrays under the microscope. *J. Clin. Mol. Pathol.* **54:**8–16.

34. Yellowlees, P. M., and P. M. Brooks. 1999. Health online: the future isn't what it used to be. *Med. J. Aust.* **171:**522–525.

Glossary

Academic medical centers Hospitals associated with medical schools. (Chapter 50)

Accountability The obligation of a person to be responsible for his or her own actions. (Chapter 2)

Accounts payable Obligations or liabilities of a buyer that usually arise from normal operations of a business. They are neither backed up by a negotiable instrument nor considered overdue. Contract obligations owed by individuals or the business on an open account. (Chapter 41)

Accounts receivable Money that is owed to the firm by outsiders (Chapter 31). Balances due from debtors on current accounts (Chapter 41).

Accreditation Approval, generally for a limited time, of an institution or program based on a review of the institution or program by one or more independent examiner(s) who determine that specific requirements or standards have been met. (Chapter 43)

Accreditation Council for Graduate Medical Education (ACGME) Professional organization responsible for accrediting post-medical school training, encompassing more than 7,000 residency programs in 110 specialty and subspecialty areas. (Chapter 6)

Accrediting agencies Organizations that validate the ability of a laboratory to perform laboratory testing. In the United States, the federal government is charged by statute (CLIA '67 and CLIA '88) with the task of regulating diagnostic laboratory testing on human subjects. CMS (Centers for Medicare and Medicaid Services, formerly Health Care and Finance Administration) is charged by Congress with the task of developing and implementing regulations. CMS can "deem" other organizations to issue accreditation if their standards substantially meet or exceed those of CMS. Testing of animals and research subjects is not covered by these regulations. (Chapter 43)

Accrual accounting System that records revenue and expenses as they occur. (Chapter 31)

Accuracy Agreement between the best estimate of a quantity and its true value. (Chapter 20)

Active inertia Insensate repetition of the same behavior pattern without regard to the magnitude of the paradigm shift. (Chapter 40)

Active listener One who listens to the whole message, including facts and feelings. (Chapter 11)

Activity fit Interlocking and reinforcing business practices that define and defend a strategic position. (Chapter 29)

Activity-based costing A method being used by some laboratories that assigns a cost to every activity throughout the organization. (Chapter 3)

Actor The self; the one doing the acting, the speaking, and the gesturing. (Chapter 8)

Actual charge The amount of money a doctor or supplier charges for a certain medical service or supply. This amount is often more than the amount Medicare approves. (Chapter 35)

Actuarial data Information used by an actuary to make projections regarding service utilization in order to determine the financial risk of providing the service. (Chapter 7)

Adaptive approach An intervention that seeks to learn how to fix the system, with the understanding that the system for fixing includes the intervenor's own style, priorities, and values. Generally, an adaptive approach consists of an iterative cycle as follows: (i) plan the intervention, (ii) make the intervention, (iii) hold steady to analyze the effect of the intervention, and (iv) plan the next cycle of intervention. (Chapter 8)

Adaptive challenge A problem that does *not* subside to satisfy the current values in the organization even when management applies the best-known methods and procedures. Generally, the resolution of an adaptive challenge requires a shift in values. For example, at least two competing values might shift to resolve a budget crisis. On the one hand, the "problem" would be resolved if the employees shifted their values to take less pay and still be satisfied. On the other hand, the "problem" might be resolved if management shifted the values in the organization to direct the business to new profitable markets, perhaps global markets. (Chapters 8, 9)

Adaptive work Effort that produces the organizational learning required to tackle tough problems, the problems that often require an evolution of values. The learning in adaptive work often requires (i) addressing the conflicts in the values that people hold or (ii) diminishing the gap between the values people espouse and the reality they face. For example, dealing with reduced budgets may require (i) addressing the conflict between "We are doing a good job" and "We could do better" together with (ii) diminishing the gap between "We are doing the best that is possible" and current reality, which may be "The public will not pay for quality service." (Chapters 8, 9)

Add-on Test that is added on by a physician after the initial laboratory order is received. (Chapter 42)

AdminaStar Federal Medicare contractor handling the review of procedure codes to determine if two or more different codes are appropriately ordered on the same date of service. This service was initiated in 1996; these edits are available on the Centers for Medicare and Medicaid Services (CMS) website. (Chapter 36)

Administration Managerial work with a service orientation. (Chapter 1)

Administrative law judge The National Labor Relations Board (NLRB) has a corps of judges who conduct hearings at which the parties present evidence. These judges work for the NLRB. Decisions of administrative law judges can be appealed to the five-member Board in Washington, D.C. (Chapter 19)

Advance beneficiary notice (ABN) A "waiver of financial liability" form used by the provider to notify Medicare beneficiaries prior to receiving services that the services in question may not be covered services and that they may have to assume financial responsibility. (Chapters 5, 33, 34, 36, 37, 39, 42)

Aerosol A system of respirable particles dispersed in a gas, smoke, or fog that can be retained in the lungs. (Chapter 26)

AFL-CIO (American Federation of Labor-Congress of Industrial Organizations) Voluntary federation of unions that provide education, lobbying, public relations, and consultation services for unions; currently has 65 member unions covering >13 million employees. (Chapter 19)

Agency shop Requires non-union members of the bargaining unit to pay a "collective bargaining service fee" to the union; however, the person is not required to join the union. Other terms are collective bargaining service fees, and fair-share arrangements. (Chapter 19)

Agenda A list of things to be discussed and acted on at a meeting. (Chapter 12)

Age/Sex Rating A method of structuring capitation payments based on membership enrollee age and sex. (Chapter 7)

Airborne transmission The spread of infection by inhalation of droplet nuclei containing an infectious agent. (Chapter 26)

Algorithm A binary decision tree using patient response to intervention and other information to guide stepwise treatment of a specific problem. (Chapter 7)

Allogeneic blood Blood donated by a person other than the recipient. (Chapter 5)

Allowances Amounts to be subtracted from gross billings (along with bad debt) in the calculation of net revenue, including contractual and cost-based reimbursements, reductions in payments based on discounted charges, and charity care. (Chapter 41)

Ally doctrine Acceptance by a neutral employer of work normally performed by striking employees of a struck employer; thus the neutral employer becomes an "ally" of the struck employer. The neutral or ally employee may be legally picketed by the striking employees of another employer. "Ally doctrine" does not apply within healthcare settings (example: hospital). (Chapter 19)

Alpha The individual in the community to whom the others defer. Both humans and their nearest species relatives, the chimpanzees, show deference to the alpha of the community by ritualized gestures such as bowing, allowing the alpha to walk first in a procession, or standing aside when the alpha challenges. Furthermore, both humans and chimpanzees select an alpha of the community in a competition of (i) physical displays of confidence and (ii) coalition building. Accordingly, among humans and chimpanzees alike, the alpha of the community often is not the strongest, but rather the one who projects confidence, gives gifts, and strategically curries favor. (Chapter 9)

Ambulatory patient classification (APC) A method of determining payment for outpatient services based on a predetermined rate for outpatient services (similar to the inpatient DRG system). Certain services like radiology and blood products have their own APCs; others include supplies bundled into the 345 APCs. Diagnostic laboratory services are paid on a fee schedule and are not assigned an APC. (Chapters 4, 5)

American Association of Blood Banks (AABB) A professional organization that provides a voluntary inspection and accreditation program for blood banks and transfusion services. (Chapter 4)

American Board of Medical Specialties (ABMS) Organization of 24 medical specialty boards certifying physicians. (Chapter 6)

American National Standards Institute The claim adjustment "reason codes" indicate why a claim for service was "adjusted" (e.g., paid differently from expected) and are maintained by the American National Standards Institute; "remark codes" add greater specificity and additional explanatory narrative to the "reason codes" and are maintained by CMS. (Chapter 36)

American Osteopathic Association A professional association of doctors of osteopathy that also provides laboratory accreditation services, primarily for physician office laboratories. (Chapter 23)

American Society for Microbiology (ASM) The American Society for Microbiology is the world's largest educational, professional, and scientific society dedicated to the advancement of the microbiological sciences and their application for the common good. The Society represents more than 40,000 microbiologists, including scientists and science administrators working in a variety of areas including biomedical, environmental, and clinical microbiology. (Chapters 15, 17, 25, 26, 27, 43, 45)

American Society of Health Care Risk Management Organization for healthcare risk management professionals. (Chapter 6)

Americans with Disabilities Act (ADA) A federal law prohibiting discrimination in hiring and retention based on disability of qualified individuals. Applies to institutions with 15 or more employees. (Chapters 5, 15, 16)

Amperometry Measurement of current produced upon application of voltage potential. (Chapter 49)

Analyte Sample to be measured. (Chapter 20)

Analyte-specific reagents (ASR) If the ASR is used in accordance with the ASR rule and all other reasons for medical necessity are met, assays may be reimbursed at the discretion of a contractor. (Chapter 36)

Analytic activity Pertaining to actual performance of test procedure on a specimen. (Chapter 24)

Analytical error The difference between the result of an analytical method and the true value. (Chapter 20)

Analytical method Set of written instructions that describe the procedure, materials, and equipment necessary for the analyst to obtain a result. (Chapter 20)

Analytical range The range of concentration or other quantity in the specimen over which the method is applicable without modification. (Chapter 20)

Analytical time Time for the labor required to analyze the specimen or specimens and to perform all routine procedures up to reporting of results. This time includes any required calculations and checking but does not include test repeats. (Chapter 38)

Appraisal type Formal and informal appraisals, self-appraisals, peer-to-peer appraisals, 360-degree appraisals. (Chapter 16)

Approved amount The fee Medicare sets as reasonable for a covered medical service. This is the amount a doctor or supplier is paid by the beneficiary and Medicare for a service or supply. It may be less than the actual amount charged by a doctor or supplier. The approved amount is sometimes called the "approved charge." (Chapter 35)

Arbitration A process during which a neutral party decides the outcome of a dispute between labor and management, typically regarding a collective bargaining agreement. (Chapter 19)

Asset (and asset accounts) Represent the resources owned or used by the firm. (Chapter 31)

Asset management ratios Measure how effective the firm is at managing its assets. (Chapter 31)

Assets All money, property, or valuables that are owned by an individual or organization. Assets may be used in whole or in part to pay off liabilities (debts). (Chapter 41)

Association of American Medical Colleges (AAMC) Association of medical schools, teaching hospitals, and academic societies dedicated to improvements in medical education, research, and healthcare. (Chapter 6)

Attribution theory The reasons a person assigns to success and failure. Those reasons may be internal or external and either fixed or variable. (Chapter 10)

Authority Power granted to perform a service. The exchange of power for a service may be formal or informal. Formal authority arises where the officeholder promises to meet a set of explicit expectations, such as a job description or professional standards. Informal authority arises where employees confer power on a person based on implicit expectations; for example, "If Sally were here, she would know what to do." (Chapters 8, 9)

Authorization Allows the use or disclosure of protected health information for purposes other than patient treatment, payment, or healthcare operations. (Chapter 5)

Authorization card A card that authorizes the union to represent the employee during the collective bargaining process, once the card is signed by the employee. (Chapter 19)

Authorization card, required percentage Union must obtain authorization cards from at least 30% of the employees within a bargaining unit as proof of "employee interest" before the National Labor Relations Board will allow an election for union representation. (Chapter 19)

Autologous blood Blood donated by a person with the anticipation of its being later transfused back to the donor. (Chapter 5)

Automated Complaints/Incidents Tracking System Tracks and processes complaints and incidents reported against laboratory providers in a federal payor program. (Chapter 37)

Average cost Full cost divided by the unit of service. (Chapter 31)

Average rate of return (ARR) The average dollar return on a project divided by the average dollar investment it represents, usually calculated on an annual basis. (Chapter 41)

Bad debt Billings that are unpaid and uncollected and/or uncollectible. Recorded as an expense for gross charges that are deemed uncollectable from self-payors. (Chapters 31, 41)

Balance sheet Shows assets on the left side and liabilities and claims against assets on the right side. The balance sheet shows a firm's financial position at a particular point in time. (Chapters 31, 38)

Balanced Budget Act of 1997 (BBA) Package of spending reductions designed to balance the federal budget by 2002. Changes in Medicare financing of graduate medicine education (GME) included a cap on number of residents counted for reimbursement and a reduction in indirect graduate medical education payment (IME). This bill included provisions for numerous healthcare issues such as civil penalties for fraud and abuse, anti-kickback violations, guidelines for exclusion from the Medicare program, diagnostic information on medical necessity, coverage for additional screening tests, and Prospective Payment of Part B services to patients in a skilled-nursing facility. (Chapters 5, 6)

Balanced Budget Refinement Act of 1999 Legislation that offset or revised some of the GME funding provisions of the Balanced Budget Act of 1997. (Chapter 6)

Bargaining topics Include wages, hours, and conditions of employment; neither labor nor management can refuse to bargain on these issues. (Chapter 19)

Bargaining unit Group of employees (approved by the National Labor Relations Board) that share a community of interest and can vote in a union representation election; they will be the group represented by the union and are covered by the terms of the collective bargaining agreement if the union wins the election and negotiates a contract with the employer. (Chapter 19)

Bargaining unit, employees Usually composed of a family of closely associated jobs. (Chapter 19)

Barr's model of laboratory utilization A model that identifies the factors that affect the clinician's decisions or actions at each step of the laboratory utilization process. (Chapter 47)

Behaviorally anchored rating scale (BARS) Assessment of performance requiring input from other observers based on how employees behaved in a given situation. (Chapter 16)

Benchmark A standard against which performance is measured. The standard typically represents performance that is considered the best in the field or the gold standard of possible performance. Various internal, external, industry-wide, and non-industry performance measures may all be used as benchmarks. (Chapter 43)

Benchmarking A management tool that involves comparing one's performance with peers. The goal is to identify a "best performer" and understand how one deviates from the ideal. (Chapters 43, 45)

Beneficiary Term used for a person who has health insurance through the Medicare or Medicaid program. (Chapter 5)

Benefit The value a feature of the product or service brings to the customer. (Chapter 3)

Bias Systematic error that describes difference between measured and true or assigned value. (Chapter 20)

Bilingual A term which defines all people because all people speak two languages: one language with their words and another, more loudly, with their actions. (Chapter 10)

Billable test (Current Procedural Terminology, 4th edition, codable tests) Tests performed and charged to a patient, physician, or third-party payor account that generates revenues. The billable test is the focal point in laboratory cost accounting for laboratories that generate revenue. Usually defined in benchmarking parlance as a test for which there is a CPT-4 code and that could, therefore, be billed to Medicare (and most other insurers). (Chapters 38, 43)

Billed test A test that is actually billed to an insurer or client. Billable test is the parameter usually preferred by benchmarking programs because institutions vary in what they actually bill. (Chapter 43)

Billing Presenting a statement of charges to another healthcare provider, such as a hospital or physician office (account bill or client bill), or to a patient (patient bill). (Chapter 41)

Billing code Standardized designation for medical procedures (like laboratory tests) that are billable under federal government reimbursement rules, e.g., the Current Procedural Terminology (CPT) code assigned by the American Medical Association and updated annually. (Chapter 41)

Biohazard An agent of biological origin that has the capacity to produce deleterious effects on humans, e.g., microorganisms, toxins. (Chapter 27)

Bioinformatics The science of developing computer databases and algorithms for the purpose of speeding up and enhancing biological research. (Chapter 7)

Biologics Substances derived from living sources (such as humans, animals, and microorganisms), in contrast to drugs that are chemically synthesized. Most biologics are complex mixtures that are not easily identified or characterized, and many biologics are manufactured using biotechnology. Biological products often represent the cutting edge of biomedical research and, in time, may offer the most effective means to treat a variety of medical illnesses and conditions that presently have no other treatments available. (Additional information is available at the website for the Centers for Biologics Evaluation and Research, http://www.fda.gov/cber [accessed March 2, 2004].) (Chapter 5)

BIOS (basic input/output system) The program a computer uses to start its operations when it is turned on (booted up). The BIOS also coordinates the flow of data between the operating system (OS) and peripheral devices such as the hard disk, video adapter, keyboard, mouse, and printer. (Chapter 22)

Blood bank A facility that collects and dispenses blood products, also known as a transfusion medicine service. (Chapter 5)

Blood center A facility that collects and manufactures blood and blood products. (Chapter 5)

Blood-borne pathogens Pathogenic microorganisms that are present in human blood and can cause disease in humans. (Chapter 26)

Book costs Outstanding liabilities counted against the assets of a business as shown on its account books, and reflecting allocations of past outlays to the current period. (Chapter 41)

Bottom-up microcosting Estimating the unit cost of a laboratory test by summing the estimated unit costs of each of the input components (materials, labor, etc.) for a single performance of that test (also called job order costing). (Chapter 41)

Brand A name, term, sign, symbol (logo), design, or combination used to identify and differentiate the products of one firm from the competition. (Chapter 3)

Break-even or crossover point The point in the lifespan of a business or project at which the revenue it generates equals its cost, and thus represents a net contribution margin or profit of zero. (Chapter 41)

Break-even point The level of activity at which revenue and total costs are exactly equal. Point at which net income equals total costs. (Chapters 31, 35)

Bundling To place codes together in a panel. (Chapters 33, 37)

Bureaucracy Organizational hierarchies and defined lines of control. (Chapter 1)

Business associate A person or organization to whom a covered entity discloses protected health information to perform a function or activity on behalf of a covered entity, but who is not part of the covered entity's workforce. A business associate can also be a covered entity in its own right. (Chapter 5)

Business ethics Learning and doing the right thing in the workplace, directly relating to products, services, and stakeholders. (Chapter 1)

Business plan A financial and operational analysis of the feasibility of the implementation of a program. (Chapter 39)

Cabal A group of people working secretly and underhandedly to overthrow a regime. An acronym for a group of ministers chosen by Charles II of England in 1667: Clifford, Arlington, Buckingham (of *Three Musketeers* fame), Ashley Cooper (later Earl of Shaftesbury), and Lauderdale. (Chapter 30)

Calibration Process of using standards of known concentration to establish a relationship between measured signal from the instrument and analyte concentration. (Chapter 20)

Capital The cash required to purchase the firm's property, plant, and equipment. (Chapter 31)

Capital budget The financial plan for the acquisition of capital assets. (Chapter 31)

Capital budgeting The process of planning for the expenditures expected to generate income to flow into the organization. (Chapter 3)

Capital item A fixed asset that is expected to provide service (i.e., have a useful life) of more than 1 year. (Chapter 41)

Capital lease A lease that cannot be canceled during its term and that typically includes an option to purchase. It is accounted as a form of capital borrowing for a purchase and is accounted for as a capital acquisition within the capital budget. A lease in which the firm retains ownership of the asset at the end of the lease period. (Chapters 31, 41)

Capital markets The markets for long-term debt and corporate stocks. (Chapter 31)

Capitation A predetermined, fixed amount paid to providers in return for rendering a specified set of health services. The payment is usually on a per-member-per-month basis related to the number of patients enrolled in the health plan. The payment does not fluctuate with the level of activity. (Chapters 7, 31, 33, 34, 35)

Carcinogen Substance capable of causing a malignant tumor in humans or animals. (Chapter 26)

Carrier Primary third-party contractor with the Center for Medicare and Medicaid Services which administers Part B payments according to the local medical review policies (LMRP) to physicians, ancillary services, and clinical laboratory providers. (Chapters 5, 33, 35, 36)

Carrier Advisory Committee Local medical review policies (LMRP) are generally developed through a systematic approach with review by the Carrier Advisory Committee. (Chapter 36)

Carve out Services and procedures that are defined by contract to be separate and apart from the negotiated capitation rate that are typically paid on a fee-for-service basis. To exclude from a capitated contract and bill as fee for service (Chapters 7, 33, 35)

Cash accounting Records revenue and expenses when the cash has either been paid out or collected. (Chapter 31)

Cash budget The cash management plan for how the operational and capital budgets will be supported. (Chapter 31)

Cash flow The patterns of receipts and expenditures of a company (or other entity) resulting in the availability or nonavailability of cash; excludes non-cash expenses such as depreciation. (Chapters 31, 38, 41)

Cash flow statement Reports the impact on cash flow of a firm's operating, investing, and financing activities over a period of time. (Chapters 31, 38)

Catchment/market/service area A specific service area defined by geographic boundaries targeted by health plans, providers, and service networks to market products and services. (Chapter 7)

Ceiling limit The airborne concentration of a substance that cannot be exceeded at any time during the workday. (Chapter 26)

Ceiling-of-effort theory My contention that a leader's perceived level of effort sets a ceiling above which no follower's level of effort can be expected to go. (Chapter 10)

Centers for Disease Control and Prevention (CDC) The federal agency within the Department of Health and Human Services with broad responsibility for disease monitoring and prevention, epidemiology and statistics, and laboratory practice. (Chapter 46)

Centers for Medicare and Medicaid Services (CMS) Formerly known as the Health Care Financing Administration (HCFA), CMS administers the Medicare program, Medicaid program, and State Children's Health Insurance Program (SCHIP) and enforces the CLIA '88 regulations by conducting laboratory inspections, determining test reimbursements, auditing billing for medical necessity, and contracting with carriers and fiscal intermediaries to provide reimbursement. CMS is the primary federal body responsible for the oversight of clinical laboratory activity and licensure. (Chapters 4, 5, 24, 39)

Central processing unit (CPU) The main information processor in a computer that interprets and implements instructions. The CPU performs calculations, makes logical decisions, and stores information transiently. (Chapter 22)

Cerebrospinal fluid Venereal Disease Research Laboratory (CSF-VDRL) test A serologic test for neurosyphilis that is performed on a cerebrospinal fluid specimen rather than on a peripheral blood specimen. (Chapter 44)

Certification election Conducted by the National Labor Relations Board to determine whether employees do or do not want to be represented by the union that wants to represent them. (Chapter 19)

Certified union Has the exclusive right to bargain on behalf of the employees it represents; individual employees within the represented group are not allowed to enter into separate agreements with the employer. (Chapter 19)

Chain of trust agreement (COT) A pattern of agreements that extends protection of healthcare data by requiring that each covered entity that shares healthcare data with another entity require that entity to provide protections comparable to those provided by the covered entity, and that that entity, in turn, require any other entities with which it shares the data to satisfy the same requirements. (Chapter 5)

Change The process of transforming the way in which an organization or individual acts from one set of behaviors to another. (Chapter 14)

Charge coupled device (CCD) camera A video camera that uses a silicon detector as sensor. (Chapter 49)

Charge for a given test In the context of outpatient fee-for-service within the hospital, the charge for a given test is the amount associated with it in the institution's charge description master (CDM), representing the amount the hospital theoretically bills all fee-for-service payors for the test. (Chapter 41)

Charge related to unfair labor practice An allegation made by an individual, employer, or labor organization of an unfair labor practice (ULP) under the National Labor Relations Act (NLRA); charges are filed at the National Labor Relations Board's regional offices. (Chapter 19)

Checklist adjectives evaluation At least three adjectives (e.g., aggressive, articulate, meticulous) from a checklist are selected to describe desirable as well as undesirable characteristics of an employee. (Chapter 16)

Chemiluminescence Luminescence or a flash of light resulting from a chemical reaction. (Chapter 49)

Civil False Claims Act and the Civil Monetary Penalties Law Authorizes the Secretary of Health and Human Services to impose civil monetary penalties (CMPs) for violations of Medicare rules and regulations, as well as additional assessments for statutory violations of Medicare law. (Chapter 37)

Civilian Health and Medical Program of the Uniformed Services (CHAMPUS) Administered by the Department of Defense, CHAMPUS provides medical care to active-duty members of the military, military retirees, and their eligible dependents. (This program is now called TRICARE.) (Chapter 5)

Clad A coin consisting of an outer layer of one metal bonded to a core of a different metal. (Chapter 40)

Claim A request for payment for services rendered to beneficiaries by providers; the claim form or invoice, which allows transmission of the bill to a payor. (Chapters 5, 33, 35, 36)

Claim denial management Can enhance revenue; denials usually arise from process problems leading to inadequate documentation. (Chapter 34)

CLIA '88 The Clinical Laboratory Improvement Amendments of 1988 (q.v.) and their implementing regulations, as published since 1992. (Chapter 28)

CLIA-waived testing A category of laboratory test complexity under CLIA (q.v.) which applies to tests which (i) are cleared by the U.S. Food and Drug Administration for home use; (ii) employ methods that are so simple and accurate as to render the likelihood of erroneous results negligible; or (iii) pose no reasonable risk of harm to the patient if the test is performed incorrectly. (Chapter 28)

Client The computer/workstation that requests an action from a server in a client/server relationship. (Chapter 22)

Client bill Bill sent to the client for payment of laboratory services as opposed to billing the patient or the patient's insurance. (Chapter 42)

Clinical laboratory consultation Providing advice on test strategy and interpretation of test results. (Chapter 50)

Clinical laboratory consultative services Services that provide direct communications to healthcare providers regarding appropriate testing protocols. (Chapter 47)

Clinical Laboratory Improvement Act Amendments of 1988 (CLIA '88) Passed by Congress in 1988 to establish quality standards for laboratory testing and to ensure the accuracy, reliability, and timeliness of patient test results. Laboratory tests were categorized as being waived, of moderate complexity, or of high complexity. Laboratories performing tests in the latter two categories had to register and comply with a set of regulatory rules to become certified (licensed). In 2003, a Final Rule was issued in the Federal Register that defined some new regulations and changed the categorization of tests into two categories (waived and nonwaived tests). In total, CLIA covers approximately 175,000 laboratory entities. The Division of Laboratory Services, within the Survey and Certification Group, under the Center for Medicaid and State Operations has the responsibility for implementing the CLIA program. The objective of the CLIA program is to ensure quality laboratory testing. Although all clinical laboratories must be properly certified to receive Medicare or Medicaid payments, CLIA has no direct Medicare or Medicaid program responsibilities. CLIA requires an objective system to document competency of employees performing

testing on patient specimens. The final rules were first published in *The Federal Register* on February 28, 1992. (Chapters 4, 16, 24, 39, 46)

Clinical Laboratory Improvement Act of 1967 (CLIA '67) First published in 1967 and amended in 1988, CLIA '67 is a statute requiring all laboratories performing clinical testing on human specimens to comply with specific federal certification regulations. (Chapters 5, 43)

Clinical Laboratory Improvement Amendments (CLIA) complexity categories Complexity categories based upon analyst training and experience as well as operational characteristics of testing that is performed. They include (i) high complexity, e.g., histopathology, cytopathology, cytogenetics, blood banking, histocompatibility, and complicated chemistry, hematology, and microbiology procedures; (ii) moderate complexity, for the bulk of routine hematology and chemistry procedures; (iii) provider-performed microscopy, encompassing a limited number of procedures (e.g., microscopic urinalysis) commonly performed in physician offices in conjunction with patient visits; and (iv) waived testing, performed in any location with minimal quality control and personnel requirements and without any inspection requirement. In 2003, a Final Rule was issued in the Federal Register that defined some new regulations and changed the categorization of tests into two categories (waived and nonwaived tests). (Chapter 46)

Clinical Laboratory Improvement Amendments of 1988 (CLIA '88) technical consultant One who is responsible for the technical and scientific oversight of laboratory testing in moderate-complexity laboratories. (Chapter 47)

Clinical Laboratory Management Association (CLMA) A professional organization concerned with all aspects of laboratory management. Many local chapters have been organized. (Chapter 43)

Clinical Laboratory Scientist (CLS) Term generally used to refer to a person who has completed a four-year college-level program that requires specific training in the clinical laboratory sciences. In recent years, CLS has replaced the older term Medical Technologist (MT). The designation of MT also indicates a specific level of professional certification by the American Society for Clinical Pathology. A CLS can perform a full range of laboratory tests. (Chapter 4)

Clinical pathology That branch of pathology which deals with laboratory testing, as opposed to anatomic pathology, which deals with gross and microscopic diagnosis of surgical and autopsy tissues. (Chapter 50)

Clinical pathways Practice guidelines for patient care that have been adapted to local conditions to standardize treatment. (Chapter 7)

Clinical practice guideline (CPG) A set of recommendations for addressing selected clinical problems. (Chapter 48)

Clinical scientist A title that currently represents the clinical laboratory scientist/medical technologist. (Chapter 47)

Clinical trial A research study that looks at a similar group of patients selected using strict criteria and assesses the impact of changes of single variables. (Chapter 6)

Clinical utility Economists refer to the ability to satisfy needs as utility. In medicine it is more commonly referred to as clinical utility. (Chapter 3)

Closed shop Illegal; employment site where all employees must join the union prior to employment. (Chapter 19)

CMS-1450 form (formerly UB-92) Form used for institutional (e.g., hospitals, nursing homes) claims for Medicare Part A services. (Chapter 36)

CMS-1500 Claim form authorized by the Health Care Financing Administration (now CMS) for filing Medicare Part B claims with carriers. (Chapter 36)

Coaching Providing an employee with the direction, support, and self-assurance to improve performance on the job. (Chapter 2)

Code jamming Inserting a code that was not provided by the ordering provider but which will justify payment. (Chapter 37)

Code set Under the Health Insurance Portability and Accountability Act (HIPAA), a code set is any set of codes used to encode data elements, such as tables of terms, medical concepts, medical diagnostic codes, or medical procedure codes. This includes both the codes and their descriptions. Under HIPAA, the Code Set Maintaining Organization creates and maintains the code sets adopted by the Secretary for use in the transactions for which standards are adopted. (Chapter 5)

Code steering Providing lists of diagnostic codes that are known to justify payment. (Chapter 37)

Coefficient of variation A measure of variance expressed as a percentage of the mean ([standard deviation/mean] $\times$ 100). (Chapter 20)

Coinsurance The percentage split of the agreed-upon cost sharing ratio between a health plan participant and the insurer or employer. Usually the employer assumes 80% and the employee assumes 20%. (Chapter 7)

COLA (formerly the Commission on Office Laboratory Accreditation) A national nonprofit physician-directed organization that provides continuing medical education programs, accreditation standards, and accreditation of physician office laboratories. (Chapters 16, 23)

Collective bargaining Contract negotiations between union and employer; mandatory topics include wages, hours, and conditions of employment. (Chapter 19)

College of American Pathologists (CAP) A medical society of board-certified pathologists that provides proficiency testing samples, continuing medical education programs, accreditation standards, and accreditation of pathology and laboratory services. CAP also provides services such as Q-Probes and Q-Tracks (q.v.). (Chapters 4, 6, 16, 23, 39, 44)

Commission on Laboratory Accreditation Administers the College of American Pathologists Laboratory Accreditation Program, which is approved to inspect laboratories in lieu of the Centers for Medicare and Medicaid Services. (Chapter 6)

Commission on Office Laboratory Accreditation (COLA) An organization that was granted "deemed" status by CMS to inspect physician office laboratories for accreditation. (Chapter 4)

Commission plan A written plan for calculation and distribution of commission payment to marketing staff and other individuals. (Chapter 42)

Commoditization The process by which a product provided by one firm becomes indistinguishable from products provided by other firms. (Chapter 29)

Common purpose A state that is achieved when team members fully understand the team's purpose or reason for existing, and there is significant goal congruence. (Chapter 18)

Communication Exchange of thoughts, messages, or information flowing in all directions within the organization (through speech, signals, writing, or behavior); art and technique of using words effectively to impart information or ideas; system, such as mail, telephone, or television, for sending and receiving messages; exchange or transmission of ideas, attitudes, or beliefs between individuals or groups. Communication can be written or spoken, verbal or nonverbal, formal or informal. (Chapters 2, 11, 21)

Communication barriers Any behavior or physical obstruction that hinders or restricts the flow of meaningful communication. (Chapter 11)

Community health information network A network formed among community healthcare providers and insurers to maintain healthcare information for patient management purposes. (Chapter 3)

Community-based rating A method of calculating insurance premiums based on the combined experience of multiple groups within a geographic region, adjusted for age, sex, and high risk. (Chapter 7)

Competency Ability to do a job correctly and safely and to recognize and solve minor problems without needing assistance. (Chapter 16)

Competitive advantage Qualities that allow a firm to outperform its rivals consistently. (Chapter 29)

Competitive benchmarking Comparing your own performance against competitors in the same industry or market rather than focusing primarily on gold standards or best practices as standards for performance. (Chapter 43)

Competitive bidding The process used by buyers to request price quotations from suppliers to get the best product and service at the lowest price. (Chapter 3)

Competitor analysis Assessment of the capabilities, goals, assumptions, and strategies of competitors, with the aim of predicting competitor behavior. (Chapter 29)

Complaint After investigating an unfair labor practice charge, if the regional office finds merit and no settlement is reached, the regional director of the National Labor Relations Board issues a complaint in the name of the Board stating the unfair labor practices and containing a notice of hearing before an administrative law judge. The complaint does not constitute a finding of wrongdoing, but raises issues to be decided by the judge. (Chapter 19)

Complex sale A complex sale is one that requires more than one signature/authorization for approval or more than one decision maker. (Chapter 3)

Compliance Program Guidance for Clinical Laboratories (1998) Updated Model Clinical Laboratory Compliance Plan (1997); designed to ensure that appropriate reimbursement is made through federal programs, to ensure that payors "pay it right"; provides guidance for doing the right thing (through compliance with all regulatory and statutory rules). (Chapter 37)

Composite rate A uniform premium that applies to all eligible members in a subscriber group regardless of the number of dependents covered. Commonly used with labor unions and large employer groups. (Chapter 7)

Comprehensive Error Rate Testing (CERT) Program A designated CERT contractor has responsibility for random review of selected claims processed by federal payors to verify that contractor decisions were accurate and based on sound policy compliant with statutes and regulations; the purpose is to generate national paid claim error rates (benchmark data). (Chapter 37)

Computerized physician order entry (CPOE) A computer-based system for placing clinical orders. Some systems have the ability to integrate orders with pharmacy and laboratory data, to make recommendations for drug dosage and timing, and to alert the ordering physician of issues such as drug allergy. (Chapter 44)

Confidence interval Expected range of values within a group with a specified probability. (Chapter 20)

Conflict A disagreement over goals or methods to achieve them. (Chapter 13)

Conflict of interest A situation in which a person has a private or personal interest sufficient to appear to influence the objective exercise of his or her duties. (Chapter 1)

Conflict resolution The process of identifying, analyzing, and eliminating conflict. (Chapter 13)

Conflict resolution styles Five approaches to resolving conflict. (Chapter 13)

Consent A document signed by an individual that allows the use or disclosure of the individual's protected health information for the purpose of treatment, payment, or healthcare operations. (Chapter 5)

Consolidation An internal laboratory system strategy to reduce cost by eliminating the duplication of services and excess capacity, restructuring the work flow, implementing changes in staff resources, and centralizing operation management. (Chapter 7)

Constant systematic error An error that is always in the same direction and of the same magnitude even as the concentration of analyte changes. (Chapter 20)

Constraints Factors that limit the flexibility of action. (Chapter 30)

Constructive conflict Disagreements that are acknowledged and lead to resolution. (Chapter 13)

Consultants Individuals with recognized expertise who are asked by a client, in this case a healthcare provider, to apply their knowledge and skills to a given situation. (Chapter 47)

Consumer In healthcare, the consumer is the patient. The patient is sometimes also an employee, a subscriber, or a beneficiary. (Chapter 7)

Contaminated Describes the presence or reasonably anticipated presence of blood or other potentially infectious materials on an item or surface. (Chapter 26)

Context-appropriate real-time knowledge support (CARTKS) Knowledge support that is directed specifically to the clinical problem at hand and is presented in such a way that it does not interrupt the normal flow of work. (Chapter 48)

Contingency workforce Employees not defined as permanent or regular employees, usually assigned jobs based on short-term needs. (Chapter 17)

Continuous quality improvement A more human-focused quality management theory, relying heavily on worker involvement in the product improvement process. (Chapter 1)

Continuous/lifelong learning A self-empowering theory that the employee will throughout his or her life learn and strive to improve and move on to new things. (Chapter 1)

Continuum of care A patient's continuum of care would include the hospital, physician office, skilled-nursing facility, outpatient surgery, primary care, specialty care, and any other health service the patient might need. (Chapter 42)

Contract A legal agreement between two parties that can be enforced through legal channels and that creates an obligation. (Chapter 6)

Contract mix The distribution of enrollees by number of dependents (single, double, family). (Chapter 7)

Contractual allowances Discounts on gross charges given to third-party payors who have a negotiated contract with the billing provider. (Chapter 31)

Contribution margin The excess of revenue over variable costs. (Chapter 31)

Control limit A range of expected values that, if exceeded, warns of random and/or systematic error in an analytical process. (Chapter 20)

Control material Specimen which is repeatedly analyzed and test results are statistically analyzed to monitor method performance. (Chapter 20)

Controllable costs Fixed or variable costs that can be influenced by a specific individual's decision making. (Chapter 41)

Coordination of benefits (COB) A program that determines which plan or insurance policy will pay first if two health plans or insurance policies cover the same benefits. If one of the plans is a Medicare health plan, federal law may decide who pays first, in a written statement that states which health plan or insurance policy is primary when two health plans or insurance policies cover the same benefits. (Chapter 5)

Copayment (copay) A fixed dollar amount paid by the subscriber to the provider at the time of services. (Chapters 7, 34)

Core laboratory This term may have several meanings. It may refer to a main (central) laboratory within a multiple laboratory system, or it may refer to a dedicated section within a single laboratory that does the majority of routine and stat testing. (Chapter 4)

Corporate compliance program The development of effective internal controls that promote adherence to applicable federal and state laws and the program requirements of federal, state, and private health plans. The program is aimed at the prevention of fraud, abuse, and waste in these healthcare plans while at the same time furthering the fundamental mission of all hospitals, which is to provide quality healthcare to patients. (Chapter 6)

Corporate integrity agreement (CIA) A settlement agreement between a healthcare provider and the Office of the Inspector General (OIG) that sets forth the terms and conditions for continued participation in the Medicare program following investigation and conviction of fraud and abuse. (Chapter 5)

Corrosive Any substance that causes visible destruction of human tissue at the site of contact. The U.S. Environmental Protection Agency defines a corrosive as a substance that is highly acidic (pH $<$ 2.1) or highly alkaline (pH $>$ 12.4). (Chapter 26)

Cost accounting A system of measuring and reporting information about costs. (Chapters 31, 38)

Cost per billable result Unit cost of production of all the reportable results that are included in a unit of service, such as a test panel or battery that is made up of multiple individual analyte results, but billed as a group. (Chapter 41)

Cost per reportable result Unit cost of production for all the items necessary to report a test result, including the individual analyte test result itself and all the quality control, calibrator, waste, and repeat results that are necessary to be able to report it. (Chapter 41)

Cost per test (or cost per result) Unit cost of production of a single individual analyte test result, representing both fixed and variable direct costs, as well as allocations of certain indirect costs most closely associated with production: reagents, disposable supplies, equipment, and labor. (Chapter 41)

Cost-benefit analysis A projection of the resources needed to implement a program and the benefits derived from such a program. (Chapter 39)

Council on Graduate Medical Education (GME) Congressionally authorized body charged with evaluating physician workforce and graduate medical training and financing. (Chapter 6)

Covered lives Population insured by a managed-care contract. (Chapters 33, 35)

Credit rating The creditworthiness of a firm based on past and projected financial performance, an assessment of the management, and the external business environment. (Chapter 31)

Creeping inflation A pricing strategy that uses modest price increases over time that are typically not noticeable to the consumer. (Chapter 3)

Criterion Standard of judging task performance. (Chapter 16)

Critical (clinical) pathways Standardized, multidisciplinary approach to a specific problem. Traditionally more detailed than practice guidelines, though the difference may not be distinct. Written criteria to guide care based on standards of practice, delineating necessary treatment and facilitating appropriate use of resources (also referred to as clinical pathway). (Chapters 6, 7)

Critical incident evaluation Written notations of exceptional performance are summarized in the performance appraisal. (Chapter 16)

Cross-training Training of individuals to perform more than one task. (Chapter 30)

Cross-walking When a new test is determined to be similar to an existing test, multiple existing test codes, or a portion of an existing test code, the new test code is assigned the related existing local fee schedule amounts and resulting national limitation amount. In some instances, a test may equate only to a portion of a test, and in those instances, payment at an appropriate percentage of the payment for the existing test is assigned. The fee is set at the same rate as that for another CPT code (or codes) deemed "equivalent" and to which it is "mapped." (Chapters 5, 35)

Cultural lag The gap between technologic advances and the ability of society to control and work with them. (Chapter 1)

Current procedural code (CPT-4) Test codes recognized by the American Medical Association and required for filing claims and billing of Medicare. (Chapter 24)

Current procedural terminology codes Systematic five-digit codes maintained and copyrighted by the American Medical Association, defining medical procedures or services and required for filing claims and billing of Medicare. (Chapters 5, 33, 35, 36, 37, 50)

Custom panel Grouping of several independent codes made available as a single, orderable procedure, usually as an ordering convenience. (Chapter 37)

Data mining A practice in which large organized repositories of information (databases) are examined to extract knowledge. The detailed analysis of data by looking at progressively increasing detail in the data ("drilling down"). Data mining parameters include the following (Chapters 7, 45, 48):

- *Association.* Looking for patterns where one event is connected to another event. (Chapter 7)
- *Classification.* Looking for new patterns (may result in a change in the way the data are organized, but that's okay). (Chapter 7)
- *Clustering.* Finding and visually documenting groups of facts not previously known. (Chapter 7)
- *Forecasting.* Discovering patterns in data that can lead to reasonable predictions about the future. (Chapter 7)
- *Sequence or path analysis.* Looking for patterns where one event leads to another later event. (Chapter 7)

Debt management ratios Measure both the extent to which the firm is financed with borrowing and its likelihood of defaulting on its debt obligations. (Chapter 31)

Decertification Election in which bargaining-unit employees vote to rescind the union's certification as their representative. (Chapter 19)

Decertification requirement Petition for decertification election requires a minimum of 30% of the employees within the bargaining unit. (Chapter 19)

Decision theory The study of how decisions are made and what guides a manager to a good decision. (Chapter 1)

Decontamination A procedure that eliminates or reduces microbial or toxic agents to a safe level with respect to the transmission of infection or other adverse effects. (Chapter 26)

Deductible The amount of medical expense that the insured must pay before the insurer assumes liability for all or part of the remaining cost of the covered service. (Chapter 7)

Deemed authority The approval by the Centers for Medicare and Medicaid Services (CMS), as agent for the federal government, of another organization to represent the government in accrediting clinical laboratories that evaluate human specimens, whether they be hospital laboratories, commercial laboratories, or physician office laboratories. Deemed status is time-limited, so each deemed organization must document that it holds a valid certificate of certification. The standards of each deemed organization must be reviewed and accepted by CMS. (Chapter 43)

Deficit Reduction Act of 1984 Public law that authorized the Medicare clinical laboratory fee schedule and mandated that only the laboratory actually performing the testing, not the physician who ordered the testing, may bill Medicare for the services directly (direct billing requirement). (Chapter 7)

Delegate Appoint someone to act in a particular role. A principal delegates to an agent portions of the principal's authority, the power to perform a service. (Chapter 8)

Delegation Assigning a specific task to an accountable subordinate. (Chapter 2)

Delta check Rule-based method to compare a patient's current test result to previous measurements to check for unexpected differences that might be due to analytical or nonanalytical errors in the testing process. It is also used to compare results of two or more analytes reflecting a particular pathology or organ dysfunction, such as blood urea nitrogen and creatinine, which are both expected to be elevated in renal disease. If only one of the analytes, such as creatinine, is elevated, the elevation would be suggestive of drug interference. On the other hand, an elevation of blood urea nitrogen alone would rule out renal involvement. (Chapters 20, 49)

Demand The relationship between the price and the quantity needed for a particular product or service. Demand is the quantity of goods that the customers are willing to buy at a given price. (Chapter 3)

Depreciation An annual charge of an asset's cost into each year of the asset's useful life, for assets that have a useful life of greater than 1 year. Estimated allowance made in accounting for the decrease in value of a fixed asset through wear, deterioration, or obsolescence during its useful life; may be calculated by different standard methods. (Chapters 31, 41)

Destructive conflict Disagreements that are not addressed or resolved. (Chapter 13)

Diagnosis code Medical diagnoses are assigned a number code from a book titled International Classification of Diseases, Ninth Revision (Clinical Modification) (ICD-9-CM). The ICD-9-CM code refers to the patient's medical diagnosis established after study to be chiefly responsible for causing the patient to receive medical care. (Chapters 5, 33, 36)

Diagnosis-related group (DRG) Classification system developed at Yale University that defines 467 major diagnostic categories and places patients into case types based on the International Classification of Diseases Ninth Revision (Clinical Modification) (ICD-9-CM) code classifications. A classification system that groups patients according to diagnosis, type of treatment, age, and other relevant criteria and is a method of determining payment for hospital services, calculated on a predetermined rate per discharge for inpatient hospital services based on the discharge diagnosis. Under the prospective payment system (PPS), hospitals are paid a set fee for treating patients in a single DRG, regardless of the actual cost of care for the individual. (Chapters 4, 5, 7, 33, 34, 35, 36, 37)

Differential or incremental costs The change in future fixed and/or variable costs projected to result from changes in production methods, costs of inputs, or other events or specific courses of action. (Chapter 41)

Diminishing return When additional volume reaches a point that instruments and people are performing at their maximum throughput, the operational efficiency achieved by economy of scale begins to decline. An infinite number of tests cannot be performed in a finite amount of time and space without ultimately reaching the point of diminishing returns. (Chapter 3)

Direct allocation Allocates costs of each service department directly and only to revenue-producing responsibility centers. (Chapter 31)

Direct billing Medicare mandate that claims for laboratory services be submitted by the laboratory rendering the service and not billed by the provider that ordered the test. (Chapter 7)

Direct cost A cost that can be traced to, or caused by, a particular service, product, segment or activity of the department. Examples are labor and consumables. All costs that are incurred directly as a result of producing test results, e.g., technical, supervisory, and clerical wages; overtime; on-call payments; and chemicals and supplies specifically expended to perform the test. (Chapters 31, 38, 41)

Direct Graduate Medical Education Payment (DGME) Medicare payment to teaching hospitals for costs directly related to training programs, including residents' stipends, faculty supervision costs, and overhead. (Chapter 6)

Direct observation A marketing research technique that yields the fastest and most reliable information about the prospective market segments, customer base, and competition. (Chapter 3)

Directed donor blood Blood that is donated at the request of a potential recipient by a friend or family member and designated for transfusion to that specific recipient. Many people think that this is safer than volunteer, allogeneic blood, though scientific data do not support this notion. (Chapter 5)

Directing Planning specific action and actively overseeing the execution of a plan. (Chapter 2)

Disaster Any incident that interferes with a facility's ability to operate in a normal manner. (Chapter 27)

Disclosure Release, transfer, provision of access to, or divulgence of information by an entity to persons or organizations outside of that entity. (Chapter 5)

Discount rate The rate used to calculate the present value of future cash flows. (Chapter 31)

Disease management A system of coordinated interventions and communications for populations with conditions in which patient self-care efforts are significant. (Chapter 48)

Disinfectant An agent intended to destroy or irreversibly inactivate all microorganisms, but not necessarily their spores, on inanimate surfaces, e.g., work surfaces or medical devices. (Chapter 26)

Disinfection A procedure that kills pathogenic microorganisms but not necessarily their spores. (Chapter 26)

Disproportionate share payment (DSH) Payment to teaching hospitals to offset costs of treating a relatively large proportion of uninsured patients. (Chapter 6)

DNA sequencing A method used to determine the order of base pairs along a stretch of DNA. (Chapter 7)

Downcode The use of a lower-reimbursed test, generally coupled with rebundling, to induce unnecessary utilization. (Chapters 33, 37)

DRG creep Use of a DRG code that provides a higher level of reimbursement than the code that accurately reflects the patient's condition. (Chapter 5)

Due diligence A confidentiality agreement exercised between two competing businesses during discussions related to partnership and joint ventures. (Chapter 3)

Dues Paid by the union members, usually on a monthly basis; with employee signed authorization, can be paid through automatic payroll deduction. (Chapter 19)

Dumb terminals Devices that consist of a monitor and a keyboard and serve solely as a client of the laboratory information system. (Chapter 22)

DWYPYWD A customer service phrase: "do what you promised you would do." (Chapter 3)

Economy of scale The reduction in the cost to produce a unit of product when the level of production increases. (Chapters 3, 7, 29, 41)

Effort The only internal and variable cause to which one can attribute success or failure. It is the variable which, if attributed to success or failure, most often leads to success. (Chapter 10)

Ego The picture of ourselves we want to see. (Chapter 10)

Electrochemiluminescence Luminescence that is produced when a chemical reaction occurs at the surface of an electrode upon application of a voltage potential. (Chapter 49)

Electronic medical record Documentation of the patient care treatment experience in an electronic format. (Chapter 7)

Eligibility/Medicare Part A Federally managed health insurance plan covering Americans over age 65 and Americans under age 65 who have certain disabilities and for most patients with end-stage renal disease (ESRD); established by a 1965 amendment to the Social Security Act. Part A covers hospitalization. (Chapter 33)

Eligibility/Medicare Part B Federally managed health insurance plan covering Americans over age 65 and Americans under age 65 who have certain disabilities and for most patients with end-stage renal disease (ESRD); established by a 1965 amendment to the Social Security Act. Part B provides supplementary coverage for medical service and supplies, including physician services, outpatient services, and certain home healthcare services, as well as diagnostic laboratory tests and services, X rays, and the purchase and rental of durable medical equipment. (Chapter 33)

Emergency A natural or human-caused event that suddenly or significantly disrupts the environment of care, disrupts care and treatment, or changes or increases demands for the organization's services. (Chapter 27)

Employee Assistance Program (EAP) Psychological assessment and brief treatment; considered an employee benefit. (Chapter 16)

End-stage renal disease (ESRD) Terminology used by Medicare to designate beneficiaries having permanent kidney dysfunction and requiring dialysis treatment. (Chapters 5, 33, 34, 35, 36, 37)

Engineering controls Controls (e.g., sharps disposal containers, self-sheathing needles, safer medical devices) that isolate or remove the hazard from the workplace. (Chapter 26)

Entrepreneur A person within a corporation who takes direct responsibility for turning an idea into a profitable finished product through assertive risk taking and innovation. (Chapter 40)

Environmental analysis A thorough and systematic review of the external and internal factors that affect the functioning and performance of the laboratory. (Chapter 2)

EOB, EOMB Explanation of (medical) benefit form. (Chapter 34)

Equal Employment Opportunity Commission (EEOC) The EEOC was established by Title VII of the Civil Rights Act of 1964 and began operating on July 2, 1965. The EEOC enforces the following federal statutes (Chapters 15, 39):

- Section 501 and 505 of the Rehabilitation Act of 1973, as amended, prohibiting employment discrimination against federal employees with disabilities (Chapter 39)

- The Age Discrimination in Employment Act (ADEA) of 1967, as amended, prohibiting employment discrimination against individuals 40 years of age and older (Chapter 39)

- The Civil Rights Act of 1991, providing monetary damages in cases of intentional discrimination and clarifying provisions regarding disparate impact actions (Chapter 39)

- The Equal Pay Act (EPA) of 1963, prohibiting discrimination on the basis of gender in compensation for substantially similar work under similar conditions (Chapter 39)

- Title I and Title V of the Americans with Disabilities Act (ADA) of 1990, prohibiting employment discrimination on the basis of disability in the private sector and state and local governments (Chapter 39)

- Title VII of the Civil Rights Act of 1964, as amended, prohibiting employment discrimination on the basis of race, color, religion, sex, or national origin (Chapter 39)

Equal Employment Opportunity Commission of 1972 Enforces Americans with Disabilities Act (ADA). (Chapter 16)

Equity Claims against, or interests in, the assets of a company, divided into liabilities and owners' equity. (Chapter 31)

Equity financing Results from the sale of stock, and therefore, a portion of the ownership in the company. (Chapter 31)

Ergonomics The science of fitting the job task to the individual in order to reduce exposure to musculoskeletal disorders and repetitive motion injuries. (Chapter 5)

Error Deviation of measured concentration from expected or true value. (Chapter 20)

Evaluative listener A listener who hears the words but makes no attempt to understand the feelings of the speaker. (Chapter 11)

Evidence-based medicine The application of medical data (evidence) that have been analyzed using rigorous criteria for clinical decision making, taking into account patient preferences and the physician's experienced judgment. An approach to the teaching and practice of medicine that utilizes literature review and outcome-based studies of effectiveness and possible harm to patients, rather than tradition or anecdotal experience, to guide diagnostic and treatment interventions. (Chapters 6, 7, 44, 46)

Example All aspects of a leader's observable behavior. It is the one aspect of a leader which people will follow, or won't. (Chapter 10)

Executive Order 11246 of 1965 Created affirmative action programs requiring employers to establish plans to address racial disparities in hiring and promotion. (Chapter 15)

Expense budget The amount of resources that will be required to produce the forecasted activity. (Chapter 31)

Experience rating A method of calculating insurance premiums based on the experience of one group in terms of claims submitted. (Chapter 7)

Expert system A computer program that emulates the decision-making capability of an expert human in a limited area. (Chapter 48)

Explanation of benefits A notice that is sent to beneficiaries after a provider files a claim for Part A or B services under the original Medicare plan to explain what the provider billed for, the Medicare-approved amount, how much Medicare paid, and what the beneficiary must pay. This is being replaced by the Medicare Summary Notice, which sums up all the services (Part A and B) that were provided over a certain period of time, generally monthly. (Chapter 5)

External benchmarking Benchmarking activities that include comparison of the performance of one laboratory with that of its peers. The comparisons may be made through the intermediary of an external organization or by informal arrangement among laboratories. (Chapter 43)

External communication Occurs with entities outside of the organization (e.g., insurance companies, regulatory agencies, accreditation organizations). (Chapter 21)

External disaster An event external to the physical laboratory location that may affect operations by limiting available staff or supplies or changing laboratory workload (e.g., influx of patients, uncommon tests required). Examples include major storms, earthquakes, transportation accidents, or acts of terrorism. (Chapter 27)

External locus of control The belief that the requirement for success exists outside people in the form of luck, fate, other people, or task difficulty. (Chapter 10)

External sources of conflict Issues and concerns in the environment. (Chapter 13)

Facilitation The process of assisting participants to move through material in a logical and structured way. (Chapter 2)

Facility A healthcare organization (hospital, clinic, physician's office) that includes an on-site laboratory. (Chapter 27)

Failure A necessary step on the road to success. (Chapter 10)

Featherbedding Union having employees paid for work not actually performed. (Chapter 19)

Feature Characteristic of your product or service that adds value or benefit to the end user. (Chapter 3)

Fee for service (FFS) The method of reimbursing providers a fee for each unit of service provided rather than by capitation, case rate, or per-diem payment. Payment may be based on a percentage of charges or an agreed-upon fee schedule. (Chapters 7, 40)

Fee schedule Listing of the prices charged for tests by an outreach laboratory in fee-for-service situations, i.e., in billing individuals who are nonpatients of the laboratory or its parent institution or in billing clients representing nonpatients. (Chapter 41)

Fiscal intermediary A primary third-party contractor with the Centers for Medicare and Medicaid Services that administers Part A payments according to the local medical review policies for hospitals and rehabilitation and skilled-care facilities. (Chapters 5, 33, 36)

Fiscal polices Use of taxation and government spending as a means of controlling the economy. (Chapter 3)

Fiscal year The year on which the general ledger is based. It can be different from the calendar year. The fiscal year used by a firm is usually based on the norm of the industry to which it belongs. (Chapter 31)

Fixed assets The items of physical property (equipment, buildings and/or land) owned by a business or other entity; also known as tangible or nonliquid assets. (Chapter 41)

Fixed budget A budget in which the budgeted amounts do not fluctuate with the volume. (Chapter 31)

Fixed costs Costs that remain constant in total regardless of changes in the level of activity, e.g., supervisory and custodial wages and benefits required regardless of volume, building maintenance and utilities, and depreciation. Fixed costs are only fixed in relation to the given time period and are only fixed within a relevant range of activity. (Chapters 31, 38, 41, 42)

Fixed rate The negotiated payment rate for a service or group of services linked to a diagnosis code or procedure that is paid either prospectively or retrospectively. (Chapter 7)

Flexible budget A budget in which the variable portion of the budget fluctuates with the level of volume. (Chapter 31)

Food and Drug Administration (FDA) One of the administrative components of the Department of Health and Human Services of the federal government. The FDA regulates the laboratory instruments, reagents, and systems provided by the medical device industry. The FDA also regulates blood and blood products and can inspect laboratory blood banks and donor centers. Responsible for the oversight of commercial tests and for their approval and licensure for use in clinical health laboratories. The FDA Modernization Act of 1997 (PL 105-115) affirmed FDA's public health protection role and defined the agency's mission as follows (Chapters 4, 5, 24, 39):

- As determined to be appropriate by the Secretary, to carry out paragraphs (1) through (3) in consultation with experts in science, medicine, and public health and in cooperation with consumers, users, manufacturers, importers, packers, distributors, and retailers of regulated products

  1. To participate through appropriate processes with representatives of other countries to reduce the burden of regulation, harmonize regulatory requirements, and achieve appropriate reciprocal arrangements
  2. To promote the public health by promptly and efficiently reviewing clinical research and taking appropriate action on the marketing of regulated products in a timely manner
  3. With respect to such products, to protect the public health by ensuring that foods are safe, wholesome, sanitary, and properly labeled; human and veterinary drugs are safe and effective; there is reasonable assurance of the safety and effectiveness of devices intended for human use; cosmetics are safe and properly labeled; and public health and safety are protected from electronic product radiation

Food and Drug Administration clearance Failure to have Food and Drug Administration clearance or approval for a particular test is generally justification for claim denial. (Chapter 36)

Forced distribution Rater distributes a certain percent of employees in each category (e.g., outstanding, above average, average, below average, unsatisfactory). (Chapter 16)

Formal channels of communication Communication networks designed to follow the structure (lines of authority) of the organization. (Chapter 11)

Fraud The intentional deception or misrepresentation that an individual knows, or should know, to be false, or does not believe to be true, and makes, knowing that the deception could result in some unauthorized benefit to himself or some other person(s). (Chapter 5)

Fraud and abuse Fraud is purposely billing for services that were not rendered or billing for a service that has a higher reimbursement than the service actually performed or provided. Abuse occurs when payment is accepted for items or services that are billed by mistake by providers but should not have been paid by Medicare. This is not the same as fraud. (Chapters 5, 37)

Fraud and abuse provisions Portions of the Medicare and Medicaid regulations pertaining to definitions of prohibited laboratory business practices, such as physician self-referral, and other forms of inducement and conflict of interest. (Chapter 41)

Full-time employee (FTE) A measure of the workforce. Part-time employees are counted as fractions of an FTE. Generally, FTEs are calculated by dividing total paid hours by 2,080 (52 weeks of 40 h each). (Chapters 4, 17, 23, 31, 38, 42, 43)

Full-time workers Workers who usually work 35 h or more per week at their sole or main job. (Chapter 19)

Fund accounting A form of accounting in which revenues and expenses must always be equal and expenses are stopped when revenue is exhausted. (Chapter 31)

Future costs Anticipatable costs that potentially can be affected by current budget and capital-acquisition decisions and thus represent the most appropriate focus of planning. (Chapter 41)

Future value (FV) The amount to which a given amount of cash will grow at the end of a given period of time when compounded at a given rate of interest. (Chapter 31)

GainManagement GainManagement in the laboratory has three major elements: LabPlanning (GainPlanning), LabMaking (GainMaking), and LabSharing (GainSharing). (Chapter 25)

GainSharing A financial plan in which improved group productivity determines the amount of money that is shared among the company, investors, and members of the group. (Chapter 18)

Gap analysis A study of the differences between systems, procedures, or applications, often for the purpose of determining how to get from the current state to a new state. The analysis defines the space between where we are and where we want to be, bridging the gap. (Chapter 7)

Gap filling Method used to detemine payment for medical services when no comparable, existing test code is available. A new code is deemed novel and not adequately described by an existing code. Payments are set by individual contractors based on existing charges, and these payments are then used to subsequently set a national limitation amount (NLA). (Chapters 5, 35)

Gatekeeper The primary care provider (PCP) responsible for managing the healthcare of a health maintenance organization (HMO) enrollee. (Chapter 7)

Gaussian distribution A random distribution of values described by their average and variance (standard deviation); used to described analytical imprecision. (Chapter 20)

Gene therapy The introduction of therapeutic genes into cells to treat or cure disease. (Chapter 7)

General competencies Six domains of competency adopted by the ABMS and ACGME as requisite for physicians: patient care, medical knowledge, interpersonal and communication skills, professionalism, practice-based learning, and systems-based practice. (Chapter 6)

General ledger The system that records all accounting activity. (Chapter 31)

General Professional Education of the Physician and College Preparation for Medicine AAMC project panel charged with developing improved educational strategies. (Chapter 6)

General rule of supply The production of a good or service increases when the price goes up and decreases when the price goes down. (Chapter 3)

Generalist One trained in multiple areas of the laboratory. (Chapter 17)

Generally accepted accounting principles (GAAP) A widely recognized set of standard accounting procedures and definitions, which are used to compare one firm's financial statements with other firms' statements. (Chapters 31, 41)

Genotype All or part of the genetic constitution of an individual. (Chapter 7)

Germicide A general term for an agent that kills pathogenic microorganisms on inanimate surfaces. (Chapter 26)

Give-get-merge-go model A communications model used to resolve conflict. (Chapter 13)

Global economy In a global economy, businesses are forced to shift from being multinational (a national company with foreign subsidiaries) to being transnational (where there is one economic unit, the world). (Chapter 3)

Goal An outcome that the organization hopes to attain. (Chapter 2)

Goal congruence The degree to which team (or group) members' individual goals coincide with the team's (or group's) goals. (Chapter 18)

Goal setting The process by which team and/or individual goals are determined, communicated, and agreed upon. (Chapter 18)

Goals Specific, measurable, attainable, relevant, and timed (SMART) providers of direction. (Chapter 10)

Good faith bargaining To bargain collectively is the performance of the mutual obligation of the employer and the representative of the employees to meet at reasonable times and confer in good faith with respect to wages, hours, and other terms and conditions of employment, or the negotiation of an agreement or any question arising thereunder, and the execution of a written contract incorporating any agreement reached if requested by either party, but such obligation does not compel either party to agree to a proposal or require the making of a concession. (Chapter 19)

Graduate medical education (GME) Specialty or subspecialty training occurring after medical school. (Chapter 6)

Graphic rating scales A quality or characteristic rated by choosing a point along a horizontal axis. The scale may be discrete (1-2-3-4-5, excellent-good-fair-poor-unacceptable) or continuous. (Chapter 16)

Graphical user interface (GUI) A "picture-oriented" paradigm for using software applications that depends on use of a pointing device (e.g., a mouse) rather than on key strokes for issuing commands. (Chapter 22)

Grievance Allegation, typically by a union or bargaining unit employee, that the employer has acted improperly, usually by violating a provision(s) of the collective bargaining agreement. (Chapter 19)

Gross revenue Gross revenue is derived by multiplying the volume or quantity of services used by the unit price for the service. Gross revenue is the actual billed charges or fees for products and services before applying any adjustment for contractual arrangements for volume discounts, third-party limits of allowance, or direct and indirect expenses. (Chapter 3)

Gross revenue or gross billed revenue The amount of gross income that would theoretically result if a hospital or laboratory could bill and collect all its charges from all its payors. (Chapter 41)

Group effectiveness The sum of the group member's individual capabilities, plus process gain, minus process loss. (Chapter 18)

Group practice without walls When two or more physician groups share the costs of a lease for an office space. Each group has assigned days of the week for use of the space. This time-sharing business arrangement enables physician groups to expand their service area and eliminates the duplication of lease expenses for the entire month. (Chapter 7)

Group process The way groups get things done, including communication patterns, decision-making methods and techniques, leader behavior and interaction, power dynamics, conflict resolution methods and techniques, and the way members interact with each other. (Chapter 18)

Group purchasing organization A large group of users banding together to increase their purchasing power and lower procurement costs. (Chapter 25)

Guidebook A book that provides comprehensive information about the laboratory and its operations, policies (including forms), testing, specimen preparation, result reporting, billing, staff, and licensure. (Chapter 42)

Halo effect Appraiser gives all employees an acceptable rating, regardless of their performance. When an employee is outstanding in one area, an evaluator ignores performance problems in other areas. Opposite of the "pitchfork effect." (Chapter 16)

Hard disk A peripheral device, also known as a "disk drive," "hard drive," or "hard disk drive," that stores and provides ready access to large amounts of recorded data. (Chapter 22)

Hawthorne effect The proven, positive effect that attention and feelings of importance have on production. (Chapter 10)

Hazardous material A substance or material that has been determined by the U.S. Department of Transportation to pose an unreasonable risk to health, safety, and property when transported in commerce. (Chapter 27)

Hazmat Team Group of individuals who are trained to respond to and clean up hazardous material spills. (Chapter 27)

HCFA-1450 The basic form prescribed by the Medicare program for claim submission for all facility billing, except for the professional component of physician services. Also known as CMS-1450 or UB-92. (Chapter 5)

HCFA-1500 Claim form authorized by the Health Care Financing Administration (now CMS) for filing Medicare Part B claims with carriers (*see* CMS-1500). (Chapters 5, 33, 36)

Health Care Financing Administration (HCFA) Now renamed Centers for Medicare and Medicaid Services (CMS); the Federal agency within the Department of Health and Human Services with primary responsibility for payment and payment standards for the Medicare and Medicaid programs. (Chapters 5, 46)

Health information Any information, whether oral or recorded, in any form or medium, that is created or received, and that relates to the past, present, or future physical or mental health or condition of a patient or the past, present, or future payment for the provision of healthcare to a patient. (Chapter 5)

Health Insurance Portability and Accountability Act of 1996 (HIPAA) Title I protects health insurance coverage for workers and their families when they change or lose their jobs. Title II requires the Department of Health and Human Services to establish national standards for electronic healthcare transactions and national identifiers for providers, health plans, and employers. It also addresses the security and privacy of health data. Adopting these standards will improve the efficiency and effectiveness of the nation's healthcare system by encouraging the widespread use of electronic data interchange in healthcare. (Chapters 5, 6, 33, 36, 37, 42, 46)

Health level 7 (HL-7) Near-universal standard adopted for healthcare information management. The HL-7 domain is limited to clinical and administrative data; specifications identify the appropriate location and sequence of data elements in messages between healthcare information systems. (Chapter 22)

Health Maintenance Organization (HMO) A prepaid system of healthcare with emphasis on the prevention and early detection of disease and on continuity of care. HMOs generally offer a package of services; however, the choice of physician is frequently limited to those working within the HMO. (Chapters 34, 35)

Health Resources and Services Administration Agency of the U.S. Department of Health and Human Services charged with ensuring access to quality healthcare for uninsured and low-income populations. (Chapter 6)

Healthcare Benchmarking System International (HBSI) HBSI is a benchmarking tool used by many healthcare facilities to compare specific departmental operations, including the laboratory, to other similar healthcare facilities. (Chapter 4)

Healthcare Common Procedural Coding System (HCPCS) A medical code set that identifies healthcare procedures, equipment, and supplies for claim submission purposes. (Chapter 5)

- HCPCS procedure modifier codes can be used with all three levels, with the WA to ZY range used for locally assigned procedure modifiers.
- Level I codes contain numeric CPT codes which are maintained by the American Medical Association.
- Level II codes contain alphanumeric codes used to identify various items and services to supplement services that are not included in the CPT medical code set. These are maintained by CMS, the Blue Cross and Blue Shield Association, and the Hospital Insurance Association of America.
- Level III codes contain alphanumeric codes that are assigned by Medicaid state agencies and local Medicare intermediaries to identify additional items and services not included in level I or II. These are usually called local codes and must have "W," "X," "Y," or "Z" in the first position.

Healthcare Employer Data Information Set Monitors for effectiveness of healthcare under various payor plans. (Chapter 38)

Healthcare Integrity and Protection Data Bank National data collection program mandated by the Health Insurance Portability and Accountability Act of 1996 (HIPAA) to combat fraud and abuse in healthcare delivery. Collects and discloses adverse actions against practitioners, including civil judgments, criminal convictions, injunctions, federal or state licensing and certification actions, and other adjudicated actions. (Chapter 6)

Healthplan Employer Data and Information Set (HEDIS) A survey methodology developed by the National Committee for Quality Assurance (NCQA) that standardizes the quality performance data the managed care organizations provide to NCQA. HEDIS allows NCQA to compare managed care organizations and issue report cards on the quality of services they offer. (Chapter 7)

Heterogeneous immunoassays Immunoassays with multiple separation or washing steps, in contrast to homogeneous immunoassays, where no separation steps are involved. (Chapter 49)

Hierarchy A group of individuals organized or classified according to rank or authority. (Chapter 21)

Hierarchy of needs Defined by Maslow, from the most basic to the highest level, these are needs that must be addressed to motivate the employee. (Chapter 1)

Historical costs Costs incurred by a business in the form of payments that are accounted for and recorded at the time of actual cash outlay (also known as sunk costs). (Chapter 41)

Hospital information system (HIS) This term usually refers to a hospital computer system and its support personnel. Total hospital computer system that is often linked to the laboratory information system or a third-party order-entry system. (Chapters 4, 22)

Human relations movement An approach to management, focusing on the worker and his individual needs. (Chapter 1)

Hunger Strong desire or craving. Some hungers may be genetic, such as the strong desire to take another breath. Other hungers may have a cultural source, such as the craving for music. (Chapter 9)

Hygiene factors Tangible, physiological factors whose absence causes employee dissatisfaction but whose presence does not create satisfaction (e.g., salary, working conditions, benefits). (Chapter 10)

Image analysis An evaluation of the customer's beliefs, ideas, and impressions of an organization. (Chapter 39)

Impasse A deadlock in negotiating between management and union over terms and conditions of employment. According to the National Labor Relations Board, whether an impasse in bargaining exists "is a matter of judgment" and depends on such factors as "bargaining history, the good faith of the parties in negotiations, the length of the negotiations, the importance of the issue or issues as to which there is disagreement, the contemporaneous understanding of the parties as to the state of negotiations." (Chapter 19)

Impedance The resistance offered by nonconducting cells in blood suspended in an electrolyte as they pass through the aperture of a hematology analyzer. (Chapter 49)

Imprecision Analytical variance, usually expressed as the standard deviation or coefficient of variation ([standard deviation/mean] $\times$ 100). (Chapter 20)

Imputed costs Costs incurred by a business in any form that does not involve actual outlay of cash, such as opportunity costs, depreciation, etc., which are not explicitly listed in accounting records but must be derived by calculation. (Chapter 41)

Income statement Reports the financial results of a firm's operations over a period of time. (Chapters 31, 38)

Incremental budgeting Uses prior year results as a basis for building the current year budget. (Chapter 31)

Independent Provider Association (IPA) An independent association of multiple healthcare providers organized to negotiate contracts with an insurer for the provision of healthcare services within a specified service area at a negotiated cap rate or fee schedule. (Chapter 3)

Indirect cost All expenses that cannot be directly assigned to a billable test but contribute to the production of a test and the provision of an adequate work environment. Examples are lease or rental contracts, maintenance contracts, maintenance for physical plant, utilities, etc. (Chapters 31, 38)

Indirect costs (or overhead) All general laboratory costs not easily or directly traceable to the production of individual test results but included in total laboratory operating expense, e.g., depreciation; building and equipment maintenance; insurance; utilities; housekeeping; and costs associated with purchasing and billing services, sales, marketing, and development. (Chapter 41)

Indirect Graduate Medical Education payment (IME) Medicare payment to teaching hospitals to compensate for higher costs related to severity of patient illness. (Chapter 6)

Indirect provider Under the HIPAA regulations, an indirect provider is an entity or individual (e.g., laboratory or pathologist) without a direct treatment relationship to a patient. The indirect provider delivers healthcare based on the orders of another provider and typically provides services or reports the diagnosis or results to another provider. (Chapter 46)

Individual The person (adult, emancipated minor, or legal representative) who is the subject of the protected health information. (Chapter 5)

Individually identifiable health information Certain health information that identifies the individual or provides a reasonable basis to identify the individual. (Chapter 5)

Inducement Offering incentives to nonfederal payors to encourage them to also submit federal program testing; violation of the Stark legislation. (Chapter 37)

Industry analysis An evaluation of an industry that recognizes unique factors within the industry that have an impact on the survival of an organization. It includes barriers to entry, determinants of supplier power, determinants of substitution threat, determinants of buyer power, price sensitivity, and rivalry determinants. (Chapter 39)

Industry Connectivity Consortium A group that has developed engineering standards for electronic communication between POCT devices. (Chapter 23)

Infectious waste Waste containing or assumed to contain pathogens of sufficient virulence and quantity that exposure to the waste by a susceptible host may result in a communicable disease. (Chapter 26)

Inflation The result of increases in the price of goods that reduce the consumer's purchasing power (Chapter 3). Effective relative increase in the amount of money in circulation, resulting in a fall in its value and a rise in prices over time. (Chapter 41)

Informal channels of communication Informal routes that people use to spread information to one another. (Chapter 11)

Information revolution in laboratory medicine A change in laboratory services that includes tasks related to gathering, distributing, and adding value to the information provided by clinical laboratories. (Chapter 47)

Inherent reasonableness CMS may employ "reasonable charge methodology" to arbitrarily reduce or increase a national limitation amount (NLA) deemed grossly excessive or grossly deficient. (Chapter 35)

Inside-out approach A product development strategy that develops the product first and then identifies the market. (Chapter 3)

Institute of Medicine (IOM) Private, nongovernmental organization, associated with the National Academy of Sciences, whose mission is to advance science and healthcare policy. (Chapter 6)

Institutional Review Board (IRB) Reviews research proposals and monitors human research conducted in healthcare organizations. Required for healthcare organizations receiving federal funding for such research. (Chapter 6)

Instrument interface A hardware and software connection between a server and a laboratory instrument that facilitates communication between the two. (Chapter 22)

Integrated delivery system A system that is formed when payors and healthcare providers (including acute-care providers, physicians, home healthcare agencies, nursing homes, primary care offices and others) combine forces to extend their service lines to improve the coordination and quality of care while controlling costs. (Chapter 3)

Interdepartmental communication Occurs between the laboratory and other organizational departments, clients, and healthcare providers. Tends to be structured and formal. (Chapter 21)

Interest rate The amount charged by lending institutions for the use of the money borrowed by a firm. (Chapter 31)

Interference One or more specimen constituents that cause bias by affecting the analytical method. (Chapter 20)

Internal benchmarking Benchmarking activities within an organization, usually by tracking the performance of a laboratory over time. (Chapter 43)

Internal disaster An internal event within the laboratory or facility that affects patient care and facility operation, including power failure, hazardous chemical spill, fire, or lack of personnel. (Chapter 27)

Internal locus of control The belief that the ingredients needed to succeed exist within people in the form of effort, persistence, intelligence, energy, and/or talent. (Chapter 10)

Internal rate of return (IRR) The rate that equates the present value of a project's expected cash inflows to the present value of the project's costs. (Chapter 31)

Internal sources of conflict Issues and concerns within the individual. (Chapter 13)

International Air Transport Association (IATA) A body of the commercial airline industry that governs international aviation. Publishes *Technical Instructions for the Safe Transport of Dangerous Goods by Air* and regulates dangerous goods for member airlines and anyone who tenders dangerous goods to those airlines. (Chapter 26)

International Classification of Diseases, Ninth Revision (ICD-9) A medical code set maintained by the World Health Organization (WHO). ICD-9 classifies morbidity and mortality information for statistical purposes and for the indexing of hospital records by disease and operations for data storage and retrieval. (Chapter 5)

International Classification of Diseases, Ninth Revision, Clinical Modification (ICD-9-CM) The American Medical Association's ICD-9-CM is based on the official version of the World Health Organization's ICD-9. The term "clinical" is used to emphasize the modification's intent: to serve as a useful tool to classify morbidity data for indexing medical records, medical care review, and ambulatory and other medical care programs, as well as for basic health statistics. To describe the clinical picture of the patient, the codes must be more precise than those needed only for statistical groupings and trend analysis. ICD-9-CM is totally compatible with ICD-9, thus meeting the need for comparability of morbidity and mortality statistics at the international level. (Chapters 5, 39)

International Classification of Diseases, Version 10, Procedure Coding System (ICD-10-PCS) Laboratory coding system intended for use as an alternative to current procedural terminology (CPT) codes. (Chapters 33, 35, 36)

International Organization for Standardization (ISO) International organization that establishes common voluntary standards for manufacturing, trade and communications. ISO standards previously applied to manufacturing are now being applied to blood manufacturing. (Chapter 5)

Interview A two-way discussion between employee and manager about employee's performance (*inter* "between"; *view* "look"). (Chapter 16)

Intradepartmental communication Occurs within the laboratory between management, sections or divisions, and work shifts. Tends to be informal. (Chapter 21)

Intrinsic motivation A redundancy, because all motivation is intrinsic. All motivation is internal. All motivation is a fire within. (Chapter 10)

Intuitive decisions Utilization of hunches, subjective values, and personal or emotional factors in deciding what actions to take. (Chapter 1)

Job description Written delineation of the title, duties, responsibilities, and reporting relationships of a position and the requisite qualifications needed to meet these. (Chapter 15)

Job enrichment The deliberate upgrading of responsibility, scope, and challenge as they apply to a position, title, or employee. (Chapter 10)

Job order costing *See* Bottom-up microcosting. (Chapter 41)

Joint Commission on the Accreditation of Healthcare Organizations (JCAHO) JCAHO evaluates and accredits nearly 17,000 healthcare organizations and programs in the United States. An independent, not-for-profit organization, JCAHO is the nation's predominant standards-setting and accrediting body in healthcare. JCAHO's evaluation and accreditation services are provided for the following types of organizations (Chapters 4, 5, 6, 16, 23, 39):

- Ambulatory-care providers, for example, outpatient surgery facilities, rehabilitation centers, infusion centers, and group practices, as well as office-based surgery

- Assisted-living facilities that provide or coordinate personal services, 24-hour supervision and assistance (scheduled and unscheduled), activities, and health-related services

- Behavioral healthcare organizations, including those that provide mental health and addiction services, and services to persons with developmental disabilities of various ages, in various organized service settings

- Clinical laboratories, including independent or freestanding laboratories, blood transfusion and donor centers, and public health laboratories

- Critical access hospitals

- General, psychiatric, children's, and rehabilitation hospitals

- Healthcare networks, including managed-care plans, preferred-provider organizations, integrated delivery networks, and managed behavioral healthcare

- Home-care organizations, including those that provide home health services, personal care and support services, home infusion and other pharmacy services, durable medical equipment services, and hospice services

- Nursing homes and other long-term-care facilities, including subacute-care programs, dementia special-care programs and long-term-care pharmacies

Joint venture Term used to describe management agreements, partnerships, strategic laboratory arrangements, or conglomerates formed to share risk or expertise. (Chapter 3)

Judgmental decisions Conclusions reached after data are gathered, facts are analyzed, and concrete examples are explored. (Chapter 1)

Kanban A Japanese system that monitors production line, inventory, consumer demand, and feedback to deliver goods and services just in time (8). (Chapter 7)

Key results area An aspect of a job on which employees must concentrate time and attention to ensure that they achieve the goal for that job. Forces manager to focus only on those activities that add value. Although this concept is motivational, staff may be slow to accept. (Chapter 16)

Kickback The provision of any item of value in exchange for referral of federal business to a laboratory. (Chapter 37)

Knowledge support (clinical decision support) Computer software that is able to present key factual information in such a way that it speeds or enhances the accuracy of a clinical decision. (Chapter 48)

Knowledge work Work that begins with data analysis and the use of personal intellectual capital and includes consultation with other clinical service providers. (Chapter 47)

Knowledge workers Those who fulfill expanded roles by gathering, distributing, and adding value to information. (Chapter 47)

LabMaking The process of involving all employees in a structured process with the goal of making continuous performance improvements. (Chapter 25)

Labor laws, agency (Chapter 19):

- 1935, National Labor Relations Act (Wagner Act): federal law passed in 1935; gives employees the right to organize, select their representative(s), and bargain with the employer regarding wages, hours, and working conditions; established the authority of the National Labor Relations Board.

- 1947, Labor-Management Relations Act (Taft-Hartley Act): federal law passed in 1947; amended National Labor Relations Act and established the authority of the Federal Mediation and Conciliation Service.

- 1954, Labor-Management Reporting and Disclosure Act (Landrum-Griffin Act): designed to close loopholes in the Taft-Hartley Act pertaining to internal union affairs and provides amendments to the National Labor Relations Act.

- 1974, Amendments to the NLRA: provides NLRA notice requirements in the healthcare industry.

- 1978, Civil Service Reform Act: established the Federal Labor Relations Authority (FLRA) for administration of federal sector labor relations.

- Federal Mediation and Conciliation Service (FMCS): federal agency that provides mediation services to labor and management to resolve bargaining impasse situations or to assist in securing arbitrators.

Laboratory A facility that provides services including specimen collection, testing, and results reporting. (Chapter 27)

Laboratory file (LF) The laboratory information system counterpart to the master patient index; contains patient demographics and information about laboratory tests ordered and resulted. (Chapter 22)

Laboratory information services (or system) (LIS) This term usually refers to a laboratory computer system and its support personnel. (Chapter 4)

Laboratory information system (LIS) A computer system used to report laboratory test results. A large number of commercial systems are available. Most can be interfaced directly with instruments to facilitate test result reporting and to minimize the need for manual data entry. Some systems have added functionality such as order entry. (Chapters 22, 44)

Laboratory Management Index Program The LMIP is a benchmarking tool managed by the College of American Pathologists (CAP). It allows a clinical laboratory to compare its operational effectiveness to that of other similar laboratories using ratios from operational management data. (Chapter 4)

Laboratory medicine Virtually synonymous with "clinical pathology," with the exception that the term is more commonly used when referring to academic medical centers as opposed to community hospitals. (Chapter 50)

Laboratory network A system (formal or informal) of clinical laboratories spread over a geographical area to provide laboratory services in a coordinated, integrated manner. A laboratory network can include commercial laboratories. (Chapter 4)

Laboratory supervisor Individual responsible for staffing and scheduling the laboratory. (Chapter 17)

Laboratory utilization The frequency with which laboratory tests are ordered and performed. (Chapter 50)

LabPlanning The work managers do to lead and focus the laboratory on continuous gains and to organize for a high level of employee involvement. (Chapter 25)

LabSharing The process of sharing laboratory and organizational gains as overall or specific performance measures improve. (Chapter 25)

Latex allergy Allergic reaction associated with latex glove use. The two types of allergic reactions are contact dermatitis (type IV delayed hypersensitivity), due to chemicals used in processing latex, and the more serious immunoglobulin E/histamine-mediated allergy (immediate or type I hypersensitivity), due to latex proteins. (Chapter 26)

Law of demand As the price for a product or service increases, the demand for the product decreases. (Chapter 3)

Leadership Influencing others to attain group, organizational, and societal goals. The activity of mobilizing employees to tackle tough problems, the problems that often require an evolution of values. Generally, any employee in the organization can exercise leadership, but the actions of those with authority in the organization can inadvertently discourage employees from exercising leadership. Alternatively, those with authority can exercise leadership by mobilizing employees generally to exercise their own leadership. (Chapters 1, 8, 9)

Leadership legitimacy The degree to which a team or group leader is accepted by both the team or group members and the employing organization. (Chapter 18)

Lease A written agreement or contract by which one party (the lessor) gives to another (the lessee) the use and possession of property for a specified time (the term) and for fixed payments. (Chapter 41)

Length of stay (LOS) The number of days a patient is hospitalized from admission to discharge for a specific diagnosis. This metric has been used by managed-care organizations to compare institutions and their utilization of services. (Chapters 3, 6)

Leukoreduction The process of reducing the number of leukocytes in a unit of blood to $<5 \times 10^6$. Leukoreduction decreases the risk of febrile, nonhemolytic transfusion reactions, cytomegalovirus transmission, and development of alloantibodies to HLA antigens in transfusion recipients. (Chapter 5)

Liabilities (and liability accounts) Represent the debts or obligations owed to outsiders. (Chapter 31)

Liaison Committee on Medical Education (LCME) Accrediting authority for U.S. and Canadian medical schools. (Chapter 6)

Ligase chain reaction A DNA sequence amplification reaction using thermostable DNA ligase. (Chapter 7)

Liquidity ratios Measure the firm's ability to meet its immediate obligations; thus, the relationship between a firm's current assets and its current liabilities. (Chapter 31)

List price The price of a test listed in a laboratory's fee schedule and representing the nominal price charged to its fee-for-service clients (nonpatients and clients representing nonpatients). The actual price is typically negotiated to include a discount off of the fee schedule list price. (Chapter 41)

Local area network (LAN) A group of several computers or workstations that are connected to a server. The server manages client use of software applications and often serves as a repository for the networked client's data. The LAN enables client workstations without storage capabilities to be operational at a much lower cost than for full-fledged, stand-alone workstations. (Chapter 22)

Local medical review policies (LMRPs) Local policies outline how contractors will review claims to ensure that they meet Medicare coverage requirements. CMS requires that LMRPs be consistent with national guidance (although they can be more detailed or specific), that they be developed with scientific evidence and clinical practice, and that they be developed through certain specified federal guidelines. Contractor Medical Directors develop these policies. (Chapters 5, 39)

Lockout Employer closes the business or dismisses employees in order to deny current employees access to the workplace. (Chapter 19)

Locum tenens A position, usually temporary, for a healthcare professional often in an underserved area. (Chapter 6)

Locus of control The location of the events, traits, circumstances, or people that determine someone's success or failure. (Chapter 10)

Logical Observation Identifier Names and Codes (LOINC) LOINC is considered a universal laboratory language which is based on the systematic breakdown of the components of a service into more specific units, ultimately creating a highly standardized, typically seven-digit, number, with each possible result from a procedure being mapped to a specific code. Unlike CPT, LOINC is publicly available and can be used with no license fee. It is widely used by commercial laboratories to track specific procedures from order to result. (Chapter 33)

Long-term debt The firm's obligations that are due more than a year later. (Chapter 31)

Lookback A process in which blood product recipients are notified of possible transmission of human immunodeficiency virus or hepatitis C virus by a unit that tested negative at the time of donation. The blood donor subsequently tested positive for one of these viruses, creating concern that the unit could have contained virus not detectable by the original test. (Chapter 6)

Loss leader A test sold to a client at a price discounted below cost in order to meet an overall service need or provide "one-stop shopping." Note that it is not legal to loss-lead entire accounts, but only individual tests within an account. *See also* Predatory pricing *and* Fraud and abuse provisions. (Chapters 35, 41)

Macrocost analysis Analysis of costs by breaking down overall budgetary costs. (Chapter 23)

Macroeconomics Macroeconomics examines the interaction of income, employment, and inflation on the economy as a whole. (Chapter 3)

Manageable components A parameter over which a manager has control. Scheduling and use of overtime are manageable. Vacation time and work breaks are defined by government or the institution and are thus not manageable (although the number of employees eligible for these benefits may be). (Chapter 30)

Managed-care organization (MCO) An organization formed by a third-party insurer as an alternative healthcare delivery system in an attempt to control the escalating costs of healthcare to large employer groups and the government. An organization that provides medical insurance to beneficiaries within a framework that manages patients' access to certain healthcare services with the goal of providing care at a lower cost. The amount of healthcare coverage varies from one MCO to another depending on the program and fee paid by the client (patient). (Chapters 3, 4, 40)

Management Getting things done through other people. The act or practice of supervision and control. (Chapters 1, 8, 9)

Management by objectives Setting goals for the individual to achieve, dovetailing with larger organizational objectives. (Chapter 1)

Management by walking about (MBWA) A process that promotes informal communication between managers and employees. (Chapter 21)

Management reporting A process of communicating actual versus budgeted performance throughout the organization to identify necessary corrective actions and help make decisions. (Chapter 31)

Management science Management techniques based on mathematic models. (Chapter 1)

Management's rights clause Contract clause in a bargaining agreement that states that anything not covered in the contract remains within the purview of management. (Chapter 19)

Mapping The method used to determine the chromosomal location of a gene. (Chapter 7)

Marginal cost The change in total cost relative to the change in volume, i.e., the cost of producing one more unit of service; incremental cost. (Chapters 31, 41)

Marginal listener One who hears the words but does not comprehend the intent. (Chapter 11)

Market potential The total anticipated revenue potential for volume of services during a defined period. (Chapter 3)

Market price The actual price at which a commodity is commonly purchased. (Chapter 3)

Market research A marketing strategy utilized by companies to identify the need for new products and services in new and existing markets. (Chapter 3)

Market segment A portion of the market where consumers share a group of common characteristics. (Chapter 39)

Market share The estimate of the share of the specific market or territory that you expect to capture. (Chapter 3)

Market surveys Market surveys are techniques typically used to obtain valuable market information, for example, direct mail surveys, telephone surveys (telemarketing), and personal interviews. (Chapter 3)

Marketing Determining the customers' needs and wants. (Chapter 39)

Maslow's other theory The theory that the more influence and power you give to someone else, the more you have for yourself. (Chapter 10)

Master patient index (MPI) Contains data related to current and past patients who receive medical care from the system. Usually contained in the hospital information system. (Chapter 22)

Material Safety Data Sheet (MSDS) Provides detailed information about hazards and protective measures relative to hazardous chemical substances. (Chapter 26)

Matrix Total constituents of the specimen that may affect the analytical process. (Chapter 20)

Maximum allowable error (MAE) Amount of error associated with an analytical method that can be tolerated without invalidating the medical usefulness of the result. (Chapter 20)

Mean Arithmetic average of a set of values. (Chapter 20)

Medicaid Program established under Title XIX of the Social Security Act, which provides health insurance to the impoverished; the state and federal governments fund it jointly. (Chapters 5, 33, 36, 40)

Medical Laboratory Technician (MLT) An MLT can perform general tests under the supervision of a Clinical Laboratory Scientist (CLS). (Chapter 4)

Medical necessity Services that are "covered, reasonable and necessary for the beneficiary, given his or her clinical condition" (P. Talbee, HHS Office of Inspector General's Compliance Program Guidance for Clinical Laboratories, 1998). The determination of ICD-9-CM codes for which a CPT code will be reimbursed as reasonable and necessary. (Chapters 33, 36, 37, 42)

Medical School Objectives Project (MSOP) Association of American Medical Colleges (AAMC) project to examine learning objectives and assessment methods in medical education. (Chapter 6)

Medical Technician Also known as Clinical Laboratory Technician; a person with an associate's degree in Medical Laboratory Technology (or equivalent). (Chapter 17)

Medical Technologist Also known as Clinical Laboratory Technologist; a person with a bachelor's degree in Medical Technology or in a selected health science and who has completed a 1-year practicum. (Chapter 17)

Medical usefulness limits Quality control limits derived from clinical application of results rather than statistical imprecision of the method. (Chapter 20)

Medically necessary Services or supplies that are proper and needed for the diagnosis or treatment of a medical condition; are provided for the diagnosis, direct care, and treatment of a medical condition; meet the standards of good medical practice in the local area; and are not mainly for the convenience of the beneficiary or the provider. (Chapter 5)

Medicare Federally managed health insurance plan covering Americans over age 65 and Americans under age 65 who have certain disabilities and for most patients with end-stage renal disease; established by a 1965 amendment to the Social Security Act. (Chapters 33, 36, 40)

Medicare Part A Part A is the hospital insurance portion of Medicare. Medicare was established by §1811 of Title XVIII of the Social Security Act of 1965, as amended, and covers inpatient hospital care, skilled-nursing-facility care, some home health agency services, and hospice care. (Chapter 5)

Medicare Part B Part B is the portion of Medicare insurance that pays for physician services and covered outpatient services, also referred to as supplemental medical insurance. It was established by §1831 of Title XVIII of the Social Security Act of 1965, as amended, and covers services of physicians or other suppliers, outpatient care, medical equipment and supplies, and other medical services not covered by Part A of Medicare. (Chapter 5)

Medicare Payment Advisory Commission Independent advisory group assessing physician workforce and graduate medical education funding. (Chapter 6)

Medicare secondary payor (MSP) A Medicare provider, whether a physician, nonphysician practitioner, laboratory, or other supplier (durable medical equipment supplier, etc.), is required to indicate if there is other insurance that may be primary to Medicare when submitting a Medicare claim for payment. The purpose of this questionnaire is to determine whether Medicare or the other insurance has primary responsibility for meeting the beneficiary's healthcare costs. The goal of these MSP information-gathering activities is to identify MSP situations rapidly, thus ensuring correct primary and secondary payments by the responsible parties. Information that is collected from the patient to determine when Medicare is not the primary payor. (Chapters 5, 39, 42)

Meeting When two or more people come together to discuss something; usually implies a face-to-face meeting but could be a telephone or electronic meeting; examples are departmental or staff meeting, committee or task force meeting, and training meeting. (Chapter 12)

Metrics Specific, quantifiable measurements used as an indicator of progress. (Chapter 2)

Microcost analysis Analysis of costs by adding up costs for performing an individual test. (Chapter 23)

Microcosting Calculating the unit costs of test production to account for each and every category of expense involved at the laboratory's current test volume; performed in either a bottom-up or top-down fashion. (Chapter 41)

Microeconomics Economic information that focuses on individual behavior and the interaction of companies. (Chapter 3)

Miniaturization The use of smaller and smaller "micro" components, which allows the number of analytes in a device to increase, replacing larger analyzers. This facilitates point-of-care testing (POCT). (Chapter 6)

Minutes An official record of the meeting of an organization. (Chapter 12)

Mission statement A written statement that clearly defines what the organization does and why it is important. (Chapter 2)

Mixed costs Costs that are somewhat, though not totally, dependent on volume, i.e., are difficult to classify definitively as either fixed or variable, e.g., clerical staff. (Chapter 41)

Model Laboratory Compliance Program (MLCP) A statement of expectations published by the Centers for Medicare and Medicaid Services (CMS) for laboratories to use as a model for behavior. (Chapter 42)

Modifier Modifiers are composed of two-digit numbers which are attached to a specific code prior to the billing process. They are "used to indicate that a service or procedure has been altered by some specific circumstance but not changed in its definition or code." (Chapters 33, 36, 37)

Modular automation A process in which only certain components of laboratory work flow or laboratory functions are automated. This process allows the flexibility to add additional automated modules as workload requirements increase and future automation can be cost justified. (Chapter 49)

Moment of truth The moment when a business recognizes that the customer has developed an impression or perception about their products and services and the organization through encounters that happen over time. (Chapter 3)

Monetary policies Policies related to the management of the money supply and the market rates of interest. (Chapter 3)

Monitoring devices Devices that are attached directly to a patient and that provide periodic or continuous measurements. (Chapter 23)

Motivation An inner force that causes behavior; a fire from within. Inspiration or stimulation to perform in a desired way or to achieve a desired result. (Chapters 2, 10)

Motivators Internal factors that relate to the nature of work and the egos of employees. If properly addressed, these factors can create employee satisfaction (e.g., recognition, appreciation, self-actualization). (Chapter 10)

Myth Inaccurate information perceived as truth by major administrative decision makers. (Chapter 40)

Myth of motivation A long-lived, often believed falsehood that people can motivate other people. (Chapter 10)

Narrative rating Includes concise, specific illustrations. Easy to construct, but subjective and difficult to compare employees' ratings. (Chapter 16)

National Accrediting Agency for Clinical Laboratory Sciences (NAACLS) An international agency responsible for accrediting educational programs in the clinical laboratory sciences and related healthcare fields. (Chapter 4)

National Correct Coding Initiative (NCCI) Review of procedure codes to determine if two or more different codes are appropriately ordered on the same date of service. This service was initiated in 1996 through a contract with a Medicare contractor, AdminaStar Federal. These edits are available on the Centers for Medicare and Medicaid Services (CMS) website. (Chapters 36, 37)

National Coverage Decisions (Determinations) (NCDs) National coverage policies developed by CMS that indicate whether and under what circumstances certain services are covered under the Medicare program. They are published in CMS regulations, published in the *Federal Register* as a final notice, contained in a CMS ruling, or issued as a program instruction. An NCD sets forth whether Medicare will cover, or not cover, specific services, procedures, or technologies on a national basis. Medicare contractors are required to follow NCDs. If an NCD does not specifically exclude an indication or circumstance, or if the item or service is not mentioned at all in an NCD or in a Medicare manual, it is up to the Medicare contractor to make the coverage decision (*see* Local medical review policies). (Chapters 5, 39)

National Limitation Amount (NLA) The national fee cap for a particular test. (Chapter 35)

National Patient Safety Foundation Nonprofit organization whose mission is to improve patient safety in the delivery of healthcare. (Chapter 6)

National Practitioner Data Bank Established through Title IV of Public Law 99-660, the Health Care Quality Improvement Act of 1986, to collect reports regarding medical malpractice payments, adverse licensure actions, clinical privilege actions, and professional society membership actions against healthcare practitioners. Restricts the ability of practitioners to move from state to state without disclosure of adverse actions or incompetent performance. (Chapter 6)

National Technical Information Service Publishes the NCCI procedure code edit documents on a quarterly basis. (Chapter 36)

Natural credit balance accounts General ledger accounts that have negative balances as established by GAAP rules. (Chapter 31)

Natural debit balance accounts General ledger accounts that have positive balances as established by GAAP rules. (Chapter 31)

NCCI edits National Correct Coding Initiative edits fall into two major categories, (i) comprehensive/component, and (ii) mutually exclusive. Edits indicate the code pairs in these edit categories for which a modifier (generally -59) may be appropriate. (Chapter 36)

NCCLS Voluntary consensus standards-developing organization disseminating standards and guidelines to the healthcare community (especially laboratory practice); previously known as the National Committee for Clinical Laboratory Standards. (Chapters 17, 23)

Need Something required for performance. Different goals of performance may require different resources, different environments, and different attitudes. (Chapter 9)

Neg Reg Negotiated Rulemaking Committee for diagnostic clinical laboratory tests. (Chapters 33, 36)

Negative language Words or phrases used to communicate thoughts and feelings by using excessive criticism and confrontation. (Chapter 11)

Negative predictive value Probability that a negative result indicates absence of disease. (Chapter 24)

Negotiated rule making The process of federal agency representatives and other special interest groups convening to negotiate the text of a proposed rule. (Chapter 5)

Net contribution margin For all hospital inpatient and outpatient testing, the total net test revenue generated by the laboratory, minus the total cost of test production (both direct and laboratory-related indirect) for which the laboratory is responsible, constitutes its contribution to the hospital's bottom line. (Chapter 41)

Net present value (NPV) The present value of all the cash flows created by a project minus the dollar amount of the initial investment in it (also known as the time value of money associated with the investment). The present value of future net cash flows, discounted at the cost of capital. (Chapters 31, 41)

Net profit For all true outreach nonpatient testing, the total net revenue generated by the laboratory, minus the total cost of test production (direct and indirect) for which the laboratory is responsible, constitutes the laboratory's profit. (Chapter 41)

Net revenue Gross revenue minus contractual allowances and sales discounts is net revenue. (Chapter 3)

Net revenue or net collected revenue The amount either the hospital or the outreach program actually gets paid for a given test is equal to the billed amount minus allowances and bad debt. (Chapter 41)

New laboratory model A model that describes the total testing process as an interactive process; the focus is not only on the quality of test data generated (process/analytical) but also on the clinical appropriateness of test requests (input/preanalytical) and the correct interpretation of and response to laboratory information (output/postanalytical). (Chapter 47)

New style of leadership Noticing in real time the effects that you have on the quality in an organization. From this view, anyone in the organization can exercise "leadership" by mobilizing employees to tackle tough problems. But the actions and words of those with authority and power can discourage the "leadership" of others without intending that result. (Chapters 8, 9)

New variant Creutzfeldt-Jakob disease A disease of the central nervous system, transmitted through a conformational protein change, transmitted by eating by-products of infected cows. (Chapter 5)

Niagara syndrome The condition affecting all people whose life or work suffers from a lack of direction. (Chapter 10)

Noncontrollable costs Costs outside the scope of a specific individual's control. (Chapter 41)

Noncovered service A service that does not meet the requirements of a Medicare benefit category, is statutorily excluded from coverage on other grounds, or is deemed not reasonable and necessary. (Chapter 5)

Nonlistener A person who does not hear anything that is said. (Chapter 11)

Nonproductive FTE Commonly used to describe those personnel who are not involved directly in generation of test results. This category includes supervisory personnel, support personnel (marketing, customer service, washroom, etc.), and the portion of line personnel devoted to activities such as quality control and maintenance. (Chapter 43)

Nonproductive time Paid time for non-job-related activities such as vacation, holidays, and sick time. (Chapter 31)

Nonprogrammed decisions Unusual or atypical situational solutions. (Chapter 1)

Nonstaff physicians Physicians that are not part of the hospital medical staff. (Chapter 42)

Normal range *See* Reference range. (Chapter 20)

Norms Informal behaviors which are generally acceptable in a workplace. (Chapter 16)

No-solicitation rule Rule instituted by management in order to prevent solicitation of employees for union membership at the workplace. Rules that are too broad are often found to be invalid by the National Labor Relations Board and the courts. (Chapter 19)

No-strike, no-lockout clause During the life of the contract, a clause in which the union agrees not to strike and management agrees not to lock employees out or keep them from reporting to work. (Chapter 19)

Not medically necessary The determination that an ICD-9-CM code does not justify payment for a service. (Chapters 33, 36)

Not-for-profits Companies whose primary purpose is something other than generating a profit. Typical not-for-profits are hospitals and charitable organizations. These organizations may make more money than they spend (excess revenue over costs), but there are no shareholders to receive that money, which instead may be donated or reinvested in the business. (Chapters 31, 38)

Notice of proposed rule making The document that describes and explains a regulation that the federal government proposes to adopt at some future date and invites interested parties to submit comments related to it. These comments can then be used in developing a final regulation. (Chapter 5)

Nucleic acid testing (NAT) Testing that relies on measuring specific sequences of nucleic acid. Amplifying genetic material to detect the smallest amount of a substance. This allows earlier detection of infectious agents and malignancy recurrence. (Chapters 5, 6)

Nutrition Balancing hungers and needs. (Chapter 9)

Objective A specific aim directed toward achieving a goal. (Chapter 2)

Occupational exposure Reasonably anticipated skin, eye, mucous membrane, or parenteral contact with a hazard that may result from the performance of an employee's duties. (Chapter 26)

Office for Protection from Research Risks (OPRR) Section of the Department of Health and Human Services now known as the Office for Human Research Protections. (Chapter 6)

Office of Safety and Health Administration (OSHA) The mission of OSHA is to save lives, prevent injuries, and protect the health of America's workers. OSHA and its state partners have approximately 2,100 inspectors, plus complaint discrimination investigators, engineers, physicians, educators, standards writers, and other technical and support personnel spread over more than 200 offices throughout the country. This staff establishes protective standards, enforces those standards, and reaches out to employers and employees through technical assistance and consultation programs. (Chapter 39)

Office of the Inspector General (OIG) The mission of the OIG, as mandated by Public Law 95-452 (as amended), is to protect the integrity of Department of Health and Human Services programs, as well as the health and welfare of the beneficiaries of those programs. The OIG has a responsibility to report to the Secretary and the Congress program and management problems and recommendations to correct them. The OIG's duties are carried out through a nationwide network of audits, investigations, inspections, and other mission-related functions performed by OIG components. (Chapters 5, 39)

Old style of leadership Expecting to build sufficient power, expertise, and reputation so that people will see the wisdom in your decisions. (Chapters 8, 9)

Omnibus Reconciliation Act (OBRA) of 1989 Prohibits physicians from referring laboratory testing for Medicare beneficiaries to a laboratory in which the physician has an ownership interest. Also known as the Stark Law. (Chapter 5)

Omnibus Reconciliation Act of 1990 Denies Medicare reimbursement to a laboratory for a test performed off-site unless at least 70% of the tests for which the laboratory receives requests and submits claims are performed on-site. Also known as the "shell lab" act. (Chapter 5)

Operating budget The financial plan for managers with direct responsibility for managing the operations of a responsibility center(s). The operating budget is made up of a statistical budget, a revenue budget, and an expense budget. (Chapter 31)

Operating lease A lease that can be canceled during its term and that typically does not include an option to purchase. It is accounted as a form of operating expense. (Chapter 41)

Operating system (OS) The software that makes a computer operational. The OS prompts users (or peripheral devices) for input and/or commands, takes actions, and then reports back the results of these actions. It stores and manages data and oversees the sequence of software and hardware operations. (Chapter 22)

Operational assessment An evaluation of the organization's ability to provide the types and levels of services defined by prior market needs. (Chapter 39)

Operations management Applied management technique, utilizing mathematic modeling and industrial engineering to promote efficiency and effectiveness. (Chapter 1)

Opportunity costs Imputed costs representing missed opportunity, i.e., the potential financial gain that is missed when a more profitable use of resources (materials, labor, facilities, or capital) is rejected or abandoned in favor of a less profitable one. They are lost revenue, not expenditures, and they represent variable costs whose amounts depend on the alternatives under consideration. (They are related to the concepts of time value of money or net present value, i.e., best use of funds among competing investments.) (Chapter 41)

Organizational chart A diagram that shows hierarchical and authority relationships among functional areas in an organization. Defines the formal lines of reporting and communication. (Chapters 2, 40)

Organizational culture Social and artistic expression characteristic of a community or population that pertains to behavior patterns, arts, beliefs, institutions, and all other products of human work and thought. (Chapter 11)

Organizing The process of structuring resources and activities in a way that promotes the accomplishment of specific activities. (Chapter 2)

Other potentially infectious material (OPIM) Human body fluids including semen; vaginal secretions; urine; cerebrospinal fluid; synovial fluid; pleural fluid; pericardial fluid; peritoneal fluid; amniotic fluid; saliva; body fluids which may be contaminated with blood; unfixed tissue; human immunodeficiency virus- or hepatitis virus-containing cell or organ cultures; blood or tissue from an infected animal; reagents; infectious waste; and cultures. (Chapter 26)

Outcome An outcome is a measured change or event that reflects the status of a patient during a defined period (for example, death, the onset of symptoms, the disappearance of symptoms, discharge, readmission, complications, or diagnosis). (Chapter 7)

Outcome assessment The process of determining whether a particular measure will have a positive clinical, and presumably financial, impact on patient care. (Chapter 38)

Outcome Project Accreditation Council for Graduate Medical Education (ACGME) initiative emphasizing educational outcomes in the accreditation of resident training programs. (Chapter 6)

Outcome research Research that looks at diverse patient groups to determine which medical interventions or diagnostic tests have an effect on patients. (Chapter 6)

Out-of-pocket costs Costs involving immediate expenditures, i.e., incurred as cash outlays occurring at or near the time of purchase; potentially important in capital budgeting. (Chapter 41)

Outpatient prospective payment system (PPS) The method of payment used by Medicare to determine how much Medicare pays and how much the Medicare beneficiary pays for outpatient services at hospitals or community mental health centers under Medicare Part B. Medicare does not pay for all outpatient services under the new PPS begun August 1, 2000 (for example, procedures Medicare considers inpatient procedures, such as fixing a fractured hip). (Chapter 5)

Outreach program Marketing laboratory services to physician offices, nursing homes, and other hospitals. (Chapter 40)

Outside-in approach A frequently utilized product development method that first identifies a need in the marketplace, then develops the product or service to meet the need. (Chapter 3)

Outsourcing Contracting with consultants, reference laboratories, or other clinical laboratories to provide services. (Chapter 17)

Overhead costs Costs that are from non-revenue-generating departments. (Chapter 31)

Overtime Time worked before or after regularly scheduled working hours or pay for such time worked. (Chapter 38)

Owners' equity The ownership claim against the total assets of a company (also called stockholders' equity). (Chapter 31)

"P and L" (profit and loss) responsibility Individual financial accountability for a business or portion of a business implies that all of its costs are controllable, either directly or indirectly, by that individual. (Chapter 41)

Paid hours The number of employee hours actually paid by the laboratory. It includes those hours that were worked and those that are due the employee as part of a benefit package (sick leave, vacations, etc.). (Chapter 43)

Paradigm shift Change from one way of doing things to another; often encompasses a change in an entire concept, model, or standard. (Chapter 14)

Parenteral Piercing mucous membranes or the skin through events such as needlesticks, human bites, and abrasions. (Chapter 26)

Pareto principle (80/20 rule) Used in many industries; states that 80% of an entity's total revenues are produced by 20% of its products. (Chapter 24)

Pareto Principle (Law) A total quality management principle used by W. Edwards Deming that demonstrates that cause and effect are not linearly related; for example, approximately 20% of the causes account for 80% of the effect. (Chapter 3)

Participative selection A process in which team members choose new members of their team based on team-related criteria that were determined and agreed upon prior to candidate identification. (Chapter 18)

Part-time workers Workers who usually work less than 35 h per week at their sole or main job. (Chapter 19)

Path of work flow Combined sequential activities in the laboratory, beginning with the clinician's ability to order a test and culminating in data being generated and reported for use in patient care. (Chapter 24)

Patient service centers Phlebotomy sites or draw stations located off-site in service areas convenient to medical office buildings are referred to as patient service centers. The employees are often cross trained to offer a variety of services including electrocardiograms and chain-of-custody drug abuse screening collections for private industry. (Chapter 3)

Patients Individuals receiving care (and laboratory testing) after being registered and seen in clinic (hospital outpatients), after being registered and admitted to the hospital (hospital inpatients), or as clients of the laboratory's outreach business with no other connection to the hospital per se (hospital nonpatients). (Chapter 41)

Pay it right Pay the right amount to the right provider for the right service to the right beneficiary. (Chapter 37)

Payback period The period of time that a capital investment takes to be completely recovered from its resulting cash flows. (Chapter 41)

Payor Any entity that assumes the risk of paying for medical treatments for an uninsured patient, a self-insured employer, a

health plan, or an HMO. Any third-party insurance company that sells traditional indemnity and managed-care products to group purchasers, large and small employers, and private individuals for healthcare coverage. (Chapters 5, 7)

Payor mix Describes those entities that have fiscal responsibility for payment of services. The distribution of the different forms of healthcare financing in place among the population served by a healthcare provider, e.g., Medicare, Medicaid, private pay, managed care, uninsured, etc. Revenue realized from different types of payors (Chapters 34, 40, 41)

PCR (polymerase chain reaction) A technique for amplifying millions of times a single target DNA sequence using thermostable DNA polymerase so it can be detected and studied more easily. (Chapter 7)

People message A value judgment made by a manager and perceived by staff members as relating to the quality of the staff members themselves. (Chapter 10)

Per diem The negotiated daily reimbursement rate for services provided for inpatient hospital services. The rates are negotiated specific to the type of service rendered (for example, general medical, surgical, or intensive care). (Chapter 7)

Per member per month (PMPM) rate For services provided under a managed-care arrangement, the managed-care organization's per capita payments to the hospital for its members' care. Under such arrangements, laboratory tests are most typically bundled; i.e., there is no separate billing for tests, which are regarded as being reimbursed as part of the overall capitated payment. (Chapter 41)

Performance appraisal A planned, formal, and periodic management activity in which an employee's on-the-job behavior is evaluated to enable salary and promotion decisions, change an employee's behavior, determine competence, improve work skills, identify training needs, and determine progress toward goals and career development. (Chapter 16)

Performance evaluation Feedback regarding current performance on job tasks and responsibilities that is used as a guide for future performance. (Chapter 2)

Performance standards Defined performance expectations that are specific and measurable. (Chapter 16)

Period costs Costs that represent fixed outlays for the whole laboratory or the whole hospital per unit time. (Chapter 41)

Permissible exposure limit (PEL) Maximum allowed exposure during a time-weighted average period (e.g., 8-h workday or 40-h workweek). (Chapter 26)

Personal digital assistant (PDA) A small computer that fits into a shirt pocket. (Chapter 48)

Personal protective equipment (PPE) Equipment or garments used to protect employees from exposure to workplace hazards. (Chapters 5, 26)

Physician hospital organization An organization formed by hospitals and physicians to negotiate managed-care contracts with third-party payors. (Chapter 3)

Physician Office Connectivity System that allows clients access to the laboratory information, usually via the Web. The system should also provide the client the ability to register patients, order tests, and print results. (Chapter 42)

Physician office laboratory (POL) A clinical laboratory operation located on-site in a healthcare provider's office. The testing performed by a physician office laboratory is regulated by the Clinical Laboratory Improvements Amendment and is limited to waived, moderate, or complex test services. A laboratory run by a physician who performs laboratory tests on his or her own patients. (Chapters 3, 4)

Physician-performed microscopy (*see*** Provider-performed microscopy)** Microscopic examinations such as KOH preps and wet preps performed by primary care physicians outside the laboratory setting. (Chapter 23)

Pitchfork effect Poor performance in an isolated instance that adversely affects the employee's assessment. (Chapter 16)

Point-of-care testing (POCT) An industry term used to describe user-friendly instrumentation developed for use in near-patient testing or bedside testing sites versus traditional laboratory sites. Often performed by a nonlaboratorian. POCT is often managed or overseen by clinical laboratory personnel. (Chapters 3, 4, 6, 23, 50)

Point of service A managed-care plan with reduced benefits that allows the enrollee to select services and benefits at the point of service for a network, prepaid plan and an out-of network, fee-for-service (FFS) plan. The out-of-network plan usually carries a copayment that is a percentage of the FFS charges to the health plan. (Chapter 7)

Policies Internally generated rules that set expectations for behaviors within the laboratory. (Chapter 2)

Positive language Words or phrases used to communicate thoughts and feelings by using positive actions and consequences. (Chapter 11)

Positive predictive value (PPV) Probability that a positive result indicates presence of disease. (Chapter 24)

Postanalytic activity Pertaining to the period after the actual testing of a specimen. Includes phases such as reporting of results, storage and retention of specimens and data, and assessment of effect of results on patient outcomes. (Chapter 24)

Postanalytical time Time for labor required to report results, as well as the sorting, filing, and telephoning related to final reports. (Chapter 38)

Potentiometry Measurement of potential that develops at the surface of an electrode, which is measured against a standard reference potential. This principle is the basis for the measurement of hydrogen ion concentration (pH) and pCO_2. (Chapter 49)

Practice guidelines Systematically defined statements to assist practitioner and patient decisions about appropriate healthcare for specific clinical circumstances. (Chapter 6)

Practice management systems Computer systems that handle all the paperwork (both medical charts and organization aspects) in a physician's office. (Chapter 48)

Preanalytic activity Pertaining to period prior to actual testing of specimen. Includes phases such as test selection and implementation, appropriate test utilization, and specimen collection, transport, and storage, as well as test ordering. (Chapter 24)

Preanalytical time Time for specimen collection, work list and label preparation, start-up, sample-cup, and daily quality controls and standards. (Chapter 38)

Predatory pricing Discount of the full fee schedule to a client below the laboratory's cost, and done for the purpose of excluding competition, is unethical and illegal. (Chapter 41)

Preferred provider organization (PPO) A healthcare organization composed of physicians, hospitals, and other providers which provides healthcare services at a reduced fee. In a preferred provider organization, care is paid for as it is received, rather than as a scheduled fee in advance as with an HMO. A healthcare organization that negotiates set rates of reimbursement with participating healthcare providers for services to insured clients; a type of prospective payment system. (Chapters 5, 34)

Present value (PV) The value today of a future cash flow. (Chapter 31)

Present value (PV) or time value of money The dollar amount which, if it were invested now at a given rate of return, would accumulate to a given specified value at a specified time in the future. (Chapter 41)

Price variance The difference between the price of a supply or service versus the price that was budgeted. (Chapter 31)

Primary container A vessel, including its closure, that contains a specimen. (Chapter 26)

Prions Infectious, abnormal host proteins that cause transmissible spongiform encephalopathies and are resistant to a number of standard disinfection and sterilization procedures. (Chapter 26)

Priority Weighing the importance of the tasks at hand to determine which have the highest level of immediate precedence. (Chapter 2)

Probing A sales technique used to gather information and uncover customer needs. An open probe asks a direct question, while a closed probe limits a customer's answers to yes or no and helps to confirm a need. (Chapter 3)

Procedure A prescribed way to carry out an activity. (Chapter 24)

Process Systematic course of definitive actions or activities culminating in a desired end product. (Chapter 24)

Process costing A method of microcosting in which unit costs are estimated from aggregate expenses divided by units of service. Also called top-down microcosting. (Chapter 41)

Process loss (gain) The degree to which group processes inhibit (enhance) the successful completion of group objectives. (Chapter 18)

Product message A value judgment made by a manager that relates to the quality of something produced or accomplished by one or more staff members. (Chapter 10)

Productive FTE Usually employed to define those laboratory workers who actually produce test results. In practice, defining who these individuals (or parts of individuals) are becomes very difficult, and even more difficult to calculate. For instance, do you count those people who enter the specimen into the system or enter results into the information system? (Chapter 43)

Productive time Paid time for job-related activities. (Chapter 31)

Productivity measures Raw numbers or calculations that describe work performed relative to hours worked, tests billed, revenue generated, reagents used, etc. (Chapter 17)

Professional employees Employees meeting the National Labor Relations Act (amended) criteria; generally professionals and nonprofessionals are not included in the same bargaining unit. (Chapter 19)

Profit Earnings above the expenditures for salaries, benefits, and direct and indirect costs. (Chapter 3)

Profitability ratios Ratios that measure the combined effects of liquidity, asset management, and debt management policies on operating results. (Chapters 31, 38)

Program Memoranda National coverage decisions have been updated with technical corrections on a regular basis through Program Memoranda issued by CMS. (Chapter 36)

Progressive discipline Stepwise process to address deficiencies in job-related activities or attitudes. (Chapter 15)

Progressive rates A method used by some health maintenance organizations (HMOs) in which they implement new rates monthly, quarterly, or semiannually when contracting with large employer subscriber groups. (Chapter 7)

Promotion The function of informing, persuading, or otherwise influencing the consumer's buying decision. (Chapter 3)

Proportional systematic error An error that is always in one direction and whose magnitude is a percentage of the concentration of analyte being measured. (Chapter 20)

Prospective payment system (capitated payment) Payment is received prior to the delivery of services. Profit results from care delivered at a total cost below the contract payment; loss results from care delivered at a total cost above the contract payment. (Chapter 33)

Prospective payment system (PPS) A method of reimbursement in which Medicare payment is made based on a predetermined, fixed amount. The payment amount for a particular service is based on the classification of that service (for example, diagnosis-related groups) for inpatient hospital services, enacted by the Social Security Amendments of 1983 (Public Law 98-21). (Chapters 5, 7)

Protected health information (PHI) Individually identifiable health information, transmitted or maintained in any form or medium, which is held by a covered entity or its business associate, identifies the individual or offers a reasonable basis for identification, is created or received by a covered entity or an employer, and relates to a past, present, or future physical or mental condition, provision of healthcare, or payment for healthcare. (Chapter 5)

Protocols A set of prescribed actions that control the way an activity is performed. (Chapter 48)

Provider Any entity (for example, hospital, skilled-nursing facility, home health agency, outpatient physical therapy, comprehensive outpatient rehabilitation facility, end-stage renal disease facility, hospice, physician, nonphysician provider, laboratory, supplier) providing medical services. (Chapter 5)

Provider mix Describes those entities that actually perform and/or bill the services. (Chapter 34)

Provider-performed microscopy (PPM) A category of moderate-complexity tests under CLIA (q.v.) involving a patient care provider using a microscope for testing, such as urine microscopic examinations. (Chapter 28)

Provider-performed microscopy procedures (PPMP) CLIA '88 term for a limited number of moderate-complexity, microscope-based tests that may be performed by a physician, midwife, or nurse practitioner operating under a PPMP certificate. (Chapter 5)

Pull-through The testing that is sent to a laboratory because the client already has to use the laboratory for other testing. Usually associated with a laboratory that has a health maintenance organization (HMO) contract. Clients that have a large volume of testing for that HMO may send the laboratory testing for other patients whose insurance does not require a specific laboratory. (Chapter 42)

Pulse oximetry A portable spectrophotometric device that can be applied to a heel or fingertip to obtain a continuous measurement of oxygen saturation. In principle, two specific wavelengths in the near-infrared region are used, with one wavelength dedicated to the measurement of deoxyhemoglobin while the other wavelength measures all forms of hemoglobin. (Chapter 49)

Purchasers Buying groups, employers, or individuals who purchase healthcare policies from third-party payors (insurers). (Chapter 7)

Q-Probes A program provided by the College of American Pathologists that allows laboratories to collect data regarding laboratory processes and to compare their data with data collected from peer organizations. The data are collected for one time only. (Chapter 44)

Q-Tracks A program provided by the College of American Pathologists that allows laboratories to collect data *through time* regarding laboratory processes and to compare their data with data collected from peer organizations on a quarterly basis. (Chapter 44)

Quality assurance (QA) A process to ensure that all services involved in the delivery of patient care have been accomplished in the appropriate manner that will maintain excellence in medical care. The U.S. Food and Drug Administration defines quality assurance as planned and systematic activities to ensure a laboratory will meet certain requirements for quality (from the FDA website http://www.fda.gov). A systematic approach to continuously analyzing, improving, and reexamining the total testing process. The sum of activities planned and performed to provide confidence that all systems and their elements that influence quality of the product are functioning as expected and relied upon. Systematic approaches to assessing and improving the quality of care within a specific healthcare setting (e.g., a hospital or clinic) or healthcare program. (Chapters 5, 20, 21, 43, 44)

Quality control (QC) A process for monitoring assay performance to detect deviations from expected outcomes. (Chapter 20)

Quality improvement (QI) Involves outcomes, results, ends, and information rather than just concerns with specific processes. Whereas quality assurance is focused on providing a quality test result, QI is concerned with improving the entire process so that the results are more accurate, more timely, and presented in a more useful and informative manner to the clinician. Thus, QI is concerned with all aspects of testing including the preanalytic, analytic, and postanalytic phases. (Chapter 43)

Quality-adjusted life year (QALY) Used as a standardized measure of the quality of life. It is a year of life, adjusted for its quality. The measure takes into account both longevity and the quality of life lived. One year of perfect health is 1.0 QALY. (Chapter 5)

Quantity variance The difference between the amount of inputs (labor and/or supplies) used to produce each unit of service versus the quantity that was budgeted. (Chapter 31)

RACE Acronym describing the appropriate approach by first responders to a fire or disastrous situation: rescue, alarm, confine, evacuate/extinguish. (Chapter 27)

Railroad Retirement Act A federal insurance program similar to Social Security, designed for workers in the railroad industry. The provisions of the Railroad Retirement Act provide for a system of coordination and financial interchange between the Railroad Retirement program and the Social Security program. (Chapter 5)

Random access memory (RAM) The component of a computer in which the operating system, the application software, and the data in current use are stored so that they can be quickly accessed by the central processing unit. Accessing or storing data in RAM is much faster than accessing or storing it on a hard disk, a floppy disk, or a CD-ROM drive, but the data are present in RAM for only as long as the computer is turned on. (Chapter 22)

Random error A variance from expected that is not reproducible or predictable. (Chapter 20)

Ranking system Evaluates employees based on comparison with their peers (e.g., paired comparison, person-to-person comparison). This system does not allow all employees to be ranked as excellent, even if all employees have an excellent work performance. (Chapter 16)

Rating system Compares employee performance to some set of criteria and produces either a number or a letter grade that represents the employee's level of performance (e.g., graphic scale, free form, critical incident, behaviorally anchored scale, checklist of adjectives, forced choice, or distribution). Allows everyone to be rated highly, if they deserve it. (Chapter 16)

Real-time correction An intervention that, based on a comparison of the desired versus actual progress, seeks to cancel the effects of the excessive interventions you have made and to bolster the effects of the interventions you have made that were too weak. One important feature of a real-time correction is holding steady long enough to collect the data and information you need to evaluate actual progress. For example, in driving a car, if you do not hold steady long enough to see what effect you have had, you may oversteer by swinging too much first to the left and then to the right. (Chapter 9)

Reasonable charge methodology Based on inherent reasonableness, authority to arbitrarily increase or decrease payment. (Chapter 36)

Recovery Amount (usually expressed as percentage) of known quantity of an analyte that is measured when added to a specimen. (Chapter 20)

Reference laboratory An on- or off-site laboratory performing tests on behalf of a clinical laboratory or facility, typically including rare or esoteric test menus. (Chapter 27)

Reference range Test results that are within expected parameters for about 95% of all individuals in a defined healthy population. Values outside of the range are classified as abnormal and may be associated with a pathological condition. (Chapter 20)

Referral A recommendation by the primary-care physician that a member receive services from another network provider. It is a notification process and not a review to establish medical necessity. (Chapter 7)

Reflection The actor's careful consideration of the effects that follow from the actor's words and deeds. Reflection is like an instant replay in which the actor can watch, from a wide-angle camera view, the coordination of the actor's deeds with the deeds of others to create the organizational outcome. (Chapter 8)

Reflex test Second related, codable test, performed automatically when initial tests are positive or abnormal (e.g., susceptibility test on pathogen). (Chapters 35, 37)

Reflex testing A process in which a primary test reflective of organ dysfunction or pathology is chosen, and only if that test result is abnormal are additional tests performed to confirm or rule out a diagnosis. A typical example is the use of thyroid-stimulating hormone as a primary thyroid function test. If thyroid-stimulating hormone is abnormal, additional laboratory tests are performed to establish diagnosis. (Chapter 49)

Regionalization A system of laboratories capable of providing services to a larger geographic area. Regional systems allow the aligned laboratories to market the combined strengths of the collective testing menus to keep more tests within the regional system and eliminate referrals outside of the system, positioning the regional laboratory system to compete for managed-care contracts. (Chapter 7)

Regulated waste Liquid or semiliquid blood or other potentially infectious material (OPIM); contaminated items that would release blood or OPIMs in a liquid or semiliquid state if compressed; items that are caked with dried blood or OPIMs and are capable of releasing these materials during handling; contaminated sharps; and pathological and microbiological wastes containing blood or OPIMs. (Chapter 26)

Regulation Legally binding rules developed to implement a statute. (Chapters 34, 36)

Relative value unit (RVU) Workload units accounted under any of several weighting systems devised and implemented by professional organizations to account for a labor component involving significant professional time spent on cognitive interpretative tasks in the production of certain test results, like surgical pathology reports, in order to equitably bill for them. The laboratory costs associated with these billables can be accounted as cost per RVU. (Chapter 41)

Repertoire The collection of tested problem-solving procedures that the organization is prepared and competent to perform. (Chapter 8)

Represented by unions Employees who may or may not be union members, but whose jobs are part of a bargaining unit represented by a union. (Chapter 19)

Required rate of return Known as the hurdle rate or cost of capital, it represents the minimum return on investment a firm requires on capital expenditures. (Chapter 31)

Resistance to change Force active in groups and individuals that limits the amount of change that occurs. (Chapter 14)

Resource utilization group Payment for services rendered to a Medicare beneficiary in a skilled bed of a nursing home facility; also known as consolidated billing. (Chapter 5)

Resource-based relative value scale A scale of national uniform relative values for all physicians' services. The relative value of each service must be the sum of relative value units representing physicians' work, practice expenses, net of malpractice expenses, and cost of professional liability insurance. (Chapter 5)

Resource-based relative value system A system of reimbursement that reimburses providers for the true cost or value of the services they provide. True cost and value are determined using a formula that multiplies a relative value unit by a monetary conversion factor. The relative value unit rates the value of the actual cost of the service based on a physician cost component (work), a practice cost component (overhead), and a malpractice cost component. The cost-based approach more closely approximates a normal, competitive market than charge-based systems. (Chapter 7)

Responsibility The state or fact of being accountable. Generally, people exercise leadership when they have a feeling of personal responsibility for improving quality in the organization. (Chapter 8)

Responsibility When given, responsibility is a visible, active expression of trust. When accepted, it is the true source of power. (Chapter 10)

Restriction fragment length polymorphism (RFLP) Variations in the base sequence of a short DNA segment are the basis for the formation of RFLPs. Restriction enzymes that cleave DNA at a specific sequence can be used to uncover RFLPs. The name RFLP derives from the fact that fragments of various lengths are obtained on electrophoresis depending on whether the polymorphism was within or outside the restriction enzyme cleavage site. RFLPs can be used to type microbial organisms. (Chapter 49)

Restructuring Tactical measures used in laboratory consolidation include downsizing, point-of-care testing, consolidating work at benches, and interdisciplinary teams on utilization. (Chapter 7)

Results-based evaluations (RBEs) Evaluations performed by managers who focus on attainment of specific, measurable results. (Chapter 16)

Return on investment (ROI) The tangible and intangible returns received from an investment, minus the fixed, variable, and capital expenditures for the venture. Calculation (involving a variety of different methods) of a specified payback amount (also known as the required rate of return, or discount rate) on a given investment. ROI analysis shows how much profit (or loss) will be made on an investment (usually capital dollars) for laboratory equipment, projects, or programs. (Chapters 3, 4, 41)

Revenue Actual or expected cash inflow due to the outreach program's major business. (Chapter 40)

Revenue budget The revenue that will be generated by the forecasted activity for a responsibility center. (Chapters 31, 38)

Revenue code Uniform Bill 92 requires submission of a "revenue code." This code is used to identify specific accommodation charges, ancillary service charge, or a type of billing calculation. Revenue codes are maintained by the National Uniform Billing Committee. (Chapter 5)

Revenue cycle Sequence of events that the provider must monitor to maximize the amount and timeliness of payment from payors. (Chapter 40)

Risk The chance or possibility of loss. (Chapters 5, 6)

Risk management A process to identify, reduce, and eliminate exposure to risk that results in financial loss. (Chapter 5)

Risk pool A portion of provider fees or capitation payments that are withheld as financial reserves to cover unanticipated utilization of services. (Chapter 7)

Risk sharing The process of establishing financial arrangements, utilization controls, and other mechanisms to share the financial risks of providing care among providers, payors, and users. (Chapter 7)

Robotics Computerized, mechanical equipment that automates specimen handling and delivery to automated laboratory analyzers. (Chapter 4)

Role The character or part played by an actor. Each adult person has experienced at least playing the role of child. In addition, many adults have experienced playing the role of mother or father. (Chapter 8)

Root cause analysis Team based problem-solving tool used to determine how or why something happened. Asking "why?" five times or using cause-and-effect diagrams are common methods employed. (Chapter 5)

Rotation Movement of personnel through the tasks for which they have been trained, often on a regular, sequential basis. (Chapter 30)

Rule of 78 A formula used in sales projections based on the premise that a new account sold in the first month of the fiscal year will add revenue for 12 months, while an account brought on board in the second month will only add revenue for 11 months, and so on. The sum of 12 + 11 + 10 + 9 + 8 + 7 + 6 + 5 + 4 + 3 + 2 + 1 is 78. (Chapter 3)

Sample Part of specimen that is measured. (Chapter 20)

Sanctioned physicians Physicians who have been barred from billing Medicare, Medicaid, or other government payors, usually for compliance/billing issues. Other providers and persons can also be barred from the government programs. (Chapter 42)

Sanctions Administrative remedies and actions (for example, exclusion, civil monetary penalties) available to the Office of the Inspector General to deal with questionable, improper, or abusive behaviors of providers under the Medicare, Medicaid, or any state health programs. (Chapter 5)

Satellite laboratory A laboratory separated from the main laboratory, usually with a limited test menu, that is dedicated to a specific set of patients and locations in a medical facility. (Chapter 4)

Secondary container A vessel into which the primary container is placed for transport within an institution; will contain a specimen if the primary container breaks or leaks in transit. (Chapter 26)

Secondary payor Another healthcare plan that provides coverage on the balance after payment by the primary payor. (Chapter 34)

Self The actor that can take on many different roles, including mother, father, child, manager, or employee. (Chapter 8)

Semistructured interview An applicant interview using both prepared and "spur-of-the-moment" questions. (Chapter 15)

Semivariable costs Costs that include both variable and fixed-cost elements. (Chapter 31)

Send-out test Procedure not performed in any of the hospital's clinical laboratories and which, therefore, must be sent to another laboratory to be assayed. (Chapter 40)

Sensitivity Ability of test to detect a condition ([number with condition testing positive/number having the condition who are tested] $\times$ 100 = percent sensitivity). (Chapter 24)

Sensitivity analysis A method for testing premises used in decision making, i.e., determining the sensitivity of conclusions derived from calculation to the ranges of numerical values chosen as inputs with substitution of the change in one variable at a time to determine their effects (also known as what-if calculations or best- and worst-case scenarios). (Chapter 41)

Sensitivity, analytical The lowest detection limit of an assay; sometimes measured as the concentration of an analyte that can be differentiated from a blank within a 95% confidence interval. (Chapter 20)

Server A computer that has software applications installed for use by members of a local or wide area network. It also can serve as a repository for data generated by other computers or workstations on the network. (Chapter 22)

Service costs Costs that are incurred as tests are performed, representing variable costs plus those fixed costs that are most directly traceable to the testing, and related to the concept of cash flow. (Chapter 41)

Service levels Test menu, results reporting, and ancillary assistance provided by the laboratory to hospitals, clinics, physicians, and patients. (Chapter 27)

Sharps container A container approved for the containment and transport of contaminated sharps. (Chapter 26)

"Shell lab" provisions Portion of federal fraud and abuse regulations dictating an effective upper limit for the portion of a laboratory's volume (30%) that can be sent out to another laboratory. (Chapter 41)

Short-term exposure limit Maximum exposure to a hazardous substance allowed at one time (normally measured in a single 15-min period). (Chapter 26)

Situational analysis Description of the major features in a local environment which impact an organization and includes a background, current activity, normal forecast, market description, and product review. (Chapter 39)

Situational management Acting only on what needs to be addressed at that moment and recognizing that there is no best way to get a job done. (Chapter 1)

Six Sigma A highly disciplined process focusing on developing and delivering near-perfect products and services. An approach to improving quality that involves measuring defects or adverse events against "sigma," a common measure of variation. The goal is to reduce sigma to a minimum. This approach could be viewed as a variation on internal benchmarking. (Chapters 1, 43)

Skill mix The mixture of personnel with varying degrees of training, education, and certification. Examples include laboratory technicians, medical laboratory technicians, and medical laboratory technologists. The nature of the work will define the required proportion of workers of each background. (Chapters 30, 43)

Social Security Act of 1967 Provided for healthcare benefits for "the diagnosis of treatment of illness or injury or to improve the functioning of a malformed body part" in the elderly and, subsequently, in disabled individuals. (Chapter 36)

Specialist One trained and experienced in one specific laboratory discipline; formally, one who has a minimum of 5 years' experience in that discipline and has passed a qualifying examination for that discipline by an accepted accrediting organization. (Chapter 17)

Specificity Ability of test to define a true condition ([number without condition testing negative/total number without condition who are tested] $\times$ 100 = percent specificity). (Chapter 24)

Specificity, analytical The ability of an analytical method to determine solely the component(s) it purports to measure. (Chapter 20)

Standard Material of known or assigned concentration used for assay calibration. (Chapter 20)

Standard cost A measure of how much an item should cost, rather than a record of how much it actually did. (Chapter 31)

Standard deviation A statistic that describes the amount of variance of a set of measurements about the mean value. It is used to describe random error of an analytical method. (Chapter 20)

Standard operating procedure (SOP) Organizational approved protocol that defines step-by-step instructions for all staff to follow when performing a particular test or activity to ensure a consistent and accurate result or outcome. A written set of instructions that codify technical and administrative activity in the laboratory. (Chapters 2, 16)

Standard Precautions Set of precautions applied to all patients; designed to reduce risk of transmission of microorganisms in the healthcare setting. (Chapter 26)

Standard transaction The transmission of any health information in electronic form in connection with a transaction. (Chapter 5)

Standards of conduct Standards should promote commitment to the accurate, ethical, and legal practice of laboratory medicine. (Chapter 37)

Stark I Amendment A federal law prohibiting physicians from referring a Medicare patient to an entity for the furnishing of laboratory services if the physician, or the physician's immediate family member, has a direct or indirect financial interest in the entity providing the laboratory services. (Chapter 5)

Stark II Amendment An extension of the Stark I Amendment that prohibits physicians from referring Medicare and Medicaid patients for certain types of services known as "designated health services" to entities if the physician, or the physician's immediate family member, has a direct or indirect financial interest in the entity. (Chapter 5)

Stark legislation (regulations) The Stark legislation prohibits a physician from referring his or her patients to entities with which the physician or his or her family members have a financial relationship, such as an ownership interest or compensation arrangement. Designed to ensure that laboratories provide services to ordering providers without any evidence of inducement or kickback. The initial Stark legislation, known as Stark I, was enacted in 1989 and applies only to clinical laboratory services. In 1993, Congress enacted the Stark II legislation, which extends the prohibition to referrals made by a physician to an entity for the furnishing of "certain designated health care services" if the physician or his or her family member has a financial relationship with that entity. (Chapters 35, 39, 46)

Statistical budget The forecast of activity for a responsibility center. (Chapter 31)

Statute A law passed by the U.S. Congress or a state legislature. (Chapters 34, 36)

Step-down allocation Distributes the costs of the service departments providing the most services to all departments. All remaining service departments' costs are then allocated in descending order determined by the amount of service they render. (Chapter 31)

Step-fixed costs Costs that are fixed over a range of activity and are then increased when activity levels go up. (Chapter 31)

Sterilant An agent intended to destroy all microorganisms (viruses, vegetative bacteria, fungi, and a large number of highly resistant bacterial endospores) on inanimate surfaces. (Chapter 26)

Sterilization A procedure that effectively kills all microbial life, including bacterial spores, on inanimate surfaces. (Chapter 26)

Steward Individual within a union who serves as the union's counterpart of the employer's manager or supervisor. (Chapter 19)

Stockholder equity accounts Represent the difference between a firm's assets and liabilities (claims against assets). The accounts are reported on the balance sheet and have natural credit balances. (Chapter 31)

Stop-loss A provision within a health plan that limits the members' or providers' out-of-pocket expense to a maximum allowance. (Chapter 7)

Straddling The attempt to execute several distinct business strategies or to hold several strategic positions at once. (Chapter 29)

Straight-line depreciation Standard accounting method of calculating depreciation of fixed assets that involves equal weighting of time periods. (Chapter 41)

Strategic alliance/partnership An arrangement that enables companies to combine their resources to share risks, reduce cost, and solidify customer and supplier relationships. (Chapter 3)

Strategic decision Focus on an organization's relationship with the external environment, competitive posture, and major policies. (Chapter 1)

Strategic plan Documentation of a process which develops the organization's future goals and programs within the context of a changing industrial and market environment. The plan includes a mission statement, goal development, strategy formulation, and control procedures. (Chapter 39)

Strategic planning A methodical and structured process whereby an organization defines its mission, identifies directions, develops a unified approach, prioritizes long- and short-term goals, assigns accountabilities, and allocates financial resources. An organized process for developing a business strategy. (Chapters 2, 29)

Strategic position Serving a particular set of customers or meeting a defined set of needs, usually in a manner that is unique. (Chapter 29)

Strategy An artful means to a defined objective or goal. The technique, approach, or mechanics developed by the management team in order to facilitate the organization's ability to perform successfully. Quest for sustainable competitive advantage by means of analysis of industry structure and competitors, identification of a strategic position, and adoption of business practices that defend that position. (Chapters 2, 3, 29)

Structured interview An applicant interview in which all of the interviewer's questions are prepared in advance. (Chapter 15)

Style The personal details and mannerisms that an actor adds to the text and stage directions. Within a modern organization, the actor must invent even the text and stage directions for doing the job. Furthermore, for anyone who attempts leadership—mobilizing employees to tackle the tough problems in the organization—there may be controversies over what the "job" is. Accordingly, leadership is mainly "style," the personal details and mannerisms that a responsible person invents and adds to the routine of the organization. (Chapter 8)

Substantially in excess Defined as 120% of the average charge to all payors for each test. (Chapter 37)

Sum of the years' digits (SYD) method Standard accounting method of calculating depreciation of fixed assets that involves unequal weighting of time periods. (Chapter 41)

Sunk costs *See* Historical costs. (Chapter 41)

Supply The quantity of goods and services that a company is willing to produce and sell at a specific price. (Chapter 3)

SWOT analysis A careful consideration of the laboratory's *s*trengths, *w*eaknesses, *o*pportunities, and *t*hreats. In most analyses, strengths and weaknesses are internal to the organization, while opportunities and threats derive externally. See Chapter 2 for a detailed description. (Chapters 2, 3, 39)

Tactical decision Steps toward the implementation of organizational strategy. (Chapter 1)

Target market The market segment(s) chosen by the organization to focus on. (Chapter 39)

Task interdependence The degree to which a task's progression or completion is influenced by, determined by, or subject to the progression or completion of one or more other tasks. (Chapter 18)

Tax Equity and Fiscal Responsibility Act of 1982 Public Law 97-248, which established payment for inpatient stays for Medicare beneficiaries based on diagnosis-related groups and introduced the clinical laboratory competitive bidding demonstration project. (Chapter 7)

Taylorism and scientific management An approach to work and the workplace where every job is divided into the smallest possible segments and each segment is examined and improved. (Chapter 1)

Technical problem A problem that *does* subside to satisfy the current values in the society when management applies the best-known methods and procedures. (Chapter 8)

Technical solution An intervention plan that includes (i) a fixed statement of the problem and (ii) fixed standards for success defined before the intervention was made. (Chapter 8)

Technical work The physical and mental effort that applies known methods for achieving a goal. (Chapter 8)

Telecommunication Voice, video, or data information is transmitted from one location to another using integrated services, digital networks, phone lines, T1 (fiber optic) lines, or digital subscriber lines or various forms of wireless communications. (Chapter 7)

Telemarketing A market research technique employed by representatives using a predefined list of questions to gather vital information on the market potential. The survey, conducted by telephone, is directed to a specific staff member in a prospect's office. (Chapter 3)

Telemedicine The practice of medicine using telecommunication technology to transmit data, sound, and images between two or more distant sites. (Chapter 7)

Telepathology The practice of pathology using telecommunication technology to link patients with pathologists and other healthcare providers. (Chapter 7)

Testing FTE *See* Productive FTE. (Chapter 43)

Theory X and theory Y Defined by McGregor, a theory highlighting the difference between those who believe that people need to be forced to work and those who believe that people want to work. (Chapter 1)

Third-party administrator An entity required to make or responsible for making payment on behalf of a group health plan. An unrelated third-party entity that administers and pays claims for multiple small insurers in a geographic region. (Chapters 3, 5)

360-Degree evaluations Multilevel assessment adopted by AT&T, IBM, and other Fortune 500 corporations. May be used to identify how a manager is viewed by his or her supervisor, peers, subordinates, and customers. Full-circle feedback. (Chapter 16)

Time value of money A concept that recognizes that a dollar of cash today is worth more than a dollar of cash to be received at some time in the future. (Chapter 31)

Time-resolved fluorescence Fluorescence is energy released at a longer wavelength upon excitation of a molecule at a relatively shorter wavelength. In time-resolved fluorescence the lifetime of fluorescence is longer and there is a wide separation (in nanometers) between the excitation and fluorescence emission wavelengths (nearly 250 nm) compared to conventional fluorescence labels. (Chapter 49)

Top-down microcosting *See* Process costing. (Chapter 41)

Tort A legal term for a wrongful act that is done on purpose and causes injury or harm. (Chapter 6)

Total automation The process of automating all the functions of the laboratory (preanalytical, analytical, and postanalytical data reporting steps) at one time. (Chapter 49)

Total FTE The total number of FTEs employed in the laboratory, regardless of their duties. (Chapter 43)

Total quality management (TQM) Designed-in product quality, with the focus on customer wants and needs as the key drivers in product and process improvement. An approach to integrating multiple activities revolving around quality improvement. (Chapters 1, 43)

Trademark A brand that has received legal protection for the exclusive use of the sole owner. (Chapter 3)

Transfusion medicine service Department or laboratory that provides compatibility testing, labeling and release of blood to patients. Also provides consultative services to clinicians. (Chapter 5)

TRICARE TRICARE is the healthcare program for active duty members of the military, military retirees, and their eligible dependents. TRICARE was called CHAMPUS in the past. (*See* Civilian Health and Medical Program of the Uniformed Services.) (Chapter 5)

Troponin A component of cardiac muscle. Blood levels rise after myocardial damage. (Chapter 6)

Trust The currency of all leadership. Leaders earn followers by earning their trust. Trust is reciprocal; leaders must give it to get it. (Chapter 10)

Turnaround time The interval between the beginning of one event to the end of another event in the total testing process. Typically measured as the collection to reporting time or as the time from phlebotomy or receipt of specimen in laboratory to reporting time. (Chapters 20, 21, 25)

UB92/HCFA-1500 Standard billing forms: UB92 is the billing form used by hospitals; HCFA-1500 is the billing form used by physicians and other ancillary nonhospital providers. (Chapter 42)

Unbundling Submission of bills for various tests in a piecemeal or fragmented fashion. Generally this practice is illegal if done to maximize reimbursement. To code individual tests rather than using an approved CMS panel. (Chapters 5, 33, 37)

Undergraduate Medical Education for the 21st Century National demonstration project funded by the Health Resources and Services Administration to foster medical school training in primary care and in ambulatory-care settings. (Chapter 6)

Uniform Bill-92 (UB-92) A uniform institutional claim form, developed by the National Uniform Billing Committee, that has been in general use since 1993. The form, also known as HCFA-1450 or CMS-1450, is used by facilities when filing Medicare claims with fiscal intermediaries. (Chapter 5)

Union shop Site where all employees must join the union after short introductory period. (Chapter 19)

Unit costs Costs per unit of production or unit of service provided (test, reportable result, billable result, or relative value unit), accountable as total of fixed plus variable costs per unit. (Chapter 41)

Unit of service (UOS) The denominator in ratios used to analyze cost or productivity. The most commonly used UOS is the billable test. The logical measure of work for a given area. In the laboratory, it is usually either the number of billed tests or the number of procedures performed. (Chapters 31, 38, 43)

Universal access The concept that all persons, regardless of health or economic status, have access to a minimal, standard package of healthcare benefits that provides quality healthcare. (Chapter 7)

Universal Precautions Set of precautions designed to reduce risk of transmission of human immunodeficiency virus, hepatitis B virus, and other blood-borne pathogens in the healthcare setting. (Chapter 26)

Unrelated business income tax (UBIT) An income tax that must be filed and paid annually for net income that is not related to the hospital. Laboratory testing and revenue generated from physician office, clinics, and employers that do not have a corporate relationship with the laboratory or parent company would be considered unrelated. The income tax rate is 40% of the unrelated net income. (Chapter 42)

Unstructured interview An applicant interview in which no interview questions are prepared in advance. (Chapter 15)

Upcoding Performing a related test for which the CPT-4 code pays at a higher level; using a higher-paying code than justified to maximize reimbursement. (Chapters 5, 33, 37)

Up-selling The practice of informing clients of a new or improved laboratory test that may have improved sensitivity and specificity over the routine screening assay. These new or im-

proved assays may be applicable to patients with a well-defined subset of a certain disease or for patients who have failed the usual therapeutic strategies. (Chapter 40)

Usual, customary, and reasonable fees Fees paid to a physician under one of the following conditions (Chapter 7):

- If the charge does not exceed the "usual" charge from his office
- If the charge does not exceed the amount "customarily" charged by other physicians in the area
- If the charge is otherwise "reasonable"

Utility The satisfaction derived from using a product or service. (Chapter 3)

Utilization management The concurrent or prospective process of monitoring, assessing, and controlling the utilization of healthcare services to promote efficiency and quality. The process includes review of length of stay, admission rates, coordination of physician and nonphysician services, and use of services like emergency room, laboratory, pharmacy, and radiology. (Chapter 7)

Utilization review A retrospective healthcare assessment tool used by managed-care organizations to ensure that their members have received appropriate quality services. Admissions, length of stay, and utilization of services are included. (Chapter 7)

Validation Establishing documented evidence which provides a high degree of assurance that a specific process will consistently produce a product meeting its predetermined specifications and quality attributes. A process is validated to evaluate the performance of a system with regard to its effectiveness based on intended use. (Chapter 5)

Value A desirable standard or quality for which a person will sacrifice what others consider to be of higher importance. (Chapters 8, 9)

Value-added service Laboratory service which addresses effectiveness as well as cost and efficiency. (Chapter 47)

Variable costs Direct or indirect costs that vary in direct proportion to test volume or level of activity changes, e.g., technologist wages and benefits, reagents, glassware, disposable supplies, and forms. (Chapters 31, 38, 41)

Variance Standard deviation squared. Assuming all sources of error are independent of each other, total error is the sum of variances of individual sources of error. (Chapter 20)

Variance analysis The process of analyzing differences in actual versus budgeted performance to identify necessary corrective actions and help make decisions. (Chapter 31)

Video adapter An integrated circuit board in a computer that enables digital-to-analog conversion of a video signal so that data can be displayed on a monitor. (Chapter 22)

View from a "wide-angle zoom lens" Metaphorically, a series of snapshots that encompass most of the organization as a whole. The operation of a zoom lens at a sports event illustrates the metaphor. The zoom lens adjusts to provide just enough of the field of action but not too much. In particular, when the player looks up at the instant replay of the view from the wide-angle zoom lens, the player can see more than the player saw when running the play. That is, from the view of the wide-angle zoom lens, the player can see enough of the system to determine how the player's actions coordinated with the actions of others to create the final organizational outcome. (Chapter 9)

Vision statement A written statement that defines not what an organization is, but what the organization expects to become. A vision statement should inspire the organization to achieve its mission. (Chapter 2)

Volume variance The difference between the volume of services performed versus the volume that was budgeted. (Chapter 31)

Waived testing Laboratory testing with the lowest level of complexity that can be performed under a certificate of waiver rather than a full laboratory license. Certain simple laboratory tests meet requirements for waived testing as outlined in CLIA '88. Waived testing may be performed without concern for personnel standards or written procedures. Some of these tests are approved by the FDA for home use (such as blood glucose monitoring), are simple, and supposedly have little chance for error or major effect on the patients if an error occurs. (CMS, available at http://cms.hhs.gov/clia/waivetbl.pdf [accessed March 3, 2004].) (Chapters 4, 23)

Wide area network A group of several personal computers or workstations connected via a geographically dispersed telecommunications network. (Chapter 22)

Window period The period when blood tests are negative for a pathogen though the individual is infected and able to transmit the agent. Lookback and postdonation information are designed to identify recipients of blood who might have been transfused during the window period. (Chapter 5)

Win-win outcome A resolution that works well for all parties. (Chapter 13)

Withhold A payment method that withholds a percentage of a negotiated payment in a reserve fund for specialty provider contracts. Annually, if the negotiated quality and cost criteria have been met, the portion of the fee that was withheld is returned according to the risk-bearing terms of the contract. (Chapter 7)

Work flow Tasks organized in a particular way to accomplish a specified result. (Chapter 2)

Work group Two or more individuals who interact primarily to share information and to make decisions that help each other perform within his or her area of responsibility. (Chapter 18)

Work team Two or more individuals whose individual efforts result in a performance that is greater than the sum of those individual parts and who have different tasks but work together adaptively to achieve specified and shared goals. (Chapter 18)

Worked hours The number of hours actually worked by employees (compare paid hours). (Chapter 43)

Workload recording A means of measuring laboratory output and consequently productivity by tallying individual components of laboratory tests quantitatively. The most prominent national program that provided norms for quantifying effort was eventually abandoned because of the difficulty in maintaining a viable system. (Chapter 43)

Workstation A computer intended for use by an individual for professional purposes rather than for home or recreational purposes. Since processing speed is usually important, it tends to have a fast microprocessor, a large amount of RAM, and a high-speed video adapter. (Chapter 22)

Writeoffs Recorded reductions in revenue for gross charges that are deemed uncollectable from third-party payors. (Chapter 31)

Zero defections A customer service strategy that strives for no lost customers, or zero defections. The goal is to keep every customer the company can serve, and this strategy empowers the organization to achieve the goal. (Chapter 3)

Zero tolerance The Office of the Inspector General's position that a healthcare institution will promote and adhere to compliance at all levels and that noncompliance will not be tolerated. (Chapter 5)

Zero-based budgeting A budgeting methodology in which every expenditure must be justified regardless of the prior year's results. (Chapter 31)

Zero-sum game When one person wins by making the other person lose. (Chapter 13)

Index